# MEDICAL MANAGEMENT OF THE THORACIC SURGERY PATIENT

# MEDICAL MANAGEMENT OF THE THORACIC SURGERY PATIENT

## Michael I. Lewis, MD

Director, Cedars-Sinai Multi-Campus Pulmonary/Critical Care Fellowship Program
and Respiratory Intensive Care Unit
Cedars-Sinai Medical Center
Professor of Medicine
David Geffen School of Medicine at UCLA
Los Angeles, California

## Robert J. McKenna Jr., MD

Director, Division of Thoracic Surgery
Cedars-Sinai Medical Center
Professor of Surgery
David Geffen School of Medicine at UCLA
Los Angeles, California

## Associate Editors

## Jeremy A. Falk, MD

Associate Medical Director, Lung Transplant Program
Division of Pulmonary and Critical Care Medicine
Women's Guild Lung Institute, Cedars-Sinai Medical Center
Assistant Clinical Professor of Medicine
David Geffen School of Medicine at UCLA
Los Angeles, California

## George E. Chaux, MD

Medical Director, Lung Transplant Program
Division of Pulmonary and Critical Care Medicine
Women's Guild Lung Institute, Cedars-Sinai Medical Center
Assistant Clinical Professor of Medicine
David Geffen School of Medicine at UCLA
Los Angeles, California

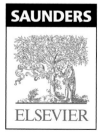

SAUNDERS

ELSEVIER

**SAUNDERS**
ELSEVIER

1600 John F. Kennedy Blvd.
Ste 1800
Philadelphia, PA 19103-2899

MEDICAL MANAGEMENT OF THE THORACIC SURGERY PATIENT ISBN: 978-1-4160-3993-8

---

**Notice**

Knowledge and best practice in this field are constantly changing. As new research and experience broaden our knowledge, changes in practice, treatment and drug therapy may become necessary or appropriate. Readers are advised to check the most current information provided (i) on procedures featured or (ii) by the manufacturer of each product to be administered, to verify the recommended dose or formula, the method and duration of administration, and contraindications. It is the responsibility of the practitioner, relying on their own experience and knowledge of the patient, to make diagnoses, to determine dosages and the best treatment for each individual patient, and to take all appropriate safety precautions. To the fullest extent of the law, neither the Publisher nor the Editors assumes any liability for any injury and/or damage to persons or property arising out of or related to any use of the material contained in this book.

The Publisher

---

**Library of Congress Cataloging-in-Publication Data**
Medical management of the thoracic surgery patient / [edited by]
Michael I. Lewis, Robert J. McKenna Jr. – 1st ed.
    p. ; cm.
    Includes bibliographical references.
    ISBN 978-1-4160-3993-8
1.  Chest–Surgery.   2.  Chest–Diseases–Diagnosis.   3.   Therapeutics,
Surgical. I. Lewis, Michael I. II. McKenna, Robert J., 1925-
    [DNLM: 1.   Thoracic Diseases–surgery.   2.   Thoracic Surgery–methods.   3.   Patient Care–methods.
4.   Perioperative Care–methods.   5.   Thoracic Surgical Procedures–methods. WF 980 M489 2009]
    RD536.M365 2009
    617.5′4–dc22                            2008034700


*Acquisitions Editor:* Dolores Meloni
*Design Direction:* Louis Forgione

Printed in United States of America

Last digit is the print number: 9  8  7  6  5  4  3  2  1

*We dedicate this book to our families whose love and support
sustained us during the creation of this book.*

*Lewis family*: Carol (Ariella-Shira), Samantha, Josh, Elyssa
*McKenna family*: Kathy, Kelley, Rob, Kirsten
*Falk family*: Karine, Max, Jordan
*Chaux family*: Luca, Nicole

# CONTRIBUTORS

**Fereidoun Abtin, MD**
Assistant Professor, Thoracic Imaging, Department of
Radiological Sciences, David Geffen School of Medicine at
UCLA, Los Angeles, California
*Radiofrequency Ablation of Lung Tumors*

**Kamyar Afshar, DO**
Assistant Professor of Clinical Medicine, Division of Pulmonary
and Critical Care Medicine, Keck School of Medicine,
University of Southern California, Los Angeles, California
*Lung Transplantation: Perioperative Management and Early
Complications*

**William R. Auger, MD**
Professor of Clinical Medicine, Division of Pulmonary and
Critical Care Medicine, University of California,
San Diego, Medical Center, San Diego, California
*Clinical Features and Evaluation of Chronic Thromboembolic
Pulmonary Hypertension*

**David Balfe, MBBCh, FCP(SA)**
Attending Physician, Division of Pulmonary and Critical Care
Medicine, and Medical Director, Pulmonary Stepdown Unit,
Women's Guild Lung Institute, Cedars-Sinai Medical Center;
Assistant Clinical Professor of Medicine, David Geffen School of
Medicine at UCLA, Los Angeles, California
*Role of Lung Biopsy in Diffuse Lung Disease*

**Bruce M. Barack, MD**
Chief, Thoracic Radiology, Department of Imaging, Veterans
Administration Greater Los Angeles Healthcare System,
Los Angeles, California
*Evaluation and Management of the Solitary Pulmonary
Nodule*

**Ross Bremner, MD, PhD**
Surgical Director, Center for Thoracic Disease; Chief,
Division of General Thoracic Surgery, The Heart and Lung
Institute, St. Joseph's Hospital and Medical Center,
Phoenix, Arizona
*Surgical Techniques and Options*

**Kathleen Brown, MD**
Professor of Radiology, Department of Radiological Sciences,
David Geffen School of Medicine at UCLA, Los Angeles, California
*Imaging of the Thoracic Surgery Patient*

**George E. Chaux, MD**
Medical Director, Lung Transplant Program, Division of
Pulmonary and Critical Care Medicine, Women's Guild Lung
Institute, Cedars-Sinai Medical Center; Assistant Clinical
Professor of Medicine, David Geffen School of Medicine at
UCLA, Los Angeles, California
*Patient Evaluation and Selection; Lung Transplant Donor
Selection and Management; Lung Transplantation: Perioperative
Management and Early Complications; Intermediate and Late
Complications of Lung Transplantation; Transplant Pharmacology*

**Steve C. Chen, MD**
Director, Division of Pediatric Surgery, Cedars-Sinai Medical
Center; Assistant Clinical Professor of Surgery and Pediatrics,
David Geffen School of Medicine at UCLA, Los Angeles,
California
*Congenital and Developmental Lung Malformations*

**Wen Cheng, MD**
Surgical Director, Lung Transplant Program, Cedars-Sinai
Medical Center, Los Angeles, California
*Surgical Techniques and Options*

**John Cho, MD**
Senior Pulmonary/Critical Care Fellow, Cedars-Sinai Multi-
Campus Fellowship Program, Cedars-Sinai Medical Center,
Los Angeles, California
*Masses of the Middle Mediastinum*

**Henri G. Colt, MD, FCCP**
Professor of Medicine, Director, Clinical Programs,
UCI Pulmonary and Critical Care Medicine, and Director,
Interventional Pulmonology, University of California, Irvine,
Irvine, California
*Diagnostic Bronchoscopy; Therapeutic Bronchoscopy*

**Allan Conlan, MD**
Thoracic Surgery Division, University of Massachusetts Medical
School, Worcester, Massachusetts
*Massive Hemoptysis*

**David Tom Cooke, MD**
Formerly Cardiothoracic Surgery Resident, Section of Thoracic
Surgery, University of Michigan, Ann Arbor, Michigan;
Division of Cardiothoracic Surgery, University of California,
Davis, Medical Center, Sacramento, California
*Carcinoma of the Esophagus*

## Jennifer Cutler, MD

Attending Anesthesiologist, Department of Anesthesiology, Cedars-Sinai Medical Center, Los Angeles, California

*Anesthetic Considerations in Thoracic Surgery*

## Jean Deslauriers, MD

Attending Thoracic Surgeon, Laval Hospital; Professor of Surgery, Laval University, Quebec, Canada

*Thoracic Surgical Anatomy and Procedures*

## Ashraf Elsayegh, MD

Director, Medical Intensive Care Unit, Women's Guild Lung Institute, Cedars-Sinai Medical Center, Los Angeles, California

*Chest Wall Invasion in Lung Cancer*

## Jeremy A. Falk, MD

Associate Medical Director, Lung Transplant Program, Division of Pulmonary and Critical Care Medicine, Women's Guild Lung Institute, Cedars-Sinai Medical Center; Assistant Clinical Professor of Medicine, David Geffen School of Medicine at UCLA, Los Angeles, California

*Emphysema: Lung Volume Reduction Surgery; Patient Evaluation and Selection; Lung Transplant Donor Selection and Management; Lung Transplantation: Perioperative Management and Early Complications; Intermediate and Late Complications of Lung Transplantation; Transplant Pharmacology*

## Peter F. Fedullo, MD

Clinical Professor of Medicine, Division of Pulmonary and Critical Care Medicine, University of California, San Diego, Medical Center, San Diego, California

*Clinical Features and Evaluation of Chronic Thromboembolic Pulmonary Hypertension*

## Richard H. Feins, MD

Professor of Surgery, Division of Cardiothoracic Surgery, University of North Carolina, Chapel Hill, North Carolina

*Tube Thoracostomy; Pleural Effusions and Complications*

## Mark K. Ferguson, MD

Director, Thoracic Surgery Service, The University of Chicago Hospitals; Professor, Department of Surgery, The University of Chicago, Chicago, Illinois

*Preoperative Evaluation of Thoracic Surgery Patients*

## Daniel L. Fortes, MD

Resident, Thoracic Surgery, Mayo Clinic, Rochester, Minnesota

*Other Neoplastic Lesions: Benign and Malignant*

## Éric Fréchette, MD

Attending Thoracic Surgeon, Laval Hospital; Clinical Professor of Surgery, Laval University, Quebec, Canada

*Thoracic Surgical Anatomy and Procedures*

## Clark Fuller, MD

Attending Thoracic Surgeon, Cedars-Sinai Center for Chest Diseases; Surgical Director, Esophageal Center, Cedars-Sinai Medical Center, Los Angeles, California

*Superior Vena Cava Syndrome; Superior Sulcus Tumors*

## Sara Ghandehari, MD

Assistant Director, Lung Transplant Program, Cedars-Sinai Medical Center, Los Angeles, California

*Patient Evaluation and Selection*

## S. Melanie Greaves, MBBS

Department of Radiology, South Manchester University Hospital NHS Trust, Manchester, United Kingdom

*Imaging of the Thoracic Surgery Patient*

## Leland Green, MD

Attending Hematologist/Oncologist, Cedars-Sinai Medical Center, Los Angeles, California

*Small Cell Lung Cancer*

## Dani Hackner, MD

Associate Chair, Department of Medicine, and Director, Translational Critical Care Services, Cedars-Sinai Medical Center, Los Angeles, California

*Masses of the Middle Mediastinum; Posterior Mediastinal Masses*

## Benjamin E. Haithcock, MD

Assistant Professor of Surgery, Division of Cardiothoracic Surgery, University of North Carolina, Chapel Hill, North Carolina

*Pleural Effusions and Complications*

## Alex Hakim, MD

Resident, UCLA-San Fernando Valley Internal Medicine Residency Program, Los Angeles, California

*Masses of the Anterior Mediastinum*

## Michael E. Halkos, MD

Resident in Cardiothoracic Surgery, Division of Cardiothoracic Surgery, Department of Surgery, Emory University School of Medicine, Atlanta, Georgia

*Pneumothorax and Bronchopleural Fistula*

## John E. Heffner, MD

Garnjobst Chair of Medicine, Providence Portland Medical Center; Adjunct Professor of Medicine, Oregon Health and Science University, Portland, Oregon

*Tracheotomy*

## Kay E. Hermes, BS

Biomedical Analyst, Clifton F. Mountain Foundation, Houston, Texas

*Staging of Lung Cancer*

## Michael T. Jaklitsch, MD

Attending Thoracic Surgeon, Division of Thoracic Surgery, Brigham and Women's Hospital, Harvard Medical School, Boston, Massachusetts

*Pleural Masses*

**Stuart W. Jamieson, MB, FRCS, FACS**

Division of Cardiothoracic Surgery, University of California, San Diego, Medical Center, San Diego, California

*Chronic Thromboembolic Pulmonary Hypertension and Pulmonary Thromboendarterectomy*

**Heather D. Jones, MD**

Medical Director, Saperstein Intensive Care Unit, Division of Pulmonary and Critical Care Medicine, Cedars-Sinai Medical Center, Los Angeles, California

*Preoperative Assessment of High-Risk Patients for Lung Cancer Resection*

**Stanley C. Jordan, MD**

Professor of Pediatrics and Medicine, David Geffen School of Medicine at UCLA; Director, Nephrology and Transplant Immunology, and Medical Director, Kidney Transplant Program, Comprehensive Transplant Center, Cedars-Sinai Medical Center, Los Angeles, California

*Transplant Immunology*

**Peter J. Julien, MD**

Director of Thoracic Imaging, Cedars-Sinai Medical Center, Los Angeles, California

*Lung Cancer Screening*

**Nader Kamangar, MD, FACP, FCCP**

Director, Hospitalist/Intensivist Program, Olive View-UCLA Medical Center; Associate Director, Cedars-Sinai Multi-Campus Pulmonary/Critical Care Fellowship Program, Cedars-Sinai Medical Center; Associate Professor of Medicine, David Geffen School of Medicine at UCLA, Los Angeles, California

*Masses of the Anterior Mediastinum*

**Samer Kanaan, MD**

Thoracic Surgery Fellow, Division of Thoracic Surgery, Brigham and Women's Hospital, Harvard Medical School, Boston, Massachusetts

*Pleural Masses*

**Robert M. Kass, MD**

Surgical Director, Heart Transplant Program, and Co-Director, Cardiothoracic Surgery, Cedars-Sinai Medical Center, Los Angeles, California

*Surgical Techniques and Options*

**Steven S. Khan, MD**

Attending Cardiologist, Department of Cardiology, Kaiser Sunset Medical Center; Clinical Associate Professor, David Geffen School of Medicine at UCLA, Los Angeles, California

*Preoperative Evaluation of Thoracic Surgery Patients*

**C. Joyce Lee, MD**

Pulmonary/Critical Care Fellow, Cedars-Sinai Multi-Campus Fellowship Program, Cedars-Sinai Medical Center, Los Angeles, California

*Intermediate and Late Complications of Lung Transplantation*

**Michael I. Lewis, MD**

Director, Cedars-Sinai Multi-Campus Pulmonary/Critical Care Fellowship Program and Respiratory Intensive Care Unit, Cedars-Sinai Medical Center; Professor of Medicine, David Geffen School of Medicine at UCLA, Los Angeles, California

*Congenital and Developmental Lung Malformations; Staging of Lung Cancer; Superior Vena Cava Syndrome; Superior Sulcus Tumors; Chest Wall Invasion in Lung Cancer; Intermediate and Late Complications of Lung Transplantation; Masses of the Middle Mediastinum; Posterior Mediastinal Masses; Other Mediastinal Disorders: Fibrosing Mediastinitis, Acute Mediastinitis, and Mediastinal Hemorrhage; Pleural Effusions and Complications; Diaphragm Disorders: Paralysis, Hernia, Eventration*

**Moishe Liberman, MD**

Clinical Fellow in Thoracic Surgery, Division of Thoracic Surgery, Massachusetts General Hospital, Harvard Medical School, Boston, Massachusetts

*Tracheal Stenosis; Tracheoesophageal Fistula; Tracheal Masses*

**Atikun Limsukon, MD**

Senior Pulmonary/Critical Care Fellow, Cedars-Sinai Multi-Campus Fellowship Program, Cedars-Sinai Medical Center, Los Angeles, California

*Other Mediastinal Disorders: Fibrosing Mediastinitis, Acute Mediastinitis, and Mediastinal Hemorrhage*

**James D. Luketich, MD**

Chairman and Professor, Division of Thoracic and Foregut Surgery, Department of Surgery, University of Pittsburgh School of Medicine, UPMC Health System, Pittsburgh, Pennsylvania

*Benign Esophageal Disease; Management of Esophageal Perforation*

**Michael M. Madani, MD, FACS**

Division of Cardiothoracic Surgery, University of California, San Diego, Medical Center, San Diego, California

*Chronic Thromboembolic Pulmonary Hypertension and Pulmonary Thromboendarterectomy*

**Ali Mahtabifard, MD**

Attending Thoracic Surgeon, Cedars-Sinai Center for Chest Diseases, Cedars-Sinai Medical Center, Los Angeles, California

*Mediastinoscopy and Mediastinotomy; Surgical Management of Non-Small Cell Lung Cancer*

**Alberto M. Marchevsky, MD**

Department of Pathology and Laboratory Medicine, Cedars-Sinai Medical Center; Clinical Professor of Pathology, David Geffen School of Medicine at UCLA, Los Angeles, California

*Pathologic Classification of Lung Malignancies and Special Pathologic Procedures*

**Daniel R. Margulies, MD**

Director of Trauma and Surgical Critical Care, Department of Surgery, Cedars-Sinai Medical Center, Los Angeles, California

*Initial Trauma Management; Management of Thoracic Trauma*

### Douglas J. Mathisen, MD

Chief, General Thoracic Surgery, Massachusetts General Hospital; Hermes C. Grillo Professor of Thoracic Surgery, Department of Surgery, Harvard Medical School, Boston, Massachusetts

*Tracheal Stenosis; Tracheoesophageal Fistula; Tracheal Masses*

### Robert J. McKenna Jr., MD

Director, Division of Thoracic Surgery, Cedars-Sinai Medical Center; Professor of Surgery, David Geffen School of Medicine at UCLA, Los Angeles, California

*Mediastinoscopy and Mediastinotomy; Video-Assisted Thoracoscopic Surgery; Emphysema: Lung Volume Reduction Surgery; Surgical Management of Non-Small Cell Lung Cancer; Chest Wall Invasion in Lung Cancer; Masses of the Anterior Mediastinum; Masses of the Middle Mediastinum; Posterior Mediastinal Masses; Pleural Effusions and Complications*

### Ciaran McNamee, MD

Division of Thoracic Surgery, Brigham and Women's Hospital, Harvard Medical School, Boston, Massachusetts

*Massive Hemoptysis*

### Reza J. Mehran, MD

Associate Professor, Department of Thoracic and Cardiovascular Surgery, University of Texas M.D. Anderson Cancer Center, Houston, Texas

*Resection for Pulmonary Metastases*

### Joseph I. Miller Jr., MD

Professor of Surgery, Division of Cardiothoracic Surgery, Department of Surgery, Emory University School of Medicine, Atlanta, Georgia

*Pneumothorax and Bronchopleural Fistula*

### Amin J. Mirhadi, MD

Attending Physician, Department of Radiation Oncology, Samuel Oschin Comprehensive Cancer Institute, Cedars-Sinai Medical Center, Los Angeles, California

*Overview of Radiation Therapy Terms and Procedures in the Management of Thoracic Malignancies*

### John D. Mitchell, MD

Chief, General Thoracic Surgery, Division of Cardiothoracic Surgery, and Associate Professor, University of Colorado Denver School of Medicine, Aurora; Consultant, National Jewish Health, Denver, Colorado

*Thoracic Surgical Considerations in Infectious and Inflammatory Diseases of the Lung*

### Christopher R. Morse, MD

Instructor in Surgery, Division of Thoracic Surgery, Massachusetts General Hospital, Harvard Medical School, Boston, Massachusetts

*Tracheal Stenosis; Tracheoesophageal Fistula; Tracheal Masses*

### Zab Mosenifar, MD

Executive Vice Chair, Department of Medicine, Director, Division of Pulmonary and Critical Care Medicine, and Medical Director, Women's Guild Lung Institute, Cedars-Sinai Medical Center; Professor of Medicine, David Geffen School of Medicine at UCLA, Los Angeles, California

*Emphysema: Lung Volume Reduction Surgery; Preoperative Assessment of High-Risk Patients for Lung Cancer Resection*

### Clifton F. Mountain, MD*

Clinical Professor of Surgery, Department of Cardiothoracic Surgery, University of California, San Diego, San Diego, California

*Staging of Lung Cancer*

### Tej Naik, MD

Senior Pulmonary/Critical Care Fellow, Cedars-Sinai Multi-Campus Fellowship Program, Cedars-Sinai Medical Center, Los Angeles, California

*Masses of the Anterior Mediastinum*

### Ronald Natale, MD

Senior Research Advisor and National Director, Lung Cancer Research Program, Aptium Oncology, Inc.; Attending Physician, Cedars-Sinai Outpatient Cancer Center, Samuel Oschin Comprehensive Cancer Institute, Cedars-Sinai Medical Center, Los Angeles, California

*Adjuvant and Neoadjuvant Chemotherapy in Non-Small Cell Lung Cancer*

### Tina T. Ng, MD

Department of Surgery, Cedars-Sinai Medical Center, Los Angeles, California

*Congenital and Developmental Lung Malformations; Initial Trauma Management; Management of Thoracic Trauma*

### Francis C. Nichols, MD

Consultant, Division of General Thoracic Surgery, and Associate Professor of Surgery, Mayo Clinic, Rochester, Minnesota

*Other Neoplastic Lesions: Benign and Malignant; Chest Wall*

### Vijay K. Nuthakki, MD

Fellow, Minimally Invasive Thoracic Surgery, Cedars-Sinai Medical Center, Los Angeles, California

*Mediastinoscopy and Mediastinotomy*

### Scott Oh, DO

Pulmonary/Critical Care Fellow, Cedars-Sinai Multi-Campus Fellowship Program, Cedars-Sinai Medical Center, Los Angeles, California

*Intermediate and Late Complications of Lung Transplantation*

### Yoko Ozawa, MD

Senior Pulmonary/Critical Care Fellow, Cedars-Sinai Multi-Campus Fellowship Program, Cedars-Sinai Medical Center, Los Angeles, California

*Nuclear Medicine Imaging in Thoracic Surgery*

*Deceased

**Alden M. Parsons, MD**
Thoracic Surgery Resident, University of North Carolina
Hospitals, Chapel Hill, North Carolina
*Tube Thoracostomy*

**Isabel Pedraza, MD**
Director, Surgical Consult Service, Cedars-Sinai Medical Center,
Los Angeles, California
*Superior Vena Cava Syndrome*

**Richard D. Pezner, MD**
Associate Chair, Division of Radiation Oncology, City of Hope
Medical Center, Duarte, California
*Adjuvant and Neoadjuvant Radiation Therapy for Lung
Cancer*

**Allan Pickens, MD**
Assistant Professor of Surgery, Section of Thoracic Surgery,
University of Michigan, Ann Arbor, Michigan
*Carcinoma of the Esophagus*

**George Rakovich, MD**
Thoracic Surgery Fellow, Laval Hospital, Quebec, Canada
*Thoracic Surgical Anatomy and Procedures*

**Hari Reddy, MD**
Pulmonary/Critical Care Fellow, Cedars-Sinai Multi-Campus
Fellowship Program, Cedars-Sinai Medical Center, Los Angeles,
California
*Intermediate and Late Complications of Lung Transplantation*

**T. Brett Reece, MD**
Cardiothoracic Surgery Fellow, Division of Cardiothoracic
Surgery, University of Colorado Denver School of Medicine,
Aurora, Colorado
*Thoracic Surgical Considerations in Infectious and
Inflammatory Diseases of the Lung*

**Curtis Sather, MD**
Pulmonary/Critical Care Fellow, Cedars-Sinai Multi-Campus
Fellowship Program, Cedars-Sinai Medical Center, Los Angeles,
California
*Masses of the Anterior Mediastinum*

**Sinan Simsir, MD**
Surgical Director, Heart Transplant Program, Division of
Cardiothoracic Surgery, Cedars-Sinai Medical Center,
Los Angeles, California
*Lung Transplant Donor Selection and Management*

**Peter Smethurst, MD**
Senior Pulmonary/Critical Care Fellow, Cedars-Sinai
Multi-Campus Fellowship Program, Cedars-Sinai Medical
Center, Los Angeles, California
*Superior Sulcus Tumors*

**Harmik J. Soukiasian, MD**
Attending Surgeon, Division of Cardiothoracic Surgery,
Cedars-Sinai Medical Center, Los Angeles, California
*Benign Esophageal Disease; Management of Esophageal
Perforation*

**Robert D. Suh, MD**
Associate Professor, Director, Thoracic Interventional Services,
and Director, Residency Training Program, Thoracic Imaging,
Department of Radiological Sciences, David Geffen School of
Medicine at UCLA, Los Angeles, California
*Radiofrequency Ablation of Lung Tumors*

**John D. Symbas, MD**
Division of Cardiothoracic Surgery, Department of Surgery,
Emory University School of Medicine, Atlanta, Georgia
*Management of Thoracic Trauma*

**Panagiotis N. Symbas, MD**
Division of Cardiothoracic Surgery, Department of Surgery,
Emory University School of Medicine, Atlanta, Georgia
*Management of Thoracic Trauma*

**Mieko Toyoda, PhD**
Comprehensive Transplant Center, Cedars-Sinai Medical Center,
Los Angeles, California
*Transplant Immunology*

**Brian Tzung, MD**
Senior Radiology Resident, Cedars-Sinai Medical Center,
Los Angeles, California
*Lung Cancer Screening*

**Ashley A. Vo, PharmD**
Program Director, Transplant Immunotherapy, Comprehensive
Transplant Center, Cedars-Sinai Medical Center; Assistant
Professor of Pediatrics, David Geffen School of Medicine at
UCLA, Los Angeles, California
*Transplant Pharmacology*

**Alan Waxman, MD**
Director of Nuclear Imaging, Cedars-Sinai Medical Center,
Los Angeles, California
*Nuclear Medicine Imaging in Thoracic Surgery*

**Carol C. Wu, MD**
Thoracic Imaging Fellow, Department of Radiological Sciences,
UCLA Medical Center, Los Angeles, California
*Evaluation and Management of the Solitary Pulmonary
Nodule*

**Phillip Zakowski, MD**
Senior Infectious Disease Consultant, Cedars-Sinai Medical
Center; Associate Professor of Medicine, David Geffen School
of Medicine at UCLA, Los Angeles, California
*Thoracic Surgical Considerations in Infectious and
Inflammatory Diseases of the Lung*

# PREFACE

The concept and motivation behind developing a new textbook of this nature was born in the weekly Thoracic Surgery Case Conferences and Thoracic Tumor Boards held at Cedars-Sinai Medical Center. As an academic pulmonary/critical care physician, it became abundantly obvious week after week that the "pearls of knowledge" emanating from our thoracic surgical colleagues and the other disciplines present were not readily available, if at all, in outstanding standard pulmonary and critical care texts. Furthermore, thoracic surgery texts deal in detail with operative techniques and fail to cover the key principles of workup and management relevant to pulmonary/critical care specialists who deal with these patients, often prior to any thoracic surgical considerations. These "pearls of knowledge" often deal with key issues and concepts that should be known but are not readily available or taught to trainees in pulmonary/critical care medicine and other specialties interacting with thoracic surgeons. This is even more pertinent in the current era of medicine in which 24/7 ICU care by intensivists and multidisciplinary approaches to complex patient care are standard practice or expectations. This textbook thus fills a necessary void.

The format of the book is also somewhat unique. This format is driven by the guiding principle that the textbook should be *action packed with facts and concepts, but easy to read and retain,* as opposed to selecting the key facts from a lengthy, albeit well-written narrative. With this in mind the text configuration chosen was that of a "bullet" format. Each chapter is well illustrated with figures, tables and algorithms (where appropriate) to enhance visual clarity and retention. Further, video images (e.g., illustrating video-mediastinoscopy, VATS, etc.) are provided online via a designated ExpertConsult.com website. In addition, all references are accessed online at the designated website and hyperlinked to PubMed. (This includes all numbered citations in each chapter, key or classic references highlighted for ready reference, and additional recent suggested reading.)

Finally, where possible, each chapter is illustrated by one or more cases relevant to that subject. Key pearls are included in the analysis of these brief illustrative cases, which serve to emphasize key facts highlighted in the text.

The textbook is broad in scope and was written by more than 80 leading experts in all topics covered, culminating in an authoritative and up-to-date work that will certainly fill that "void" highlighted above. The book is divided into eleven major sections. These include: "Diagnostic Workup of the Thoracic Surgery Patient"; "Thoracic Surgical Procedures and Management"; "Upper Airway"; "Disorders of the Lung"; "Lung Transplantation"; "The Mediastinal"; "Diseases of the Pleura"; "Diseases of the Chest Wall and Diaphragm"; "Pulmonary Vascular Conditions"; "Thoracic Trauma"; and "Disorders of the Esophagus".

This textbook is a resource well suited to pulmonary and critical care specialists and their trainees, as well as those disciplines and their trainees that interact or consult on thoracic surgical patients, including oncologists, radiation oncologists, internists, general surgeons, thoracic and interventional radiologists, and pulmonary pathologists. We are most grateful to the numerous authors who put so many hours into writing outstanding chapters. The invaluable assistance of the associate editors, Jeremy Falk and George Chaux, is also much appreciated. Having experienced teachers in pulmonary/critical care medicine and thoracic surgery as co-editors worked well in balancing the "surgical side" with the "medical needs" deemed necessary for this endeavor and its intended readership.

It has been a long road from the *initial seeds and concept* of such a textbook, to fruition. We believe that this text fills a much needed void and look forward to it becoming a standard text for pulmonary and critical care clinicians, their trainees and other specialties involved in the care of such patients.

*Michael I. Lewis, MD*
*Robert J. McKenna Jr., MD*

# ACKNOWLEDGMENTS

We wish to acknowledge the uplifting environment and culture of Cedars-Sinai Medical Center whose pursuit of excellence in teaching, patient care, research and community service, inspired the creation of this new text.

We also wish to acknowledge the outstanding contributions and hard work of our many contributors. Sharing their unique expertise in a comprehensive and thoughtful manner was much appreciated.

We also acknowledge the encouragement and tireless assistance of a wonderful group of editorial staff at Elsevier: Dolores Meloni, Elena Pushaw, and Kim DePaul.

# CONTENTS

# DIAGNOSTIC WORKUP OF THE THORACIC SURGERY PATIENT

## 1 IMAGING OF THE THORACIC SURGERY PATIENT

S. Melanie Greaves, MBBS and Kathleen Brown, MD

## THE THORAX: RADIOLOGIC-ANATOMIC CORRELATIONS

### IMAGING MODALITIES

#### General Considerations

- A variety of imaging options are available to thoracic surgeons for evaluation of the thorax.
- The choice of imaging examination should be based on the clinical question, recommendations in the literature, and expertise of the radiologist.
- Cost-effective practice requires selection of procedures that increase diagnostic yield and minimize costs. (Common indications for thoracic computed tomography [CT, Table 1-1].)

#### Chest Radiographs

- Plain chest radiographs (Fig. 1-1) are the most commonly performed radiologic investigation for the diagnosis of thoracic disease. The standard projection is an erect posteroanterior (PA) chest radiograph taken in full inspiration. The patient stands with the front of their chest against the imaging plate and the x-ray beam passes from posterior to anterior, limiting magnification of the heart and mediastinal structures. A lateral examination is useful in identifying abnormalities in regions not clearly seen on the frontal view.
- Patients who are unable to have a PA chest radiograph may have a portable examination at the bedside. The imaging plate is positioned against the patient's back, with the x-ray beam passing from anterior to posterior. The beam diverges around the heart and mediastinum, resulting in magnification of these structures and often creating difficulties with interpretation. Images are made with lower energy x-rays and exposure times are longer. Ill patients often have difficulty with breath holding and the resultant respiratory motion artifact may degrade image quality.
- Lateral decubitus views may help in the diagnosis of a pleural effusion and expiratory views may aid diagnosis of a small pneumothorax.

- Traditional film-screen methods are being widely replaced by digital imaging. Digital systems have several advantages over film-screen systems. Images may be electronically manipulated such that an interpretable image can be generated even if the x-ray exposure is suboptimal. Images can be transmitted and stored electronically, and utilizing a picture archiving and communications system (PACS), digital images are available to referring clinicians and radiologists simultaneously both on and potentially off the hospital site.[1]

#### Computed Tomography

- CT scanners (Figs. 1-2 and 1-3) generate a cross-sectional image of the patient with a very narrow beam of x-rays. This beam passes through the patient to strike electronic detectors. During the scan, the beam rotates around the patient and multiple measurements are made. Data are processed by computers, and digital images are reconstructed, free from superimposition of overlying structures.
- The majority of CT scanners are now multislice machines with multiple rows of detectors (currently ranging from 4 to 256) within the doughnut-shaped gantry.[2] The patient lies on the scanner table and is moved through the gantry as it continuously rotates, with each of the rows recording information. A large volume of data can now be acquired extremely quickly. There is a degree of tradeoff between resolution of the images and the speed of scanning. Most patients can hold their breath for 20 seconds, the approximate time required to image the thorax. If very thin slices are required for improved resolution, the scan will take longer to perform.
- Scanners reconstruct sets of images in the axial plane for routine clinical work. Volume data acquisition allows for high-quality two- and three-dimensional reformations along multiple planes without additional radiation exposure. These additional reconstructions are helpful for diagnosis and surgical planning. Surface rendering is a particular form of three-dimensional imaging that is particularly useful for visualizing anatomic structural lumens such as those of the bronchial tree (Fig. 1-4).
- Tissues are displayed in terms of their attenuation of the x-ray beam. A small volume of tissue, a voxel, is displayed on a

---

**TABLE 1-1 ■ COMMON INDICATIONS FOR THORACIC COMPUTED TOMOGRAPHY**

Determination of presence and extent of neoplastic disease
Diagnosis of pulmonary embolism
Diagnosis of bronchiectasis, diffuse lung disease, emphysema and small airways disease.
Guidance for interventional procedures
Localization of loculated collections of fluid if ultrasound is not diagnostic
Evaluation of suspected mediastinal abnormalities seen on chest x-ray examination

---

CT image as a two-dimensional pixel. The pixel is given a Hounsfield unit (HU) value depending on the density of its contained tissues. Water has a HU of 0, dense bone up to +2000 and air -1000. The Hounsfield unit values of the multiple pixels in the image are then mapped to a gray scale. Windowing is the process used to display the data to the full advantage. For image display purposes, no single window setting can adequately show all of the information available on a chest CT scan. The display of the CT image on the monitor is determined by the window width and level. Typically for thoracic CT examinations, one setting is used to optimally display the lungs and a second setting is used for the soft tissues.

## Iodinated Contrast

- Thoracic CT scans are often performed to specific protocols and can be performed with and without iodinated intravenous and oral contrast. Intravenous contrast is required in patients with suspected vascular abnormalities and is typically used for staging of carcinomas and in patients with suspected mediastinal, hilar, or pleural abnormalities.

- Intravenous contrast administration is not without risk, and although adverse reactions occur at low rates, reactions are not infrequently encountered given the widespread use of iodinated contrast. Reactions range from mild urticaria to anaphylactic shock and death. The incidence of severe reactions with nonionic agents is 0.4% and of very severe reactions is 0.004%.[3-6] Patients with an increased risk of contrast reaction include those who have had a previous contrast reaction, those with asthma, and those with multiple, well-documented allergies. In these individuals, unenhanced CT or a different imaging modality may suffice diagnostically.

- Some institutions advocate premedication with steroids and antihistamines before further contrast administration, but there is no conclusive evidence of benefit for the prophylactic use of steroids in the prevention of severe reactions to contrast media.

- Iodinated contrast media has nephrotoxic potential but rarely cause significant renal failure in patients with normally functioning kidneys. Contrast should be avoided in patients with existing renal impairment, with diabetes, with congestive heart failure of class III or IV, in patients with reduced effective arterial volume (e.g., nephrotic, cirrhotic), or those receiving drugs that may impair renal function or increase contrast nephrotoxicity.

## Radiation Dose

- Radiation exposure should be kept as low as reasonably achievable (ALARA). CT has made an enormous impact on diagnostic imaging; however, the radiation dose for CT is far greater than for conventional radiographs. In addition, the use of CT has markedly increased over time.

- In a recent United Kingdom survey, CT scans constituted 7% of all radiologic examinations, but contributed 47% of the total collective dose from medical x-ray examinations in 2000/2001; in the United States, CT accounts for approximately

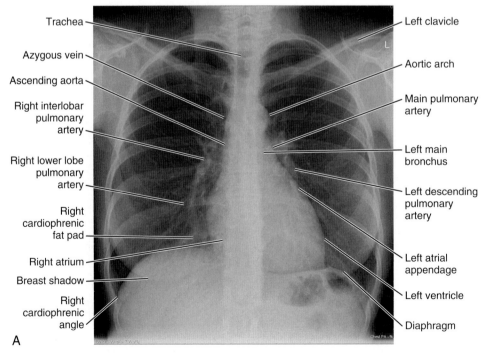

**Figure 1-1:** **A,** Normal PA and **B,** lateral chest radiographs: anatomic features.

*(Continued)*

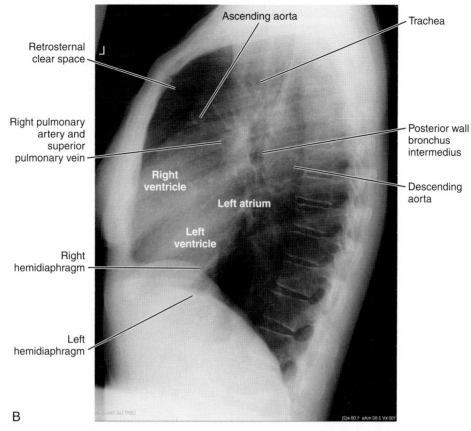

B

**Figure 1-1—cont'd.**

11% of all radiology procedures and almost 70% of the total effective radiation dose.[7,8] Increased CT use has led to an overall increase in the total amount of medical radiation used, despite reductions in other areas.[7-9]

■ The increase in radiation exposure via CT scanning may represent a public health issue in the future. A recent report in the *New England Journal of Medicine* suggested that the radiation from current CT scan use may cause as many as 1 in 50 future cases of cancer.[10] The risks are greater in children because of their increased radiosensitivity and because of the greater

years of life during which a radiation-induced cancer could develop.

■ Possible strategies to address the above-mentioned issues include decreasing the absolute number of CT examinations by using other imaging modalities such as ultrasound and magnetic resonance imaging (MRI) and altering scan parameters to decrease the dose of individual examinations.[11] Education of patients and physicians regarding radiation dose and potential risks is critical in order to address the issue of increasing radiation exposure.

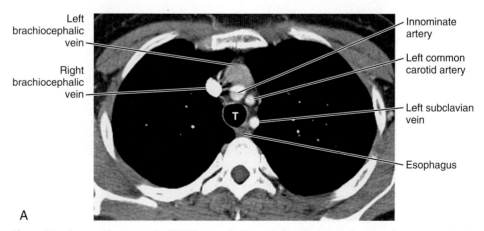

A

**Figure 1-2:** Computed tomography (CT) thorax soft tissue windows demonstrating normal anatomy. **A,** At the level of the great vessels, the brachiocephalic vein is crossing the mediastinum from left to right anterior to the innominate, carotid, and subclavian arteries. The esophagus can be identified posterior to the trachea (T).

*(Continued)*

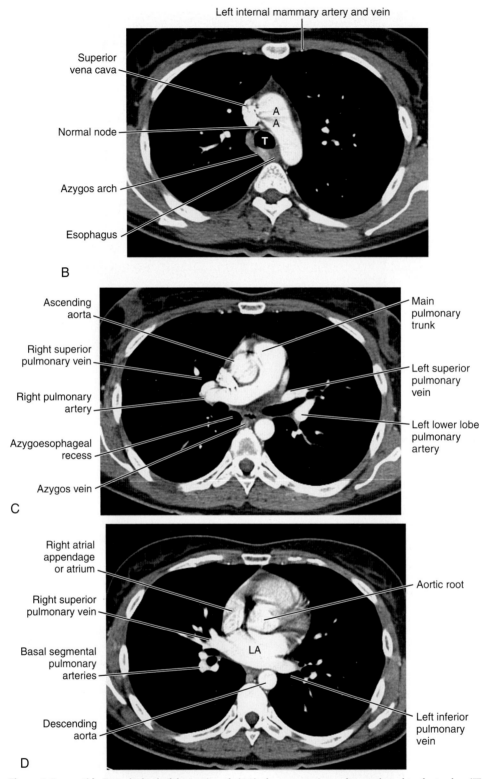

**Figure 1-2—cont'd: B,** At the level of the aortic arch (AA), the azygos vein can be seen lateral to the trachea (T) as it ascends in the posterior mediastinum and arches forward to join the superior vena cava (SVC). The right paratracheal region contains a normal size node. The internal mammary arteries and veins are clearly seen in the parasternal regions bilaterally. **C,** Just below the carina, the right pulmonary artery is crossing the mediastinum. The azygoesophageal recess can be identified, with the lung contacting pleural overlying the esophagus and azygos vein. **D,** Right superior and left inferior pulmonary veins can be seen entering the left atrium (LA).

*(Continued)*

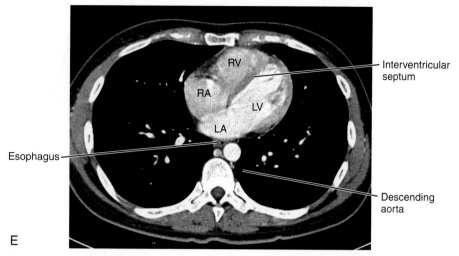

**Figure 1-2—cont'd: E,** At this level, the right ventricle (RV), right atrium (RA), left ventricle (LV) and left atrium (LA) can be clearly identified.

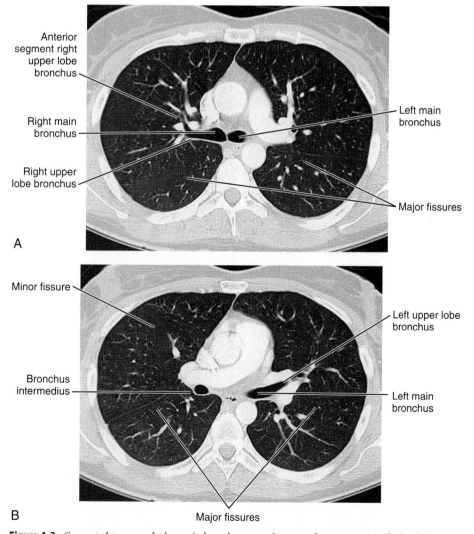

**Figure 1-3:** Computed tomography lung windows demonstrating normal anatomy. **A,** At this level, the right upper lobe bronchus can be seen along its length as it originates from the right main stem bronchus. The major fissures separate the upper lobes anteriorly from the lower lobes posteriorly. **B,** The bronchus intermedius is visible as an oval lucency. Its posterior wall should be smooth and thin. The left main and upper lobe bronchus can also be identified. The minor fissure is seen as a relatively avascular region.

*(Continued)*

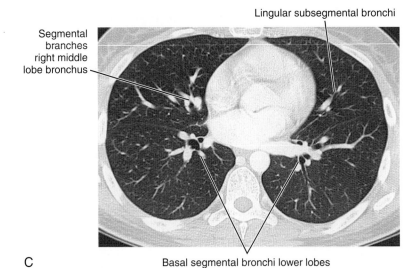

Segmental branches right middle lobe bronchus

Lingular subsegmental bronchi

Basal segmental bronchi lower lobes

**Figure 1-3—cont'd: C,** Image through the basal segmental bronchi of the lower lobes showing both the bronchi and their associated vessels.

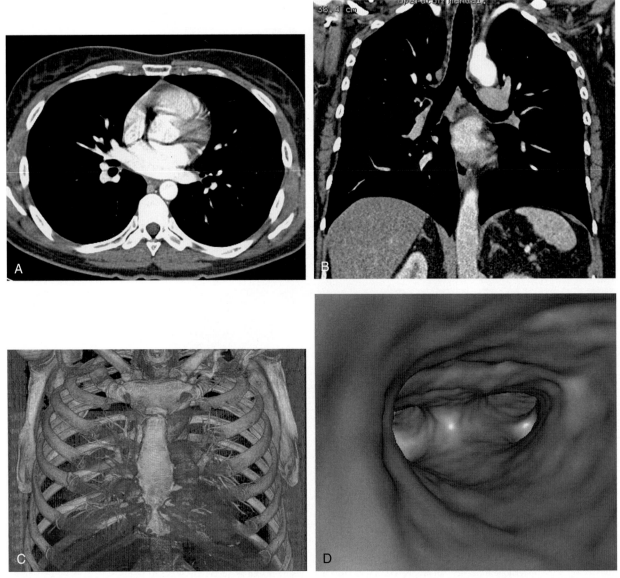

**Figure 1-4:** Images demonstrate axial (**A**), two-dimensional multi-planar reconstruction (MPR) (**B**), three-dimensional (**C**), and endoluminal (**D**) reconstructions of a standard thoracic computed tomography volume data set.

## Positron Emission Tomography

- Positron emission tomography (PET) and CT scanners can be combined in the same gantry to optimize the localization of PET abnormalities (Fig. 1-5).
- Patient preparation is required for PET. High glucose levels can compete with fluorodeoxyglucose (FDG) uptake and can degrade image quality; patients are typically not permitted to eat or drink for approximately 4 hours before the scan. Diabetics require special preparation. Caffeine, nicotine, and alcohol should be avoided for 24 hours before the scan. Oral hydration may be helpful.
- Appropriate timing of the PET examination following procedures is required to prevent false-positive studies. The following guidelines are suggested[12]:
  Post biopsy 1 week
  Post surgery 6 weeks
  Post chemotherapy 4 to 6 weeks
  Post radiation 4 to 6 months
- Solitary pulmonary nodules
  1. PET scanning is well established for the evaluation of solitary pulmonary nodules with an intermediate pretest probability of malignancy.[13]
  2. If the pretest probability is high, biopsy or resection should be considered. If the pretest probability is low, observation should suffice.
  3. A negative PET scan indicates that a nodule is highly likely to be benign, although it is important to take the pretest probability of malignancy into account.
  4. A positive PET scan indicates that the lesion is most likely to be malignant.
     Although false-positive results can occur, PET has higher specificity than CT or MRI scanning alone.
  5. A negative PET scan is usually more accurate than a positive PET scan.
     If the lesion does prove to be malignant, PET is the most accurate modality for staging mediastinal lesions (see Fig. 1-5).
  6. False-positive results have been described in active granulomatous/inflammatory disease. False-negative results

occasionally occur in patients with bronchioloalveolar carcinoma, carcinoid, and in small (less than 1 cm) nodules. Therefore, PET scanning is usually reserved for lesions larger than 1 cm in size. PET can be considered in lesions smaller than 1 cm, but negative nodules should be closely observed.

## Magnetic Resonance Imaging

- MRI scanners generate a strong magnetic field around the patient, who is then exposed to short bursts of radio waves called radiofrequency (rf) pulses. The motion of protons in the body is altered by the rf pulses, which when they return to their original states, emit rf signals of their own, which are detected by the scanner and are used to construct a cross-sectional image of a slice of tissue.
- The main advantage of MRI over CT is the lack of ionizing radiation and the superior soft tissue contrast resolution. The ability of MRI to produce images in multiple planes is less of a differentiating factor because excellent multi-planar images can now be reconstructed with multidetector computed tomography (MDCT).
- MRI is not generally useful for imaging the pulmonary parenchyma but can provide excellent images of the mediastinum and chest wall. It is particularly useful for imaging superior sulcus tumors.
- Nephrogenic systemic fibrosis (NSF), a rare multisystemic fibrosing disorder, has recently been described in patients receiving gadolinium-based MRI contrast agents.[14-16] Initially termed nephrogenic fibrosing dermopathy because of the skin involvement, the disease has been shown to demonstrate systemic fibrosis involving skeletal muscle, bone, lungs, pleura, pericardium, myocardium, kidneys, testes and dura. Although the etiology of NSF is unclear, several contributing factors have been described, including renal insufficiency, major tissue injury such as arterial or venous thrombosis or surgery, and exposure to gadolinium-based contrast agents. At present, dialysis after the administration of gadolinium-based agents or a lower dose of agent has not been shown to decrease the incidence of NSF. The US Food and Drug Administration issued a public health advisory regarding gadolinium-based contrast agents in patients with renal failure in June 2006, which was updated in May 2007.[17] The use of gadolinium-based contrast agents should be avoided unless the diagnostic information is not available with non–contrast-enhanced MRI in patients with acute or chronic severe renal insufficiency (glomerular filtration rate <30 mL/min/1.73m$^2$, or acute renal insufficiency of any severity due to hepato-renal syndrome or in the perioperative liver transplantation period.
- Contraindications to MRI scanning are:
  Metallic foreign bodies in the eye.
  Implanted electronic devices such as pacemakers.

## Ultrasound

- Ultrasound uses high-frequency sound waves to image tissue. Reflected echoes are detected and used to create an image.
- Thoracic ultrasound is most useful for the detection and characterization of pleural disease, particularly pleural effusions (Fig. 1-6), and is often helpful in guiding thoracentesis and drain placements.
- In selected circumstances, peripheral lung lesions may be localized and biopsied using ultrasound for guidance.
- Ultrasound may be useful in evaluating the diaphragm in cases of suspected diaphragmatic paralysis.
- Ultrasound may also be used to assist in placement of central venous lines.

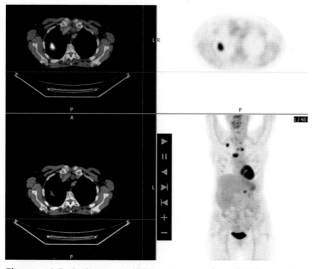

**Figure 1-5:** Positron emission tomography (PET)/computed tomography (CT) images in a patient with a right upper lobe non–small cell lung carcinoma with right hilar and mediastinal nodal metastases. CT (*bottom left*) and PET (*top right*) images are fused (*top left*) to provide an image with both anatomical and physiological information. Note the normal cardiac uptake and FDG activity in the bladder.

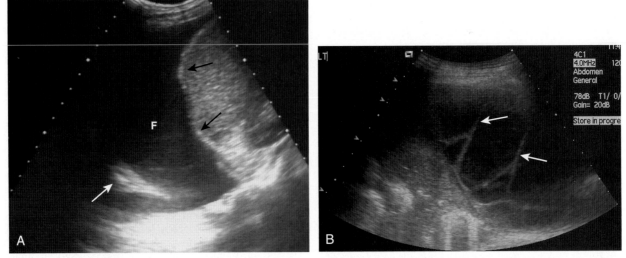

**Figure 1-6: A,** Free-flowing effusion and fluid with septa. Thoracic ultrasound of a free-flowing pleural effusion. The fluid (F) is hypoechoic (*black*) adjacent to the diaphragm (*black arrows*). A small triangular tongue of collapsed lung is also visible (*white arrow*). B. Thoracic ultrasound of a complex effusion containing fine septae (*arrows*).

## Esophageal Imaging

- The esophagus can be imaged using barium esophagrams, CT, MRI, and endoscopic ultrasound. Barium esophograms provide useful information about mucosal surface lesions and esophageal motility. CT does not show the mucosa in detail but demonstrates tissues surrounding the esophagus and can evaluate extension of tumor and the presence of lymph nodes. Endoscopic ultrasound is the investigation of choice for the T staging of esophageal tumors but is still not universally available.
- Esophageal trauma is usually diagnosed on the basis of chest radiographs and contrast swallows. If clinical evaluation and traditional radiographic studies are equivocal, CT should be performed.
- Esophageal endoscopic ultrasound (EUS) may also be useful for that staging of lung cancer. In particular, lower level 7 (subcarinal), 8 (paraesophageal), and 9 (inferior pulmonary ligament) lymph nodes may be better visualized or biopsied by EUS than by endobronchial ultrasound (EBUS) or mediastinoscopy.

## KEY RADIOLOGIC PRINCIPLES IN IMAGING THE THORACIC SURGERY PATIENT: THORACIC NEOPLASMS

### General Principles

Knowledge of the lymphatic drainage pattern in the thorax is useful in the staging of a variety of thoracic neoplasms, and for the accurate assessment of nodal involvement which is a critical factor in staging of malignancy.[18]

Nodal short axis has been shown on autopsy studies to be a more accurate predictor of nodal size than long axis. Although the size of normal nodes may vary depending on the region of the medistinum, in general, lymph nodes in the paratracheal, aortopulmonary window, hilar, subcarinal, and paraesophageal regions are considered abnormal if the nodal short axis is greater than 1 cm. Peridiaphragmatic and internal mammary nodes are considered abnormal if the nodal short axis is greater than 5 mm. Nodes within the retrocrural and extrapleural regions are not normally visible, and should be considered abnormal

when present. However, accurate staging requires pathologic examination of enlarged nodes, because nodal size alone is not reliable in the assessment of neoplastic involvement.

## Imaging Principles in Lung Cancer

- Accurate staging is critical in determining the most appropriate therapy and prognosis. Familiarity with the current staging system for lung cancer is a requirement for those involved in the assessment of these patients.[19]
- The goal of the surgeon is to surgically resect all patients with a resectable tumor who are medically able to tolerate resection, yet avoid unnecessary thoracotomies.
- The radiologist is critical in helping to determine whether the patient is resectable with accurate descriptions of T status to include primary tumor size and extent; N status to include location, size, and number of nodes; and M status to include presence and location of metastases.
- Roadmapping of the primary tumor, nodes and metastases can be performed to aid biopsy (Fig. 1-7).
- Radiographic features that indicate unresectability or stage IIIB or IV disease include T4 disease with invasion of mediastinum or diaphragm, ipsilateral pleural metastatic disease, N3 disease with contralateral mediastinal, contralateral or ipsilateral supraclavicular nodes, and M1 disease with distant metastases.

### Primary Tumor

- The main role of CT in the assessment of the primary tumor is in differentiation of T3 from T4 lesions.
- A CT diagnosis of T4 tumor can be made if
  1. Tumor is involving the trachea or narrowing the carina.
  2. Tumor is surrounding, distorting, or attenuating, or having greater than 180 degrees of contact with the superior vena cava, the aorta, the main pulmonary artery, right or left pulmonary artery within the mediastinal pleural reflection, or the central pulmonary veins.
  3. Tumors abutting the superior vena cava with elevation of the diaphragm to indicate invasion of the phrenic nerve.
  4. Tumor results in the destruction of a vertebral body (Fig. 1-8) or involvement of the brachial plexus.
  5. The presence of pleural carcinomatosis as confirmed on CT by soft tissue pleural nodules.

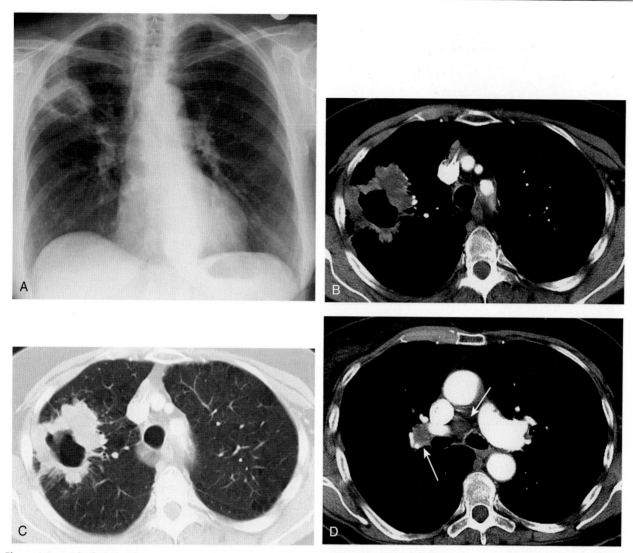

**Figure 1-7: A,** The frontal radiograph demonstrates a large, irregularly marginated, mass in the right upper lobe with some adjacent distortion of the superior right hilum. **B** to **C,** CT images confirm the presence of a thick-walled, irregularly marginated, cavitating tumor in the right upper lobe. **D,** Right hilar and low right paratracheal nodes are greater than 1 cm in short axis diameter (*arrows*). The right paratracheal nodes were positive for malignancy at mediastinoscopy precluding surgery.

- In selected cases, CT or MRI can reliably identify involvement of major thoracic structures, that is, T4 disease, precluding surgery (Figs. 1-9 and 1-10). Findings suggesting mediastinal invasion include extensive contact between the tumor and the mediastinum, loss of a fat plane between tumor and the mediastinum, mass effect on adjacent mediastinal structures, and pleural and pericardial thickening.[20]

- The assessment of mediastinal invasion can however be very difficult using CT alone because inflammation and desmoplastic reaction can simulate tumor invasion, and microscopic extension may be missed. Minimal invasion of pericardium, fat, vagus, and phrenic nerves are generally considered resectable disease. Radiologic determination of the proximity of lesions to the tracheal carina may also be problematic, although the ability to view CT reconstructions in multiple planes is often very helpful.

- Chest wall invasion does not rule out surgery unless there is invasion of the subclavian artery or of a vertebral body. CT is limited in assessing chest wall invasion, with reported sensitivities and specificities ranging from 38-87% and 40-89%, respectively.[21-23] The only reliable findings of chest wall invasion are the presence of rib destruction and a chest wall mass (Fig. 1-11). However, these findings are present in only 20% to 40% of patients with surgically proven chest wall invasion.[22,23] Although the sensitivity and specificity of MRI is greater than those of CT, MRI is also of limited value. When a lung tumor abuts the parietal pleura, the presence of chest wall pain is a better predictor of chest wall invasion than the appearance on the CT scan, unless there is rib destruction.

- Invasive tumors arising in the lung apex may produce the characteristic clinical findings of Horner's syndrome and pain involving the shoulder and arm. CT can provide anatomic information regarding the local extent of the tumor, and demonstration of this region has improved with the multiplanar views made possible with multislice CT. The superior contrast resolution of MRI makes it the preferred modality for assessment of the extent of local tumor invasion, particularly with respect to brachial plexus and vascular involvement (Fig. 1-12).

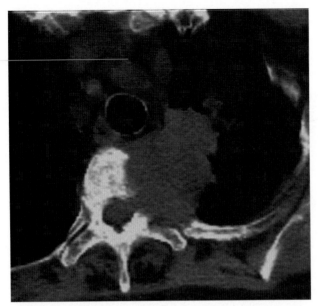

**Figure 1-8:** Computed tomography image of a large T4 tumor in the posterior left upper lobe invading the adjacent vertebral body.

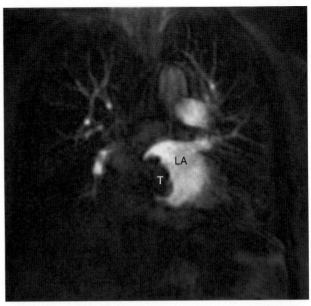

**Figure 1-10:** Magnetic resonance imaging scan demonstrates filling defect within the left atrium (LA) from direct tumor (T) invasion.

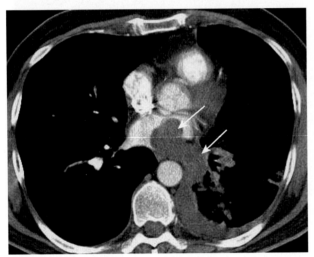

**Figure 1-9:** Computed tomography image of an unresectable T4 tumor that is invading the left atrium via the left inferior pulmonary vein (*arrows*).

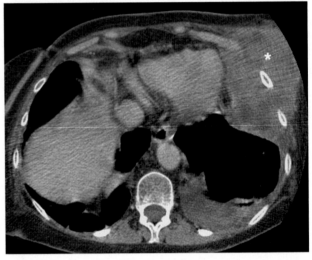

**Figure 1-11:** Computed tomography image of a large left sided tumor that is invading the chest wall, producing an obvious chest wall mass (*asterisk*).

### Nodal Disease

- Prognosis in lung cancer is influenced by the number and size of nodes, and intracapsular versus extracapsular and microscopic versus macroscopic disease.
- CT is limited in its ability to stage mediastinal nodes accurately because it relies on nodal size alone. Nodes are considered enlarged when they measure greater than 10 mm in short axis. However, benign hyperplastic nodes may be enlarged, and normal size nodes may contain microscopic foci of malignant disease. In a study by McLoud and colleagues, 13% of nodes less than 1 cm contained metastases, and nearly one third of nodes 2 to 4 cm were hyperplastic nodes and did not contain metastases.[24] As such, the most important role of CT in the assessment of nodal disease is in determining the presence of enlarged nodes, and CT is the best method of directing nodal sampling for histological evaluation (Fig. 1-13). The sensitivity and specificity for the CT evaluation of mediastinal nodal metastases are both about 65%.

### Metastatic Disease

- Extrathoracic metastases are present in approximately 40% of patients with newly diagnosed lung cancer (Fig. 1-14).
- Clinical evaluation and laboratory tests are usually performed to evaluate for metastatic disease; the use of CT in the assessment of extrathoracic metastases in asymptomatic patients with normal biochemistry remains controversial.

### Positron Emission Tomography in the Staging of Non–Small Cell Lung Carcinoma

- PET is now standard for staging of non–small cell carcinoma of the lung. The addition of PET to the conventional workup of lung cancer patients will prevent unnecessary surgery in one out of five patients and will change the stage of more than half of the patients.[25,26] PET mediastinal staging has a reported sensitivity of 81%, and specificity 90%; PET/CT has

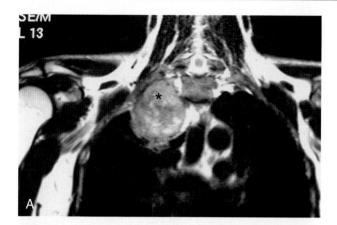

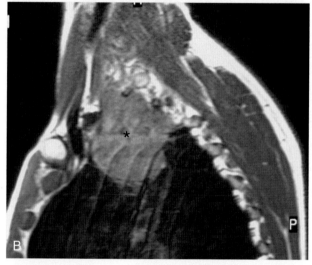

**Figure 1-12:** Coronal (**A**) and sagittal (**B**) MRI scans of the thoracic inlet show a rounded mass at the right lung apex that is invading the chest wall at the right lung apex (*asterisk*).

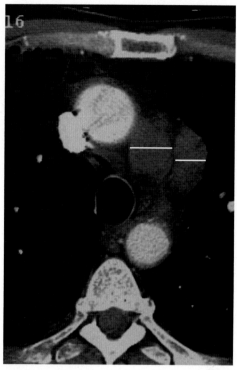

**Figure 1-13:** Contrast-enhanced computed tomography image demonstrating enlarged subaortic (station 6 nodes). The short axis diameter of these nodes (lines) measured greater than 1 cm.

superior accuracy compared with that of CT or PET alone[25,26] (Fig. 1-15).

- PET is useful in patients with potentially operable disease and no abnormal mediastinal nodes or distant metastases on CT. If the PET scan is negative, mediastinoscopy can potentially be avoided. In patients with enlarged mediastinal nodes, the false-negative rate of PET is approximately 5% to 9%, compared with an estimated false-negative rate for mediastinoscopy of 9%.[27] Understanding the standard pattern of lymphatic spread of lung lesions by location is helpful in avoiding false-positive results both in CT and PET scanning.
- Positive PET results should be confirmed by mediastinoscopy or lymph node sampling before excluding surgery, because the false-positive rate of PET in the mediastinum is 13% to 22%.[27] Mediastinoscopy may be avoided if the pretest probability is very high. However, patients who have dual pathology such as tuberculosis may have false-positive results.
- PET detects unsuspected distant metastases in approximately 10% of patients. PET has equal or greater sensitivity and is more specific for the diagnosis of bone metastases from lung carcinoma, and 100% sensitivity and 80% specificity for adrenal metastases has been reported.[28] Adrenal hyperplasia may have increased uptake and can mimic bilateral adrenal metastases in patients with carcinoid or small cell lung carcinoma.[28] However, PET has only a 60% sensitivity for brain metastases due to the high background metabolic activity of the brain

and, therefore, cannot be used in place of CT or MRI for evaluation of brain metastases.[28]

- PET can be used to differentiate malignant from benign pleural disease with a sensitivity of 97% and a specificity of 89%.[29] Intense uptake is highly predictive of malignancy; moderate uptake should be interpreted with caution because inflammatory disorders may result in this appearance. A prior talc pleurodesis can also cause increased pleural uptake.
- PET can be helpful in the post-thoracotomy chest for diagnosing recurrent malignant disease. PET can differentiate between local recurrence and post-treatment change with a sensitivity of 97% to 100% and a specificity of 62% to 100%.[30] False-positive results may occur from inflammatory reactions following therapy. PET is more accurate than CT for the detection of local disease recurrence, and PET/CT is substantially more specific than PET alone.[30]

## Imaging Principles in Mesothelioma

- Mesothelioma is the most common primary neoplasm of the pleura but is still a relatively rare disease. The vast majority of cases are secondary to asbestos exposure. Presenting symptoms include chest pain and shortness of breath.
- The presence of unilateral effusion, volume loss, nodular pleural thickening, and pleural thickening involving mediastinal or fissural pleura suggests mesothelioma (Fig. 1-16). Calcified plaques suggesting asbestos exposure are seen only in the minority of mesothelioma patients. CT is currently the imaging investigation of choice for diagnosis and staging of this disease. MRI and PET scanning have useful complimentary roles in making treatment decisions.
- Mesothelioma is staged using a system from the International Mesothelioma Interest Group. This system emphasizes criteria used to determine the extent of local tumor and lymph node involvement.

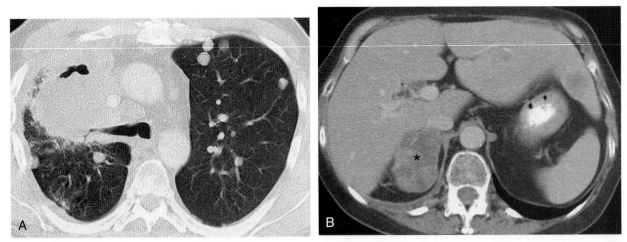

**Figure 1-14:** **A** and **B,** M1, stage IV lung carcinoma with metastases. **A,** Computed tomography (CT) lung window demonstrating a large right upper lobe tumor with multiple round nodules bilaterally, which is consistent with metastases. **B,** CT soft tissue image through the upper abdomen showing a large, heterogeneous attenuation, adrenal metastasis (*asterisk*).

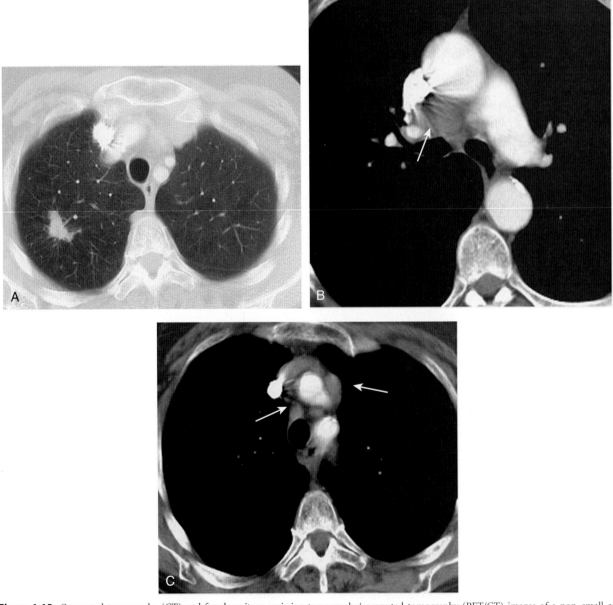

**Figure 1-15:** Computed tomography (CT) and fused positron emission tomography/computed tomography (PET/CT) images of a non–small cell lung cancer in a 45-year-old woman. **A,** CT lung window demontrates the primary lesion in the right upper lobe. CT soft tissue image (**B**) shows enlarged nodes in the low right paratracheal region (*arrow*) and (**C**) small (less than 1 cm) short axis diameter nodes in the high right paratracheal region and in the contralateral mediastinum (*arrows*).

*(Continued)*

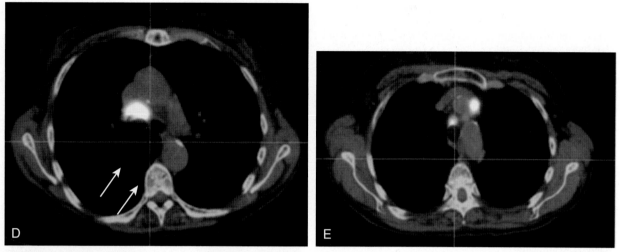

**Figure 1-15—cont'd:** Fused PET/CT (**D&E**) images reveals avid fluorodeoxyglucose uptake in both the enlarged right paratracheal nodes but also in the smaller nodes, upstaging the patient from N2 to N3.

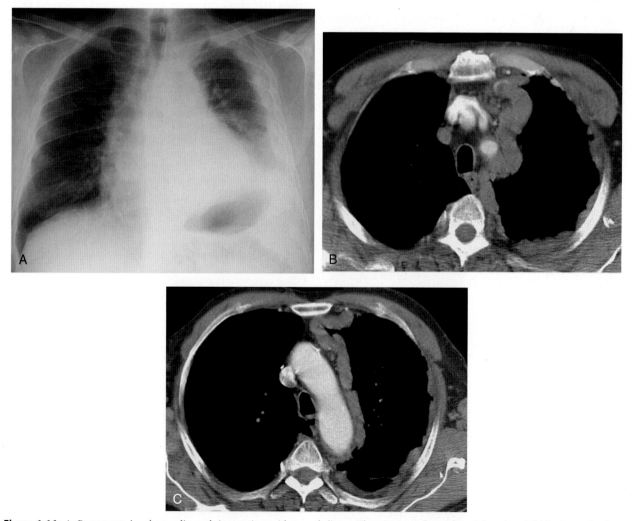

**Figure 1-16: A,** Posteroanterior chest radiograph in a patient with mesothelioma. There is circumferential, nodular, pleural thickening and volume loss of the left hemithorax. **B,** Contrast-enhanced axial computed tomographic images confirm the presence of circumferential thickening of the pleura. The mediastinal pleura is involved, and the pleural thickening exceeds 1 cm; both are indicators of pleural malignancy. **C,** Similar findings of pleural mass/thickening at lower level.

- It is important to distinguish between the potentially resectable T3 tumor and the unresectable T4 tumor. As in non–small cell lung carcinoma, the presence of N3 nodal disease and distant metastases precludes surgery.
- Mesothelioma is locally aggressive and can involve intercostal muscles and adjacent bone. It can extend into the chest wall along chest tube tracts and biopsy sites.
- Pericardial involvement may be seen at CT as nodular pericardial thickening or pericardial effusion. Chest CT may demonstrate pulmonary metastases or rarely extrathoracic spread.
- Metastases to lymph nodes are present at autopsy in approximately 40% to 45% of patients. As in lung carcinoma staging, the evaluation of lymph nodes by CT has a relatively low sensitivity and specificity because it relies on size alone. CT can also underestimate chest wall involvement and peritoneal disease.[31]
- The superior contrast resolution of MRI may allow for improved detection of tumor extension, especially to the chest wall and diaphragm.[31]
- PET can distinguish mesothelioma from benign pleural processes and can be useful in staging and preoperative evaluation of the disease. Areas of high standardized uptake value (SUV) within diffuse pleural disease may guide biopsy. PET has increased accuracy in the detection of mediastinal nodal metastases when compared with CT. PET may predict prognosis in that higher FDG activity is associated with a poorer prognosis. A high level of uptake is associated with the presence of N2 disease and poor outcome. PET is very useful in the identification of distant metastases that preclude thoracotomy.

## Imaging Principles in Esophageal Carcinoma

- Cross-sectional imaging is used to stage esophageal cancer but is somewhat suboptimal. Current T staging emphasizes the depth of invasion of the primary tumor. CT and MRI scanning cannot reliably delineate the individual layers of the esophageal wall and therefore cannot be used to differentiate between T1 and T2 lesions. Accurate T1/T2 staging relies on esophageal ultrasound, which has an overall accuracy of 85% to 95%.[32]
- The accuracy of CT in identifying mediastinal invasion varies between 59% and 82%.[32] Loss of intervening fat planes may be helpful. If the esophageal mass is displacing or indenting the posterior wall of the trachea or bronchus, the tumor is probably invading the structure.
- Involvement of the aorta or tracheobronchial tree signifies inoperable, T4 tumor.
- CT findings include
  1. Irregular thickening of the esophageal wall
  2. An intraluminal polypoid mass
  3. Eccentric narrowing of the lumen
  4. Dilatation of the esophagus proximal to the narrowing
  5. Tumor invasion of adjacent structures
- Nodal spread is typically to paraesophageal, other mediastinal, gastrohepatic ligament, and left gastric nodes (Fig. 1-17). As in the staging of other carcinomas, CT is limited by its reliance on anatomic size of the nodes. It can be difficult to differentiate enlarged paraesophageal nodes from contiguous tumor spread.
- Distant metastases can be identified by CT. PET scanning is limited in T staging but may show distant sites of metastatic disease.[33]
- Complications after esophageal resection are not uncommon and include anastomotic leaks, torsion of the pulled-up segment, hemorrhage, wound infections, and subphrenic abscesses.[34,35] Late complications include anastomotic strictures and reflux esophagitis.

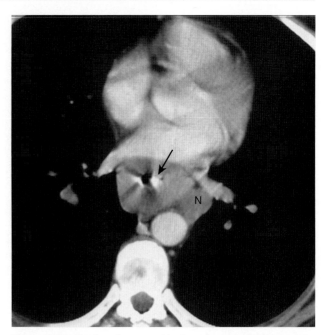

**Figure 1-17:** Esophageal cancer with circumferential thickening of the esophageal wall (*arrow*) and adjacent paraesophageal lymphadenopathy (N).

## Imaging Principles in Mediastinal Masses

A variety of primary and secondary neoplasms can produce masses in the mediastinum. These neoplasms can often be detected on plain chest radiographs because they alter the normal mediastinal contours. A relatively large mediastinal mass may result in only subtle chest radiographic abnormalities, and knowledge of normal mediastinal anatomy is required to detect subtle mediastinal abnormalities. Several lines and stripes are helpful in identifying the presence or absence of mediastinal disease on chest radiographs (Fig. 1-18).

- The right paratracheal stripe is an easy-to-identify linear opacity resulting from the combination of the right lateral tracheal wall and adjacent pleura. The right paratracheal stripe should be less than 4-mm thick. Right paratracheal lymphadenopathy will result in widening of the right paratracheal stripe.
- The azygoesophageal recess is a curved interface extending from the azygos vein inferiorly, usually concave to the right and projected over the thoracic spine. The azygoesophageal recess is formed by the interface between the right lung and the azygos vein and esophagus in the mediastinum. Loss of the interface or new convexity may result from lymphadenopathy or mediastinal tumor within the middle mediastinum.
- The paraspinal lines parallel the thoracic spine. Abnormal convexity of these lines implies disease within the posterior mediastinum.
- The aorticopulmonary or aortopulmonary window is the space between the aortic arch and the main pulmonary artery. A convexity in this region is usually abnormal and is most commonly due to lymphadenopathy.

On the lateral view, anterior mediastinal pathology can cause increased opacity behind the sternum.

For diagnostic purposes, the radiologist typically divides the mediastinum into anterior, middle, and posterior compartments (Fig. 1-19), because many mediastinal masses have characteristic locations.

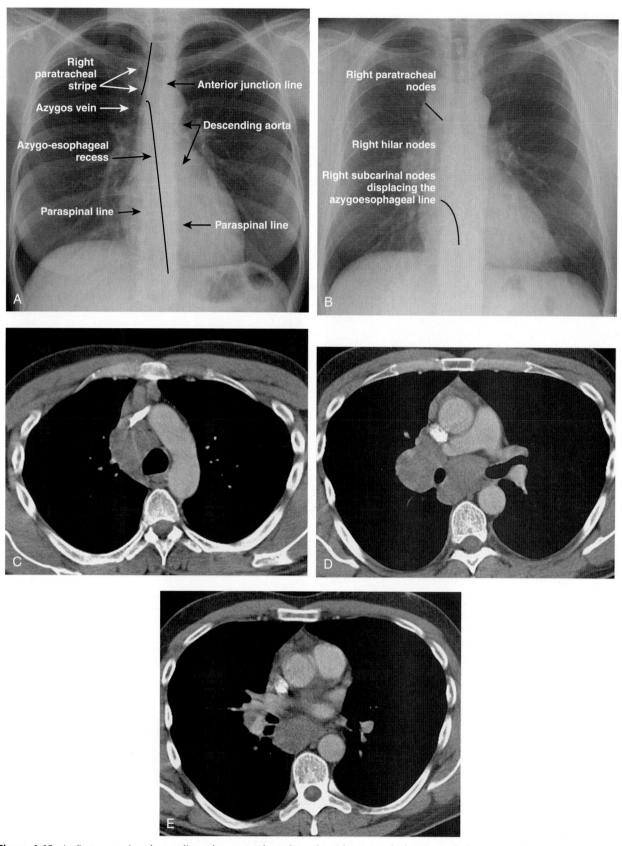

**Figure 1-18: A,** Posteroanterior chest radiograph annotated to show the right paratracheal stripe and the azygoesophageal recess interface. **B,** Posteroanterior chest radiograph in a different patient demonstrates mediastinal and right hilar adenopathy, with widening of the right paratracheal stripe, displacement of the azygoesophageal line, and lobulated appearance to the right hilum. **C-E,** Computed tomography scan confirms the presence of right paratracheal, right hilar, prevascular, subcarinal and paraesophageal adenopathy.

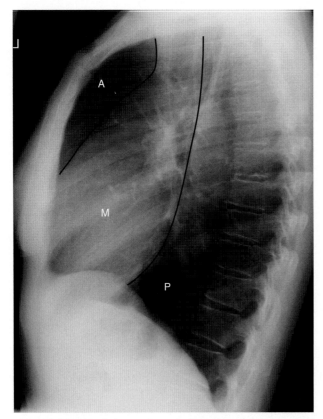

**Figure 1-19:** Lateral chest radiograph demonstrates the mediastinal compartments. Anterior mediastinum (A), middle mediastinum (M), posterior mediastinum (P).

■ The anterior mediastinum can be defined as the area bounded by the sternum anteriorly and the anterior surfaces of the heart and great vessels posteriorly.

■ The middle mediastinum is bordered by the anterior and posterior mediastinum.

■ The posterior mediastinum is bounded by the posterior surface of the pericardium anteriorly and the vertebral bodies, and paravertebral gutters posteriorly.

CT is almost invariably used to localize and characterize mediastinal abnormalities further. CT diagnosis is usually based on the location of the mass, its shape, its constituent tissues and additional features such as its interaction with surrounding structures. The presence of fat in a mediastinal lesion on CT or MRI usually points to a diagnosis of teratoma or thymolipoma. Diffuse fatty infiltration in the mediastinum occurs in mediastinal lipomatosis. Calcification in a mediastinal tumor narrows the differential down to thyroid goiter, thymoma or teratoma. CT is helpful in guiding biopsy and for surgical planning.

Lesions in the anterior mediastinum include

■ Lesions originating from the thymus (thymoma, thymic carcinoma, thymic cysts, thymic carcinoid, thymolipoma)
■ Lesions originating from thyroid tissue
■ Lymph node masses, including lymphoma
■ Teratomas and other germ cell tumors

Lesions in the middle mediastinum include

■ Lymph nodes
■ Bronchogenic carcinoma
■ Foregut duplication cysts
■ Pericardial, aortic and cardiac lesions

Lesions in the posterior mediastinum include

■ Lesions arising from the esophagus
■ Descending aortic aneurysm
■ Neurogenic tumors
■ Vertebral body abnormalities (abscess, myeloma, metastases)

## Anterior Mediastinal Masses
### Thymic Tumors

■ The normal thymus is concave outward and becomes replaced by fat with increasing maturity. The most common primary thymic tumor is a thymoma, and these tumors account for approximately 15% of primary mediastinal masses.[36]

■ Thymomas are usually seen on CT in the prevascular space but may also be paracardiac (Fig. 1-20). They are typically homogeneous soft tissue masses, although calcification (10% to 40%) and cystic degeneration can be present. Usually the tumor grows asymmetrically to one side of the mediastinum.

■ Thymomas are staged at the time of surgery based on the presence and extent of invasion. Approximately 30% of thymomas are invasive and infiltrate adjacent structures or have spread locally as pleural or pericardial implants (Fig. 1-21). Thymomas rarely metastasize outside the thorax.

■ It can be difficult to differentiate invasive from non invasive thymomas preoperatively. Indicators of invasive thymomas on CT scans include
  1. Invasion of mediastinal structures
  2. Poorly defined tumor margins
  3. Obliteration of fat planes
  4. The presence of a large lobulated tumor
  5. CT can identify nodules of tumor arising from the pleural and pericardial surfaces. Pleural implants are usually unilateral and are frequently not associated with a pleural effusion.

### Primary Germ Cell Tumors

■ Primary germ cell tumors account for 10% to 15% of primary mediastinal metastases, and more than 80% are benign. Teratomas are much more common in children and young adults.

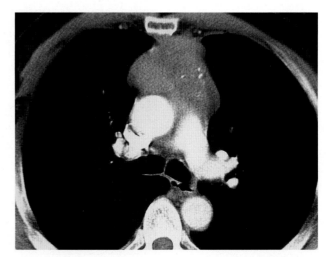

**Figure 1-20:** Contrast-enhanced computed tomography of a noninvasive thymoma. A large soft tissue mass is visible in the prevascular space. It contains small foci of calcification. The fat planes between the tumor and the vessels are indistinct, but there was no evidence of invasion at surgery.

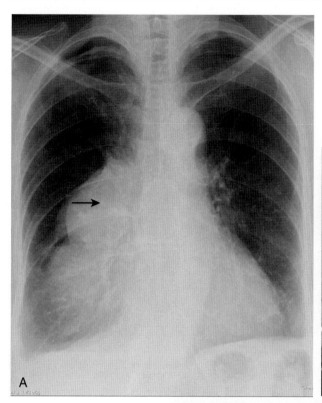

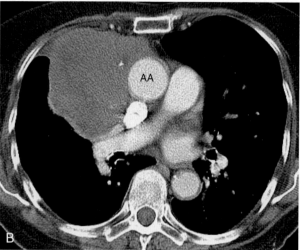

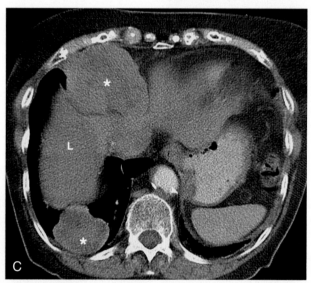

**Figure 1-21:** Invasive thymoma. **A,** The posteroanterior chest radiograph demonstrates abnormal right mediastinal contours, suggesting a mediastinal mass. The right hilum (*arrow*) is visible through the mass, suggesting that the mass lies anterior or posterior to the hilum but not engulfing the hilar vessels. **B,** Contrast-enhanced computed tomography image showing a bulky soft tissue mass in the prevascular space extending preferentially to the right side. There is loss of the fat planes between the tumor and the ascending aorta (AA). **C,** Pleural implants (*asterisk*) can be seen anterior and posterior to the liver (L) in the costophrenic sulci.

■ Mature teratomas may demonstrate a combination of fluid, fat, soft tissue, and calcification; pleomorphism and particularly the presence of fat are clues to diagnosis. A typical lesion would be a predominantly cystic, thin-walled lesion in the anterior mediastinum.

■ Malignant germ cell tumors are less likely to contain areas of calcification and fat. They are often large and grow rapidly with areas of cystic necrosis.

### Thyroid Goiters

■ Thyroid lesions commonly result in deviation and distortion of the trachea (Fig. 1-22). On a chest radiograph, the upper margins of a thyroid goiter become indistinct above the clavicles. This is termed the cervicothoracic sign, and occurs because above the clavicles the thyroid gland lies adjacent to other soft tissues in the neck rather than aerated lung. A clearly marginated soft tissue/air interface is therefore no

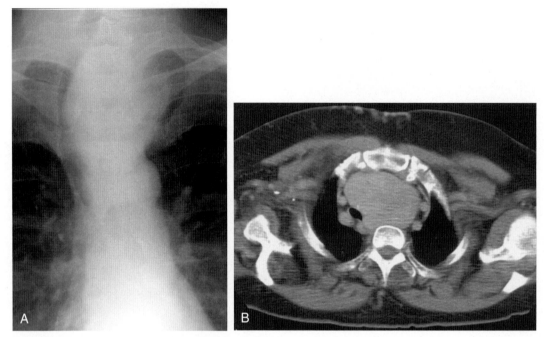

**Figure 1-22: A,** Coned-down view of the thoracic inlet in a patient with a thyroid goiter. This shows a large mediastinal mass with smooth margins displacing the trachea to the right and narrowing its transverse diameter. The lateral margins of this mass fade out above the level of the clavicles indicating that the mass is in the anterior mediastinum. **B,** Computed tomography confirms the anterior mediastinal location of the mass. Its attenuation is above that of adjacent muscle because of its iodine content. The mass compresses the trachea.

longer seen (Fig. 1-23). A mass in the posterior portion of the mediastinum such as a neurogenic tumor remains in contact with lung above the clavicles, and its borders can therefore still be clearly identified (see Fig. 1-23).
- CT can demonstrate the extent of a thyroid mass and its relationship to other structures. CT can be useful in the preoperative assessment of substernal extent.
- Thyroid goiters are usually seen to be contiguous with the thyroid gland in the neck, although a goiter may be separate from the thyroid. At least a portion of the goiter will

be of high attenuation because thyroid tissue is usually of high soft tissue attenuation due to the intrinsic presence of iodine. Mediastinal thyroid masses are often inhomogeneous and may contain cystic regions and areas of calcification.
- Irregularity of contour, lack of distinct surrounding fascial planes, and mediastinal/cervical lymphadenopathy raise the suspicion of malignancy.
- A radionuclide thyroid scan can be very useful in further confirming that an anterior mediastinal mass is thyroid in origin.

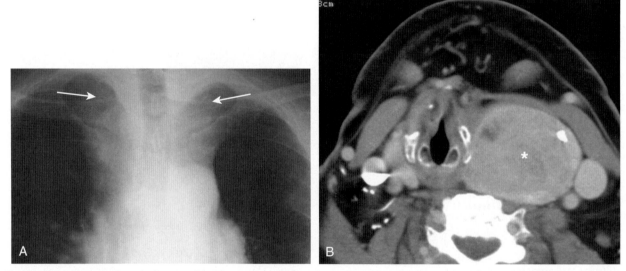

**Figure 1-23:** The cervicothoracic sign. **A** and **B,** The margins of an anterior mediastinal mass such as a thyroid goiter (**A**) will fade out above the clavicles on a chest radiograph (*arrows*). This is because the mass lies anteriorly, adjacent to the soft tissues of the neck, as shown on the computed tomography image (*asterisk*). **B,** In contrast, a mass in the posterior mediastinum will still lie adjacent to lung parenchyma above the level of the clavicles and will have sharply defined lateral margins.

*(Continued)*

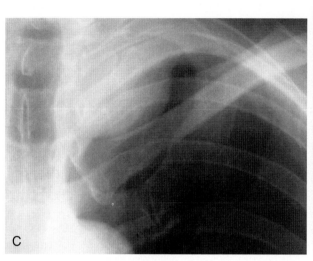

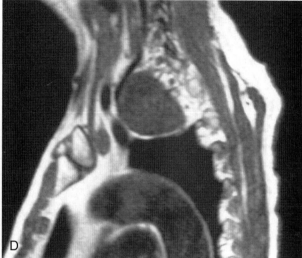

**Figure 1-23—cont'd: C,** Coned-down image of a posteroanterior chest radiograph in a patient with a posteriorly located neurogenic tumor as confirmed by magnetic resonance imaging (**D**). The margin is very well defined laterally because its border remains in contact with aerated lung parenchyma.

### *Lymphoma*

- Both Hodgkin's and Non-Hodgkin's lymphomas can cause mediastinal masses. Hodgkin's lymphoma is most likely to result in an anterior mediastinal mass.
- Fifty to eighty percent of patients with Hodgkin's disease present with mediastinal lymphadenopathy, typically seen on CT as a homogeneous anterior mediastinal soft tissue mass without calcification or cavitation. Paratracheal and hilar lymphadenopathy is often present, and disease may involve the adjacent lung.

## Middle Mediastinal Masses

- **Malignant lymph nodes** are the most common cause of a middle mediastinal mass. In a cigarette smoker, these are most likely to be from a primary lung carcinoma.
- **Mediastinal cysts** are usually congenital in origin and include foregut duplication cysts and pleuropericardial cysts. Bronchogenic cysts are the most common and are usually easily diagnosed on chest radiographs and CT (Fig. 1-24). They can occur in any part of the mediastinum but are typically located near the carina (52%) or in the paratracheal region (19%). Bronchogenic cysts contain fluid and, on CT, are usually rounded or elliptical with thin and almost imperceptible walls, and are sharply marginated and smooth in contour. The attenuation of the contained fluid is highly variable. Approximately half will contain fluid of water density, but contents may be of high attenuation when milk of calcium is present. MRI can be used to confirm their cystic nature with an invariably high signal on T2-weighted images. The presence of a homogeneous fluid containing smoothly marginated subcarinal mass is almost diagnostic of a bronchogenic cyst.

## Posterior Mediastinum

- Vascular lesions are usually easy to diagnose on contrast enhanced CT.
- Neurogenic tumors are typically identified with CT, but MRI can be useful in confirming connection to the spinal cord or nerves.

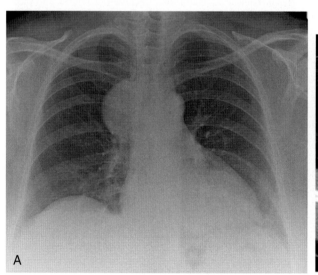

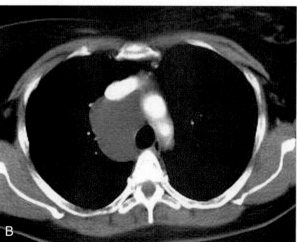

**Figure 1-24:** Chest radiograph (**A**) and computed tomography (**B**) of a mediastinal bronchogenic cyst. The chest radiograph demonstrates an abnormality in the right paratracheal region. A well-marginated, low-attenuation bronchogenic cyst is visible on a contrast-enhanced computed tomography. Its wall cannot be seen.

■ Both tuberculous and pyogenic paraspinal abscesses may present as posterior mediastinal masses and are usually associated with spinal osteomyelitis and discitis. Plain radiographs typically show extensive destruction of the margins of the vertebral bodies adjacent to the infected disc space.

## KEY RADIOLOGIC PRINCIPLES IN IMAGING THE THORACIC SURGERY PATIENT: NON-NEOPLASTIC DISEASES

### Imaging Principles in Emphysema

■ Chest radiographs are relatively insensitive for diagnosis, but in advanced disease (Fig. 1-25), the following may be seen:
1. Hyperinflation with flattening of the hemidiaphragms
2. Increased AP diameter of the thorax
3. Increased retrosternal space
4. Small heart size
5. Attenuation of the normal vascular pattern in the periphery with enlargement of the central pulmonary vessels

■ HRCT is much more sensitive than chest radiographs and correlates with macroscopic pathologic findings of emphysema (Fig. 1-26). It is superior even to pulmonary function tests.

■ The main use of CT is in the preoperative assessment of patients being considered for bullectomy or for lung volume reduction surgery (LVRS). CT can determine the extent and severity of bullae and emphysema, and accurately localize disease before surgery. Bullectomy is most effective in patients with large bullae, absence of generalized emphysema, and compression of normal lung adjacent to the bullae. The best surgical candidates for LVRS are those patients with severe emphysema causing hyperinflation.[37,38] The emphysema should be heterogenous in distribution with typically severe disease in the upper lungs but relatively normal lung elsewhere.

■ CT is also useful for the identification of subpleural bullae and blebs in patients with idiopathic spontaneous pneumothorax (Fig. 1-27).

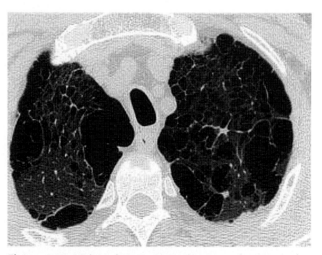

**Figure 1-26:** High-resolution computed tomography image of a different patient with severe emphysema shows focal areas of decreased attenuation with no identifiable walls. The emphysema is extensive in the subpleural regions, where bullae are present.

## Imaging Principles of Pleural Disease Pleural Effusion and Thickening

■ CT is useful in the evaluation of pleural disease, which is often complex and difficult to diagnose.

■ Pleural thickening is visualized on CT as soft tissue internal to the ribs. If the pleura can be seen on CT, it is abnormally thickened (Fig. 1-28). Abnormal pleura usually enhances following intravenous contrast.

■ Small pleural effusions can sometimes be difficult to differentiate from pleural thickening. Pleural fluid is of water density, is usually mobile, and localizes within the dependent portion of the thorax. It will not enhance following intravenous contrast (Fig. 1-29).

■ Pleural effusions are usually crescentic in shape. Effusions may extend into the fissures (Fig. 1-30). If the effusion is loculated, it may appear lenticular in shape.

■ Acute hemothorax is often of high attenuation and may demonstrate a fluid-fluid level within it. As the hemothorax begins to clot, loculations develop within the pleural fluid and fibrin balls emerge. These are of high attenuation on CT. The long-term sequelae of hemothorax include fibrothorax and pleural calcification.

■ Pleural thickening associated with an effusion suggests that the effusion is an exudate, although only about 60% of exudates are associated with pleural thickening.

■ A loculated collection of fluid in a fissure may have a confusing appearance on chest radiographs and can be mistaken for a lung mass. CT can help in the diagnosis of difficult cases.

## Empyema

■ Empyemas can be free or loculated. An empyema may have classic appearances on CT. The enhancing thickened visceral and parietal pleura separate from one another to enclose the empyema, resulting in the split pleura sign (Fig. 1-31). The presence of air within a fluid collection is usually secondary to intervention, although occasionally, it may indicate a bronchopleural fistula or infection with a gas forming organism.

■ If an empyema extends into the chest wall, this is called an empyema necessitatis. The majority of these lesions are caused by tuberculosis, but alternative organisms such as actinomycosis and nocardia should be considered.

■ Distinguishing an empyema from a lung abscess is important in deciding further treatment. When imaged with CT, empyemas typically have smooth interfaces with the lung parenchyma and make an obtuse angle with the chest wall.

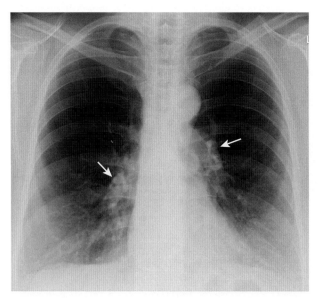

**Figure 1-25:** Posteroanterior chest of patient with smoking-related severe emphysema. There is marked hyperinflation with flattening of the hemidiaphragms and a relative paucity of vessels in the upper lobes that are thinner and fewer in number than in normal lungs. The central pulmonary arteries are large (*arrows*).

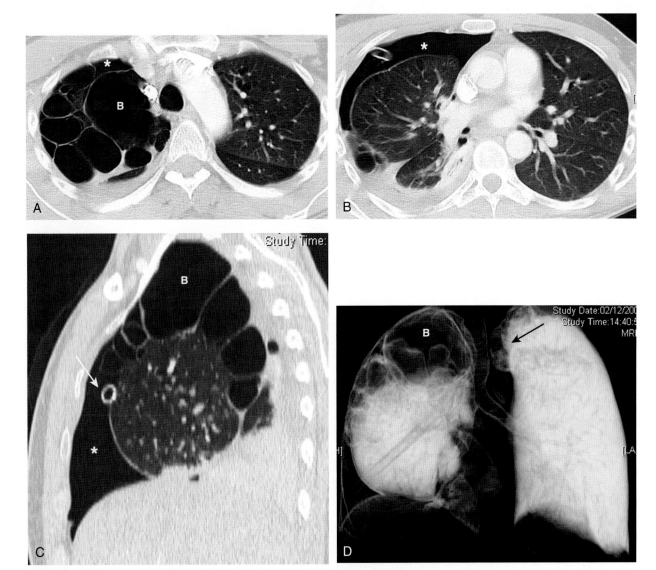

**Figure 1-27:** Computed tomography images of a 29-year-old man who presented with a spontaneous pneumothorax that was resistant to multiple chest tubes and that eventually required surgery. Two axial images (**A** and **B**) and a sagittal multi-planar reconstruction (MPR) image (**C**) show a right-sided pneumothorax (*asterisk*) and a right-sided chest drain (*white arrow*). The apical right upper lobe is almost completely replaced by large bulla (**B**). **D,** Additional blebs and bulla are also present at the left lung apex on the three-dimensional reconstruction (*black arrow*).

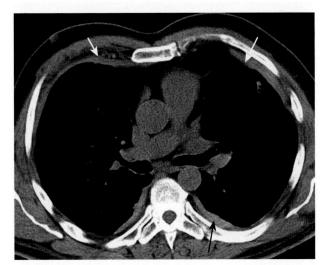

**Figure 1-28:** Computed tomography image of patient with benign asbestos–related pleural thickening (*arrows*). The pleural thickening is smooth, less than 1 cm thick, and does not involve mediastinal pleura.

Adjacent normal lung is displaced and atelectatic. In contrast, lung abscesses often manifest as irregularly marginated, thick-walled spherical cavities that have an acute angle of contact with the chest wall. They frequently contain a combination of necrotic lung, fluid, and air. Abscesses tend to destroy adjacent lung rather than displace it. Consolidated lung surrounds the cavity, and air bronchograms often extend into the abnormal region.

- Chronic empyemas are often associated with a markedly thickened fibrous pleura that requires surgical decortication. Calcification may be present if the empyema has been present for a long time.

## Malignant Pleural Disease

- Malignant pleural disease can be due to metastatic malignancy (typically adenocarcinoma), mesothelioma, or more rarely, lymphoma, sarcoma, or thymoma (Fig. 1-32). CT findings that strongly suggest the presence of malignancy include:
  1. Pleural thickening that is greater than 1 cm in thickness
  2. Circumferential pleural thickening.
  3. Nodular pleural thickening
  4. Involvement of the mediastinal pleura

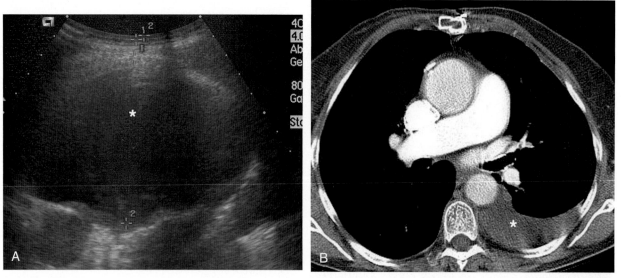

**Figure 1-29:** Thoracic ultrasound (**A**) and computed tomography (CT) image (**B**) of a patient with a small, free-flowing left-sided pleural effusion. The thoracic ultrasound shows the hypoechoic (*black*) pleural fluid. CT confirms the presence of a small left-sided pleural effusion that is layering posteriorly (*asterisk*).

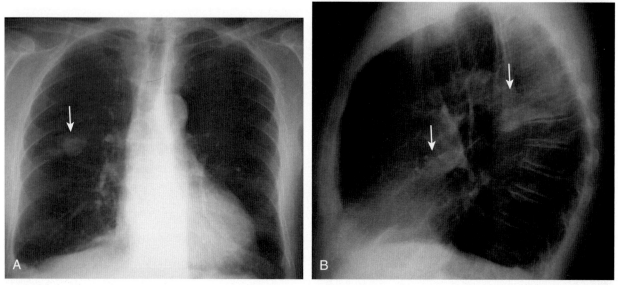

**Figure 1-30:** Pleural effusion loculating within the right major fissure that may be mistaken for pulmonary nodules in the right mid zone (*arrows*). Frontal (**A**) and lateral (**B**) examination show elliptical opacities localized to the right major fissure with sharply defined margins. There is a small right basal effusion blunting the right costophrenic angles. The effusions resolved following treatment for heart failure.

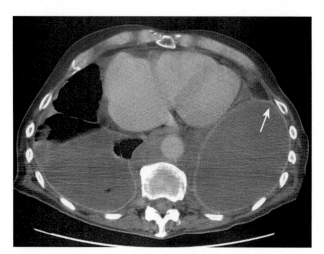

**Figure 1-31:** Computed tomography image of bilateral empyemas. Loculated pleural effusions are present in the posterior chest. The pleura is enhancing and can be seen splitting to enclose the left-sided effusion (*arrow*).

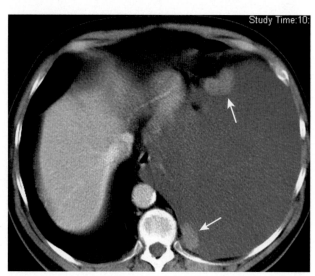

**Figure 1-32:** Contrast-enhanced computed tomography image in a patient presenting with a large left pleural effusion. There are irregular enhancing pleural nodules (*arrows*) adjacent to a large left pleural effusion. Appearances are those of malignant pleural disease.

■ Benign pleural processes that mimic malignancy on chest radiographs can often be accurately diagnosed by CT. These include rounded atelectasis, pleural plaques, loculated pleural fluid, and extrapleural fat. Rounded atelectasis in particular has classic CT findings but may be misinterpreted as a suspicious mass on chest radiographs. On CT, rounded atelectasis typically appears as a rounded, peripheral mass that abuts an area of pleural thickening, enhances following intravenous contrast, and is associated with volume loss of the affected lobe. Bronchovascular structures are seen to curve into the abnormal area.

■ Talc pleurodesis can result in areas of dense pleural thickening containing areas of high attenuation resembling calcification.

## KEY RADIOLOGIC PRINCIPLES IN IMAGING THE THORACIC SURGERY PATIENT: THE POST-THORACIC SURGERY PATIENT

### Intensive Care Unit Imaging: General Considerations

■ Rapid processing of intensive care unit (ICU) images, immediate and accurate interpretation of images by the radiologist, and ease of accessibility of images to the clinician are crucial in the care of critically ill patients.

■ Interpretation of chest radiographs in critically ill patients is the most difficult area of chest radiology. Radiographs are typically acquired with portable equipment, and patient positioning may be suboptimal. Despite its limitations, there is clear evidence that the chest radiograph is a valuable component in the management of the ICU patient.[39,40]

■ Critically ill patients are frequently imaged in the supine position. This can make the diagnosis of pleural effusions and pneumothoraces difficult. Pleural effusions will layer posteriorly, producing a diffuse increase in density of the hemithorax but no lateral meniscus (Fig. 1-33). Pneumothoraces may

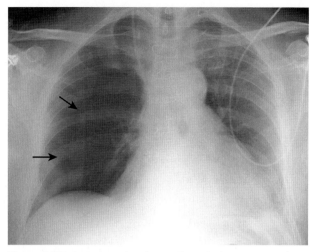

**Figure 1-34:** Anteroposterior chest radiograph demonstrates a large right pneumothorax. There are no lung markings lateral to the white (*visceral*) pleural line (*arrows*).

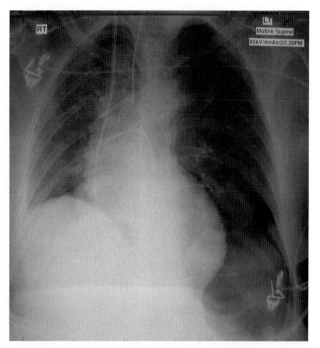

**Figure 1-35:** No lateral pleural line can be seen on this supine chest radiograph of a large left pneumothorax. There is sharp delineation of the left heart border and a deep lucent left cardiophrenic and lateral costophrenic sulcus. The inferior left hemithorax appears hyperlucent. Note the endotracheal tube (ETT), which is placed too low in the trachea just above the carina, the left subclavian central venous line, and the pulmonary artery catheter.

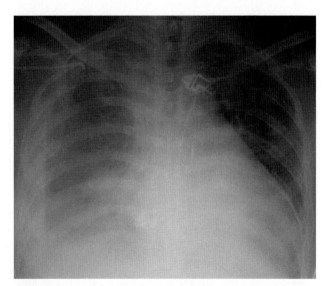

**Figure 1-33:** Supine chest radiograph demonstrates partial opacification of the right hemithorax. Pulmonary vessels can be identified through their density. Fluid can be identified laterally and over the right lung apex, suggesting that the appearances are secondary to a large pleural effusion. Note the intra-aortic balloon pump positioned within the descending thoracic aorta and the right subclavian central venous line.

manifest as an area of increased lucency in the medial basal portion of the thorax rather than the more typical apicolateral pleural line (Figs. 1-34 and 1-35).

### Support and Monitoring Devices
#### Endotracheal and Tracheostomy Tubes

■ Malpositioned endotracheal and tracheostomy tubes may cause potentially serious complications. Clinical assessment of tube location may be difficult; a chest radiograph is recommended following intubation or repositioning of a tube.

- Endotracheal tubes are fixed in position at the nose or mouth, and therefore, flexion and extension of the neck may result in motion of the tube relative to the carina, with the tube descending during flexion and ascending during extension.
- The ideal position of an endotracheal tube is 5 to 7 cm above carina with the neck in a neutral position. This equates to the T2 to T4 level if the carina is not clearly visible. The location of the tube may also be evaluated relative to the aortic arch, because the carina is typically just caudad to the arch. Hence, location of the tube just above the aortic arch is usually satisfactory.[41]
- The balloon cuff should not be greater in diameter than the trachea because cuff overinflation can cause pressure necrosis of the tracheal wall.
- Right main stem bronchial intubation occurs in approximately 9% of endotracheal intubations and may result in atelectasis of the left lung, hyperinflation of the right lung, or pneumothorax (Fig. 1-36). A double-lumen endotracheal tube may occasionally be used for selective intubation.
- Inadvertent placement of an endotracheal tube into the esophagus is uncommon but may be catastrophic. Findings suggesting inadvertent esophageal intubation include gastric or distal esophageal distension, tube location lateral to tracheal air column and deviation of trachea due to overdistended intraesophageal balloon cuff (Fig. 1-37).
- Late complications of intubation include tracheal stenosis, tracheoinnominate or tracheoesophageal fistula, stomal infection, recurrent aspiration, and nosocomial pneumonia.

### Nasogastric and Feeding Tubes

- Nasogastric and feeding tubes may be inadvertently passed into an airway, particularly in patients with neurologic impairment (Fig. 1-38).
- Other esophageal devices visible on chest radiograph include balloon tubes for treatment of varices and stents for treatment of stenosis, with gastric rupture a rare complication.

### Vascular Catheters

- Central venous catheters (central venous lines) are commonly used for administration of fluids, antibiotics, chemotherapy, or hyperalimentation, hemodialysis or hemodynamic

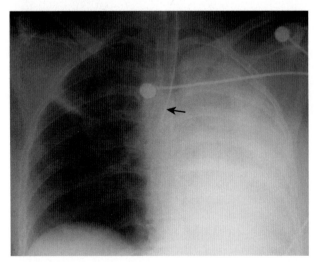

**Figure 1-36:** Malpositioned endotracheal tube is seen in the right bronchus intermedius distal to the takeoff of the right upper lobe bronchus (*arrow*). There is consequent complete collapse of the left lung and partial atelectasis of the right upper lobe.

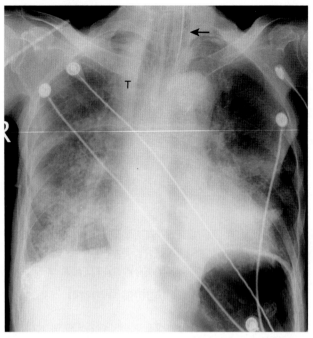

**Figure 1-37:** Esophageal intubation. The endotracheal tube (*arrow*) is within the esophagus, with the tracheal air column (T) projecting to the right of the esophagus. The esophagus and stomach are distended with air.

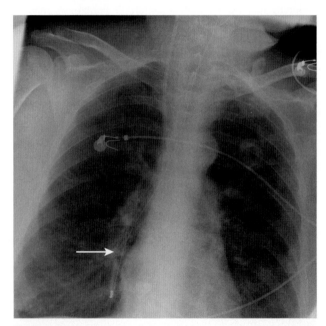

**Figure 1-38:** Supine chest radiograph from the intensive care unit following placement of a nasogastric tube. This is malpositioned within the right lower lobe bronchi (*arrow*). Tracheostomy tube and a right central venous line are appropriately positioned.

monitoring. Although the superior vena cava is most often the preferred location for the catheter tip, some authors suggest positioning the tip in the upper one-third of the right atrium.[41,42]

- Complications of placement include catheter malpositioning, catheter fracture, pneumothorax, hematoma, hemothorax, arterial puncture and air embolism or perforation of a vessel with pericardial effusion, hydrothorax, and mediastinal hemorrhage. Long-term complication of venous access devices include delayed perforation, catheter knotting, and catheter fragmentation (Figs. 1-39 and 1-40). Pinch-off syndrome, with catheter compression at the intersection of the clavicle and the rib may occur with subclavian line placement and result in catheter malfunction and possible fracture.

▪ Malpositioning of venous catheters is common and may result in venous thrombosis, perforation and inaccurate pressures.

▪ Pulmonary arterial catheters are used for hemodynamic monitoring. Complications in addition to those of central venous lines include arrhythmias, pulmonary artery perforation, and parenchymal infarction should the catheter migrate peripherally.

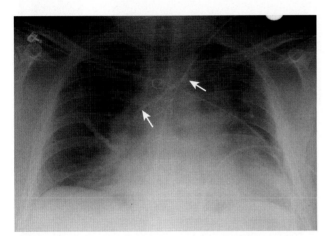

**Figure 1-39:** Anteroposterior portable chest radiograph. A left subclavian central venous line (*arrows*) has sheared off during attempted removal, leaving the distal fragment in the left brachiocephalic vein.

▪ Intra-aortic balloon counterpulsation may be used in patients with cardiogenic shock, decreasing work of the left ventricle by reducing afterload and by increasing coronary blood flow. The tip of the balloon should be located distal to the origin of the left subclavian artery.

### Chest Tubes

▪ Chest or thoracostomy tubes may vary in size. The optimal location varies depending on whether air or fluid is to be evacuated; typically, anterosuperiorly for air and posteroinferiorly for effusion. Failure of drainage may be secondary to malpositioning of tube within an interlobar fissure, chest wall, or the lung. Other causes for inadequate drainage include kinking of the tube, location of the tip of the tube against the mediastinum, or a tube side port in the chest wall.[41]

▪ CT may be helpful if there is inadequate drainage and chest radiographs are nondiagnostic.[43]

## Radiographic Appearance of the Postsurgical Chest
### Normal Appearances Postpneumonectomy

▪ In the immediate postoperative period, the postpneumonectomy space usually contains air and a small amount of fluid. The mediastinum is central, and there is mild congestion of the remaining lung.[44-46]

▪ Although the rate of accumulation of fluid in the postpneumonectomy space varies, an air-fluid level will gradually rise thereafter and the mediastinum usually shifts to the side of the pneumonectomy. Total obliteration of the pneumonectomy space takes weeks to months. The heart rotates in a clockwise fashion, and the remaining lung herniates across the midline. These factors result in an opaque postpneumonectomy space with permanent shift to the side of surgery (Fig. 1-41).

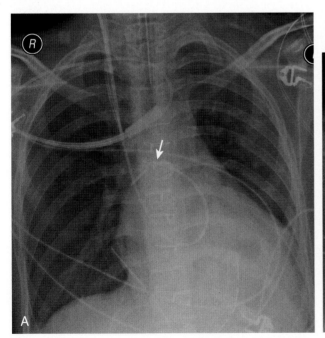

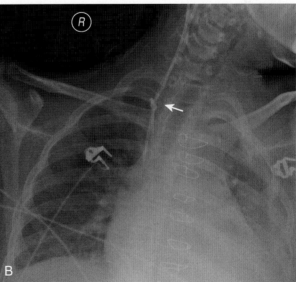

**Figure 1-40:** Portable chest radiographs of a patient after cardiac surgery. **A,** Multiple lines and tubes are in place. Close inspection of the pulmonary artery catheter reveals a knot in the distal catheter within the right main pulmonary artery (*arrow*). **B,** The majority of lines and tubes have now been removed, but note the tight knot in the distal posteroanterior catheter, which is now lodged in the right internal jugular vein adjacent to a central venous line (*arrow*).

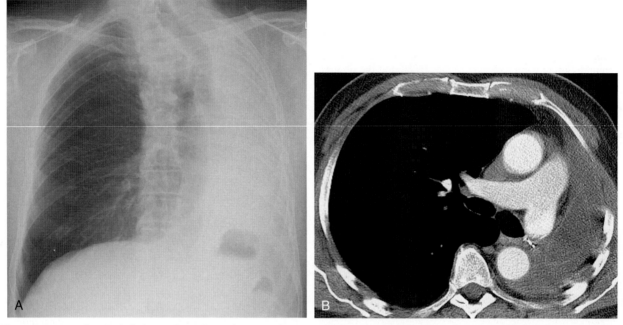

**Figure 1-41:** **A** and **B,** Typical chest radiographic and computed tomography features several months following a left pneumonectomy. There is complete opacification of the left hemithorax with mediastinal shift toward the side of the resected lung.

- It is important to evaluate the position of the mediastinum on postoperative radiographs because a shift toward the remaining lung is often a sign of a bronchopleural fistula or postoperative empyema.

### Normal Appearance Postlobectomy

- Surgical clips are typically seen at the hilum, which shifts toward the lobectomy site. Careful examination of the CT scan will show absence of a lobar bronchus with staples at

the origin of the missing bronchus, a missing major fissure after resection of a lobe on the left, or anterior displacement of the major fissure after right upper lobectomy. Chest radiographic appearance eventually resembles that of the respective lobar collapse, although the degree of volume loss after lobectomy is usually greater than with collapse (Fig. 1-42).

- Following wedge resection, multiple staples are usually seen at the resection site, with patchy air space disease adjacent to the staples representing surgical contusion. Postoperative pneumothorax due to air leak is common.

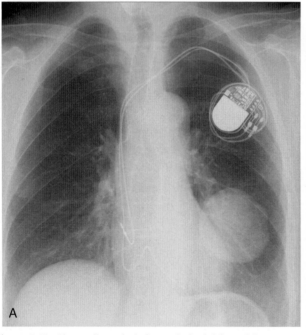

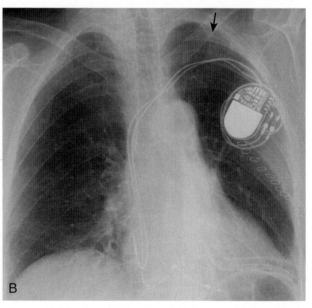

**Figure 1-42:** Chest radiographs before and after left lower lobectomy. **A,** A large, well-defined tumor lies within the left lower lobe. Note the dual-chamber pacing system. **B,** Two days after left lower lobectomy. A left basal chest drain and thoracotomy skin clips remain in place. There is a tiny left apical pneumothorax (*arrow*). There is slight volume loss of the left hemithorax, and surgical clips can be identified at the left hilum, which is now much smaller than the right.

## Postsurgical Complications Pulmonary Abnormalities

- Chest radiography and CT are especially useful in the evaluation of complications related to pulmonary resection. Air space disease may be secondary to edema, atelectasis, pneumonia, hemorrhage, or adult respiratory distress syndrome.
- **Atelectasis** results from postoperative retention of secretions and hypoventilation. It is particularly common after sleeve resection due to local edema at the anastomosis and disruption of lymphatics and cilia.
- Post-thoracotomy **pneumonia** is more common in those patients requiring prolonged ventilation. Radiographic findings vary, but typically pneumonia is seen as patchy consolidation.
- Post-thoracotomy **edema** may develop following pneumonectomy or lobectomy. It occurs most commonly after a right-sided pneumonectomy. It is usually a diagnosis of exclusion once infection and aspiration have been excluded. Interlobular septal thickening (Kerley's lines) may be visible on chest radiographs accompanied by peribronchial cuffing and loss of definition of vessels. Severe cases result in extensive consolidation identical to that seen in acute respiratory distress syndrome (ARDS).

## Hemothorax

- A rapidly enlarging pleural effusion in the immediate postoperative period usually represents a hemothorax, particularly if it contains areas of high attenuation. Later in the postoperative period, it may be secondary to a chylothorax or empyema.

## Persistent Air Leak

- Air leak is a common problem following lobectomy or segmentectomy, and it occurs more often with incomplete or absent fissures.[46]
- Pneumothorax, pneumomediastinum, and subcutaneous emphysema may be seen on chest radiograph or CT.
- The vast majority of air leaks cease within 24 to 48 hours; persistent air leaks may occur if there is a bronchopleural fistula (BPF) or bronchioloalveolar-pleural fistula.[44]

## Bronchopleural Fistula

- BPF is associated with a high mortality rate of up to 70%, the majority of deaths occurring from aspiration and ARDS. In the early postoperative period BPF is most commonly due to surgical technique or infection of the bronchial stump. BPF occurring months after surgery is most commonly due to recurrent malignancy.
- The diagnosis should be considered if there is persistence of significant pneumothorax, pneumomediastinum, or surgical emphysema greater than 24 to 48 hours after surgery.
- Radiologic findings include
  1. Persistent intrapleural air
  2. New air-fluid level
  3. Drop in a pre-existing air fluid level
  4. Movement of the mediastinum back to a more central position
- CT findings include air and fluid collections in the pleural space. A communication between the airway and pleural space may be directly visualized (Fig. 1-43).
- A lung ventilation scan is helpful to diagnose a BPF after pneumonectomy if radionucleide is seen on the surgical side. Other than that, there is no radiologic finding that is diagnostic for a BPF.

## Postpneumonectomy Empyema

- Postpneumonectomy empyema is a serious complication with a significant mortality, especially if it is associated with a bronchopleural fistula. Development of multiple air-fluid

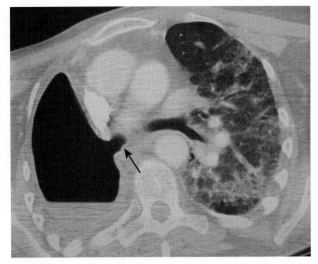

**Figure 1-43:** Bronchopleural fistula that developed 6 weeks following a right pneumonectomy for lung carcinoma. The computed tomography image demonstrates free communication between the right main bronchial stump and the right pleural cavity secondary to infection (*arrow*). Air and a small amount of fluid now occupy the right thoracic cavity. Patchy consolidation is present within the remaining left lung secondary to recurrent aspiration of infected material.

levels on chest radiographs in the early postoperative period is highly suggestive of this complication. If postpneumonectomy empyema develops later in the postoperative course, it may manifest as movement of the mediastinum away from the pneumonectomy, reflecting the space occupying nature of the empyema.

## Acute Pulmonary Embolism

- The choice of imaging tests depends on the pretest clinical probability. CT angiography (CTA) is usually the investigation of choice for suspected pulmonary thromboembolism (Fig. 1-44). CT can provide additional diagnostic information that may provide an additional or alternative diagnosis.

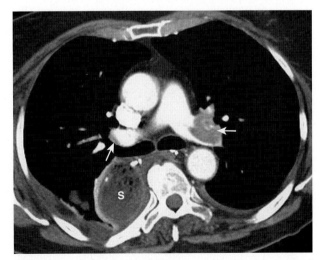

**Figure 1-44:** Contrast-enhanced axial computed tomography image of pulmonary emboli following esophagectomy for esophageal carcinoma. Emboli can be identified as filling defects within the left main and left upper lobe pulmonary arteries. A subtle filling defect is also present adjacent to the lateral wall of the distal right main pulmonary artery (*arrows*). The stomach is now intrathoracic and contains food residue (S). There are small postoperative pleural effusions.

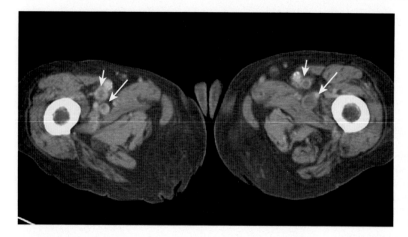

**Figure 1-45:** Axial computed tomography (CT) image from a CT leg venogram demonstrating extensive bilateral deep venous thrombosis. Filling defects are present in the superficial femoral veins (*short arrows*) and the deep femoral veins (*long arrows*). The veins are enlarged and have thickened walls. There is bilateral leg swelling and edema.

- Multidetector CT has a sensitivity of between 83% and 100% and a specificity of 89% to 97%.[47,48] In most protocols for CTA, the effective dose is between 3 and 5 mSv, which is equivalent to 1 to 2 years of background radiation.
- CT venography (CTV) can be performed as part of the CT examination, with scanning of the pelvic and leg veins taking place approximately 3 minutes after the injection of contrast for the CTA component (Fig. 1-45). The recently completed Prospective Investigation of Pulmonary Embolism Diagnosis (PIOPED) II study of 711 CT venograms showed 95% concordance between US and CTV.[47] This study concluded that CT angiography with a sensitivity of 83% and a specificity of 96% was not adequate to exclude PE but that CT angiography with CTV (sensitivity 90%, specificity 95%) was adequate. The additional radiation burden of CTV can be decreased by scanning from the acetabulum to the tibial plateau because isolated clot in the pelvic veins is rare.
- MR angiography can potentially serve as a second line examination for the diagnosis of PE in patients who are unable to receive contrast or for whom exposure to ionizing radiation is of particular concern. MR examination times are however much longer than those of CT and unstable patients are very difficult to access and safely monitor in the magnet.
- A normal perfusion scan excludes pulmonary embolism (PE) with a negative predictive value close to 100%. However, most patients will not have a definitive diagnosis made by scintigraphy. The restriction of ventilation perfusion scans to those patients with normal chest radiographs can increase the likelihood of a diagnostic scan. A ventilation perfusion scan was shown to be diagnostic in 91% of patients suspected of having PE with a normal chest radiograph.[49]

## Lobar Torsion

- Torsion of the lung, with the rotation of the bronchovascular pedicle, is a rare complication following lung resection.[50,51] Torsion may also occur spontaneously in the presence of a lung abnormality, such as a mass, or after traumatic pneumothorax.
- Torsion may involve one or more lobes, and results in airway and vascular compromise, and if uncorrected, pulmonary infarction. In the reported literature, torsion most often involves the right middle lobe. The degree of torsion is typically 180 degrees, and the rotation of hilar structures results in impaired circulation, interstitial edema, and alveolar exudates.
- Clinical findings are nonspecific, and may include fever, tachycardia, and abnormal breath sounds.
- Radiographic findings include rapid, partial, or complete lung opacification and change in position of the affected lobe.

- CT findings include increased soft tissue attenuation at the hilum, tapered, kinked or obliterated pulmonary artery and bronchus, consolidation, poor enhancement, increased volume, septal thickening, and ground glass attenuation of the involved lobe.

## Cardiac Volvulus

- Cardiac herniation and volvulus are rare but potentially catastrophic events. Most cases reported in the literature have occurred following right intrapericardial pneumonectomy in the early postoperative period, but cardiac herniation has also been described following severe chest trauma and as a consequence of a congenital pericardial defect.[52-54] The rotation of the heart on the vascular pedicle results in kinking of the superior vena cava at the right atrial junction.
- Signs and symptoms may mimic myocardial infarction, massive pulmonary embolism, or hemorrhage.
- Radiographic findings include displacement of the heart from the midline, displacement of the cardiac apex into the right hemithorax, a notch between the rounded cardiac border and the great vessels, and air within the pericardium (Fig. 1-46).

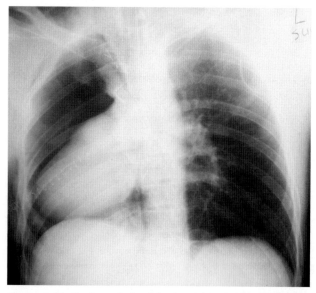

**Figure 1-46:** Cardiac volvulus following right pneumonectomy. Left central line is kinked at the superior vena cava and the cardiac apex is in the right hemithorax. The volvulus was emergently repaired and the patient recovered completely.

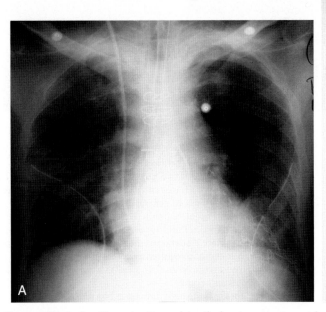
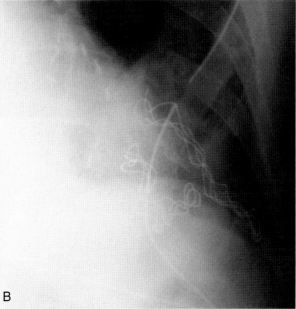

**Figure 1-47: A,** Curvilinear density overlying the heart represents a retained sponge. Cone-down view (**B**) better demonstrates the marked foreign body. Sternal wires; endotracheal, nasogastric, and right-sided chest tubes; mediastinal drains; and pulmonary artery catheter are present.

Changes in the appearance of postsurgical devices may occur, with displacement of chest tubes, rotation of the pulmonary artery catheter, or a sharp kink in a central venous catheter. Signs of impending herniation include the "snow cone sign," with an unusual bulge along the right side of the heart due to partial herniation preceding complete herniation.
■ An echocardiogram is also helpful in making this diagnosis.

## Postpneumonectomy Pulmonary Artery Stump Thrombosis

■ Thrombosis of the pulmonary artery stump may occur following pneumonectomy. In one study, stump thrombi were identified on CT in 12.4% of postpneumonectomy patients.[55] In 82% of patients, the thrombus was present on the initial CT scan. No propagation of thrombus was seen outside the stump.

## Postpneumonectomy Syndrome

■ Postpneumonectomy syndrome is a rare long-term complication of pneumonectomy. The profound mediastinal shift that often accompanies a pneumonectomy can distort and compress the remaining central airways, leading to recurrent pneumonia and bronchiectasis. Risk factors include young age of the patient and right pneumonectomy. Children or adolescents following right pneumonectomy are at greatest risk of this complication.
■ CT is useful to demonstrate the mediastinal shift and counterclockwise rotation of the mediastinum, and the site of airway obstruction.

## Retained Surgical Sponges (Gossypiboma)

■ A retained surgical sponge or swab may be known as a gossypiboma, derived from *gossypium* (Latin, cotton) and *boma* (Swahili, place of concealment).

■ The true incidence is unknown; it is estimated that 1500 cases of a retained foreign body occur annually in the United States.[56] In one study of retained instruments and sponges after surgery, 7.4% of retained foreign bodies were found in the thorax. Risk factors include emergency operations, unexpected change in procedure, and higher patient body-mass index.[56]
■ Retained sponges may be asymptomatic or may elicit a granulomatous response with development of abscess, intestinal obstruction, or fistula.
■ Most surgical sponges have an incorporated radiopaque marker because the body of a sponge is typically not visible. Radiographs are the most commonly used tool to evaluate for a retained sponge or other foreign body (Fig. 1-47). CT scan may reveal a well-circumscribed soft tissue mass with a spongiform pattern with bubbles of air.[57,58] The retained surgical foreign body may mimic an abscess in the early post operative period.
■ The American College of Surgeons has published guidelines for the prevention of retained foreign bodies after surgery (see the appendix to this chapter).

## References

Interactive references and additional readings for this chapter can be accessed online at *expertconsult.com*.

## Appendix

Appendices for this chapter can be accessed online at *expertconsult.com*.

# 2 NUCLEAR MEDICINE IMAGING IN THORACIC SURGERY

Alan Waxman, MD and Yoko Ozawa, MD

## TERMINOLOGY

- Ventilation/perfusion lung scan (V/Q)
- 2-deoxy-2($^{18}$F)fluoro-D-glucose (FDG)
- Positron emission tomography (PET)
- Standardized uptake value (SUV)
- Positron
- Coincident event

## DEFINITIONS

- *SUV*: Refers to the ratio of the concentration of radiopharmaceutical (usually FDG) in a volume of tissue in microcuries of injected agent per volume to concentration in the body if uniformly distributed (determined by a standard body phantom). The SUV has no units. An SUV of 1.0 is achieved in any tissue volume when the count rate is equal to the count rate of the uniformly distributed activity in the body phantom. The results are usually normalized to body weight.
- *Positron*: Positive electron
- *Coincident event*: Annihilation of matter when positron combines with a negative electron resulting in two 511 keV photons originating at 180 degrees from each other. The two photons are detected by the PET scanner as a coincident event if they strike the detector within a narrow time window (7–10 nanoseconds) with a 511 keV energy
- *FDG*: Glucose analog that is transported across the cell membrane similar to glucose by transporters such as GLUT-1. FDG is phosphorylated by hexokinase similar to glucose and cannot leave the cell (Fig. 2-1). FDG is not able to be metabolized in the glycolytic pathway like glucose. In highly metabolic tumors with a high requirement for glucose, an FDG concentration far greater than normal background is usually achieved.[1-5]

## IMAGING CONSIDERATIONS IN THE SOLITARY PULMONARY NODULE

- FDG PET
  - Malignant solitary pulmonary nodules (SPNs) tend to have positive PET when they are greater than 10 mm
    - Sensitivity for nodules greater than 10 mm is 95% to 98%.[6-12]
  - Spiculated nodules on computed tomography (CT) with strongly positive PET (SUV > 2.5) usually malignant
    - Specificity for malignancy increases with increasing SUV (Fig. 2-2).[6-12]
- *Sensitivity*
  - Small (<10mm) malignant pulmonary nodules seen on CT may be negative on FDG-PET or have a reduced SUV due to a partial volume effect.[13-14]

- Partial volume effect will lower the perceived activity of small objects (size below system resolution).
    - Lesions as small as 4 to 5 mm are detectable with FDG-PET, but accurate SUVs are not available unless corrections are made using phantom generated solutions (Fig. 2-3)
  - Sensitivity and negative predictive values for indolent malignancies such as carcinoid tumors, and bronchoalveolar and well-differentiated adenocarcinomas are less than tumors with high metabolic requirements (Fig. 2-4).[15-18]
  - Sensitivity is reduced in "stunned" tumors during or following chemotherapy.
  - Tumor uptake is strongly influenced by glucose and insulin levels. High glucose levels may significantly reduce tumor SUV (Fig. 2-5).
- Specificity
  - Specificity and positive predictive value of 50% to 80% are influenced by patient selection, regional influence with endemic fungal disease, exposure to tuberculosis, environmental exposures, medication, as well as criteria used to define a positive study.
- Accuracy
  - FDG-PET accuracy is greater than that of CT for characterizing SPN.[19,20]
- Prognosis
  - SUV values for an SPN of 2.5 have been suggested as a dependable marker for malignancy[10]; however, many benign lesions will have SUVs at this level, and sensitivity and specificity values at this level may be unreliable, especially in regions with high prevalence of tuberculosis or fungal disease.
  - SUV values of 5 to 10 for malignant SPNs are highly associated with a poor prognosis.[21-24]
    - Reports indicate that FDG-PET is more accurate than pathology in predicting survival or recurrence.[23,24]
  - Staging with FDG-PET is effective in offering prognostic information. However, even with a PET-negative study other than the pulmonary nodule (Stage I PET), an SUV greater than 5 is associated with poor patient outlook.[23]
- Problem areas in SPN evaluation with FDG-PET
  - False-positive studies for FDG-PET are seen in many conditions.[25-27]
    - Infectious granulomas including fungal, tuberculosis
    - Other infections; aspergillosis, bacterial, viral
    - Noninfectious granulomas; sarcoid, rheumatoid nodules, Wegener's
    - Benign neoplasms; hamartoma, fibroma
    - Inhalation disease; silicosis, lipoid pneumonia
    - Other pathology; pulmonary infarction, sequestration, inflammatory alveolitis
- Dual-time point imaging
  - Increasing SUV over time (60 versus 180 minutes) suggests malignancy.
  - Decreasing SUV over time suggests benign nodule.[28,29]

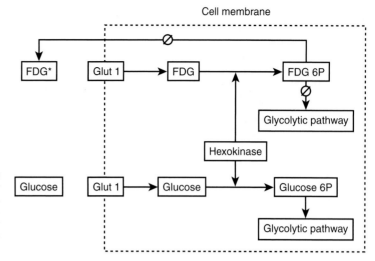

Cell membrane

**Figure 2-1:** A schematic of glucose and fluoro-deoxyglucose (FDG) uptake by a tumor cell. Note the GLUT-1 transporter recognizing both for cell entry while both are phosphorylated by hexokinase. Glucose is able to be metabolized, whereas FDG cannot enter the glycolytic pathway and is trapped within the cell, resulting in a high concentration of the radiotracer and is easily detected using the modern PET scanners.

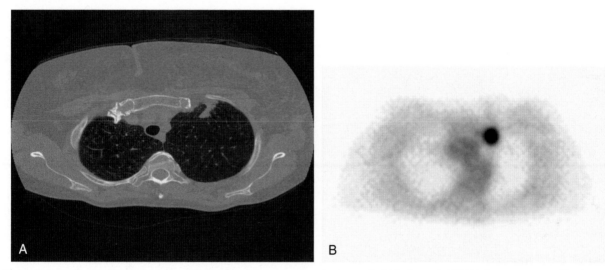

**Figure 2-2:** A 68-year-old woman, with a history of smoking, living in endemic area for histoplasmosis. CT (**A**) demonstrates scar-like abnormality in the left upper lobe. FDG-PET (**B**) demonstrates intense activity (SUV = 6.8) suggesting malignancy. Pathologic diagnosis is squamous cell cancer of the lung.

## Key Facts

- Probability of malignancy for SPN increases with increasing FDG-PET activity
- Any FDG activity in a spiculated nodule on CT suspicious for malignancy especially if nodule increases in size on serial x-ray study or CT within 90 days
- High sensitivity for 15 mm or larger pulmonary nodules due to non–small cell lung cancer (NSCLC) (95–98%)
- Specificity of FDG PET for NSCLC pulmonary nodule 50-75% dependent on multiple factors
- Indolent pulmonary malignancies have low SUVs and may be visually PET negative (bronchoalveolar cancer, carcinoid, well-differentiated adenocarcinoma)
- Correct patient preparation (low-carbohydrate diet for a minimum of 6 hours before injection of FDG and no exercise for 24 hours recommended for optimum results).
- Dual-time point imaging may be helpful in differentiating a benign from a malignant nodule.

## *FDG-PET/CT IN STAGING OF NON–SMALL CELL LUNG CANCER*

- Accurate staging of subjects with NSCLC is required for optimum patient management.[30,31]
- CT staging for NSCLC is inaccurate due to size criteria of 10 mm for positive node.[32-38]
- FDG-PET, especially with CT fusion, has emerged as the most accurate noninvasive approach to staging.[16,39-46]
- FDG-PET has been shown to be a more accurate indicator of nodal or distant metastatic disease than imaging with CT or MRI alone.[39-44]
- FDG-PET sensitivity for detection of nodal spread of NSCLC has been reported to range from 75% to 95%. Variability varies due to instrumentation, patient selection bias, and surgical and pathologic sampling (Fig. 2-6).[39-44]
- Probability of nodal malignancy is greatest when positive nodes are larger than 10 mm (Fig. 2-7), followed by FDG-positive

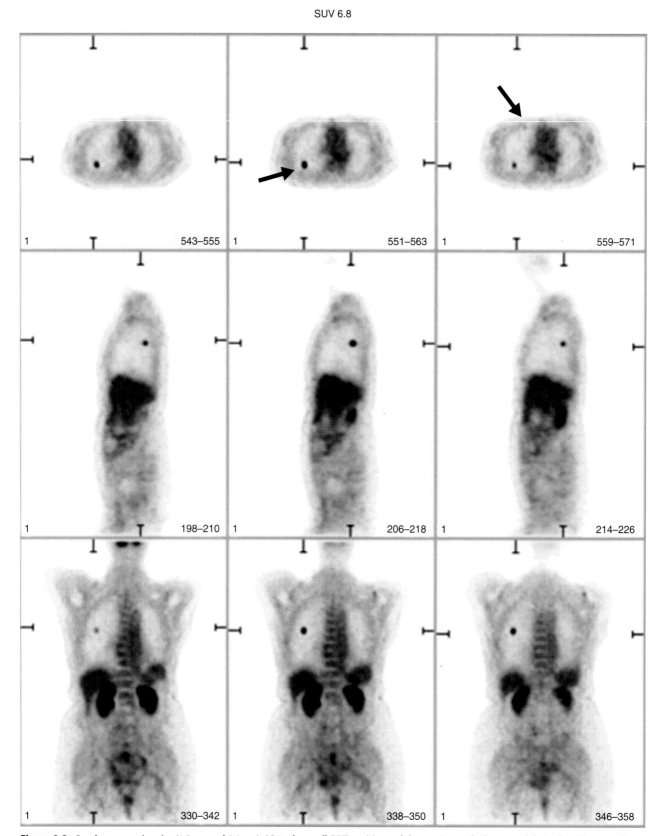

**Figure 2-3:** Synchronous primaries (1.2 cm and 0.9 cm). Note the small PET-positive nodule anterior to the larger nodule in the right upper lung. SUVs in small nodules (<10 mm) may be artificially reduced due to partial volume effects.

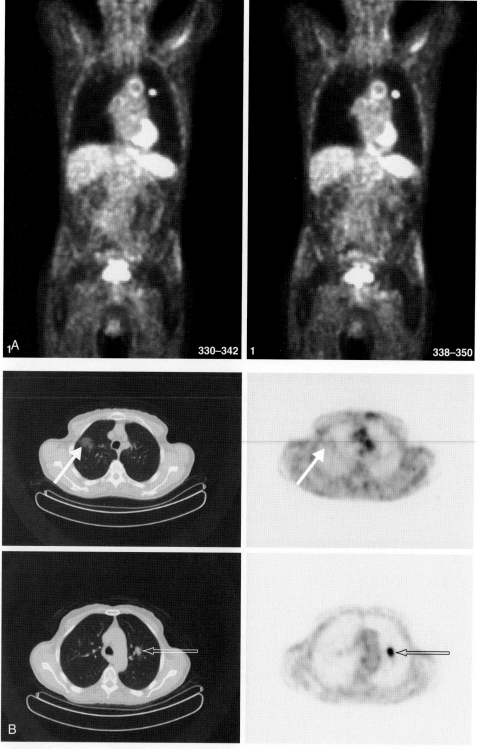

**Figure 2-4:** **A,** Coronal FDG-PET views of patient with a ground-glass opacity (3.5 cm) in the right upper lung and a 2.0-cm nodule in the left upper lung. Pathology is hamartoma on the left, with inflammatory cells and bronchoalveolar cancer of the right upper lung. **B,** CT with PET axial slices in same patient as Figure 2-4A.

ELEVATED GLUCOSE (210 mg/dL)          NORMAL GLUCOSE (110 mg/dL)

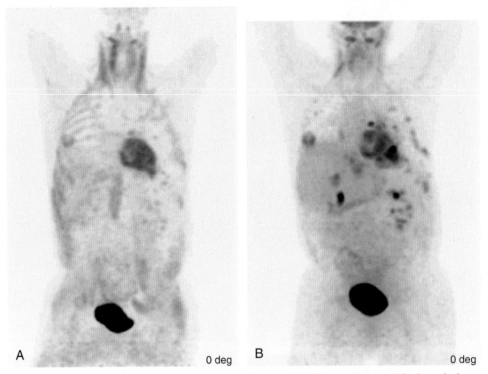

**Figure 2-5:** Importance of proper patient preparation before FDG-PET scan. Patient with elevated glucose demonstrates low-level activity in right lower lung primary adenocarcinoma. Patient properly prepared (no carbohydrate for a minimum of 6 hours before injection of FDG) demonstrates increased intensity in primary with additional foci in both right and left lung.

LUNG CANCER SUV 4.1

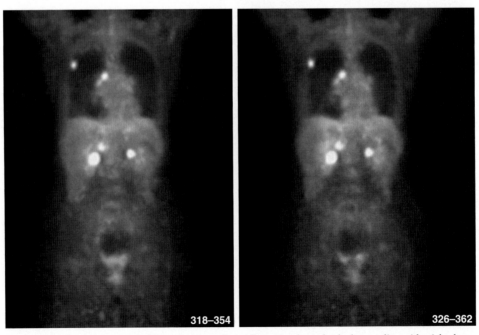

**Figure 2-6:** Coronal FDG-PET views demonstrating right upper lung focal abnormality with right lower paratracheal focus as well. Pathology is adenocarcinoma with mediastinal metastasis (Stage 3A).

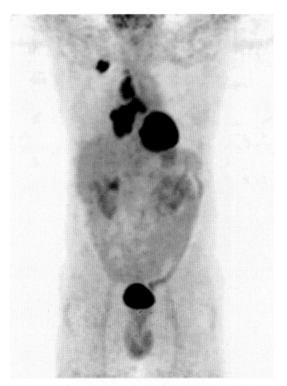

**Figure 2-7:** Maximum Intensity Projection (MIP) FDG-PET image in a patient with right upper lung adenocarcinoma and extensive mediastinal metastasis. Primary tumor SUV = 12.4. Higher SUV values of primary generally correlate with poor prognosis and increased frequency of metastasis.

nodes smaller than 10 mm, followed by FDG-negative nodes larger than 10 mm, and least probable when FDG-PET is negative in nodes smaller than 10 mm.[45]

- FDG-PET is more accurate than CT in nodal staging; however, use of combined PET/CT systems or software fusion is more accurate than PET or CT alone (Fig. 2-8).[40,42-44]
- Specificity may be reduced in regions of endemic tuberculosis (TB) and fungal disease.
- PET correctly alters staging 20% to 30% of the time and changes patient management 14% to 37% of the time (Fig. 2-9).[41,47–49]
- PET staging is a better predictor of time to death than clinical or CT staging.

## Surgical Resectability
- Accurate staging important in determining resectability for cure.
- $T_3$ lesions (extension into chest wall, diaphragm, mediastinal pleura, pericardium or main bronchus) may have curative surgical potential.
- $T_4$ lesions (invasion of mediastinum, great vessels, heart, trachea, esophagus, vertebra, or other vital structures) generally not amenable to surgery.
- PET specificity and positive predictive values are unreliable for mediastinal evaluation with unacceptable false-positive results (Fig. 2-10). Tissue confirmation is required in most cases of positive mediastinal PET results. Usually, this is done with mediastinoscopy when possible.[45,50-52]
  - ○ PET will help to determine the best biopsy approach and also may determine if stage IV disease is present.
  - ○ Central primary tumor may obscure mediastinal nodal activity, especially with high SUV values (mediastinoscopy suggested).

## Detection of Extrathoracic Metastases
- FDG-PET and PET/CT whole body scan is effective in detecting stage IV disease (Fig. 2-11).[53-62]
- The frequency of extrathoracic metastases is 10% to 15%.[63-64]
- Lytic or trabecular metastases best detected with FDG-PET compared with conventional technetium-99m methylene diphosphonate (Tc99m MDP) bone scans.[59]
- Osteoplastic bone metastases are best detected with conventional bone scans.[59]
- Response to therapy is best assessed with FDG-PET as false-positive increases often seen with conventional bone scans due to healing effect (FLARE).
- Nonosseous metastases (adrenal and liver most common sites).[55,61-62]
- Brain metastasis may be detected; however, due to high concentration of FDG, MRI is the test of choice

## Restaging Following Therapy (Chemotherapy)
- Traditional response assessment by size changes with radiography, CT, or MRI.
- New response assessment uses morphology and function (tumor viability).
- Reduction in metabolic activity after one to three cycles of chemotherapy correlates with clinical response in most reports (Fig. 2-12).[67-71]
- Management changes due to results of FDG-PET are as high as two thirds of cases.[47]

## Radiation Therapy Planning
- FDG-PET/CT allows contouring of target volumes using both anatomic and metabolic borders. Regions that are not detected with planning CT often are detected with PET allowing inclusion in radiation field (Fig. 2-13).[72-75]
- Changes in target volumes may increase or decrease depending on results[74] of the FDG-PET scan
- Response to radiation therapy can be successfully monitored with FDG-PET.
  - ○ Post-therapy inflammation, however, may persist for months, resulting in an inaccurate interpretation.

## *MESOTHELIOMA*
- CT conventional imaging is the main imaging technique for assessment of malignant pleural mesothelioma.
- Limitations of CT
  - ○ N staging is limited: enlarged nodes (>1 cm) are often benign. Small nodes (<1 cm) may harbor metastases.
  - ○ Pleural thickening may be benign scarring.
  - ○ Underestimates extent of chest wall involvement and peritoneal involvement.[76-78]
- PET and PET/CT identifies malignant sites (Fig. 2-14).[79]
  - ○ SUV higher in malignant sites than in most benign processes.
  - ○ Superior to CT alone in nodal staging.[79]
  - ○ Identifies extrathoracic metastases.[80]
  - ○ Directs biopsy to most appropriate site.[81]
  - ○ High SUV is associated with a poor prognosis.[82]

## *VENTILATION/PERFUSION LUNG SCANS*
### Ventilation Scans
- Ventilation studies with gaseous radiopharmaceuticals
  - ○ Xenon 133
  - ○ Xenon 127
  - ○ Krypton 81m

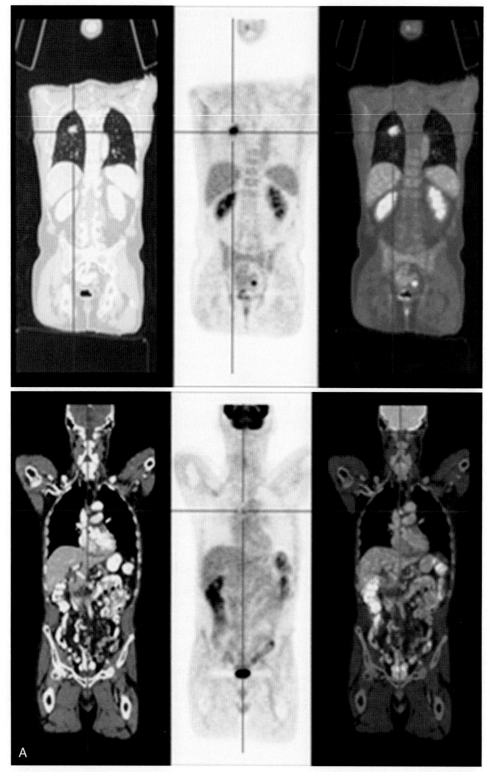

**Figure 2-8: A,** Patient with 3.5-cm spiculated right upper lung lesion on CT scan, and borderline precarinal lymph node, otherwise normal. FDG-PET demonstrated intense activity in the lesion (SUV = 9.2) and also detected a small mediastinal node. Staging increased from 2A to 3A. Pathology is adenocarcinoma with positive precarinal lymph node.

*(Continued)*

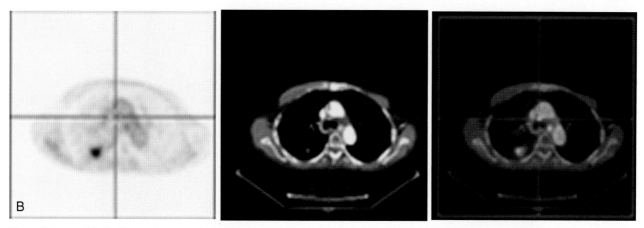

**Figure 2-8—cont'd: B,** CT scan demonstrating borderline precarinal lymph node with definite FDG activity on FDG-PET.

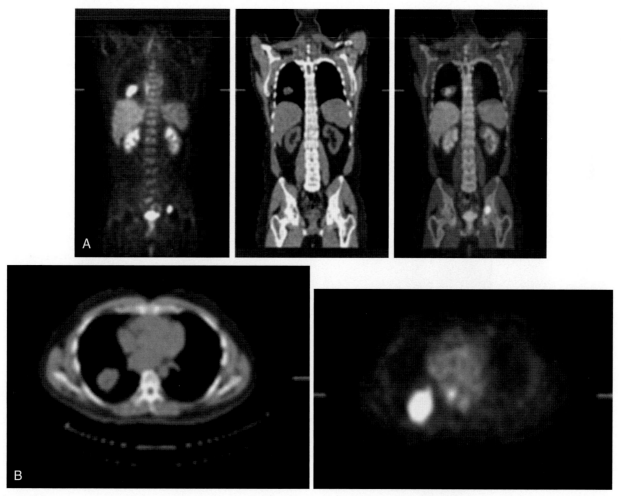

**Figure 2-9: A,** Large right lower lung nodule 4.2 × 3.5 cm. SUV is 10.4. Note metastasis to the left acetabulum. Pathology is squamous cell cancer of the lung. **B,** Same patient in Figure 2-8A. Note metastatic focus adjacent to spine and posterior mediastinum.

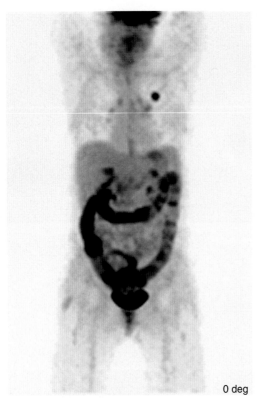

0 deg

**Figure 2-10:** MIP image with solitary left upper lung pulmonary nodule. Multiple small foci in bilateral hilum and mediastinum. Pathology for nodule is adenocarcinoma. Pathology for mediastinal nodes is noncaseating granulomas. FDG-PET detects small lymph nodes with granuloma or other inflammatory/infectious processes and is therefore not specific for tumor. The distribution pattern in this patient is typical for granuloma.

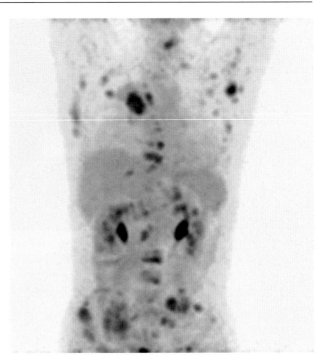

**Figure 2-11:** Patient with metastatic squamous cell cancer (Stage 4). Note multiple metastatic sites including mediastinum, axilla, and multiple osseous sites. Patient was asymptomatic, with no history of bone pain. FDG-PET has been shown to be an excellent test for staging of distant metastasis, and is superior to x-ray and CT imaging.

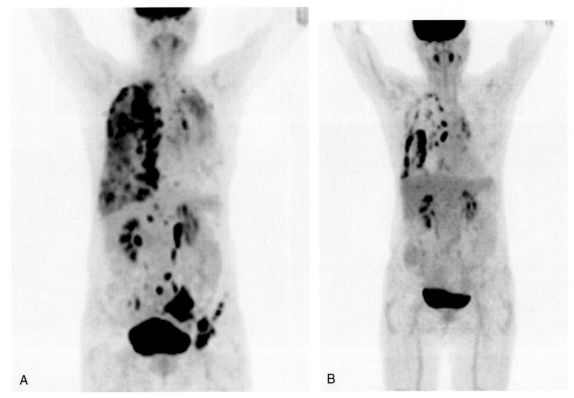

A                                                                    B

**Figure 2-12:** FDG-MIP images in a patient with widespread lung cancer pre- and postchemotherapy. **A,** Baseline prechemotherapy. **B,** After three cycles of chemotherapy.

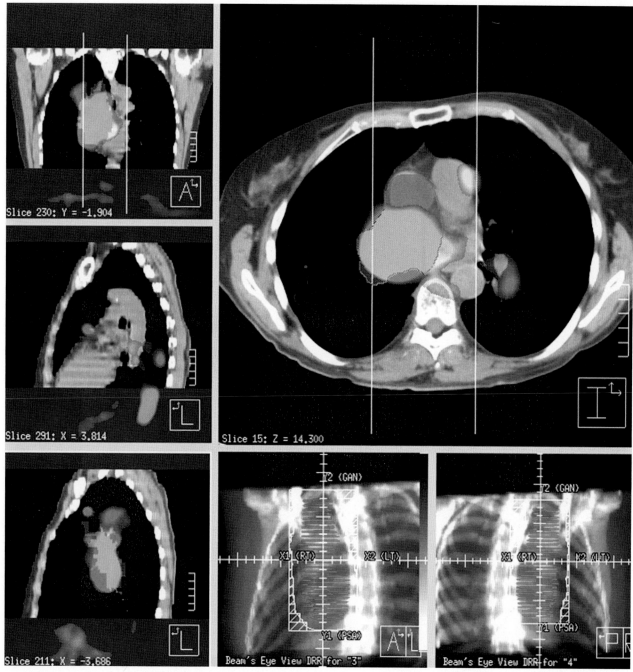

**Figure 2-13:** FDG-PET fused with radiation therapy planning CT. Red areas on axial image indicate the target volume determined by contouring of CT. Green areas represent FDG-PET distribution. Orange regions represent overlap of CT contour and FDG-PET distribution. Note the tumor sites not included in the original CT contour map. FDG fusion mapping is frequently included in determining target volumes for radiation therapy.

- Xenon 133 advantages
  - May be used pre or postperfusion.
  - Readily available commercially.
  - Inexpensive.
  - Wash-in, washout information.
  - Useful to establish postpneumonectomy stump leak.
- Xenon 133 disadvantages
  - Limited views
  - May be difficult for seriously ill or elderly patients to cooperate for study
  - Leakage from face mask may cause local contamination

- Xenon 127 advantages
  - Photopeak energy (keV) ideal for postperfusion ventilation studies
- Xenon 127 disadvantages
  - Not readily available
  - Expensive
  - Other as per Xenon 133
- Krypton 81m advantages
  - Short half life (13 sec) approximates alveolar distribution
- Krypton 81m disadvantages
  - Production generator (Rb81) required

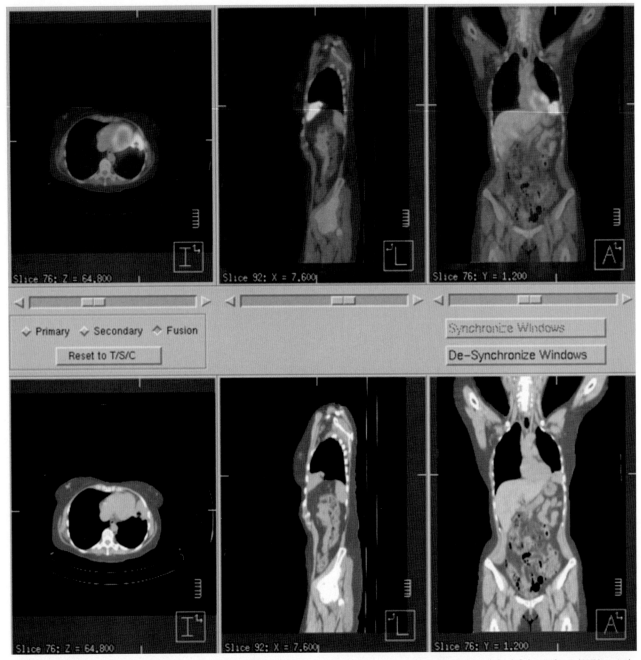

**Figure 2-14:** FDG-PET/CT in a patient with malignant mesothelioma (epithelioid type) involving the pleura of the left lower lung (SUV = 9.1). Fusion imaging is helpful in defining the extent and location of malignant mesothelioma. Pleurectomy via thoracoscopy demonstrated a malignant pleural mesothelioma. The pericardium was not involved.

   ○ Expensive
   ○ Not readily available
   ○ Not adequate to evaluate obstructive airway disease
 ■ Ventilation studies with submicronic particles
   ○ Technetium-99m diethylenetriamine-pentacetic acid (Tc 99m DTPA)
   ○ Tc 99m sulfur colloid
 ■ Tc 99m DTPA advantages
   ○ Multiple views are easy to obtain.
   ○ Study is inexpensive.
   ○ Patient cooperation is usually satisfactory.
   ○ Nebulizer kit and radiopharmaceutical are readily available.
   ○ Obstructive airway disease is really diagnosed.

 ■ Tc 99m DTPA disadvantages
   ○ Difficult to use when performing a V/Q study with quantitation of perfusion unless perfusion is done before ventilation.
 ■ Tc 99m sulfur colloid advantages
   ○ Similar to Tc 99m DTPA
 ■ Tc 99m sulfur colloid disadvantages
   ○ Higher patient dose than Tc99m DPTA (slower clearance)
   ○ Slightly higher cost than Tc99m DTPA

### Perfusion Lung Scan

 ■ Radiopharmaceutical Tc 99m macroaggregated albumen (MAA) particles (30–60 μ size)

## Perfusion Lung Scan: Clinical Applications

- Evaluation of pulmonary embolus (PE)
- Preoperative assessment before lung resection for tumor or parenchymal disease
- Prediction of postresection pulmonary function
- Evaluation of lung transplant candidate
- Evaluation of post-transplant pulmonary function in suspected rejection
- Evaluate right-to-left cardiac shunts
- Evaluate congenital heart disease

## V/Q Evaluation of Pulmonary Embolus

- Prospective investigation of pulmonary embolism diagnosis (PIOPED): widely used in original or modified form to evaluate V/Q studies
  - Probability of PE assigned based on criteria established by V/Q scan correlation with angiography[83-87]

### Interpretation of V/Q Scan for PE Diagnosis

- Normal: No PE
- Near-normal: less than 5% probability
- Low probability (5–19%)
- Intermediate (20–79%)
- High probability (≥80%)

- Normal
  - Uniform activity throughout both lungs (Fig. 2-15)
- Low probability
  - Small scattered defects
  - V/Q multiple matched findings with no infiltrates on chest x-ray study (Fig. 2-16)
  - Single matched moderate or large defect may be low or intermediate
  - Perfusion defects smaller than chest x-ray study findings
- Intermediate probability
  - Neither high or low probability
  - Mismatched defects less than 2 segmental equivalents
  - Matched V/Q and chest x-ray study
  - Knowledgeable interpreter should stratify within intermediate category (low to high intermediate)
- High probability
  - Two or more mismatched segments or segmental equivalents (Fig. 2-17)
- False positive V/Q for PE
  - Vasculitis
  - Central tumor involving pulmonary artery segments directly or nodal enlargement with vascular compression
  - Fibrosing mediastinitis
  - Chronic or prior PE with residual fibrinous webs
  - Primary pulmonary hypertension
  - Congenital defects involving pulmonary artery

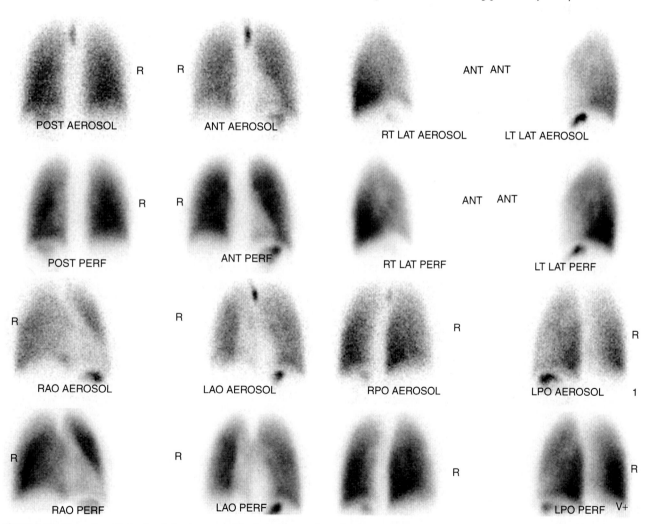

**Figure 2-15:** Normal ventilation/perfusion lung scan. Ventilation was performed using a submicronic mist of Tc-99m DTPA (1 millicurie). Note the homogeneous appearance throughout both lungs. A perfusion lung scan is then performed with 4 millicuries of Tc-99m macroaggregated albumin particles (30–50 μ). Note the homogeneous appearance.

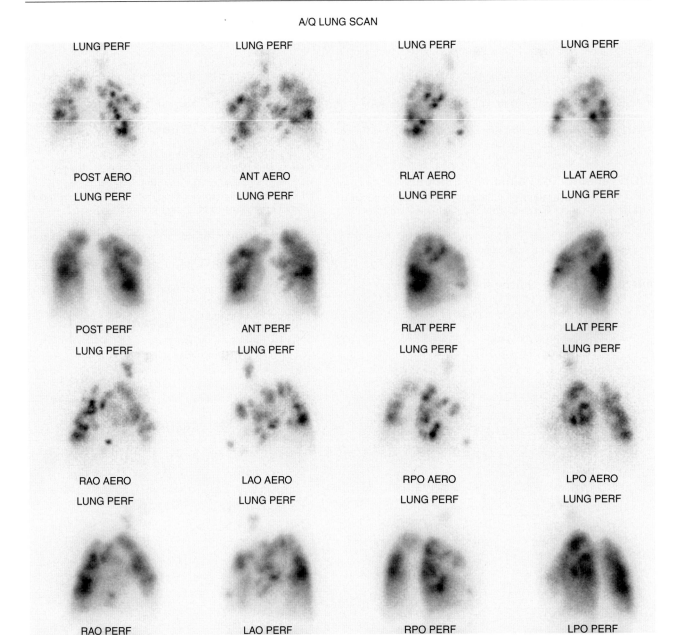

**Figure 2-16:** Low-probability V/Q scan in a patient with extreme shortness of breath. Note the severe nonhomogeneous pattern on ventilation consistent with obstructive pulmonary disease and probable parenchymal disruption. Perfusion is mainly matching but overall appears more uniform. There are no mismatches. This finding is representative of patients with a pulmonary parenchymal process with an obstructive component.

## Preoperative Assessment Before Resection with Perfusion Lung Scan

- Prediction of residual lung function postresection (calculation of percentage perfusion remaining approximates residual lung function).[88-92]
- Identifies regional abnormalities where resection may give favorable results (upper lobe hypoperfusion identifies patients who are likely to improve with upper lobe resection allowing expansion).[92]
- Quantitation techniques variable
  ○ Three-zone technique is not anatomic and unreliable.
  ○ Identify and quantitate upper lobe, lower lobe, middle lobe, and lingula.

○ Give percentage perfusion for each lung (normal 55–60% right, 40–45% left)
○ Within each lung, calculate percentage perfusion for each lung (lateral and oblique views helpful) (Fig. 2-18A to D)

## Right-to-Left Intracardiac Shunt Evaluation with Perfusion Lung Scan

- Pulmonary to systemic shunt usually interatrial or interventricular defect.[92-96]
- Normally more than 95% of injected macroaggregated particles are trapped in lung capillaries.

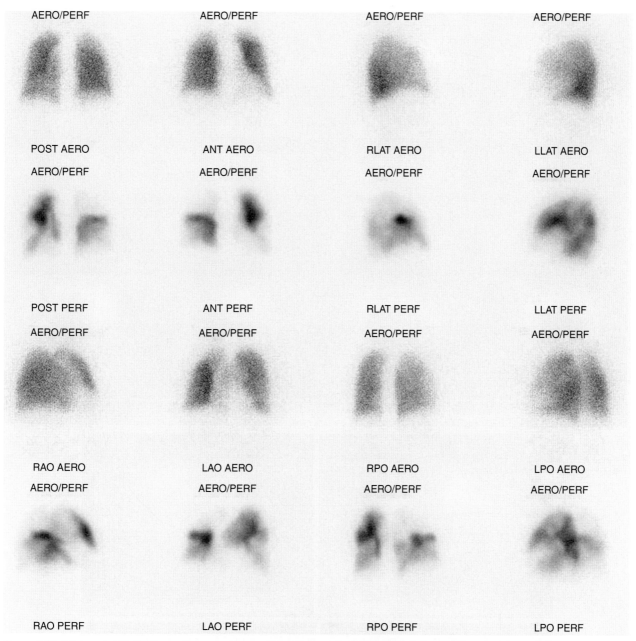

**Figure 2-17:** High-probability V/Q scan demonstrating normal ventilation and multiple segmental and large subsegmental perfusion abnormalities. Mismatched segments or large subsegments greater than 2 segmental equivalents are considered a high probability for pulmonary emboli (greater than 80%).

- If right to left shunt is present, particles are trapped in extra-pulmonary sites in proportion to blood flow, mainly kidneys and brain (Fig. 2-19A and B)
- Imaging with 4 mCi Tc 99m-MAA in a preparation containing fewer than 600,000 particles suggested
- Percent of right to left shunt equals counts for total body (usually lung + brain + kidney) minus lung counts divided by total body counts. This value is multiplied by 100 to achieve percent of right to left shunt. Time to acquire counts must be identical for all sites
- Nuclear medicine techniques for shunt evaluation are complimentary to primary modality of Echo-Doppler. MRI using gated, dynamic techniques is excellent but requires special equipment and is difficult to perform.

## Differential Diagnosis
- Interatrial or intraventricular defects
- Intrapulmonary shunt
- Congenital defects
- Hepatopulmonary syndrome

## Lung Transplantation Evaluation with Ventilation Perfusion Scans
- Pre transplant[97,98]
  ○ Identifies most severely compromised lung for single lung transplant.
  ○ Quantitation is mandatory.
  ○ Always used in conjunction with pulmonary function studies.

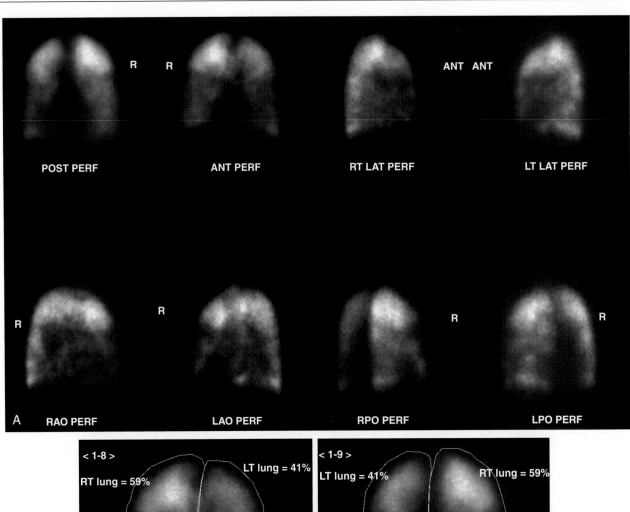

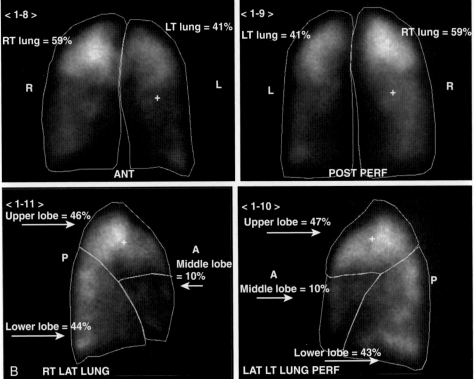

**Figure 2-18:** **A,** Perfusion lung scan with 4 mCi Tc-99m MAA particles in a 66-year-old patient with chronic obstructive pulmonary disease and emphysema for possible lung reduction surgery. **B,** Quantitative perfusion analysis in same patient; note the nonhomogeneous pattern throughout the lungs, with greater activity in the upper lung zones than in the mid and lower regions. Patient is not a candidate for a lung reduction surgery.

*(Continued)*

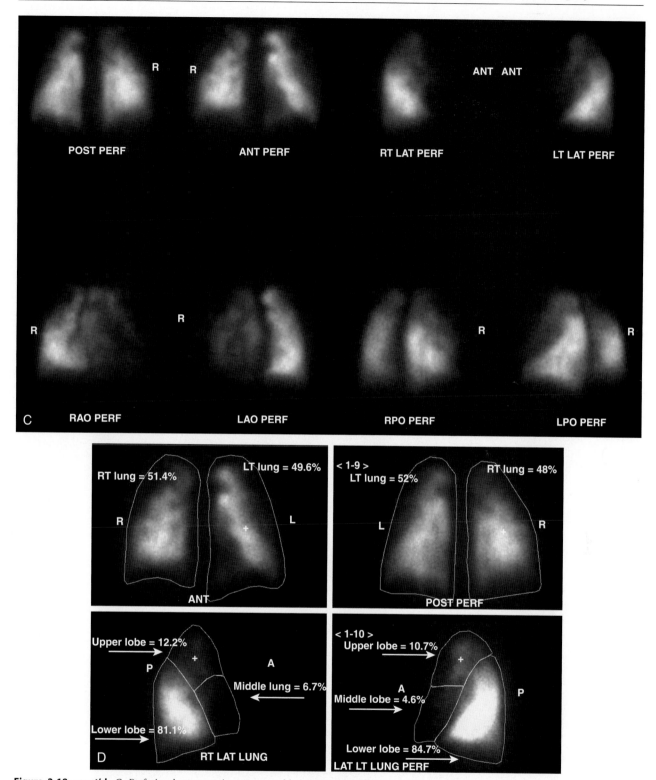

**Figure 2-18—cont'd: C,** Perfusion lung scans in a 61-year-old patient with emphysema. Note the bilateral reduction of upper lobe perfusion. **D,** Quantitative perfusion analysis of same patient demonstrates severe reduction in upper lobe perfusion bilaterally (right upper lobe, 12% of total right lung perfusion; left upper lobe, 11% of total left lung perfusion).

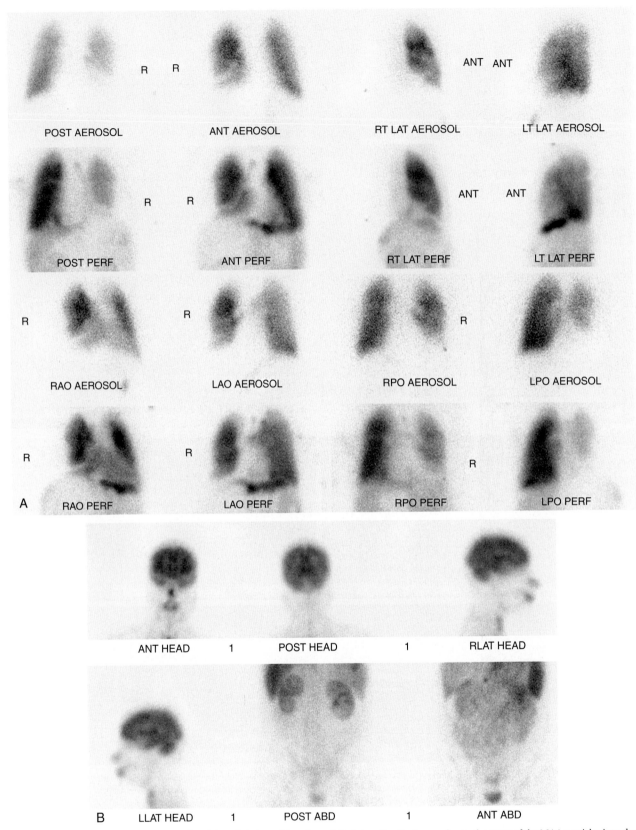

**Figure 2-19:** **A,** V/Q scan in a patient with a right to left shunt. Note the activity below the diaphragm due to the entry of the MAA particles into the systemic circulation after bypassing the pulmonary vasculature. **B,** Same patient as in Fig. 2-16A. High-resolution images of the brain and kidneys demonstrate increased activity due to the MAA particles, which have entered the systemic circulation. The degree of shunt can be calculated by measuring the counts in the whole body and individually within the lungs.

■ Post-transplant
  ○ Successful transplant demonstrates return of normal or near-normal scan patterns for both ventilation and perfusion.
  ○ Early rejection demonstrates mild reduction in ventilation with more 20% discordance between ventilation and perfusion (single lung transplant).
  ○ Ventilation declines more rapidly than perfusion.
  ○ Serial studies are helpful to evaluate rejection, especially with dual lung transplantation.

## Postpneumonectomy Leak Evaluation

■ Determine if air leak is present in the bronchial stump post pneumonectomy
■ Xenon 133 using a long rebreathing protocol will detect an airway defect in the bronchial stump as trapping of Xenon gas occurs over time (Fig. 2-20)

## NUCLEAR MEDICINE EVALUATION OF THYMUS AND THYMIC TUMORS

■ Radiopharmaceuticals that may demonstrate thymic activity include F18-deoxyglucose, gallium 67 citrate, In 111 pentetreotide, and I 131 post-therapy for thyroid cancer
■ Thymic hyperplasia
  ○ Increased gallium and FDG thymic activity are often seen in children and young adults following chemotherapy (thymic rebound). Finding may be present in older subjects at times and occasionally as a normal variant (Fig. 2-21).[99-101]
  ○ Thymic activity usually diffuses and fades by 6 months post-chemotherapy but may persist especially in younger subjects.
  ○ Activity is thought to be secondary to reactive thymic medullary epithelial cells and regional lymphocytes stimulated during recovery phase following chemotherapy.
  ○ May be present in activated lymphocytes in patients with systemic lupus erythematosus.[102]

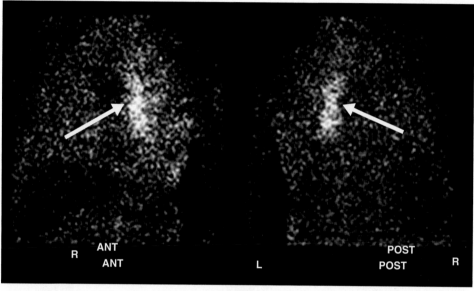

**Figure 2-20:** Xenon 133 anterior and posterior images of the thorax in a subject following left pneumonectomy and suspected leak of the bronchial stump. Note the collection of xenon in the medial left thorax (*arrows*) following 3 minutes of rebreathing from a spirometer containing xenon 133.

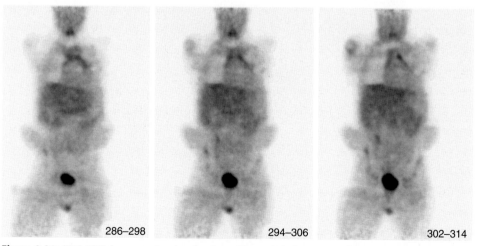

**Figure 2-21:** FDG-PET demonstrating thymic rebound/hyperplasia in a patient following chemotherapy. Note the characteristic pattern of an inverted "cap" in the anterior superior mediastinum. Thymic hyperplasia is most common in young individuals; however, the condition may occasionally be seen in older subjects. Findings have also been described using gallium-67 citrate.

- Thymoma
  - Highly likely to be positive on FDG-PET.[103-105]
  - FDG-PET will not differentiate a benign from a malignant thymoma because both may have similar spectrum of activity (malignant overall slightly higher).[106]
  - Additional FDG focus in mediastinal nodes increases probability of malignancy.
  - Approximately a third of patients with thymoma will develop symptoms of myasthenia gravis.

## Thymic Epithelial Tumors
- Multiple histologic subtypes: A, AB, B1, B2, B3.

### Thymoma and Thymic Carcinoma
- A, AB considered benign
- B1 considered low-grade malignancy with 10-year survival rate higher than 90% (low-risk thymoma),
- B2 and B3 are higher grade tumors with progressively worse prognosis (high-risk thymomas).
- Thymic carcinoma (poor prognosis).
- FDG-PET imaging.
  - MRI and CT are the established primary imaging modalities.
  - PET/CT is rapidly emerging as a primary modality for diagnosis, staging, restaging, and monitoring of therapeutic response
  - Benign and low risk thymoma (A, AB, B1) have slightly lower SUV than high risk (B2, B3) thymoma but difference not statistically significant
  - Both low- and high-risk thymoma have lower SUV values than thymic carcinoma (P < 0.001).[105,106]
  - Scan pattern of homogeneous FDG uptake more frequent in thymic carcinoma than high-risk (P = 0.027) or low-risk (P = 0.001) thymoma.
  - Presence of FDG in mediastinal fat, mediastinal nodes, pleural or pericardial implants, or distant metastases indicates aggressive thymic neoplasm.[106]
  - PET/CT is most helpful in characterizing lymph node or distant metastases than either PET or CT alone (Fig. 2-22A to C).[106]
  - PET/CT is useful in differentiating thymic tumor subtypes and staging.[105,106]

## Differential Diagnosis of Thymic Masses with FDG-PET
- Thymoma including high- and low-risk subtypes: SUVs usually proportional to grade but considerate overlap prevents precise separation.[106]
- Thymic carcinoma: SUVs high (>5.0) can usually separate thymoma from thymic carcinoma.[105,106]
- Thymic cyst (third bronchial pouch) usually negative on FDG-PET unless inflamed or infected.
- Hypermetabolic brown fat: may have high SUVs. Characteristic distribution in cervical, axillary, and paraspinal regions (Fig. 2-23).
- Thymolipoma: variable size, negative on FDG-PET
- Metastatic involvement: variable SUV. Primary may be detected.
- Systemic lupus erythematosus: may have diffuse homogeneous activity.[102]
- Substernal thyroid: nonhomogeneous low-level activity (Fig. 2-24).
- Germ cell tumor
  - Variable FDG acivity, low in teratoma and higher in seminoma.
- Melanoma
- Lymphoma (Fig. 2-25)
  - Most common anterior mediastinal malignancy.
  - SUVs usually high. Low-grade lymphoma less active.
  - FDG-PET good for post-therapy follow-up (Fig. 2-26)
- Thymic carcinoid
  - Usually low SUV.[107]
  - Increased In 111 pentetreotide activity.

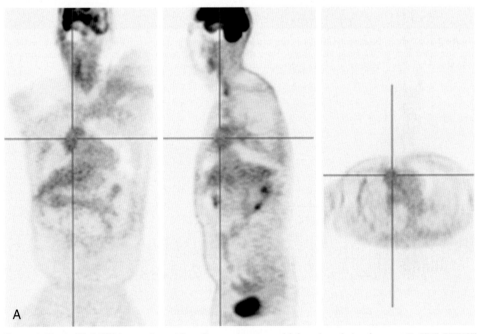

**Figure 2-22: A,** FDG-PET in a patient with malignant thymoma with lymph node involvement. **B,** FDG-PET/CT fusion image. Same patient as Figure 2-20A.

*(Continued)*

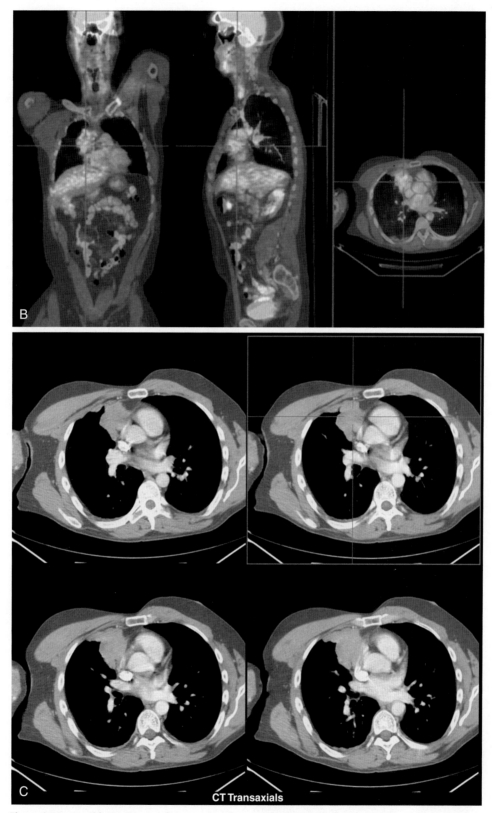

**Figure 2-22—cont'd:** C, CT scan of same patient demonstrating mediastinal tumor involvement.

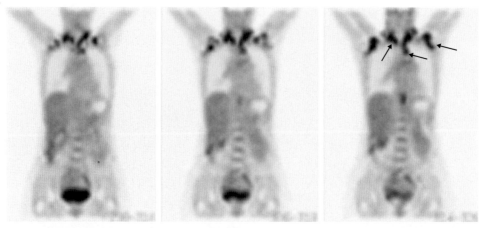

**Figure 2-23:** FDG-PET demonstrating hypermetabolic regions in the neck, supraclavicular regions, axilla, and mediastinum corresponding to low-density regions on CT scan. Study was performed for restaging of thymoma in a patient determined to have no residual disease. Findings are typical for detection of brown fat using FDG-PET imaging.

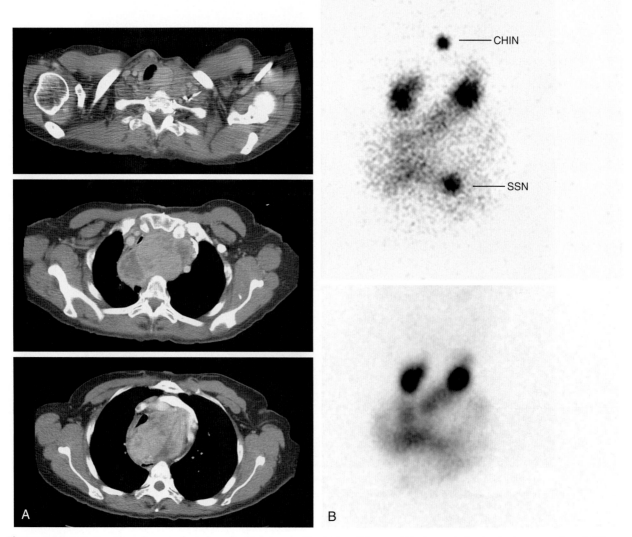

**Figure 2-24:** Patient with a large neck and mediastinal mass with stridor. CT scan (**A**) demonstrates tracheal compression. I-123 scan (**B**) demonstrates large thyroid goiter with substernal extension.

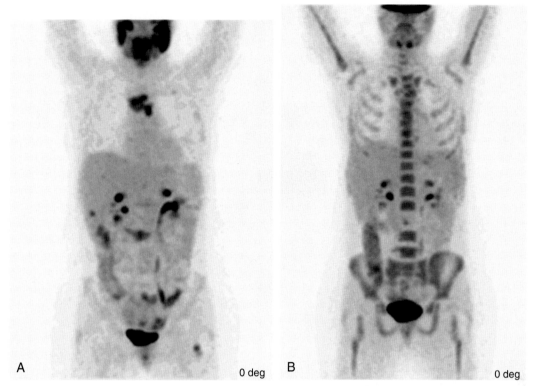

**Figure 2-25:** FDG-PET in a patient with Hodgkin's lymphoma, baseline scan (**A**) and post-therapy scan (**B**). Note the intense mediastinal and minimal marrow activity on baseline and complete resolution of mediastinal activity with markedly increased bone marrow activity following chemotherapy. Increased marrow activity commonly seen following chemotherapy (chemotherapy rebound) especially when colony stimulating factors are administered.

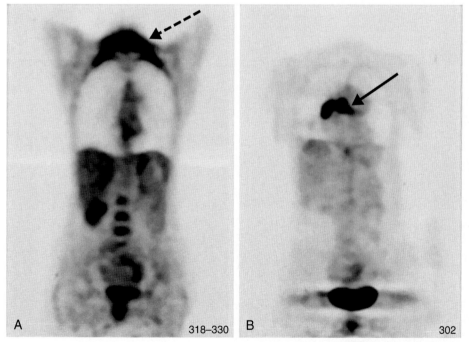

**Figure 2-26:** FDG-PET in patient with Hodgkin's lymphoma in clinical remission (NED) (**A**) and 14 months later with recurrence. Solid line points to recurrence (**B**). Note the brown fat (broken arrow **A**) is often associated with a cold environment and can be minimized or prevented by keeping patient warm following FDG injection. Beta blockers or benzodiazepines will also reduce or prevent FDG uptake in brown fat.

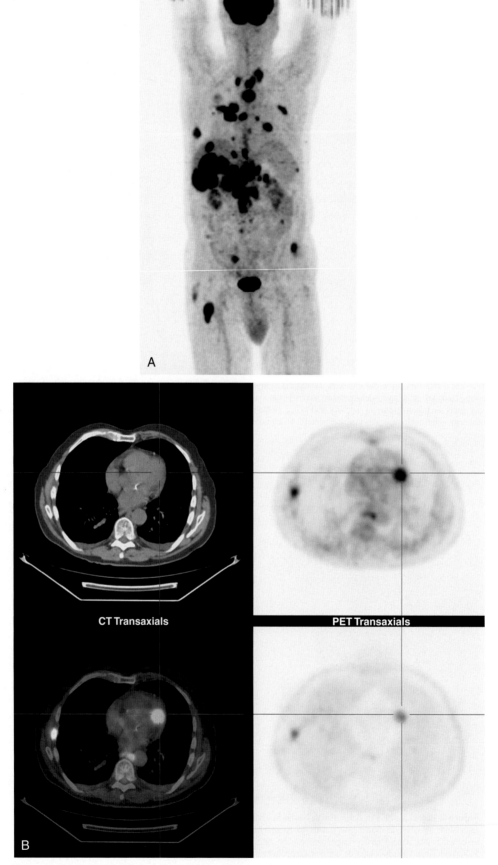

**Figure 2-27:** FDG-PET/CT in patient with metastatic melanoma. MIP image (**A**). PET/CT (**B**). Note the metastatic focus to the left ventricular wall and extensive mediastinal node involvement.

- Melanoma
  - May present with mediastinal adenopathy (Fig. 2-27).
  - Metastases are often widespread.
  - Usually high SUVs.

## NUCLEAR MEDICINE EVALUATION OF ESOPHAGEAL CANCER

- FDG-PET: General
  - Both squamous and adenomatous forms of esophageal cancers are highly FDG avid.[108-110]
  - Preferred technique is now combined PET/CT with fusion.[111,112]
    - Enhanced detection and localization with improved sensitivity and specificity compared with either test done independently.
  - Approved by Centers for Medicare and Medicaid Services (CMS) for staging and restaging
  - FDG PET excellent for staging, restaging, prognosis and monitoring response to therapy[113-123]
- FDG PET: Preoperative Assessment
  - Primary tumor
    - Sensitivity for detection of primary tumor is >90% in symptomatic patients. Limitations present in small T1 lesions (Fig. 2-28A and B).
    - Specificity for primary tumor of 80% to 90% with false positive findings due to inflammation or physiologic uptake common in distal portion especially GE junction.
  - Nodal staging
    - Endoscopic ultrasound (EUS) accuracy 70% to 80%. Difficulty in separating benign from malignant nodes.[124-126]

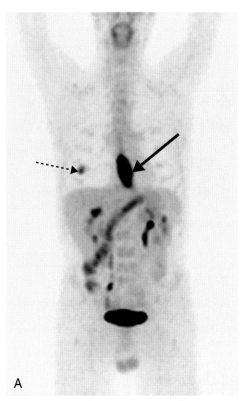

A

**Figure 2-28:** FDG-PET in a patient with an esophageal cancer (*bold arrow*) and solitary pulmonary nodule (*dotted arrow*). Maximum intensity projection image (**A**) and orthogonal projections (**B**).

(*Continued on page 54.*)

- EUS is not useful in detection of distant meta-stasis.[127]
- CT accuracy for mediastinal nodes is less than that of EUS; 50% to 70% with cut off less than 10 mm.[128]
- FDG-PET accuracy for mediastinal nodes 75% to 80%. Accuracy increases to more than 90% with PET/CT.[111,112]
- Specificity of FDG-PET is 60%. Specificity improves to more than 80% with PET/CT
- Best imaging test for nodal metastasis is FDG-PET/CT using combined hybrid systems and contrast CT. Endoscopic ultrasound may be superior in immediate peritumoral region.
  - Overall staging
    - Accuracy for CT staging is 50% to 60%.[128-131]
    - CT is good for hepatic and adrenal metastases but poor for locoregional nodes.
    - Accuracy of PET alone is 80% to 85%. Accuracy improves to 85% to 90% with PET-CT.[111,112]
    - PET/CT is the most accurate modality in detection of nodal and distant metastases.
    - Management changes due to PET or PET/CT 14% to 34%.[121]

## NUCLEAR MEDICINE EVALUATION OF INFECTION

### Introduction

- Nuclear medicine plays an important role in the evaluation of patients suspected of harboring infection.
- Several tracers are available for imaging infection.
  - 67Ga citrate
  - 111In-labeled autologogous leukocytes
  - 99m Tc-hexamethylpropyleneamine oxime (HMPAO)-labeled autologous leukocytes
  - 99m Tc-Fanolesomab—in vivo leukocyte label
  - 18F-FDG-PET
- Labeled leukocyte imaging is the current radionuclide gold standard for imaging most acute infections.
- Datz has identified characteristics of the ideal radiopharmaceutical: low in cost, widely available, easily prepared, low in toxicity, high in specificity, and have a high target to background ratio of activity.[10]
- No such agent is available now, so the clinician must choose the most appropriate study in each clinical situation while minimizing risks.
- Fusion imaging of metabolic PET study along with anatomic CT or MRI study is gaining wide acceptance and improves localization of inflammatory foci.

### 67Ga citrate

- 67Ga citrate is an analog of iron, of which 90% circulates in plasma bound to transferrin.
- Increased blood flow and vascular permeability, as part of the immune response, results in increased delivery and accumulation of transferrin-bound 67Ga at inflammatory foci.
- Typical adult dose: 5 uCi of intravenous 67Ga citrate.
- Imaging typically performed 48 to 72 hours after injection.
- Normal biodistribution of 67Ga: bone, bone marrow, liver, genitourinary and gastrointestinal tracts, and soft tissues.
- Advantages: easy to prepare, low toxicity and low target-to-background ratio.
- Disadvantages: Need for delayed images, low specificity often requiring other radiopharmaceuticals to confirm.
- Detects both bacterial and nonbacterial infections, and therefore, is useful in immunosuppressed patients (Fig. 2-29).
- Preferred in neutropenic patients because they do not have sufficient leukocytes to be radiolabeled.

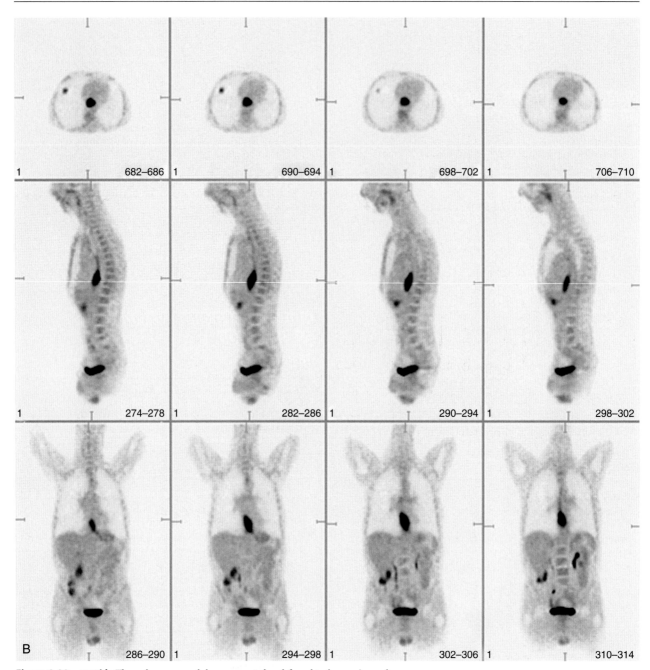

**Figure 2-28—cont'd:** The pulmonary nodule was resected and found to be a primary lung cancer.

- Also preferred in patients with a blood-borne communicable disease such as human immunodeficiency virus (HIV) because it does not require the direct handling of blood products.
- Most commonly used for imaging chronic osteomyelitis, suspected vertebral osteomyelitis, lung infections, and fevers of unknown origin (FUO), especially in immunocompromised patients.
- Normal 67Ga study for the chest virtually excludes opportunistic infections in the chest.
- In HIV-positive patient, lymph node uptake of 67Ga is most often due to mycobacterial disease or lymphoma.

- Focal, or localized, pulmonary parenchymal uptake is usually associated with bacterial pneumonia.
- Diffuse pulmonary uptake is indicative of *Pneumocystis carinii* pneumonia, especially when uptake is intense

## Labeled Leukocytes

- Current radionuclide gold standard for imaging infections in immunocompetent patients.
- Limitations: labor intensive in vitro labeling process, is not always available, and involves direct handling of blood products.

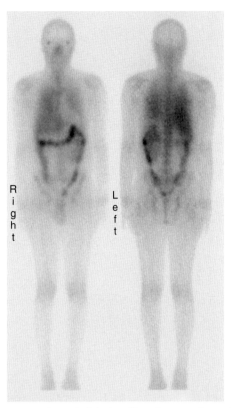

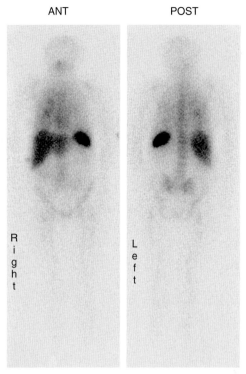

**Figure 2-29:** A 48-hour whole body gallium citrate scan in a patient with HIV and cough. Note the diffused pulmonary activity equal to the liver (3+/4+ rating). Patient was found to have *pneumocystis carinii* infection. Also note the activity in the ascending, transverse, and descending colon often seen in patient with HIV.

**Figure 2-30:** Indium-111 white blood cell study in a patient with pulmonary infection. Note the focal increase in the right lung corresponding to infiltrate on chest x-ray. No other source was found for the pt's febrile illness.

- Radiolabeling procedure takes about 2 to 3 hours. Involves withdrawal of 40 mL of whole blood, which is kept upright for about 1 to 2 hours for gravity sedimentation or undergoes hypotonic lysis of red cells in order to separate out the leukocytes. After centrifugation, the leukocyte "pellet" is washed and incubated with the radiolabel, and then reinjected into the patient.
- Uptake of labeled leukocytes is dependent on intact chemotaxis, crawl (diapedesis) into the tissues in between postcapillary endothelial cells, the number and types of cells labeled, and the cellular component of a particular inflammatory response.
- Total white count of at least 2000/mm$^3$ needed to obtain satisfactory images.
- Majority of leukocytes labeled are neutrophils, and therefore, they are most useful for identifying neutrophil-mediated inflammatory processes, such as bacterial infections.
- Limited utility in immunocompromised patients because leukocytes generally do not detect viral and parasitic infections.
- Images obtained shortly after injection are characterized by intense pulmonary activity, which clears rapidly, likely due to leukocyte activation during labeling that impedes movement through pulmonary vascular bed.[12]
- Images obtained the day after injection reflect migration from the blood into tissues or airspaces indicative of ongoing neutrophil trafficking associated with inflammation, such as occurs in bronchiectasis. (Fig. 2-30)
- Patients with lobar pneumonia seldom have a positive leukocyte scan, although neutrophils are abundant in the lung.[10]
- Most commonly used in vitro leukocyte-labeling techniques include 111In-oxime and 99m Tc-HMPAO.

- 111In-label
  - Usual dose is 300 to 500 uCi.
  - Maximal uptake reached at 30 minutes and remains until 24 hours.
  - Usual imaging time is 24 hours after injection.
  - Normal distribution of activity limited to liver, spleen, and bone marrow.
  - Advantages of 111In label: stable label with constant normal distribution; long half-life allows for delayed images which is valuable for musculoskeletal infection.
  - Disadvantages of 111In label: low photon flux, less-than-ideal photon energies, 24 hours interval between injection and imaging required, difficult to prepare leokocytes, expensive, and difficult to obtain radiolabel.
  - Best suited for imaging indolent conditions such as prosthetic joint infections and chronic osteomyelitis. Also preferred for investigation of inflammation in kidneys, bladder, and gallbladder. Use in FUO or occult fever is controversial. May be useful in detection of endocarditis (Fig. 2-31A and B)
- 99m Tc-HMPAO label
  - Usual dose is 5 to 10 mCi.
  - Usual imaging time is within a few hours after injection.
  - Normal biodistribution is the liver, spleen, bone marrow, genitourinary tract, and gastrointestinal tract.
  - Advantages of 99m Tc label: ability to detect abnormalities within a few hours after injection, cheaper and more readily available than 111In label, higher photon flux allowing improved visualization and lower radiation dose.
  - Disadvanatages: genitourinary tract and colonic activity; instability and short half-life of tracer when delayed 24-hour imaging is needed.

ANT          POST

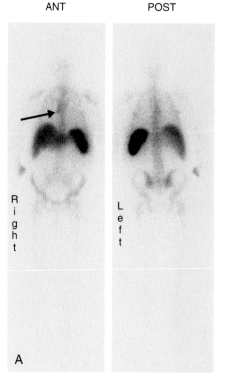

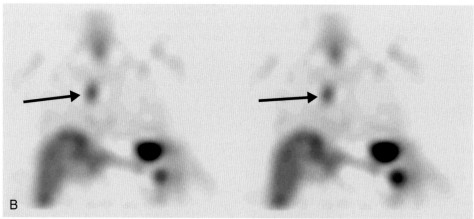

**Figure 2-31: A,** Indium-111 whole body planar scan in a patient with suspected endocarditis. Note the slight increase in the mediastinum to the right of the midline (*arrow*). **B,** Same patient with single photon emission computed tomography (SPECT) imaging of the chest demonstrating intense activity in the region of the aortic valve. Patient was found to have aortic valve endocarditis. SPECT imaging increases contrast resolution and is more sensitive than planar images.

○ Best suited for imaging acute inflammatory conditions, such as inflammatory bowel disease, osteomyelitis, soft tissue sepsis, and to a lesser extent, occult fever.

## 99m Tc-Fanolesomab

- Murine monoclonal antigranulocyte antibody that is currently under investigation for in vivo leukocyte labeling.
- Presumably binds both to circulating neutrophils that may migrate to focus of infection, or neutrophil debris already sequestered in area of infection.
- In contrast to in vitro labeled leukocytes, no increased retention of activity in lungs.
- Usual imaging time is 25 to 35 minutes after injection.

- Normal biodistribution: liver, spleen, bone marrow, and blood pool
- Transient drop in number of circulating leukocytes occurs within 20 minutes after injection. Recovery occurs within 45 minutes.
- Based on available date, agent is safe, with little toxicity, and eliminated from blood with mean half-life of 8 hours. No serious adverse effects occurred among 400 patients enrolled in multicenter trial.

## 18F-FDG-PET

- Desirable modality because it allows fast, sensitive, high-resolution tomography.

- 18F-FDG is carried via glucose transporters into cells. Inflammatory cells have an increased expression of glucose transporters when they are activated. Cytokines and growth factors also increase the affinity of glucose transporters for deoxyglucose.
- FDG normal distribution includes brain, myocardium, and genitourinary tract with inconsistent activity in the bone marrow, stomach, and bowel. Mild diffuse uptake in liver and spleen.
- Pros include high-resolution tomographic images that are quantifiable, availability of agent, rapid completion of procedure, and high sensitivity.
- Cons: Although sensitive for localizing abnormalities, cannot distinguish benign from malignant disease.
- Radionuclide imaging of choice in the evaluation of the patient with FUO. Superior to labeled leukocyte imaging or 67Ga imaging due to increased sensitivity (Figs. 2-32 to 2-34).[4]

- Limited data of prospective studies indicate that PET has the potential to play a central role as a second-line procedure in the management of patients with FUO.[13] PET scan contributed to the final diagnosis in 25% to 69% of the patients. Infectious diagnoses obtained included focal abdominal, thoracic, soft tissue infections, and chronic osteomyelitis with a high degree of certainty. Noninfectious diagnoses included large vessel vasculitis, inflammatory bowel disease, sarcoidosis, and painless subacute thyroiditis. Common malignancies detected included Hodgkin's disease and aggressive non-Hodgkin's lymphoma, colorectal cancer, and sarcoma.
- Compared with labeled leukocytes, 18F-FDG PET allows diagnosis of a wider spectrum of diseases. Compared with 67Ga-citrate scanning, 18F-FDG PET seems to be more sensitive.[13]

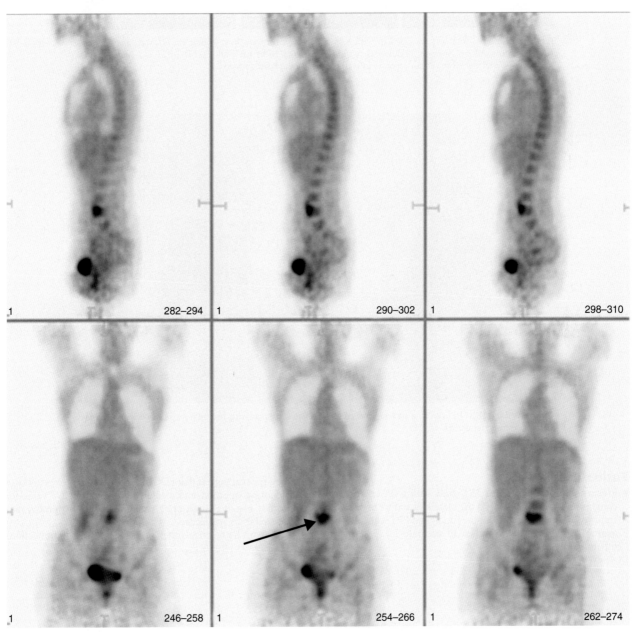

**Figure 2-32:** FDG-PET scan in a patient with prior history of lymphoma presenting with back pain. Biopsy demonstrated osteomyelitis of the L4 vertebral body.

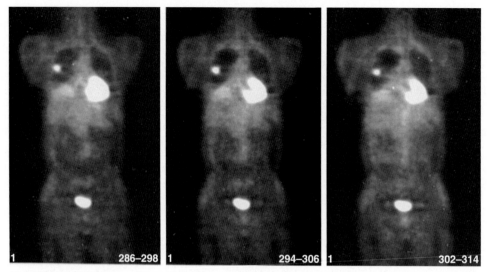

**Figure 2-33:** FDG-PET scan in a patient with a spiculated 2.5 cm right lung nodule on CT scan. Patient was suspected of neoplasm, however, nodule was found at pathology to be tuberculosis. FDG-PET is a sensitive test for infection and therefore cannot separate infection from a neoplastic process.

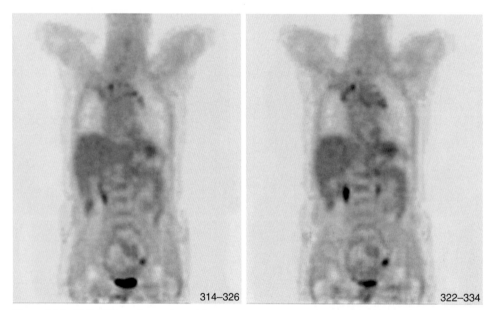

**Figure 2-34:** FDG-PET scan in a patient with reactivation tuberculosis with multiple mediastinal lymph nodes demonstrating granuloma.

## Fusion Imaging

- Efficacy improved by fusing PET study with a CT or MRI by combining anatomic data with the metabolic nature of disease.
- Improved data obtained from the functional PET scan and the anatomic CT scan have resulted in accurate localization of inflammatory foci.

- Dumarey et al suggest that FDG-PET/CT has a high sensitivity in diagnosing infection and a high negative predictive value for infection in a small study of 21 patients.[12] Larger prospective randomized trials are needed.
- May help characterize other diseases that are noninfectious such as sarcoidosis (Fig. 2-35)

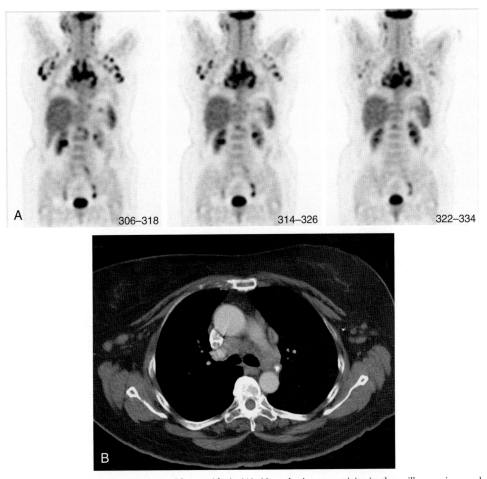

**Figure 2-35:** FDG-PET in a patient with sarcoidosis (**A**). Note the intense activity in the axillary regions and mediastinum. CT scan (**B**) demonstrates multiple axillary and mediastinal lymph nodes. Specificity for mediastinal detection of cancer is limited by the sensitivity for detection of inflammation/infection. Multiple scattered sites of relatively low SUV values generally is associated with granuloma/inflammation.

## References

 Interactive references and additional readings for this chapter can be accessed online at *expertconsult.com.*

# 3 PREOPERATIVE EVALUATION OF THORACIC SURGERY PATIENTS

Mark K. Ferguson, MD and Steven S. Khan, MD

## RATIONALE

- Provide a rational basis for discussing risks and outcomes with patients.
- Help with issues surrounding informed consent.
- Assist in patient selection for major surgery.
- Enable discussions among caregivers and with referring physicians about risks and expectations.
- Populate databases to enable development of risk models that will assist with all of the above.

## DEFINITIONS

The preoperative evaluation of thoracic surgery patients includes a general assessment of the patient's status, knowledge of the diagnosis or possible diagnoses for which surgery may be performed, and a set of focused tests that evaluate the patient's physiologic ability to undergo the proposed operation. This chapter will not deal with diagnostic or staging studies that are aimed at determining the appropriateness of surgery for a specific condition or whether the operation is feasible from a technical aspect.

## HISTORY

- The association between lung function and long-term survival was initially described in 1846 by Hutchinson.
- Gaensler first introduced the concept of timed expiratory function as a means for assessing pulmonary insufficiency and its relation to postoperative outcomes after lung surgery (1951).
- As lung resection for cancer became commonplace in the 1960s and 1970s, and additional measures of pulmonary reserve were introduced
  - Maximum ventilatory volume in 1 min (MVV)
  - Postoperative predicted FEV1
  - FEV1 expressed as a percent of predicted for age, height, and gender.
- Lung spirometric function currently used to develop actuarial tables for life insurance purposes and for estimating survival after lung cancer resection.[1,2]
- In the 1980s, gas exchange, oxygen consumption, and other forms of exercise testing were introduced as additional measures to assess risk after lung resection.
  - Single-breath diffusing capacity for carbon monoxide (DLCO)[3]
  - Maximum oxygen consumption during exercise (VO2max)[4]
  - Stair climbing test and other measures of exercise capacity[5,6]
- In the 1980s and 1990s, clinical databases were first used to identify individual risk factors for complications and mortality after major lung resection; databases for esophagectomy were slower to develop.
- In the 1990s and subsequently, risk models were first developed for prediction of outcomes after major lung resection; predictive models for esophagectomy outcomes were infrequent. No predictive models were developed for other major thoracic surgery.

## AGE

- Historically, advanced age confers increased risk of mortality after major thoracic surgery.
- There is no specific age cutoff for prohibitive risk.
- Recent reports suggest that age is declining in importance as a risk factor for mortality, possibly because of improved patient selection and perioperative management.[7]
- Advanced age continues to be associated with an increased risk of postoperative complications.
- A recent systematic review[8] of pulmonary risk stratification in mainly noncardiothoracic surgery (but included major esophageal and aortic surgery) reported that advanced age conferred higher odds for postoperative pulmonary complications (age 60 to 69 years: odds ratio 2.09 [1.66-2.64]; age 70 to 79 years: odds ratio 3.04 [2.11 to 4.39]).

## PERFORMANCE STATUS

- Performance status should be assessed in every patient considered for major thoracic surgery.
- It is a fundamental element in decision making about major thoracic surgery.
- Measures of performance status include the Eastern Cooperative Oncology Group (ECOG) performance status criteria (Table 3-1)[9] and Karnovsky performance status criteria (Table 3-2)[10]

## THORACIC SURGERY: PERIOPERATIVE PULMONARY PATHOPHYSIOLOGY

A number of physiologic aberrations occur perioperatively in the thoracic surgical patient (see later).

---

### TABLE 3-1 ■ EASTERN COOPERATIVE ONCOLOGY GROUP PERFORMANCE STATUS CRITERIA

| Score | Description |
|---|---|
| 0 | Fully active, able to carry on all predisease performance without restriction |
| 1 | Restricted in physically strenuous activity but ambulatory and able to carry out work of a light or sedentary nature, e.g., light housework, office work |
| 2 | Ambulatory and capable of all self-care but unable to carry out any work activities. Ambulatory more than 50% of waking hours |
| 3 | Capable of only limited self-care; confined to bed or chair more than 50% of waking hours |
| 4 | Completely disabled. Cannot carry on any self-care. Totally confined to bed or chair |
| 5 | Dead |

---

### TABLE 3-2 ■ KARNOVSKY PERFORMANCE STATUS CRITERIA

| Score | Description |
|---|---|
| 100 | Normal: no complaints, no evidence of disease |
| 90 | Able to carry on normal activity; minor symptoms |
| 80 | Normal activity with effort; some symptoms |
| 70 | Cares for self; unable to carry on normal activities |
| 60 | Requires occasional assistance; cares for most needs |
| 50 | Requires considerable assistance and frequent care |
| 40 | Disabled: requires special care and assistance |
| 30 | Severely disabled: hospitalized but death not imminent |
| 20 | Very sick: active supportive care needed |
| 10 | Moribund: fatal processes are progressing rapidly |
| 0 | Dead |

---

*Note: In patients with pre-existing pulmonary conditions, these sequelae can compound the already abnormal lung mechanics and gas exchange evident in these patients.*

- **Diaphragm dysfunction:**
  - Impaired force production and endurance capacity due to[11-14]:
    - Direct injury to diaphragm or phrenic nerve
    - Lengthening contraction-induced muscle injury
    - Impaired force due to prolonged mechanical ventilation
    - Altered chest wall/lung compliance with increased work of breathing
    - Reduced shortening fraction of the diaphragm
    - Reduced central drive (reflex; opioids)
    - Contiguous inflammatory process
    - Sepsis
    - Metabolic derangements
  - Diaphragm dysfunction can last several weeks
  - Diaphragm dysfunction is similar with thoracotomy and with video-assisted thoracoscopic surgery (VATS), except that recovery time is shorter with VATS
- **Abnormal lung function**
  - In early postoperative period, FEV1 and forced vital capacity (FVC) reduced about 35 to 50%.[15-19] From those predicted values according to extent of resection.
  - Slightly greater decrement in FVC with thoracotomy compared with VATS.

○ By discharge, values approach 80% of predicted values according to extent of resection.

○ Functional residual capacity (FRC) is reduced about 30% in the early postoperative period.

○ It can take up to 3 to 4 months to approach postoperative predicted values.

■ **Gas exchange**

○ Microatelectasis contributes to hypoxemia (reduction in lung volumes; abnormal mucociliary clearance)

○ Hypercapnia can occur due to central respiratory depression (opiate analgesia, residual effects of anesthetic agents), incomplete reversal of neuromuscular blockade, diaphragm dysfunction, splinting and abnormal rapid-shallow breathing pattern

## PULMONARY FUNCTION

■ Definitions and determinants

○ **FVC** (forced vital capacity): the amount of air that can be forcefully exhaled from total lung capacity to residual volume, in a single breath, is determined by several factors aside from height (positive correlation) and age (negative correlation).

*Determinants are:*

■ Inspiratory muscle strength
■ Elastic recoil forces of the lung
■ Chest wall compliance
■ Dynamic closure of airways (and thus the balance between lung recoil and airways resistance upstream of a flow limiting collapse point)
■ Expiratory muscle strength
■ Patient cooperation and ability

○ **FEV1** (forced expiratory volume in one second): the amount of air that can be forcefully exhaled in the first second of an FVC maneuver.

*Determinants are:*

■ Factors determining flow, such as lung recoil and airways resistance upstream of a flow limiting collapse point

■ Reduced in the presence of restriction of lung volume (in proportion to curtailment of FVC or increased in relation to FVC, in the presence of increased lung recoil)

○ **MVV** (maximum ventilatory volume): the total volume of air that can be cycled during 1 min of maximum ventilation (extrapolated from a 12- or 15-second maneuver)

*Determinants are:*

■ Elastic and flow resistive factors determining flow
■ Respiratory muscle strength
■ Respiratory system coordination
■ Can be disproportionately reduced relative to the FEV1 (lower limit = FEV1 × 32.8) with neuromuscular weakness, upper airways obstruction, and poor effort

○ **DLCO:** single breath diffusing capacity for carbon monoxide (also termed transfer factor)

*Determinants are:*

■ Total surface area available for gas exchange
■ Membrane thickness a minor factor
■ Total capillary blood volume
■ Hemoglobin concentration
■ Maldistribution of gas
■ Carboxyhemoglobin concentration

○ **VO2max:** highest oxygen consumption *achievable* during maximal effort for an incremental exercise test and fails to increase further, i.e., plateaus. Usually we measure the maximum VO2, which is the highest VO2 *achieved* with a maximal effort (this may equal or be similar to VO2max, but not in all cases).

○ **Evaluation**

○ Essential before major lung resection

○ Recommended for many patients undergoing esophagectomy

○ Of little value in patients undergoing lesser operations unless respiratory status is tenuous

○ **Impaired pulmonary function is associated with**

○ Preoperative chemoradiotherapy[20]

○ Increased risk of pulmonary complications and mortality after major lung resection[3]

○ Increased risk of pulmonary complications after esophagectomy[20-22]

○ **Assessment of pulmonary function prior to major lung resection**[23]

○ Use of spirometric values in predicting risk of major lung resection

■ Preoperative threshold values for increased risk:
○ FEV1 less than 2 L or less than 60% predicted
○ MVV <50% predicted

■ **Predicted postoperative (ppo) threshold values for increased risk**
1. ppoFEV1 less than 800 to 1000 mL
2. ppoFEV1 less than 40%

■ **Estimates of ppo** values calculated using percentage of functioning lung postoperatively based on[24]:
○ Percentage of functioning lung segments remaining after resection based on location of primary tumor
○ Quantitative ventilation/perfusion scan
○ Quantitative computed tomography (CT) densitometry

○ **Oxygen exchange/consumption** in predicting risk of major lung resection

■ Some assessment should be performed routinely, not just in patients with impaired spirometry

■ **Lowest cost** technique is measurement of oxygen saturation during two-flight stair climb[25]
○ Maintenance of saturation in normal range indicates of low risk
○ Desaturation or inability to complete stair climb indicates high risk
○ Inability to complete stair climb test indicates of prohibitive risk

■ A **moderate-cost**, high-accuracy technique is DLCO; DLCO predicts operative outcomes even in patients with normal spirometry[26]; high risk is associated with[3]
○ DLCO less than 60%
○ ppoDLCO less than 40%

■ **Highest cost**, high-accuracy assessment is measurement of VO2max[27]:
○ Normal risk VO2max: higher than 15 to 20 mL/kg/min (>60% to 70% predicted)
○ High risk VO2max: 10 to 15 mL/kg/min (50% to 60% predicted)
○ Prohibitive risk VO2max: less than 10 mL/kg.min [less than 40% to 50% predicted]

○ An algorithm for assessing pulmonary status before major lung resection is shown in Figure 3-1

○ **Assessment of pulmonary function before esophagectomy**

○ Measurement is appropriate in patients who are elderly, have substantial tobacco exposure, or who have chronic obstructive pulmonary disease (COPD).

○ Increased risk of pulmonary complications associated with impaired pulmonary function is evidenced by decreased FEV1 or decreased DLCO, or both.[20-22]

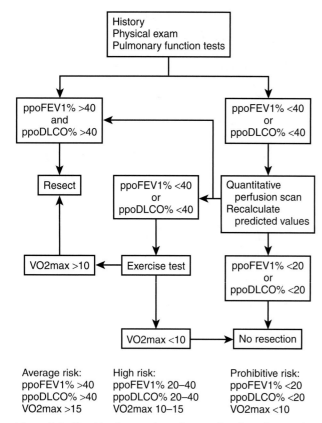

**Figure 3-1:** Algorithm for assessing pulmonary function prior to major lung resection.

## CARDIOVASCULAR STATUS

- The **incidence of cardiovascular events** after major thoracic surgery varies depending on the presence of prior known heart disease
  - The 2002/2006 American College of Cardiology and American Heart Association Perioperative Clearance Guidelines (ACC/AHA) classify thoracic surgery as an intermediate risk procedure with a cardiac risk of 1% to 5%.[28,29]
    - Risk of perioperative myocardial infarction (MI) is 0.13% in patients with no prior cardiac history versus 2.8% to 17% in patients with a prior history of MI.[30]
  - Patients who require major thoracic surgery often have risk factors for cardiovascular complications.[31]
  - Low incidence of such complications[32] likely a result of:
    - Careful patient screening
    - Correction of specific problems preoperatively
    - Improved perioperative management
- **Preoperative cardiac approach to patient**
  - Determine patient's cardiac risk
  - Evaluate for the four major cardiac risk factors: (1) unstable coronary syndromes, (2) decompensated heart failure, (3) significant arrhythmias, (4) severe valvular disease
  - Determine cardiac risk of planned thoracic procedure
  - Preoperative testing, if appropriate
  - Preoperative drug therapy to minimize cardiac risk
  - Recommend appropriate intraoperative monitoring and therapy
- **Perioperative management**
  - Prophylactic therapy for arrhythmias, if appropriate
  - Surveillance for myocardial infarction if appropriate
  - Continuation of perioperative beta blockade if appropriate
  - Predischarge cardiac risk factor optimization

- **Cardiac factors associated with increased cardiac risk** of major thoracic surgery[28]
  - **Major**
    - Unstable coronary syndromes defined as:
      - Acute or recent MI (MI within prior 30 days) with evidence of important ischemic risk (by clinical symptoms or noninvasive testing criteria)
      - Unstable angina (acceleration or change in pattern within prior 6 weeks) or severe angina (Canadian class III or IV angina)
    - Decompensated congestive heart failure
    - Significant arrhythmias: supraventricular tachycardia (SVT), atrial fibrillation or flutter with uncontrolled ventricular rate; uncontrolled or symptomatic ventricular tachycardia; high-grade atrioventricular block
    - Severe valvular disease, particularly severe aortic stenosis or mitral stenosis.
  - **Intermediate**
    - Mild angina pectoris (Canadian class I or II)
    - Prior MI by history or pathologic Q waves
    - Compensated or prior congestive heart failure
    - Renal insufficiency
    - Diabetes mellitus, particularly the insulin-dependent type
  - **Minor**
    - Low functional capacity (e.g., inability to climb one flight of stairs with a bag of groceries)
    - Advanced age
    - Abnormal electrocardiogram (left ventricular hypertrophy, left bundle-branch block, ST-T abnormalities)
    - Rhythm other than sinus rhythm (e.g., atrial fibrillation)
    - Uncontrolled systemic hypertension
    - History of stroke
- **Presence of a major factor precludes any elective operation until situation is resolved.** Formal evaluation of intermediate factors is warranted. Evaluation of minor factors is patient and procedure dependent.
- **American College of Cardiology/American Heart Association Algorithm for assessing and managing cardiac risk associated with possible coronary artery disease**[29,32]
  - **General points**
    - Patients with no or only minor risk factors can go to operating room without further testing.
    - Thoracic surgery patients (noncardiac, nonvascular thoracic surgery) with only intermediate risk factors and good exercise tolerance (greater than 4 metabolic equivalent tasks [METS] exercise tolerance: i.e., can climb one or more flights of stairs with groceries, walk uphill, run a short distance, walk on level ground at 4 mph) can undergo surgery without further cardiovascular testing
    - Asymptomatic patients who have undergone recent revascularization (less than 5 years) can undergo surgery without further testing
    - **All patients with a single major risk factor require further evaluation (Fig. 3-2)**

## OTHER SYSTEM DISORDERS

- **Nutritional status**
  - Impaired immune function
  - Impaired wound healing
  - Little can be done to correct this in the short term
- **Renal dysfunction**
  - Difficult fluid management
  - Increased risk of bleeding
  - Impaired wound healing
  - Impaired immune function

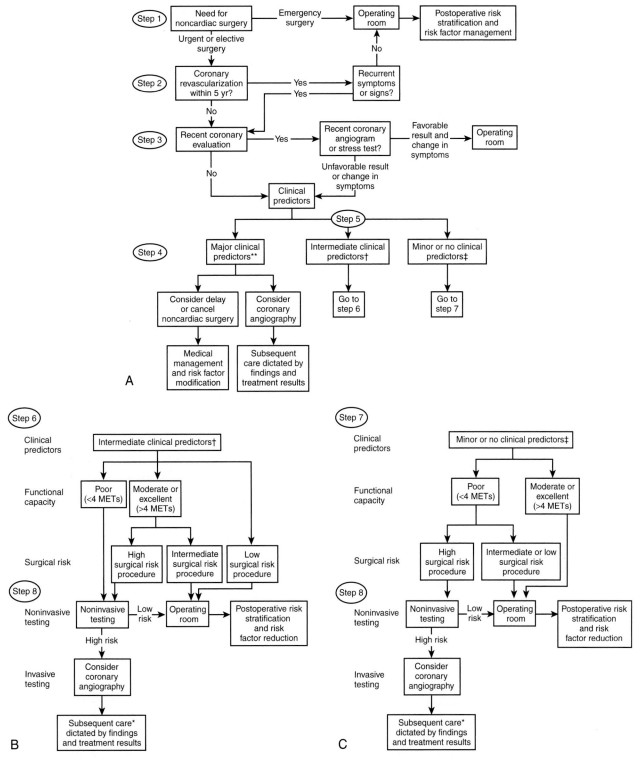

**Figure 3-2:** American College of Cardiology/American Heart Association Algorithm for evaluation and management of possible coronary artery disease. **A,** Major predictors or Recent Revascularization. **B,** Intermediate predictors. **C,** Minor or no clinical predictors. *(From Eagle KA, Berger PB, Calkins H, Chaitman BR, Ewy GA, Fleischmann KE, et al. ACC/AHA guideline update for perioperative cardiovascular evaluation for noncardiac surgery—executive summary: a report of the American College of Cardiology/American Heart Association Task Force on Practice Guidelines [Committee to Update the 1996 Guidelines on Perioperative Cardiovascular Evaluation for Noncardiac Surgery.] J Am Coll Cardiol 2002;39:542-553.)*

- **Hepatic dysfunction**
  - Increased risk of bleeding
  - Increased risk of postoperative confusion
- **Coagulopathy**
  - Management of anticoagulation can be challenging, particularly regarding timing and costs
    - Coumadin
    - Lovenox
  - Increased risk of thromboembolic disease in patients with malignancy
  - Correction of noniatrogenic clotting deficiencies is mandatory

## RISK ASSESSMENT/SCORING

- **Why assess risk?**
  - Patient selection
  - Informed consent
  - Preoperative preparation
  - Resource assignment
  - A tool for standardizing outcomes
  - A method for assessing performance
- **Formal assessment** of risk is appropriate
  - Assess each potential risk factor for each patient
  - Do not ignore warning signs of increased risk; there is rarely a need for urgent surgery precluding a formal and careful evaluation of risk factors
- **Risk scoring systems**
  - Published systems[33-37]
    - Apache II
    - Predictive respiratory quotient (PRQ)
    - Cardiopulmonary risk index (CPRI)
    - POSSUM (Physiologic and Operative Severity Score for the Enumeration of Mortality and Morbidity)
    - Estimation of physiologic ability and surgical stress (E-PASS)
    - Predicted postoperative product (PPP)
    - Charlson index
    - Expiratory volume, age, diffusing capacity (EVAD)
    - European Thoracic Society systems (ETS 1 and ETS 2)
  - **Current systems lack utility** and thus are not in routine use
    - Large databases are very accurate for identifying globally important predictive variables
    - Applicability to individual institutions, surgeons, or patients is limited
      - Inverse relationship between database size and individual applicability
      - Risk factors that are specific to a patient population, institution, or surgeon are overlooked
    - Insufficient predictive power to be generally useful
    - Importance of surgeon's judgment is not recognized by current scoring systems

## RISK REDUCTION

- **Cardiopulmonary rehabilitation**[38,39]
  - Increases functional capacity
  - Enhances quality of life
- **Preoperative pulmonary toilet instruction**[40]
  - Increases inspiratory muscle strength
  - Improves postoperative lung function
- **Correction of cardiovascular deficits**

## RISK MANAGEMENT

- **Change approach to operation**
  - Muscle-sparing thoracotomy rather than posterolateral thoracotomy
  - Consider minimally invasive (VATS) approach
- **Parenchymal sparing resection**[41]
  - Wedge resection
  - Segmentectomy
  - Sleeve lobectomy
- **Volume reduction surgery**[42-44]
  - In addition to lesser resection
  - Lobectomy as volume reduction surgery
  - Improved lung function evident only in patients with the most marginal lung function
- **Provides additional resources for perioperative management**
  - Experienced anesthesiologist
  - Experienced, high-volume surgeon
  - High-volume institution
  - Experienced intensive care specialist
  - Consider referral to regional center of expertise
- Consider both the short-term (operative mortality, operative morbidity) and long-term (survival, quality of life) outcomes in assessing risk.

## PERIOPERATIVE CARDIOVASCULAR COMPLICATIONS

- **Cardiac Arrhythmias:** Most common perioperative cardiac complication after noncardiac thoracic surgery is cardiac arrhythmia.
  - Most common postoperative arrhythmia is atrial fibrillation.[45] Average time of onset of atrial fibrillation is 2.9 days postoperatively.
  - Atrial fibrillation prolongs discharge an average of 2.4 days[46] after thoracic surgery
  - Prophylaxis of atrial fibrillation: Recent meta-analysis of 11 trials of medications for prophylaxis after noncardiac thoracic surgery[47]
    - Drugs shown to be effective: beta blockers (two randomized trials, relative risk [RR], 0.40; 95% confidence interval [CI], 0.17–0.95), calcium channel blockers (four trials, RR, 0.50; 95% CI, 0.34–0.73), magnesium sulfate (one trial, RR, 0.4; 95% CI, 0.21–0.78). Results with a small trial of flecainide were not clear.
    - Not effective or potentially harmful: Digoxin (associated with increased risk of atrial fibrillation, RR, 1.51; 95% CI, 1.0–2.28), amiodarone (randomized trial stopped due to high risk of postoperative adult respiratory distress syndrome in amiodarone group)
    - Meta-analysis[47] concluded that calcium channel blockers and beta blockers are effective in reducing postoperative atrial arrhythmias
  - Significant ventricular arrhythmias are uncommon. In 412 pneumonectomy/lobectomy patients, 15% developed nonsustained ventricular tachycardia (VT greater than 3 beats), but none developed sustained VT (greater than 30 seconds) or required treatment for hemodynamic compromise from VT.[48]
- **Myocardial infarction/ischemia**
  - As noted earlier, the incidence of perioperative MI is low (less than 0.13%) in patients without prior history of MI.[30]
  - Mortality of perioperative MI after noncardiac thoracic surgery is high.
  - It remains unclear whether preoperative angioplasty or stenting reduces incidence of perioperative MI.

○ Monitoring for 3 days postoperatively is recommended for high risk patients.[45]
▪ **Pulmonary edema**
○ Usually noncardiac in origin: due to increased filtration gradient across pulmonary microvascular bed and increased permeability
▪ **Shunting**
○ Development of right to left shunting through patent foramen ovale (PFO) or atrial septal defect (ASD) can occur. Incidence of PFO may be as high as 20% to 35%
○ Can result in platypnea-orthodeoxia syndrome: shunt worse in upright posture or when patient dehydrated
○ More common after right sided pneumonectomy and may be due to rotation of heart with preferential direction of flow from vena cavae across atrial septum. Right atrial (RA) pressures frequently normal.
○ May not develop symptoms until several months after surgery. Diagnosis made by echocardiogram, catheterization, magnetic resonance imaging (MRI).

○ Treatment is closure of PFO or ASD using a clamshell device or suture closure on cardiopulmonary bypass.
▪ **Cardiac Herniation**
○ Rare complication when pericardium left unclosed. Heart herniates out of pericardium causing cardiac torsion and obstruction of venous inflow.[49]
○ Occurs 24 to 72 hours after surgery and presents as shock, chest pain, and cyanosis. Sixty percent of patients have superior vena cava syndrome.
○ Treatment is surgical; heart is placed back in pericardium. In cases of right-sided herniation, pericardium is closed, whereas with left-sided herniation, total pericardiectomy is performed.

## References

 Interactive references and additional readings for this chapter can be accessed online at *expertconsult.com*.

# 4 DIAGNOSTIC BRONCHOSCOPY
## Henri G. Colt, MD, FCCP

## DEFINITION

Bronchoscopy is the examination of the upper and lower airways. Procedures are performed using either a flexible or a rigid bronchoscope. Rigid bronchoscopes are a rigid stainless steel tube with a series of mirrors inside to transmit the image to the operator through an eyepiece and connected videocamera. Flexible bronchoscopy is performed using a flexible tube with a series of flexible fiberoptic bundles; however, increasingly, flexible bronchoscopy is performed using a tube with a distal charge coupled device, transmitting the image of the airways onto a videoscreen.

## HISTORY

Gustav Killian, an Otorhinolaryngologist at Freiburg, Germany performed the first rigid bronchoscopy on March 30, 1897 in order to remove a piece of bone embedded in the right main bronchus of a 63-year-old man. Until then, the indirect laryngoscope method had been used to visualize only parts of the tracheobronchial tree. A few years later, Professor Chevalier Jackson, a famous North American Otorhinolaryngologist, was instrumental in disseminating the use of the rigid bronchoscope in the United States as well as abroad.

▪ Although rigid bronchoscopy can be used for diagnostic procedures, it is most comfortably performed under general anesthesia, and thus is more frequently used for therapeutic procedures such as laser resection, stent insertion, and airway dilation of malignant and benign strictures.
▪ The rigid bronchoscope comes in various diameters and lengths. The external diameter of the rigid bronchoscope may also vary depending on manufacturer. For adults, most tubes are at least 8 mm wide.

Shigeto Ikeda of Tokyo, Japan introduced the first flexible fiberoptic bronchoscope at the Ninth International Congress on Diseases of the Chest held in Copenhagen in 1966.[1]

▪ Flexible bronchoscopy is usually performed using moderate sedation, but it can also be safely and comfortably performed in the fully awake and alert individual. The scope can vary in diameter from 3 to 6 mm, and usually it has a working channel of 1.9 to 2.4 mm. An increasing number of ancillary instruments and flexible bronchoscopic procedures are being designed to enhance diagnostic yield for a variety of indications.

## INDICATIONS

▪ **Suspected of known malignancy**
○ **Suspected bronchogenic carcinoma** is a frequent indication for diagnostic bronchoscopy. Patients are often referred because of symptoms such as cough, dyspnea, hemoptysis, a history of previous carcinoma potentially metastatic to the lungs and airways, or radiographic abnormality suggestive of neoplasm (mass, lymphangitic-type infiltrate, focal infiltrate, solitary or multiple pulmonary nodules, mediastinal adenopathy).

Small cell carcinoma:

▪ The yield of bronchoscopic procedures is excellent. Tumors are often infiltrative, and diagnosed using washing, brushings, submucosal needle aspiration, and endobronchial biopsies.

Non–small cell carcinoma:

▪ Tumors can present with normal as well as abnormal tracheobronchial mucosa. When abnormal, appearances include but are not limited to intraluminal mucosal thickening, exophytic lesions, nodules, and friable mucosal changes.

- Sometimes there are indirect signs of neoplasm and volume loss represented by focal and extensive airway narrowing, segmental bronchial strictures, extrinsic compression, large airway narrowing, carinal involvement, bronchoesophageal fistula, bronchomediastinal fistula, thickening of posterior pars membranosa, and thickening of mucosal spurs to peripheral bronchi. These changes are also seen in patients with small cell carcinoma and in patients with cancers metastatic to the airways (for example, breast cancer, colon cancer, renal cell carcinoma, malignant melanoma, thyroid cancer, esophageal cancer, adenoid cystic carcinoma, carcinoid tumors, and sarcomas).
- Resectability can be assessed by careful measurement of distance from the carina, presence of associated airway strictures, and presence or absence of synchronous or asynchronous ipsilateral or contralateral abnormalities.
- Mediastinal staging is possible using transbronchial needle aspiration (TBNA) or endobronchial ultrasound. Diagnostic yield is significantly increased when more than 4 needle passes are made; rapid on-site cytology examination (ROSE) is employed.[2]

○ **Early lung cancer detection**
  - Increasingly advocated for patients at risk for new or recurrent bronchogenic carcinoma (patients with chronic obstructive pulmonary disease (COPD), smoking history, history of lung resection for bronchogenic carcinoma, patients with history of head and neck cancer).
  - Autofluorescence bronchoscopy can be used to increase sensitivity. Numerous biopsies of abnormal areas warranted.
  - New technologies include optical coherence biopsy, high-magnification bronchoscopy, and confocal endoscopy. Goals for these new technologies are to increase specificity, but further research and technology development are still needed.[3]

○ **Lymphoma**
  Non-Hodgkin's and Hodgkin's Lymphoma:
  - Can be seen as simple airway mucosal thickening.
  - Mediastinal and hilar adenopathy

○ **Tracheal tumors**
  - Tracheal tumors are easily diagnosed using bronchoscopic procedures. Distance from the vocal cords and carina is assessed, and resectability can be determined by measuring lesion length, distance from the carina and vocal cords, and the number of cartilaginous rings involved.

○ **Metastatic tumors**
  - Tumors of the lung can be diagnosed even in the absence of airway involvement. Brushings, washings, bronchoalveolar lavage, and transbronchial lung biopsy provide diagnostic material when patients have focal or diffused infiltrates or nodular opacities.

○ **Other malignancies**
  - Solid tumors with mediastinal nodal metastases (breast cancer most common; thyroid, renal, rectal, and so on) are diagnosed.
  - Esophageal cancer can cause fistulas, as can esophageal cancer with an associated esophageal stent insertion or radiation therapy.
  - Surgical complications such as postpneumonectomy or postlobectomy stump fistula can be visualized and determinations made regarding indications for bronchoscopic or open surgical repair.

- **Benign Disease**
  ○ **Benign tracheal strictures**
    - Symptoms include cough, shortness of breath, sudden onset of respiratory insufficiency, recurrent intubation of difficulty weaning from mechanical ventilation, adult-onset asthma, or asthma symptoms unresponsive to therapy.

- Patients often have a history of difficult intubation, trauma, mechanical ventilation, or tracheostomy.
- Airway strictures should also be suspected in patients with vasculitis such as Wegener's Granulomatosis, as well as in patients with a history of tuberculosis, sarcoidosis, and other granulomatous disorders.
- Length, caliber, and type of benign stricture (simple or complex, hourglass or circumferential, focal or multifocal) can be determined.
- Resectability is determined, in part, by measuring length of the stricture as well as distance from the vocal cords.

○ **Tracheobronchial malacia and excessive dynamic airway collapse**
  - Increasingly recognized, may be primary or secondary with numerous possible etiologies[4]
  - Dynamic bronchoscopy helps make diagnosis. Patients are examined with the bronchoscope in the sitting and supine positions, and asked to inhale and exhale forcibly. Excessive dynamic airway collapse (significant intrusion of the posterior membrane) can be seen with or without associated malacia (softening of the airway cartilage) (Fig. 4-1).[5]

○ **Other causes of airway strictures**
  - Postradiation
  - Foreign body inhalation
  - Burn and inhalation injury
  - Brachytherapy, postelectrocautery, cryotherapy, laser resection, stent insertion, or airway photodynamic therapy.
  - Postsurgical (sleeve lobectomy, resection anastomosis, lung transplantation)

○ **Lung transplantation**
  - Bronchoscopy is helpful to inspect anastomoses and to diagnose anastomosis strictures or dehiscence.
  - Bronchoscopy is used to detect infection and transplantation-related complications including bronchiolitis and infectious lung disease.[6]

○ **Infectious and inflammatory lung disease**
  - Greatest yield from combined washings and bronchoalveolar lavage.
  - Transbronchial biopsy may increase yield in both intact and immunocompromised patients, but the risk/benefit ratio of biopsy must be carefully considered.

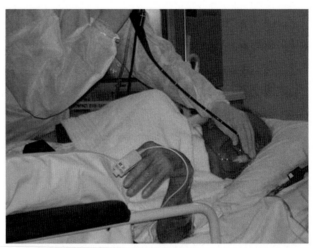

**Figure 4-1:** Patient with expiratory central airway collapse (malacia and excessive dynamic airway collapse) moved into lateral decubitus position as part of dynamic bronchoscopy performed using moderate sedation.

- Fungal, viral, bacterial diseases diagnosed, including tuberculosis; *Mycobacterium avium-intracellulare*, Pneumocystis, and Aspergillus infection; coccidioidomycosis.
- Patients usually have pulmonary infiltrates, atelectasis, and lobar consolidation, but infection can also be diagnosed by mediastinal sampling using TBNA.
- Interstitial lung diseases can be diagnosed by transbronchial lung biopsy. Yield in increased using multiple procedures such as endobronchial biopsy, transbronchial biopsy and TBNA for diseases such as Sarcoidosis.[7] In other illnesses, such as nonspecific interstitial pneumonitis, usual interstitial pneumonitis, and desquamative interstitial pneumonitis, biopsies may be nonspecific, showing only fibrosis. Bronchoalveolar lavage with cell count differential is usually reserved for research purposes. Transbronchial biopsies can be helpful to diagnose bronchiolitis and alveolitis if representative samples are obtained.

## CONTRAINDICATIONS

- According to numerous guidelines and surveys, practice patterns differ, but the only contraindication is persistent or refractory hypoxemia.[8,9]
- Risks and benefits of each procedure must be carefully weighed.
- Strategy and planning for each procedure includes indication, preprocedure evaluation, allergies, risks (respiratory failure, cough, vasovagal events, bleeding, pneumothorax, fever, procedure-related anxiety).
- Preprocedure evaluation includes examination for significant comorbidities, especially cardiac arrhythmias, bleeding or coagulation disorder, medications including anticoagulants, antiplatelet agents, history of narcotic use (may require increased dose of sedation drugs), as well as careful assessment of patient's preferences (nasal or oral bronchoscope insertion), expectations, and discussion of potential alternative diagnostic procedures.
- "Time out" can be valuable in order to ascertain that nursing team, patient, and bronchoscopists agree on procedures to be performed, that appropriate precautions are taken in case of procedure-related complications or adverse events, and that all equipment and ancillary instruments are readily available.
- Sedation should be individualized based on comorbidities, response to medication, desire for procedure recall, and need for patient collaboration during the procedure (forced cough, dynamic bronchoscopy). Synergistic effect of combined medications such as benzodiazepines and narcotics should be considered, particularly in patients with airway obstruction or poor ventilatory function.[10]
- Feeding should be held before procedures according to institutional guidelines because of risk of vomiting (cough and gag reflex) and aspiration.
- Procedures appear safe even after myocardial infarction, in the elderly, and in patients with elevated intracranial pressures or pulmonary hypertension, although routine precautions are warranted.[11-14] Some investigators suggest that bronchoscopy should be postponed, if possible, at least 4 weeks after myocardial infarction, and increased risk exists in patients with active congestive heart failure and left ventricular dysfunction.[15] Transbronchial lung biopsies should be avoided, unless absolutely necessary in patients with pulmonary hypertension.
- Bronchoscopy is usually safe in patients with asthma, although it should probably be avoided in patients with status asthmaticus. In addition, preprocedure bronchodilators and, of course, corticosteroids should be administered and procedures postponed, if possible, in patients with active asthma

or exacerbations of COPD, as demonstrated by wheezing, shortness of breath, and pulmonary hyperinflation.[16,17]
- Pregnancy is definitely associated with increased risk for bronchoscopy. This is related to the reduced cardiac preload, decreased lower esophageal sphincter tone, increased oxygen consumption, and the primary respiratory alkalosis associated with pregnancy.[18]
- Critically ill patients on mechanical ventilation should be placed on 100% oxygen during the procedure. In nonintubated patients with impending respiratory failure, consideration should be given to use of noninvasive ventilation support and also precautionary intubation (sometimes over the flexible bronchoscope) prior to performing bronchoscopy.
- Complications can be readily addressed by careful strategy and planning for each procedure. Also, necessary techniques and equipment should be known. For example, techniques of bronchoscopic intubation, bleeding control using balloons and endobronchial blockers, and emergency techniques for supplemental oxygen administration can be learned through postgraduate courses, guided reading, and simulation scenarios (Fig. 4-2).

## PROCEDURES

### Inspection, Washings, and Brushings

- Helpful for basic inspection bronchoscopy and surveillance, to exclude some infection, remove secretions, identify cause for atelectasis or consolidation, and to sample simple airway mucosal abnormalities.
- Extremely low risk. Procedures can usually be completed in less than 10 minutes
- Careful inspection of upper airway, vocal cords, and entire tracheobronchial tree and all bronchial segments is warranted. A bite block should always be used in case of oral insertion of bronchoscope. Procedures performed with supplemental oxygen and monitoring by pulse oximetry and heart rate/rhythm.

### Endobronchial Biopsy and Bronchoalveolar Lavage

- Endobronchial biopsy most helpful to diagnose malignancy, but also inflammation, granulomatous disorders, and occasionally fungal disease (tracheobronchial aspergillosis).

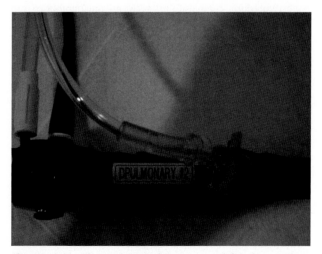

**Figure 4-2:** Supplemental oxygen being connected directly to working channel of flexible bronchoscope using three-way stopcock. This technique allows delivery of supplemental oxygen while maintaining ability to suction using suction valve of the flexible scope.

- Procedure-related bleeding is usually not consequential but may require electrocautery, placement of the patient in the lateral decubitus position (bleeding side down to enhance gravity-dependent clot formation and protection of contralateral lung), and topical administration of diluted epinephrine.
- Bronchoalveolar lavage usually performed by instillation of more than 100 mL into a focal area of lung through the bronchoscope wedged into a segmental airway. Usually only one territory needs to be sampled, and should contain less than 4 percent bronchial epithelial cells. Goal is to proceed with alveolar filling. Bronchoalveolar lavage is most effective for the diagnosis of infectious lung disease, but it is also used to detect for bronchogenic cancer, lymphangitic spread of carcinoma (breast cancer for example), bronchoalveolar cell carcinoma. It may also be helpful in the diagnosis of some peripheral nodules.[19-21]
- Particularly helpful for tuberculosis diagnosis, especially if acid fast bacilli (AFB) sputum smears are negative, and in presence of local infiltrates.
- Patients should be informed of possible postprocedure fever, which usually alleviated within 24 hours using ibuprofen.

## Transbronchial Lung Biopsy

- Effective for the diagnosis of neoplastic lung disease in patients with pulmonary nodules greater than 2 cm in diameter.
- Also effective to increase yield of infectious lung disease, but risk and benefits compared with washing-brushing-bronchoalveolar lavage must be carefully weighed and discussed with consenting patient and family.
- Transbronchial lung biopsy should be avoided in patients with possible coagulopathy or on antiplatelet agents such as Clopidogrel.[22]
- In other patients, platelets should probably be greater than 50,000 and INR corrected to normal to significantly decrease risks of fatal or uncontrollable bleeding related to transbronchial lung biopsy.
- Transbronchial lung biopsy is usually done only on one lung and in a gravity-dependent segment because of risk of pneumothorax and bleeding.
- Pneumothorax may infrequently require chest tube insertion.
- Fluoroscopy assists in avoiding biopsy-related patient discomfort, ensuring that the appropriate target pulmonary segment is being biopsied and to ascertain absence or presence of procedure-related pneumothorax.
- Postprocedure complications such as pneumothorax can occur many hours after intervention. Therefore, appropriate discharge instructions and follow-up are probably warranted.

## Transbronchial Needle Aspiration

- Most useful for diagnosis and staging of mediastinal adenopathy.[23,24]
- Yield increased with experience and with use of ROSE.
- Cytology and histology needles are available.
- Yield greatest for malignancy, less for lymphoma.[25]
- Probably extremely underused because of steep learning curve to obtain satisfactory yield similar to that of experts.
- Endobronchial needle aspiration also is possible for mucosal lesions, and usually avoids any risk for bleeding. Endobronchial needle aspiration has been shown to increase diagnostic yield for lung cancer from approximately 60% to greater than 90%, and may be diagnostic alone in more than 20% of instances.
- Procedure-related patient complications are rare but do include inadvertent puncture of a large vessel (usually of no consequence), and pneumomediastinum.

- Procedure-related complications from equipment malfunction or operator error are possible. These include inadvertent puncture of the bronchoscope,

## ENDOBRONCHIAL ULTRASOUND (EBUS)

- Increasingly used to diagnose mediastinal adenopathy (Fig. 4-3).
- Has become standard of practice in many countries because of increased yield, and ability to avoid mediastinoscopy and mediastinotomy.[26]
- Can be combined with esophageal ultrasound in selected cases.
- Is able to differentiate level of cartilaginous and peribronchial neoplastic invasion.
- Used to stage mediastinum to level 11 nodes with accuracy in experienced hands and also to identify internal structures.[27]
- Can be performed using moderate sedation in either intubated (number 8 and above endotrachal tube) or nonintubated patients.
- Can also be performed using general anesthesia.
- EBUS is a good modality for lymph node stations 8 and 9, with sensitivity 81% to 97% and specificity 83% to 100%, but the test has a high false-negative rate.[28,29]
- Use of convex probes show images in real time, allowing operator to witness needle insertion directly into target adenopathy. Doppler mode can be used to visualize blood adjacent large blood vessels.[30]
- Increasingly, multiple different modalities can be used and many bronchoscopists predict that bronchoscopic imaging will soon replace surgical exploration of the mediastinum and for the diagnosis and staging of lung cancer.[31]

## Navigational Bronchoscopy

- Allows navigation of forceps and brushes into peripheral nodules by creating an electromagnetic field around the chest. This is done using a microsensor overlaid on a previously obtained three-dimensional computed tomography (CT) scan (SuperDimension Inc., Minneapolis, MN).[32,33]
- In one recent prospective randomized study of 120 patients using surgical biopsy as the gold standard, navigational bronchoscopy sampling in addition to EBUS of lesions less than 20 mm in diameter provided greater yield than EBUS or navigational bronchoscopy alone.[34]

## Fluorescence Bronchoscopy

- Autofluorescence bronchoscopy is based on the principle that tissue fluorescence allows differentiation between normal and preneoplastic or neoplastic tissues. Malignant and early malignant tissues leads to several-fold reduction in normal fluorescence (Fig. 4-4).
- Disadvantages of this technique include high sensitivity, low specificity, frequent false-negative results, and longer procedure time because of the need for multiple biopsies.
- Fluorescence bronchoscopy allows identification of early lung cancer better than simple white light flexible bronchoscopy.[35,36]
- It can also be used to improve staging radiographically occult cancers.[37]
- Devices that have not been approved by the US Food and Drug Administration (FDA), such as the SAFE 3000 (Pentax Corp, Tokyo, Japan), allow twin images of white light (WL) and autofluorescence (AF) to be displayed simultaneously, and thus might improve specificity without compromising sensitivity.

LEVEL OF RT. MAIN BRONCHUS FOR #7 NODE

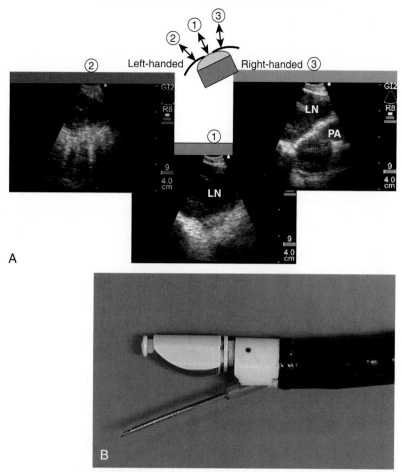

A

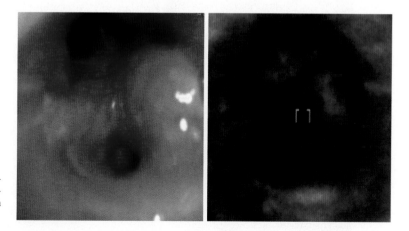

**Figure 4-3:** **A,** Photo of EBUS needle and scope. **B,** Endobronchial ultrasound examination of level 7 nodes seen from left and right sides. (*Courtesy of Olympus Corps, Japan. Courtesy Noriaki Kurimoto, St. Marianna University Hospital, Japan.*)

**Figure 4-4:** White light bronchoscopy and Autofluoroscence of bronchial tumor (note reddish brown discoloration on bronchial spur).

- *Drug-induced fluorescence*: This system uses Photofrin (Axcan Pharma, Inc., Birmingham, AL) where the hematoporphyrin derivative is preferentially retained by tumor. Photofrin in tumor emits red fluorescence when illuminated by violet light. The disadvantages of this procedure is that it requires preparation, has a high cost, and can induce skin photosensitivity.

- *Autofluorescence*: This system differentiates between normal and preneoplastic/neoplastic lesions.[38]
- Blue light (400 to 440 nm) results in green fluorescence by normal bronchial tissue. Preneoplastic and early malignant lesions lead to 10-fold reduction in fluorescence and a change in red/green (R/G) ratio.

- LIFE: Cadmium laser generates blue monochromatic light (442 nm).
- Xilix OncoLIFE: Filtered arc lamp (395 to 445 nm) for blue light.
- SAFE 3000 uses Xenon light source for white light bronchoscopy (WLB) and diode laser for AF; dark bluish red for pre-neoplastic and early neoplastic lesions, and green for normal.
- Pitfalls of AF bronchoscopy: high sensitivity and low specificity, especially for bronchitis, previous biopsy site, airway fibrosis requiring more biopsy, longer procedural time.
- Novel imaging modalities under investigation include Optical Coherence bronchoscopy,[39,40] which displays structures of airway wall and histologic imaging without excisional biopsy; Narrow Band Imaging,[40] which delineates characteristic microvascular networks; R/GH ratio bronchoscopy, which provides a numeric representation of red and green fluorescence to identify moderate dysplasia; and high-magnification bronchoscopy.
- We strongly believe that the future of bronchoscopic imaging, especially for lung cancer diagnosis and staging, will require a multiplatform apparatus from which several diagnostic modalities can be used sequentially in order to first detect suspicious lesions (with increased sensitivity) and then focus on true abnormalities (increased specificities).

## TRAINING—COMPETENCY-BASED MODELS

- Patient safety and the accountability of healthcare professionals to the public distinguish the practice of medicine today from earlier years.
- Society wants to be reassured that physicians are knowledgeable and competent in their scope of practice.
- New curricula based on a "competency-based" paradigm,[41] including competency-based education and assessment, web-based learning, and the use of simulation in medical education have enhanced procedure-related education.
- In pulmonary medicine, a paradigm shift away from the pure apprenticeship model, based on the "see one, do one, teach one" paradigm, is warranted because training programs are

required to demonstrate levels of competency achieved by their trainees.

- Patients should not bear the burden of procedure-related training when complementary alternatives such as low-fidelity and high-fidelity models and computer-based learning programs are available.[42]
- The Essential Bronchoscopist (www.bronchoscopy.org) is a free, on-line curriculum of theoretic bronchoscopic knowledge available in five different languages. It has already been officially endorsed as a complementary educational tool by several national and international bronchology and thoracic organizations.[43]
- Alongside this curriculum, validated assessment tools to measure basic bronchoscopic knowledge and technical skill have also been proposed.[44]

### Illustrative Case #1: Excessive Dynamic Airway Collapse

- *History:* A 50-year-old man with progressive shortness of breath with minimal exertion, chronic cough, difficulty in clearing secretions, and suspected intractable adult-onset asthma. Patient had a history of prolonged intubation and tracheotomy (now healed) following complicated coronary artery bypass surgery two years earlier (Fig. 4-5).
- *Examination:* Vitals: tachycardia (120 to 130/min); blood pressure, 160/90; respirations, 28/min; temperature, 99.0° F, pulse oximetry saturation (SPO$_2$), 88% (2 L/min NC O$_2$).
- *Blood tests:* Complete blood count and electrolytes were normal.
- *Imaging:* Dynamic CT scan of chest (see Fig. 4-1) shows more than 50% narrowing of the tracheal lumen during tidal exhalation due to excessive bulging of the posterior membrane.

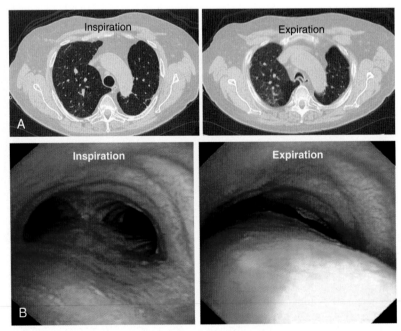

**Figure 4-5: A,** Excessive dynamic airway collapse (EDAC) diagnosed by paired inspiratory-expiratory dynamic computed tomography which shows narrowing of the airway lumen from excessive bulging of the posterior membrane. **B,** EDAC diagnosed by performing dynamic bronchoscopy. The cartilaginous structures remain intact and the narrowing is exclusively caused by excessive bulging of the posterior membrane during tidal exhalation.

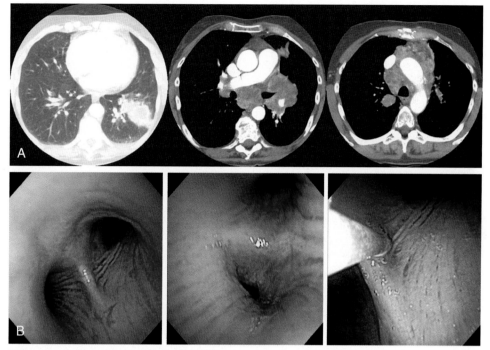

**Figure 4-6:** **A,** *Image A.* Computed tomography scan shows left lower lobe mass. *Image B.* Mediastinal windows demonstrate extensive left hilar and subcarinal adenopathy. *Image C.* Paratracheal adenopathy easily identified. **B,** *Image A.* Bronchoscopy reveals an enlarged main carina with corrugated mucosa on the posteromedial walls of both main stem bronchi. *Image B.* Enlarged LC2 with erythematous, infiltrated mucosa causing partial obstruction of the left lower lobe and upper division bronchi. *Image C.* Transbronchial needle aspiration using cytology needle at the subcarinal level.

- *Bronchoscopy:* Performed in the supine, lateral, and sitting position confirms the CT findings and documents the absence of cartilaginous abnormalities.
- *Diagnosis/pathology:* Suspected excessive dynamic airway collapse.
- *Management alternatives:* Patient to be discussed within multidisciplinary group to review treatment alternatives, which might include pneumatic splinting through the use of continuous positive airway pressure, silicone stent trial, or evaluation for possible membranous tracheoplastic surgery.

### Key Points

- Dynamic bronchoscopy helps identify type and extent of airway abnormalities.
- Etiology may be multifactorial.
- Stent insertion, although possible, can also be associated with substantial complications. Risks and benefits should be carefully weighed and explained to the patient and family.

### Illustrative Case #2: Transbronchial Needle Aspiration for Mediastinal Lymphadenopathy

- *History:* Patient is a 72-year-old woman with 120-pack per year history of smoking presented with progressive shortness of breath and wheezing. She had poor appetite and 15-pound weight loss within the last 3 months before admission (Fig. 4-6).

- *Examination:* Cachectic woman in mild respiratory distress; Vitals: tachycardia (120/min); blood pressure, 190/80; respirations, 26/min; temperature, 99.0° F, SPO$_2$, 95% (Venturi mask 50%). Lung auscultation revealed bilateral expiratory wheezes.
- *Blood tests:* Complete blood count and electrolytes were normal.
- *Imaging:* CT scan showed a left lower lobe mass with extensive left hilar, subcarinal, and paratracheal lymphadenopathy (see Fig. 4-1).
- *Bronchoscopy:* Revealed enlarged main carina and infiltrated erythematous mucosa and enlargement of LC2.
- *Diagnosis/pathology:* TBNA from the subcarinal tumor (see Fig. 4-2) with rapid onsite cytology showed small cell carcinoma.
- *Management alternatives:* Patient to be discussed within multidisciplinary group to review treatment alternatives, which might include palliative care and chemotherapy with concurrent or sequential radiation therapy.

### Key Points

- TBNA is safe and has a high yield for diagnosing mediastinal adenopathy.
- ROSE improves the yield and decreases the duration of the procedure.
- Other diagnostic bronchoscopic procedures such as endobronchial biopsy, brushing, or washings can be avoided if TBNA with ROSE provide a diagnosis.

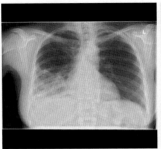
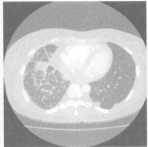
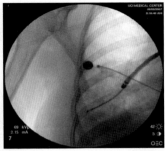

**Figure 4-7: A,** Chest radiograph reveals right lower lobe infiltrate confirmed on **B,** computed tomography scan. **C,** Fluoroscopic image of biopsy forceps in area of radiographic abnormality. Note proximity to chest wall and pleural surfaces.

## Illustrative Case #3: Transbronchial Lung Biopsy for Interstitial Disease

- *History:* The patient is a 47-year-old woman presented with new onset dry cough, shortness of breath, fatigue, and 7-pound weight loss within 1 month. She is a nonsmoker, but she had history of stage IV signet cell mucinous adenocarcinoma of the appendix. She underwent hysterectomy and bilateral oophorectomy with partial omentectomy for suspected ovarian cancer (Fig. 4-7).
- *Examination:* Vitals: tachycardia (100/min); blood pressure, 140/80; respirations, 14/min; temperature, 97.0° F, $SPO_2$, 95% (room air).
- *Blood tests:* Complete blood count and electrolytes were normal.
- *Imaging:* Chest radiograph showed interstitial changes in right mid and lower lung field (see Fig. 4-3A). CT scan revealed intralobular septal thickening and suggestive of lymphangitic spread of tumor in right lower lobe (see Fig. 4-3B)

- *Bronchoscopy:* Performed under fluoroscopy with bronchioloalveolar lavage, brushings, and transbronchial lung biopsies (see Fig. 4-3C).
- *Diagnosis/pathology:* Transbronchial biopsy showed metastatic adenocarcinoma, well differentiated, with associated mucus, consistent with origin from alimentary canal; bronchioloalveolar lavage and brushings showed numerous red blood cells but no malignant cells or infections.
- *Management alternatives:* Patient to be discussed within multidisciplinary group to review treatment alternatives, which might include palliative care, chemotherapy, and surgical resection of the right lower lobe.

### Key Points

- Transbronchial biopsy increases the yield for diagnosing lymphangitic spread of tumor.
- Fluoroscopy improves the yield and safety of bronchoscopic lung biopsy.
- Risks and benefits of all treatment alternatives will be explained to the patient and family.

## References

Interactive references and additional readings for this chapter can be accessed online at *expertconsult.com.*

# 5 MEDIASTINOSCOPY AND MEDIASTINOTOMY

Vijay K. Nuthakki, MD, Ali Mahtabifard, MD, and Robert J. McKenna Jr., MD

## TERMINOLOGY

- Cervical mediastinoscopy
- Extended cervical mediastinoscopy
- Anterior mediastinotomy (Chamberlain procedure)

## DEFINITION

**Cervical mediastinoscopy** is a surgical procedure that allows exploration of the superior mediastinum and allows for biopsy of level 2, 4, 7, and 10 lymph nodes or masses.

**Extended cervical mediastinoscopy** is a cervical mediastinoscopy during which the surgeon passes the mediastinoscope around the innominate artery to gain access to the aortopulmonary window to biopsy the level 6 and 5 nodes.

**Video mediastinoscopy** is the use of a video mediastinoscope to perform mediastinoscopy. For traditional mediastinoscopy, the surgeon looked directly through the mediastinoscope to perform the procedure. The video mediastinoscope allows better visualization of the structures in the mediastinum so that a better operation is performed.

## INTRODUCTION

Pathologic staging of the mediastinum is a crucial step in the evaluation and treatment of non–small cell lung cancer. The extent of lymph node involvement guides the therapeutic plan toward resection, neoadjuvant therapy, or nonsurgical treatment. Accurate staging of the mediastinum is, therefore, essential (Fig. 5-1).[1]

Radiographic assessment of the mediastinum is not as accurate as pathologic staging. The size of mediastinal lymph nodes on computed tomography (CT) cannot be relied on in the staging of non–small cell lung cancer.[2,3] Up to 40% of positive mediastinal nodes are less than 1 cm, and only 60% of nodes greater than 2 cm contain metastases.[2-4] Therefore, both the sensitivity and specificity for the CT evaluation of the mediastinum are 60%. The positron emission tomography (PET) scan has a higher sensitivity, but the false-positive rate is as high as 35%. Pathologic assessment of the mediastinum via mediastinoscopy is the preferred method of staging the mediastinum.[3-6]

## CERVICAL MEDIASTINOSCOPY

Carlens developed cervical mediastinoscopy to enable the passage of a mediastinoscope into the mediastinum for biopsy of nodes from the paratracheal and subcarinal regions.[7] Cervical mediastinoscopy is one of the most important procedures used in the staging and diagnosis of non–small cell lung cancer.

It also aids in the pathologic evaluation of mediastinal adenopathy not associated with lung cancer and some mediastinal masses.

Recently, other techniques have been used to biopsy mediastinal nodes. Esophagoscopy with endoscopic ultrasound–guided biopsies has been shown to diagnose level 2, 4, 7, 8, and 9 nodes; level 6 nodes may possibly also be biopsied with this technique. Endobronchial ultrasound can help biopsy level 2, 4, 7, and 10 nodes. The advantage of these techniques is that they do not necessarily require general anesthesia as mediastinoscopy does. However, mediastinoscopy remains the gold standard to which all new techniques are compared.[8-11]

■ Lymph node stations accessible to cervical mediastinoscopy.
  ○ High paratracheal, left and right (stations 2L, 2R).
  ○ Pretracheal (stations 1, 3).
  ○ Tracheobronchial angle, left and right (stations 4L, 4R).
  ○ Subcarinal (station 7).
  ○ Level 10 nodes on the main stem bronchi.
■ Lymph node stations not accessible to conventional cervical mediastinoscopy.
  ○ Para-aortic and aortopulmonary window (station 6 and 5) (see later section on extended cervical mediastinoscopy).
  ○ Paraesophageal (station 8).
  ○ Inferior pulmonary ligament (station 9).
  ○ Level 11, 12, and 13 nodes.

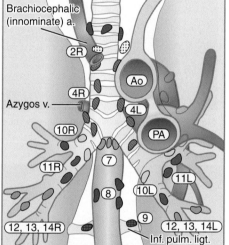

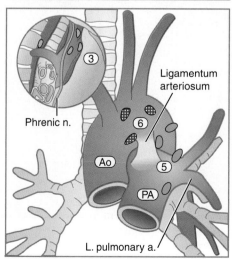

**Superior mediastinal nodes**

● 1 Highest mediastinal

☺ 2 Upper paratracheal

○ 3 Pre-vascular and retrotracheal

○ 4 Lower paratracheal (including Azygos nodes)

N₂ = single digit, ipsilateral

N₃ = single digit, contralateral or supraclavicular

**Aortic nodes**

○ 5 Subaortic (A-P window)

⊕ 6 Para-aortic (ascending aorta or phrenic)

**Inferior mediastinal nodes**

● 7 Subcarinal

● 8 Paraesophageal (below carina)

⊕ 9 Pulmonary ligament

**N₁ nodes**

○ 10 Hilar

● 11 Interlobar

○ 12 Lobar

○ 13 Segmental

○ 14 Subsegmental

**Figure 5-1:** Lymph node stations for staging of lung cancer.

## INDICATIONS

- Mediastinal staging in patients with greater than stage 1A (T1N0) non–small cell lung cancer, and patients with[7,12-14]
  - ○ Central tumors
  - ○ Adenocarcinoma
  - ○ Need for pneumonectomy
  - ○ Superior sulcus tumors
  - ○ Adenopathy or suggested invasion on CT scan
  - ○ Patients with synchronous primary lung cancers
  - ○ Patients with poor performance status
- Undiagnosed mediastinal adenopath.
- Lymphoma
- Inflammatory disease
  - ○ Sarcoidosis
  - ○ Histoplasmosis
  - ○ Drainage of abscess or lymphocele
  - ○ Tuberculosis
- Pneumoconioses
- Mediastinal tumors and cysts
  - ○ Parathyroid adenoma
  - ○ Thymoma
  - ○ Cystic hygromas, bronchogenic cysts
  - ○ Mediastinal goiter

## TECHNIQUE

- General anesthesia with a single lumen endotracheal tube.[7,12-14]
- Patient positioned supine with neck extended via a roll or pillow under the shoulders.
- Transverse 2-cm incision approximately 2 cm above the sternal notch (Fig. 5-2).
- Divide platysma transversely.
- Dissect in midline to retract the strap muscles, exposing the pretracheal fascia.
- Open the fascia, bluntly dissect on anterior surface of trachea.
- Identify and partially dissect adenopathy or mass by palpation using the index finger; this also opens the plane for introduction of the mediastinoscope.

- The right paratracheal nodes lie anterior and lateral to the trachea and inferior to the innominate artery, whereas the left paratracheal nodes lie lateral and posterior to the trachea.
- Introduce the mediastinoscope along the anterior surface of the trachea (Fig. 5-3).
- Use a metal suction catheter to mobilize nodes at the various stations (Fig. 5-4).
- Grasp and biopsy nodes with a cupped biopsy forceps (Fig. 5-5).
- If any doubt regarding the vascular nature of a structure, a 22-gauge spinal needle can be used to aspirate; however, this is rarely necessary because nodes are dissected well enough that there should be no doubt that they are nodes, not vessels.
- Small bleeding vessels can be cauterized or clipped.

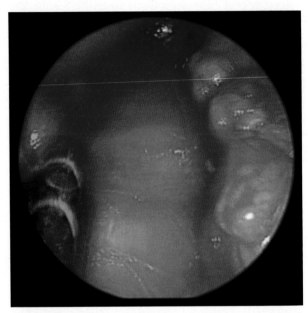

**Figure 5-3:** View of mediastinum, anterior to the trachea. Metal suction catheter along left side of trachea.

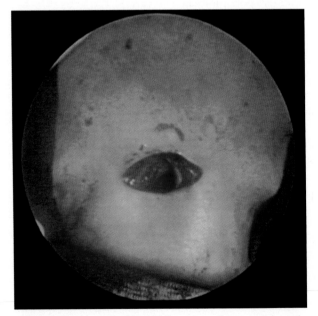

**Figure 5-2:** Transverse skin incision 2 cm above sternal notch. Patient's head is toward the bottom of the picture.

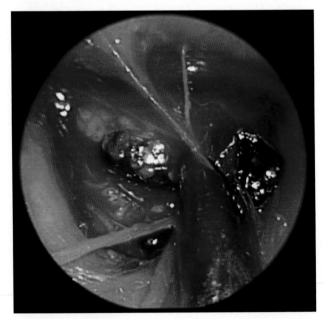

**Figure 5-4:** Metal suction catheter is used to mobilize nodes at various stations.

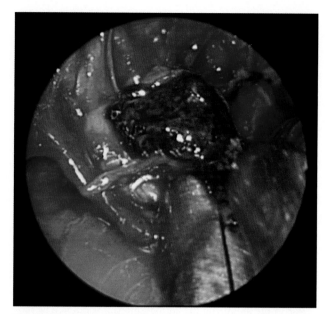

**Figure 5-5:** Cupped biopsy forceps are used to grasp and biopsy lymph nodes or a mass in the mediastinum.

- If no clear bleeding vessel is identified, then can pack with oxidized cellulose, Surgicel (Johnson & Johnson, Langhorne, PA), or long, 1-inch packing and re-evaluate after a few minutes; almost all minor bleeding will stop with packing and time.
- After adequate hemostasis, the strap muscles are reapproximated in the midline.
- The platysma is closed with interrupted stitches, followed by closure of the skin with subcuticular stitches.
  *Note: See video of procedure on accompanying DVD.*

## LIMITATIONS

- Conditions that increase difficulty but are not absolute contraindications.[12,15,16]
  - ○ Superior vena cava (SVC) obstruction because collateral veins increase the risk of bleeding with the procedure.
  - ○ Previous radiation or chemotherapy because it usually causes significant scarring that may make the dissection dangerous
- Contraindications
  - ○ Large goiter that physically precludes access to the trachea and the mediastinal nodes.
  - ○ Severe calcification or aneurysm of the innominate artery. Stroke is a well known, albeit rare, complication of mediastinoscopy because the mediastinoscope may compress the innominate artery during the procedure. Severe calcifications may break loose and travel to the brain and cause an embolism.
  - ○ End tracheostomy after laryngectomy. A permanent tracheostomy is in the surgical field and very close to the incision for mediastinoscopy so that sterility for the operation is compromised.
  - ○ Severe cervical arthritis and kyphosis preclude extension of the neck, which is necessary for the mediastinoscope to gain access to the mediastinum.
  - ○ Prior paratracheal lymph node dissection because all the tissue from the trachea to the superior vena cava is resected so that attempted dissection in that area is likely to damage either the trachea or the superior vena cava.

## COMPLICATIONS

The mortality rate for mediastinoscopy is 0 to 0.5%, and the morbidity rate is 0.6% to 2.3%. The following complications all occur in less than 1% of cases.[8-10,12,17-19]

- Massive hemorrhage
  - ○ Due to injury to the aorta or its branches, SVC, azygous, pulmonary artery or anterior pulmonary arterial branch to right upper lobe (truncus).
  - ○ If significant bleeding occurs, the mediastinum is packed and a median sternotomy is performed to control the bleeding.
- Mediastinitis requires mediastinal drainage through the cervical incision or may require a right thoracotomy
- Tracheobronchial injury can occur during dissection around the trachea and bronchi, especially when there is extensive scarring, which can occur with fibrosing mediastinitis, following radiation and chemotherapy, or with severe granulomatous disease. If the injury is in the cervical trachea, it can be repaired through a slightly enlarged mediastinoscopy incision. If the injury is in the distal trachea or in a bronchus, then a thoracotomy will likely be required for the repair.
- Esophageal injury can occur because level 7 nodes abut the esophagus in the subcarinal space and the L4 nodes abut the esophagus to the left and posterior to the trachea. Repair will usually require a right thoracotomy, although a removable esophageal stent may control the problem.
- A chylous leak will need to be drained and usually also needs thoracic duct clipping near the diaphragm via the right side of the chest.
- Recurrent nerve injury can occur during removal of the left tracheobronchial and low L4 nodes because they abut the left recurrent nerve. Also, the right recurrent nerve is at risk during the removal of the high R2 nodes, which abut the right recurrent laryngeal nerve. Very rarely, both nerves can be injured. In some cases, that will require a tracheostomy. Generally, when a laryngeal nerve injury occurs, return of function will occur but may take 6 months. If a patient with unilateral recurrent nerve injury aspirates (coughing with ingestion of thin liquids) or if the voice is very weak, then the affected vocal cord can be injected with a protein to temporarily improve the voice and protect the trachea. The protein is usually reabsorbed by about the time that the nerve function returns.
- Right-sided pneumothorax may occur because the right pleura abuts the lateral side of the R2 and R4 nodes. During mediastinoscopy, the pleura and the right lung are usually seen. If a pneumothorax occurs, the patient may need a pleural catheter and Heimlich valve or a chest tube.
- Stroke (atheroembolic or hypoperfusion) may occur due to compression of the innominate artery by the mediastinoscope.
- Myocardial infarction may occur because older smokers who develop lung cancer have increased risk for coronary artery disease.
- Tumor seeding at the incision site can occur because nodes containing cancer may be removed during mediastinoscopy. This occurs in about 0.1% of cases and should be treated with local radiation.
- Wound infections usually resolve with antibiotics but may require drainage. If a wound infection occurs, it is important to watch for mediastinitis and to remember that the erythema of the incision could represent tumor seeding at the incision site. Wound infection is an early complication and tumor recurrence is usually a late complication after mediastinoscopy.

## EXTENDED CERVICAL MEDIASTINOSCOPY

Whereas cervical mediastinoscopy aids in the evaluation of the superior mediastinum, nodes located in front of and inferior to the aortic arch in the anterior mediastinum (level 5 and level 6) are inaccessible by this method. Left upper lobe tumors have been shown to have lymphatic spread to these nodes in the anterior mediastinum. Ginsberg et al[20] described the technique of extended cervical mediastinoscopy, which involves further dissection between the innominate and left common carotid arteries to provide access to the anterior mediastinum. However, owing to the added experience needed and difficulty of this procedure, it has not become a widely used technique. Dissection for this procedure can result in a tear of the innominate or carotid artery, which causes sudden, massive bleeding. Repair requires an immediate median sternotomy. Most thoracic surgeons prefer either an anterior mediastinotomy or left video-assisted thoracic surgery (VATS) to biopsy the level 5 and 6 nodes.

## ANTERIOR MEDIASTINOTOMY

### INTRODUCTION

McNeil and Chamberlain developed the anterior mediastinotomy (the Chamberlain procedure) to allow evaluation of the lymph nodes or lesions in the anterior mediastinum.[21] This procedure is usually performed on the left, but it can be performed on the right if an anterior mediastinal mass extends to the right.[9] Left VATS can also provide access to biopsy level 5 and 6 nodes.

- Lymph node stations evaluated
  - Para-aortic (station 6)
  - Subaortic (station 5)

### INDICATIONS

- Staging of mediastinum in patients with enlarged subaortic nodes and negative results on cervical mediastinoscopy[20,21]
- Biopsy of an anterior mediastinal mass

### TECHNIQUE

- General anesthesia is administered with a single-lumen tube and the patient in the supine position.[21]
- A 4-cm incision is made over the cartilaginous portion of the second rib, just lateral to sternum.
- The pectoralis major muscle fibers are separated, exposing underlying cartilage.
- The perichondrium is divided and preserved, whereas the cartilage is resected from sternal border to the costochondral junction.
- With care taken to avoid the internal mammary artery and vein (which are 1 cm lateral to the sternum), the posterior perichondrium is divided along the sternal border. The pleura is retracted laterally with care taken to avoid opening the pleura.
- Under direct visualization, the mass or enlarged lymph nodes are biopsied.
- For better visualization, the mediastinoscope can be placed through the incision.

### LIMITATIONS

- Conditions that increase difficulty[21]
  - Prior coronary bypass surgery with patent LIMA
  - SVC syndrome with extensive collateral veins on the chest wall because significant bleeding may occur from these collateral veins.

### COMPLICATIONS

The mortality rate for an anterior mediastinotomy is less than 1%. Complications are uncommon (<1%) and include the following:

- Massive hemorrhage due to injury of the aorta or pulmonary artery during dissection. This requires emergent median sternotomy and carries a high mortality risk.
- Bleeding from internal mammary artery or vein can occur during removal of the cartilage because the vessels are under the cartilage, 1 cm lateral to the sternal border. The vessels are tied or clipped if there is an injury.
- Phrenic nerve injury may occur because the nerve runs anterior to the hilum and the aortopulmonary window. The thoracic surgeon must pass the nerve to gain access to the level 6 and 5 nodes. Nerve function will usually return but often takes 6 to 12 months.
- Recurrent laryngeal nerve injury may occur because the level 5 nodes are removed from the aorto-pulmonary window. Treatment is performed as mentioned earlier.
- Pneumothorax may occur as the pleura is mobilized away from the mediastinum to gain access for the biopsies. Occasionally, this will require temporary pleural drainage.
- Wound infection is rare.

---

### Brief Illustrative Case

- *History*: 82-year-old man with no respiratory symptoms. No headaches, weight loss, or bone pains.
- *Examination*: Well-developed man in no distress. No cervical lymphadenopathy, and no chest wall lesions.
- *Blood tests*: Complete blood count and electrolytes are normal.
- *Imaging*: CT scan of chest (Fig. 5-6): centrally located left upper lobe mass and no obvious mediastinal lymphadenopathy. PET scan: increased uptake in left upper lobe lesion and no activity anywhere else.
- *Pulmonary function tests*: FEV1: 87% of predicted; DLCO: 97% of predicted
- *Management of lung mass*: Staging cervical mediastinoscopy; if malignancy found, then neoadjuvant chemotherapy, followed by re-evaluation in 2 to 3 months for resection. If mediastinal nodes are benign, then proceed with exploratory thoracoscopy and wedge resection for diagnosis and lobectomy if malignancy is found. Given the central location of this tumor, wedge resection is not an option and the patient will need left upper lobectomy for diagnosis and treatment.
- *Diagnosis/pathology*: Subcarinal lymph node showed metastatic non–small cell carcinoma.

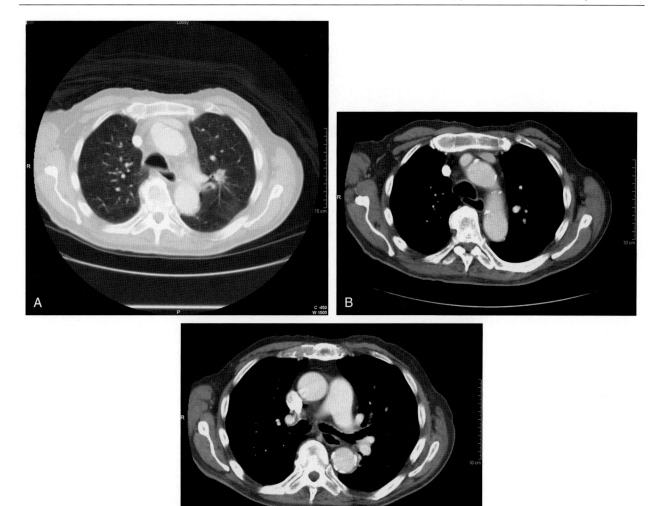

**Figure 5-6: A,** Transaxial computed tomography (CT) section showing a left upper lobe mass (lung window). **B** and **C,** Transaxial CT sections (mediastinal windows) showing no enlarged lymph nodes in pretracheal and subcarinal spaces.

## Key Points

- This illustrates the insensitivity of CT to detect mediastinal lymph node invasion (sensitivity in the mid-60s).[22]
- On the other hand, if this case with a central tumor did show enlarged mediastinal nodes on chest CT, reactive inflammatory nodes could be noted in a fair number of cases, that is those with false-positive results (specificity in the mid-60s).[22]
- Centrally located mass and high uptake on PET scan is highly suggestive of a malignancy.
- No mediastinal uptake on PET scan (sensitivity greater than CT but false-negative rate still up to 20%).[23,24]
- Staging mediastinoscopy to guide treatment in this elderly patient is thus justified.

- Pathology indicates metastases to subcarinal nodes (stage III-N2 disease).
- Patient thus needs neoadjuvant chemotherapy in view of acceptable pulmonary function and performance status.
- Patient will need re-evaluation for possible resection in 2 to 3 months.

## References

 Interactive references and additional readings for this chapter can be accessed online at *expertconsult.com.*

# 6 VIDEO-ASSISTED THORACOSCOPIC SURGERY

Robert J. McKenna Jr., MD

## INTRODUCTION

As with most surgical specialties, thoracic surgery has embraced the use of minimally invasive surgery. Video-assisted thoracic surgery (VATS) is not a specific procedure. It simply means the use of less invasive incisions to perform thoracic procedures. Compared with a traditional thoracotomy, VATS may provide patients with a lower rate of morbidity and mortality, a shorter length of stay, and earlier return to regular activities without compromising the quality of the procedures. Most types of chest operations have been performed with VATS. This chapter reviews the current state of the art for VATS procedures.

## TERMINOLOGY

**VATS** is video-assisted thoracoscopic surgery. VATS means different things to different surgeons. Some thoracic surgeons consider any thoracic procedure for which a thoracoscope looks into the chest a VATS procedure, even if the ribs are spread and the surgeon looks into the chest. However, the most common definition is that VATS is any thoracic operation using small incisions and the video camera, but without spreading the ribs. The surgeon looks at the monitor, not through the incisions.

**SPN** is a solitary pulmonary nodule.

## VIDEO-ASSISTED THORACIC SURGERY TECHNIQUES

### Anesthesia

- Usually general anesthesia, although pleural biopsies or pleurodesis can be performed with local anesthesia and sedation.
- Lung collapse is needed to see into the pleural space. That usually means that one-lung ventilation is used via a double-lumen endotracheal tube.
- A single-lumen endotracheal tube can be used for some simpler procedures, such as a lung biopsy, if the anesthesiologist hand ventilates the patient with small title volumes and occasional short periods of apnea.
- Sympathectomy can be performed with a single lumen tube. The procedure starts with apnea and $CO_2$ insufflation in the pleural space to be operated. When the lung has collapsed, ventilation is resumed.

### Visualization

- A thoracoscope is placed through a trocar into the pleural space for visualization.
  - A 2- to 3-mm scope may be used for some procedures, such as a sympathectomy
  - A 5-mm scope with a 30-degree lens is what we use for almost all of the VATS procedures that we perform.
  - Some surgeons use a 10-mm scope. Current video equipment is of such good quality that smaller scopes provide

excellent visualization. Smaller scopes cause less torsion and less trauma to the intercostal nerves.
- Visualization is on a monitor, not directly though the incisions.

### Incisions

- Incisions vary from 2 to 8 cm.
- Generally, the trocar and thoracoscope are placed low in the chest to provide good, panoramic visualization of the chest cavity.
- Additional incisions are made as needed to perform the required procedure.

### Monitors

- For most VATS procedures, the monitors are placed above the head of the bed.
- For some procedures low in the chest (e.g., Heller's myotomy), the monitors may be placed by the patient's feet.

### Indications

- VATS procedures were first performed about 1990. In the late 1980s, video equipment was developed to allow general surgeons to perform laparoscopic procedures, such as cholecystectomy. Then, endoscopic staplers were developed. The combination of these two developments created the opportunity for thoracic procedures to be performed by VATS.
- The ability to perform a procedure by VATS has not really changed the indications for an operation.
- Table 6-1 shows the simpler procedures that are commonly performed by VATS.
  - At present, most thoracic surgeons perform these procedures with VATS.
- Table 6-2 shows more complex VATS procedures that some surgeons perform.
  - These procedures are less commonly performed by VATS.
  - The first VATS lobectomy was performed in 1991. In the United States, approximately 10% to 15% of lobectomies are performed by VATS. In 2005, 94% of our lobectomies were performed by VATS. That included sleeve lobectomies, so it is possible that many thoracic operations can be performed via VATS.

### Limitations

- The limitations/contraindications to VATS procedures, as seen in Table 6-3, are related to the patient's disease, type of procedure needed, or technical capabilities of the surgeon.
- Physical limitations of the patient's disease, such as a tumor larger than 6 cm or tumors invading the chest wall require a thoracotomy to spread the ribs for removal of the tumor (e.g., Pancoast tumors).
- Severe respiratory failure ($FIO_2 = 100\%$ and high positive end-expiratory pressure) preclude one-lung ventilation for

| TABLE 6-1 ■ SIMPLER PROCEDURES THAT ARE COMMONLY PERFORMED BY VIDEO-ASSISTED THORACIC SURGERY |
|---|
| Lung Biopsy |
| Pleural Biopsy |
| Pleurodesis |
| Pericardial Window |
| Sympathectomy |
| Mediastinal Biopsy |
| Drainage of a pleural effusion or empyema |

| TABLE 6-2 ■ COMPLEX PROCEDURES THAT CAN BE PERFORMED BY VIDEO-ASSISTED THORACIC SURGERY |
|---|
| Lobectomy |
| Segmentectomy |
| Pneumonectomy |
| Esophagectomy |
| Heller myotomy |
| Thymectomy |
| Decortication of the lung |

| TABLE 6-3 ■ POSSIBLE LIMITATIONS OR CONTRAINDICATIONS TO PROCEDURES THAT CAN BE PERFORMED BY VIDEO-ASSISTED THORACIC SURGERY |
|---|
| Tumor characteristics |
|     Tumors larger than 6 cm |
|     Tumors invading the chest wall |
| Intrathoracic scarring |
|     Preoperative chemotherapy and radiation |
|     Extensive adhesions due to granulomatous disease |
|     Dense adhesions |
| Inability to tolerate on lung anesthesia |
|     Respiratory failure |
| Surgeon's skills |
|     Lack of training in video-assisted thoracic surgery |

an operation or even prevent transporting a patient to the operating room for an operation.

- Almost all thoracic surgeons can perform simpler procedures (as listed in Table 6-1), but the majority do not have the training or skills for the more complex VATS procedures (see Table 6-2).

## Workup

- The workup for a VATS procedure is the same as the workup for any thoracic procedure. The workup includes laboratory studies, such as a complete blood count (CBC), coagulation studies, electrolytes, and an electrocardiogram (EKG), as indicated.

## Imaging Studies

- Xray studies appropriate for the symptoms or diagnosis are ordered. For example, a healthy young person for a sympathectomy may not need any xray or may need a chest xray if there has been a history of pneumonia or pulmonary disease.

## Pulmonary Function Studies

- Pulmonary function studies are indicated if the patient is to undergo a pulmonary resection, such as a lobectomy, or if there is a history of pulmonary disease, such as emphysema, that needs to be assessed to determine the operative risk.

## Special Diagnostic Studies

- There are no special tests that need to be ordered for a VATS procedure.

## Video-Assisted Thoracic Surgery versus Thoracotomy

- There are few randomized studies that compare VATS and thoracotomy approaches with thoracic operations.
- Although the National Emphysema Treatment Trial was primarily a randomized trial of maximal medical management versus that plus lung volume reduction surgery, it also compared VATS with median sternotomy for the operation.[1] The morbidity, mortality, and benefits were the same for both groups, but the cost was less and the recovery was faster for the VATS group.
- Several studies have shown that patients suffer less pain after VATS than after a thoracotomy. Postoperative pain, measured by a Visual Analog Scale, total dose of narcotic, need for additional narcotic, need for intercostal blocks, and sleep disturbances, is less after VATS than after thoracotomy.[2]
- Patients who have undergone VATS have greater shoulder strength[3] at 6 months, although by 1 year, the results were comparable.
- The postoperative recovery appears to be better with the VATS approach than with a thoracotomy. Demmy[4] reported earlier returns to full preoperative activities ($P < 0.01$). Suguira[5] noted better short term and long term quality of life (QOL). Others have reported less postoperative pain ($P = 0.014$) and less shoulder dysfunction.[6,7]
- VATS procedures may be less expensive than a thoracotomy.[8]

## *POSTOPERATIVE MANAGEMENT AFTER VIDEO-ASSISTED THORACIC SURGERY*

### General Principles

- Early ambulation (three times a day in the hallways, starting on postoperative day 1)
- Laxative if no bowel movement by postoperative day 2
- No routine laboratory tests. Order laboratory tests as clinically indicated (e.g., CBC, cultures, and so on for fever workup)
- No routine x-ray studies. Presence of a chest tube is not an indication for a chest x-ray study. They are not needed after removal of the tube.
- Incentive spirometer q 1 hour during the day and evening shifts.
- Nebulizer treatments are ordered as needed.
- Patients may shower as soon as the chest tubes are removed.

### Pain Management

- Pre-emptive analgesia in the operating room with local anesthesia (usually bupivacaine [Marcaine, Wintrop Pharmaceuticals, New York, NY] with epinephrine) that provides pain relief for 12 to 16 hours.
- Postoperative analgesia with hydrocodone (Vicodin, Watson Pharmaceuticals, Inc., Corona, CA) po or Dilaudid (Abbott Laboratories, Abbott Park, IL) sq.
- In contrast to thoracotomy, rarely is an epidural catheter used after VATS.

## Chest Tube Management

- Chest drainage system usually to water seal. Air leaks are longer with chest drainage system on suction than on water seal.[9]
- Suction on drainage system for patients after pleurodesis, decortication, extensive lysis of adhesions, significant subcutaneous emphysema, and significant postoperative bloody drainage.
- The chest tube is generally removed when there is no air leak and when the drainage is less than 450 mL/day. The chest tubes are removed with lower drainage for patients with poor pulmonary function and after pleurodesis.
- If the drainage is less than 100 mL/day and the patient has a persistent air leak, then a Heimlich valve is attached to the chest tube. To collect the liquid that drains through the Heimlich valve, a Lukens's trap is placed on the Heimlich valve.
- The patient may be discharged from the hospital and the chest tube is removed when there is no longer an air leak.
- To check for an air leak, the Heimlich valve is observed as the patient coughs. When there is no longer an obvious air leak, the end of the Heimlich valve is placed under water and the patient coughs.
- When liquid accumulates in the tube proximal to the Heimlich valve, the air leak has resolved.

## Discharge Instructions

- Ambulate outside the house daily.
- Shower twice per day because warm water on the chest wall loosens the muscles and reduces postoperative pain.
- Driving is allowed when the patient feels safe to drive.
- Shoulder range of motion exercises are encouraged.
- Patients return to the office for suture removal approximately 1 week after discharge.

---

### Shoulder Range of Motion Exercises

- Climb up the wall with fingers until the arm is straight up and the chest is against the wall
- Shrug shoulders
- Hold shoulders up and back
- Hold arms together, straight out in front and rotate the arms and torso 90 degrees in each direction

---

## OPERATIVE TECHNIQUES AND PROCEDURES

- The typical VATS operation uses the incisions in Figure 6-1. Under one-lung general anesthesia, the patient is placed in the lateral decubitus position with a slight posterior tilt. The trocar and thoracoscope are placed through the eighth intercostals space in the midaxillary line.

*Note: Videos demonstrating VATS procedures are available on the accompanying DVD. (Also see video section accompanying the chapter on "Congenital and Developmental Disorders" for VATS in a pediatric patient)*

## VIDEO-ASSISTED THORACIC SURGERY PROCEDURES

### VIDEO-ASSISTED THORACIC SURGERY LUNG BIOPSY FOR INTERSTITIAL INFILTRATES

- At present, VATS has replaced an open lung biopsy as the standard method for obtaining a lung biopsy.

### Advantages

- Because all areas of the lung are accessible to VATS, it allows greater flexibility in the choice of what area of the lung to biopsy than an open lung biopsy.
- Multiple studies have shown the diagnostic yield of surgical lung biopsy to be more than 90%, with a resulting management change in 27% to 73% of patients.[10]
- Shorter operation, shorter length of stay, less pain medicine, and comparable diagnostic yield.[10-12]
- Some even report that a chest drain may not be necessary after a lung biopsy if there is no air leak; 100% diagnostic yield.[13]

### Disadvantages

- Usually requires general, one-lung anesthesia.

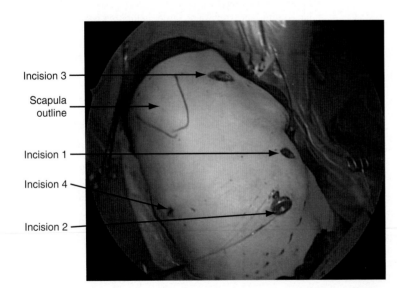

Incision 3

Scapula outline

Incision 1

Incision 4

Incision 2

**Figure 6-1:** The incisions for a VATS lobectomy: *Incision 1* is a 2-cm incision through which instruments or a stapler pass to help with the operation. *Incision 2* is a 5-mm incision for the 5-mm trochar through which the thoracoscope is passed. *Incision 3* is the 4- to 5-cm incision through which the operation is performed without spreading the ribs. *Incision 4* is a 1-cm incision through which instruments and a stapler are passed.

## VIDEO-ASSISTED THORACIC SURGERY LUNG BIOPSY FOR PULMONARY MASS

- VATS wedge resection has replaced a thoracotomy for the diagnosis of a solitary pulmonary nodule (SPN).
- Before VATS became available, it was reasonable to put the patient through the trouble, cost, and morbidity that might result from transthoracic needle biopsy, even if the chance of obtaining a specific benign diagnosis was low, because the pain and disability resulting from thoracotomy were fairly significant. However, with the advent of VATS wedge excision, which can be performed with a hospital stay of 24 to 48 hours and minimal postoperative disability, we rarely use transthoracic needle biopsy.

### Advantages

- The safety and effectiveness of VATS excision of indeterminate solitary pulmonary nodules were demonstrated by Mack and associates,[14] who performed the procedure as a primary diagnostic maneuver in 242 patients. A definitive diagnosis was obtained in all cases; two patients required thoracotomy because the lesion could not be identified at VATS. There was no mortality or major morbidity, and minor complications occurred in 3.6% (less than the 5% risk of pneumothorax requiring chest tube placement after transthoracic needle biopsy). The average hospital stay was 2.4 days. Forty-eight percent of the lesions were found to be malignant.[14]

### Disadvantages

- A thorough understanding of the correlation between computed tomography (CT) and a patient's anatomy is required and good video skills are needed to identify some pulmonary nodules.
- Some nodules (bronchioloalveolar carcinoma [BAC] <1 cm, nodules deeper in the lung, smaller nodules, and soft nodules) may be difficult to identify with VATS.

## VIDEO-ASSISTED THORACIC SURGERY FOR PULMONARY METASTASES

- In a patient with suspected pulmonary metastases, a VATS resection may be beneficial for diagnosis and treatment.
- Resection of pulmonary metastases is performed in the hopes of a cure if the primary is controlled, there is no disease elsewhere, and if all disease can be resected.
- When a patient has a history of breast cancer and a solitary pulmonary mass, the patient must not be assumed to have recurrent breast cancer. In fact, the diagnoses were primary lung cancer (48%), pulmonary metastasis from the breast cancer (34%), and benign disease (18%). Ten percent of patients had more than 1 mass found intraoperatively.[15]

### Advantages

- At least for solitary metastases, survival is the same for procedures performed by VATS or a thoracotomy.[16]

### Disadvantages

- Some authors are concerned that a procedure performed by VATS may miss nodules detected via a thoracotomy. Traditionally, in about 30% of cases, more nodules are found at thoracotomy than are found on the CT scan.

## VIDEO-ASSISTED THORACIC SURGERY PERICARDIAL WINDOW

- There is no standard surgical approach for the treatment of pericardial effusion. The options include thoracotomy, subxiphoid pericardiotomy, and VATS. The choice depends on comorbidities, patient's health status, the presence of a pleural effusion, and surgeon's skills with VATS.
- Approximately 50% of pericardial effusions that require surgical intervention are due to cancer, usually lung or breast cancer.[17]
- A VATS approach can be performed for almost any pericardial effusion, but it is particularly useful when there is a pleural effusion that needs pleurodesis,[17] after a failed subxiphoid window, loculated pericardial effusion, delayed pericardial effusion after cardiac surgery, or posterior effusions.
- The cause of the pericardial effusion is established in about 50% of cases where a window is performed.[17]
- Piehler found a direct relationship between the amount of pericardial resection and the incidence of recurrent effusion or pericardial constriction.[17]

### Disadvantages/Contraindications

- Tamponade
- Inability to tolerate one lung anesthesia
- Requires general anesthesia and single-lung ventilation

### Advantages

- Extensive resection of pericardium, both anterior and posterior to the phrenic nerve is possible (more extensive resection than with subxiphoid window).
- Less pain than a thoracotomy.
- Lower recurrence rate than subxiphoid or catheter drainage in sclerosis.[17]
- Ninety-five percent chance of control of pericardial effusion at 3 months.[17]
- A comparison with other approaches for control of a pericardial effusion is shown in Table 6-4.

## VIDEO-ASSISTED THORACIC SURGERY PLEURODESIS

- Although the first thoracoscopy for pleural disease was performed by Jacobeus in 1910, it became a much more valuable technique with the advent of video equipment.
- Ten-20% of pleural effusions remain undiagnosed after thoracentesis.[18] Of these undiagnosed effusions, about 60% are found to be caused by cancer.[19]

| TABLE 6-4 ■ RATES OF CONTROL FOR PERICARDIAL EFFUSION AFTER THE VARIOUS METHODS FOR TREATMENT[17] | |
|---|---|
| Technique | No Recurrence at 3 Months (%) |
| Pericardiocentesis | 10 |
| Pericardiocentesis plus sclerosis | 75 |
| Subxiphoid window | 86 |
| Thoracotomy for window | 90 |
| VATS window | 95 |

- Indications for VATS include undiagnosed pleural effusions, symptomatic effusions that require pleurodesis, recurrent effusion after pleurodesis, and loculated effusion,
- Talc pleurodesis can be performed through a chest tube placed under local anesthesia. One randomized study demonstrated the same efficacy for bedside pleurodesis compared with VATS pleurodesis,[20] whereas another found better outcome with VATS.[21]
- A reasonable approach is VATS to diagnose an idiopathic effusion or to treat a malignant effusion when the lung expands or the use of an indwelling catheter if the lung fails to expand.[22]

### Disadvantages/Contraindications

- Usually performed under general, one-lung anesthesia, although it can be performed with local anesthesia and sedation.

### Advantages

- Biopsies can be obtained for the diagnosis of an undiagnosed effusion.
- Loculations can be lysed to allow the lung to expand. Pleural apposition is necessary for a pleurodesis to be effective.
- The most common operation is a wedge resection and mechanical pleurodesis. Talc pleurodesis or pleurectomy is occasionally indicated.
- See section on pneumothorax.

## *VIDEO-ASSISTED THORACIC SURGERY TREATMENT OF SPONTANEOUS PNEUMOTHORAX*

- Surgical treatment of a spontaneous pneumothorax is indicated for the reasons seen in Table 6-5.
- Operation for pneumothorax involves a lung procedure (to excise the source of the air leak) and a pleural procedure (to create pleural symphysis).

## *VIDEO-ASSISTED THORACIC SURGERY THYMECTOMY*

- Thymectomy is indicated for the removal of a thymic tumor or for treatment of myasthenia gravis.
- Owing to a concern regarding possible spillage of tumor cells, many surgeons prefer an open approach for tumors in the thymus.
- Thymectomy can be performed via a cervical approach, median sternotomy, or VATS.
- VATS approach may be unilateral, bilateral, or with VATS and a cervical approach.[23]

### TABLE 6-5 ▪ INDICATION FOR SURGICAL TREATMENT OF PNEUMOTHORAX

Persistent air leak
Recurrent pneumothorax
Tension pneumothorax
Bilateral pneumothorax
Catemenial pneumothorax
Certain professions (pilot)
Patient's residence allows poor access to medical care

- We prefer to start with a 2-inch transverse cervical incision to mobilze the horns of the thymus and to dissect to the level of the innominate vein. Then we use a VATS approach for exenteration of the anterior mediastinum from the diaphragm to the thyroid, from the right to the left phrenic nerves, and from the pericardium to the posterior table of the sternum. This is a maximal thymectomy to remove all possible thymic rests.

### Advantages

- Excellent exposure and less pain than a sternotomy.
- With a VATS approach, the overall clinical improvement at follow-up was observed in 30 of 36 (83.0%) patients, with five of 36 (14.0%) patients in complete stable remission.[23]

### Disadvantages

- Requires excellent video skills.
- It may be challenging to see the phrenic nerve on the opposite side.
- Rarely, a patient with myasthenia gravis develops respiratory failure postoperatively.

## *VIDEO-ASSISTED THORACIC SURGERY/LUNG VOLUME REDUCTION SURGERY*

- Lung volume reduction surgery has been proven to be of benefit for selected patients with severe symptoms due to emphysema.
- See section on emphysema.

## *VIDEO-ASSISTED THORACIC SURGERY ESOPHAGECTOMY*

- Very advanced thoracic surgery procedures now are performed by some thoracic surgeons.
- A few current modifications of this procedure include VATS mobilization of the esophagus plus open transhiatal esophagectomy, laparoscopic mobilization of the stomach plus thoracotomy to complete the procedure, and a procedure completely performed with VATS and laparoscopy.[24] There is no evidence-based recommendation that can be made regarding the best approach.
- In general, esophagectomy carries a 5% mortality rate, and 50% of patients have postoperative complications. Risks include leak, recurrent laryngeal nerve paresis, and pneumonia.
- Recurrent laryngeal nerve paresis is important because patients aspirate so a swallowing evaluation should be performed. All patients are at risk, so aspiration precautions are reasonable.
- A feeding jejunostomy is routinely used for postoperative nutrition. Patients usually eat only about 500 calories per day when discharged. Continuous jejunal feeding is used for 10 to 12 hours at night until the patient can maintain weight without the feedings (usually about 6 weeks).
- See chapter on esophageal cancer (Chapter 56).

## *VIDEO-ASSISTED THORACIC SURGERY LOBECTOMY*

- VATS lobectomy is now recognized as a reasonable treatment for lung cancer
- See the section on treatment of lung cancer in Illustrative Case #1.

## VIDEO-ASSISTED THORACIC SURGERY DECORTICATION

- VATS is an excellent technique for the treatment of many cases of empyema. If drainage of a peripneumonic effusion is not completely drained with thoracentesis or chest tube, then decortication should be performed soon. This approach facilitates quicker recovery than nonsurgical treatment (see Illustrative Case #2).
- When Napoleon's surgeon, Dupuytren, developed an empyema in 1835, he was heard to comment that "he would rather die at the hands of God than of surgeons." He lived 12 days.
- Bronchoscopy should be performed to make sure that there is no endobronchial obstruction that would preclude expansion of the lung.
- Patients usually have pleural symphysis (no pleural space). Usually with two incisions and another incision for the trocar, the debris can be removed from the pleural space. The lung should be mobilized from the apex of the chest to the diaphragm. Then the surface of the lung is decorticated if the lung does not expand completely.
- Technique of choice for fibrinopurulent stage.
- After 3 weeks, the empyema is in an organizing phase, which is harder to treat with VATS but is still often possible even for a stage 3 empyema.
- A review concluded that VATS is superior to chest drain and fibrinolytics.[25]
- VATS may offer significant advantages over open thoracic surgery.[26-28]

### Advantages
- Most VATS decortications can be performed in approximately 1 hour.
- The approach to a parapneumonic effusion should be to attempt drainage percutaneously, unless the effusion is obviously located. If the fluid does not drain and the lung does not expand well, then prompt decortication is indicated. This reduces complication rates for the empyema and shortens hospital length of stay. Even lungs trapped by a stage 3 empyema can be decorticated by an experienced VATS surgeon.
- The operation has several components—drainage of all pockets of fluid, decorticating the lung so that it may expand fully to fill the chest, removing the parietal pleura if the expansion of the chest is inhibited by the scarring (as shown by a contracted hemithorax on CT scan), and mobilizing the diaphragm so that it can move and function properly.

## DISADVANTAGES

- At times, the dense adhesions may be very difficult to deal with during VATS.
- A high level of technical skill is needed for the VATS treatment of advanced empyema.

## KEY FACTS/"PEARLS" HIGHLIGHT

- The momentum is building for the specialty of thoracic surgery to move toward minimally invasive procedures.
- Most thoracic surgeons can perform simple procedures with VATS, and some thoracic surgeons now regularly perform advanced procedures with VATS.
- We have moved through the era of investigating the possibilities for VATS into the era of evidence-based medicine showing that VATS has many advantages for patients.

### Brief Illustrative Case #1

- A 74-year-old man patient underwent a screening chest CT to assess coronary calcification score. The screening CT scan showed a 2-cm spiculated mass in the right upper lobe (Fig. 6-2).
- He was essentially asymptomatic.
- Pulmonary function tests were near-normal with $FEV_1$ greater than 80% of predicted.
- He was classified clinically as having stage 1 disease, based on clinical workup including blood and imaging studies.
- The patient's lesion was judged to be both resectable (i.e., surgery with curative intent feasible) and operable (i.e., no comorbidities precluding surgery).
- The patient underwent a VATS right upper lobectomy and lymph node dissection.
- Final pathology showed a stage 1A (T1N0M0) pulmonary adenocarcinoma.
- He was discharged on the first postoperative day and returned to work on postoperative day 7.
- See reference 29 for analysis of 1100 cases of VATS lobectomy.

### Brief Illustrative Case #2

- A 25-year-old, previously healthy woman presented to the emergency department because of severe dyspnea, left-sided chest pain, productive cough, and fever. Her 23-day history predating this is as follows:
- She presented with tonsillitis (throat swab positive for *Streptococcus viridans*) and was treated with a 7-day course of moxifloxicin.
- After initial improvement, her symptoms recurred, so she was given another course of moxifloxicin.
- She presented to a community hospital 10 days later, where chest x-ray study revealed left lower lobe consolidation compatible with pneumonia.

*(Continued)*

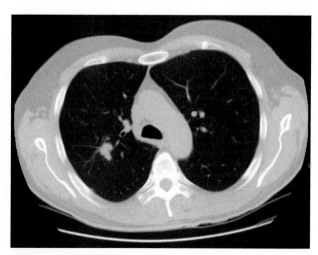

**Figure 6-2:** Computed tomography scan of the chest depicting a 2-cm mass in right upper lobe (lobular and spiculated configuration).

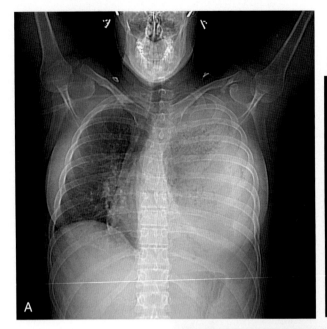

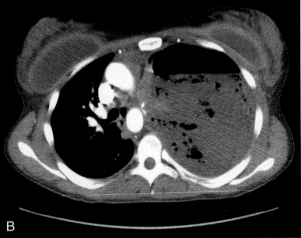

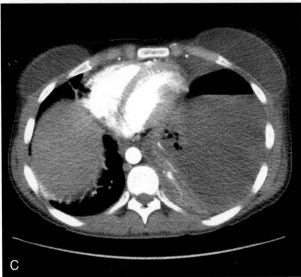

**Figure 6-3:** **A,** Computed tomography (CT) scout film showing shift of the mediastinal structures to the right side with a fluid collection with a pattern of mottled gas collections within. **B** and **C,** The chest CT revealed the very large complex fluid collection with prominent mottled gas collections within, an air fluid level, and complete collapse of the left lung.

## Brief Illustrative Case #2—cont'd

- She was again given oral antibiotics for a week.
- Three days after completing the third course of antibiotics, she presented to a major hospital emergency department as described earlier, and was immediately admitted to the intensive care unit.
- Vital signs revealed a temperature of 102° F, blood pressure of 85/50, thready pulse of 125/min, and labored respirations of 26/min. SpO$_2$ on room air was 84%.
- Minimal exudates were present in the posterior pharynx.
- Percussion revealed stony dullness over the left lung with no audible breath sounds
- White cell count was 38,000/mL with 21% bands
- Imaging studies: Chest radiograph was similar to the CT scout film (Fig. 6-3A). This showed shift of the

mediastinal structures to the right side with a fluid collection with a pattern of mottled gas collections within (shown well on the scout film). The chest CT revealed the very large complex fluid collection with prominent mottled gas collections within, an air fluid level and complete collapse of the left lung (Figs. 6-3B and C).
- A chest tube was inserted, and purulent material was removed.
- Broad spectrum antibiotics to cover methacillin-resistant *Staphylococcus aureus* (MRSA); anaerobes and gram-negative organisms were begun
- VATS drainage and decortication was planned for the next day.
- Pleural fluid cultures were positive only for *Fusobacterium necrophorum*.

## Key Points

- This patient may well have had Lemierre's syndrome.[30] The latter is a complication of tonsillitis in which septic thrombophlebitis of the internal jugular vein occurs, with septic emboli to the lungs and other organs. *Fusobacterium necrophorum* is a virulent organism that has been closely associated with Lemierre's syndrome.[30]
- It is also possible that with severe tonsillitis, the patient might well have had repeated micro-aspirations owing to a 'compromised' upper airway, resulting in an anaerobic pneumonia.
- Repeated courses of the same antibiotics, without searching for other causes of treatment failure, was unwise and resulted in severe complications.

- With the scenario depicted earlier, VATS drainage/decortication to effectively treat and clear this complex empyema is urgently required. Simple chest tube drainage and antibiotics would not have been adequate.
- The mottled gas pattern noted before any pleural intervention suggested the presence of gas-producing organisms.

## References

 Interactive references and additional readings for this chapter can be accessed online at *expertconsult.com*.

# THORACIC SURGICAL PROCEDURES AND MANAGEMENT

## 7 ANESTHETIC CONSIDERATIONS IN THORACIC SURGERY

Jennifer Cutler, MD

The anesthetic considerations for thoracic surgery that are required to provide a safe operating room outcome are (1) understanding the patient's anatomy and pathophysiology, (2) understanding the effects of general anesthesia on their pulmonary function, and (3) understanding the surgeon's treatment plan. This chapter gives an overview of the effects of anesthesia on pulmonary physiology in general, and more specifically, on patients with pre-existing lung disease. It then discusses the anesthetic management for thoracic surgery, with emphasis on equipment used and preserving patient's cardiopulmonary function intraoperatively and postoperatively. Last, the anesthetic management of specific cases in thoracic surgery are highlighted.

## OVERVIEW OF NORMAL PULMONARY ANATOMY AND PHYSIOLOGY

### Anatomy[1,2]
- Upper airway
  - Nose, nasopharynx, and oropharynx
  - Function: warm and humidify inspired gases; ciliary clearance of airway irritants and secretions.
    **Note:** *loss of this normal function needs to be remedied during anesthesia.*
- Bronchopulmonary tree
  - Each lobe subdivides into segments.
  - Each segment gives off between 10 and 25 branches.
  - Lung reflex innervation is mediated via branches of the vagus nerve.
  - Airway smooth muscle tone is mediated by the parasympathetic nervous system. Cholinergic nervous stimulation results in airway smooth muscle spasm, mucus secretion, and bronchial vasodilatation. Airway smooth muscle relaxation is mediated by inhibitory nonadrenergic non cholinergic (NANC) nerves. Exitatory NANC nerves may contribute to bronchoconstriction. Sympathetic adrenergic nerves have little or no role in regulating airway smooth muscle tone. However, note that human airway smooth muscle richly expresses

beta-adrenergic receptors, the stimulation of which produces bronchodilation.[3]
  - Tracheobronchial blood vessels are innervated by adrenergic nerves

### Physiology
During the perioperative period, significant events can occur in

- Lung mechanics
- Thoracic cage mechanics
- Respiratory muscle function
- Alveolar gas exchange
- Baseline parameters for the above-quantified by preoperative pulmonary function studies and measurement of arterial blood gases.

## OVERVIEW OF THE EFFECTS OF GENERAL ANESTHESIA ON PULMONARY FUNCTION

### Endotracheal Tubes
- Bypass the function of the upper airway resulting in the passage of dry, cold gases and buildup of secretions and irritants.[4,5]
- Reduce the size of the trachea (usually by 30-50%) which in turn increases airway resistance

### Vapors
- Smooth muscle relaxants[6,7]
  - Cause collapse and occasionally occlusion of the soft palate of the upper airway.
  - Decrease the centrally mediated respiratory response to hypercapnia and hypoxia.
- Potent bronchodilators—can be used in the management of status asthmaticus.
- Attenuate the hypoxic pulmonary vasoconstriction (HPV) response.[8,9]

## Neuromuscular Blockade

- Loss of muscle tone allows for cephalad movement of the diaphragm.[10-12]
- In most cases, neuromuscular blockade is reversed with antagonists at the termination of surgery.

## Opiates

- Centrally acting respiratory depressants
- Decrease responsiveness to $CO_2$
- Mu receptor agonists

## Positioning

- Supine position[10,11]:
  - Used during induction and emergence of anesthesia.
  - Supine position while awake decreases functional residual capacity (FRC).
  - Supine position while under anesthesia decreases FRC by another 15% to 20% due to the cephalad movement of the diaphragm
- Lateral decubitus position:
  - Used for the majority of thoracic surgical procedures.
  - In adults, there is a moderate decrease in the FRC of the dependent lung owing to compression from the mediastinum and abdominal contents.
  - In infants and young children, there is a larger decrease in FRC because there is also compression of the dependent lung from the rib cage.

## Lung Volumes

- Decreased FRC[12-14]
- Closing capacity approaches, or surpasses, FRC, which leads to alveolar collapse.

## *ATELECTASIS*

- Alveolar collapse of the lower lung fields results in atelectasis.
- High inspiratory oxygen levels result in absorption atelectasis.
- Result is shunting and impaired gas exchange.
- Positive end-expiratory pressure (PEEP) will improve atelectasis, but at the expense of decreasing cardiac output.

## Positive Pressure Ventilation

- Increases intrathoracic pressure, which, in turn, reduces venous return to the heart.[15]
- Decreased right-sided heart output impairs blood flow through the pulmonary vessels.
- Decreased left-sided heart output impairs oxygen delivery to the tissues.

## *OVERVIEW OF THE EFFECTS OF GENERAL ANESTHESIA ON PULMONARY FUNCTION IN PATIENTS WITH PRE-EXISTING LUNG DISEASE*

### Obstructive Lung Disease

- Pathophysiology[16]
  - "Irreversible"—emphysema and chronic bronchitis
  - "Reversible"—asthma
  - Have pre-existing reduced $FEV_1$
  - Have pre-existing V/Q mismatch

- Often require medications to assist pulmonary function.
  - Oral or inhaled steroids
  - Home oxygen
  - Nebulizers or metered-dose inhalers
- Patients are often former smokers or are still smoking at the time of surgery. Effects of smoking on general anesthesia include[17,18]:
  - Hypersecretions and impairment of mucociliary transport activity. It takes 4 to 8 weeks to return to normal after smoking cessation.
  - Increased plasma levels of carboxyhemoglobin shifts the oxyhemoglobin dissociation curve. It takes 4 to 6 hours to return to normal after smoking cessation.

## General Anesthesia and Obstructive Lung Disease

- Instrumentation of the airway, as in laryngoscopy, bronchoscopy and intubation may precipitate bronchospasm.[19-21]
- Vapors and local anesthetics may attenuate this response.
- Humidified circuits should be used to warm and humidify the inspired gases.
- Anticholinergics may be required to treat excess airway secretions.
- Anesthetic vapors are potent bronchodilators but will impair the HPV response, resulting in further V/Q mismatch.
- Nitrous oxide expands gas-enclosed spaces and should be avoided in patients with bullae because it can expand or rupture the bullae, resulting in a pneumothorax or tension pneumothorax.
- PEEP will minimize the atelectasis but at the expense of decreased cardiac output and risk of barotraumas.
- Beta-2 agonists used to treat bronchospasm can produce tachyarrythmias.

## Restrictive Lung Disease

- Pathophysiology[16]
  - Intrinsic restrictive lung disease (RLD)—example: interstitial lung disease
  - Thoracic restrictive disorders:
    - Morbid obesity
    - Pleural disorders, for example, fibrothorax
    - Neuromuscular respiratory disorders
    - If it is large, anterior mediastinal mass can contribute to restrictive physiology
- Have pre-existing decreased total lung capacity (TLC) +/- diffusing capacity
- Can have associated pulmonary hypertension

## General Anesthesia and Restrictive Lung Disease

- Similar precautions for patients with obstructive lung disease should be used for patients with RLD
- Increased risk for biventricular cardiac failure due to cardiac depressant effects of anesthetic vapors in patients with pre-existing pulmonary hypertension and cor pulmonale.
- Special consideration for patients with anterior mediastinal mass[22]:
  - Often symptoms are not manifested until after the patient is anesthetized.
  - Loss of muscle tone from anesthesia paralysis can result in complete airway or vascular obstruction.
  - Emergency airway equipment and ability to perform cardiac bypass should be available for large anterior mediastinal masses

## More and More Neoadjuvant Therapy is Received Prior to Surgery for Patients Who Presented with Metastatic Lung Cancer

- Multiple chemotherapy drugs (e.g., bleomycin, paclitaxel [Taxol], and so on) have been associated with postoperative adult respiratory distress syndrome (ARDS).[23,24]
- Greater risk for intraoperative bleeding if radiation therapy was given.
- Inspiratory oxygen levels must be decreased during surgery (preferably below 40%).
- Fluids are minimized.

## Surgery is Often Diagnostic, not Curative

- Examples include lung and lymph node biopsies.
- No improvement in respiratory symptoms postoperatively.

## *UNDERSTANDING THE SURGEON'S TREATMENT PLAN*

At Cedars Sinai Medical Center in Los Angeles, California, more than 1180 thoracic surgeries were performed in 2005.

Table 7-1 presents an overview of the types of cases performed and the anesthetic considerations for each case.

## *ANESTHESIA EQUIPMENT USED FOR THORACIC SURGERY*

### Endotracheal Tubes that Provide One-Lung Ventilation

- One-lung ventilation (OLV) is almost essential in thoracoscopic surgery.
- A review by Weiskopf and Campos[25] demonstrates many ways to achieve OLV in adults.
- We provide lung separation using a double-lumen tube (DLT; Mallinckrodt Medical, Inc, St. Louis, MO).
- DLTs provide excellent lung separation and allow suctioning of the nonventilated lung during the surgery.

- Most of the time, we place a R-DLT for all left-sided surgeries and an L-DLT for all right sided surgeries. The exception to this is when the right upper lobe takeoff lies proximal to the tracheal carina (incidence of 0.4%). In this case, an L-DLT would be used for a left-sided surgery.
- Most institutions only place L-DLT, citing a greater ease of use and a greater safety margin during positioning.[26,27]
  - ○ Proponents of the left-sided policy state that R-DLTs are harder to place because if the Murphy eye for the right upper lobe moves a tiny amount, the right upper lobe is not ventilated and the patient becomes hypoxic.
  - ○ We find that the L-DLTs move as much as R-DLTs.
  - ○ Right-sided tubes are needed for left sided sleeve resections and are easier to use for left pneumectomies. A L-DLT for a left pneumonectomy would require pulling back to the DLT and adjusting its position before stapling the bronchus.

### Double-Lumen Tube Size

- There is no exact science to determine which size DLT should be placed.
- Brodsky and colleagues[28] measured tracheal widths on preoperative chest x-ray studies to help determine the size of L-DLTs. This technique provided tubes too large for a mostly Asian population.[29]
- Because we select a DLT opposite to the side of the surgery, we always ventilate through the bronchial lumen. The method of ventilating through the bronchial lumen makes tube size very important:
  - ○ A tube that is too small will usually result in a leak around the bronchial cuff.
  - ○ To compensate for a bronchial leak, one often puts an excessive volume of air into the bronchial balloon, which can (1) cause airway trauma, (2) make it easier for the bronchial cuff to herniate out of the main stem bronchus, resulting in tube misalignment, and (3) rarely, rupture the main stem bronchus.
  - ○ A tube that is too large can (1) be difficult to place and (2) result in airway trauma.
- We have found good results using (for both right and left sided DLTs) 39F DLTs for men and 37F DLTs for women.

**TABLE 7-1 ▪ ANESTHETIC CONSIDERATIONS FOR THORACIC SURGERY AT CEDARS-SINAI MEDICAL CENTER**

| Procedure | Airway Management | Anesthetic Management | Considerations |
|---|---|---|---|
| VATS–wedge resection | DLT<br>Male 39 F<br>Female 37 F | PIV<br>+/- A line | T&S<br>Place DLT opposite to side of surgery |
| VATS–lobectomy | DLT | PIV<br>A line | T&C |
| VATS–edge vs lobe | DLT | PIV<br>A line | T&C<br>Do not awaken patient until biopsy is confirmed |
| VATS–evacuation of pleural effusion, hemothorax, chylothorax, with or without decortication | DLT | PIV<br>A line | T&C<br>Chest tube to suction–patient will continue to lose blood over next 24 hours.<br>Induce patient in sitting position<br>Rare complication: re-expansion pulmonary edema |

*(Continued)*

| | | | |
|---|---|---|---|
| **TABLE 7-1 ■ ANESTHETIC CONSIDERATIONS FOR THORACIC SURGERY AT CEDARS-SINAI MEDICAL CENTER—CONT'D** | | | |
| **Procedure** | **Airway Management** | **Anesthetic Management** | **Considerations** |
| VATS–talc pleurodesis | DLT | PIV | T&S |
| VATS–first rib resection | DLT | PIV | T&S |
| VATS–diaphragm plication | DLT | PIV | T&S |
| VATS–sympathectomy | Single lumen ETT | PIV<br>Temperature stickers on each hand | Patient will be supine, with arms at 90 degrees<br>Surgeon will insufflate with $CO_2$ in chest |
| Thoracotomy–lobectomy with or without chest wall resection | DLT | PIV<br>A line<br>Epidural | T&C<br>If patient received neoadjuvant therapy → keep $FIO_2$ low |
| Thoracotomy–pneumonectomy | DLT | PIV<br>A line<br>Epidural | T&C<br>ICU bed<br>Keep IVF < 1.5 L<br>Diltiazem 20 mg IV<br>Ask surgeon if lower extremity line is required<br>Rare complications: right-sided heart failure and postpneumonectomy pulmonary edema |
| VATS or thoracotomy–bronchial sleeve resection | DLT | PIV<br>A line<br>Epidural if open | T&C<br>ICU bed |
| VATS or thoracotomy–resection of posterior mediastinal mass | DLT | PIV<br>A line<br>Epidural if open | T&C |
| VATS or thoracotomy esophagectomy | DLT–left-sided DLT | PIV<br>A line<br>Central line with dopamine infusion<br>NGT<br>Keep patient warm | T&C<br>ICU bed |
| VATS or mediansternotomy–resection of anterior mediastinal mass | DLT–VATS<br>ETT–sternotomy | PIV<br>A line | T&C |
| VATS or mediansternotomy–BLVRS | DLT | PIV<br>A line<br>Epidural<br>NICO monitor<br>Pressure control ventilator | T&C<br>ICU bed<br>Bronchodilator tx immediately after surgery<br>Surgeon will ask for air leak following reduction |
| VATS or subxyphoid pericardial window | DLT–VATS ETT–subxyphoid | PIV<br>A line | Induce with etomidate<br>Have ephedrine available |
| Mediastinoscopy or medianstinotomy (Chamberlain procedure) | Single-lumen ETT | PIV | Minimum narcotics and muscle relaxant |
| Mediastinoscopy with possible VATS | DLT | PIV<br>A line | T&C |
| Laparoscopic Nissen fundoplication | Single lumen ETT | PIV<br>NGT<br>54–60 F Bougies | Keep NGT for postoperative care |
| Tracheal resection | Single lumen ETT | PIV<br>Sterile ETT for field | Patient's chin will rest against chest at end of case → be careful with extubation<br>If need to reintubate → fiberoptic intubation only |
| Esophagoscopy (stent, laser) | Single lumen ETT or no ETT | PIV | Avoid direct light for PDT patients |
| Bronchoscopy–flexible or rigid (stent, laser) | Large single lumen ETT or no ETT | PIV | Propofol infusion<br>Avoid direct light for PDT patients |

BLVRS, bilateral lung volume reduction surgery; DLT, double-lumen tube; ETT, endotracheal tube; IV, intravenous; IVF, intravenous fluid; NICO, non-invasive cardiac output; NGT, nasogastric tube; PIV, peripheral IV line; PDT, photodynamic therapy; T&C, type and cross; T&S, type and screen; tx, treatment; VATS, video-assisted thoracoscopic surgery.

## Fiberoptic Bronchoscopy

- Although some anesthesiologists position the DLT with an x-ray, that is a time consuming process.
- Our policy is to position every DLT with a fiberoptic bronchoscope.
  - This allows us to line up the ventilating slots with the appropriate bronchi and to check for any unforeseen pathology, such as intrabronchial tumors.[30]
  - Intraoperative hypoxia is usually due to misalignment of the DLT. Left-sided tubes can be too deep, so that the left upper lobe is not being ventilated. Right-sided tubes can move so that the right upper lobe is not being ventilated.
- Occasionally when direct laryngoscopy proves to be difficult, a fiberoptic bronchoscope is very helpful for intubation:
  - Fiberoptic intubations are best performed with the patient's neck hyperextended and his or her tongue pulled out of the mouth.
  - The fiberoptic bronchoscope is placed through the bronchial lumen of the DLT.
  - The bronchoscope is passed along the midline of the tongue and then under the epiglottis to visualize the vocal cords.
  - Once the bronchoscope is in the correct main stem bronchus, the DLT slides over the bronchoscope and into the main stem bronchus.

## Checking for Complete One-Lung Ventilation

- Lung surgery and especially VATS procedures depend on good isolation of the lung.
- If the operated lung stays expanded or is ventilated during the operation, the ability of the surgeon to perform the procedure is compromised and much time is wasted in repositioning the tube.
- Proper function of the DLT should be done as soon as it is placed.
  - Our policy is to position the DLT with the fiberoptic bronchoscope.
  - Because we always place our DLT opposite to the side of the surgery, we clamp off the tracheal portion of the DLT so that the surgical side is not ventilated and ventilation only occurs through the bronchial tube.
  - Distal to the clamp, the tubing to the tracheal side is opened to allow the air from the surgical lung to escape, resulting in collapse of that lung.
  - If there is evidence of ventilation in the surgical lung, the DLT may need to be adjusted or a larger tube may need to be placed for a better seal.

## Difficult Airway

- When a difficult airway is recognized in the operating room, be even more cautious regarding extubation at the end of the procedure
  - Make sure that the patient has minimal chances of postoperative respiratory distress.
  - Consider watching the patient for a longer period of time in the recovery room.
- For the remainder of the patient's hospitalization, a sign over the patient's hospital bed should state that the patient has a difficult airway. This lowers the threshold for health-care providers to electively intubate the patient if respiratory distress develops.

## Ventilators that Provide Both Volume Control and Pressure Control

- Flexibility in ventilatory modes (volume cycled; pressure preset modes) required for optimizing ventilation in different patient disease populations.

## Measurement of Both Inspiratory and Expiratory Tidal Volumes to Assess Air Leaks

- Used to assess air leak (for example, for bilateral lung volume reduction surgery).
- The inspiratory and expiratory volumes are measured before the operation and after the resection. If the difference is greater than 50 mL, then the lung is inspected for leaks.

## Invasive Monitors

- Arterial lines are usually placed.
- Central venous lines are not routinely used, but they are placed when the operation is expected to be bloody, when a pneumonectomy is performed, or when central venous pressures will be monitored postoperatively.
- A pulmonary artery catheter is required for patients with pulmonary hypertension or cor pulmonale, or for any patient with postoperative hypotension that is unresponsive to fluid boluses.

## Patient-Controlled Anesthesia versus Epidurals for Postoperative Pain Management

- Our standard practice is to place a thoracic epidural for all thoracotomies, bilateral video-assisted thoracic surgeries (VATS), patients with low pain thresholds, and patients with a marginal performance status.
  - This avoids the respiratory depressant effects of parental opiates.
  - All epidurals are placed with the patient awake, either at the start of the surgery or after surgery (for unexpected VATS converted to a thoracotomy).
  - Postoperatively patients with an epidural receive a continuous infusion of fentanyl 5 μg/mL plus bupivacaine 1/16.
- Sympathetic blockade from local anesthetics produces a small decrease in $FEV_1$ and VC, but the decrease is negligible compared with those patients who had thoracic surgery and did not receive an epidural.[31-34]
- There is no evidence to suggest the sympathetic blockade effects bronchial tone.
- For all other thoracic surgical patients, the surgeons perform intercostal nerve blocks and, when necessary, the patients receive patient-controlled anesthesia (PCA). More than 90% of lobectomies are performed by VATS, and epidural catheters are not used for those cases.

## ANESTHETIC MANAGEMENT OF THE THORACIC SURGERY PATIENT

### Goals of Thoracic Anesthesia

- Minimize cardiac depression.
  - Prevent myocardial ischemia.
  - Maintain oxygen delivery to tissues.
- Minimize increases in pulmonary artery pressure and pulmonary vascular resistance

- Minimize V/Q shunting during OLV.[8,9,35-37]
  - The body's normal response to OLV is to shunt blood away from the nonventilated lung (pulmonary vessels constrict in response to acute hypoxia).
  - Preserving HPV during thoracic anesthesia is critical to maintaining a normal $PaO_2$ and $SpO_2$ during OLV.
- Extubate the patient as soon as possible after surgery.
  - To decrease positive pressure on the bronchial anastomosis.
  - To decrease the risk of infection.
  - All patients with pre-existing lung disease are at risk for postoperative pulmonary failure.
  - Postoperatively, ensure that the patient is awake and alert, and has a strong cough.
  - Minimize factors that can lead to reintubation postoperatively (hemodynamic instability, retention of $CO_2$).

## The Effects of Thoracic Anesthesia on Intraoperative Cardiopulmonary Function

- Effects of anesthetic vapors[8,9,38]
  - All anesthetic vapors decrease cardiac output (either by direct myocardial depression or by decreasing systemic vascular resistance [SVR]). This is most common with halothane.[39]
  - All anesthetic vapors attenuate HPV in a dose-related manner.[6,38,40-43]
  - Desflurane can trigger bronchospasm.
  - Vapors may be beneficial as potent bronchodilators in patients with reactive airway disease.
- Effects of intravenous amnestic agents
  - Propofol and barbiturates (sodium thiopental) decrease cardiac output by decreasing SVR and by causing venodilation with decreased venous return.[44,45]
  - Etomidate provides hemodynamic stability because its effects on cardiac output are minimal.
  - Ketamine has sympathomimetic properties that make it advantageous to use in patients presenting with hypovolemia (e.g., emergency thoracic surgery for trauma to the chest), but should be avoided in patients with pulmonary hypertension because it increases PVR.[46,47]
  - No effect on HPV or bronchial tone by intravenous amnestic agents.
- Effects of intravenous narcotics
  - Provide hemodynamic stability.
  - Do not effect HPV.
  - Fentanyl is a good choice for thoracic surgery because it is a potent analgesic, but it is also short acting, which allows for rapid awakening from anesthesia.[48]
- Effects of neuromuscular blockade
  - Pancuronium has vagolytic properties and will produce tachycardia. It should be avoided in patients who are at risk for postoperative tachydysrhythmias.
  - Atracurium causes histamine release and can produce bronchospasm in patients with reactive airway disease.
  - All other muscle relaxants (both depolarizing and nondepolarizing) do not have either hemodynamic effects or effects on HPV.
- Effects of fluid resuscitation[49]
  - Owing to disrupted lymphatics, patients who are undergoing thoracic surgery are at risk for postoperative pulmonary edema.
  - Because of this risk, patients are kept hypovolemic, which can cause intraoperative hypotension.
- Intraoperative management
  - Our policy is to watch with noninvasive (blood pressure cuff, pulse oximeter, three-lead echocardiography [ECG])

and invasive (arterial and occasionally central venous pressure) monitors the cardiopulmonary function in all thoracic surgery patients. Patients with pulmonary hypertension or cor pulmonale require a pulmonary artery catheter.
  - Some anesthesiologists recommend using propofol or barbiturates for an amnestic agent because neither class of drug attenuates the HPV response.[38]
  - We find that by using a balanced technique of vapor plus muscle relaxant plus narcotics we can use a smaller inspiratory level of vapor. This minimizes the vapor's negative effect on both cardiac depression and attenuation of HPV, and allows for rapid recovery from anesthesia with adequate postoperative analgesia.
  - Although epidurals are often placed at the start of surgery, we do not administer them until the end of surgery. This prevents intraoperative hypotension due to a sympathectomy from local anesthetic administration, and respiratory depression from opiate administration.
  - Many thoracic surgery patients have hypertension at the time of surgery. Although beta blockers can and should be used in patients with concomitant coronary artery disease, one should be aware of their risk of bronchoconstriction.

## The Effects of Thoracic Anesthesia on Postoperative Cardiopulmonary Function

- Effects of anesthetic vapors
  - Residual vapor contributes to postoperative hypotension.
  - Residual vapor impairs the patient's ventilatory responses to both $CO_2$ and hypoxia.
  - Both hypotension and impaired ventilatory responses decrease oxygen delivery to the tissues.
  - The resulting acidosis increases the risk of reintubation.
- Effects of fluid resuscitation
  - Patients are often hypovolemic postoperatively.
  - Carefully watch chest tube output.
  - Carefully watch urine output (approximately 30 mL/h is desirable)
  - Carefully watch hemoglobin/hematocrit if the patient has had substantial blood loss during the procedure or has significant chest tube drainage
  - The routine use of x-ray studies or blood tests after lung surgery is not needed
  - Minimally invasive surgeries have decreased third space fluid requirements
- Postoperative management
  - Keep patients in a semisitting position to allow full chest expansion for deep breathing and coughing. (However, FRC remains reduced for several days after surgery.)
  - Early use of nebulizers or metered-dose inhalers (MDIs) to relieve bronchoconstriction.
  - Early use of chest physiotherapy (PT) to help patients clear secretions.
  - Delivery of humidified oxygen via face mask.
  - As early as possible, decrease oxygen flow rates on chronic obstructive pulmonary disease (COPD) patients.
  - Consider use of continuous positive airway pressure (CPAP) or bilevel positive airway pressure (BiPAP).
  - Begin epidural infusion if the patient is hemodynamically stable. Keep in mind that the local anesthetic may cause sympathectomy or block the cardiac accelerator fibers.
  - Remember that some surgeries are diagnostic and not curative. These patients will have no improvement in their pulmonary function postoperatively.

## The Effects of Thoracic Surgery on Postoperative Cardiopulmonary Function

- Risk of postoperative arrhythmias following lobectomy and pneumonectomy is approximately 20% after lung surgery:
  - Usually atrial fibrillation due to atrial stretching.[50,51]
  - Our policy is for patients to receive an intravenous bolus of diltiazem intraoperatively if they are thought to be at risk for postoperative atrial fibrillation.
  - The risk of atrial fibrillation is reduced by shorter operations, such as VATS.
- Risk of right-sided heart failure following pneumonectomy[52]
  - Right pneumonectomy poses a greater risk than a left pneumonectomy.
  - Increased intraoperative fluids increases the risk of pulmonary edema.
- Risk of pulmonary edema following re-expansion of a trapped lung[53]

## ANESTHETIC CONSIDERATIONS FOR SPECIAL CASES IN THORACIC SURGERY

### Lung Volume Reduction Surgery

- Patients have severe COPD[54]
  - $FEV_1$ less than 45%
  - Oxygen dependent
  - Can be steroid dependent
- Anesthetic considerations:
  - Patients often maintain high sympathetic tone while awake, and become hypotensive when anesthetized at induction.
  - Pressure-controlled ventilation is recommended to prevent barotraumas.
  - Patients are at risk for air leaks—compare inspiratory with expiratory tidal volumes after each reduction. If the difference is greater than 50 mL, then the lung is inspected for leaks.
  - Patients are extremely sensitive to centrally acting sedatives and narcotics—thoracic epidurals are the best route for pain management.
- Postoperatively patients are at risk for respiratory failure.
  - Our protocol is to provide respiratory therapy (nebulizers and chest PT) immediately after surgery and every 4 hours postoperatively.
  - Patients need early and frequent ambulation.

### Pulmonary Hypertension

- Introduction:
  - Pulmonary hypertension[55] presents a major challenge for the anesthesiologist.
  - With noncardiac surgery, the presence of pulmonary hypertension, was associated with a 7% early mortality rate and a 42% incidence of morbidity.[56]
  - Anesthesia increases the risk of acute right ventricular decompensation.
  - Thoracic surgical procedures confer a very high risk.
- Pathophysiologic principles guiding anesthetic care[57]:
  - Prevent excessive reduction in right ventricular (RV) preload/filling pressures.
    - Whereas appropriate diuretic management reduces RV pressure and volume overload, excessive diuresis can impair RV function and precipitate acute failure.
    - Correct any blood or fluid loss.
    - Fluid administration or diuresis should be guided by hemodynamic objective parameters.

  - Prevent myocardial depression (i.e., preserve right ventricular contractility)
    - Avoid cardiodepressant anesthetic and other agents
  - Avoid increments in right ventricular afterload.
    - Prevent hypoxia
    - Prevent hypercapnia
    - Prevent acidosis
    - Avoid light anesthesia
    - Provide adequate analgesia
    - Avoid sympathomimetic drugs that increase the pulmonary vascular resistance (PVR).
  - Avoid hypotension
    - Drug induced
    - Correct fluid and blood losses
  - Maintain sinus rhythm
    - Prevent/treat arrhythmias.
    - Atrial fibrillation is a common problem with a variety of thoracic surgical procedures and is not well tolerated in patients with significant pulmonary hypertension and RV dysfunction.
  - Continue pulmonary hypertension—specific drugs, including intravenous prostanoids.
- Anesthetic monitoring:
  - Transesophageal ECHO (TEE) is considered the best modality to assess changes in chamber sizes and filling pressures, RV function, pulmonary artery pressures, and so on.
  - Pulmonary artery catheter: useful in peri- and postoperative setting
  - Arterial catheter
- Anesthetic agents and influences on PVR[57,58]:
  - *Propofol*: data on the effects on PVR controversial in man[59,60] with enhanced response to vasoconstrictors in animals.[61] The agent has been used without adverse events in patients with severe pulmonary arterial hypertension.[62] With single-lung ventilation, propofol produced higher $PaO_2$ and reduced shunt fractions compared with some volatile anesthetic agents.[63]
  - *Etomidate*: No effect on PVR, and can be used.
  - *Ketamine*: Increases PVR via sympathetic activation.[64] Should probably avoid.
  - *Opioids*: Fentanyl, alfentanil, sufentanil, and remifentanil can be used. No effect on PVR.
  - *Thiopental*: decreases PVR with induction dose.
  - *Volatile anesthetics*: Most experience with isoflurane.[65] Can also use sevoflurane. Complex issues related to desflurane, enflurane and halothane make these less desirable.[57] In patients undergoing single-lung ventilation, baseline hemodynamics revealed significantly increased PVR and pulmonary pressures with desflurane compared with those of isoflurane.[66]
  - *Nitrous oxide (NO)*: Several reports of increased PVR, as well as no impact.[67,68]
  - *Neuromuscular blocking agents*: Both depolarizing and nondepolarizing agents can be used.
- Management of pulmonary hypertension during surgery:
  - Pulmonary vasodilators
    - Maintain use of preoperative medications and/or infusions.
    - NO must be readily available with equipment and skills to provide the gas on mechanical ventilation. Usual dose: 20 to 40 ppm.
    - Intravenous prostanoids (epoprostenil, prostaglandin $E_1$, treprostinil).
    - Adenosine infusion.
    - Inhaled prostanoids (iloprost, epoprostenil, treprostinil).

- Inotropic support
  - Used with hypotension and significantly decreased cardiac index, despite euvolemia.
  - Dobutamine: inotropic effects on the RV and modest pulmonary vasodilator properties
  - Milrinone: A phosphodiesterase-3 inhibitor. Inotropic effects on RV with reported reduction in PVR.
  - Pressors should be avoided unless there is refractory hypotension despite correction of all reversible factors and inotropic support.
- Principles of immediate postoperative care:
  - Prevent hypoxia and hypercapnia.
  - Adequate attention to analgesia (pain increases sympathetic drive).
  - Warm and prevent shivering (shivering increases sympathetic drive).
  - Avoid hypotension.
  - Avoid/treat arrhythmias.
  - Continue usual pulmonary hypertension specific regimen.
  - Wean added intraoperative pulmonary vasodilators and/or vasoactive medications gradually and with caution.
  - Elective admission to the intensive care unit.
- Pediatric pulmonary hypertension
  - A recent study addressed complications in children with pulmonary arterial hypertension undergoing anesthesia for noncardiac surgery or catheterization.[69]
  - Two hundred and fifty-six procedures in 156 patients (56% idiopathic; 21% congenital heart disease; the rest: chronic lung and liver disease).
  - Cardiac arrest and pulmonary hypertensive crisis occurred in 4.5% of patients.
  - High baseline pulmonary pressures were a major risk factor. Anesthetic management and etiology did not predict risk.
- Alternatives to general anesthesia:
  - Thoracic epidural:
    - No impact on baseline PVR.
    - Can be associated with adverse cardiac and hemodynamic effects. Hypotension can occur. High thoracic epidural anesthesia can block cardiac afferent and efferent sympathetic nerve fibers, resulting in bradycardia and myocardial depression.
    - Thoracic epidural anesthesia combined with isoflurane had less impairment of gas exchange compared with a propofol and fentanyl regimen in patients undergoing lung surgery.[70]
  - Regional nerve block:
    - When feasible.
    - Brachial or lumbar plexus nerve block.
    - Needs skilled operators because incomplete block will result in pain and anxiety, and increase pulmonary pressures and PVR.

## Lung Transplant
- Candidates[54,71,72]
  - Although single-lung transplant can be performed for patients with interstitial pulmonary fibrosis, double-lung transplants are currently preferred by most large centers.
  - Double-lung transplant is most often performed for patients with COPD, cystic fibrosis, idiopathic pulmonary hypertension, or pulmonary hypertension complicating a primary disorder.
- Lung transplant and cardiopulmonary bypass (CPB):
  - Elective use of CPB is almost always used for patients with severe pulmonary hypertension or for patients with poor right ventricular systolic function.

- CPB does increase the amount of blood lost intraoperatively or the amount of blood transfused postoperatively.
- Antifibrinolytics may help decrease the amount of blood products required.
- Anesthetic considerations:
  - At risk for biventricular failure.
  - TEE is the best intraoperative monitor to assess changes in chamber sizes, chamber filling pressures, RV function, and pulmonary artery pressures.
  - An arterial line and a pulmonary artery catheter are also required for peri- and postoperative hemodynamic monitoring.
  - Maintain sinus rhythm (consider a-v sequential pacing).
  - Avoid increases in pulmonary artery pressure and pulmonary vascular resistance:
    - Prevent hypoxia.
    - Prevent hypercapnia.
    - Prevent acidosis.
    - Avoid sympathomimetic drugs that increase pulmonary vascular resistance.
  - Inhaled NO and intravenous milrinone are often used to selectively decrease pulmonary artery pressure without decreasing systemic artery pressure.
  - Continue pulmonary hypertension–specific drugs, including intravenous prostanoids.
  - Be prepared for going on cardiopulmonary bypass.
- Postoperatively patients are at risk for:
  - Right-sided heart failure due to clamping of the pulmonary artery intraoperatively, hypoxia, hypercarbia, or hypothermia.
  - Bronchial dehiscence and respiratory failure due to rejection and/or infection.
  - Silent aspiration due to reduced cough reflex.
  - Reperfusion syndrome resulting in stiff, wet lungs.
  - High transfusion requirements if CPB was used.

## Surgery on the Upper Airway
- Careful planning with the surgeon must take place before anesthetizing these patients.[73-75]
  - For tumor debulking by laser (YAG or PDT), fire safety precautions are required.
  - For masses or stenotic tracheas that are resectable, plan with the surgeon how ventilation will take place while the airway is exposed to atmospheric pressure during resection and anastomosis (controlled apnea versus high frequency ventilation).
- Anesthetic considerations:
  - Intravenous steroids should be given at the start of surgery.
  - Tracheal stenosis and intraluminal tumors require smaller endotracheal tubes (ETT) for intubation. Rigid bronchoscopy may be performed first to dilate a stenosis or assess a tumor. Intubation may be performed by fiberoptic bronchoscopy to properly position the endotracheal tube in relation to the location of the tumor.
  - Have various sized reinforced ETTs on the surgical field for tracheal resections when ventilation is performed distal to the resection.
  - Only intravenous amnestic agents should be used because vapors will lead to operating room contamination.
  - Check for an air leak around the ETT before extubation because patients are prone to airway edema.
- Postoperatively, patients are at risk for airway edema.
  - All medical personnel must be aware that the patient may be difficult to reintubate, and a fiberoptic bronchoscope should be available.
  - Keep the patient in a sitting position to help decongest the airway

## Thoracic Surgery on Pediatric Patients

- Pediatric patients present with a number of congenital and acquired thoracic lesions.[76-78]
  - Lesions common to infants: lung hypoplasia, congenital diaphragmatic hernia, tracheal-esophageal fistula, congenital lung sequestration.
  - Lesions common to children: scoliosis, pectus excavatum.
- Methods used to achieve OLV are often dependent on the patient's age:
  - Infants: OLV is obtained by intentionally intubating the main stem bronchus of the nonsurgical side with a single-lumen ETT.
  - Children younger than 6 years of age: lung separation can be obtained using a bronchial blocker such as a Fogarty embolectomy catheter placed into, or alongside, the ETT.
  - Children 8 years of age and older: lung separation can be obtained using a univent tube, or small DLT.
- Pediatric patients are more prone to shunting and hypoxemia on OLV:
  - Infants have a greater drop in FRC in the lateral decubitus position due to compression of the dependent lung from the rib cage.
  - Children have a greater oxygen consumption (6 to 8 mL/kg/min) compared with adults (2 to 3 mL/kg/min). The increased oxygen consumption coupled with increased FRC produces more hypoxemia.
- Anesthetic considerations:
  - Often an inhaled induction is required and intravenous access is obtained after induction of anesthesia. Halothane might stimulate cardiac arrhythmias in children on beta-2 agonists. Desflurane might trigger bronchospasm at high inspiratory concentrations. Sevoflurane may be preferred agent for inhalation induction.
  - Because most methods of obtaining OLV in children do not allow for intrabronchial suctioning on the surgical side, the nonventilated lung will collapse slowly.
  - PEEP is often required.
  - Careful vigilance is required for bronchial blockers. If they become dislodged, they can move into the trachea causing an obstruction to ventilation.
  - Smaller fiberoptic bronchoscopes are required to confirm bronchial blocker positioning.
  - Thoracic epidurals often have to be placed with the children asleep.

- Postoperatively pediatric patients are at risk for:
  - Hypoxia due to the loss of FRC combined with increased oxygen consumption
  - More difficult pain control. Because most epidurals are placed while the children are asleep, a true test of the epidural can be done only after surgery, when the patient is awake.

## Thoracic Surgery on Morbidly Obese Patients

- Common comorbidities associated with morbid obesity include type 2 diabetes mellitus and coronary artery disease (CAD).[79,80]
- Morbid obesity imposes high elastic loads (simulated by placing sand bags on top of the chest of normal subjects) and increased work of breathing.
- May have obstructive sleep apnea and/or obesity hypoventilation syndrome (pickwickian syndrome).
- May have accompanying pulmonary arterial hyper-tension.
- Anesthetic considerations:
  - Lack of identifiable landmarks means that invasive monitors and thoracic epidurals can be challenging to place.
  - Early use of PEEP may lessen the intraoperative atelectasis and shunting
  - There is no evidence that morbidly obese patients require a different DLT size, but fiberoptic bronchoscopy may be required for intubation
  - There is no evidence that one amnestic agent is better than others in these patients
- Postoperatively patients are at risk for:
  - Airway obstruction due to collapse of the soft palate from residual vapor or predisposition for upper airway narrowing or obstruction in the case of sleep apnea Oral airways should be available at the bedside.
  - Profound hypercapnia and hypoxia due to atelectasis or lack of central drive.
  - Obstructive sleep apnea. CPAP or BiPAP may be required.

## References

 Interactive references and additional readings for this chapter can be accessed online at *expertconsult.com*.

# 8 THORACIC SURGICAL ANATOMY AND PROCEDURES

George Rakovich, MD, Éric Fréchette, MD, and Jean Deslauriers, MD

## *SURGICAL ANATOMY*

A detailed knowledge of surgical anatomy is of major importance in the practice of thoracic surgery. The following descriptions only summarize the basic anatomic information that every thoracic surgeon and chest physician must know.

## Chest Wall

The bony thorax includes the sternum, 12 pairs of ribs and costal cartilages, and 12 thoracic vertebrae.[1-3]

## Ribs

Ribs form bony arches that curve downward from back to front.

- Accordingly, ribs are two interspaces lower anteriorly than posteriorly.
- The point of greatest change in the curvature of a rib is called the angle of the rib.

Typical ribs (3–9) are composed of a head, neck, and shaft.

- The head (enlarged posterior portion) articulates with the corresponding thoracic vertebra and the vertebra immediately above (costovertebral joint).

- The neck connects the head to the shaft. At this junction, there is a tubercle that articulates with the transverse process of the corresponding vertebra (costotransverse joint).
- The intercostal vessels and nerve run in the costal groove on the inferomedial surface of the rib (Fig. 8-1).

The ribs are true, false, and floating.

- True ribs (1–7) articulate directly with the sternum and manubrium by way of their own costal cartilages.
- False ribs (8–10) articulate with the cartilage of the rib above, not the sternum directly.
- Floating ribs (11–12) end freely into the muscles of the anterior abdominal wall.

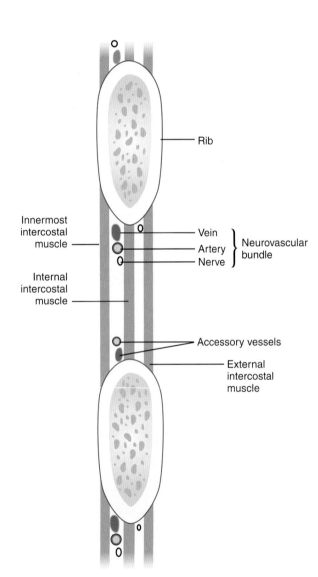

**Figure 8-1:** Cross-sectional diagram of the chest wall demonstrating the anatomic relationship of the intercostal space, rib neurovascular bundle, and accessory vessels. Observe that a chest tube inserted above the superior border of the rib will avoid trauma to the main neurovascular bundle. (*From McFadden PM, Jones JW. Tube thoracostomy: anatomical considerations, overview of complications, and a proposed technique to avoid complications. Milit Med 1985;150:681-685.*)

## Sternum

The sternum is a flat bone that consists of three parts: manubrium, body, and xyphoid process.

### MANUBRIUM

The manubrium is the most superior part of the sternum.

- The suprasternal notch is located in the midline superiorly.
- Laterally, three paired notches articulate with the clavicles, first, and second costal cartilages.
- The manubrium articulates with the body of the sternum at the sternal angle.
- The sternal angle is located at vertebral level 4 to 5 and is a useful anatomic landmark because it marks the level of the insertion of the second costal cartilages.

### THE BODY OF THE STERNUM AND XYPHOID PROCESS

- Laterally, six paired notches articulate with costal cartilages 2 to 7.
- The xyphoid process articulates with the body at vertebral level 10 to 11.

## Muscles

Major muscles of the chest wall include the pectoralis major, latissimus dorsi, serratus anterior, and trapezius muscles (Fig. 8-2). These muscles cover large portions of the chest wall and thus are frequently involved by thoracic incisions, which may affect postoperative pain, breathing mechanics, and upper limb function.

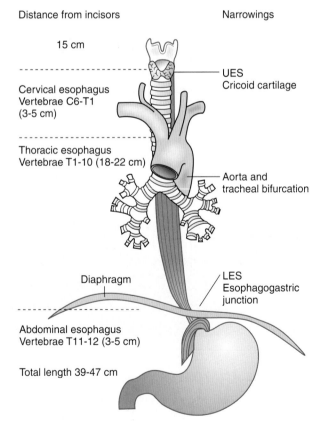

**Figure 8-2:** Classic divisions of the esophagus. UES, upper esophageal sphincter; LES, lower esophageal sphincter. (*Courtesy of Dr. Dorothea Liebermann-Meffert.*)

These muscles may be useful clinically in the reconstruction of major soft tissue defects of the chest wall and the management of intrathoracic surgical complications such as infected pleural spaces.

### Pectoralis Major

Insertions:

- Clavicular head: medial half of the clavicle.
- Sternocostal head: anterior surface of the sternum, costal cartilages 1–6, and external oblique aponeurosis.
- Lateral lip of the intertubercular groove of the humerus.
- Innervation: medial and lateral pectoral nerves.

Function: depresses the shoulder, adducts and medially rotates the arm, elevates the upper ribs during forced inspiration.

The pectoralis major is a large fan-shaped muscle which can be useful for covering soft tissue defects of the chest wall and for obliterating complicated pleural spaces.

- It can be harvested as either a muscle flap or a myocutaneous flap based on the thoracoacromial vessels. The fifth rib may be harvested with the muscle in cases where skeletal support is required. It can also be used as a turn over flap based on internal mammary perforator vessels.

### Latissimus Dorsi

Insertions: spines of the lower six thoracic vertebrae, thoracolumbar fascia, iliac crests, as well as the lower 3 to 4 ribs. Superiorly, the floor of the intertubercular groove of the humerus.

Innervation: Thoracodorsal nerve.

Function: Powerful adductor and extensor of the arm.

The latissimus dorsi is useful for the reconstruction of full-thickness chest wall defects anteriorly and laterally and can also be used intrathoracically.

- It can be harvested as either a muscle flap or a myocutaneous flap based on the thoracodorsal artery (a branch of the subscapular artery) or as a reverse flap based on multiple paraspinous perforators (from the posterior intercostal vessels).

### Serratus Anterior

Insertion: Arises from the external surfaces of first 8-9 ribs and inserts over the anterior surface of the medial border of the scapula.

Innervation: long thoracic nerve (C5–7), which courses on the anterior surface of the muscle in the midaxillary line.

Function: Applies the scapula to the chest wall. Allows elevation and abduction of the arm. Paralysis of the serratus anterior is characterized by winging of the scapula.

- It may be harvested as a muscle flap based on the lateral thoracic artery (a branch of the thoracodorsal artery). It may also be used as a composite flap of muscle, rib and skin, or together with the latissimus dorsi based on the thoracodorsal artery.

### Trapezius

Insertions: Occiput at superior nuchal line, ligamentum nuchae of neck, spinous processes of vertebrae C7–T12, spine of scapula, acromion, and lateral third of clavicle.

Innervation: Spinal accessory nerve and fibers from C3 to 4. The spinal accessory nerve is vulnerable to injury in the posterior triangle of the neck, where it may be very superficial.

Function: stabilizes the shoulder; elevates, depresses and rotates the scapula; and participates in entire the range of scapulohumeral movements.

### Intercostal Space

Main site of surgical access to the chest (thoracentesis, thoracostomy, thoracotomy) (see Fig. 8-1).

Because of the position of the intercostal vessels and nerves in the costal groove, they are vulnerable to injury by an incision along the inferior border of the rib, which may cause hemorrhage and prolonged neuralgia.

### Intercostal Muscles

Three layers of intercostal muscles span the intercostal space. They are attached to the periosteum of the rib above and the rib below.

- Fibers of the external intercosal muscle run obliquely forward and downward from the rib tubercle to the costal cartilage.
- Fibers of the inner intercostal muscles run obliquely backward and downward from the sternum to the angle of the rib. These fibers run at right angle from the external intercostal.

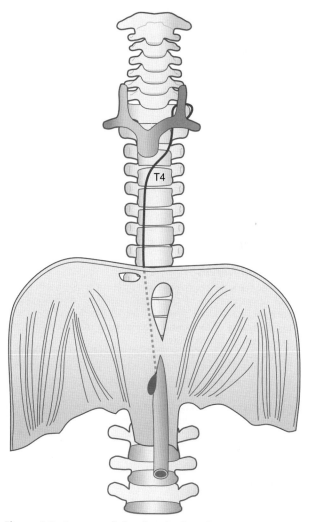

**Figure 8-3:** Anatomy of the thoracic duct. (*Courtesy of Dr. Reza Mehran.*)

- The innermost intercostal muscles are present only at the midportion of the intercostal spaces. They may be absent superiorly. Muscle fibers run backward and downward. Along with the subcostal and transversus thoracic muscles they form the most internal muscular layer.
- The neurovascular bundle is located between the inner and innermost intercostal muscle layers.

### Intercostal Arteries

The first and second posterior intercostal arteries arise from the superior intercostal arteries (branches of the subclavian artery). The other posterior intercostal arteries arise directly from the thoracic aorta.

#### BRANCHES
- A posterior branch supplies the spinal cord and soft tissues of the back.
- An anterior branch runs in the costal groove. At the midaxillary line, a lateral cutaneous branch perforates the intercostal space to supply the skin.
- A collateral branch arises near the angle of the rib and travels anteriorly along the superior border of the rib below.

#### ANTERIOR INTERCOSTAL ARTERIES
- Branches of the internal thoracic artery superiorly, and of the musculophrenic arteries inferiorly.
- They give off two segmental arteries in each space.
- One courses above (in the costal groove) and the other along the upper border of the rib below, anastomosing with branches of the posterior arteries.
- The subcostal artery (below rib 12) has a similar course but no collaterals.

### Intercostal Veins
- Follow the same course as the arteries and are mostly tributaries of the azygos and hemiazygos venous systems.
- The posterior intercostal vein of the first intercostal space may be a tributary of the brachiocephalic, vertebral, or superior costal veins.
- The superior intercostal vein drains the second, third, and fourth intercostal veins, and is a tributary of the azygos vein on the right and innominate vein on the left.

### Intercostal Nerves
- Provide the sensory innervation to the entire chest wall (1–8), and upper portion of the epigastrium (9). Anesthesia and paralysis are seldom produced by the section of only one nerve because of the considerable overlap in innervation that exists between adjacent nerves.
- Spinal nerves $T_3$ to $T_6$ have the most common pattern and are thus considered typical nerves. While exiting the intervertebral foramen, each spinal nerve divides into a ventral and a dorsal ramus. The ventral ramus communicates with the sympathetic chain via rami communicators and beyond this point, it becomes the intercostal nerve.
- In the costal groove, the intercostal nerve lie first inferior to the intercostal artery.

### DIAPHRAGM

The diaphragm is a two-dome–shaped musculotendinous structure separating the thorax from the abdomen. Each half of the muscle inserts into a central (costal part) tendon.[4,5]

Insertions: Lumbar vertebrae (L1–3) (crurae), lower six ribs and costal cartilages, xyphoid process.

Innervation: Phrenic nerves.

Function: The diaphragm is the most important respiratory muscle. Its contraction lowers the position of its central tendons, elevates the ribs, and widens the thoracic cavity.

The diaphragm three most important openings are

- The aortic hiatus. It contains the aorta, azygos vein and thoracic duct. It is limited by the body of T12 posteriorly, the diaphragmatic crura laterally, and median arcuate ligament anteriorly.
- The esophageal hiatus. It contains the esophagus, vagus nerves, and branches of the left gastric artery. It is located anterior to the aorta at T10, where the fibers from the right crux of the diaphragm form a sling around the lower esophagus.
- The caval hiatus. It contains the inferior vena cava and is located posteriorly to the right of the midline at T8.

### MEDIASTINUM

#### Trachea and Main Bronchi
- The trachea is a semirigid structure running from the cricoid cartilage to the carina; it measures 10 to 12 cm and is supported anteriorly by 16 to 20 horseshoe-shaped cartilaginous rings (Figs. 8-4 and 8-5).[6-8]
- Its posterior membranous portion is apposed against the esophagus.
- The tracheal lumen is lined by a columnar and ciliated epithelium. A submucosal layer of connective tissue contains mucous glands.
- The trachea divides into right and left main-stem bronchi at the carina, located at T5.

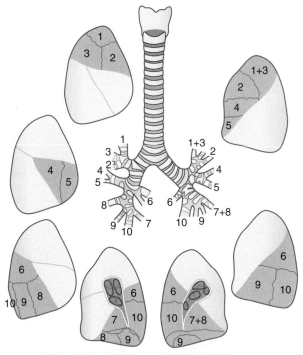

**Figure 8-4:** The lobes and segments of the lung. Right upper segments: 1, apical; 2, anterior; 3, posterior. Right middle segments: 4, lateral; 5, medial. Right lower lobe segments: 6, superior; 7, medial basal; 8, anterior basal; 9, lateral basal; 10, posterior basal. Left upper lobe segments: 1 + 3, apical posterior; 2, anterior; 4, superior lingular; 5, inferior lingular. Left lower lobe segments: 6, superior; 7 + 8, anteromedial basal; 9, lateral basal; 10, posterior basal. *(Courtesy of Dr. Thomas W. Rice.)*

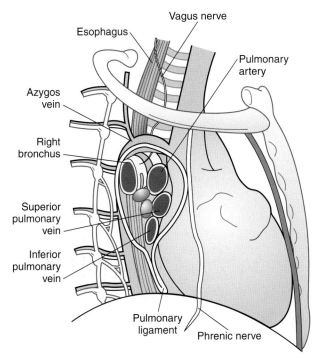

**Figure 8-5:** Right pulmonary hilum. *(Reprinted from Deslauriers J, Mehran R. Handbook of perioperative care in thoracic surgery. Philadelphia: Elsevier; 2005. p. 196.)*

- The left main stem bronchus is longer and originates at a sharper angle than the right. It measures approximately 5 to 6 cm.
- The right main stem bronchus is shorter, wider, and more vertical than the left. Thus, the right lung is particularly vulnerable to aspiration of foreign bodies or digestive secretions.

- A rich network of lymphatics accompanies the bronchi and bronchial vessels.
- These lymphatics are important pathways in the spread of bronchogenic carcinoma, and their involvement by cancer has important therapeutic and prognostic implications.

## Great Vessels
### Systemic Arteries
#### THE AORTIC ARCH
- Begins at the level of the sternal angle (Fig. 8-6)
- It arches superiorly and to the left, passing in front of the trachea and then to the left of the trachea and esophagus.
- The arch runs posteriorly behind the root of the left lung.
- It becomes the descending thoracic aorta at the level of the second sternocostal joint (T4).

#### THE BRACHIOCEPHALIC (INNOMINATE) TRUNK
- It arises from the aortic arch behind the manubrium slightly to the left of the midline.
- It ascends superolaterally on the anterior surface of the trachea and branches into the common carotid and right subclavian arteries at the level of the sternoclavicular joint.

### The Left Common Carotid Artery
- Arises from the aortic arch posterolaterally to the innominate artery.
- It ascends first anterior and then to the left of the trachea. It courses posteriorly to the sternoclavicular joint and into the neck.

#### THE LEFT SUBCLAVIAN ARTERY
- It arises from the posterior part of the aortic arch; as ascending, it lies agains the left lung and pleura laterally. It passes into the neck behind the the sternoclavicular joint posterolateral to the carotid artery.

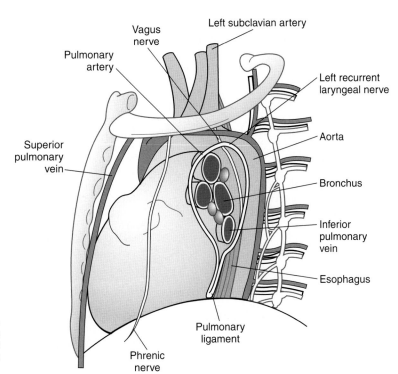

**Figure 8-6:** Left pulmonary hilum. *(Reprinted from Deslauriers J, Mehran R. Handbook of perioperative care in thoracic surgery. Philadelphia: Elsevier; 2005. p. 195.)*

## Pulmonary Arteries

### THE MAIN PULMONARY ARTERY

- Originates in the right ventricle, runs in a posterior direction, and divides into right and left pulmonary arteries behind the aortic arch.

### THE RIGHT PULMONARY ARTERY

- Crosses between the carina and ascending aortic arch and posteriorly superior vena cava anteriorly to reach the hilum of the right lung.

### THE LEFT PULMONARY ARTERY

- It is shorter and attached to the underside of the aortic arch by the ligamentum arteriosum. It reaches the hilum of the left lung, just above the left main bronchus.

## Systemic Veins

### THE BRACHIOCEPHALIC (INNOMINATE) VEINS

- They arise posterior to the medial part of the clavicles by the union of the internal jugular and subclavian veins.
- Each brachiocephalic (innominate) vein drains the corresponding internal thoracic, vertebral, inferior thyroid and superior intercostal veins. The right brachiocephalic vein descends vertically, whereas the left crosses the superior mediastinum obliquely in front of the branches of the aortic arch.
- The brachiocephalic veins unite at the inferior border of the first costal cartilage to form the superior vena cava.

### THE SUPERIOR VENA CAVA AND AZYGOS SYSTEM

- The superior vena cava (SVC) drains all venous blood from above the diaphragm except that from the heart and lungs.
- It lies anterolateral to the trachea and posterolateral to the ascending aorta, and enters the right atrium at the level of the third costal cartilage.

The azygos and hemiazygos veins are located on either side of the vertebral column, and drain the back and the thoracic and abdominal walls. Their anatomy is variable. They assume particular importance in cases of SVC obstruction where they provide important collateral pathways.

- The azygos vein arises from the right ascending lumbar vein. It drains blood from the right posterior intercostal veins. It travels close to the right side of the inferior 8 thoracic vertebrae. It arches anteriorly just above the hilum of the right lung and drains into the superior vena cava.
- The hemiazygos vein arises from the left ascending lumbar vein. It drains the lower left posterior intercostal veins and ascends on the vertebral bodies posterolateral to the descending aorta. At T8, it crosses to the right behind the aorta, thoracic duct, and esophagus, and joins the azygos vein.
- The accessory hemiazygos vein descends on the left side of vertebrae T5 to T8. It receives tributaries from the fourth to eighth intercostal veins and sometimes the left bronchial veins. It crosses to the right at T7 or T8 behind the aorta and thoracic duct to join the azygos vein.

## Nerves

### Phrenic Nerves

The paired phrenic nerves originate from C3 to 5. Although supplying mainly motor fibers to the diaphragm, some of their fibers are sensory (see Figs. 8-5 and 8-6).

In the neck the phrenic nerves course over the scalenus anterior muscle from lateral to medial.

The right phrenic nerve enters the chest between the subclavian artery and the origin of the right brachiocephalic vein. It crosses the internal thoracic artery at the thoracic inlet, runs along the right side

of the the right brachiocephalic vein and SVC, and over the pericardium anterior to the hilum of the lung all the way to the diaphragm.

The left phrenic nerve enters the chest between the subclavian artery and the left brachiocephalic vein; it crosses the internal thoracic artery and descends between the left subclavian and common carotid arteries, crosses over the aortic arch anterior to the left vagus. It continues its course over the pericardium anterior to the hilum and all the way to the diaphragm.

### Vagus Nerves

The right vagus nerve enters the thorax anterior to the right subclavian artery. It courses behind the right brachiocephalic vein and SVC and then posteroinferiorly on the right side of the trachea. The pulmonary plexus arises from the vagus nerve behind the lung hilum. The vagus then courses over the esophagus where it branches into a periesophageal plexus.

The left vagus nerve descends posterolateral to the left common carotid artery. It diverges posteriorly at the level of the aortic arch, where it lies deep to the superior intercostal vein. Distally, its course mirrors that on the right side.

The recurrent laryngeal nerves are important branches of the vagi that innervate the larynx. They may be vulnerable to injury during surgical procedures in the neck and chest.

- The right recurrent laryngeal nerve loops posteriorly around the right subclavian artery and ascends to the larynx in the tracheoesophageal groove.
- The left recurrent laryngeal nerve arises at the level of the aortopulmonary window. It arches posteriorly around the aortic arch lateral to the ligamentum arteriosum, and ascends to the larynx in the tracheoesophageal groove.

### Sympathetic Nerves

The sympathetic chain is located in the paravertebral gutter.

The stellate ganglion (lower cervical ganglion) is located at the superior border of the first rib. Traumatic injury or destruction by a malignant process causes ipsilateral Horner's syndrome (ptosis, myosis, anhydrosis of the face).

The greater splanchnic nerve is formed by branches of sympathetic ganglia to 10. It courses inferiorly over thoracic vertebral bodies, medial to the sympathetic trunk and lateral to the azygos/hemiazygos veins. It pierces the diaphragm and courses to the celiac ganglion.

## Esophagus

- The esophagus is a muscular tube extending from the pharynx cartilage to the cardia, and averaging 25 to 30 cm in length (see Figs. 8-2 and 8-5).
- It has cervical, thoracic, and abdominal segments.
- Striated muscle present in the wall of the proximal esophagus is progressively replaced by smooth muscle fibers distally.
- The esophagus is fixed to the diaphragm (phrenoesophageal membrane) and back of the cricoid cartilage. Otherwise, it is loosely attached to surrounding structures.
- Within the mediastinum, the esophagus is located posterior to the trachea and left main bronchus, posterior to the pericardium, and to the right of the descending aorta.

## Thoracic Duct

- The thoracic duct originates in the cysterna chyli in the abdomen at L2, enters the thorax through the aortic hiatus, and ascends laterally to the esophagus, between the aorta and azygos vein (see Figs. 8-3, 8-5, and 8-6).
- It crosses to the left at T4 and ascends on the left posterior side of the esophagus to the thoracic inlet.

- It arches to the left behind the innominate vein to join the venous system at the junction of the left subclavian and internal jugular veins.
- Surgical injury to the thoracic duct may result in chylothorax.

## LUNGS

### Lobes and Fissures

The right lung is larger and heavier than the left and is divided into three lobes (see Fig. 8-4).

- The upper lobe is anterior and the lower lobe is posterior.[9]
- The middle lobe is anteroinferior.
- The minor fissure is horizontal, and separates the upper and middle lobes. It is usually incomplete.
- The major fissure extends obliquely down and forward from the level of T3 posteriorly to the 6th costochondral junction anteriorly; it separates the lower lobe from the upper and middle lobes.
- The left lung is somewhat smaller than the right and is divided into two lobes.
- Only one fissure (oblique) separates the left upper and lower lobes.
- The upper lobe lies above and in front of the fissure, whereas the larger lower lobe lies below and behind.

### Bronchopulmonary Segments

- The bronchopulmonary segment is the anatomic and functional unit of the lung (see Fig. 8-4).
- Each anatomic bronchopulmonary segment consists of one bronchus, one artery, draining vein, and their associated lung parenchyma.
- The segmental bronchus and artery are in close association and located centrally, whereas the veins are peripheral and course in the intersegmental plane.
- The right lung is composed of 10 bronchopulmonary segments. The smaller left lung is composed of eight segments.

### Hilum

The hilum is the area between the lung and mediastinum, where the pulmonary artery, pulmonary veins, main stem bronchus, bronchial arteries, and lymph vessels enter and leave the lung. Hilar structures are covered by visceral pleura (see Figs. 8-5 and 8-6).

#### Right Hilum

- The superior pulmonary vein draining the upper and middle lobes is the most anterior structure in the hilum.
- The right pulmonary artery courses in a plane between the bronchus posteriorly and the superior vein anteriorly.
- The inferior pulmonary vein drains the inferior lobe and is located at the inferior aspect of the hilum, at the superior end of the inferior pulmonary ligament.
- The azygos vein arches over the superior aspect of the right hilum.

#### Left Hilum

- The superior pulmonary vein draining the upper lobe is the most anterior structure.
- The pulmonary artery is the uppermost hilar structure as it arches over the bronchus.

- The bronchus runs in a plane between the artery and superior pulmonary vein.
- The inferior pulmonary vein drains the inferior lobe and is located at the inferior aspect of the hilum, at the superior end of the inferior pulmonary ligament.
- The aorta arches over the superior aspect of the hilum.
- The space between the pulmonary artery and aortic arch is called aortopulmonary window: it contains lymph nodes as well as the left recurrent laryngeal nerve.

### Pulmonary Arteries

Familiarity with the anatomy of the pulmonary artery within the lung fissures is fundamental to performing anatomic pulmonary resections, that is, lobectomy and segmentectomy (see later) (see Figs. 8-5 and 8-6).

#### Right Pulmonary Artery

The first branch of the right pulmonary artery is the truncus anterior, which supplies the apical and anterior segments of the upper lobe.

Within the fissure, the pulmonary artery becomes the interlobar artery; the interlobar artery and its branches run anterior to and are in close association with the corresponding bronchial divisions.

Branches of the interlobar artery include the middle lobe artery, a posterior ascending artery to the posterior segment of the upper lobe, an artery to the superior segment of the lower lobe and a common trunk to the basal segments of the lower lobe.

#### Left Pulmonary Artery

The first branch of the left pulmonary artery is the anterior artery, which supplies the anterior segment of the upper lobe. One or a few additional branches to the apicoposterior segment of the upper lobe are generally seen.

Within the fissure, the pulmonary artery and its branches are in close association with the corresponding bronchial divisions.

Arterial branches within the fissure include a lingular branch, an artery to the superior segment of the lower lobe and a common trunk to the basal segments of the lower lobe.

### Pulmonary Veins

- The pulmonary veins collect arterial blood from the lungs and direct it to the left atrium.
- Usually there is one pulmonary vein for each lobe, but on the right side, the right upper and middle lobe veins join near the hilum to form the right upper vein.

### Lymphatics of the Lungs

- There is a superficial lymphatic system that is located subpleurally and a deep lymphatic system that follows the segmental bronchi.
- Both of these systems intercommunicate and their flow is toward the hilum, where they end in the bronchopulmonary nodes.
- In approximately 10% of normal individuals, there is a crossover between lymphatics of individual pulmonary segments.

## PLEURA

- The pleura is made of two serosal membranes, with one covering the lung (visceral pleura) and one covering the inner chest wall (parietal pleura); the pleural space is the space delimitated by the two layers.

- The transition between parietal and visceral pleurae is at the level of the pulmonary hilum. At this level, the reflection covers the different constituents of the hilum except inferiorly, where the reflexion extends down to the diaphragm (inferior pulmonary ligament).

## Visceral Pleura

- Covers all lung surfaces and extends into the fissure.
- Is thin, transparent, and tightly adherent to the lung.
- Is devoided of somatic innervation and is thus insensitive.

## Parietal Pleura

- Covers almost completely the inner surface of the thoracic wall and medial aspect of mediastinum.
- Is attached to inner surface of the ribs through endothoracic fascia.
- Is innervated through a rich network of somatic, sympathetic, and parasympathetic fibers.

## TECHNIQUES IN THORACIC SURGERY

### INCISIONS

Obtaining adequate exposure is one of the most important technical aspects of any surgical procedure. Because of the large spectrum of diseases treated in thoracic surgery, and because of the relatively difficult access to intrathoracic organs due to their lack of mobility and to the rigidity of the chest wall, a wide variety of incisions have been described over the years. This section reviews the main incisions used in thoracic surgery (Table 8-1). The surgeon's experience and degree of comfort with a particular approach, the exposure needed for a procedure, and the acceptability to the patient in terms of appearance, postoperative discomfort, and long-term muscular and neurologic sequelae must be carefully weighed when choosing an appropriate incision.

## Cervical Incisions

The upper trachea, thyroid gland, cervical esophagus, and peritracheal and prescalenic lymph nodes are usually best accessed through the neck (Fig. 8-7).[10,11]

- Suprasternal incisions allow access to the superior and middle mediastinum for mediastinoscopy or mediastinal abscess drainage.
- Transverse cervical incisions are used for procedures involving the upper trachea and thyroid gland.
- Oblique incisions along the anterior border of the sternocleidomastoid muscle are invaluable for exposure of the cervical esophagus (resection, reconstruction, cure of Zenker's diverticulum).
- Supraclavicular incisions may be necessary for biopsy of prescalenic nodes or access to the thoracic duct.

## Abdominal and Thoracoabdominal Incisions

- Upper abdominal incisions provide access to the esophageal hiatus, diaphragm, omentum, pericardium, and also to the abdominal viscera for reconstruction after esophagectomy.[12]
- Thoracoabdominal incisions provide extended exposure and simultaneous access to the pleural and abdominal cavities for complex procedures in the lower chest or upper abdomen, such as those involving the esophagus.
- Appropriate placement of diaphragmatic incisions is important in order to avoid injury to branches of the phrenic nerves.

## Thoracic Incisions
### Anterior Thoracic Incisions
#### MEDIAN STERNOTOMY

- Provides excellent access to the heart, anterior mediastinum and simultaneous access to both pleural cavities.[13-21]
- Exposure of posterior hilar structures is poor, particularly on the left side, and left lower lobectomies are difficult to perform.
- However upper and middle lobectomies, pneumonectomies, sleeve resections, and resections of the carina may all be carried out.

---

TABLE 8-1  ■  COMMON PROCEDURES PERFORMED THROUGH MAIN INCISIONS USED IN THORACIC SURGERY

| Anatomic Area | Type of Incisions | Example of Procedures |
|---|---|---|
| Cervical incisions | Suprasternal | Mediastinoscopy |
| | Transverse cervical | Trachea or thyroid resections |
| | Supraclavicular | Lymph nodes biopsy |
| | Oblique | Esophageal reconstruction |
| Thoracic incisions | Posterolateral thoracotomy | Anatomic lung resection |
| | Muscle-sparing thoracotomy | Anatomic lung resection |
| | Anterolateral thoracotomy | Lung nodule resection |
| | Anterior mediastinotomy | Mediastinal mass biopsy |
| | Median sternotomy | Mediastinal tumor resection |
| | "Clamshell" incision | Double lung transplantation |
| | Limited axillary thoracotomy | First rib resection |
| Abdominal incisions | Upper midline incision | Pericardial window |
| | Thoracoabdominal incision | Aortic replacement |
| | Partial sternotomy | Tracheal resection |
| | Vertical axillary thoracotomy | Anatomic lung resection |

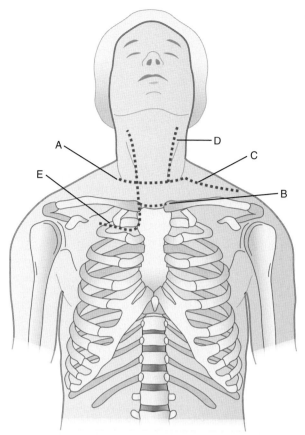

**Figure 8-7:** Variety of common cervical incisions. **A,** Transverse cervical. **B,** Suprasternal. **C,** Supraclavicular. **D,** Oblique. **E,** Anterior transcervical. *(Reprinted from Deslauriers J, Mehran R. Handbook of perioperative care in thoracic surgery. Philadelphia: Elsevier; 2005. p. 208.)*

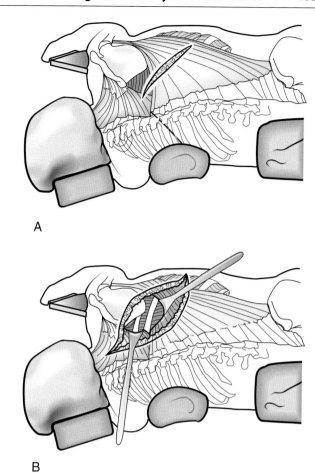

A

B

**Figure 8-8:** Muscle-sparing lateral thoracotomy. **A,** Transverse 10- to 12-cm skin incision. **B,** Latissimus dorsi retracted posteriorly and serratus anterior elevated anteriorly. *(From Mitchell R, Angell W, Wuerflein R, Dor V: Simplified lateral chest incision for most thoracotomies other than sternotomy. Ann Thorac Surg 1976;22:284.)*

- Postoperative pain is reduced and there is less effect on pulmonary function compared to a standard thoracotomy.
- Partial sternotomies may be used for the resection of anterior mediastinal tumors and for some tracheal procedures.

### ANTEROLATERAL THORACOTOMY (FIG. 8-8)
- Provides improved cosmesis and improved cardiopulmonary function (due to the patient's supine position) at the expense of more limited exposure.
- Incision of choice for lung biopsy in critically ill patients. Also useful for the resection of lung nodules and emphysematous bullae.

The clamshell incision (bilateral anterior thoracotomies joined by a transverse sternotomy) provides excellent exposure of both pleural cavities.

- It is the incision of choice for double lung transplantation, resection of bilateral pulmonary metastases or larger tumors of the anterior mediastinum, and bilateral lung volume reduction surgery.

### ANTERIOR MEDIASTINOTOMY
- Useful mostly for biopsy of lymph nodes or tumors of the anterior mediastinum.
- A mediastinoscope may be used through the incision in order to improve visualization.
- Has been recently supplanted by video-assisted thoracic surgery (VATS) which provides an excellent visualisation of this area using a minimally invasive approach.

## Posterior Thoracic Incisions
### POSTEROLATERAL THORACOTOMY (FIG. 8-9)
- Provides an excellent exposure of the lung, hilum, middle and posterior mediastinum, trachea, and esophagus.[22,23]
- The latissimus dorsi muscle is usually transected, although the serratus muscle is preserved and retracted anteriorly.
- Results in increased pain and disturbance of respiratory mechanics.
- Preserving the latissimus dorsi (muscle-sparing thoracotomy) may result in decreased pain, improved arm motion, earlier ambulation and recovery of arm function at the expense of slightly decreased exposure.

## Axillary Incisions
### AXILLARY THORACOTOMY (FIG. 8-10)
- Good access for pleurodesis, resection of upper lobe blebs, bullae or nodules, excision of some mediastinal tumors, and resection of a first or cervical rib.[24-29]
- Advantages include minimal muscle transection and reduced postoperative discomfort.
- Exposure is limited and does not allow complex procedures.
- The long thoracic nerve and intercostobrachial nerves may be vulnerable to injury.

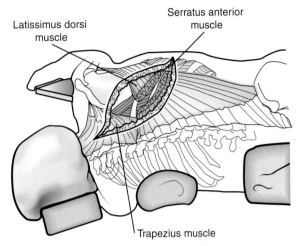

**Figure 8-9:** Posterolateral thoracotomy with division of the latissimus dorsi muscle. *(Reprinted from Deslauriers J, Mehran R. Handbook of perioperative care in thoracic surgery. Philadelphia: Elsevier; 2005. p. 217.)*

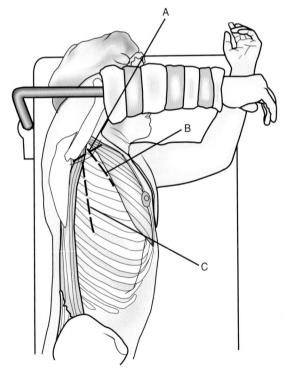

**Figure 8-10:** Axillary thoracotomies. **A,** Limited axillary thoracotomy (horizontal). **B,** Limited axillary thoracotomy (vertical incision). **C,** Vertical axillary thoracotomy. *(Reprinted from Deslauriers J, Mehran R. Handbook of perioperative care in thoracic surgery. Philadelphia: Elsevier; 2005. p. 215.)*

## LUNG RESECTION

The spectrum of lung resections varies from simple enucleation of a benign pulmonary nodule to pneumonectomy and lung resection en-bloc with surrounding structures. We summarize the different aspects of lung resection in relation to the types of resection and their clinical consequences.

## Pneumonectomy

- Involves resection of a complete lung by dissection and division of the pulmonary artery, veins, and main bronchus at the hilum. It is usually performed through a posterolateral thoracotomy.[30]
- Mostly performed for large or centrally located lung cancer. Other indications include chronic infections leading to destruction of lung parenchyma such as tuberculosis, bronchiectasis, and fungal disease.
- Because pneumonectomy is associated with higher morbidity and mortality as well as more important postoperative physiologic disturbances than lesser resections, the decision to perform a pneumonectomy instead of a lobectomy or sleeve resection (see later) must always be carefully weighed by the surgeon on the basis of preoperative and intraoperative findings.
- Because the right lung represents 55% of total lung ventilation and perfusion, physiologic disturbances following a right pneumonectomy outweigh those following a left pneumonectomy.
- Postoperatively, the postpneumonectomy space normally becomes obliterated in the weeks following surgery through elevation of the diaphragm, shift of mediastinal structures, hyperinflation of the contralateral lung, intercostal space contraction and the accumulation of serosanguinous fluid. Infection of the postpneumonectomy space by intraoperative contamination or a bronchopleural fistula is a serious complication.

## Lobectomy

- Lobectomy is the most commonly performed procedure for the surgical treatment of lung cancer. Other indications include tuberculosis, chronic lung abscess, bronchiectasis, benign tumors, fungal infections and congenital anomalies.[31]
- Lobectomy is usually performed through a posterolateral thoracotomy. Other common incisions include sternotomy (for upper and middle lobectomies), anterolateral thoracotomy, and video-assisted thoracic surgery (VATS).
- Adhesions and incomplete fissures may be found at the time of resection, particularly in cases of inflammatory lesions. Careful dissection is then necessary to avoid parenchymal trauma that could result in prolonged air leaks. The fissures are usually divided using a linear stapler. A chest tube is inserted at the end of the procedure for postoperative drainage of the pleural cavity.
- Because the remaining lobes are generally sufficient to fill the pleural cavity, management of the pleural space is straightforward, and temporary postoperative chest tube drainage usually suffices. Occasionally, a diseased residual lobe may be insufficiently large. In these cases, prevention of a postoperative pleural space may necessitate the creation of an apical pleural tent or temporary paralysis of the phrenic nerve using a local anesthetic. The creation of a postoperative pneumoperitoneum may also be valuable in an attempt to obliterate a basal space; thoracoplasties and diaphragm repositioning have been abandoned and are of historical interest only.

## Segmentectomy

- Lobectomy remains the standard operation for lung cancer. However, segmentectomy and lesser resections may have a role, especially in patients with limited pulmonary reserve.[32-35]
- Segmentectomy is an anatomic operation involving removal of a segmental bronchus, along with its associated segmental artery, lung parenchyma, and lymph nodes.
- Good surgical results have been obtained with this type of resection in cases of early lung cancer (T1N0). Thus, long-term

survival is possible in patients with poor pulmonary function, although at the expense of a higher rate of local recurrence.

- Historically, segmentectomy has also been useful in suppurative disease such as bronchiectasis and tuberculosis. Other potential indications include mycotic infections such as aspergillus, and congenital lesions such as lung cysts.
- Segmentectomy is usually performed through a posterolateral thoracotomy. The segmental artery and bronchus are sequentially isolated and divided. Parenchymal division follows along intersegmental planes where the draining veins are located.
- The immediate physiologic effects of lobectomy and segmentectomy are comparable. The benefits of parenchymal sparing become apparent during the ensuing months with progressive recovery of lung function. Potential postoperative complications resemble those after lobectomy and include prolonged air leaks, empyema, and pleural space problems; however, most space problems, when they occur, are mild. The mortality rate is low (around 1%).

## Wedge Resection

- A limited pulmonary resection may be necessary to remove lung metastases and early stage lung cancer in patients with marginal pulmonary function (as stated earlier).
- The thorax is accessed by thoracotomy or VATS and a nonanatomic resection is carried out using a mechanical stapler.
- The technique is appropriate for peripheral lesions in cases in which minimal sacrifice of normal lung tissue is required. Morbidity and mortality rates are minimal.

## Sleeve Lobectomy

- Sleeve lobectomy refers to the resection of a segment of major bronchus with subsequent bronchial reconstruction in order to preserve associated lung parenchyma.[36]
- Indications include lung cancer or metastatic lymph nodes involving the main bronchus or more than one lobar bronchus, which would otherwise necessitate a pneumonectomy for complete resection. Sleeve resection is thus an alternative to pneumonectomy, resulting in an equal oncologic outcome with decreased morbidity and mortality.
- Endobronchial tumors such as carcinoids, bronchial strictures, and other inflammatory diseases are also often amenable to this type of resection.
- A vascular sleeve resection (i.e., segmental resection of the pulmonary artery) may sometimes be necessary, particularly for proximal lesions of the left upper lobe where the artery curves over and behind the upper lobe bronchus.
- Pneumonia and atelectasis of the ipsilateral remaining lobe are common postoperative complications whose incidence can be minimized by postoperative bronchoscopy and aspiration of secretions.

## References

 Interactive references and additional readings for this chapter can be accessed online at *expertconsult.com.*

# 9 THERAPEUTIC BRONCHOSCOPY

Henri G. Colt, MD, FCCP

## DEFINITION

Therapeutic bronchoscopy consists of airway interventions performed to restore or maintain airway patency, either for palliation or cure of malignant and benign lesions of the upper and lower airways. Procedures are performed using either a flexible or a rigid bronchoscope. Procedures are often referred to as interventional bronchoscopic procedures, and indeed, societies such as the American Thoracic Society, the European Respiratory Society, and the American College of Chest Physicians have offered guidelines pertaining to the practice and training of interventional bronchoscopy as a set of procedure performed by interventional pulmonologists and thoracic surgeons.[1,2]

## HISTORY

Gustav Killian, an otorhinolaryngologist at Freiburg, Germany performed the first rigid bronchoscopy on March 30, 1897 in order to remove a piece of bone impacted in the right main bronchus of a 63-year-old gentleman. Rigid bronchoscopy, however, was rarely performed for therapeutic debulking because of the risk of bleeding, and was usually reserved for foreign body extractions until Nd:YAG laser resection became popular in the 1980s.[3]

- Therapeutic rigid bronchoscopy is always done under general anesthesia, using spontaneous assisted ventilation or jet ventilation. Therapeutic flexible bronchoscopic procedures are also usually performed under general anesthesia with endotracheal intubation but can also be performed using laryngeal mask airways.
- The rigid bronchoscope comes in various diameters and lengths. The external diameter of the rigid bronchoscope may also vary depending on manufacturer. For adults, most tubes are at least 8 mm wide.
- Shigeto Ikeda, of Tokyo, Japan introduced the first flexible fiberoptic bronchoscope at the Ninth International Congress on Diseases of the Chest held in Copenhagen in 1966.[4]
- Therapeutic flexible bronchoscopy is usually performed using moderate sedation or general anesthesia. Many therapeutic procedures can be performed through the flexible scope, including foreign body removal, argon plasma coagulation, brachytherapy catheter placement, photodynamic therapy, Nd:YAG photocoagulation and resection, electrocautery, and balloon dilation, bronchial thermoplasty, and endobronchial valve placement for emphysema. Expandable metal stents can also be inserted using a combination of Seldinger techniques, flexible bronchoscopy, and fluoroscopy.

## INDICATIONS

- Central airway obstruction[5,6]:
  - ○ **Fixed central airway obstruction** is a frequent indication for therapeutic bronchoscopy. Patients are often referred because of symptoms such as cough, dyspnea, hemoptysis, a history of previous carcinoma potentially metastatic to the lungs and airways, or a radiographic abnormality suggestive of neoplasm or benign strictures. Patients may have a history of previous intubation, tracheotomy, or suspected vasculitic disease. Other etiologies of fixed airway obstruction include idiopathic tracheal stenosis, postintubation strictures, a history of burn or inhalation injury, lung transplantation, tracheal resection and reanastomosis surgery, metal or silicone stent insertion; history of infectious airway disease, including tuberculosis, *Klebsiella rhinosleroma*, and fungal disease such as coccidiodomycosis, histoplasmosis and aspergillus.
    - Results of dilation and other bronchoscopic therapies are often satisfactory in more than 30% of cases initially.
    - Procedures may be curative or palliative.
    - Several types of neoplasms may also cause fixed airway obstruction. These include thyroid cancer, esophageal cancer invading the airway, enlarged mediastinal adenopathy from a neoplasm, carcinoid tumors, and adenoid cystic carcinoma.
    - Segmental obstruction can be caused by malignant and benign disorders, and are usually less amenable to bronchoscopic therapies, although brachytherapy, electrocautery, and photodynamic therapy should be considered.
    - Fixed strictures should be evaluated for etiology and possible cause. Before embarking on bronchoscopic therapy, particularly for patients with benign etiologies, a multidisciplinary approach is warranted. Surgical consultation is recommended, particularly for patients with potentially respectable airway strictures.
  - ○ Dynamic central airway obstruction
    - May be associated with fixed airway obstruction.
    - May be caused by variable extrinsic compression snf also by expiratory central airway collapse (tracheobronchomalacia and excessive dynamic airway collapse).
    - Should be considered in patients who present weaning difficulties.
    - Other etiologies include vascular compression, post-pneumonectomy changes, chronic obstructive pulmonary disease (COPD), chronic airway infection, ball-valve airway tumors, including bronchogenic carcinoma, metastases from kidney, colon, breast cancer and malignant melanoma, diseases such as relapsing polychondritis (that may mimic asthma, but is usually refractory to conventional therapies).
  - ○ Segmental airway obstruction
    - May be caused by a similar variety of benign and malignant disorders:
    - Can be seen as simple airway mucosal thickening.
    - May also be associated with or caused by mediastinal and hilar adenopathy.
    - Careful attention should be paid to adjacent vascular structures when bronchoscopic therapies are considered.
    - Granulation tissue formation prompted by inhaled foreign bodies can bleed easily.
  - ○ Airway-esophageal and bronchopleural fistulas
    - Fistulas are troublesome and may cause symptoms such as prolonged airleak, difficulty weaning from mechanical ventilation, recurrent aspiration, dysphagia, and recurrent pneumonia.
    - Overall prognosis is usually poor.
    - Single-airway, esophageal, or double-airway and esophageal stents often help palliate symptoms and prolong survival.
    - Stents may also be helpful to palliate bronchoesophageal fistulas that occur after thoracic surgery or radiation therapy.
    - Other techniques such as balloon occlusion and administration of fibrin sealants can be attempted.
  - ○ Procedure-related strictures
    - Insertion of metal or silicone stents can be followed by formation of granulation tissue or tumor overgrowth.
    - Metal stent rupture or excess epithelialization may cause airway stenosis.
    - Migration of a covered stent may cover the opening to a bronchus or the origin of a main stem bronchus.
    - Covering (silicone, polyurethane, polyester mesh) of metal and hybrid stents may rupture and cause airway obstruction. Careful attention is needed in case electrocautery, argon plasma, or laser is used to remove broken wire struts because airway fires can occur.
    - Electrocautery, cryotherapy, and excessive laser application can each cause collateral damage and recurrent airway strictures.
    - Vigorous dilation, especially usually overinflated balloons or large rigid bronchoscopes, can stretch airway mucosa and cause increased chance for scar tissue formation, especially in the region of the cricoid cartilage.
    - Recurrent stenosis is frequently seen after photodynamic therapy, so frequent clean out bronchoscopies are usually warranted to remove necrotic debris after photodynamic therapy (PDT).
  - ○ Other malignancies
    - Solid tumors with mediastinal nodal metastases (breast cancer most common; thyroid, renal, rectal, and so on) are diagnosed.
    - Esophageal cancer can cause fistulas, as can esophageal cancer with associated esophageal stent insertion or radiation therapy.
    - Surgical complications such as postpneumonectomy or postlobectomy stump fistula can be visualized and determinations made regarding indications for bronchoscopic or open surgical repair.
- Systemic diseases:
  - ○ Asthma and emphysema
    - Symptoms include recalcitrant cough, shortness of breath, respiratory insufficiency which are refractory to treatment, and recurrent intubation.
    - Bronchial thermoplasty remains "experimental" and should be performed as part of clinical trials and special protocols.
    - Endobronchial valves can be considered as part of clinical trials and special protocols. This method of bronchoscopic lung volume reduction can cause pneumothorax and recurrent pneumonia. Information pertaining to procedure-related risks should be shared with patients.
  - ○ Tracheobronchial malacia and excessive dynamic airway collapse
    - Increasingly recognized; may be primary or secondary with numerous possible etiologies
    - Stent trial may be warranted in selected cases, but information pertaining to increased risks of stent-related complications should be shared with patients, families, and referring physicians.[7]
    - Definitive treatment for malacia is often a tracheoplasty and bronchioplasty, but benefit from stenting may confirm that a patient is a good candidate for tracheoplasty.

○ Other illnesses
  ■ Airway strictures should also be suspected in patients with vasculitis such as Wegener's granulomatosis, as well as in patients with a history of tuberculosis, sarcoidosis, and other granulomatous disorders.
  ■ Length, caliber, and type of benign stricture (simple or complex, hourglass or circumferential, focal or multifocal) can be determined.
  ■ Bronchoscopic treatment is determined, in part, by measuring length of the stricture as well as distance from the vocal cords, risk of airway perforation, availability of appropriately seized stents, operator experience, risk of bleeding, capacity to control airway compromise, and respiratory failure.

## CONTRAINDICATIONS

■ Risks and benefits of each procedure must be carefully weighed.
■ Strategy and planning for each procedure includes indication, preprocedure evaluation, allergies, risks (respiratory failure, prolonged hypoxemia, bleeding, pneumothorax, fever, procedure-related anxiety).
■ Preprocedure evaluation includes examination for significant comorbidities, especially cardiac arrhythmias, a bleeding or coagulation disorder, medications including anticoagulants, antiplatelet agents, history of narcotic use (may require increased dose of sedation drugs), as well as careful assessment of patient's preferences (nasal or oral bronchoscope insertion), expectations, and discussion of potential alternative diagnostic procedures.[8]
■ "Time out" can be valuable in order to ascertain that nursing team, patient, and bronchoscopists agree on procedures to be performed, that appropriate precautions are taken in case of procedure-related complications or adverse events, and that all equipment and ancillary instruments are readily available.
■ Sedation should be individualized based on comorbidities, response to medication, desire for procedure recall, need for patient collaboration during the procedure (forced cough, dynamic bronchoscopy). Synergistic effect of combined medications such as benzodiazepines and narcotics should be considered, particularly in patients with airway obstruction or poor ventilatory function.
■ Feeding should be done before procedures according to institutional guidelines because of risk of vomiting (cough and gag reflex), and aspiration.
■ Special precautions are warranted in patients with heart disease, in the elderly, and of course, in case of bleeding diathesis.
■ Careful examination of teeth, gums, and neck flexion and extension is warranted to avoid injury.
■ Patients with C-collars, limited neck mobility, and comorbidities such as advanced rheumatoid arthritis or ankylosing spondylitis may be especially difficult to manage, particularly for rigid intubations (Fig. 9-1).
■ Intubation of patients with congenital deformities may also be especially difficult or impossible to intubate with a rigid bronchoscope.
■ In patients with evidence of hyperreactive airway disease or COPD, preprocedure bronchodilators and corticosteroids should be administered.
■ In patients with tracheal strictures or evidence of laryngeal edema, postprocedure corticosteroids are usually administered.
■ Pregnancy is definitely associated with increased risk for therapeutic bronchoscopy, which should be performed only if absolutely necessary. Careful obstetric consultation is warranted, and often, obstetrics should stand by at the time of the bronchoscopic intervention.

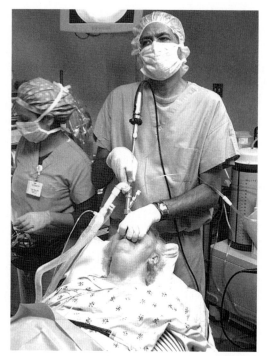

**Figure 9-1:** Patient with ankylosing spondylitis could not be placed supine for rigid intubation because of cervical spine ankylosis.

■ Care should always be taken when rigid bronchoscopy is performed in critically ill patients on mechanical ventilation. Intubation with the rigid tube should probably be done under direct visualization as the endotracheal tube is being removed, so that the rigid tube can be seen entering the upper tracheal.
■ Complications can be readily addressed by careful strategy and planning for each procedure. Also, necessary techniques and equipment should be known. For example, techniques of bronchoscopic resection required in-depth knowledge of laser-tissue interactions, or effects of electrocautery, and knowledge of stent-related complications.
■ The bronchoscopist and team should be practiced and experienced with techniques for (1) emergency intubation; (2) regaining an airway in case of laryngeal obstruction, laryngeal spasm or inability to intubate; (3) bleeding control using balloons and endobronchial blockers. Some of these techniques can be learned in postgraduate courses, guided reading, and simulation scenarios. All should be practiced by the interventional team before embarking on operative cases.

## SUMMARY OF RESULTS OF LASER, STENTS, AND PHOTODYNAMIC THERAPY

■ Risks and benefits of each procedure must be carefully weighed.
■ Demonstrated survival benefit, improved dyspnea scores, and improved quality-of-life scores directly related to bronchoscopic treatment.[9,10]
■ Patients who undergo successful re-establishment of airway patency usually survive longer than those who have continued partial obstruction or in whom attempts at restoring airway patency are unsuccessful.[11,12]
■ Pulmonary function has been shown to improve by as much as 300 mL, Karnofsky scores often improve from 40 to 60, but median survival after stent insertion, for example, is only about 5 months. This reinforces the fact that the airway

disease is simply one manifestation of an end-stage disease, or that life-threatening symptoms of airway obstruction may occur as a terminal or near-terminal event. However, palliation of airway obstruction is justified to provide improved comfort, diminished breathlessness, and increased ability to interact with family and friends.

- In patients with superficial early lung cancer and carcinoma in-situ, potentially curative bronchoscopic treatment should also be considered. Photodynamic therapy may be a valuable treatment for such early in situ cancers (rarely), especially in patients who are not surgical candidates.[13]
- PDT may also treat the extension of a lung cancer out of a bronchus so that a standard lobectomy may be performed, rather than a more complex sleeve lobectomy or to shrink a tumor away from the carina.
- Procedures are also safe in the elderly and elder elderly, although anesthesia-related events such as hypoxemia and unstable blood pressure must be controlled.[14]
- Although surveillance bronchoscopy is probably not necessary, any new or recurrent symptoms in patients with indwelling stents warrant bronchoscopy.[15]
- Patients can be given a medical alert document indicating type and location of stent, and also providing instructions in case of emergency. A model is freely downloadable from the www.bronchoscopy.org.

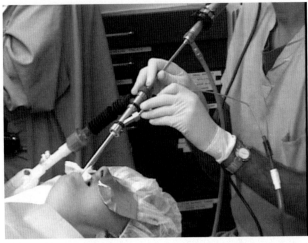

**Figure 9-2:** The rigid bronchoscope is freely mobile, with a suction port and port for introduction of laser fibers. A side-port allows connection to anesthesia machine.

## PROCEDURES

### Rigid Bronchoscopic Dilation and Coring Out

- The beveled edge of the rigid scope is used to core out tumor after laser or electrocautery coagulation.
- Technique needs to be learned and practiced.
- Operator must be able to control mucosal bleeding, and must recognize appropriate time for coring out, depending on assessment of necrosis and lack of vascularization of the target tissues.

### Rigid Bronchoscopic Neodymium YAG Laser Resection

- Most frequently used laser is the neodymium YAG (Nd:YAG) laser, with a wavelength of 1064 nm. This laser provides deep tissue effects, with laser energy penetrating up to 10 mm into target or adjacent tissues.
- Careful attention should be paid to risks of collateral damage, such as airway wall or vascular perforation.
- Air- or water-cooled, or bare fibers can be used. Laser precautions are always warranted (Figs. 9-2 and 9-3).
- All airway procedures can be safely performed using less than 40 watts. Tissue effects will also depend on power density (laser power in watts and distance of the laser fiber from the target tissue). The longer the distance, the lower the power density, and the greater is the deep penetration, and less is surface absorption.
- Note that Nd:YAG laser energy is highly absorbed by pigmented (dark, or red) tissues.[16]

### Rigid Bronchoscopic Insertion of Silicone Stents

- Ideally suited for central airway obstruction (trachea and main bronchi, including carina).
- Excellent safety record with numerous operators having more than twenty years experience.[17]
- Disadvantages include risk of migration (6-20%), obstruction by retained secretions, infection, and obstruction by tissue overgrowth.[17]

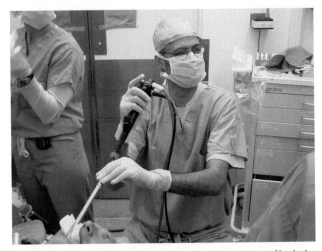

**Figure 9-3:** Interventional bronchoscopy often requires use of both the rigid and the flexible bronchoscope.

- Poorly tolerated when placed within the subglottis. Also, higher risk of migration in these cases.
- Stent-related complications are frequent when stents are used in patients with malacia or excessive dynamic airway collapse.
- Relatively safe even when electrocautery or Nd:YAG laser is used on tissues surrounding the stent. Lower power density and few pulses should be used especially in case of blood or discoloring of the stent.
- Chronic infections have been reported and may warrant stent replacement.
- Patients with indwelling stents and new or increased symptoms of cough or dyspnea are likely to have stent-related complications and warrant flexible bronchoscopy for diagnosis.
- External beam radiation and brachytherapy can be used without difficulty in patients with indwelling silicone stents.
- Several shapes, sizes, and lengths are available, including Y-shaped stents, L-shaped stents, and custom-made stents.
- Requires rigid bronchoscopy and general anesthesia. Specific skills are needed to manage stent-related complications and also to manage occasional difficulties encountered during stent insertion (stent not unfolding, stent placed too low or

too high). Y-stents can be more difficult to insert than straight stents.

▪ Anesthesia techniques include spontaneous assisted ventilation and jet ventilation.

▪ High-riding, subglottic stents should be kept, when possible, more than 2 cm from the vocal cords to avoid granulation tissue formation (Figs. 9-4 and 9-5).

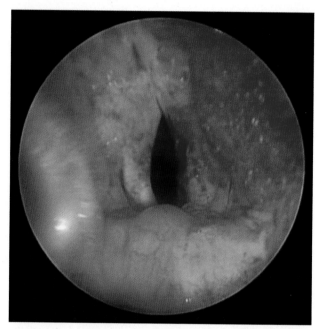

**Figure 9-4:** Patient with upper tracheal stricture second to prolonged intubation and tracheostomy.

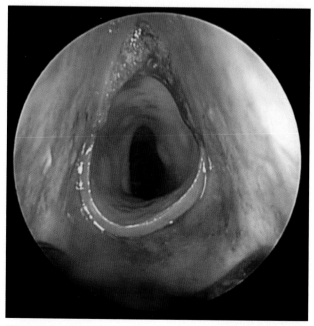

**Figure 9-5:** A large silicone stent has been deployed in the airway. Its proximal extremity is approximately two centimeters from the vocal cords.

## Rigid or Flexible Bronchoscopy-Assisted Self-Expanding Metal Stent Insertion

▪ Indications include malignant central airway obstruction but also benign conditions such as anastomotic stricture after lung transplantation, external compression from thoracic aortic aneurysm, airway strictures related to tuberculosis, recurrent bronchial infection, lobectomy, radiation therapy, and disorders such as antineutrophil cytoplasmic antibody–positive vasculitis or relapsing polychondritis, as well as in patients after lung transplantation.[18,19]

▪ Major dangers include epithelialization and formation of granulation tissue through the stent lattice, which make removal or repositioning difficult.[20]

▪ Epithelialization can occur within 6 weeks of stent insertion.

▪ Other complications include stent rupture, perforation of vessels or airway wall from protruding metal stents, and stripping of polyurethane or silicone stent covering. Migration and obstruction from granulation tissue or tumor overgrowth may also occur.[21]

▪ Removal of metal stents, especially when placed inappropriately in the subglottis, can be difficult and may require open surgery.

▪ Careful attention should be paid when using Nd:YAG or electrocautery in and around covered and uncovered metal stents, because metal wires will be broken easily, stent covering may catch fire, and metal itself conducts thermal energy.

## Flexible Bronchoscopic Resections, Dilation, and Stent Insertion

▪ Usually reserved for insertion of self-expanding covered and uncovered metal stents using fluoroscopic guidance to assist in proper stent positioning.

▪ Preliminary dilation using angioplasty or urology dilating balloons may or may not be necessary and adds additional costs to the procedure.

▪ Best performed using large-channel flexible video-bronchoscopes.[22]

▪ Careful measurement of airway diameter and length of stricture is necessary to avoid restenosis in case of shortening of the metal stent after deployment.

▪ Stents are made of stainless steel wire mesh, shape-memory nitinol. Stents may be covered by polyurethane membrane but also may be manufactured from polyester wire mesh embedded in silicone.

▪ Determining the caliber of the airway lumen can be difficult. Measurements can be made using multislice computer tomography but also with specifically designed luminal measuring devices. Morphometric bronchoscopy techniques are also being studied and simplified in order to be made more easily applicable to practitioners.[23,24]

▪ Stent removal may require rigid bronchoscopy; the beveled edge of rigid tube is inserted between stent surface and airway wall, grasping stent with forceps, rotating I, and removing it through the rigid tube. This technique is possible before and even after minor epithelialization of the metal stent.

▪ Recurrent stenosis may require insertion of a second larger self-expanding stent, or insertion of a larger silicone stent with the metal stent.

▪ Indications of potential complications should be carefully discussed with the patient, especially in case of benign airway strictures. The results of the published US Food and Drug Adminstration (FDA) warning should be shared with the patient.

## Brachytherapy

▪ Delivery of ionizing radiation from a source placed within or very near the tissues being treated.

- Rapid fall-off of radiation dose concentrates the tissue effect to tissues surrounding the radioactive implant.
- Most commonly performed by first placing afterload catheters by bronchoscopy and subsequently inserting Ir$^{192}$ in the radiation oncology suite.
- Low-, medium-, and high-dose brachytherapy can be delivered. The low dose is usually 3000 cGy every 20 to 30 hours via a single implant.
- Results are satisfactory for early-stage lung cancer, with excellent 5-year survival times in patients who are not surgical candidates.
- For late-stage lung cancer, results are less satisfactory, and brachytherapy is usually reserved for patients with segmental obstruction who have exhausted attempts at external beam radiation and for whom laser treatments are not indicated.
- Can be combined with photodynamic therapy, but also with Nd:YAG laser resection and airway debulking.[25]
- Most recently, electromagnetic navigational techniques are being described to guide fiducial placement for robotic stereotactic radiosurgery.[26,27]

## Cryotherapy

- Possible through both the flexible and rigid bron-choscopes.
- Depth of penetration and collateral tissue damage can be difficult to control.
- Consists in freezing target tissues using liquid nitrogen or liquid nitrous oxide. Tissue is exposed for at least 10 to 20 seconds, causing an ice ball to form. This destroys vessels and causes tumor necrosis.
- Follow-up bronchoscopy is required to remove necrotic tissues. Therefore, the procedure is not warranted for patients with airway obstruction requiring emergent or urgent restoration of airway patency.
- Cryotherapy is also useful for removal of certain foreign bodies and blood clots.
- Usually not performed for benign airway strictures

## Electrocautery and Argon Plasma Coagulation

- Techniques of electrosurgery each with its advantages and disadvantages (Figs. 9-6 and 9-7).
- Depth of penetration and collateral tissue damage can be difficult to control.
- Argon plasma allows noncontact mode of electrosurgery.
- Consists in electrical energy delivery to target tissues. Surface tissues are thus cauterized. Depth of penetration is low (less than 5 mm) compared with Nd:YAG laser.[28]
- Smoke evacuation is necessary.
- Can be used to help debulk airway tumors but is best used for smaller tumors and granulation tissue. Can also be used for benign airway strictures, but care should be taken to avoid circumferential applications, which might cause collateral tissue damage and worsen airway strictures.
- Can be cost effective compared with laser surgery.[29]

## Photodynamic Therapy for Early and Advanced Lung Cancer

- Well described technique that is FDA approved and that may be an excellent adjunct to early lung cancer treatments diagnosed using a variety of bronchoscopic screening techniques.[30]
- Can be performed with both curative and palliative intent (Figs. 9-8 and 9-9).
- Tissue effects are dependent on photoderivatives used and also on light activation wavelength (for example, red light with 630-nm wavelength has depth of penetration of only 4 mm).[31]

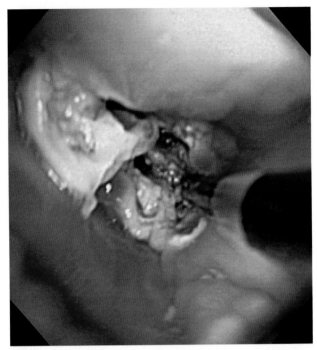

**Figure 9-6:** Electrocautery probe in position in area of granulation tissue formation and significant airway narrowing.

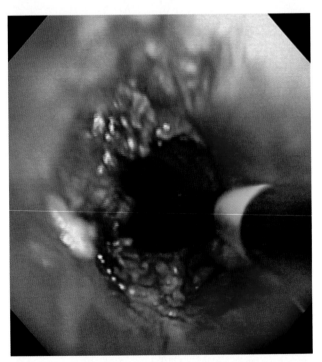

**Figure 9-7:** Airway patency has been restored after electro-cautery.

## Microdissector

- An alternative to the above-mentioned techniques is the microdissector, which is a drill with a knife blade.
- Performed through a rigid bronchoscope
- Can quickly core out a malignant or benign stricture of the trachea or main stem bronchus.
- Bleeding is usually minimal.
- Avoids the need for radiation or the photosensitivity associated with PDT.

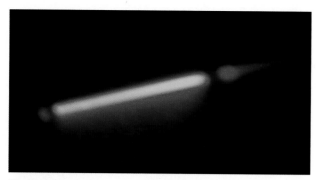

**Figure 9-8:** Cylindrical probe for photodynamic therapy.

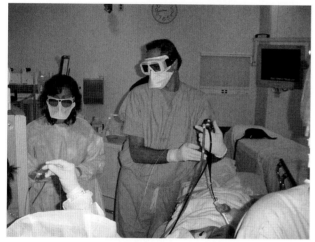

**Figure 9-9:** Photodynamic therapy being performed during flexible bronchoscopy. Note red light (630 nm) delivered through flexible laser fiber.

## Bronchial Thermoplasty

- As of this writing, bronchial thermoplasty remains an investigative, outpatient procedure for patients with severe asthma.[32]
- Treatments performed using the Alair Bronchial Thermoplasty System (Asthmatx, Inc, Mountain View, CA), with applications in segmental airways 3 to 10 mm in diameter.
- The Alair thermoplasty electrode is introduced through a catheter. Once expanded inside the airway, the electrode has four wires that each touch the airway wall, repositioning the electrode every 5 mm after electrical current is applied, avoiding overlap, and taking care to airway motion with respiration.
- Under direct bronchoscopic visualization, radio-frequency electrical energy is applied to subsegmental and segmental airways in a systematic fashion, usually beginning distally and moving proximally.
- Usually only one lobe is treated per session, for a maximum of three sessions, usually separated by several weeks to avoid prompting asthma exacerbations or life-threatening diffuse airway edema.
- Careful attention is paid to patient selection and preparation. Patients should not have indwelling pacemakers or neurostimulators, and should have asthma symptoms despite stable maintenance medication.[33]

## Bronchoscopic Lung Volume Reduction Treatments

- Performed with the hope that bronchial blocking can create atelectasis that would mimic lung volume reduction surgery.

- Based on the premise using unidirectional valves that block inhaled airway from entering disease portions of lung, while allowing air and secretions to escape during exhalation.[34]
- Still under investigation in the United States, although several clinical trials are ongoing with apparently satisfactory safety profiles.
- Several different valve designs are being proposed and tested. Usually, several bronchial segments in the target lobe need to be treated.
- Procedures usually possible using flexible bronchoscopy and moderate sedation or general anesthesia.
- Bronchial blocking is usually reserved for patients with target areas assessed using computed tomography scans, and low forced expiratory lung volumes but without evidence of hypercapnia.
- Preliminary results show minimal improvements in $FEV_1$, 6-minute walk, and respiratory-related quality of life.[35]
- Airway bypass is a different procedure that involves placing a stent in a hole created in a segmental airway. This procedure is currently under investigation for the use in homogeneous emphysema. Preliminary results are encouraging when the stent remains patent. Drug-eluding stents appear to have better patency rates.

## Bronchoscopy-Assisted Percutaneous Dilatational Tracheotomy

- Can be performed using flexible bronchoscopy at the bedside or using rigid bronchoscopy in the operating suite.
- Multiple and single dilator techniques have been described. The incidence of complications is low, but problems include oxygen desaturation, bleeding (usually easily controllable), and stomal strictures.
- Safety profile is satisfactory compared with open surgical techniques of tracheotomy.[36]
- The incidence of late sequela is difficult to determine because of a high mortality rate in critically ill patients in the intensive care unit.
- Care should be taken to avoid fracture of the cricoid cartilage.
- Bronchoscopic assistance helps avoid inappropriate placement of the percutaneous tracheal stoma. The bronchoscope is used to visualize stomal dilation and tube insertion.
- Rigid bronchoscopic guidance should be considered instead of flexible bronchoscopic guidance in patients with a history of previous tracheostomy, risk of difficult airway or bleeding, abnormal neck anatomy, or in patients with indwelling tracheal stents.[37]
- Rigid bronchoscopy helps avoid complications, avoids damaging a flexible bronchoscope, and allows continuous confirmation of correct intratracheal placement of needles, wires, dilators, and catheters and the tracheotomy tube without risk of damage to the posterior tracheal membrane. In addition, any airway bleeding that might occur is readily controlled.[38]

## *TRAINING*

## Guidelines, Simulation-Based Models, and Performance-Based Evaluations

- Not all interventional bronchoscopists will be expert in all techniques.
- Bronchoscopists should be aware of a variety of techniques of anesthesia, including laryngeal mask airway, jet ventilation, and spontaneous assisted ventilation. Teamwork with experienced anesthesiologists is essential.[39,40]
- Procedural guidelines advocate competency based on number of procedures. These numbers, for all procedures, are probably not achievable for most practitioners.[31]

■ Interventional bronchoscopy appears to a subspecialty field requiring dedicated training and experience.

■ A paradigm shift away from the pure apprenticeship model, based on the "see one, do one, teach one" paradigm, is warranted, and new educational techniques are needed so that trainees can demonstrate competency.

■ Simulation-based scenarios are helpful for teams and for interventional bronchoscopists practice their techniques (Fig. 9-10).

■ A formalized curriculum with specific procedure-related guidelines can be helpful to help programs and national organizations focus on core interventional training.

■ Greater participation from national organizations is probably warranted. Validated assessment tools introduced and validated for diagnostic bronchoscopy can be modified and then tested as part of validation studies in order to create a set of instruments and exercises that might be used to measure interventional bronchoscopic knowledge and technical skill acquisition.[41]

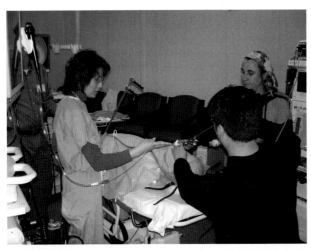

**Figure 9-10:** Example of simulation exercise using airway mannequin and rigid equipment in order to simulate rigid bronchoscopic resection, including communication skills with anesthesiologist and nurse assistant.

## Brief Illustrative Case #1: Dyspnea and Cough in a 75-Year-Old Man with Squamous Cell Carcinoma

• *History:* 75-year-old man with progressive shortness of breath cough and difficulty in clearing secretions presented to the emergency department. He has a history of unresectable squamous cell carcinoma involving the left side of the chest and mediastinum, and he has partially completed external-beam radiation therapy.

• *Examination:* Vitals: barrel chest (Fig. 9-11A) tachycardia (120–130/min); BP 160/90; respirations 28/min; temp: 99.0° F, SPO$_2$ 86% (2 l/min NC O$_2$). Patient has a known FEV$_1$ of 1.0 liters.

• *Blood tests:* Complete blood count and electrolytes—normal.

• *Imaging:* Computed tomography scan reveals a large subcarinal mass infiltrating the medial and posterior wall of the left main bronchus, extending to the take off of the left upper lobe bronchus (LC1). The mass is causing significant extrinsic compression of the mid and distal left main bronchus (Fig. 9-11B).

• *Bronchoscopy:* Confirms radiographic findings. The patient is taken to the operating suite, where rigid bronchoscopy is performed. The patient is intubated with a 12-mm ventilating EFER-Dumon rigid bronchoscope (Bryan Corp, Woburn, MA). After flexible bronchoscope inspection, the rigid tube is used to dilate the left main bronchus and to remove exophytic tumor infiltrating through the posterior membrane of the proximal and mid left main bronchus. Laser photocoagulation and resection is not performed in order to avoid further mucosal necrosis or creation of a bronchoesophageal fistula. With the bronchus dilated, a large 12-mm by 50-mm silicone stent is inserted. In this case, a smooth-walled silicone stent with rounded flanges at both extremities was used rather than a studded stent. One hypothesis was that the smooth walls might help prevent airway wall perforation in this

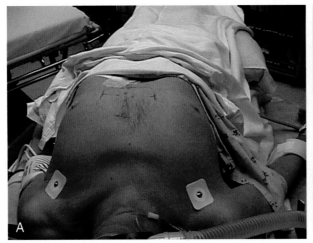

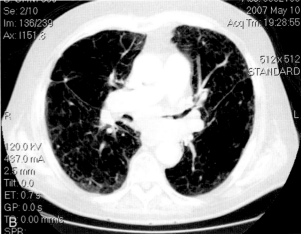

**Figure 9-11:** Vitals: barrel chest (**A**) a large subcarinal mass (**B**) infiltrating the medial and posterior wall of the left main bronchus, extending to the take off of the left upper lobe bronchus (LC1). The mass is causing significant extrinsic compression of the mid and distal left main bronchus.

already necrotic, friable and easily torn posterior left main bronchus (caused by tumor and recent radiation therapy).
- *Diagnosis/Pathology:* Central left main bronchial obstruction by recurrent squamous cell carcinoma and mediastinal adenopathy. (See attached video.)
- *Management alternatives:* As described, once airway patency is restored, patient could be discharged and resume external beam radiation therapy.

**Key Points**

- Comorbidities such as COPD, asthma, significant metastatic carcinoma, cardiac disease, unstable cervical spine, neuromuscular disease, skeletal deformities involving the spine, and of course neck or jaw deformities can increase procedure difficulty and warrant appropriate precautions and management strategies.
- Airway stents improve quality of life and survival in patients with bronchogenic carcinoma.
  - Careful consideration should be given to laser-tissue interactions before performing laser or electrosurgical bronchoscopic resection.
  - Stent selection is important. In this case, in view of significantly altered airway anatomy, a covered metal stent, or hybrid stent could also have been inserted.

## Illustrative Case #2: Dyspnea and Impending Respiratory Failure in a Patient with Relapsing Polychondritis Three Months after Stent Insertion

- *History:* Patient is a 40-year-old woman with a 4-year history of increasing cough and wheezing. Treatment for presumed hyperreactive airways disease has been unsuccessful, and patient had been on high-dose oral corticosteroids for several months. She also has a history of respiratory insufficiency requiring hospitalization in the intensive care unit and intubation on two separate occasions. Following referral to a tertiary institution, for presumed asthma exacerbation, flexible bronchoscopy revealed diffuse circumferential airway narrowing with thickened bronchial and lower tracheal mucosa. The patient's working diagnosis was relapsing polychondritis, later confirmed by supplemental tests and rheumatology consultation. To restore airway patency, a large silicone Y-stent was inserted, and the patient was discharged with instructions to use nebulized saline solution three times daily in order to maintain fluid secretions and assist with expectoration. Two months after discharge, the patient is admitted with increasing shortness of breath and wheezing.
- *Examination:* A large, cushingoid woman in moderate respiratory distress; Vitals: tachycardia (116/min); BP 190/100 respirations 26/min; temp: 99.0° F, SPO$_2$ 90% (Venturi mask 50%). Lung auscultation revealed bilateral expiratory wheezes.
- *Blood tests:* Complete blood count and electrolytes—normal.

- *Imaging:* Chest radiograph revealed indwelling silicone Y-stent.
- *Bronchoscopy:* Revealed thick airway secretions partially occluding the tracheal limb of the Y-stent, as well as both bronchial limbs. Distal to the stent, airway mucosa was thick and circumferentially narrowed (Fig. 9-12).
- *Diagnosis/Pathology:* Recurrent obstruction by tenacious secretions lodged within silicone Y-stent.
- *Management alternatives:* This patient needs urgent bronchoscopy to remove thick and tenacious respiratory secretions and to restore airway patency. Rigid bronchoscopy is probably warranted in order to minimize airway compromise and perform the procedure quickly. Careful attention should be paid to saline administration to liquefy secretions, and to using large diameter suction device and forceps in order to remove thick sticky and partially impacted secretions. Electrocautery or laser resection may be required to remove stent-related granulation tissue proximal or distal to the silicone stent. Precautions are necessary in this case to avoid airway fires. (See attached video.)

**Key Points**

- Patients with indwelling stents usually do well, but stent-related complications do occur and usually require repeat intervention.
- The role of surveillance bronchoscopy remains unclear, but at least one study suggests that it is not necessary so long as patients are rapidly undergoing bronchoscopy in case of new or recurrent airway symptoms.
- Obstruction of Y-stents can be life-threatening when tumor or secretions completely obstruct the tracheal limb of the stent, preventing airflow distally. Careful informed consent should always be obtained before

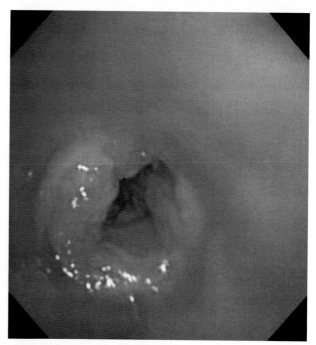

**Figure 9-12:** *Bronchoscopy: Revealed thick airway secretions partially occluding the tracheal limb of the Y-stent, as well as both bronchial limbs. Distal to the stent, airway mucosa was thick and circumferentially narrowed.*

stent insertion. Patients should be given specific instructions regarding medical management in case of an emergency, and also a stent alert document (a template is freely downloadable, for example, from the Bronchoscopy International website *www.bronchoscopy.org* on the downloads menu).

## Illustrative Case #3: Fixed Obstruction by Extrinsic Tracheal Compression from Esophageal Stent

- *History:* 67-year-old smoker with a history of esophageal cancer requiring stent insertion, now presenting with increasing shortness of breath and cough.

- Dysphagia is well controlled following insertion of large covered ultraflex esophageal stent.
- *Examination:* Vitals: tachycardia (120/min); BP 130/68; respirations 24/min; temp: 97.0° F, SPO$_2$ 95% (room air).
- *Blood tests:* Complete blood count and electrolytes—normal.
- *Imaging:* Computed tomography scan revealed extrinsic compression of midtrachea by metal esophageal stent. No evidence of fistula (Fig. 9-13A)
- *Rigid bronchoscopy:* Performed using general anesthesia and spontaneous ventilation. Bronchoscopic image reveals evidence of fixed obstruction by extrinsic compression (Fig. 9-13B).
- *Management alternatives:* Alternatives include insertion of covered metal stent, hybrid stent, or large silicone stent into mid trachea to restore airway patency and relieve symptoms of dyspnea and cough. Rigid bronchoscopy was performed and a 16-mm wide by

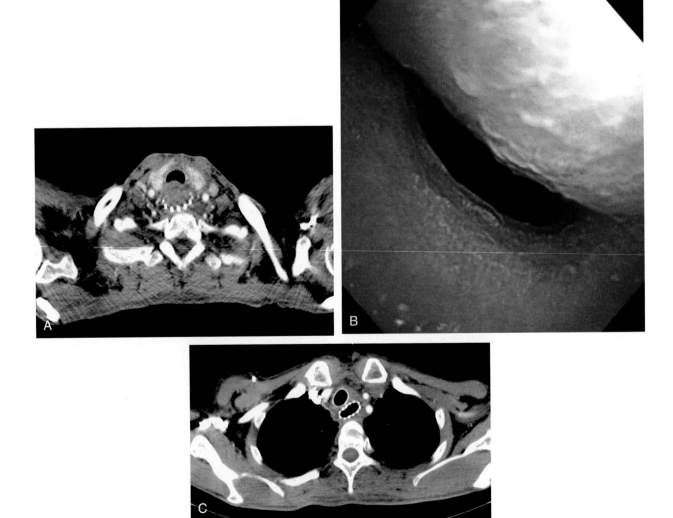

**Figure 9-13: A,** Computed tomography scan revealed extrinsic compression of midtrachea by metal esophageal stent. No evidence of fistula. **B,** Bronchoscopic image reveals evidence of fixed obstruction by extrinsic compression. **C,** Rigid bronchoscopy was performed and a 16-mm wide by 50-mm long silicone stent thoracs inserted sinto the trachea.

50-mm long silicone stent was inserted into the trachea (Fig. 9-13C). (See attached video.)

## Key Points

- Esophageal stent insertion can cause airway compromise
- Careful examination for extrinsic compression or spread of esophageal tumor through posterior membrane into the airway, or a search for evidence of tracheoesophageal or bronchoesophageal fistula should be performed. May require swallow study, repeat esophagoscopy, and bronchoscopy in supine and sitting positions.
- Airway stenting usually provides palliation and significantly improves quality of life and survival. Stents are usually well tolerated, and complications are very rarely life-threatening. Symptoms of recurrent cough, dyspnea, pneumonia suggest stent-related complications such as migration, obstruction by secretions, or obstruction by tumor regrowth, and should warrant flexible bronchoscopy for diagnosis.

## References

 Interactive references and additional readings for this chapter can be accessed online at *expertconsult.com*.

# UPPER AIRWAY

## 10 TRACHEOTOMY

John E. Heffner, MD

## TERMINOLOGY

- Tracheotomy
- Tracheostomy
- Standard surgical tracheotomy
- Percutaneous tracheotomy
- Cricothyroidotomy

## DEFINITIONS

- *Tracheotomy* refers to a procedure that creates an opening in the trachea.
- *Tracheostomy* refers to the opening created by tracheotomy and to the artificial airways inserted into the opening.
- An *open surgical tracheotomy* entails surgical dissection of pretracheal tissue with incision of the trachea to create an opening by varying techniques that include the removal or incision of anterior tracheal rings and the creation of a tracheal wall (Björk) flap. The tracheostomy tube is inserted under direct vision.
- *Percutaneous tracheotomy* refers to differing procedures wherein a tracheostomy tube is inserted by a guidewire Seldinger technique below the first or second tracheal rings using a dilator or a forceps-like device to cut and spread the trachea.
- *Cricothyroidotomy* allows[1] insertion of an artificial airway through the cricothyroid membrane either by percutaneous or surgical techniques.

## INDICATIONS

Tracheotomy is performed in critically ill patients for the following indications:

- Airway control and suctioning for patients with incompetent glottic function or poor clearance of tracheobronchial secretions;
- Functional or mechanical upper airway obstruction;
- Airway access for continuing mechanical ventilation after an initial period of translaryngeal endotracheal intubation.
- Emergency airway access:
- Some centers report high complication rates for emergency surgical tracheotomy in nonintubated patients[1] and prefer cricothyroidotomy.[2,3] Surgeons with specialized otolaryngologic skills report good outcomes with emergency tracheotomy.[4]
- Emergency percutaneous tracheotomy has use in the emergency setting in experienced hands.[5,6]
- Selection of a preferred approach for emergency airway access depends on available expertise, team-based training and drilling, and demonstrated outcomes.

## SURGICAL VERSUS PERCUTANEOUS TRACHEOTOMY

Surgical tracheotomy is usually performed in the operating room but can be done in an intensive care unit (ICU) if an operating milieu is created (appropriate staff, lighting, sterility, and equipment).[7]

- Advantages of surgical tracheotomy:
  - Traditional procedure with long-term experience with techniques and outcomes.
  - Low early complication rates for critically ill patients.
  - Direct access to deep cervical structures to control bleeding and ensure proper placement of standard or specialized airways for patients with abnormal cervical anatomy.
- Disadvantages of surgical tracheotomy:
  - Most performed in the operating room with attendant high hospital-based costs and charges[8] and risks of patient transport.
  - Procedure delays because of operating room availability.
  - Stoma infection and bleeding.
- Advantages of percutaneous tracheotomy:
  - Low early complication rates in the critical care setting when performed by experienced operators.
  - Avoids deep neck dissections and provides a tamponading effect of the tracheostomy tube on vascular structures to decrease bleeding.
  - Nonsurgeons can perform the procedure to expand available operators, increase access, and avoid operating room (OR) delays to decrease the duration of translaryngeal intubation before tracheotomy.
  - Can be performed at the bedside to avoid OR-related risks of patient transport[9] and costs.[10]
  - Few contraindications, which allows its wide application for critically ill patients.

- Disadvantages of percutaneous tracheotomy:
  - Airway misplacement when performed without bronchoscopy.
  - Few long-term outcome studies to define late airway complications.
- Comparative advantages and disadvantages of surgical versus percutaneous tracheotomy:
  - Percutaneous tracheotomy has lower costs and delays in scheduling when compared with surgical tracheotomy performed in the operating room.[8-11] Costs may be similar if surgical tracheotomy is performed at the bedside.[12]
  - Large-scale randomized studies do not exist to compare short-term and long-term outcomes between the two procedures. Available studies and meta-analyses vary in their conclusions. Recent critical appraisals[11] suggest:
    - Most clinically important complications are comparable between the two procedures.
    - The overall mortality rate is similar but may be lower when percutaneous tracheotomy is compared with surgical tracheotomy performed in the operating room.
    - Percutaneous tracheotomy has a lower incidence of stoma wound infection.
    - Percutaneous tracheotomy has a lower incidence of clinically relevant bleeding.
    - Long-term follow-up studies with comparative quality-of-life measures are few but show no differences between procedures.[13]
  - Better neck cosmesis with percutaneous tracheotomy after decannulation.
  - Conclusions: Although most major outcomes appear similar between the two procedures, percutaneous tracheotomy is becoming the preferred procedure in centers with adequately skilled operators.
- Patient selection for percutaneous tracheotomy:
  - Early trials of percutaneous tracheotomy excluded potentially complicated patients and proposed contraindications, such as obesity, thyroid disease, use of positive end-expiratory pressure (PEEP), and bleeding disorders, based on lack of experience with these clinical settings.
  - Increased experience with the procedure indicates that few absolute contraindications exist and that only 5% of critically ill patients require an open procedure.[14]
  - Absolute contraindications include:
    - Active infections over the tracheotomy site;
    - Uncontrolled bleeding disorders;
    - Unstable cardiopulmonary status (hypotension on pressors or extreme ventilation and oxygenation requirements that worsen with a brief interruption of ventilation or oxygenation);
    - Uncontrollable patient movement or agitation.
    - Inability to identify tracheolaryngeal structures due to cervical anatomic abnormalities.
  - Special considerations:
    - Obesity—Some reports[15] note more complications (44% versus 18%) in obese patients, but others report no differences in outcomes.[16]
    - Repeated tracheotomy—Retrospective reviews support the safety of percutaneous tracheotomy after previous tracheotomies.[17]
    - Bleeding disorders—5% bleeding risk in thrombocytopenic patients with thrombocytopenia transfused with platelets before the procedure.[18]
    - Neutropenia—Reported safe.[19]
    - Spinal cord injury—Reported safe in trauma patients before cervical spine clearance and in those with stabilized cervical spine injuries.[20]
    - Sternotomy—No relationship exists between early tracheotomy and mediastinitis after median sternotomy.[21-27]
    - PEEP—Reported safe in patients with severe hypoxic respiratory failure that requires high levels of PEEP (15–20 cm $H_2O$).[28]

## SPECIALIZED TRACHEOSTOMY TUBES

- Obese patients have a deep stoma tract from skin to tracheal lumen and benefit from a long tube (extra-length tubes) with an adjustable or fixed flange (Fig. 10-1).[29-31] Some extra-length tubes are flexible and wire reinforced.
- Dual-cannula tracheostomy tubes have a removable inner cannula that can be removed for cleaning.
- Localized tracheomalacia where tube cuff rests against the tracheal wall benefits from a long tube that places the cuff below the area of tracheal injury or tubes with multiple cuffs.
- Tracheostomy tubes with proximal suction ports allow aspiration of tracheal sections to lower risk of pneumonia; no data exist regarding benefit in contrast to studies with endotracheal tube suction ports.
- After removal of an inner cannula, fenestrated tubes allow breathing through the native upper airway on exhalation to promote speech. Deflation of the cuff allows breathing through the fenestrations and around the tube for patients undergoing spontaneous weaning trials.
- Pneumatic speaking tubes have ports to stream air above the cuff to allow speech.
- Many manufacturers can provide customized tracheostomy tubes to meet specialized needs with a 1-week response to requests.

## AIRWAY PLACEMENT TECHNIQUES

- Surgical tracheotomy:
  - Extend the neck
  - 1-cm incision transversely just above the sternal notch
  - Blunt dissection in the midline, directly to the trachea. With a normal sized thyroid, nothing needs to be done with the thyroid
  - Transverse tracheal incision to excise an 8-mm portion of the fourth tracheal ring.

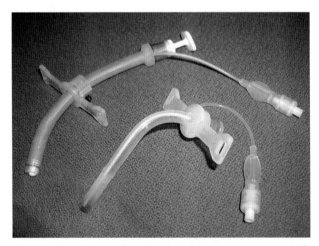

**Figure 10-1:** Extra-length tubes for placement in patients with abnormal cervical anatomy, such as obesity. The tubes may be flexible and wire reinforced with an adjustable flange (*left*) or rigid with a long intratracheal length (*right*).

○ Tube size equals two thirds the tracheal diameter at level of stoma.

○ Specialized dissections and excision of subcutaneous fat can be performed for obese patients.[32]

○ A Björk flap in the anterior tracheal wall can be placed to facilitate tube replacement before the stoma tract matures.[33]

■ Percutaneous tracheotomy can be performed by several techniques. Consensus and available studies do not support the superiority of one procedure over another in expert hands.

○ Ciaglia Blue-Rhino—Seldinger guidewire insertion of a single progressive dilator, followed by insertion of a tracheostomy tube.

• One can visualize proper insertion of the needle/guidewire and tube in the trachea through bronchoscopy to avoid tube misplacement or perforation either of the posterior tracheal wall or the endotracheal tube.[34]

• Ultrasound can also assist in placement of the needle or guidewire, especially in obese patients, and can aid in evaluation of the surgical site for abnormal vascular anatomy before the procedure.[35]

• The procedure is performed in some centers as a blind technique,[14] whereas others guide tube placement by capnography.[36]

• Postprocedure chest radiographs are not necessary when bronchoscopy guides insertion.[37]

○ A Griggs forceps technique inserts a forceps with a groove that allows loading of a guidewire onto the forceps, which is used to dilate the trachea, thread the wire, and insert a tracheostomy tube by a Seldinger technique.

○ Frova and Quintel described a single-step dilator that threads a screw-type dilator between tracheal rings.[38]

○ Fantoni described translaryngeal tracheotomy that places a tracheostomy tube in a reverse direction from within the airway through the tracheostomy tract.[39] The procedure is commonly performed in Europe.[13]

## TIMING OF TRACHEOTOMY IN PATIENTS ON MECHANICAL VENTILATION

■ Expert opinion and limited comparative studies propose multiple potential advantages for tracheotomy as compared with prolonged translaryngeal intubation (Table 10-1)[7,40,41]:

○ Enhanced patient comfort, mobilization, oral hygiene, and decreased sedative requirements.[42]

○ More secure airway, which may improve outcome for difficult-to-reintubate patients, such as those in halo fixation.[43]

○ Accelerated transfer from the ICU to intermediate care for ventilator-dependent patients.

| TABLE 10-1 ■ **COMMONLY CITED BENEFITS OF TRACHEOTOMY** |
| --- |
| Spares larynx from direct injury |
| Accelerates ventilator weaning |
| Does not promote sinusitis |
| Facilitates nursing care and secretion removal |
| Enhances patient mobility |
| Provides secure airway |
| Facilitates transfer from the intensive care unit |
| Improves patient comfort |
| Permits speech |
| Facilitates oral nutrition |
| Improves psychological wellbeing |

○ Some[44] but not all[45] studies note decreased airway resistance (inspiratory load) for patients undergoing weaning from ventilators.

○ Improved airway suctioning and secretion removal.

○ Avoidance of laryngeal injury from prolonged translaryngeal intubation. Nearly 90% of patients with subglottic stenosis have a history of translaryngeal intubation with a mean duration of intubation of 17 days.[46]

○ Ability to speak and feed orally.

○ Decreased anatomic dead space has been proposed as an advantage, but clinical studies demonstrate no measurable change in dead space after tracheotomy.[47]

■ Limited data exist, however, to determine the relative risks and benefits of tracheotomy as determined by duration of translaryngeal intubation to identify the ideal timing of tracheotomy.[48]

■ Studies in specific patient cohorts report conflicting results or no benefit from early tracheotomy for trauma[49-51] or burn patients.[52] Brain-injured patients may experience fewer complications and earlier weaning with early tracheotomy.[53]

■ Important clinical outcomes to establish ideal timing include mortality rate, risk of hospital-acquired pneumonia, duration of mechanical ventilation, and length of ICU stay.

○ Mortality rate—Timing of tracheotomy does not appear to affect the mortality rate in general populations of patients. One recent study in medical intensive care patients with APACHE II scores greater than 25 noted a decreased mortality rate with early percutaneous tracheotomy largely due to a decreased risk of ventilator-associated pneumonia.[54]

○ Pneumonia—Timing of tracheotomy does not alter the risk of ventilator-associated pneumonia in most studies. One study of critically ill medical patients demonstrated marked decreases in pneumonia rates with early tracheotomy,[54] but the degree of benefit appears unprecedented and requires confirmation by future studies. Other studies have observed an increase in pneumonia rates after tracheotomy.[55,56]

○ A Cochrane meta-analysis reported that the duration of mechanical ventilation may be decreased in patients undergoing early tracheotomy.[57]

○ The overall length of ICU stay is decreased by early tracheotomy.[57-59] This outcome may represent "care shifting," with transfer of ventilator-dependent patients to non-ICU settings or other facilities, such as long-term acute care centers.[60] This factor may account for the increase in application of tracheotomy observed in some regions.[60]

■ It is difficult to draw conclusions regarding impact of early versus late tracheotomy because studies use different definitions of "early" versus "late," failure to control for other important treatment variables (e.g., glucose control, sedation use, and low tidal volume ventilation), lack of blinding, small study sizes, and other inadequacies in study designs.

■ **Recommendations:** Clinicians should base decisions for timing tracheotomy on multiple factors and individualize the decision by anticipating probable duration of mechanical ventilation and incorporating patient and family viewpoints.

○ Some patients may be so critically ill (APACHE II > 25,[54] severe head injuries, severe shock on admission,[61] advanced underlying cardiopulmonary disease with severe trauma or severe complications of major surgery) that early tracheotomy can be performed after initial stabilization.

○ Other patients should be evaluated after 5 to 7 days of intubation to anticipate the likely duration of continued ventilation.[62,63] Patients who appear unlikely to achieve extubation within the next 7 to 10 days (e.g., high ongoing $FIO_2$ requirements in adult respiratory distress syndrome [ARDS][64]) can undergo tracheotomy when stable. Other patients can be continued with translaryngeal intubation with daily assessments for extubation with recurrent consideration for tracheotomy based on subsequent course.

○ Avoid "calendar watching" wherein an arbitrary duration limit for translaryngeal intubation determines timing of tracheotomy.[65,66]

## PERIOPERATIVE/EARLY COMPLICATIONS

Both the percutaneous and surgical routes for tracheotomy have low rates of early complications (Table 10-2), but those complications that occur can be life-threatening; close monitoring is required.[67]

Important early complications include

■ Stoma infection.
   ○ Incidence—Low rate of tissue infection because wound is open and drainage. Necrotizing tracheostomal infections very rare.
   ○ Risk factors—Diabetes.
   ○ Clinical clues—Indurated tissue or cellulitis surrounding the stoma; breakdown of the stoma track.
   ○ Summary workup—Aspiration for culture of spreading cellulitis; culture of necrotic tissue.
   ○ Summary principles of treatment—Purulent drainage alone requires stomal care rather than antibiotics. Systemic antibiotics needed for actual tissue infection.
■ Stomal hemorrhage.
   ○ Incidence—Clinically important bleeding in 3% to 5% of patients.
   ○ Risk factors—Bleeding disorders, open surgical tracheotomy, vascular anomalies.
   ○ Clinical clues—Bloody drainage or tracheal suctioning aspirate.
   ○ Summary workup—Exclude early a tracheoinnominate fistula, then examine the stoma track for bleeding source.
   ○ Summary principles of treatment: Tamponade bleeding site with packing but do not interfere with security of airway. Examine wound for bleeding site if bleeding persists. Serious bleeding needs to be evaluated in the operating room.

## TABLE 10-2  ■  MAJOR COMPLICATIONS OF TRACHEOTOMY

| Early | Late |
|---|---|
| Death <1% | Abnormal speech or voice |
| Cardiopulmonary arrest | Tracheocutaneous fistula |
| Stoma infection | Tracheal stenosis |
| Stoma hemorrhage | Tracheoinnominate fistula |
| Pneumothorax | Tracheal ring rupture and herniation |
| Pneumomediastinum | Tracheoesophageal fistula |
| Subcutaneous emphysema | Tube obstruction |
| Aerophagia | Aspiration |
| Aspiration | Swallowing dysfunction |
| Tube misplacement | Infection of adjacent structures |
| Tube displacement | ■ Clavicle |
| Laceration or perforation of adjacent structures (esophagus or posterior tracheal space) | ■ Mediastinum |

## LATE COMPLICATIONS

It is difficult to separate the late complications of tracheotomy from those that result from prolonged translaryngeal intubation.

Manifestations of delayed complications may simulate symptoms due to an underlying condition (e.g., heart failure, COPD) or delayed resolution of critical illnesses (e.g., ARDS, critical care myopathy with poor cough).[68]

To lower risk of complications, maintain cuff pressures between 20 and 25 mm Hg; pressures that are too low allow aspiration, and pressures that are too high cause muscosal ischemia.

Use clinical judgment: a small air leak around a tracheostomy does not have to be eliminated by injecting more air into a tracheostomy cuff. As long as the patient is being ventilated and oxygenated well, ignore the small air leak around the cuff.

Recommendations to routinely change tracheostomy tubes are controversial, but one study noted fewer complications due to granulation tissue after implementation of tube changes every 2 weeks.[69]

Major late complications include

■ Difficulties with speech and voice.
   ○ Incidence—Few studies carefully examine patients for alterations in speech, but incidence appears to be significant.
   ○ Risk factors—Uncertain.
   ○ Clinical clues—Patient reported symptoms.
   ○ Summary workup—Otolaryngologic examination of sinuses and glottic function.
   ○ Summary principles of treatment—Speech therapy.
■ Tracheal stenosis—Clinically important degrees (>50% loss of tracheal caliber) of tracheal stenosis rarely occurs.[70] Chest radiograph and standard computed tomography (CT) protocols have low diagnostic sensitivity. Symptomatic patients benefit from spiral CT with three-dimensional airway reconstruction[71] or bronchoscopy. Please see Chapter 11 entitled Tracheal Stenosis.
■ Tracheoesophageal fistula
   ○ Incidence—Less than 1% of patients.
   ○ Risk factors—Rigid nasogastric tube that impinges on the esophagus and posterior tracheal wall against an inflated tracheostomy tube cuff, high cuff pressures, extensive tube movement, high ventilator pressures, prolonged intubation, and diabetes.
   ○ Clinical clues—During mechanical ventilation, signs are increased secretions, pneumonia, increased gastrointestinal gas, and gastric contents aspiration. Symptoms after decannulation include chronic cough, cough after swallowing, and increased sputum production, which simulates chronic bronchitis or aspiration.
   ○ Summary workup—Evaluation requires barium swallow imaging, bronchoscopy and esophagoscopy.[72]
   ○ Summary principles of treatment—Universally fatal unless surgically repaired. Insert specialized tubes with cuffs below the level of the fistula. A covered esophageal stent can temporarily control the problem. A single-stage surgical repair after weaning from mechanical ventilation has a high success rate.
■ Tracheoinnominate fistula—Control of hemorrhage by tube cuff overinflation or digital arterial compression can be lifesaving. Patients require urgent surgery of the innominate artery and insertion of viable tissue between the trachea and divided artery.[73]
   ○ Incidence—Less than 1% of patients.
   ○ Risk factors—Cuff overinflation; tracheotomy performed low, below the fourth tracheal ring; long tracheotomy tube, with the tip positioned to impinge the anterior tracheal wall.

○ Clinical clues—Any tracheal bleeding after tracheotomy requires prompt evaluation for a tracheoinnominate fistula. Most patients have sentinel small hemorrhages, followed by massive hemoptysis.

○ Summary workup—Bedside manipulation of a tracheostomy tube to evaluate sentinel hemorrhages can induce massive hemoptysis. Evaluations should be done in the operating room, where urgent sternotomy can be performed. Bronchoscopy should examine the entire region around and adjacent to the tracheostomy cuff.

○ Summary principles of treatment—High lethality unless bleeding is quickly controlled. Overinflation of the tracheostomy tube cuff may tamponade fistula. Intubation with an endotracheal tube with positioning of the cuff over the fistula may tamponade the site. A suprasternal incision may allow blunt finger dissection and finger tamponade of the innominate artery. Intravascular occlusion of the innominate with a Fogarty catheter has been described to stabilize for surgery. Definitive therapy is sternotomy with ligation and resection of the innominate artery segment involved because vascular infection obviates a repair.

■ Tracheocutaneous fistula—Failure of the stoma tract to seal requires a stomaplasty for cosmesis.
   ○ Uncommon after decannulation
   ○ An operation is required to close the fistula

■ Tracheal ring fracture and herniation—Rare reports after percutaneous tracheotomy.[74]

## WEANING PATIENTS TOWARD AIRWAY DECANNULATION

■ After recovery from critical illness, many patients with tracheostomies are transferred to non-ICU settings, where physicians and nurses may not have adequate knowledge of tracheostomy care.[75,76]

■ Successful management toward decannulation is enhanced by a team-based approach with the necessary expertise and access to specialists.[77]

■ Multiple approaches to decannulation are available.
   ○ Patients who regain good ventilatory mechanics and upper airway control may tolerate capping of the tracheotomy tube (decannulation cap), with removal of the tube within 24 to 48 hours if cough and breathing remain adequate.

○ Patients with underlying ventilatory compromise (COPD, poor cough, muscle weakness) may not tolerate a capped tracheostomy tube because the tube's obstructing effect in the trachea. These patients may benefit from a Montgomery tube or Olympic Tracheostomy button, which clear the trachea but maintain the stoma tract patent in case recannulation of the airway is needed later.

○ The Montgomery tracheal cannula comes in short-term (Fig. 10-2) and long-term varieties. Short-term cannulas are generally used for up to 6 weeks, if needed; thus, use of long-term cannulae is rare.

○ Montgomery tubes are used to replace a tracheostomy tube with the following goals in mind:
   ● Maintain the tracheotomy stoma should a tracheostomy tube need to be replaced, especially in patients deemed to have limited ventilatory reserve
   ● Provide a means of tracheal suction
   ● Provide a means for short-term emergency ventilation.

○ The advantages of this Montgomery transition tube are
   ● No tube projecting into the trachea because the distal angulated flat flange fits snuggly against the anterior tracheal wall (see Fig. 10-2); thus, the entire tracheal lumen is patent, reducing flow resistance and work of breathing
   ● There is a groove system with safety ring maintaining position
   ● The length can be trimmed to fit any neck size
   ● A large variety of cannula sizes are available to tailor to needs for each patient; thus, it is suitable for adult and pediatric populations
   ● Can be plugged as part of the de-cannulization process.

○ Patients who tolerate a stoma plug for 24 to 48 hours undergo removal of the plug.

○ Progressively downsizing the tracheostomy tube with insertion of a cuffless tube can also maintain airway access and assess the ability of the patient to cough and breathe through the native airway. A cuffless tube had less airway resistance than a cuffed tube with the cuff deflated.

○ For patients with marginal ventilatory reserve, removal of the inner cannula of a dual-cannula tracheostomy tube decreases airway resistance.[78]

○ Occasional patients with good ventilatory mechanics but poor secretion clearance may benefit from prolonged tracheal buttons or a placement of a mini-tracheostomy tube (4.0 mm inner diameter), which allows intermittent airway suctioning.[77,79]

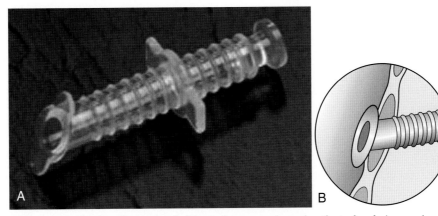

**Figure 10-2:** A Montgomery stoma plug that allows removal of the tracheostomy tube to clear the trachea during weaning and decreasing resistance to spontaneous breathing. The plug keeps the stoma patent in case the tracheostomy tube needs to be reinserted. Tracheal suctioning can be performed through the tube. **A,** A short-term cannula with angled flange, together with groove system and safety ring for maintaining position. **B,** Schematic whereby angled flange fits snuggly against the anterior tracheal wall, thus not impinging on tracheal lumen. (*Figures reproduced from Boston Medical Products brochure; web access: http://www.bosmed.com/trachtubes/montgomery.html.*)

- *History:* 45-year-old woman was brought to the trauma center after a motor vehicle accident. She had a long history of advanced chronic obstructive pulmonary disease from a life-long smoking history. She required intubation in the field for loss of consciousness and cyanosis.
- *Examination:* Vitals: tachycardia (120/min); BP 90/50; respirations 16/min; temp: 99.8 F, SPO$_2$ 95% (70% FIO$_2$). Intubated and unresponsive to painful stimuli. Chest—bilateral expiratory wheezes, crackles, and rhonchi. Emesis returns with tracheal suctioning.
- *Blood tests:* ABG (70% FIO$_2$) pH 7.32, pCO$_2$ 60 mm Hg, pO$_2$ 70 mm Hg.
- *Imaging:* Chest radiograph: intubated trachea with hyperinflated lung fields, bullous emphysematous changes, bilateral airspace consolidation, multiple rib fractures. Head CT scan normal.
- *Diagnosis:* Advanced COPD with baseline hypercapnia and acute hypoxic and hypercapneic respiratory failure due to bilateral lung contusions, chemical aspiration pneumonitis, and underlying severe COPD.
- *Hospital course:* After 2 days of treatment with mechanical ventilation and general critical care that included antibiotics, the patient remained unconscious and ventilator dependent with stable ventilator settings. The diffuse airspace consolidation was improved, but airspace consolidation in the superior segment of the right lower lobe became more predominant.

- *Airway Management:* After 2 days of critical care, the underlying COPD and development of a probable aspiration pneumonia in the setting of unconsciousness from a cerebral contusion made extubation unlikely in the next 7 days. The advanced COPD indicated that the patient would require prolonged weaning from airway and ventilatory support. The patient underwent percutaneous tracheotomy the next day rather than waiting until she fulfilled an arbitrary number of days of translaryngeal intubation.

**Key Points**

- Individualization of timing tracheotomy on the basis of anticipated duration of mechanical ventilation and benefits expected.
- Percutaneous tracheotomy can be performed safely in the ICU without delays that occur with scheduling the OR for a surgical tracheotomy.

Tracheotomy provides comfort-related benefits and may shorten the duration of ICU stay. Other benefits, such as decreased mortality, lower pneumonia risk, and decreased airway complications, are less clear.

**References**

Interactive references and additional readings for this chapter can be accessed online at *expertconsult.com*.

---

# 11 TRACHEAL STENOSIS

Christopher R. Morse, MD, Moishe Liberman, MD, and Douglas J. Mathisen, MD

## TERMINOLOGY

- Tracheal stenosis
- Tracheal stricture

## DEFINITION

- Tracheal stenosis is a benign stricture of the trachea.

## ETIOLOGY

- Idiopathic
  - Primarily in women
  - Short stenosis in proximal airway/subglottic larynx (Fig. 11-1)
  - No history of trauma, infection, inhalation injury, or intubation
  - Autoimmune workup (e.g., Wegener's granulomatosis) negative
- Post-traumatic
  - Blunt trauma
    - May go unnoticed; often initially treated with tube thoracostomy for presence of pneumothorax
  - Inhalation injury
    - Chemical and thermal burns
    - Injury often begins below vocal cords with minimal damage to the supraglottic larynx.
    - Resection is difficult, and patients are often managed with silicone T-tube.
  - Postintubation/post-tracheostomy
    - Circumferential erosion of the trachea at the level of inflatable cuff
      - Preventable with low-pressure cuffs and vigilant monitoring of pressure in tracheostomy cuff. Goal is to keep pressures lower than 20 to 25 mm Hg.
      - A small leak of air around an endotracheal tube when the balloon pressure is in the appropriate range is not a problem and should be accepted when the patient is well oxygenated and well ventilated. In that situation, increasing the balloon pressure leads to tracheal damage.
    - Symptoms may present within days of extubation.

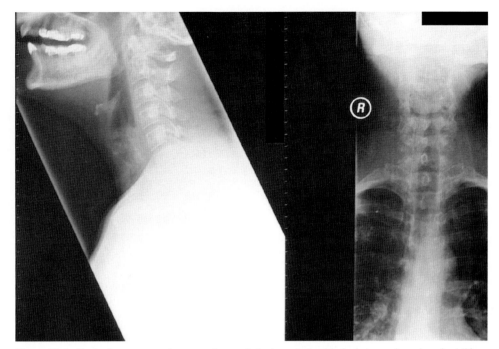

**Figure 11-1:** Tracheal tomograms demonstrating a subglottic stenosis with the lesion and vocal cords visible.

- At a previous tracheostomy site, granuloma may develop.
  ○ Subglottic injury occasionally caused by cricothyroidotomy
 ○ Post-therapeutic/stenosis following tracheal resection
  - Following attempts at tracheal reconstruction, restenosis is most often caused by tension at the anastomosis.
  - Disturbance of tracheal blood supply, postoperative radiation, and granulation tissue can also lead to restenosis.[1]
- Extrinsic lesions
 ○ Goiter
  - Often gradual compression of airway.
  - Even large goiters with tracheal deviation and/or mild stenosis are well tolerated and do not require treatment.
  - Following removal of goiter, trachea may remain distorted, but significant airway obstruction rarely appears.
 ○ Vascular
  - Congential ring
  - Innominate artery aneurysm
  - Anomalous subclavian artery passing behind trachea and esophagus
 ○ Mediastinal mass
  - Mediastinal masses causing tracheal compression are usually malignant (thymoma, lymphoma, germ cell tumors)
  - Rarely bronchogenic cyst
 ○ Postpneumonectomy syndrome
  - Following right pneumonectomy, with rotation of mediastinum, compression of remaining tracheobronchial tree
 ○ Infectious
 ○ Tuberculosis
  - Principally appears in the lower trachea and main bronchi.
  - Acute ulcerative tuberculosis leads to chronic, lengthy scarring of the airway.
  - Active disease must be addressed prior to any surgical intervention.

 ○ Histoplasmosis
  - Mediastinal fibrosis leading to airway compression
  - Erosion of calcified nodes into airway (broncholith)
 ○ Inflammatory/miscellaneous
  ○ Wegener's granulomatosis
  - Inflammatory lesions may affect larynx and trachea.
  - Most commonly produces subglottic stenosis, but can affect other upper airway sites.
  - With medical management, stable tracheal stenosis may result.
 ○ Sarcoidosis
  - Airway obstruction secondary to massive lymph node enlargement and fibrotic changes to airway
  - Usually not amenable to surgical reconstruction

## CLINICAL FEATURES

### Symptoms and Signs
- Patients often present with a long history of coughing progressing to wheezing
  ○ Lesions often recognized late.
  ○ Patients initially treated for adult onset asthma or chronic obstructive pulmonary disease (COPD).
  ○ Wheezing progressing to stridor as the caliber of the airway continues to narrow.
  ○ Chest radiographs will often demonstrate clear lung fields.
  ○ Chest tomograms will occasionally demonstrate the tracheal lesion.

## DIAGNOSTIC WORKUP

### History
- Important components of the history include
  ○ Progressive shortness of breath
  ○ Progressive dyspnea
  ○ Wheezing unresponsive to bronchodilators

- ○ Hemoptysis
- ○ Recurrent pneumonia/pneumonitis
- ○ Change in voice/increasing hoarseness

## Physical Examination

- ▪ Confirm airway patency.
- ▪ Ensure trachea is midline.
- ▪ Check bilateral breath sounds.
- ▪ Perform pulmonary auscultation.
- ▪ Head and neck exam including
  - ○ Thyroid examination
  - ○ Cervical lymph nodes, masses
  - ○ Palpate tracheal rings, and thyroid and cricoid cartilages
  - ○ Jugular venous distension
  - ○ Oral and pharyngeal examination

## Radiographic Evaluation

- ▪ Chest radiograph
  - ○ Clear chest radiograph in majority of cases
- ▪ Tracheal tomograms (see Fig. 11-1)
  - ○ Plain films of the trachea demonstrate tracheal air column **and location of lesion with respect to larynx**
- ▪ Computed tomography CT scan
  - ○ Occasionally will demonstrate a tracheal mass. Addition of high-resolution CT images and three-dimensional and multiplanar two-dimensional reconstructions increases sensitivity and specificity
  - ○ Virtual bronchoscopy CT scan (high-resolution, rapid-sequence CT scanning with computer software to reconstruct the tracheal at inspiration and expiration) can be helpful to define the location and the extent of the tracheal pathology.
  - ○ Tracheomalacia is an underdiagnosed and underappreciated disease. This is best diagnosed by virtual bronchoscopy CT scan and can be treated with a tracheoplasty via right thoracotomy.
  - ○ Useful with goiter, vascular malformations, histo-plasmosis

## Bronchoscopy

- ▪ Procedure is essential in the diagnosis and management of tracheal stenosis.
- ▪ Bronchoscopy should be performed with general anesthesia in an operating room (Fig. 11-2).

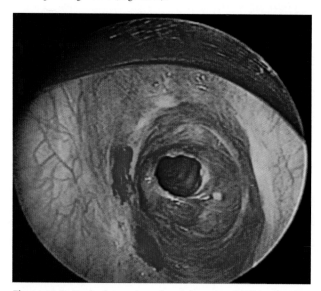

**Figure 11-2:** Tracheal stenosis as viewed through a rigid bronchoscope before dilatation and subsequent resection.

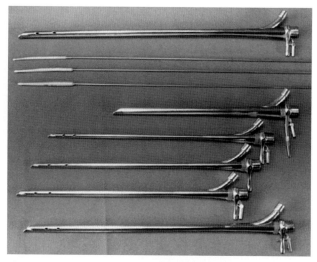

**Figure 11-3:** Rigid bronchoscopes of varying sizes, which allow for better visualization of the airway and airway pathology. In addition, the rigid bronchoscope allows for dilatation of stenosis before surgical resection.

- ▪ Potential for loss of airway in outpatient setting, so equipment for an emergent tracheostomy must be available.
- ▪ Flexible bronchoscopy is adequate
  - ○ If performed through an endotracheal tube, the tube must be pulled back and the airway examined from the level of the vocal cords
- ▪ Rigid bronchoscopy with general anesthesia superior to flexible bronchoscopy (Fig. 11-3)
- ▪ Allows for better visualization of anatomy and tracheal measurements (distance form the vocal cords to the tracheal pathology, distance of the tracheal pathology, and distance from the distal margin of the tracheal pathology to the carina). This is a key factor for proper planning of the tracheal surgery.
  - ○ Superior biopsy specimens
  - ○ Potential for airway management and improvement through maneuvers such as dilatation
- ▪ If imaging suggests a focal lesion amenable to resection, bronchoscopy can be deferred until general anesthesia can be used when resection planned.

## Pulmonary Function Tests

- ▪ Anatomic and physiologic considerations[2]:
  - ○ The coronal diameter of the trachea is 13 to 25 mm in men and 10 to 21 mm in women, with the length 10 to 11 cm.
  - ○ With inspiration, changes in length and diameter decrease airflow resistance. At functional residual capacity (FRC), the pressure within the upper airways (extrathoracic and intrathoracic) is atmospheric (referenced as 0)
- ▪ Sensitivity of pulmonary function studies and limitations:
  - ○ The most sensitive test is the flow volume loop. The classic paper by Miller and Hyatt[3] described three patterns: variable extrathoracic, variable intrathoracic and fixed. Abnormalities may not be appreciated until the airway is narrowed to about 8 to 10 mm.[4,5]
  - ○ Variable refers to dynamic narrowing of the airway diameter during either inspiration (variable extrathoracic obstruction) or expiration (variable intrathoracic obstruction). Fixed refers to no change in airway size, despite changes in transmural pressures during the different phases

of respiration, and can result from both intrathoracic or extrathoracic lesions. A *plateau pattern* of the expiratory loop only, is seen with variable intrathoracic obstruction, of the inspiratory loop only, with variable extrathoracic obstruction, and both phases of respiration with fixed obstruction.[6]

○ Fixed or variable intrathoracic patterns may be seen with tracheal stenosis, although fixed is much more likely. The variable intrathoracic pattern (e.g., with tracheal mass or tracheomalacia), occurs because on expiration, turbulent expiratory flow across the obstruction causes a fall in airway pressure, so that the pleural pressure at the obstructing site is greater than tracheal pressure, resulting in further narrowing of the airway. (During inspiration, the negative intrathoracic pressure, 'tethers open' the trachea at the site of the lesion).

○ Forced expiratory flow at 50% of vital capacity (VC) (forced expiratory flow [FEF]$_{50\%}$) to FIF$_{50\%}$ (forced inspiratory flow at 50% of VC) ratios:
  ▪ Fixed: close or equal to 1
  ▪ Variable intrathoracic: reduced to usually 0.3
  ▪ Variable extrathoracic: less than 2

○ Figure 11-4 shows an example of tracheal stenosis due to a thyroid cancer (A), with a fixed upper airway pattern noted on the flow volume loop (B).

○ Obstruction at the thoracic inlet: This can show different patterns on the flow volume loop ranging from intrathoracic to extrathoracic patterns on different days or with change in body position or neck flexion. It classically can also demonstrate a double-hump pattern on the expiratory limb (due to serial change from intrathoracic to extrathoracic position of the obstruction as end expiration approaches).

○ Reduced peak flow and maximum voluntary ventilation (MVV) may also be noted with tracheal stenosis

○ FEV$_1$ is very insensitive and is commonly in the normal range, when the above-mentioned tests are clearly abnormal. Decrements may be seen only with extreme levels of obstruction.[7,8] Thus, screening spirometry is an insensitive test for tracheal stenosis.

○ Note: Although a recent study reported that correlations exist between effort limitation and pulmonary function abnormalities, no good correlation was found between lung function abnormalities and radiologic stenosis on CT or x-ray imaging.[8,9]

▪ Concluding remarks regarding pulmonary function studies:
  ○ **Pulmonary function studies** may be of value to primary physicians and pulmonary specialists in aiding in establishing the diagnosis of tracheal stenosis. Note: The condition is often misdiagnosed as (1) asthma or COPD or (2) progression of underlying diseases (e.g., severe obstructive lung disease in which previous intubation or tracheostomy was needed).
  ○ May not be of significant value to the thoracic surgeon where the diagnosis is already established, especially in determining treatment approaches.
  ○ Despite a patients baseline pulmonary function, all will benefit from relief of central airway obstruction.

## *TREATMENT*

### Surgery

With current techniques of tracheal resection and reconstruction, surgery is the primary intervention for resectable lesions:

▪ Must be able to resect lesion and primarily reconstruct the trachea without tension.
▪ Patients must be capable of extubation after the tracheal resection.
▪ Principal contraindications to surgery include:
  ○ Extensive linear involvement of the airway such that primary end-to-end resection would not be possible without excessive tension.
  ○ Extensive patient comorbidities (i.e., morbid obesity, chronic steroid use)
  ○ Ventilator dependence
  ○ Previous radiation to the neck/chest
  ○ Quadriplegia
▪ Idiopathic tracheal stenosis
  ○ Often amenable to surgical resection (Figs. 11-5 and 11-6)
  ○ No progression of disease/recurrence following surgery
  ○ Excellent functional outcomes: For 73 patients who underwent resection at the Massachusetts General Hospital (MGH) for idiopathic subglottic stenosis,[10] 26% reported excellent results, 64% good results, and 5% fair results with respect to voice and airway.
▪ Postintubation/post-traumatic lesions
  ○ Surgical results were excellent.
  ○ Stenosis is usually focal.

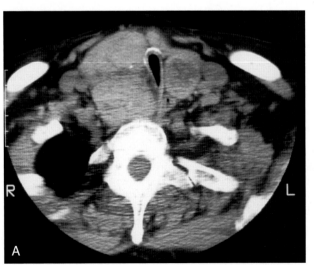
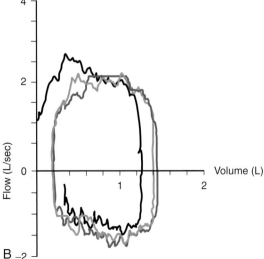

**Figure 11-4: A,** Computed tomography scan showing significant tracheal stenosis due to a thyroid carcinoma. **B,** Flow volume loop in this patient demonstrating a fixed upper airway obstructive pattern with plateaus of flow evident in both expiratory and inspiratory limbs.

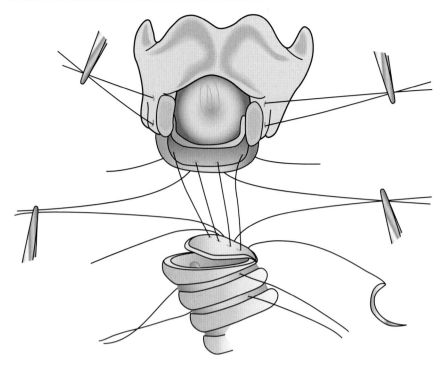

**Figure 11-5:** Resection of subglottic stenosis. The anterior cricoid has been resected and the mucosa over the posterior cricoid removed as the stenosis was circumferential. The membranous wall of the distal trachea is going to be used to resurface the posterior cricoid.

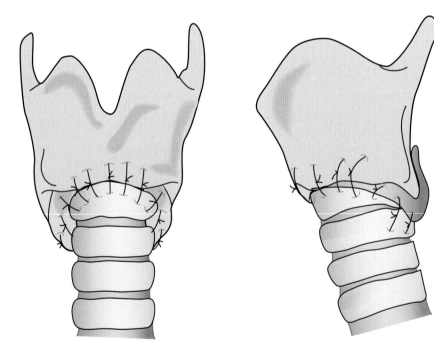

**Figure 11-6:** Completed resection of subglottic stenosis. The anterior wall of the distal trachea has been shaped to fit into the resected anterior cricoid.

- Other injuries affecting repair and outcomes include tracheoinnominate artery fistula and tracheoesophageal fistula.
- Between 1965 and 1992, 503 patients underwent tracheal resection and reconstruction for postintubation lesions at MGH.[11]
  - Two hundred and fifty-one lesions were the result of an endotracheal or tracheostomy tube, 178 were at the site of a tracheostomy, and 38 had evidence of both endotracheal cuff trauma and tracheostomy (stomal)–induced stenosis.
  - Results were good in 440 patients and satisfactory in 31 patients, and there were 20 failures and 12 deaths.

Of the patients in which therapy failed, 11 were treated with a tracheostomy, 7 with a T-tube, and 2 with dilations.
- Inhalational injuries
  - Surgical intervention is rarely indicated.
  - Initial management is often with tracheostomy, with conversion to a silicone T-tube as inflammation subsides.
  - In 18 patients with chronic airway compromise after inhalation burns, there were 18 tracheal stenoses, 14 subglottic strictures, and 2 main bronchial stenoses.[12]
- Goiter
  - Relief of extrinsic compression by thyroidectomy often eliminates the need for tracheal procedure.[13]

- Post-therapeutic stenosis
  - Optimal results from re-resection more than 6 months after initial surgery
  - Patients often palliated with silicone T-tube
  - Reoperation is difficult, but in experienced centers, 92% of patients have good or satisfactory outcomes.[14]

## Summary Principles of Surgical Procedure

- Tracheal surgery begins with bronchoscopy to assess the extent of the disease and obtain a biopsy if tumor is suspected. If there is a significant benign stenosis, rigid bronchoscopy is performed to dilate the stenosis. This allows the anesthesiologist to then place an endotracheal tube.
- Most tracheal surgery is performed through a cervical incision. Occasionally, a partial sternotomy with split of the manubrium can be helpful. Distal tracheal pathology and carinal resections are approached through a right thoracotomy.
- When the trachea is opened, ventilation is either intermittent via an endotracheal tube that is in the surgical field. The tube is placed in the distal trachea for hyperventilation and then removed for brief periods of time for dissection and suturing.
- The length of trachea that can be mobilized for resection with primary end-to-end anastomosis is generally up to 6 cm. Various mobilization techniques may be employed, including laryngeal release to reduce anastomotic tension. A cervical surgical approach is most commonly used. In a large surgical series of post intubation tracheal stenosis, the range of tracheal lengths resected was 1 to 7.5 cm.[11]
- Figure 11-7 depicts several CT images (above, at, and below the region of tracheal stenosis) in a patient who required prolonged intubation following smoke inhalation. At surgery, 3 cm of trachea was resected.

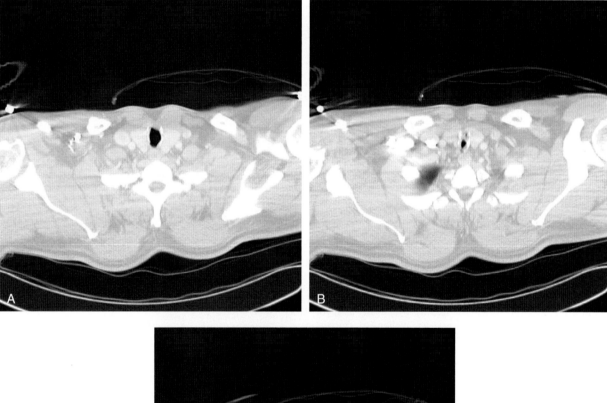

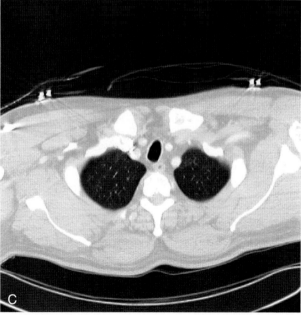

**Figure 11-7:** Computed tomography scan depicting severe tracheal stenosis complicating smoke inhalation and prolonged mechanical ventilation. **A,** above stenosis; **B,** area of maximal stenosis; **C,** below stenotic region.

### Postoperative Care

- Patients are almost always extubated at the end of the procedure.
- Following a tracheal resection, all patients have a "guardian suture" to maintain neck flexion.
- Patients stay in the intensive care unit overnight for airway monitoring.
- Patients initially kept NPO, and diet is advanced slowly over several days.
- Warm, humidified oxygen helps mobilize secretions.
- Vomiting is avoided by liberal use of antiemetics.
- Repeat bronchoscopy on postoperative day 7.
- If stridor develops at anytime postoperatively, the patient needs emergent evaluation and likely needs bronchoscopy.

### Complications

- Although anastomotic complications are rare, edema, granulation tissue and complete separation of the anastomosis are all potentially adverse outcomes.
- With an unstable airway, the patients should be intubated from above with a small endotracheal tube and with bronchoscopic assistance.
- With a stable airway, a CT scan of the neck may be obtained to look for extraluminal air and fluid collections.
  - Bronchoscopy can then be performed to evaluate the anastomosis.
- It is rare that an anastomotic separation can be repaired primarily and are best managed by either a T-tube or tracheostomy.

### Stenting/Silicone T-Tube

- Tracheal stents and T-tubes are used in situations in which the lesion is not amenable to surgery and the patient does not require ventilatory support
  - Placed with bronchoscopic guidance
  - Tracheal T-tube
    - Side arm extends through trachea
    - Can be custom fitted to patients
  - Little trauma to airway
  - Allow for speech and the patient to clear secretions with humidification of air through the nose
  - In a series of 140 patients, a silicone T-tube was used for postintubation lesions, burns, or malignant tracheal tumors.[15]
    - In 14 patients, it preceded later reconstruction, and in 16 patients, it was the solitary treatment for lesions.
    - In 43 patients, T-tubes were inserted for unreconstructable benign stenoses.
    - The tube was used as palliation in 49 patients
- TY and Y stents
  - Functional with strictures involving the trachea and the main bronchi
  - Y stents for patients who do not have a proximal tracheal stenosis
- Metal stents
  - Available with both bare metal and covered versions
  - We strongly advise consideration of all therapeutic options for each patient with benign and malignant airway obstruction before moving to stent placement.[16]
    - Stent placement will likely complicate future airway resection reconstruction in amenable lesions.

### Bronchoscopic Approaches

- Nd:YAG laser photoresection:
  - Although mostly employed for malignant upper airway lesions, laser treatment for benign tracheal stenosis has been reported in case series.[17-21]
  - Often reported in combination with gentle rigid bronchoscopic dilatation
  - In general lesions should be short (i.e., <4 cm) with a visible endobronchial lumen. Simple weblike lesions are ideal.
  - Indications include inoperable patients due to surgical considerations or significant comorbidities, patients who refuse surgical treatment, simple lesions such as postintubation granulation tissue that are easily and effectively handled by laser resection
  - Note: Laser treatment is not the treatment of choice for tracheal stenosis
- Cryotherapy:
  - Data for benign lesions are limited to several small case series.[22,23]

---

**KEY POINTS**

- Often delay in diagnosis.
- Imaging important, but bronchoscopy is essential for diagnosis, and initial management.
- Significant experience necessary to determine whether lesion is amenable to surgical management, timing of surgical management, and for good outcomes.
- A comprehensive state of the art review on central airway obstruction has recently been published.[24]

---

## Brief Illustrative Case

- *History:* 55-year-old woman with a 5-year history of progressive shortness of breath. Treated initially for adult-onset asthma with no relief of symptoms. Bronchoscopy revealed a subglottic stenosis 1.5 cm below vocal cords. No history of intubation, trauma, mediastinal mass, anti-neutrophil cytoplasmic antibody (ANCA) negative
- *Examination:* Vitals: HR, 60-70; BP, 120/68; respirations, 16/min; temp, 98.6° F, SPO$_2$, 99% (room air). Physical exam unremarkable and patient breathing comfortably at rest.
- *Imaging:* Chest radiograph normal, Chest CT imaging normal. Tracheal tomograms demonstrate subglottic stenosis 1.5 cm below vocal cords
- *Rigid Bronchoscopy:* Normal vocal cords, tight subglottic stenosis (5–7 mm) with sufficient distance below vocal cords to allow for resection. Distal tracheobronchial tree normal.
- *Management Idiopathic Tracheal Stenosis:* Patient serially dilated in the operating room with rigid bronchoscopes. Through a collar incision, tracheal resection and reconstruction performed with resection of anterior cricoid. Postoperative course unremarkable and patient discharged on postoperative day 7 following repeat bronchoscopy.

## References

 Interactive references and additional readings for this chapter can be accessed online at *expertconsult.com*.

# 12 TRACHEOESOPHAGEAL FISTULA

Christopher R. Morse, MD, Moishe Liberman, MD,
and Douglas J. Mathisen, MD

## *TERMINOLOGY*

**Acquired tracheoesophageal fistula** (TEF): Acquired communication between trachea and esophagus classified by etiology, site of fistula, and timing of onset

## *PATHOGENESIS*

### Iatrogenic
- Following esophageal resection
  - Anastomotic leakage
  - Following dilatation of esophagogastric anastomosis
  - With devascularization of trachea[1]
- Laryngectomy
- Esophageal dilation for benign stricture
- Esophageal/tracheal stenting
  - Secondary to erosion
  - Following difficult removal of existing esophageal or tracheal stent
- Following radiation therapy of esophageal or lung carcinomas

### Infectious
- Histoplasmosis/broncholiths
- Tuberculosis/granulomatous disease
  - Often limited to the membranous wall of the trachea[2]
- Immunodeficiency syndromes
  - Can lead to devastating necrotizing infections of the esophagus

### Malignancy
- Direct invasion by esophageal carcinoma
  - 78% of cases of malignant TEF secondary to esophageal carcinoma[3]
  - Located in the upper third of esophagus
  - Primarily squamous cell carcinoma
- Direct invasion by bronchogenic carcinoma or thyroid carcinoma
- Mediastinal Hodgkin's and non-Hodgkin's lymphoma

### Mechanical
- Prolonged ventilation
  - Pressure across membranous tracheal wall and esophagus secondary to cuff of endotracheal tube/tracheostomy and nasogastric tube
  - Circumferential damage to the trachea secondary to cuff injury
  - Often minimal contamination of the mediastinum as chronic process
- Esophageal foreign body

### Trauma
- Often with extensive mediastinal contamination

## *CLINICAL FEATURES*

### Symptoms and Signs
- Wide variety of signs and symptoms
- In patients on ventilator:
  - Significant increase in pulmonary secretions
  - Return of gastric feeds with suctioning of airway
  - Difficulty maintaining seal with cuff of endotracheal/tracheostomy tube
  - Development of pulmonary infiltrates and pneumonia
  - Distended abdomen on physical examination. This reflects gas insufflation of the entire gut due to positive pressure gas delivery by the ventilator (Fig. 12-1)
- Patients taking oral intake
  - In patients who are swallowing, violent coughing following oral intake is suggestive of fistula
  - Patients may expectorate food with cough
  - Occasionally hemoptysis
  - Fever and recurrent pneumonia
  - Important to distinguish direct communication (fistula) from aspiration

## *DIAGNOSTIC WORKUP*

### Radiographic Evaluation
- Chest radiograph
  - Initially normal in majority of cases but will develop a spectrum of findings associated with fistula
    - In patients on ventilator, chest radiograph often with dilatation of stomach and esophagus distal to fistula
    - Pulmonary infiltrates
    - Aspiration pneumonia
    - Adult respiratory distress syndrome
- Barium swallow
  - Preferable to use thin, dilute barium rather than hyperosmolar, water-soluble agents that can cause a severe pneumonitis (Fig. 12-2)
  - Barium swallow also useful in evaluating esophageal pathology
- Helical computed tomography scan
  - Seldom useful in the diagnosis of tracheoesophageal fistula
    - More helpful in characterizing and staging a underlying malignancy

### Endoscopy (Bronchoscopy and Esophagoscopy)
- Essential in the diagnosis and management of tracheoesophageal fistula
- Bronchoscopy most valuable to locate fistula and determine extent
  - In ventilated patients, flexible bronchoscopy can be performed through endotracheal tube (tube pulled back under direct vision) (Fig. 12-3)
  - Rigid bronchoscopy provides complete inspection of airway

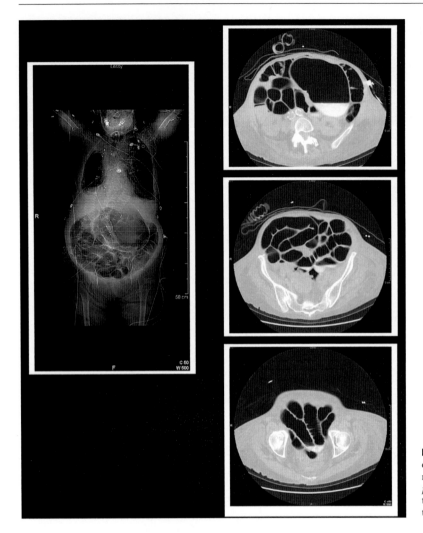

**Figure 12-1:** Computed tomography (CT) scout film of chest and abdomen/pelvis (*left panel*) and representative axial CT slices at varying levels (*right 3 panels*), showing gas dilated bowel throughout the gastrointestinal tract, in a patient with a tracheoesophageal fistula on mechanical ventilation.

- ○ Measurements should be taken of fistula and remaining normal airway (distance from the vocal cords to the TEF, diameter of the TEF, and the distance from the TEF to the carina). Documention of the measurements in the bronchoscopy note are important for future comparison and for evaluation of possible operative intervention (resection or stenting).
  - ○ Biopsies of membranous wall of the trachea should be performed if malignancy is suspected.
  - ○ Entire tracheobronchial tree to be examined and cultures sent to guide antibiotic therapy
  - ○ Tricks to identify the TEF: simultaneous bronchoscopy/esophagoscopy instill air, methylene blue
- ▪ Esophagoscopy may reveal fistula, but less reliable than bronchoscopy
  - ○ Difficult with smaller fistulas
  - ○ Bulky tumor in esophagus may make identification complex
  - ○ Essential in guiding any endoluminal interventions

## *TREATMENT*

### Initial Management
- ▪ Depends on variety of factors
  - ○ Location of fistula
  - ○ Etiology of fistula
  - ○ Degree of pulmonary contamination
  - ○ Need for ventilatory support
  - ○ Overall nutritional status of the patient

## Intervention
### *Benign Fistula-Patient Not Ventilated*
- ▪ Resolution of pulmonary issues and adequate nutritional reserve must be achieved
  - ○ Patient made NPO; enteral access obtained for feeding
  - ○ Antibiotic therapy for any pneumonia
- ▪ Single-stage repair often appropriate
  - ○ Principles include complete dissection of fistula, tension free closure of membranous wall of trachea and two layer closure of esophagus[4]
  - ○ Interposition of pedicled, healthy tissue between tracheal and esophageal suture lines (e.g., intercostal muscle flap, strap muscle)
- ▪ Exposure through variety of incisions
  - ○ Most often a low collar incision (incorporating tracheostomy)
  - ○ Left lateral neck incision anterior to sternocleidomastoid muscle
    - ▪ Both incisions can be extended to include an upper sternotomy if more exposure is required
    - ▪ Right posterolateral thoracotomy provides good exposure to distal trachea, carina, and esophagus, although it is rarely required.

### *Postintubation Tracheoesophageal Fistula*
- ▪ Before any corrective surgical intervention
  - ○ Cuff of endotracheal tube/tracheostomy tube positioned below fistula to minimize pulmonary contamination/soilage

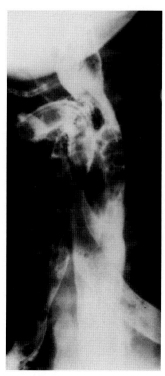

**Figure 12-2:** Barium swallow demonstrating a tracheoesophageal fistula with contrast filling both the esophagus and outlining the tracheobronchial tree.

○ Nasogastric tube is removed and gastrostomy tube placed to decompress stomach and reduce reflux
○ Jejeunostomy placed for enteral nutrition
○ Pulmonary contamination aggressively treated with a combination of pulmonary toilet, liberal bronchoscopy and antibiotic therapy
○ Nutritional status improved
■ Single-stage repair almost always possible
■ Tracheal resection may be required with circumferential tracheal damage (Fig. 12-4)
○ Trachea must not be devascularized
○ Trachea must come together without tension
○ Esophagus is closed in two layers
○ Healthy, pedicled tissue interposed between tracheal and esophageal suture lines (Fig. 12-5)
■ Results of repair benign fistula
○ Three large series composed of 78 patients[4-6]
■ 73 patients with single-stage closure
■ Forty-four of 73 with associated tracheal resection
■ Five esophageal diversions
■ Tracheoesophageal fistula recurred in approximately 7% of patients and mortality equals 9%

## Traumatic Tracheoesophageal Fistula
■ Extensive local contamination is often present
■ Management is determined by the patient's other medical problems
■ Low threshold for esophageal diversion (cervical esophagostomy)

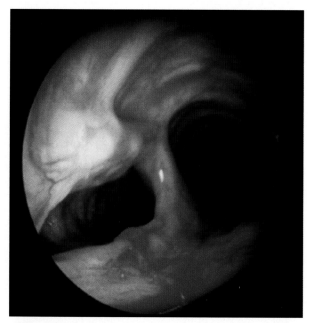

**Figure 12-3:** Bronchoscopic view of large, nonmalignant tracheoesophageal fistula encompassing the entire membranous wall of the trachea.

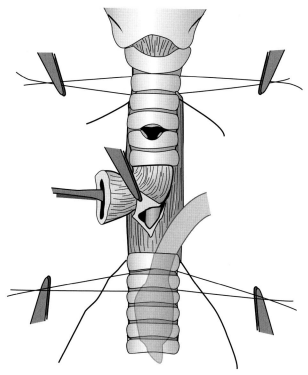

**Figure 12-4:** The most common cause of nonmalignant tracheoesophageal fistula is erosion by tracheostomy tubes or endotracheal tube cuffs that press against an in-lying, hard nasogastric tube. With circumferential tracheal damage, the injured tracheal segment is resected, along with the esophageal fistula. Here, the trachea is divided and the fistula exposed.

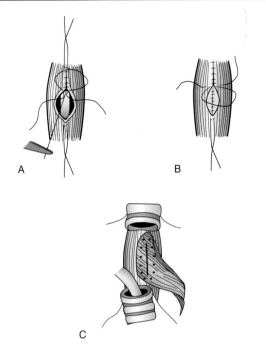

**Figure 12-5:** The esophagus is closed in two layers with fine interrupted sutures and a pedicled muscle flap placed over the esophageal repair before completion of the tracheal anastomosis.

### *Tracheoesophageal Fistula Following Esophageal Resection*

- Managed based on size, location, cause, and extent of mediastinal contamination
- Options include conservative management, buttressed repair, and takedown of neoesophagus and diversion

### *Necrotizing Esophagitis and Tracheoesophageal Fistula*

- Most often requires esophagectomy

### *Malignant Tracheoesophageal Fistula*

- Palliative stenting
  - Useful with incurable malignancies (esophageal, tracheal, bronchogenic carcinoma)
    - Prevents ongoing pulmonary contamination
    - Restores swallowing
    - May require airway stenting, esophageal stenting, or a combination of both
    - Esophageal stents migrate unless a stricture at the site of the TEF holds the stent in place
- Operative intervention
  - Airway and esophageal resections with primary anastomosis and muscle flap
  - Esophageal diversion (cervical esophagostomy, oversew the proximal thoracic esophagus, stapling of the gastroesophageal junction, and gastrostomy).
  - Operations are rarely advised because the mortality rates are high (25%–50%), patients' prognoses are poor, and stenting options with low morbidity and mortality are available

RESULTS OF TREATMENT OF MALIGNANT TRACHEOESOPHAGEAL FISTULA

- Burt et al. found 5-week survival in patients receiving all modes of therapy,[3] with pulmonary sepsis as the primary cause of death in 80%

- Many different stents have been available over the years (going back to the Celestine tube), but, currently, expandable, covered metallic stents are usually used.
- Ross and colleagues placed self-expanding metal stents (SEMS) in 97 patients, 22 with malignant TEFs. They reported improvement in symptoms in 90% of patients with a mean survival of 72 days[7]

---

**KEY POINTS**

- Variety of causes including benign, malignant, and infectious.
- Repair often not emergent and attempts to wean the patient from the ventilator (if necessary) as well as improving nutritional status should be pursued.
- With benign tracheoesophageal fistulas, single-stage repair often possible by maintaining the principles of complete dissection of fistula, tension-free closure of membranous wall of trachea, two-layer closure of esophagus and tissue interposition between the two suture lines.
- Malignant tracheoesophageal fistulas are often managed with stenting, and palliative surgical procedures are rarely pursed.

---

## Brief Illustrative Case

- *History:* 65 year-old man involved in motor vehicle accident (MVA) with prolonged intubation. Tracheostomy performed following 2 weeks of endotracheal intubation. Three weeks following tracheostomy, tube feeding identified on blind endotracheal suctioning. Patient had both a postpyloric Dobhoff feeding tube and a nasogastric tube for gastric drainage
- *Examination:* Vitals: Heart rate, 70–80; blood pressure, 120/68; Pressure control ventilation. Physical examination remarkable for decreased breath sounds bilaterally and a slightly distended abdomen.
- *Imaging:* Chest radiograph with distended stomach bubble, air-filled distal esophagus, and bilateral pulmonary infiltrates.
- *Flexible Bronchoscopy:* Tracheostomy tube pulled back and membranous wall of the trachea at the level of the cuff with significant inflammation and a small 1-cm × 1.5-cm defect noted. Circumferential inflammation of the trachea at the level of the fistula.
- *Flexible Esophagoscopy:* Significant inflammation noted in the proximal esophagus, with small defect noted in the wall of the esophagus. Remainder of the esophagus and stomach normal.
- *Initial Management:* Patient brought to the operating room, where more extensive measurements were made of the airway and fistula with a rigid bronchoscope. Repeat esophagoscopy was performed. A longer, custom tracheostomy tube was placed, with the cuff below the level of the fistula. A draining gastrostomy tube and a feeding jejunostomy tube were placed. Both the Dobhoff feeding tube and nasogastric tube were removed.

- *Definitive Management:* The patient was weaned from mechanical ventilation and remained strict NPO. When his nutrition was adequately improved, he was brought back to the operating room. Through a low, transverse collar incision, the fistula was exposed and completely dissected. A short, segmental tracheal resection was performed and the esophagus closed in layers. Strap muscle from the neck was interposed between the suture lines. His diet was eventually advanced and both the gastrostomy and jejunostomy tubes were removed.

## References

 Interactive references and additional readings for this chapter can be accessed online at *expertconsult.com*.

# 13 TRACHEAL MASSES

Christopher R. Morse, MD, Moishe Liberman, MD, and Douglas J. Mathisen, MD

## *TERMINOLOGY*

- Benign tracheal neoplasms
- Tracheal neoplasms

## *ETIOLOGY*

### Etiology—Key Facts

Squamous cell carcinoma and adenoid cystic carcinoma compose the majority of malignant tracheal neoplasms

### Malignant

- Squamous cell carcinoma
  - Approximately 40% of malignant tracheal neoplasms[1]
  - Can present as either an exophitic or ulcerative lesion and may occur anywhere in the trachea or bronchial tree
  - May invade adjacent structures (recurrent laryngeal nerve/esophagus), but distant metastasis are rare early in presentation
  - Associated with tobacco abuse
- Adenoid cystic carcinoma
  - Approximately 40% of malignant tracheal neoplasms[1]
  - Formally known as a cylindroma
  - May present as a mass in the trachea but may extend significant distances within the submucosa
  - Extremely radiosensitive, and positive margins following surgery are treated with postoperative radiotherapy
  - Can present in any age range and not associated with smoking
- Other primary malignant tracheal masses (rare)[2]
  - Adenocarcinoma
  - Adenosquamous carcinoma
  - Small cell carcinoma
  - Basaloid squamous cell carcinoma
  - Atypical carcinoid
  - Malignant fibrous histiocytoma
  - Melanoma
  - Chondrosarcoma
  - Spindle cell sarcoma
  - Rhabdomyosarcoma
  - Fibrosarcoma
  - Leiomyosarcoma
  - Kaposi's sarcoma
  - Lymphoma
  - Lymphoepithelial carcinoma
  - Angiosarcoma
  - Invasive thyroid carcinoma
  - Invasive esophageal carcinoma

### Benign

- Benign squamous papilloma
- Multiple solitary pleomorphic adenoma
- Granular cell tumor (myoblastoma)
- Glomus tumor
- Fibroma
- Fibrous histiocytoma (pseudotumor, plasma cell granuloma, xanthoma)
- Lipoma
- Leiomyoma
- Hamartoma
- Chondroma
- Chondroblastoma
- Schwannoma
- Neurofibroma
- Paraganglioma
- Hemangioma
- Hemangioendothelioma
- Vascular malformation

## *CLINICAL FEATURES*

- Symptoms and Signs:
  - Initially, patients often present with a long history of coughing progressing to wheezing. They are frequently treated for adult onset asthma or chronic obstructive pulmonary disease before the diagnosis of a tracheal mass.
  - Wheezing can progress to stridor as the caliber of the airway continues to narrow. Chest radiographs will often continue to demonstrate clear lung fields. Chest tomograms will occasionally reveal the tracheal mass.
  - Hemoptysis is a late finding and more often occurs with squamous cell carcinoma than adenoid cystic carcinoma.
  - With low lesions abutting the carina, postobstructive pneumonia can occur and needs to be evaluated with bronchoscopy
  - Late findings in the course of tracheal tumors are increasing hoarseness from invasion of the recurrent laryngeal nerves and dysphagia from esophageal invasion or compression.

## *DIAGNOSIS*

- History
  - Important components of the history include
    - Cough
    - Progressive shortness of breath
    - Progressive dyspnea
    - Wheezing unresponsive to bronchodilators
    - Hemoptysis
    - Recurrent pneumonia/pneumonitis
    - Change in voice/increasing hoarseness
    - Dysphagia
    - Thoracic/cervical malignancies
      - Lung
      - Esophageal
      - Thyroid
      - Parathyroid
      - Laryngeal
      - Squamous cell carcinoma of the head and neck
      - Carcinoid tumor
- Physical examination
  - Confirm airway patency
  - Ensure that trachea is midline
  - Bilateral breath sounds
  - Pulmonary auscultation
  - Tracheal auscultation
  - Head and neck exam including:
    - Thyroid examination
    - Cervical lymph nodes, masses
    - Palpate tracheal rings, thyroid and cricoid cartilages
    - Jugular venous distention
    - Oral and pharyngeal exam
- Radiographic evaluation:
  - Plain chest radiograph
    - Normal in majority of patients
    - Often leads to continuation of current therapy (i.e., bronchodilators), rather than guiding intervention to look for tracheal mass
  - Helical computed tomography (CT) scan
    - Occasionally will demonstrate a tracheal mass. Addition of high-resolution CT images with thin cuts and three-dimensional and multiplanar two-dimensional reconstructions increases sensitivity and specificity (Fig. 13-1)
    - Assists with staging of malignancy
    - Virtual bronchoscopy further provides imaging of the trachea and tracheobronchial tree but does not allow for intervention or diagnostic biopsy (see Fig. 13-1)
  - Bronchoscopy
    - Essential in the diagnosis and management of tracheal masses (Fig. 13-2)
    - Flexible bronchoscopy adequate
      - If performed through an endotracheal tube, the tube must be pulled back and the airway examined from the level of the vocal cords
    - Rigid bronchoscopy with general anesthesia superior to flexible bronchoscopy
      - Allows for better visualization of anatomy
      - Superior biopsy specimens
      - Potential for airway management and improvement through maneuvers such as dilatation
    - If imaging suggests a focal lesion amenable to resection, bronchoscopy can be deferred until general anesthesia when resection planned
  - Upper gastrointestinal endoscopy
    - Essential in the management of a squamous cell cancer of the trachea as essential to rule out a synchronous lesion of the esophagus
  - Pulmonary function tests
    - Not of significant value

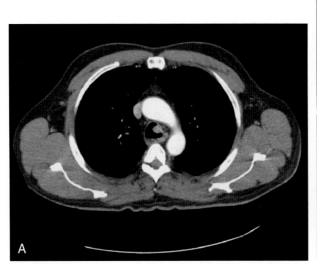

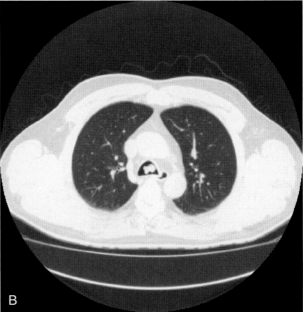

**Figure 13-1:** Computed tomography scans demonstrating tracheal papilloma. **A** and **B,** axial views.

*(Continued)*

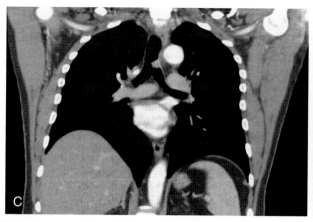

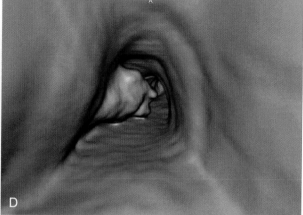

**Figure 13-1—cont'd: C,** coronal reconstruction; **D,** virtual bronchoscopy.

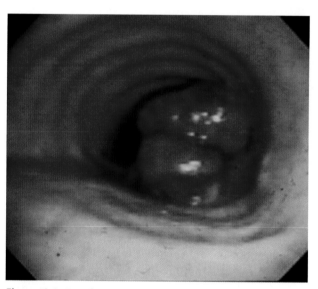

**Figure 13-2:** Bronchoscopic view of tracheal squamous cell carcinoma.

- Despite the baseline pulmonary function of a specific patient, all patients will benefit from relief of central airway obstruction

## TREATMENT

- Surgery
  - With current techniques of tracheal resection and reconstruction, surgery is recommended if primary intervention is for resectable lesions.
    - Must be able to resect the lesion, reconstructing the trachea primarily, without tension (Fig. 13-3)
    - Will occasionally sacrifice a recurrent laryngeal nerve to complete an on block resection of the tumor
    - Radical resection difficult given limitations to amount of trachea that can be resected and limitations with lateral margins (Fig. 13-4)
  - Principal contraindications to surgery include
    - Extensive linear involvement of the airway such that primary end-to-end resection would not be possible without excessive tension

    - Mediastinal invasion of nonresectable organs
    - Remote metastases
  - Rarely, palliative resection may be used with adenoid cystic carcinoma (ACC) or differentiated thyroid carcinoma, to remove a potentially obstructing lesion even in the face of pulmonary metastases[3]
- Surgical results
  - In a large Massachusetts General Hospital (MGH) series of 270 patients with ACC or squamous cell carcinoma (SCC) (135 each), 191 (71%) were resected and 79 were not resected for a variety of reasons.
    - Five and 10-year survival rates in patients with resected ACC was 52% and 29% (unresectable 33% and 10%), and in resected SCC, 39% and 18% (unresectable 7.3% and 4.9%)[4]
  - Pearson reported 29 resections in 44 patients with primary tracheal tumors. Nine patients with ACC were alive at 1 to 20 years, three died of other causes. four of six patients with SCC were alive 6 to 56 years following resection[5]
- Radiation therapy
  - Almost all patients receive postoperative radio-therapy.
  - With ACC, positive margins occasionally have to be accepted to adequately reconstruct trachea
  - Survival appears to be superior with resection followed by radiotherapy versus radiotherapy alone[4]
  - Primary radiotherapy for SCC and ACC of the trachea in doses from 4000 to 6000 cGy have been demonstrated to be ineffective in obtaining local control[6]
- Postoperative care
  - Following a tracheal resection, all patients have a guardian suture to maintain neck flexion.
  - The patient is placed in the intensive care unit overnight for airway monitoring, then he or she is moved to regular floor on postoperative day 1.
  - Patients are kept NPO, with diet advanced slowly over several days.
  - Warm, humidified oxygen helps mobilize secretions.
  - Vomiting is avoided by the use of antiemetics.
  - Repeat bronchoscopy on postoperative day 7.
  - If stridor develops at anytime postoperatively, the patient needs to be emergently evaluated and to undergo bronchoscopy.
- Complications
  - Although anastomotic complications are rare, edema, granulation tissue, and complete separation of the anastomosis are all potentially adverse outcomes.

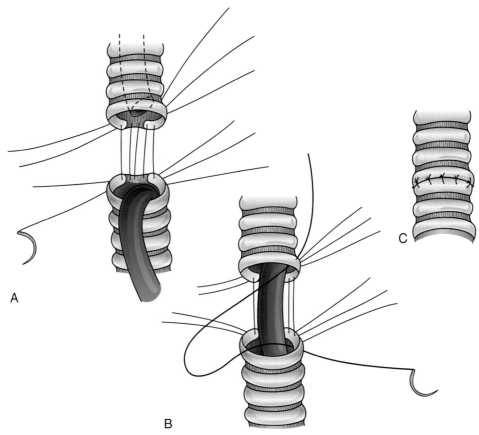

**Figure 13-3:** Tracheal resection with the tracheal mass resected and crossfield ventilation being used in the distal trachea (**A**). After the anastomotic sutures have been placed, the endotracheal tube is advanced across the anastomosis (**B**). The completed anastomosis with the trachea coming together under no tension (**C**).

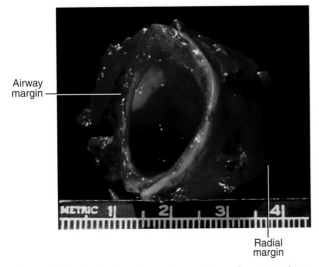

Airway margin

Radial margin

**Figure 13-4:** Tracheal specimen demonstrating the gross airway margin, limited by the amount of trachea that can be resected and the radial margin, limited by vital structures. Occasionally a recurrent laryngeal nerve will be scarified to complete an on block resection of the tumor.

   ○ With an unstable airway, the patients should be intubated from above with a small endotracheal tube and with bronchoscopic assistance.
   ○ With a stable airway, a CT scan of the neck may be obtained to look for extraluminal air and fluid collections

   ○ Bronchoscopy can then be performed to evaluate the anastomosis.
   ○ It is rare that an anastomotic separation can be repaired primarily, and the anastomosis is best managed by either a T-tube or tracheostomy.

---

**KEY POINTS**

- Almost all tracheal neoplasms are composed of either SCC or ACC.
- A high index of suspicion is needed in patients with wheezing or stridor that is unresponsive to bronchodilators.
- Tracheal resection is feasible in patients with short-segment lesions, no metastatic disease, and no local invasion.
- Tracheal resection should be performed in an experienced high volume center.

---

## Brief Illustrative Case

- *History:* A 32-year-old woman with 3-year history of chronic cough and shortness of breath with exertion. Treated with bronchodilator therapy, with no improvement of symptoms.

- *Examination:* Vitals: Heart rate 80 bpm; BP 120/68; respirations 16/min; temp: 98° F, SPO$_2$ 99% (room air). Physical examination unremarkable
- *Blood tests:* Complete blood count and electrolytes- normal
- *Imaging:* Chest radiograph with clear lung fields, no tracheal deviation. Contrast CT scan of the neck and chest unremarkable, with question of a filling defect in the proximal trachea.
- *Flexible Bronchoscopy:* Focal mass noted 2 cm below the vocal cords, approximately 2 cm in length. Partially obstructing (<50% of circumference). Biopsy demonstrated adenoid cystic carcinoma.
- *Surgery:* Patient brought to operating room, rigid bronchoscopy performed to further delineate lesion, deemed resectable. Four centimeters of trachea resected with primary anastomosis. Microscopically positive margins.

- *Postoperative course:*
- Discharged from hospital on postoperative day 7 following flexible bronchoscopy to evaluate anastomosis.
- Postoperative radiation therapy planned. Extremely radiosensitive tumor.

## References

 Interactive references and additional readings for this chapter can be accessed online at *expertconsult.com*.

# DISORDERS OF THE LUNG

## 14 CONGENITAL AND DEVELOPMENTAL LUNG MALFORMATIONS

Tina T. Ng, MD, Michael I. Lewis, MD, and Steve C. Chen, MD

### KEY WORDS

- Pulmonary agenesis
- Pulmonary hypoplasia
- Congenital pulmonary arteriovenous malformation
- Congenital cystic adenomatoid malformation (CCAM)
- Pulmonary sequestration
- Bronchogenic cyst
- Congenital lobar emphysema (CLE)
- Swyer-James syndrome (SJS)

### EMBRYOLOGY OF LUNG

#### Stages of Lung Development

- Embryonic period (0 to 7th weeks): lung bud branches off from the embryo's primitive foregut.[1]
- Pseudoglandular period (8th to 16th weeks): conducting airways form with differentiation including blood supply and mucus glands.
- Cannalicular period (17th to 24th weeks): gas exchange units form including terminal bronchioles, alveolar ducts, and alveoli.
- Terminal sac period (25th weeks to term): gas exchange units increase in number along with alveolar capillaries and differentiate into type I and II alveoli.

### PULMONARY AGENESIS

- **Definition: Pulmonary agenesis or aplasia** is complete absence of one or both bronchi in which the lung tissue also fails to develop.
- Bilateral disease is a rare condition with only few cases described in literature.
- Unilateral disease is reported with higher incidence.
- Commonly associated with multiple anomalies, frequently cardiac malformation.
- Chest usually appears symmetric, although the trachea and mediastinum are deviated to the affected side.
- Lung function is impaired by agenesis.
- There can be severe respiratory distress if the normal lung is further impaired by infection, atelectasis, or immaturity.

- Radiographic features:
  - Plain radiography: defective side is opacified; remaining lung extends across the midline to the contralateral chest.
  - Computed tomography (CT) scan, echocardiography: only one bronchus and one pulmonary artery.

### PULMONARY HYPOPLASIA

- **Definition: Pulmonary hypoplasia** is low-volume lung development resulting in small lung size and low ratio of lung-to-body weight. There is also decreased number of bronchial generations and alveoli number.
- The hypoplastic lung is seen in association with other congenital anomalies that take up space in the chest, such as congenital diaphragmatic hernia or eventration and lung malformations.
- Pulmonary hypertension and persistent fetal circulation may be presenting clinical conditions that require intensive respiratory support.
- Radiographic features: similar to those of pulmonary aplasia.

### PULMONARY ARTERIOVENOUS MALFORMATIONS

#### Definition and Epidemiology

- An arteriovenous malformation (AVM) is an anomalous direct communication between the pulmonary artery and vein.[2,3]
- Connection vessels are thin walled and resemble aneurysmal sacs that can rupture.
- The male-to-female ratio is 1:2; it is a rare condition (about 4 cases/year at a large academic center).[4]
- Peak age of presentation: 4th to 6th decades of life (90% identified in adults).

#### Pathobiology

- Most cases are congenital in nature. Approximately 70% to 90% are associated with hereditary hemorrhagic telangiectasia (HHT; also called Osler-Weber-Rendu disease). HHT is an autosomal dominant condition associated with gene mutations for ALK-1, a member of the tumor growth factor (TGF) β-1 superfamily of receptors, and endogolin.[5] However, the precise pathobiology remains unknown. Note: In patients with HHT, pulmonary AVMs are found in 15% to 30%.

■ A third of patients have multiple lesions, with bilateral lesions in a quarter.[4,6] AVMs are located in the lower lobes in more than 50% and vary in size from 1 cm to giant 10-cm lesions. Diffuse microvascular lesions are rare.

■ Classified morphologically as simple (single sac with single feeding vessel; 70%), complex (>1 feeding vessel), or multiple-type lesion (multichannel plexiform mass). Occasionally, a saccular tortuous connection. A rare presentation is a profusion of pulmonary AVMs throughout one or both lungs. This is termed diffuse or telangiectatic variety.

■ Histology reveals a single layer of lining endothelial cells.

■ Natural history is to slowly enlarge over time.

## Clinical Features

■ Classic triad: dyspnea on exertion, cyanosis, and clubbing of the fingers. This triad is no longer a common feature on more recent series.

■ Epistaxis, related to associated HHT, is a common feature. This becomes manifest many years before clinical presentation of pulmonary AVMs per se.

■ Exertional dyspnea is common (>50% of symptomatic cases). *Mechanisms include*: hypoxemia with right-to-left shunting,

high-output cardiac decompensation and, occasionally, the development of pulmonary arterial hypertension.[7,8]

■ Platypnea (increase in dyspnea when upright) and orthodeoxia (increase in desaturation in the upright posture) has been described, owing to increased blood flow and shunting when upright.

■ Bruits, which are loudest on inspiration and over dependent regions, can occasionally be heard arising from underlying AVMs.

■ Hemoptysis complicates about 12% of cases and can be massive.

■ Hemothorax described due to rupture of pleural AVMs.

■ Mucocutaneous telangiectasia noted in patients with HHT

## Diagnosis

■ Imaging:
  ○ *Plain chest radiograph*: well-defined round or oval, sometimes lobulated, lesion. Feeding vessel shadow or shadows (linear, curvilinear) and draining vein may be seen.
  ○ *CT scan*: ultrafast contrast CT and noncontrast helical CT with three-dimensional reconstruction are sensitive tests used to detect feeding vessels and AVM morphology, and are the procedures of choice (Fig. 14-1).[9,10]
  ○ *Magnetic resonance imaging (MRI):* a variety of MRI techniques are sensitive and specific for detecting AVMs and feeding vessels larger than 5 mm and 3 mm respectively.[11,12]

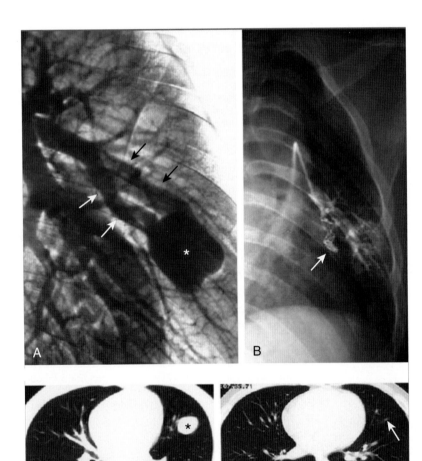

**Figure 14-1:** A series of figures related to diagnosis and treatment of a solitary pulmonary AVM. **A,** Original pulmonary angiogram showing large atrioventricuar malformation (AVM) (*) in the lingula with feeding vessel (*white arrows*) and draining vein (*black arrows*) well depicted. **B,** Follow-up angiogram following successful deployment of several occluding coils. **C,** Computed tomography (CT) scan depicting same lesion (*) before intervention. **D,** Follow-up CT scan 11 years later confirming long-lasting efficacy of initial coiling intervention. (*From Remy-Jardin M, Dumont P, Pierre-Yves B, Dupuis P, Duhamel A, Remy J. Pulmonary arteriovenous malformations treated with embolotherapy: helical CT evaluation of long-standing effectiveness after 2-21 year follow-up. Radiology 2006;239:576-585.*)

○ *Lung perfusion scan:* can show uptake systemically over the brain and kidney.[13]
○ *Conventional pulmonary angiography:* can delineate the AVM, together with a therapeutic intervention (see later) (see Fig. 14-1)
▪ **Echo:** *Contrast bubble study* shows contrast in left atrium after three to eight cardiac cycles
▪ **Shunt study:** 100% oxygen study detects an elevated shunt fraction in the majority of patients (sensitivity 87.5%).[14]

### Treatment

Treatment should be considered in all symptomatic cases, as well as in asymptomatic patients with sizable AVMs (>20 mm) or large feeding vessels (>3 mm).

#### Percutaneous Embolization Approach

▪ Employs conventional selective angiography to visualize AVM and to deploy either coils, balloons, or polyvinyl alcohol wool coils to obstruct the feeding vessel or vessels and is the procedure of choice (see Fig. 14-1).[15]
▪ More limited experience in children.[16]
▪ Multiple AVMs can be embolized at a single session or in serial sessions.
▪ Immediate impact on gas exchange and symptoms can occur.
▪ Procedure of choice, particularly with multiple AVMs, AVMs in multiple lobes, and bilateral disease.
▪ Large and complex lesions may be technically chal-lenging.
▪ Microvascular diffuse AVMs are not amenable.
▪ Air embolism, pulmonary infarction, and balloon migration can rarely complicate the procedure.
▪ Effects of embolotherapy can be long-lasting (see Fig. 14-1)

#### Surgical Approach

▪ Rarely performed electively in adults
▪ May be required with failed attempts at embolization; with a single large, often complex, or plexiform tangle; or in emergent cases.
▪ A variety of ligation and resectional procedures may be required.

### Complications

▪ Neurologic
○ Occur in up to 40%.
○ Stroke, transient ischemic attack, and brain abscess are likely secondary to paradoxical embolism.
○ Seizure, migraine
▪ Cardiovascular:
○ Pulmonary arterial hypertension (HHT).
○ High-output cardiac failure
▪ Respiratory:
○ Massive hemoptysis
○ Massive hemothorax

## CONGENITAL CYSTIC ADENOMATOID MALFORMATION

▪ **Definition:** A CCAM is considered a hamartomatous lesion of the lung with excessive proliferation of the bronchial structures with alveoli.[17] CCAMs are connected to the tracheobronchial tree because the conducting airways have already formed.

▪ As described by Stocker, lesions are classified based on the appearance of the cysts according to the size and shape.[18,19]
○ Type I (70%): single or multiple large cysts larger than 2 cm in diameter without adenomatoid tissue.
○ Type II (20%): mixture of intermediate sized cysts between 0.5 cm and 2 cm in diameter with some adenomatoid tissue.
○ Type III (10%): multiple small cysts less than 0.5 cm in diameter, almost solid like with predominately adenomatoid tissue.
▪ Most patients are diagnosed prenatally with antenatal care. Development of hydrops fetalis, which is essentially fetal congestive heart failure, is a poor prognostic sign.
▪ Newborns typically present with poor feeding, respiratory distress, or recurrent pneumonias.[20]
▪ Pulmonary hypoplasia and mediastinal shift are frequently presented.
▪ Prognosis: related to the lesion's size and the compression on the remaining lung.
○ Type I CCAMs have good prognosis.
○ Type II and III lesions have mortality rate greater than 50%.
▪ Radiographic features:
○ Prenatal ultrasound (US): detects CCAM as early as the 12th to 14th week of intrauterine life; distinguishes type I lesion from other CCAMs.
○ Plain radiography: single or multicystic structure.
○ CT scan: highlights lung markings and septations within cystic lesion (Fig. 14-2).

## PULMONARY SEQUESTRATION

### Definitions

▪ Sequestration refers to nonfunctioning lung tissue that has no connection to the tracheobronchial tree and that receives its blood supply from a systemic artery.[21,22]
▪ *Intralobar sequestration* (75%–90%):
○ Abnormal tissue within the lung parenchyma with no separate visceral pleural lining.

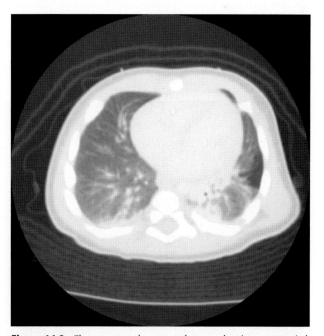

**Figure 14-2:** Chest computed tomography scan showing a congenital cystic adenomatoid malformation in the left side of the chest.

○ Arterial supply typically arises from the aorta; venous drainage is via the pulmonary vein or azygos vein (see below for more details).[23]
■ Extralobar sequestration (10%–25%):
  ○ Abnormal tissue has its own separate visceral pleural lining and therefore is separate from the normal lung
    ■ The arterial supply typically arises from the aorta; venous drainage is mainly into systemic veins.[23]

## Epidemiology

■ Low prevalence: 0.15% to 6.4% of congenital lung malformations.[21]
■ No gender preference for intralobar; male dominance for extralobar.
■ Intralobar: presents in patients older than age 20 in 50%, but can present in patients from infancy to 65 years.[24]
■ Extralobar usually presents in early childhood

## Pathobiology

■ Intralobar sequestration:
  ○ May be congenital (a branch of the developing bronchial tree becomes cut off and retains its systemic blood supply) or acquired (bronchial obstruction with repeated infection and parasitization of hypertrophied systemic vessels to maintain viability of the segment).
  ○ Histology reveals normal lung elements but with the added presence of inflammation, cysts, and fibrosis
  ○ Blood supply details: lower thoracic aorta: 75%; abdominal aorta: 20%; intercostal artery: 5%. Note: multiple vessels in 16% to 32%.[25] Venous drainage is into pulmonary veins. Rarely into systemic veins (e.g., azygos, inferior vena cava, superior vena cava, intercostals, and so on).
■ Extralobar sequestration:
  ○ Congenital in origin
  ○ Associated abnormalities include diaphragm disorders (eventration, congenital hernia), congenital heart disease, congenital vertebral disorders, and so on.
  ○ Although mainly in the thorax, it can be situated within or below the diaphragm. Extrapulmonary sequestrations in the retroperitoneum have also been reported.

**Note:** Distinguishing feature: anomalous vascular supply (Fig. 14-3).

## Clinical Features

■ Diagnosis is often missed. In a large cohort of patients with intralobar sequestration (n = 540), the diagnosis was not included in the differential diagnosis in half of the patients.[22]
■ Can be an incidental finding (15%–20%) on imaging studies with patient asymptomatic
■ Cough with or without sputum, pleuritic chest pain
■ Episodes of recurrent pneumonia (transmission of organisms through the pores of Kohn)
■ Hemoptysis
■ Extrapulmonary sequestration: often presents with respiratory distress or feeding intolerance early in life, recurrent pneumonia, or complications of associated congenital anomalies, especially diaphragmatic hernia.

## Diagnosis
## Imaging: Intralobar Sequestration[26]

■ Plain chest radiograph:
  ○ Mass lesion in lower lobes. Two thirds on the left (posterior basal segment most common location; next medial basal segment)
  ○ Can be cystic
■ CT scan:
  ○ Mass lesion containing tissue and cystic elements (often opacified) (Fig. 14-4)
  ○ CT angiogram commonly demonstrates systemic arterial supply. Note: failure to visualize does not exclude the diagnosis.
  ○ Air-fluid levels or air within the mass may be seen.[27] The mechanism likely reflects the development of some bronchial connections.
■ MRI:
  ○ Similar to CT
  ○ $T_2$-weighted images best
  ○ Hemorrhage within the lesion produces a higher signal
■ Conventional angiogram:
  ○ Replaced now by CT

## Imaging: Extralobar Sequestration

■ Ninety percent are located on the left side (Fig. 14-5).
■ Imaging can identify associated abnormalities.
■ CT with or without MRI is the procedures of choice.

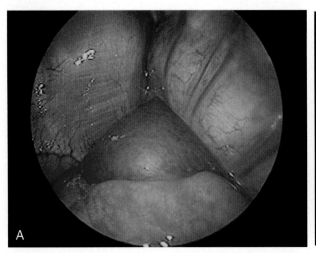 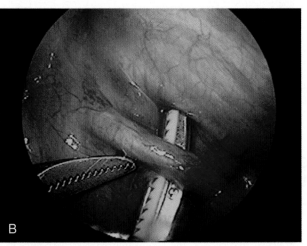

**Figure 14-3: A,** An operative view of a pulmonary sequestration mass (*center*). **B,** Pulmonary sequestration lesion and its anomalous vascular pedicle (as defined by the instruments).

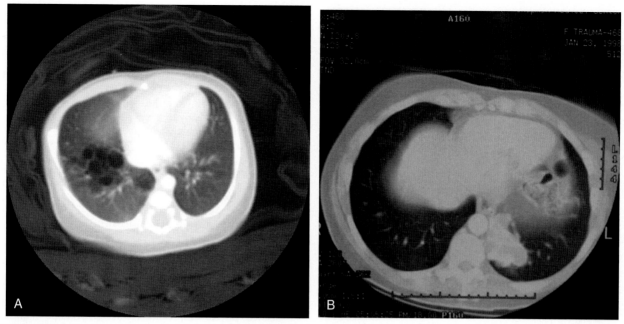

**Figure 14-4:** **A,** Computed tomography (CT) scan of the chest of a young patient with intralobar pulmonary sequestration. Note the unusual location of the lesion in this patient. **B,** CT scan of the chest depicting the more classic location of an intralobar pulmonary sequestration (posterior segment of left lower lobe).

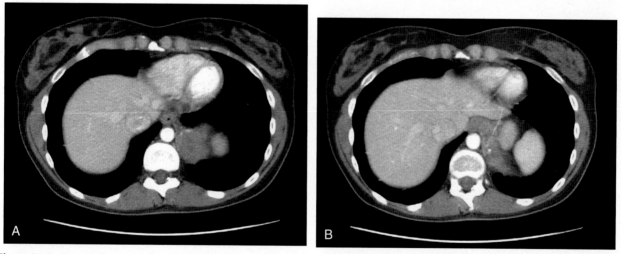

**Figure 14-5:** Computed tomography scan depicting an extralobar pulmonary sequestration. The lesion appears to arise from the region of the diaphragm (**A** and **B**). The feeding vessel of systemic origin (likely aorta) is well depicted in **B.**

## Surgical Treatment

- Intralobar sequestration:
  - The anatomic location of arterial supply (single or multiple) should always be identified before surgical resection to avoid massive hemorrhagic complications.
  - Lobectomy is usually indicated, because the sequestration usually crosses segmental divisions.
  - Resection is indicated for hemoptysis or history of recurrent infection.
  - In asymptomatic patients, surgery is usually recommended to prevent future infections.
- Extralobar sequestration
  - Resection is indicated when symptomatic.
  - If an incidental finding and asymptomatic, can follow. Some advocate resection

## BRONCHOGENIC CYST

- **Definition: Bronchogenic cyst** is an abnormal, generally noncommunicating tissue arising from aberrant budding of the foregut.[28] The histologic characteristics are much like foregut duplication cysts and can include smooth muscle, cartilage, and glands.
- Lesion is located centrally in the mediastinum or pulmonary hilum or peripherally, such as the abdomen.[29]
- Symptoms can present anytime in life:
  - Respiratory distress from airway compromise.
  - Dysphagia due to compression on the esophagus.
  - Infection secondary to abnormal mucus secretion drainage.
- Radiographic features:
  - Plain radiography (Fig. 14-6)

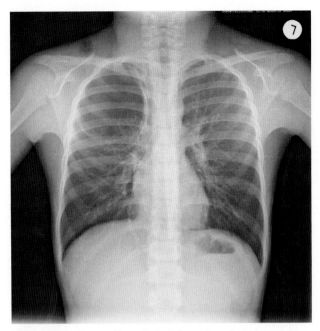

**Figure 14-6:** Chest radiograph depicting a large bronchogenic cyst, which fills up the right upper chest.

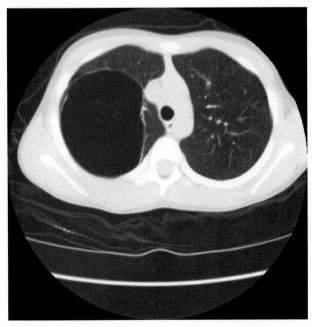

**Figure 14-7:** A chest computed tomography scan highlights the cystic structure of a bronchogenic cyst shown in Figure 14-6.

- Solid mass.
- Cystic structure with air-fluid levels if the lesion communicates with the esophagus.
  ○ CT scan delineates cystic structure and provides definitive diagnosis (Fig. 14-7).

## CONGENITAL LOBAR EMPHYSEMA

- **Definition:** CLE is a condition in which the lung has an over-distension of one lobe, resulting in compression and atelectasis of remaining lung and possibly the contralateral lung by mediastinal shift. The etiology may be due to failure of cartilage

development in the bronchus, leading to collapse and air trapping like a ball-valve effect.[30]
- Commonly affected locations are the left upper or the right middle lobe.[31]
- Two main pathologic subtypes:
  ○ Congenital lobar overinflation involves markedly dilated alveoli.
  ○ Polyalveolar lobes have increased number of alveoli.
- Symptoms present early in life:
  ○ Poor feeding, coughing, tachypnea, cyanosis
  ○ Respiratory distress, rapidly progressing to respiratory failure
- CLE may present like tension pneumothorax, but chest tube placement can be catastrophic; emergent thoracotomy with lobectomy is necessary.
- High incidence of cardiac anomalies.
- Bronchoscopy shows site of cartilage deficiency.
- Radiographic features[32]:
  ○ Prenatal US, prenatal MRI: hyperinflated portion of lung.
  ○ Plain radiography: hyperinflated, hyperlucent lung portion.
  ○ CT chest: distinguishes from other lung cysts.
  ○ Ventilation-perfusion (VQ) scan: poor perfusion and delayed uptake and clearance of radioisotope indicate affected lung portion.

## SWYER-JAMES SYNDROME
### Definition
- SJS was first described in 1953 by Swyer and James[33] in a 6-year-old child as unilateral pulmonary emphysema (unilateral hyperlucent lung) associated with a small pulmonary artery. Also called MacLeod syndrome (nine patients reported in 1954).[34]

### Pathogenesis
- SJS is thought to be the end result of a postinfectious insult culminating in obliteration of small airways, parenchymal destructive changes, and decrease in vascularity.
- Adenoviral infection in infancy is implicated. Other organisms include measles, pertussis, and mycoplasma.
- Bronchiolitis occurring in early childhood impairs lung development, resulting in a small affected lung. Bronchiolitis occurring in late childhood may be associated with a normal size lung.
- Ongoing recurrent infection can produce bronchiectatic changes proximal to the bronchiolitis obliterans

### Clinical Features
- Dyspnea on effort[35,36]
- Chronic productive cough
- Hemoptysis
- Wheezes
- Recurrent lower respiratory tract infections
- Can be complicated by pulmonary hypertension[37]
- Rarely asymptomatic
- Pulmonary function studies often reveal combined obstructive and restrictive ventilatory defects.

### Imaging
- Plain chest radiograph (Fig. 14-8)
  ○ Hyperlucency: unilateral, lobar, and rarely, bilateral
  ○ Lung size on inspiration: reduced or normal with mediastinal shift to affected side
  ○ Expiration: evidence of air trapping on affected side.

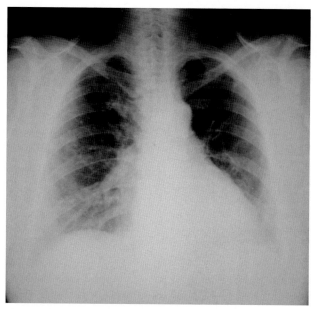

**Figure 14-8:** Swyer-James syndrome: Chest radiograph depicting left lung hyperlucency and decreased pulmonary vasculature (left hilum).

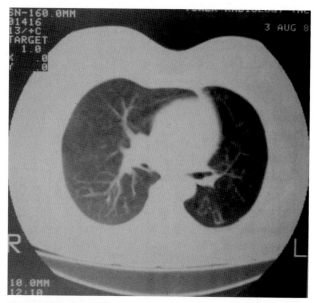

**Figure 14-9:** Swyer-James syndrome: Chest computed tomography scan depicting hyperlucency in the left side of the lung, as well as evidence of bronchiectasis. Decreased pulmonary vasculature and left hilum are also noted.

○ Decreased pulmonary vasculature and ipsilateral hilum, together with reduced vascular markings on affected side.
■ *CT scan* (Fig. 14-9)
  ○ High-resolution CT scan (HRCT) is the imaging procedure of choice[38,39]
  ○ Clearly demonstrates hyperlucencies on affected side; commonly shows contralateral patchy disease not evident on plain films. Lucencies commonly had irregular poorly defined margins
  ○ Mosaic pattern of perfusion and air trapping on expiration important features.
  ○ May show evidence of bronchiectasis
■ VQ lung scan (Fig. 14-10)
  ○ Demonstrates unilateral large matched ventilation and perfusion defects[40,41]

## Differential Diagnosis
■ Includes congenital absence of pulmonary artery, pulmonary artery occlusion, partial/ball-valve main or lobar bronchial obstruction, congenital lobar emphysema

## Treatment
■ Supportive: oxygen if indicated, bronchial toilet, treatment of infections, pulmonary rehabilitation, and exercise. Bronchodilators, steroids, and so on may have limited use, and there are no trials on which to base pharmacologic treatment principles.
■ Surgical resection may be considered in the management of complications, in select patients.
■ Lung volume reduction surgery has been reported.[42]
■ With severe end-stage disease, lung transplantation is a theoretic consideration.

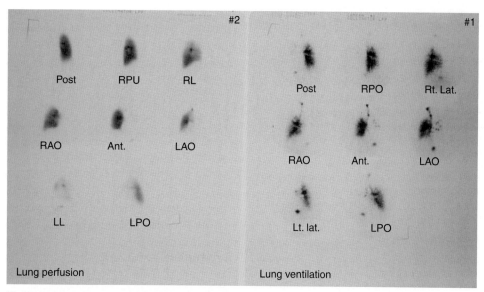

**Figure 14-10:** Swyer-James syndrome: Ventilation/perfusion lung scan (same patient as depicted earlier in Figure 14-9) showing absence of both ventilation and perfusion of the left lung.

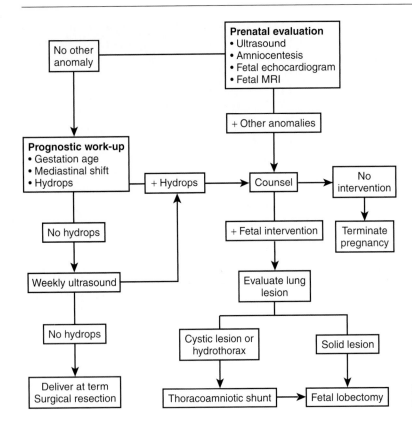

**Figure 14-11:** A proposed algorithm for the management of a prenatally diagnosed pulmonary lesion.

## SPECIAL TREATMENT CONSIDERATIONS IN CHILDREN AND PRENATAL STATE

Early detection is critical to the outcome of congenital lung disorders. The management is a multidisciplinary approach involving extensive prenatal care, adequate follow-up, and timely intervention (Fig. 14-11).

Prenatal US permits early detection of congenital lung anomalies. Plain chest radiography is the first imaging choice. CT, MRI, angiography, echocardiography, VQ scan, and bronchoscopy contribute to the correct diagnosis.

Indications for surgery include the presence of symptoms, the lesion's radiographic appearance, and the potential for malignancy.

- Operation should not be delayed for infants with symptomatic congenital lung malformation.
- Management of asymptomatic lung anomaly remains controversial. Some surgeons advocate observation because some lesions have been reported to spontaneously regress.[43-45]
- CCAM, pulmonary sequestration, bronchogenic cyst, and CLE have potential for malignant transformation. Surgical resection is recommended to avoid risk of malignancy.[43]
  - ○ CCAM-associated neoplasms include pleuropulmonary blastomas in infants and young children, and bronchioloalveolar carcinoma in older children and adults.[46-53]
  - ○ In a large review, 8.6% of malignant tumors were associated with previously documented cystic malformations.[54,55]

Surgery remains the cornerstone of treatment.

- In experienced hands, thoracoscopic surgery has successful outcomes in the pediatric population.[56]
- *Note:* A *video demonstration* of thoracoscopic resection of a congenital lung lesion is featured in the accompanying textbook DVD.

### TABLE 14-1 ■ MANAGEMENT OPTIONS FOR CHILDREN WITH CONGENITAL LUNG MALFORMATIONS

| Lung Lesion | Treatment Options |
|---|---|
| Congenital pulmonary arteriovenous malformation | Wedge resection vs. lobectomy<br>Catheter embolization (limited reports) |
| Congenital cystic adenomatoid malformation | Fetal surgery to prevent fetal demise<br>Lobectomy |
| Pulmonary sequestration | Intralobar lesion: lobectomy<br>Extralobar lesion: observe versus segmentectomy |
| Bronchogenic cyst | Segmentectomy versus lobectomy |
| Congenital lobar emphysema | Asymptomatic lesion: observe versus lobectomy<br>Symptomatic lesion: lobectomy |

- Fetal intervention is indicated only in select cases to prevent fetal demise.[57]
- Treatment options vary depending on the anomaly (Table 14-1).[43,58-61]
- In the absence of other congenital anomaly or lung disease, the prognosis is generally good. Surgical resection is well tolerated by children given their compensatory lung growth.

## References

 Interactive references and additional readings for this chapter can be accessed online at *expertconsult.com*.

# 15 EMPHYSEMA: LUNG VOLUME REDUCTION SURGERY

Jeremy A. Falk, MD, Robert J. McKenna Jr., MD, and Zab Mosenifar, MD

## DEFINITIONS

- According to the Global Initiative for Chronic Obstructive Lung Disease (GOLD), "Chronic Obstructive Pulmonary Disease (COPD) is a preventable and treatable disease with some significant extrapulmonary effects... Its pulmonary component is characterized by airflow limitation that is not fully reversible. The airflow limitation is usually progressive and associated with an abnormal inflammatory response of the lung to noxious particles or gases."[1]
- COPD has many phenotypes related to varying degrees of small airway disease and emphysema, each of which may prove to have a distinct pathogenesis and clinical course.
- Emphysema, which represents a specific phenotype of COPD is defined as "...a condition of the lung characterized by abnormal, permanent enlargement of airspaces distal to the terminal bronchiole, accompanied by the destruction of their walls, and without obvious fibrosis."[2]
- Patients with emphysema typically have loss of lung elastic recoil, leading to airflow limitation, lung hyperinflation, and air trapping. Destruction of alveolar-capillary membranes leads to reduction in diffusion capacity.
- Cigarette smoking accounts for the majority of cases of emphysema (80%–90%), however, other etiologies including $\alpha_1$-antitrypsin deficiency, occupational exposures, environmental pollution, female gender, childhood infections, and poor socioeconomic status have also been implicated.[1,3]

## PHYSIOLOGIC CONSIDERATIONS

Loss of elastic recoil: A key component in pathogenesis of emphysema is a loss of lung elastic recoil.[4] Abnormally reduced recoil leads to airway collapse and is likely a major determinant of flow limitation in the airways. Expiratory airflow limitation in the setting of poor elastic recoil then leads to gas trapping, the phenomenon of "auto-peep," and ultimately hyperinflation.[5]

- Hyperinflation: Abnormal lung elastic recoil and parenchymal lung destruction with bulla formation typically seen in emphysema ultimately lead to pulmonary hyperinflation. Hyperinflation impairs proper diaphragmatic function and may result in abnormal hemodynamics related to alterations in intrathoracic pressure and "auto-peep."[5-8]
- Airflow obstruction: The severity of airflow obstruction, as measured by the forced expiratory time in 1 second ($FEV_1$), has been shown to be inversely proportional to survival.[1,9] The underlying mechanism of increased airflow resistance is variable and ultimately related to the predominant COPD phenotype (i.e., emphysema versus chronic bronchitis). Mechanisms include mucus hypersecretion, airway inflammation, and airway collapse due to loss of recoil.
- Dynamic hyperinflation: Increases in minute ventilation that occur normally in response to exercise is accompanied by an increase in gas trapping, hyperinflation, and hemodynamic derangements in many patients with COPD. The phenomenon

of "breath stacking" is often sited as a likely mechanism of exercise limitation in this patient population.[5,6] In fact, a decreased ratio of the inspiratory capacity to total lung capacity (IC/TLC), a sensitive predictor of the development of dynamic hyperinflation during exercise, inversely correlates with mortality and exercise capacity.[10,11] Additionally, IC/TLC may signal those at risk for cardiac dysfunction as measured by the oxygen pulse, a noninvasive estimate of stroke volume.[12]

- Gas exchange abnormalities: Both hypoxemia and hypercapnea are common in severe emphysema and loosely correlate with severity of airflow obstruction.
- Pulmonary vascular disease: Mild to moderate and rarely severe pulmonary hypertension has been associated with severe emphysema.[13] Possible mechanisms include chronic hypoxia, mechanical obstruction of small pulmonary arteries from hyperinflation, vascular inflammation, and destruction of the pulmonary vascular bed.[13]
- Diaphragm dysfunction: Inspiratory muscle function, in particular diaphragm function, can be severely limited in patients with emphysema and lung hyperinflation.[14-17] Diaphragm flattening and thus, shortening of diaphragmatic muscle fibers, creates a mechanically disadvantageous condition resulting in reduced inspiratory force generation.[15] Additionally, the development of intrinsic positive end-expiratory pressure creates increased load on the muscles of ventilation.[4]
- Systemic disease: COPD is now well known to have systemic manifestations in addition to its debilitating effects on the lungs. Weight loss, cardiovascular disease, skeletal muscle dysfunction, depression, osteoporosis, sleep disorders, and sexual dysfunction are all common in patients with COPD.[18]

## RATIONALE FOR LUNG VOLUME REDUCTION SURGERY

- Improved lung elastic recoil[19-23]
  - May lead to improvements in peak expiratory flow and $FEV_1$
  - Variable effects on airway resistance
  - Does not explain improvements observed in vital capacity
- Improved lung volumes
  - Although both total lung capacity (TLC) and residual volume (RV) are increased in patients with emphysema, there is a disproportionate increase in RV, thus resulting in a significant increase in RV/TLC.[24]
  - Lung volume reduction surgery (LVRS) decreases RV moreso than TLC, resulting in an overall decrease in RV/TLC
  - Attempts made at time of surgery to remove only severely emphysematous lung that is unlikely to participate in significant gas exchange and functions primarily to compress potentially viable lung tissue.
- Improved diaphragm function
  - LVRS results in an overall lengthening of the diaphragm, thus improving diaphragmatic force generation and improving maximal inspiratory and transdiaphramatic pressures.[25-27]

○ Acute histologic changes in the diaphragm after LVRS, in contrast, have shown evidence of sarcolemmal injury, suggesting no improvement in contractile qualities of individual muscle fibers.[28]

## SELECTION OF THE CANDIDATE LUNG VOLUME REDUCTION SURGERY

- History of LVRS
  ○ Early attempts that predate modern LVRS at reducing thoracic volume have included:
    - Phrenectomy[29]
    - Whole lung radiation[30]
    - Abdominal binders[24]
    - Induction of pneumoperitoneum[29]
  ○ Modern LVRS
    - First reported in a study in 1959 by Otto Brantigan in which most severely affected lung tissue on one side was removed with hilar denervation. The procedure was repeated on the contralateral side if symptoms persisted. Despite reports of symptomatic improvement, the procedure was largely abandoned, primarily for its high mortality rate.[29]
    - In 1994, Cooper et al.[31] published a series of 20 patients who underwent bilateral LVRS via median sternotomy. Significant improvements in pulmonary function testing included a 22% decrease in TLC, a 39% decrease in RV, and an 82% increase in $FEV_1$.
    - Cooper's report of significant physiologic improvements, improved symptoms, with no deaths after 15 months after LVRS led to a renewed interest and popularity in the procedure.
    - Optimal techniques for LVRS were defined with several studies:
      ○ A randomized, prospective comparison of laser versus resection with staples showed that the staple procedure provided greater average improvement, improvement in a higher number of patients, and longer duration of benefit.[32]
      ○ A bilateral procedure, compared with a unilateral procedure, showed greater benefit, with no increased morbidity or mortality.[33]
    - Several small randomized, prospective, placebo controlled studies comparing lung volume reduction surgery to standard medical therapy with pulmonary rehabilitation showed variable benefits of LVRS.[34-36]
    - In 1996, pressured by the enormous potential cost of Medicare reimbursement for LVRS, a joint venture sponsored by the Health Care Financing Administration and the National Heart, Lung, and Blood Institute was initiated to study the efficacy, safety, and cost effectiveness of LVRS.[29]
    - Eighteen institutions were chosen to participate in the National Emphysema Treatment Trial (NETT), which was a prospective multicentered, placebo-controlled study comparing LVRS with maximal medical therapy.[29]
    - The primary outcome measures for NETT were survival and maximal exercise capacity.[29]
  ○ Entry criteria for the NETT (summary)[29]
    ○ Evidence of bilateral emphysema on high-resolution CT chest (HRCT)
    ○ Body mass index (BMI) $\leq 31.1$ kg/m$^2$ (men) or $\leq 32.3$ kg/m$^2$ (women)
    ○ Taking 20 mg prednisone daily
    ○ $FEV_1 \leq 45\%$ predicted, TLC $\geq$s 100% predicted, RV $\geq$ 150% predicted

○ $PCO_2 \leq 60$ mm Hg, $PO_2 \geq 45$ mm Hg on room air
○ Postrehabilitation 6-minute walk test $\geq 140$ meters
○ Nonsmoker for 4 months before initial interview and throughout screening, verified with plasma cotinine levels
○ Completion of a formal pulmonary rehabilitation program
- Exclusion criteria for NETT (Summary)[29]
  ○ Prior thoracic surgery (lung transplant, LVRS, median sternotomy, lobectomy)
  ○ Significant cardiac arrhythmias
  ○ Exercise induced syncope
  ○ Myocardial infarction (MI) within 6 months with left ventricular ejection fraction less than 45%
  ○ Congestive heart failure
  ○ Uncontrolled hypertension
  ○ Recurrent pulmonary infections
  ○ Significant bronchiectasis
  ○ Pleural or interstitial pulmonary disease that precludes surgery
  ○ Pulmonary nodule requiring surgery
  ○ Giant bullae (>1/3 volume of lung) discussed separately later in chapter
  ○ Pulmonary hypertension (peak systolic $\geq 45$ mm Hg or mean $\geq 35$ mm Hg)
    - Right-sided heart catheterization required if peak systolic pulmonary artery pressure on echocardiogram $\geq 45$ mm Hg
  ○ >6 L/min oxygen requirement
  ○ Computed tomographic (CT) evidence of diffuse emphysema
  ○ Unexplained weight loss
  ○ Systemic or oncologic illness with expected survival <5 years
  ○ 6-minute walk distance $\leq 140$ meters after rehabilitation

## SURGICAL TECHNIQUE

- LVRS involves resection of approximately 30% of the apices of both lungs for upper lobe disease and the lower lobes (possibly sparing the superior segments) for lower lobe disease.
- The lung tissue does not hold sutures or staples well, so the staples are buttressed with bovine pericardium.
- The procedure may be performed through either VATS or a median sternotomy.
  ○ Results are comparable for the two surgical approaches.
  ○ VATS is associated with shorter length of stay, quicker return to independent existence and less total cost of all health care services for the 6 months that follow LVRS.[3]

## POSTOPERATIVE CARE

- Patients are almost always extubated in the operating room after LVRS.
- Early ambulation and aggressive pulmonary toilet are critical to minimize postoperative complications.[38,39]
- Mortality rate for LVRS is less than 5%.[38]
- Complications are seen in Table 15-1.[37]
- Interim analysis of NETT
  ○ In 2001, an interim analysis of the NETT identified a subgroup of patients who were at an unacceptably high risk of death after undergoing LVRS.[40]
  ○ Patients with an $FEV_1 \leq 20\%$ predicted and had either a homogenous distribution of emphysema on CT or a carbon monoxide diffusing capacity (DLCO) $\leq 20\%$ predicted had a 30-day mortality rate after surgery of 16% compared with 0% in the medical arm.
  ○ Patients meeting these criteria were excluded from further enrollment in the NETT and should not be considered for LVRS in clinical practice.

**TABLE 15-1 ■ SHOWS COMPLICATION RATES AFTER LUNG VOLUME REDUCTION SURGERY BY MEDIAN STERNOTOMY (MS) OR VIDEO-ASSISTED THORACIC SURGERY (VATS)[37]**

| Postoperative Complications | MS (%) | VATS (%) | *P* value |
|---|---|---|---|
| None | 41 | 48 | 0.06 |
| Atrial fibrillation | 3 | 1 | 0.68 |
| Arrhythmias | 22 | 20 | 0.43 |
| Failure of early extubation | 3 | 6 | 0.30 |
| Tracheostomy | 10 | 6 | 0.33 |
| Failure to wean | 6 | 3 | 0.06 |
| Prolonged air leak | 1 | 1 | 0.62 |
| Reoperation for air leak | 2 | 6 | 0.05 |

## NETT OUTCOMES

- Survival benefit
  - Overall 90-day mortality rate in the LVRS group was 7.9%, compared with 1.3% in the medical group (*P* < 0.001).[41]
  - The mortality rate for all patients in the NETT, which was based on a mean follow-up of 29.2 months, was identical in the surgical and medical arms (0.11 death/person-year)
  - Patients in the previously described high-risk group (see earlier) had a 28.6% 90-day mortality rate with surgery compared with 0% for medical therapy (*P* < 0.001)
  - Surgical patients who were identified as having low exercise capacity and upper lobe predominant emphysema had a significant improvement in total mortality when compared with medical treatment (0.07 versus 0.15 death/person-year [risk ratio 0.47], *P* < 0.005)
    - Low exercise: < 40 watts exercise capacity for men, <25 watts for women.[41]
    - Upper lobe predominant emphysema: Each lung divided into three zones on HRCT (apical, middle, lower) and assigned a grade 0 (no emphysema) to 4 (>75% emphysema). A difference of 2 or more in grade among the three zones in one lung was indicative of heterogeneous disease and, if most predominant, in upper zone defined as upper lobe predominant (Fig. 15-1).[41]
  - Long-term outcomes based on a median follow-up of 4.3 years actually revealed a small but significant reduction in total mortality rate for all patients in the surgical arm versus medical arm (0.11 versus 0.13 deaths/person-year, *P* = 0.02) and the benefit was even more pronounced in the low exercise/upper lobe predominant group (relative risk [RR] = 0.57, P = 0.01).[42]
- Quality of life (QOL) and physiologic benefits (Fig. 15-2)
  - QOL
    - There was a significant overall benefit in health-related QOL at 24 months as defined by a decrease of 5 points or more on the St. George's Respiratory Questionnaire (SGRQ) in patients receiving LVRS (33% vs. 9%, *P* < 0.01).[41]
    - Significant improvements in the SGRQ in patients undergoing LVRS were also observed for all patients when stratified by preoperative predictors (baseline exercise capacity and pattern of emphysema) with the exception of patients with high-baseline exercise capacity and non–upper lobe emphysema as well as patients at high risk for death as defined earlier.
  - Physiologic benefits[41]
    - More patients randomized to LVRS had improvements in exercise capacity of 10 W or more than patients randomized to medical treatment at 6, 12, and 24 months (28%, 22%, and 15% vs. 4%, 5%, and 3%; *P* < 0.001 for each time point)
    - Improvements in lung function as measured by $FEV_1$ were observed at 6, 12, and 24 months, with 65%, 56%, and 43% showing improvement with LVRS as opposed to 27%, 26%, and 19% in the medical arm (*P* < 0.001 for each time point)
    - Subgroup analysis revealed significant improvements at all time points in exercise capacity for patients with upper lobe–predominant emphysema regardless of baseline exercise capacity, although benefits were more pronounced in those with lower exercise capacity.
    - Patients with non–upper lobe–predominant emphysema showed a significant improvement in exercise capacity only at 6 months and only for those with low baseline exercise.
    - Long term benefits for LVRS up to 3 years for exercise capacity and lung function were sustained for both the group as a whole as well as for non–high-risk patients with upper lobe–predominant emphysema.
- LVRS versus lung transplantation
  - Because both LVRS and lung transplantation are viable surgical options for patients with COPD who have been maximally medically treated, uncertainty exists as to which procedure is most appropriate for an individual patient.

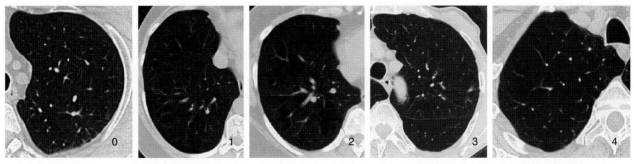

**Figure 15-1:** Examples of qualitative grading of emphysema severity. 0: no emphysema, 1: 1% to 25%, 2: 26% to 50%, 3: 51% to 75%, 4: 76% to 100%. A difference in grading of 2 or more in one lung is indicative of heterogeneous emphysema.

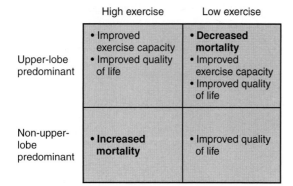

|  | High exercise | Low exercise |
|---|---|---|
| Upper-lobe predominant | • Improved exercise capacity<br>• Improved quality of life | • **Decreased mortality**<br>• Improved exercise capacity<br>• Improved quality of life |
| Non-upper-lobe predominant | • **Increased mortality** | • Improved quality of life |

**Figure 15-2:** Major outcomes in the National Emphysema Treatment Trial in patients undergoing lung volume reduction surgery stratified by baseline exercise capacity and pattern of emphysema.

○ Factors favoring LVRS[43]
  ■ Heterogeneous pattern of emphysema
  ■ Advanced age, which may preclude transplantation at some centers
  ■ Chronic medical conditions
  ■ Malignancy
  ■ Inability to maintain long-term follow-up
  ■ Psychiatric factors
  ■ Lack of social support
○ Factors favoring lung transplantation
  ■ Homogeneous pattern of emphysema
  ■ Patients at high risk for death after LVRS (FEV$_1$ ≤ 20% predicted and either DLCO ≤ 20% predicted or homogenous emphysema)
  ■ Lack of emphysema phenotype
  ■ TLC < 100% predicted
  ■ RV < 150% predicted
  ■ Severe gas exchange abnormalities (PCO$_2$ > 60 mm Hg, PaO$_2$ < 45 mm Hg)
  ■ 6-minute walk test ≤ 140 m
  ■ Pulmonary hypertension
  ■ Bronchiectasis or recurrent infection
○ No prospective data exist that compare LVRS with lung transplantation; however, limited, retrospective data suggest worse early and late survival with lung transplantation. These data must be viewed skeptically, however, because patients undergoing lung transplantation have tended to have more severe disease and had more urgent need for intervention.
○ The magnitude of physiologic benefits and QOL measures in patients undergoing lung transplantation as compared with LVRS tend to be greater; however, this must be weighed against a likely increase in mortality.[44]
○ LVRS followed by lung transplantation is a viable option for some patients, and limited data suggest no impact on transplant outcomes. This strategy may delay the need for transplantation and perhaps improve outcomes and survival than when compared to a single procedure.
■ Recommendations for LVRS candidate selection (Fig. 15-3)
  ○ Meets NETT inclusion and exclusion criteria described earlier
  ○ Patients have received maximal medical treatment, including pulmonary rehabilitation.
  ○ Does not fall into high-risk group
  ○ Upper lobe predominant disease

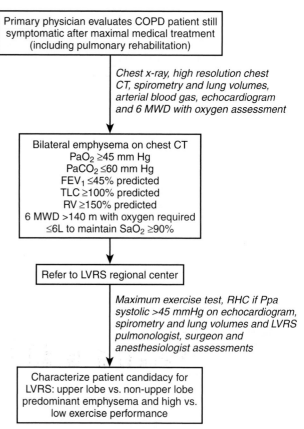

**Figure 15-3:** Proposed approach for patient consideration for lung volume reduction surgery. (*Reproduced with permission from Criner GJ, Sternberg AL, National Emphysema Treatment Trial Research Group. A clinician's guide to the use of lung volume reduction surgery. Proc Am Thorac Soc 2008;5:464.*)

## *OTHER LUNG VOLUME REDUCTION TECHNIQUES/ISSUES*

■ Giant bullae (Figs. 15-4 and 15-5)
  ○ Resection (bullectomy) considered if [45,46]:
    ■ Resultant compression of "normal" lung tissue by bullae is thought to be contributing to symptoms of dyspnea
    ■ Recurrent pneumothorax
    ■ Hemoptysis
    ■ Recurrent infection
  ○ Greatest benefit observed in those patients with >50% of hemithorax involved and those <30% are not recommended
  ○ Size of bullae may be estimated by difference in total lung capacity as measured by plethysmography and helium dilution methods.
  ○ Improvements in cardiac function after bullectomy have been described.[47]
  ○ Bullectomy can be done by standard lateral thoracotomy, midline sternotomy, or VAT.
■ Bronchoscopic lung volume reduction: With the success of LVRS, the concept of a less invasive procedure to achieve similar physiologic results has had growing interest. Several approaches with limited data are currently under investigation.
  ○ Endobronchial valves and blockers
    ■ Create a blockage of air into three segmental bronchi and allows air to escape around the blocker or through valve to produce selective lung collapse.[48]

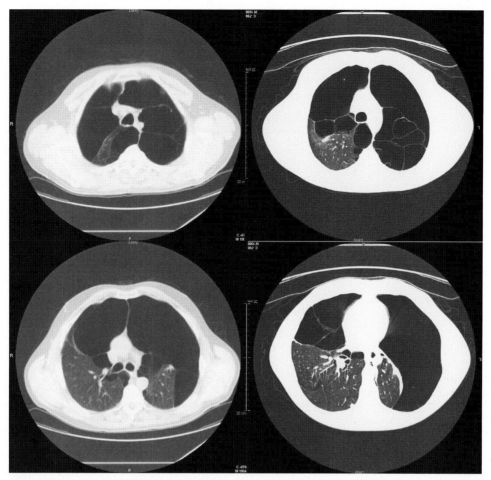

**Figure 15-4:** A patient with bilateral, giant bullae, with the left greater than the right.

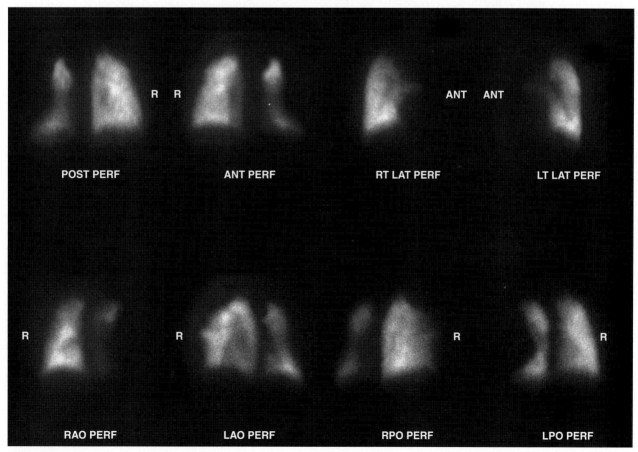

**Figure 15-5:** Perfusion scan of same patient in Figure 15-4.

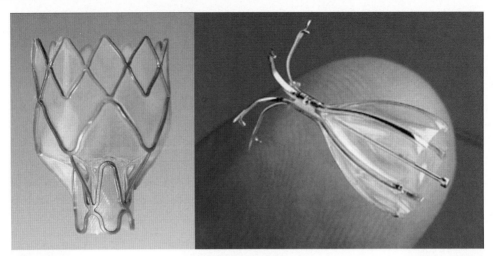

**Figure 15-6: Left Panel,** Emphasys Zephyr Endobronchial valve. *(Photo courtesy of Emphasys Medical, Inc., Investigational Device in the U.S.)* **Right Panel,** Spiration IBV valve. *(Photo courtesy of Spiration, Inc., Redmond, WA.)*

- Placed in segments with most severe disease
- Intended for use in heterogeneous emphysema, as in LVRS
- Two systems under evaluation (Fig. 15-6)
  ○ Emphasys medical (Redwood City, CA)
  ○ Spiration Incorporated (Redmond, WA)
- Limited data have shown variable response to treatment.
- Most data exist for unilateral placement.
- Pooled data of 98 patients who received the Emphasys endobronchial valve (EBV) showed modest improvements in pulmonary function (RV decreased by $4.9 \pm 17.4\%$ [$P = 0.025$], $FEV_1$ increased by $10.7 \pm 26.2\%$ [$P = 0.007$], FVC increased by $9.0 \pm 23.9\%$ [$P = 0.024$], and 6-minute walk distance increased by $23.0 + 55.3\%$ [$P = 0.001$]).[49]
- Preliminary data for the Spiration implantable intrabronchial valve (IBV) for 30 patients showed it to be safe and well tolerated with significant improvements in QOL but no significant physiologic changes in measured variables.[50]
- Benefits are likely very modest because although blockers/valves effectively block passage of air to selected areas of the lung, collateral ventilation frequently prevents the desired volume loss.
- Greatest atelectasis and benefits occur in patients with complete minor fissure
- Complications have included pneumothorax (ipsilateral and collateral), COPD exacerbation, pneumonia, and prolonged air leaks.[48]
- The mortality rate has been low at approximately 1%.
- Other clinical applications for endobronchial valves have included their use in persistent bronchopleural fistulas with pneumothorax, although this procedure is still under investigation.
○ Airway bypass
  - Bronchoscopically created communication between areas of trapped gas and the native airways in patients with emphysema.[51-53]
  - Drug-eluting stents placed in the fenestrations to maintain patency

- In decreasing the volume of trapped gas in lungs of patients with severe emphysema, theoretical benefits would include a reduction in RV, improved vital capacity, decreased end expiratory lung volume, improved diaphragm function, and a reduction in airflow obstruction and resistance.
- Used primarily for homogeneous emphysema
- Ex vivo data in emphysematous lungs explanted at the time of lung transplant have shown improvements in end expiratory lung volume, vital capacity, expiratory flow, and flow resistance.[51]
- No in vivo human data currently exist, and the durability of physiologic benefits remains unknown at this time.
○ Biologic lung volume reduction (BLVR)[54]
  - Fibrinogen and thrombin solution are injected simultaneously through a flexible bronchoscope into the distal airway of a targeted area of emphysema.
  - Inclusion criteria similar to that of the NETT, including presence of heterogeneous disease
  - Fibrinogen/thrombin solution ultimately creates a "glue" producing, over time, an area of scar with resultant volume reduction (Fig. 15-7)
  - There are currently published data for only six human patients, all of whom have had unilateral procedures.
  - Preliminary data suggest that its use is safe but with only modest benefit.

## Brief Illustrative Case

- A 71-year-old man with a 60 pack-year smoking history presented with progressive and limiting exertional dyspnea, despite maximal medical therapy. He had stopped smoking more than 10 years ago.
- He was generally sedentary and had dyspnea with activities of daily living over the previous 9 months

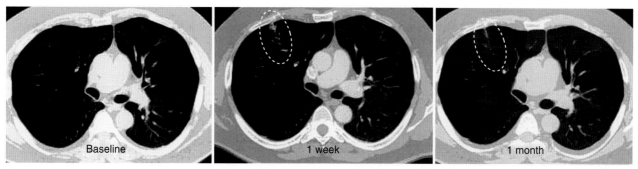

**Figure 15-7:** Computed tomography scan from a patient showing localized infiltrates 1 week after BLVR at the treatment site, changing into linear density by 1 month after BLVR. *(Reproduced with permission from Reilly J, Washko G, Pinto-Plata V, Velez E, Kenney L, Berger R, et al. Biological lung volume reduction: a new bronchoscopic therapy for advanced emphysema. Chest 2007;131:1112.)*

- He had no symptoms of chronic bronchitis and exhibited wheezing only with acute exacerbations, the last episode of which occurred 14 months previously.
- There was no history of coronary heart disease. A long history of essential hypertension was well controlled on a calcium channel blocker.
- Examination revealed a somewhat thin individual (weight 118; height 62.5 inches) in no respiratory distress at rest. There was no cyanosis. Chest: markedly diminished intensity of breath sounds in upper lobes.
- A high-resolution CT of the chest showed grade 4 emphysematous change in the upper lobes compared to 2 in the lower zones (Fig. 15-8). A V/Q scan also demonstrated heterogeneity.
- Pulmonary function studies following a 6-week pulmonary rehabilitation program revealed: FEV1: 0.57 L (25% of predicted) ; FEV1/FVC ratio: 27%; TLC: 8.85 L

(184% of predicted); RV: 6.61 L (389% of predicted); RV/TLC: 74%; DLCO: 5 ml/min/mmHg (22% of predicted)
- Blood gases: pH: 7.40; $PCO_2$: 43; $PO_2$: 67; $HCO^3$: 27 on room air
- Cardiopulmonary exercise test: Maximum work rate: 30 Watts; $VO_2$ max: 0.7 L (36% of predicted). 6-minute walk: 320 meters
- Cardiac workup: Stress thalium was negative; Echo: no evidence of pulmonary hypertension
- Bilateral LVRS via a VATS approach was performed. Apart from transient bilateral air-leaks the post-operative course was unremarkable. The patient was mobilized and ambulated perioperatively.
- On serial follow-up, the patient's symptoms, exercise tolerance, and QOL assessments were significantly improved. However, over a 3-year period, there was a progressive decline in several parameters (Table 15-2)

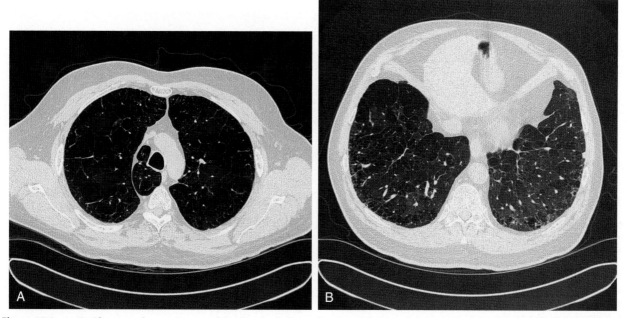

**Figure 15-8: A,** Significant emphysema in upper lobes (grade 4); **B,** emphysema grade is much lower in the lower lobes (grade 2). This indicates heterogeneous disease.

| TABLE 15-2 ▪ SERIAL MEASUREMENTS POST LUNG VOLUME REDUCTION SURGERY (LVRS) | | | | | |
| --- | --- | --- | --- | --- | --- |
| Measurement | Baseline | 6 Months Post LVRS | 12 Months Post LVRS | 24 Months Post LVRS | 36 Months Post LVRS |
| FEV1 (L) | 0.57 | 1.21 | 0.96 | 0.96 | 0.86 |
| IC (L) | 1.19 | 2.15 | 2.29 | 1.79 | 1.68 |
| TLC (L) | 8.85 | 6.58 | 6.29 | 6.70 | 6.55 |
| RV(L) | 6.61 | 2.98 | 2.81 | 3.31 | 3.81 |
| PaO$_2$ (mm Hg) | 69 | 77 | 72 | 72 | 74 |
| PaCO$_2$ (mm g) | 43 | 40 | 39 | 37 | 40 |
| Watts | 30 | 50 | 40 | 40 | 30 |
| VO$_2$ max (L) | 0.7 | 1.15 | 1.17 | 0.84 | 0.79 |
| 6-minute walk (meters) | 320 | 410 | 434 | 325 | Not performed |
| Health survey | 4 | 1 | 1 | 3 | 3 |

## Key Points

- This patient fits several criteria as defined in the results of the NETT trial that suggest benefit (heterogeneous disease; low work rate). Also, acceptable blood gases and absence of pulmonary hypertension were additional encouraging data.

- The diffusing capacity was close to the level in which increased mortality was reported (i.e., <20% of predicted)
- The case illustrates that improvement in a variety of clinical and physiologic variables decline serially over time. Other options in appropriate cases could be entertained if patients revert back to "baseline status." This includes bronchoscopic approaches and, where appropriate, lung transplantation.

## References

Interactive references and additional readings for this chapter can be accessed online at *expertconsult.com*.

# Inflammatory, Infectious, and Other Diseases

# 16  THORACIC SURGICAL CONSIDERATIONS IN INFECTIOUS AND INFLAMMATORY DISEASES OF THE LUNG

T. Brett Reece, MD, Phillip Zakowski, MD, and John D. Mitchell, MD

## TOPICS

- Bronchiectasis
- Lung abscess
- Mycobacterial disease
  - Tuberculosis
  - Nontuberculous mycobacteria
- Swyer-James syndrome
- Pulmonary fungal infections
- Hydatid lung disease

Note: For all topics covered in this chapter, the focus will be on the *possible roles of thoracic surgical interventions*. For more detailed coverage of other aspects of each topic, the reader is referred to classic references and recent review articles cited.

## BRONCHIECTASIS

### Terminology

- Bronchiectasis[1]

### Definitions

- Abnormal permanent dilatation of airways, usually subsegmental airways.
- Multiple types of bronchiectasis
  - *Cylindrical*–communicate with lung parenchyma, do not end blindly, with bronchi uniformly dilated
  - *Saccular/cystic*–dilated bronchi ending in saccular structures. Can be as proximal as the 5th generation of bronchi, with more distal bronchi destroyed.

- ○ *Varicose*–combination of saccular and cylindrical with beaded appearance
- ○ *Pseudobronchiectasis*–can be seen acutely after pneumonia but resolves in weeks to months
- ○ The above-mentioned types can be *focal* (i.e., localized to a segment or lobe) or *diffuse.*

## Etiology

- ■ Infection[1,2]
  - ○ Bacterial organisms: such as *Pseudomonas aeruginosa, Haemophilus influenza, Escherichia coli, Klebsiella,* and *Staphylococcus aureus.*[3]
  - ○ *Mycobacterium tuberculosis*
  - ○ Nontuberculous mycobacteria: *Mycobacterium. avium complex, Mycobacterium kansasii,* or *Mycobacterium abscessus*
  - ○ Note: Allergic bronchopulmonary aspergillosis (ABPA) is due to an immune reaction to aspergillus, and is associated with proximal bronchiectasis and mucoid impaction.
  - ○ Viral infections (e.g., adenovirus, influenza, measles, and so on).
- ■ Airway scarring/obstruction
  - ○ Extrinsic compression of bronchi (e.g., middle lobe syndrome due to compression by enlarged lymph nodes)
  - ○ Intrinsic bronchial obstruction (e.g., foreign body, tumor, and so on)
  - ○ Bronchial angulation after lobar resection
  - ○ Sequelae of toxic inhalation (e.g., chlorine)
- ■ Congenital
  - ○ Cystic fibrosis–predilection for upper lobes[4-8]
  - ○ Ciliary dyskinesia (e.g., Kartagener's syndrome; primary ciliary dyskinesia; Young's syndrome [secondary ciliary dyskinesia], and so on).[9]
  - ○ Tracheobronchomegaly (Mounier Kuhn)
  - ○ Cartilage deficiency (Williams-Campbell)
  - ○ Alpha 1 antitrypsin deficiency
- ■ Immune deficiency states/disorders predisposing to recurrent bacterial infection
  - ○ Hypogammaglobinemia: congenital or acquired. Includes specific immunoglogulin deficiencies, as well as subset deficiencies (for example, immunoglobulin G [IgG] subset deficiencies).
  - ○ Other rare disorders exhibiting combined humoral and cell-mediated immune deficiency states
  - ○ Chronic granulomatous disease; lazy leukocyte disorders; complement deficiency states
- ■ Autoimmune disorders
  - ○ Rheumatoid arthritis, Sjögren's syndrome, systemic lupus erythematosis
  - ○ Relapsing polychondritis
  - ○ Inflammatory bowel disease
- ■ Miscellaneous
  - ○ Yellow nail syndrome (dystrophic nails, lymphedema, pleural effusions)

## Pathogenesis/Pathophysiology

- ■ Bronchiectasis requires an infectious process plus impairment of bronchial drainage, airway obstruction, or a defect in host defenses. In cystic fibrosis, the process begins in the bronchioles.[10]
- ■ Causes of this combination include foreign body aspiration, external bronchial compression, ciliary dyskinesia, abnormal airway immune effector cells, excess neutrophils, proteases, and high levels of inflammatory cytokines
- ■ Inflammation results in destruction of muscle, elastic tissue, and cartilage of the bronchial wall by infected mucopus within. Weakened bronchial walls become dilated and are also subject to traction forces.

- ■ Bronchial arteries enlarge (up to 3 times normal), proliferate, and become tortuous to form an extensive network with anastomoses to the pulmonary circulation.

## Clinical Features

- ■ Clinical Presentation
  - ○ Recurrent pneumonia, chronic productive cough, foul-smelling sputum
    - Symptoms persist for months to years despite antibiotic treatment.
    - Nonproductive cough may be indicative of upper lobe involvement.
  - ○ Hemoptysis
    - Owing to erosion of infectious process into hypertrophied bronchial circulation
    - Less common in children than adults
  - ○ Typically affects basilar or dependent lung segments in most patients
  - ○ Preponderance for right middle lobe/lingular disease with nontuberculous mycobacterial (NTM) infection (Lady Windermere syndrome)
- ■ Complications
  - ○ Recurrent infection
  - ○ Hemoptysis, occasionally massive in nature
  - ○ Progressive lung destruction (e.g. severe cystic bronchiectasis)
- ■ Diagnostic Workup
  - ○ Full history, physical examination, and screen for underlying cause[1]
  - ○ Patients commonly clubbed; auscultation reveals crackles, wheezes, or rhonchi in the majority of patients
  - ○ Full pulmonary function tests; screening blood work and quantitative immunoglobulins with IgG subsets.
  - ○ Sputum cultures typically grow mucoid *P. aeruginosa, H. influenza, E. coli, Klebsiella,* and early on in the course, *S. aureus* (as well documented in children with cystic fibrosis). In later stages, *Burkholderia cepacia* may complicate the microbiologic milieu, because several gemovars are highly resistant to antibiotic therapies.
  - ○ NTM, most commonly *M. avium* complex or *M. abscessus*, also frequently isolated
  - ○ Chest radiographs classically demonstrate evidence of thickened and dilated bronchi, as noted by the presence of ring shadows (seen on end) and tram tracks (seen longitudinally) (Fig. 16-1).
  - ○ Sites of involvement: with cystic fibrosis, the lower zones are typically spared or less involved. In other causes of bronchiectasis, the most common sites of disease was reported as left lower lobe, right lower lobe, lingual, and right middle lobe. However, distribution depends on the etiologic factors causing bronchiectasis.
  - ○ Bronchography using contrast medium, once the standard for establishing the diagnosis of bronchiectasis, has been replaced by computed tomography (Fig. 16-2).
  - ○ High-resolution chest computed tomography (CT) is now the most common diagnostic tool with high accuracy. This clearly shows dilated bronchi, which also demonstrate ring shadows and tram tracks (Fig. 16-3), diffuse or localized disease (Fig. 16-4), or severe destruction and cystic bronchiectasis (Fig. 16-5).
  - ○ Other tests depend on etiologic considerations (e.g., cystic fibrosis, dyskinetic cilia, and so on).
  - ○ Bronchoscopy can help localize a source of hemoptysis or provide secretion clearance in cases with significant atelectasis that are unresponsive to bronchial toilet and other measures.

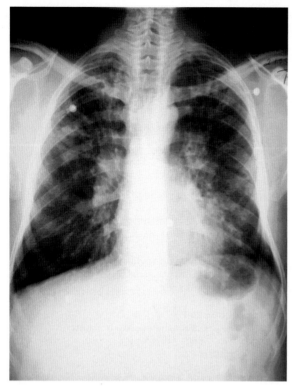

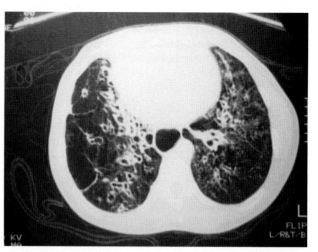

**Figure 16-3:** Computed tomography scan of the chest showing classic bronchiectasis (dilated bronchi exhibiting tram track and ring shadow appearance) in a bilateral diffuse manner.

**Figure 16-1:** Chest radiograph of a patient with cystic fibrosis, showing clear evidence of tram tracks (thickened parallel bronchial walls of dilated bronchus) especially in the right upper lobe, as well as *ring shadows* (cross-sectional equivalent of tram tracks). Relative sparing of the lung bases is evident.

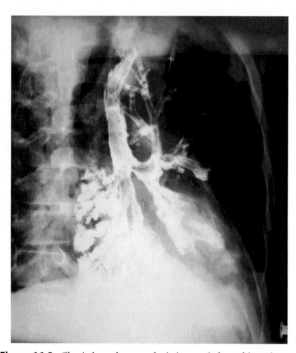

**Figure 16-2:** Classic bronchogram depicting cystic bronchiectasis.

## Treatment

- Medical[11-14]
  - ○ Remains the mainstay of therapy
  - ○ Targeted antibiotic therapy–avoid excessive rounds of monotherapy, which tend to promote resistance

  - ○ Pulmonary toilet/hygiene is key feature of medical therapy
    - Postural drainage
    - Percussive therapy
    - Flutter valves
    - High frequency chest vibrators
    - Humidification
    - Mucolytics (e.g., DNAase of value in cystic fibrosis)
    - Hypertonic saline inhalation (cystic fibrosis)
    - Bronchodilators
- Surgical[15-18]
  - ○ The rationale for surgery is to remove areas of permanently damaged lung parenchyma, into which the antibiotic therapy penetrates poorly. These areas have little impact on gas exchange, and serve as a reservoir to breed antibiotic resistance and seed later recurrence of the infection.
  - ○ Patients may benefit from resection when there is
    - Localized symptomatic disease
    - Failure of medical management
    - Persistent and debilitating symptoms
    - Multidrug resistance
    - Drug intolerance
    - Recurrent pneumonias
    - Hemoptysis
  - ○ Localized, focal areas of bronchiectasis most amenable to resection
  - ○ "Debulking" of severe areas of lung destruction in setting of generalized disease may alleviate symptoms
  - ○ Resection may involve segmentectomy or lobectomy, or rarely pneumonectomy. Nonanatomic resections are less effective. Many resections are amenable to a thoracoscopic approach.
  - ○ Bronchial artery embolization may provide temporary relief of significant hemoptysis in setting of bronchiectasis. (See Chapter 17 on Massive Hemoptysis.)
  - ○ With late-stage generalized bronchiectasis, bilateral lung transplantation may be considered.[19] (See Chapter 35 on Patient Evaluation and Selection.)

## Principles of Peri- and Postoperative Management

- Optimization of medical therapy before surgery is important. Surgery alone is not advised or curative.
- Preoperative antimicrobial therapy is based on preoperative cultures and in vitro sensitivities when appropriate, and is

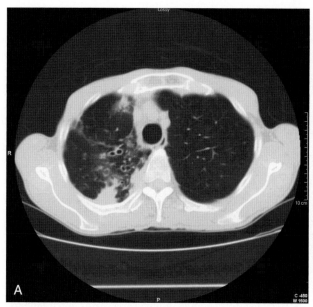
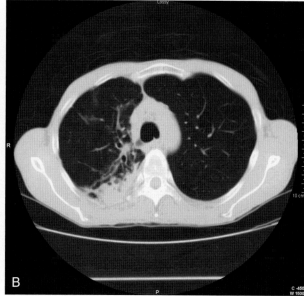

**Figure 16-4:** Computed tomography scan of the chest showing classic localized bronchiectasis. **A,** Obvious "ring shadows" noted. **B,** Lower axial cut showing well demarcated "tram tracks."

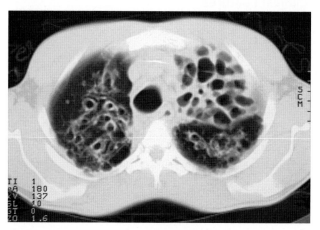

**Figure 16-5:** Computed tomography scan of the chest showing severe cystic bronchiectasis.

extended for a few weeks (bacterial) to few months (mycobacterial) before surgery.

■ Culture-negative sputum is preferable but not always possible in severe cases before surgery
■ Antimicrobial therapy is continued through perioperative period; the extent of postoperative antimicrobial therapy is not well defined

## Prevention and Management of Complications

■ Use of double-lumen tubes and toilet bronchoscopy immediately before surgery for bronchiectasis is recommended.
   ○ Avoidance of spillage within thoracic cavity and contact with chest wall/soft tissues, particularly in setting of certain mycobacterial infections such as *M. abscessus*
■ An extrapleural dissection plane may be advantageous in the setting of significant pleural symphysis
■ Active infection with positive sputum culture at the time of surgery may suggest the need for bronchial stump reinforcement with autologous tissue flap, most commonly transposed chest wall muscle or omentum, to minimize risk of bronchopleural fistula.

■ An intrathoracic "space" is common after resectional surgery for infectious lung disease, will become smaller over time, and is not necessarily indicative of pneumothorax/parenchymal air leak.

## Natural History/Prognosis

■ Surgery is used as a therapeutic adjunct to remove permanently damaged areas of lung tissue that act as a reservoir for persistent organisms, leading to antibiotic resistance and recurrent infection.

| KEY FACTS |
| --- |
| ■ Usually chronic infection in the setting of impaired bronchial drainage. |
| ■ Dependent areas, as well as right middle lobe/lingular, are commonly involved. |
| ■ Surgical resection used in select cases as an adjunct to medical therapy. |
| ■ Culture negative sputum is preferable before surgery but not always possible. |
| ■ "Debulking" of most severe areas is occasionally helpful for symptom relief and to prevent progressive lung destruction of uninvolved areas. |
| ■ Buttressing of bronchial stump is recommended for major resection (particularly pneumonectomy) in the setting of active infection. |

### Brief Illustrative Case 1

• A 47-year-old woman with 12-year history of recurrent pulmonary infections, consisting of productive cough, fever, and occasional scant hemoptysis. Has been placed on a rotating antibiotic therapy course for suppression. Previous cultures have grown *P. aeruginosa*

*(Continued)*

## Brief Illustrative Case 1—cont'd

- She now describes a several-month history of productive cough, malaise, and 10 lb. weight loss. Workup including chest CT (Fig. 16-6) demonstrates focal bronchiectasis involving the right middle lobe and lingula. Bronchoscopy with BAL demonstrate *Mycobacterium avium* complex (MAC). In vitro susceptibility testing demonstrates no macrolide resistance.
- She is placed on a four-drug regimen (azithromycin, rifampin, ethambutol, and IV amikacin). At 12 weeks after initiation of therapy, she undergoes thoracoscopic right middle lobectomy, with continuing antibiotic coverage. Testing of tissue obtained at operation show no AFB (MAC) by smear or culture.
- With continuing antibiotic coverage, 6 weeks later, she has thoracoscopic lingulectomy. Pathologic specimens remain smear and culture negative. The IV antibiotics are discontinued, and the oral regimen is continued for another nine months.
- Subsequent testing by sputum culture and radiologic imaging demonstrate no recurrence of MAC or recurrent parenchymal disease at 4 years from termination of therapy

## *LUNG ABSCESS*

### Terminology
- Abscess within the lung parenchyma[20-22]

### Definition
- Abscess cavity in the lung parenchyma secondary to localized suppuration with parenchymal destruction. Central necrosis tends to liquefy and communicate with the bronchial tree. Communication with the airway leads to classic air-fluid level seen on radiologic studies

### Etiology
- Aspiration
  - Predilection for dependent areas, that is, the posterior segment of the right upper lobe (RUL), the superior segments of both lower lobes and other lower lobe segments.

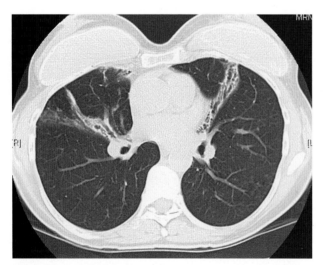

**Figure 16-6:** Computed tomography scan of the chest of patient in first illustrative case, depicting focal bronchiectasis involving the right middle lobe and lingula.

- May occur in setting of impaired consciousness, alcoholism, gastroesophageal reflux disease, other dysphagia syndromes (stricture, Zenker's diverticulum, and so on). Poor dental hygiene, gingival disease, and high bacterial counts in gingival crevices are common.
  - Bacteriology: anaerobes (most common) and aerobes (e.g., *Streptococcus. milleri*); commonly mixed anaerobe and aerobic flora. The environment in which aspiration occurs also impacts. For example hospital or nursing home flora colonization.[23]
- Endobronchial obstruction: neoplasms, foreign bodies, and external bronchial compression can result in distal infection and abscess formation
- Following necrotizing lung infection
  - Bacteriology: Staphylococcus, Streptococcus, Klebsiella, other gram-negative organisms, Legionella, Actinomyces.
  - More prevalent in the immunocompromised host. In the setting of cell-mediated immune dysfunction, consider bacterial organisms as above, Nocardia, Rhodococcus, mycobacterial, fungal and parasitic
- Secondary infection of pre-existing lung cavity (emphysema, resolving infarct, cavitating neoplasm)
- Hematogenous seeding of lung parenchyma, often multifocal

## Clinical Features
- Clinical Presentation
  - Fever, chills, severe cough, hemoptysis, and copious, foul-smelling sputum
  - Leukocytosis with left shift
  - Tachypnea, consolidation, local chest wall tenderness
  - Hemoptysis occurs rarely
  - Contributing factors can include, but are not limited to, sub-optimal dental hygiene, alcohol abuse, seizure disorders, immunosuppression, neuromuscular disorders with bulbar dysfunction, esophageal dysmotility, bronchial obstruction.
- Complications
  - Bronchopleural fistula and/or empyema can develop if abscess communicates with the pleural space.
  - Systemic infection/sepsis

## Diagnostic Workup
- Chest radiograph: pneumonitis pattern appears early, followed by air/fluid level once airway has been invaded/eroded
- Chest CT delineates the exact anatomic features and location of the abscess and its relation to adjacent structures
- Culture: aerobic, anaerobic, fungal, acid-fast bacteria can play role
  - Can direct therapy based on culture growth
  - Percutaneous sampling often yields best results
- Bronchoscopy is indicated to rule out obstructing foreign bodies or neoplasm.[24]

## Treatment
  - Medical
  - Most abscesses respond to appropriate medical treatment.
  - Empiric antibiotic therapy often used until cultures define pathogen.
  - Duration of antibiotic therapy in typical bacterial lung abscess is controversial. The duration is commonly at least 4 to 6 weeks and most often longer (months) depending on pathogen, clinical response, and if there is substantial radiologic improvement
  - Drainage of the cavity may be possible with aggressive chest physiotherapy, postural drainage

○ Bronchoscopic and percutaneous drainage, in addition to appropriate antimicrobial therapy, have also been used in certain circumstances.[25-28]
○ The complications of percutaneous drainage (empyema, pneumothorax, hemothorax) occur in less than 10% of cases.
■ Surgery
  ○ Indications include
    • Failure of medical therapy
    • Significant hemoptysis
    • Empyema secondary to abscess erosion into pleura space
    • Suspicion of underlying malignancy
  ○ Most commonly involves anatomic resection, usually lobectomy
  ○ In cases of abscess perforation into pleural space, simple unroofing of abscess, decortication, and wide drainage usually suffice
  ○ Special measures should be taken during surgery to avoid endobronchial spillage into contralateral lung
  ○ Pulmonary gangrene[29,30]
    • Definition: severe lung infection with extensive devitalization of lung tissue and necrosis. Often is secondarily infected.[29,30]
    • Surgery in such conditions is controversial. Failure of medical therapy and ongoing sepsis is a consideration
    • A case series of 35 cases reported an 8.5% postoperative mortality.[30] Lobectomy was most commonly performed.
    • Surgical complications could include bronchopleural fistula, empyema, and mediastinitis.
    • Reinforcement of the bronchial stump is advised.

## Principles of Peri- and Postoperative Management

■ Obtain good cultures and allow them to direct antimicrobial therapy
■ Address underlying cause of abscess

## Prevention and Management of Complications

■ Broad-spectrum antibiotics until cultures identify specific pathogen

## Natural History/Prognosis

■ Good prognosis once drained and treated with anti-biotics.[31]
■ Antibiotic duration may last for 6 to 8 weeks
■ Radiologic resolution may take 4 to 5 months
■ Identify predisposition–chronic aspiration, airway obstruction, and so on that could lead to recurrence

---

**KEY FACTS**

■ Medical therapy depends on adequate drainage and appropriate antibiotic selection.
■ Surgery mainly reserved for failure of medical therapy and complications of primary condition.
■ Underlying cause of abscess must be addressed to minimize recurrence.

---

## *TUBERCULOSIS*

## Terminology

■ Tuberculosis (TB)
■ Multidrug resistant tuberculosis (MDR-TB)
■ Extensive drug resistant tuberculosis (XDR-TB)

## Definition

■ Variety of infections caused by *Mycobacterium tuberculosis*, most commonly pulmonary. Other organ systems are occasionally involved.
■ MDR-TB is resistant to at least isoniazid and rifampin
■ Extensive (extremely) drug-resistant tuberculosis (XDR-TB) is resistant to at least isoniazid, rifampin, fluoroquinolones, and either aminoglycosides, capreomycin, or both.
■ Primary resistance occurs in patients never before treated
■ Secondary resistance is the development of resistance in a previously susceptible strain during or after treatment

## Etiology

■ Mycobacterium tuberculosis

## Pathogenesis/Pathophysiology

■ Most commonly begins with pulmonary transmission with inhalation of droplet nuclei (5 to 10 μ), which are deposited in the lung midzones on either side to produce the Ghon focus. Spread to regional lymph nodes produces the Ghon complex (primary TB), which is contained by the development of cell mediated immunity over 2 to 6 weeks.
■ With the initial innoculum, if innate immunity fails to contain (before the development of full cell-mediated immunity), the organisms will continue to proliferate and a few organisms may seed and then remain dormant in several organs (i.e., apices of the lung; kidneys, bones, and so on).
■ Failure to contain the primary infection results in continued proliferation and invasion of blood vessels and lymphatics to produce generalized miliary dissemination, erosion into a bronchus to produce a bronchopneumonic process, and so on.
■ Reactivation TB occurs when latent bacilli start to proliferate, often many years later. The exact mechanisms that maintain a dormant state and reactivation are not fully understood, but impairment of cell-mediated immunity under different circumstances plays a role. Figure 16-7 shows a chest radiograph of reactivation TB in the right upper lobe.
■ In general, with exposure and infection, about 3% to 5% of patients develop clinical disease within 1 year, with a 3% to 5% lifetime chance of late disease thereafter.

## Clinical Features

■ Demographic[32,33]
  ○ There were an estimated 9.2 million cases of TB worldwide in 2006
  ○ Approximately 5% of cases MDR-TB.
  ○ About 12,000 cases of TB were reported in the United States during same time period.
■ Clinical presentation
  ○ Night sweats, fever, cough, and occasionally hemoptysis
  ○ See classic texts and papers for more details, such as references 34 and 35.
■ Complications
  ○ A cause of severe hemoptysis (see Chapter 17 on Massive Hemoptysis)
  ○ See classic texts and papers for more details, such as references 34 to 36.

## Diagnostic Workup

■ Diagnosis is confirmed with acid-fast staining and culture of the sputum or other fluids/tissue sources
■ Susceptibility to first- and second-line agents should be tested
■ See classic texts and papers for more details, such as references 37 to 40.

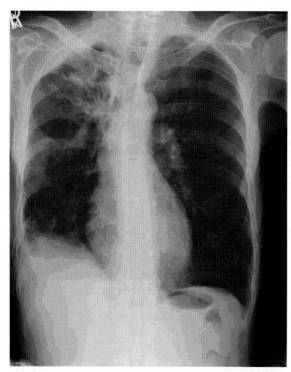

**Figure 16-7:** Chest radiograph of a patient with reactivation tuberculosis. Extensive cavitary disease is noted in the right upper lobe.

## Treatment

- Medical[41-43]
  - First-line therapy: isoniazid, ethambutol, pyrazinamide, and rifampin.
  - The (current) preferred regimen is isoniazid and rifampin for 6 months, with ethambutol and pyrazinamide administered for the first 2 months.
  - If the sputum is positive after 3 months of treatment, either the patient is noncompliant, the organism is resistant, or the diagnosis is incorrect; the patient should be recultured
  - Never add a single drug to a failing regimen
  - Pure tuberculous effusions almost always resolve spontaneously or respond promptly to chemotherapy
    - Tube thoracostomy rarely provides a cure because dense pleural reaction interferes with full re-expansion of the underlying lung
  - MDR-TB regimens should include at least four drugs (usually five or more), ranging from 18 to 24 months of treatment.[44-46]
    - Regimen can be dictated by a specific pattern of resistance.
    - Most commonly an aminoglycoside and a fluoroquinolone are used for this situation, among others. These regimens need to be given with direct observation of the patients for effectiveness and side effects, which can be common
    - With fluoroquinolones, take 2 hours after meals to optimize absorption
    - Consider drug levels at 2 and 6 hours postingestion when delayed absorption or malabsorption is suspect. Low levels can also induce resistance
  - XDR-TB use all first-line agents to which there is susceptibility and at least two second-line agents for a minimum of four to five drugs.
  - See American Thoracic Society statement on hepatotoxity of antituberculous therapy.[47]

- Surgical[48-52]
  - Indications for surgical resection[53]
    - Localized resistant TB
    - Persistent cavitary disease after extended treatment with ≥2 drugs
    - Continued positive sputum
    - MDR-TB or XDR-TB with destroyed lobe or lung
    - Massive (>600 mL/24 hours) or recurrent severe (>200 mL/24 hours) hemoptysis
    - Bronchopleural fistula
    - Bronchial stenosis secondary to endobronchial TB
  - Contraindications to resection
    - Widespread, diffuse pulmonary parenchymal involvement
    - Inadequate pulmonary reserve
    - Active endobronchial disease, because this interferes with healing of bronchial stump (preoperative bronchoscopy in all patients before resection)
  - Surgical Goals
    - Surgery remains adjunct to medical therapy, which remains primary treatment modality
    - Obliterate cavities, excise damaged lung
    - Lobectomy or pneumonectomy necessary with active disease
    - Extrapleural pneumonectomy required in cases of extensive pulmonary parenchymal disease and chronic empyema
  - Surgical outcomes in drug-resistant TB
    - A retrospective analysis of 205 patients treated for MDR-TB reported long-term success rates of 75%. Surgical resection and the use of fluoroquinolones was associated with improved outcomes.[46]
    - In a recent report of surgery in 121 patients for drug-resistant TB who had failed medical therapy with a median of seven drugs, sustained culture-free status among survivors was 74.8%.[54] Postoperative complications were noted in 22.6% of patients.
    - Other reports of surgery for MDR-TB similarly show improved outcome and low relapse rates.[55-58]

## Principles of Peri- and Postoperative Management

- Continue multidrug therapy until sputum clear (usually 6 to 9 months)
- Nutritional supplementation is very important because malnutrition is rampant in this population

## Prevention and Management of Complications

- Complications include empyema, bronchopleural fistula, and bronchogenic spread of mycobacterial disease.
  - These are more frequent when the sputum is positive at the time of operation.
  - Some believe that eradication of the disease requires obliteration of all space with latissimus or pectoralis free flap, or with thoracoplasty to reduce residual pleural space.
- Prevention: complications may be limited but not completely avoided in these patients with buttressing of the divided airway with tissue flap.
  - Omental or muscle flaps are most common.

## Natural History/Prognosis

- Progression common
- Resistance organisms are important and significant public health issue
- A recent study of 48 patients with XDR-TB treated with aggressive appropriate therapy reported a 60% cure rate, with the cure rate for 603 patients with MDR-TB reported as 66%.[59]

Thoracic surgical procedures were performed in five out of 28 patients with XDR-TB after a median of 31 months of chemotherapy and in 87 out of 603 patients with MDR-TB.[59]

---

**KEY FACTS**

- Delivery of therapy remains major stumbling block to effective eradication of infection.
- Indications for surgery much more common with MDR-TB and XDR-TB.
- Know local patterns of resistance (or where the patient contracted the infection).

---

## Brief Illustrative Case 2

- A 22-year-old woman who emigrated from the far east presents with fever, night sweats, and productive cough of several months duration.
- Skin PPD is positive.
- Chest CT is performed (Fig. 16-8), demonstrating severe bronchiectatic and cavitary parenchymal disease involving the right lung. The majority of the right lung is essentially destroyed. The left lung is relatively free of damage
- Induced sputum and BAL yield a positive AFB smear; TB resistant to isoniazid and rifampin is isolated
- Treatment is initiated with IV amikacin, ethambutol, pyrazinamide, and moxifloxacin.

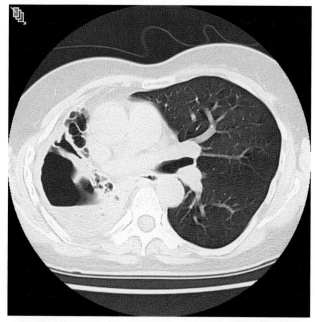

**Figure 16-8:** A chest computed tomography scan of the patient in second illustrative case, demonstrating severe bronchiectatic and cavitary parenchymal disease involving the right lung. The majority of the right lung is essentially destroyed. A hydropneumothorax is evident. The left lung is relatively free of damage.

- At 6 months, the patient is clinically improved but still AFB positive on sputum smear. Workup is undertaken for right pneumonectomy. Adequate pulmonary reserve is demonstrated
- A right pneumonectomy is performed using an extrapleural approach. The right main stem bronchial stump is covered with intercostal muscle flap. The postoperative course is uneventful. Conversion to smear and culture negative status was confirmed.
- Antibiotics are continued for another 18 months, with no recurrence of symptoms.

# NONTUBERCULOUS MYCOBACTERIAL INFECTIONS

## Terminology
- Also known as atypical mycobacteria, mycobacteria other than tuberculosis (MOTT), environmental mycobacteria
- See monograph on NTM infections.[60]

## Definition
- A spectrum of pulmonary infections with mycobacteria other than *M. tuberculosis*

## Etiology
- NTM organisms are ubiquitous in the environment
  - Found in water, soils, food, and on surfaces
  - Resistant to chlorination, disinfectants
  - Not obligate pathogens
- Increased incidence of infection in Gulf Coast states, but infection can be seen in all states.
- Cause of increased susceptibility in some individuals is unclear but likely genetic in nature.
- No person-to-person transmission.
- Actual incidence is unknown but appears to be on the rise.

## Pathogenesis/Pathophysiology
- Risk factors for pulmonary infection[60,61]
  - Geographic location (Gulf Coast)
  - Occupational exposure to soils (possibly water)
  - Pre-existing lung disease
  - Chronic obstructive pulmonary disease (COPD)
  - Gastroesophageal reflux
  - Cavitary disease
  - Bronchiectasis
  - Cystic Fibrosis
  - Female gender
  - Interferon gamma pathway defects
  - Scoliosis, pectus excavatum
- Transmission is not from person to person.
- Main NTM pathogens include
  - Slow-growing organisms
    - MAC
      - *M. avium*
      - *M. intracellulare*
    - *M. xenopi, M. malmonense, M. simiae, M. kansasii*
  - Rapid-growing organisms, so named because of their rapid isolation in vitro
    - *M. abscessus*
    - *M. chelonae*
    - *M. fortuitum*

## Clinical Features

- Demographic[60,61]
  - Not communicable, and thus true incidence not tracked by the Centers for Disease Control and Prevention.
  - May be associated with COPD, pulmonary fibrosis, and rheumatoid arthritis.
  - Rising incidence of certain phenotypes, such as middle-aged, slender white women.
- Clinical Presentation[60-63]
  - Chronic productive cough, dyspnea, hemoptysis, fatigue, recurrent pneumonias, fever
  - Two main clinical presentations
    - Middle-aged or elderly men, often with history of smoking and underlying COPD. Resembles TB with upper lobe cavitary disease. May progress to complete lung destruction.
    - Women older than 50 years of age, thin, white, nonsmokers, with right middle lobe and lingular disease—typically fibronodular bronchiectasis with occasional consolidation or cavity formation.
- Complications
  - Chronic infection can lead to significant lung destruction and nonfunctional parenchyma
  - Lung destruction may progress to other areas not initially involved with infection
  - Cachexia and malnutrition
  - Hemoptysis, rarely massive

## Diagnostic Workup

- Distinction between colonization, contamination, and true infection can be difficult[60,61,63]
- Culture testing
  - Cultures placed on both solid and liquid media.
  - Growth can take 4 to 6 weeks.
  - Liquid media is faster (10 to 14 days) but less sensitive.
  - Rapid growers may take less than 1 week in culture.
  - Decontamination required to prevent bacterial overgrowth.
  - Tissue specimens "double cultured."
  - Nucleic probes used to identify precise organism
- Routine sensitivity testing discouraged.
  - MAC: macrolide testing.
  - *M. kansasii*: rifampin testing
- Radiologic studies demonstrate typical patterns of disease
  - Fibronodular bronchiectasis
  - Cavitary lung disease
  - Destroyed lung
- Diagnosis usually requires presence of symptoms, characteristic radiologic findings, and repeated (two to three) positive cultures/smears after malignancy, TB, and fungal disease excluded

## Treatment

- Medical[60,61]
  - Primarily involves multidrug antibiotic therapy, often for 18 months
  - Therapy directed in part by susceptibility testing, and should be continued 12 months after culture negative
  - Examples include
    - MAC: macrolide, rifampin, ethambutol, with or without amikacin
    - *M. kansasii*: rifampin, ethambutol, isoniazid
    - *M. abscessus*: macrolide, amikacin, cefoxitin, and imipenem. The regimen for combination therapy is ultimately based on sensitivities to include several of these agents.
  - Multidrug combination therapy can be difficult to take, and therefore, compliance with medical therapy can be poor

- Surgical[61,64]
  - Rationale for surgery is to remove areas of devitalized lung tissue that do not "see" the delivered antibiotic therapy, and thus serve as a reservoir for the offending organism, promoting recurrence of the infection at a later date
  - Indications for surgery similar to those for bronchiectasis—persistent, focal (cavitary or bronchiectatic) parenchymal disease after recurrent antimicrobial treatment
  - Occasionally, "debulking" procedures in setting of nonfocal disease may slow disease progression and reduce symptoms
  - Pretreatment with targeted antimicrobial therapy for at least 2 to 3 months is essential before surgical intervention.
  - Anatomic lung resection (segment, lobe) is preferable.
  - Thoracoscopic approach is possible in many cases; bilateral thoracoscopic resections are usually staged 6 to 8 weeks apart
  - In cases of significant pleural symphysis, extrapleural dissection may be needed.
  - Severe disease may require pneumonectomy

## Principles of Peri- and Postoperative Management

- Nutrition is key to good outcomes
- Antibiotics continue throughout perioperative course. Culture results from surgical specimens guide further antibiotic management. Medical therapy often continued for many months after surgery

## Prevention and Management of Complications

- Morbidity and mortality of these procedures is generally low
- Common misconceptions/mistakes include
  - Inadequate pretreatment with targeted antimicrobial therapy
  - Lack of focal disease
  - Nonanatomic or incomplete resection
  - Expect an intrathoracic space after anatomic resection
  - Buttress pneumonectomy stumps or in setting of poorly controlled infection
  - Create an open thoracostomy if pleural contamination occurs
- Bronchopleural fistula most serious complication, associated with
  - MAC infection
  - Right pneumonectomy
  - Positive sputum at operation
- Certain rapid growers, such as *M. abscessus*, can cause troublesome skin and soft tissue infections

## Natural History/Prognosis

- Long-term surgical outcomes remain unknown
- Treatment goal is suppression or remission, not cure, because determinants of susceptibility remain unknown

| KEY FACTS |
| --- |
| ■ Environmental organisms without person-to-person transmission<br>■ Diagnosis can be difficult to establish<br>■ Prolonged multidrug antibiotic regimen is mainstay of therapy<br>■ Surgery used in select cases of focal, recurrent disease |

## *SWYER-JAMES SYNDROME*

### Terminology

- Unilateral hyperlucent lung syndrome
- Bret's syndrome
- Janus' syndrome
- Macleod's syndrome
- Swyer-James-Macleod syndrome
  - See Chapter 14 on "Congenital and Developmental Lung Malformations"

## PULMONARY FUNGAL INFECTIONS

## *HISTOPLASMOSIS*

### Definition

- Histoplasmosis in the systemic manifestation of disease caused by *Histoplasma capsulatum*
  - Found in soil as a mold, and in yeast form at body temperature

### Etiology

- Infection is caused by the dimorphic fungus *Histoplasma capsulatum*
- Microspores from the mycelial phase act as the transmitted agent, inhaled into the lung
- No transmission through direct human contact

### Pathogenesis/Pathophysiology

- Cell-mediated immunity is critical for host response.
- Granulomas form within lung and lymph nodes, with central necrosis and calcification.
- Progressive disseminated infection may develop in those with impaired cell-mediated immunity.
  - Liver, spleen, lymphatic system, adrenal glands
  - Diffuse pulmonary infiltrates
- Cavitary pulmonary histoplasmosis occurs in 10% of patients with symptomatic disease, usually in those with COPD
- Fibrosing mediastinitis results from excessive scarring from chronic disease (see Chapter 45 on Fibrosing Mediastinitis)

### Clinical Features
#### Demographic

- Endemic in the Mississippi, Missouri, and Ohio river valleys.
- Farmers, construction workers, and people who enjoy outdoor activities are the most at risk by inhaling spores.
- Outbreaks have been documented following construction, cleaning attics or barns, demolition, and cave exploration.
- 1 in 2000 people will develop chronic pulmonary disease.
- Disseminated infection occurs in approximately 1 in 100000.

#### Clinical Presentation

- Most patients are asymptomatic or have a mild flu-like syndrome[65,66]
  - Pulmonary manifestations include
  - *Histoplasmoma:* nodule usually smaller than 3 cm; commonly calcified; may be mistaken for a tumor
  - *Acute pneumonia:* lobar consolidation with or without mediastinal and hilar adenopathy
  - *Isolated hilar and mediastinal adenopathy* (can simulate sarcoidosis)

- *Massive inhalational histoplasmosis:* multilobar consolidation and adenopathy
- *Chronic histoplasmosis:* chronic cavitary disease that can simulate TB. Occurs in middle-aged men often with underlying lung disease (e.g., emphysema)
- *Disseminated histoplasmosis:* produces miliary disease. Progressive disseminated histoplasmosis is a risk for patients with deficiencies in cellular immunity (medically immune suppressed, lymphatic or hematopoetic malignancy, or acquired immunodeficiency syndrome [AIDS])
- *Mediastinal disease:* Fibrosing mediastinits; superior vena cava (SVC) syndrome, and so on.
- *Broncholith:* this refers to erosion of calcified lymph nodes through a bronchus. Can result in postobstructive pneumonia, atelectasis, hemoptysis (Fig. 16-9)
- *Pericardial disease with or without adenopathy*

### Diagnostic Workup

- Imaging: chest radiograph/CT[65,67]
- Stain and culture of pulmonary secretions/bronchoalveolar lavage (BAL)
- Histopathology: Occurs as an intracellular yeast and is seen best on methenamine silver stain (Fig. 16-10)
- Antigen testing: tests a histoplasma glycoprotein. Can be done on urine, blood, and BAL fluid.
- Serology: Complement fixation and immunodiffusion tests are commonly used. The sensitivity of both are 95% and 90% respectively, with immunodiffusion testing exhibiting higher specificity.
- Skin testing: with histoplasmin antigen confirms exposure to the pathogen not disease
- Suggested tests in specific circumstances:
  - *Acute pneumonia:* serology; antigen testing positive in only about 20% if low fungal burden; BAL antigen testing better; BAL with or without biopsy depending on circumstances, culture.
  - *Acute diffuse pneumonia:* antigen (sensitive because of high fungal burden), cultures; BAL with or without biopsy depending on circumstances; serology negative early on (up to 4 weeks), culture
  - *Chronic/cavitary disease:* cultures; BAL with or without biopsy depending on circumstances; urine antigen less sensitive (BAL antigen may be better)

### Treatment

- Medical
  - See Table 16-1 for indications for antifungal therapy for the different pulmonary manifestations of *H. capsulatum.*
  - See 2007 IDSA guidelines for management of histoplasmosis.[68] In summary:
    - *Mild-to-moderate acute pulmonary histoplasmosis:* Most commonly, no treatment is required. In patients who have persistent symptoms for more than 1 month, treatment is offered. Itraconazole 200 mg tid for 3 days and then 200 mg once or twice daily for 6 to 12 weeks.
    - *Moderate-to-severe acute pulmonary histoplasmosis:* Lipid amphotericin IV for 1 to 2 weeks, then itraconazole 200 mg tid for 3 days, followed by 200 mg twice daily for 12 weeks. In patients with severe respiratory distress and hypoxemia, IV methylprednisolone (0.5-1.0 mg/kg) can be considered for the first 1 to 2 weeks.
    - *Chronic cavitary pulmonary histoplasmosis:* Itraconazole 200 mg tid for 3 days and then 200 mg once or twice daily for at least 1 year. Can give for 18 to 24 months to avoid relapse. Relapse occurs in about 15% of cases.

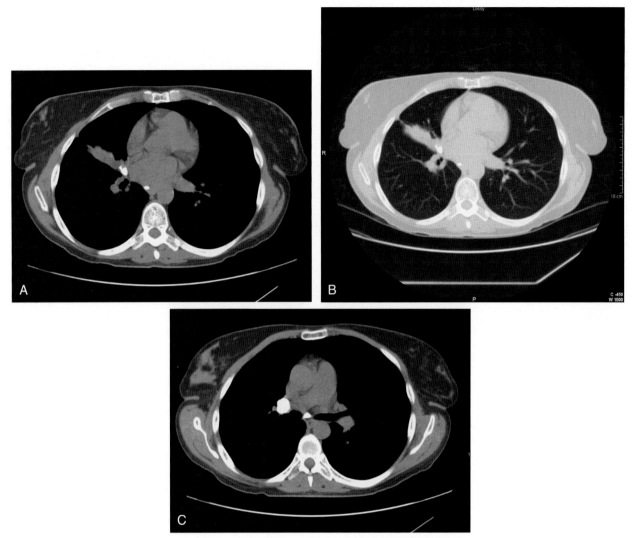

**Figure 16-9:** **A** and **B,** Chest computed tomography scan depicting calcified lymph nodes, together with a broncholith in the right middle lobe (RML) bronchus with RML collapse. **C,** Extensive hilar and mediastinal calcification in CT slice from same patient.

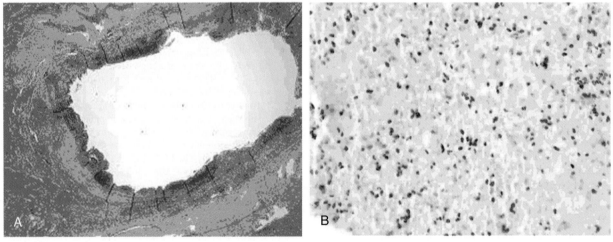

**Figure 16-10:** **A,** Histopathology from case depicted in Figure 16-9 showing bronchiectasis in the right middle lobe with chronic inflammation. **B,** Gomori methenamine silver (GMS) stain of a hilar lymph node from patient above, showing numerous histoplasma organisms in an old hyalinized granuloma.

## TABLE 16-1 ■ INDICATIONS FOR ANTIFUNGAL THERAPY IN HISTOPLASMOSIS PULMONARY DISEASE

**Definite Indication, Proven or Probable Efficacy**

Acute diffuse pulmonary infection, moderately severe symptoms, or severe symptoms
Chronic cavitary pulmonary infection
Progressive disseminated infection
Central nervous system infection

**Uncertain Indication, Unknown Efficacy**

Acute focal pulmonary infection, asymptomatic case, or mild symptoms that persist for 11 months
Mediastinal lymphadenitis
Mediastinal granuloma
Inflammatory syndromes, treated with corticosteroids

**Not Recommended, Unknown Efficacy, or Ineffective**

Mediastinal fibrosis
Pulmonary nodule
Broncholithiasis
Presumed ocular histoplasmosis syndrome

*From Wheat JL, Freifeld AG, Kleiman MB, Baddley JW, McKinsey JS, Loyd JE, Kauffman CA. Clinical practice guidelines for the management of patients with histoplasmosis: 2007 Update by the Infectious Diseases Society of America. Clin Infect Dis 2007;45:807-825, with permission.*

- *Progressive disseminated histoplasmosis*: Amphotericin B (lipid or other formulations) for 1 to 2 weeks, followed by itraconazole 200 mg two to three times daily for at least 1 year (or longer with persistent immunodeficiency).
- Monitoring of therapeutic drug levels of itraconazole recommended with severe disease and prolonged administration.
- Surgical
  ○ Anatomic resection reserved for complications or failed medical therapy
    - Chronic cavitary pulmonary disease–persistent thick-walled cavity
  ○ Surgery to remove or bypass obstruction in mediastinal granuloma. In fibrosing mediastinitis, surgery is most often unrewarding and should be avoided. Stents are commonly used in this setting (see Chapter 45 on Fibrosing Mediastinitis)

## Principles of Peri- and Postoperative Management

- Antimicrobials must be continued as adjunct to surgery.

## Prevention and Management of Complications

- Prevention of recurrent or persistent infection remains the most important management for these patients.
- Remove as much of the damaged/infected tissue as possible through anatomic lung resection.

## Natural History/Prognosis

- Early medical management has excellent outcomes
- Patients with the most complicated conditions undergo surgery; outcomes are varied but cure is likely with surgical intervention in most complicated cases.

## KEY FACTS

- Endemic to Mississippi and Ohio river valleys.
- Affects many more people than have complicated infection.
- Surgical therapy is reserved for complicated infection.

# COCCIDIOIDOMYCOSIS

## Definition

- Coccidioidomycosis is the illness caused by the pathogenic fungus *Coccidioides immitis*.[69-71]

## Terminology

- Coccidioidomycosis
- San Joaquin Valley fever
- Desert or Valley fever

## Etiology

- Causative agent is the dimorphic fungus *C. immitus*
  ○ Resilient, can withstand periods of drought and high salinity
  ○ Intolerant of cold
  ○ Found in soil as mold
- Infection occurs after spore inhalation

## Pathogenesis/Pathophysiology

- Infecting structures are arthroconidia (spores), released from mold stalk and inhaled.
- Spherules develop in distal alveolar sacs, liberating further spores and perpetuating invasive process.
- Cell-mediated immunity is critical to limit infection.

## Clinical Features

- Demographic
  ○ Endemic areas are the Southwestern United States and Mexico
  ○ Inhalation of spore laden dust places agricultural and construction workers, as well as those with avid outdoor pursuits, at risk
- Clinical presentation[69-71]
  ○ Acute valley fever is characterized by cough, fever, fatigue, dyspnea, chest pain, headache.
  ○ Development of erythema nodosum, and arthralgias suggest excellent immune response.
  ○ Symptoms occur 1 to 4 weeks after exposure.
  ○ Infection is usually self-limited and remits in several days.
  ○ A minority of patients develop persistent disease or complications.
- Pulmonary manifestations[70]:
  ○ *Acute uncomplicated pneumonia*
  ○ *Acute progressive pneumonia*
  ○ *Diffuse reticulonodular/miliary pneumonia* (often in immunocompromised hosts; fungemia)
  ○ *Adult respiratory distress syndrome* (ARDS)
  ○ *Chronic fibrocavitary pneumonia*
  ○ *Residual pulmonary nodule or nodules*
  ○ *Thin-walled cavities* can be complicated by check valve expansion, rupture, pneumothorax, hemorrhage, rupture into pleural space with bronchopleural fistula and empyema, secondary infection of cyst (Fig. 16-11)

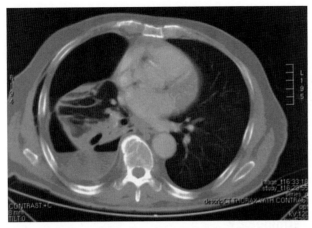

**Figure 16-11:** Computed tomography (CT) scan chest of a patient with a known enlarging cavity due to coccidioidomycosis. The patient presented with acute onset chest pain, dyspnea, and hypoxemia. The CT study reveals a hydropneumothorax due to rupture of the cyst.

○ The most important *extrapulmonary* manifestation is meningitis as a result of *disseminated disease*. Other areas confirming dissemination include bone and skin disease.
○ Risk factors for disseminated disease include the following:
  • Cell-mediated immune compromise is the greatest risk factor.
  • African Americans, Filipinos, American Indians, and Hispanics may be more susceptible to disseminated disease.
  • Men may have higher risk than women.
  • Pregnancy has been considered a risk for disseminated disease but is controversial.
  • Extremes of age
  • Diabetes mellitus

## Diagnostic Workup
■ Chest radiography and CT may demonstrate[69-72]:
  ○ Patchy, nonspecific infiltrates: segmental, lobar, multilobar (Fig. 16-12)
  ○ Diffuse miliary/reticulonodular infiltrates
  ○ Chronic upper lobe infiltrates and cavitation
  ○ Nodule or nodules
  ○ Thin-walled cavities

○ Hilar with or without mediastinal adenopathy
○ Pleural effusions
■ Diagnosis is made by serologic testing for immunoglobulin M (IgM) or IgG antibodies
  ○ IgM antibodies can be measured by tube precipitin tests or more commonly now, by immunodiffusion. These become positive within the first 3 weeks in 90%. It becomes negative usually by 3 months.
  ○ IgG antibodies are measured with the complement fixation test. It is positive by 8 weeks in symptomatic patients and remains positive for longer than the immunodiffusion test.
  ○ High-complement fixation titers such as 1:32 suggest severe disease. Rising serial titers of 1:16 or greater suggest dissemination and should be further investigated (bone scan, cerebrospinal [CSF] examination).
  ○ Enzyme-linked immunosorbent assay (ELISAs) and latex tests are sensitive but exhibit false positive results (particularly latex assays).
  ○ Note: Negative serology does not exclude a diagnosis of coccidioidomycosis, especially early on.
■ Sputum culture can provide definitive diagnosis in a minority of cases.
■ The spherules have a thin wall containing endospores, which are seen on wet mount slides
■ Bronchoscopy: BAL with or without transbronchial biopsy far more sensitive. (Positive with multilobar disease in two thirds of patients.) Open biopsy rarely necessary (Fig. 16-13)

## Treatment
■ Medical[73]
  ○ Most patients require no therapy with uncomplicated primary pulmonary infection. However, some authorities recommend treatment of all symptomatic patients. The presence of immune compromise should prompt treatment in all patients.
  ○ Amphotericin B is antifungal of choice for severe disease
  ○ Azole therapy with fluconazole 400 to 800 mg/day (PO or IV) or itraconazole (200 mg bid) can be used initially. Azole therapy can also be used for continuing maintenance therapy (following initial amphotericin) with severe disease.
  ○ For acute pneumonia, treatment courses are usually for 3 to 6 months.
  ○ For diffuse severe pneumonia, therapy is given for at least 1 year. This may be continued indefinitely in immunocompromised patients.

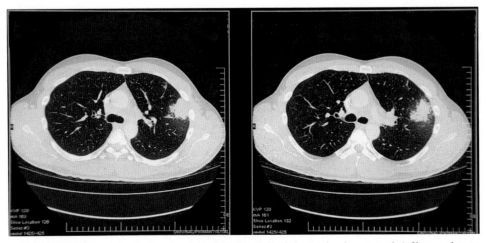

**Figure 16-12:** Computed tomography chest depicting left-sided peripheral segmental infiltrates due to coccidioidomycosis.

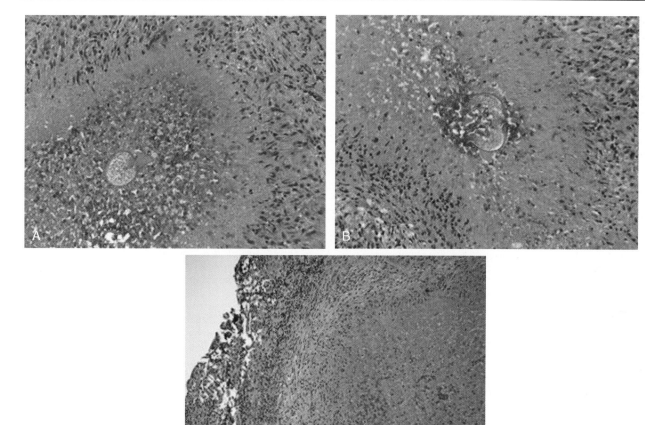

**Figure 16-13:** Histopathology from case depicted in Figure 16-12. **A,** Granuloma with coccidioides spherule. **B,** Ruptured spherule. **C,** Necrotizing granuloma.

○ Prolonged treatment is usually given (1 year) with chronic fibrocavitary disease.
○ Indications for medical therapy:
  ● Immunocompromised patients with pneumonia
  ● Severe, prolonged pulmonary disease
  ● Chronic fibrocavitary disease
  ● Risk of dissemination (see risk factors above)
  ● Disseminated disease; neurologic disease
  ● Chronic symptomatic cavitary disease
  ● Adjunct to surgical resection in setting of active disease
■ Surgical
  ○ Reserved for complications or failed medical therapy
    ● Enlarging cavitary lesion
    ● Refractory chronic fibrocavitary disease that is well localized.
    ● Hemoptysis
    ● Secondary infection
    ● Early treatment of bronchopleural fistula due to cavity rupture
  ○ Chronic nodules may mimic carcinoma, requiring resection to settle issue.

## Principles of Peri- and Postoperative Management

■ Perioperative amphotericin B is recommended for these patients with active disease; excision of a chronic nodule or nodules does not require antifungal therapy.

## Prevention and Management of Complications
■ Nutritional support and antimicrobial therapy are critical

## Natural History/Prognosis
■ For most, infection is self-limited.
■ Disseminated or pulmonary disease requires medical treatment.
■ Surgery is limited to complications of cavitary disease and suspicious nodules.

---

**KEY FACTS**

---

■ In the vast majority of cases, infection does not require treatment.
■ Disseminated disease and certain pulmonary manifestations require medical treatment.
■ Infection in the immunocompromised host can be very difficult to clear.

---

## *BLASTOMYCOSIS*
### Definition
■ Blastomycosis is a suppurative and granulomatous pulmonary disease caused by *Blastomyces dermatitidis*

## Etiology

- Causative agent is dimorphic fungus *B. dermatitidis*

## Pathogenesis/Pathophysiology

- Infecting microconidia are inhaled to alveolar level.
- Replicating yeast generates cell-mediated immune reaction.
- Pneumonitis forms with regional lymph node invol-vement.
- Granuloma formation ensues, with fibrosis and less commonly, calcification.
- Disseminated disease rare in absence of cell-mediated immune deficiencies.

## Clinical Features

- Demographic[74]
  - The endemic areas are the southeastern and central United States.
  - Fungus frequently found in soil near bodies of water making those with outdoor occupation and recreational duties at risk.
- Pulmonary manifestations[75]
  - *Asymptomatic/minor disease:* Can be asymptomatic or result in influenza-like syndrome - fever, chills, myalgias, arthralgias, and dry cough.
  - *Acute pneumonitis:* Most symptomatic patients recover in 2 to 3 weeks.
  - *Acute severe and progressive pneumonia:* multilobar; can progress to respiratory failure and ARDS.
  - *Chronic infection:* involves the upper lobes with a pyogranulomatous process.
  - *Disseminated disease:* involves multiple organs.
  - The most common extrapulmonary manifestation is cutaneous ulcers or verrucous lesions.

## Complications

  - Infiltrates may solidify along with the formation of granulomas to create a mass that is suggestive of lung carcinoma
  - Fungal dissemination involving the skin, bones, meninges, prostate, and adrenals may occur in the setting of immune deficiencies and compromised states

## Diagnostic Workup

- Imaging: chest radiograph, CT[76]
  - Nonspecific consolidation most commonly involves the upper lobes, particularly with acute disease.
  - Multilobar consolidation with or without cavitation (10% to 15%)
  - Chronic fibrocavitary disease of upper lobes (can simulate TB)
  - Mass lesions: can be large (e.g., >6 cm).
  - Nodules with or without consolidation
  - Miliary pattern
  - Pleural effusion in 20%; often in conjunction with pleural thickening
- Culture and pathology:
  - Sputum stains (potassium hydroxide [KOH]; periodic acid–Schiff [PAS], Papanicolou): can demonstrate large round organisms with double refractile thick cell walls and multiple nuclei. Can have high yield (78% in one study with Papanicolou); yield increases with repeat sputum samples. Culture takes 1 to 3 weeks.
  - Stains and culture of other fluids: aspirated pus, pleural fluid, urine
  - Bronchoscopy: BAL with or without transbronchial biopsy

- Serodiagnosis:
  - Complement fixation, immunodiffusion, and enzyme immunoassay
  - Highly variable reported results make serology not reliable

## Treatment

- Medical[77]
  - For moderately severe to severe pulmonary disease or disseminated disease, treatment is typically initiated with lipid amphotericin or amphotericin B for 1 to 2 weeks. This is followed by itraconazole (200 mg bid) for 6 to 12 months.
  - For mild to moderate pulmonary or disseminated disease, itraconazole (200 mg once or twice daily) is given for 6 to 12 months
  - For persistent immunocompromised states, lifelong suppressive treatment is required.
  - Serum itraconazole levels should be measured after 2 weeks of therapy to ensure that therapeutic levels are achieved.
- Surgical
  - Surgical excision is primarily used to exclude malignancy and establish the diagnosis.
  - Rarely, surgical intervention is needed for complications of pulmonary disease (empyema, hemoptysis, fistula)

## Principles of Peri- and Postoperative Management

- Resection is simply a diagnostic adjunct; it plays little role in treatment.
- Antifungal coverage in perioperative period is advised, if possible.

## Prevention and Management of Complications

- Correct diagnosis is key.
- Itraconazole is the antimicrobial of choice, except in moderately severe to severe pulmonary or disseminated disease.

## Natural History/Prognosis

- Subclinical disease requires no treatment
- Medical therapy is mainstay

---

**KEY FACTS**

---

- Surgery is mainly aid in diagnosis and is used to rule out malignancy.

---

## *CRYPTOCOCCUS*

### Definition

- Cryptococcosis is a subacute or chronic infection caused by *Cryptococcus neoformans*
- Often associated with cryptococcal meningitis

### Etiology

- Causative agent is the encapsulated yeast *C. neoformans*

## Clinical Features

- Demographic[78]
  - No known demographic area, but different serotypes are thought to be responsible for infection in normal and immunocompromised hosts
  - May be present in pigeon droppings.
- Clinical presentation
  - The portal of entry in humans is the respiratory tract.
  - Pulmonary symptoms are usually nonspecific or absent.
  - Cough, hemoptysis, low-grade fever, weakness, and lethargy can occur

## Complications

- Always examine CSF if *C. neoformans* is isolated from sputum or surgical specimen.
- Ten percent of patients develop cryptococcal meningitis after resection of a pulmonary lesion.

## Diagnostic Workup

- Chest radiograph and CT can show lobar consolidation, infiltrates, a mass or masses, nodules, hilar and mediastinal adenopathy, or pleural effusions.[79]
- Antigen testing: Serum cryptococcal antigen is positive in most patient with AIDS and cryptococcal meningitis, and is also useful in other conditions of immune compromise. Tests can also be performed on pleural fluid, CSF, and so on.
- Stain and culture of sputum, BAL fluid, pleural fluid can be diagnostic.
  - India ink staining reveals round budding yeast, which has gelatinous polysaccharide capsule.
- CSF should always be examined (stain, culture, antigen testing).
- Culture of cutaneous lesions can provide a definitive diagnosis.
- Bronchoscopy as needed (BAL; transbronchial biopsy).

## Treatment

- Medical[80]
  - For immunocompetent patients with only pneumonia, fluconazole therapy (200 to 400 mg/day for 3 to 6 months if asymptomatic and 6-12 months with mild-moderate symptomatic disease) is prudent as the risk of dissemination even in this group is not zero. Itraconazole also has activity.
  - With meningitis, amphotericin B and 5-flucytosine (100 mg/kg/day) is the treatment of choice for induction (2 weeks of therapy), followed by fluconazole (400 mg/day) for 10 weeks.
  - For severe pulmonary disease or pneumonia in the immunocompromised host, treat as for meningitis.
  - In patients with HIV and other states in which persistent immune compromise may be observed, lifelong suppressive therapy is required (e.g., fluconazole 200 mg/day).
- Surgical
  - Rule out malignancy (unsure diagnosis)

## Principles of Peri- and Post-Operative Management

- Usually encountered as an incidental finding following resection of pulmonary mass, which should trigger further workup including CSF examination.

## Prevention and Management of Complications

- Remain cognizant of meningeal predilection.

## Natural History/Prognosis

- Complete resection can cure infection
- Meningeal involvement suggests less optimal outcome

---

**KEY FACTS**

- Can be incidental finding.
- Do not overlook central nervous system (CNS) infection, incidental finding necessitates lumbar puncture (LP) for CSF.
- Spontaneous remission occurs in many patients with mild disease.

---

## *ASPERGILLOSIS*

### Definition

- Pulmonary disease secondary to *Aspergillus* species presents in several main forms.
  - Aspergilloma (mycetoma)
  - Chronic necrotizing aspergillosis
  - Invasive aspergillosis
  - ABPA
  - Hypersensitivity pneumonitis

### Etiology

- More than 200 species of *Aspergillus*, a ubiquitous soil-dwelling organism
- Small conidiophores released, which are easily inhaled
- *Aspergillus fumigatus*, *Aspergillus flavus*, and *Aspergillus niger* are the most common, with *A. fumigatus* dominating in human disease

### Pathogenesis/Pathophysiology

- An *aspergilloma* (mycetoma) is a mass of fungal elements, inflammatory cells, and mucus/tissue debris which forms in a pre-existing lung cavity
- *Chronic necrotizing aspergillosis (subacute invasive aspergillosis)* is a locally invasive form of aspergillosis that is usually associated with chronic underlying lung disease (e.g., COPD) with or without milder degrees of immune compromise (low-dose steroid exposure, poor nutrition, diabetes, and so on).
- *Invasive pulmonary aspergillosis* is a rare but rapidly progressive infection that occurs in the setting of[81]:
  - Myelosuppression therapies
  - Neutropenia (prolonged; >3 weeks) or neutrophil dysfunction
  - Cell-mediated immune dysfunction
  - Solid organ (especially lung) and blood stem cell transplants
  - AIDS
  - Corticosteroid therapy
  - Multiple antibiotics
  - Anti-tumor necrosis factor (TNF) agents
- *ABPA* is a hypersensitivity reaction to *Aspergillus* antigens, usually in those with long-standing asthma or cystic fibrosis. This is not a surgical condition and will not be discussed further. (See review papers for more details.[82-84])
- *Hypersensitivity pneumonitis*: a hypersensitivity response to aspergillus allergens that produces acute, subacute, or chronic presentations. Biopsy classically shows loosely formed granulomas. This is not a surgical condition and will not be discussed further. (See review papers for more details.[85])

## Clinical Features

- Demographic
  - No known demographic area but found in soil and on decaying vegetation

## Clinical Presentation

- *Aspergilloma*: frequently asymptomatic but can present with hemoptysis (minor to massive; likely related to friction of the mycetoma against cavity blood vessels); cough, sputum, and so on.[86,87]
- *Chronic necrotizing aspergillosis*: symptoms are often those of the underlying chronic lung disorder. Patients are often middle aged or elderly. Symptoms are fever, cough, sputum production, and weight loss.
- *Invasive pulmonary aspergillosis*: fever, nonproductive cough, dyspnea, hemoptysis, pleuritic chest pain (due to pleural based lung infarction caused by the vessel invasion) are frequently present.

## Complications

- Aspergilloma: hemoptysis, occasionally massive
- Chronic necrotizing aspergillosis: "worsening of underlying lung disease." Can simulate TB. May have associated fungus balls within the involved area with associated complications.
- Invasive aspergillosis: Diffuse progressive infection with vascular invasion culminating in lung destruction; respiratory compromise, hemoptysis, and so on. The mortality rate remains high in this setting despite treatment.

### Diagnostic Workup

- Radiologic studies[88]:
  - *Aspergilloma*: thick-walled cavity, usually upper lobe, with mobile mass or "fungal ball" within. Associated pleural thickening is not uncommon (Fig. 16-14).
  - *Chronic necrotizing aspergillosis*: nodule or infiltrate/consolidation most commonly in the upper lobe or superior segments of the lower lobe; cavitation; may have associated mycetoma/s (up to 50%); evidence of underlying chronic lung disease.
  - *Invasive pulmonary aspergillosis*: often nonspecific, but may show pleural infiltrates/consolidation, nodules including ground-glass opacities and peripheral densities suggestive of

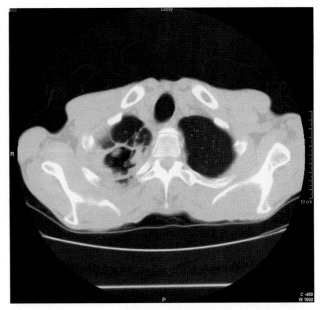

**Figure 16-14:** Chest computed tomography scan in a patient with chronic cystic lung disease in which a small aspergilloma is evident. Note also associated pleural thickening.

infarction. The Halo sign is a nodule with surrounding ground-glass opacification due to hemorrhage; it is an important CT sign suggestive of invasion. The air crescent sign on CT is another important indicator and results from circumferential lung necrosis (Fig. 16-15).

- Other diagnostic studies:
  - Aspergilloma:
    - Aspergillus precipitins is present in almost 100% of patients. Negative studies suggest nonfumigatus species
    - Culture of sputum may show *Aspergillus* but results are negative in at least half of cases.
  - Chronic necrotizing aspergillosis:
    - Sputum or BAL culture
    - Pathology: Transbronchial biopsy has poor yield and high risk; video assisted thoracoscopic surgery (VATS)/open biopsy showing tissue invasion is best but is limited often by poor pulmonary reserve of patients.

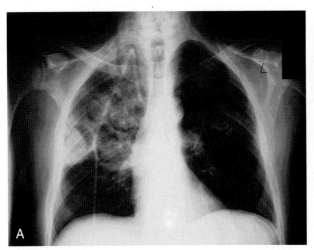

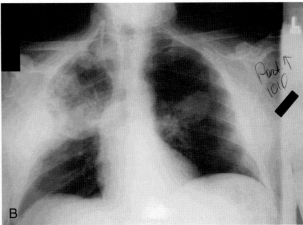

**Figure 16-15:** Chest radiographs of two different patients with invasive pulmonary aspergillosis. In both **A** and **B,** clear crescent signs are evident. In **B,** some ground-glass opacification is faintly evident around the nodule noted on the left.

- As with aspergilloma, precipitins can be positive.
- Galactomannan: fungus wall antigen. Limited data for this entity (see later).
- Compatible clinical and radiologic features, together with aspergillus isolated in sputum and exclusion of other disorders in the differential, are often all that can be done for diagnosis in patients with poor reserve.
○ Invasive pulmonary aspergillosis:
- Sputum cultures are often negative (50% to 70%). In patients at high risk who are sputum positive, empiric treatment pending further studies is prudent. In patients with hematologic malignancies, for example, positive sputum studies were reported to have positive predictive values of 80% to 90%.[86] In other patient groups not at high risk, specificity may be much lower (in part because of colonization).
- Bronchscopy: BAL particularly with diffuse lung disease.
- Lung biopsy: transbronchial biopsies are subject to sampling error and, thus, false-negative results. VATS/open lung biopsy is considered the gold standard to demonstrate hyphae with acute angles in lung tissue. Even open lung biopsy can be subject to sampling error. Silver stains produce best discrimination. Biopsy carries risks and risk/benefit should be considered on a case by case basis.
- In rare instances, transthoracic needle aspiration of a lung "mass" under CT guidance can be of value
- Serology: unhelpful
- Antigen studies:
  ○ Galactomannan, is a glycoprotein found on the aspergillus cell wall by an ELISA.
  ○ Recent studies have produced encouraging but variable results in different patient populations with invasive aspergillosis.[89-91] A recent meta-analysis in proven cases of invasive aspergillosis reported a sensitivity of 71% and a specificity of 89%. The test was most useful in patients with hematologic malignancies or following blood stem cell transplants. The test was less sensitive in patients with solid organ transplants.[89]
  ○ Galactomannan assay in BAL fluid increases sensitivity over serum asays in critically ill patients and lung transplant recipients.[92,93]
  ○ False-positive results have been reported with the use of piperacillin/tazobactam and amoxicillin/sulbactam.[94,95] Collection before an infusion of the antibiotic and using a cut off of greater than 0.7 will reduce this issue significantly.

## Treatment

- Medical[96]
  ○ Aspergilloma:
  - Usually no treatment is required.
  - Systemic antifungal therapy including intracavity installation has been reported in patients with limited pulmonary reserve (due to underlying disease such as late-stage sarcoidosis). These reports are anecdotal. The role of antifungal treatment is limited.
  - With massive hemoptysis in a patient with limited reserve, bronchial artery embolization can be tried. The presence of large collateral vessels may limit success.
  ○ Chronic necrotizing aspergillosis:
  - Treat underlying chronic lung disease.
  - Antifungal therapy: Voriconazole is the drug of choice. Recent data using voriconazole for an average of 6.5 months are encouraging.[97] Long-term and perhaps lifelong therapy may be required.
  ○ Invasive pulmonary aspergillosis:
  - Voriconazole (IV) is the treatment of choice (6 mg/kg every 12 hours for the first day, followed by 4 mg/kg every 12 hours. The oral dose is 200 to 300 mg every 12 hours).

- Liposomal amphotericin can be an alternative treatment.
- Combination therapy is not recommended for primary therapy.
- Salvage therapy can include posaconazole, itraconazole, caspofungin, and micafungin
- Duration of therapy: 6 to 12 weeks. For immunosuppressed patients, therapy is given until resolution of immunosuppression and the disease process. With ongoing immune compromise, maintenance suppressive therapy is recommended.
- Surgical
  ○ Aspergilloma:
  - Asymptomatic mycetomas should be left alone
  - Resection of aspergilloma is indicated for symptoms, particularly hemoptysis
  - Complete resection of cavity and fungal ball, usually through anatomic resection, is curative. A single mycetoma is optimal.
  - In up to 50% of cases after resection of an aspergilloma, the remaining lung does not expand well to fill the remaining chest cavity.
  - Other reported surgical complications include hemorrhage, bronchopleural fistula, and aspergillus empyema
  - In patients with poor pulmonary reserve, respiratory compromise can ensue.
  ○ Invasive and semi-invasive disease:
  - Diagnostic thoracoscopic or open lung biopsy
  - Therapeutic indications are unusual. These may include the following depending on circums-tances.[96,98]
    ○ Disease contiguous with great vessels or pericardium
    ○ Severe hemoptysis from a single cavitary lesion
    ○ Chest wall invasion
    ○ Relative: single pulmonary lesion before intensive chemotherapy or blood stem cell transplant

## Principles of Peri- and Postoperative Management

- Perioperative antifungal therapy adds little to aspergilloma resection

## Prevention and Management of Complications

- Same strategy for most pulmonary resections

## Natural History/Prognosis

- Resection of aspergilloma can have good outcomes
- The mortality rate for invasive aspergillosis remains high despite aggressive therapy

---

### KEY FACTS

- Immunocompromised status and cavitary lung disease predispose patients to Aspergillus pulmonary diseases.
- Medical therapy should be started as soon as possible with invasive disease.
- Most aspergillomas are asymptomatic but should be removed, if possible, if symptoms present and pulmonary reserve permits.

---

## *MUCORMYCOSIS*

### Definition

- Rhinocerebral or pulmonary infection caused by a number of genera such as Mucor, Rhizopus, Absidia, and others.

## Etiology

- Caused by fungi of the subclass Zygomycetes[99]
- Ubiquitous fungi found in soil and decaying organic debris.

## Pathogenesis/Pathophysiology

- Infection occurs by inhalation of spores, which travel through pharynx and usually cleared by the gastrointestinal tract. In at risk individuals, spores settle in and invade the nasal turbinates as a portal of entry or are inhaled into the lungs.
- Grows best in acidic, hyperglycemic environments, thus accounting for the susceptibility of patients with diabetic ketoacidosis.
- Risk factors include:
  - Diabetes
  - Metabolic acidotic states (e.g., ketoacidosis, renal tubular acidosis, and renal failure)
  - Hematologic malignancies
  - Cell-mediated immune dysfunction
    - Corticosteroid therapy
    - Solid organ transplant
    - AIDS
  - Desferoxamine therapy
  - In a large series and literature review, leukemia/lymphoma accounted for 37%, diabetes for 32%, renal failure 18%, transplantation 7.6%, and solid tumor 5.6%.[100]

## Sites of Involvement

- *Rhinocerebral:* nasal passage, palate, sinuses, orbits, erosion into cranium (most common in diabetics)
- *Pulmonary:* see features later (most common in hematologic malignancies and cell-mediated immune dysfunction).[101]
- *Other sites:* cutaneous, gastrointestinal, and the CNS.
- *Breakdown:* Depends on risk factors. Rhinocerebral (>50%), thoracic (20%), abdominal (15%), mixed organs (10%).

## Clinical Features

- Clinical presentation
  - *Rhinocerebral:* classic features include visible black eschars from tissue necrosis in the nasal turbinates and palate. Sinus involvement, periorbital swelling, opthalmoplegia, headache, cranial nerve involvement (5th, 7th)
  - *Pulmonary*[101]:
    - Pulmonary involvement presents as bronchopneumonia with progressive invasion, including pulmonary vessels, causing infarction.
    - Presentation similar to that of invasive aspergillosis.
    - Hemoptysis, sometimes massive not uncommon.
    - Direct invasion of chest wall and mediastinal structures can occur.
    - Disseminated disease can occur by hematogenous spread.

## Diagnostic Workup

- Imaging:
  - Chest radiograph/CT: progressive infiltrate/consolidation; peripheral wedge-shaped infiltrates suggestive of infarction; nodule or nodules, cavitation; effusions.
  - CT/magnetic resonance imaging (MRI) of the brain and sinuses: with rhinocerebral involvement to demonstrate the extent of disease and tissue invasion
- Sputum/BAL: can demonstrate characteristic hyphae but not sensitive. Cultures are rarely positive.

- Tissue diagnosis of involved sites:
  - Direct examination of infected tissue shows broad, usually nonseptate hyphae with short side branches at 90-degree angles invading tissue
  - Sites: lung, sinuses, nasal, snf palate
  - Presence of positive culture strongly supports diagnosis of invasive infection

## Treatment

- Medical[100]
  - No therapy to date is uniformly effective
  - High-dose amphotericin B (most commonly with lipid formulations) most commonly used
  - Can consider "maintenance" therapy with posaconazole as a step down following an adequate course of amphotericin and clinical response or as salvage therapy[99]
  - Note: other azoles and echinocandins are not effective.
- Surgical
  - Aggressive surgical resection to remove involved lung and soft tissue, when possible, combined with antifungal treatment likely offers the best chance for cure.[100]

## Principles of Peri- and Postoperative Management

- Aggressive approach is critical to survival in most patients.

## Prevention and Management of Complications

- Early diagnosis and treatment imperative

## Natural History/Prognosis

- The mortality rate for pulmonary mucormycosis is high.
- In a large series, the overall mortality rate was 80% (isolated 65% versus 96% for disseminated disease). Patients treated surgically in addition to antifungals had the best outcome.[100]

---

### KEY FACTS

- Rare pulmonary fungal infection often requiring aggressive therapy (i.e., antifungal therapy plus surgery).

---

# HYDATID PULMONARY DISEASE

## Definition

- Hydatid disease (also called echinococcosis) results from tapeworm infestations caused by the larvae of several species of *Echinococcus* (see excellent review by Morar and Feldman[102]).

## Etiology

- In humans, most disease is caused by *E. granulosus* and to a much lesser extent by *E. multilocularis.*
- *E. granulosus* is present wordwide (with endemic areas in the Mediterranean and Middle East, Central and South America, Africa, Australia, Russia, China), whereas *E. multilocularis* is reported in the northern hemisphere to include North America, Central Europe, parts of Asia and North Africa.
- The majority of this section will first deal with *E. granulosus*, to be followed by a short description of disease due to *E. multilocularis.*

# PULMONARY DISEASE DUE TO E. GRANULOSUS (CYSTIC FORM)

## Pathogenesis

- Humans are accidental intermediate hosts with dogs as the definitive host.[102]
- Eggs from worms in the dog small intestine are excreted in the stool and can remain attached to the dog's fur and viable for up to 1 year. Eggs can be transferred to grass or spread by wind or insects such as flies.
- Eggs are subsequently ingested by the intermediate host.
- Eggs hatch to release embryos, which traverse the intestinal wall and enter the portal circulation and are transported to capillary beds of the liver, lung, and other tissues, where they mature into cystic metacestodes containing protoscolices, each of which can develop into secondary daughter cysts in the intermediate host.

## Clinical Features

- Sites of involvement
  - The liver is the most common organ involved followed by the lung in adults; in children, the lung is most commonly involved
  - With lung parenchymal involvement, concomitant liver cysts are noted in about a third of cases.
  - Other sites of thoracic disease include: endobronchial, mediastinum, cardiac, pulmonary vasculature (with resultant pulmonary hypertension), diaphragm, pleural cavity and chest wall.[103,104]
- Clinical details
  - Pulmonary hydatid cysts can progressively enlarge by 1 to 5 cm per year to massive size over time.
  - Frequently asymptomatic for many years.
  - Symptoms can occur because of compression of adjacent structures and lung tissue, cyst rupture, secondary infection and hemorrhage.
  - With spillage of cyst contents, immunologic reactions including anaphylactic shock has been reported. However, severe anaphylaxis is fortunately very rare.
  - In a case series of 206 patients with pulmonary hydatid disease treated surgically, reported clinical features included cough (54%), chest pain (36%), dyspnea (25%), hemoptysis (19), fever/chills (10%), expectoration/emesis of cyst contents (10%), pleuritis (5%), pneumothorax (3%).[105]

## Diagnostic Workup

- Imaging:
  - Chest radiograph and CT[105-107]
    - Pulmonary cysts of varying size up to as large as 20 cm. They appear round to oval with homogeneous attenuation. Calcification common with liver cysts but rare with pulmonary.
    - More than half of patients have solitary cysts. Most are in the right lung (60%), with about a third with multiple cysts and a fifth with bilateral involvement.
    - Air between cyst wall layers to produce a crescent appearance is a radiologic sign of impending rupture (Cumbo's sign)
    - Radiologic signs of cyst rupture include: partial collapse with membranes evident within the cyst (Serpent sign); complete collapse with endocyst floating in cystic fluid (Water-Lily sign). Rupture and communication with endobronchial tree produces a fluid level, whereas rupture into the pleural space leads to a hydropneumothorax.
  - MRI: can show high signal intensity in T2-weighted images
- Serologic and other tests[108,109]
  - A variety of serologic tests are available. Results tend to be better with liver disease compared to pulmonary disease

  - Sensitivity in descending order: IgG ELISA (84%), IgM ELISA (62%), passive hemagglutination (61%), latex agglutination (58%), immunoelectrophoresis (51 percent), specific IgE ELISA (44%). Specificity of all tests: 98% to 100%. Specific IgG ELISA is the most sensitive measure of response to treatment
  - Casoni skin test: sensitivity 70% and specificity 87%
  - Eosinophilia is unusual and can be seen with cyst rupture.

## Treatment

Surgery is the treatment of choice for pulmonary hydatid disease, when feasible (see later)

- Medical treatment
  - Indications include:
    - Poor surgical candidate
    - Disseminated disease
    - Pleural disease
    - Spillage during surgery
    - Perioperative/adjuctive therapy
    - Contraindicated in pregnancy because of drug teratogenesis
  - Albendazole is drug of choice (better bioavailability than mebendazole). Praziquantal is an alternative agent.
  - Therapy is prolonged (generally >3 to 6 months for benzimidazoles)
- Surgical treatment[106,107,110–113]
  - Principle: Maximal preservation of lung tissue. Avoid spillage.
  - Surgical access: most reports describe classic thoracotomy. With bilateral disease, median sternotomy can be employed. More recently, a VATS approach has been described in both adults and children.[114,115]
  - Surgical approaches: cystectomy (peri- or endo-), cystotomy and capitonnage (i.e., surgical closure of a cyst by applying sutures to completely approximate the opposing surfaces), wedge resection, lobectomy (avoid, if possible).
  - Spillage is avoided by intact cyst resection with or without cyst aspiration with or without 15-minute installation of a scolicidal agent (e.g., hypertonic saline)
  - In treating complicated cysts, a modified capitonnage procedure can be used because it has a low morbidity rate. However with surrounding destroyed/suppurative lung, anatomic resection may be required.
  - Perioperative albendazole therapy (4 days prior and 1 to 3 months of treatment post surgery) often given. With surgery on complicated pulmonary hydatid cysts, some advocate avoidance of preoperative drug therapy (rationale: increases risk of perforation)

## Natural History/Prognosis

- Complete excision can result in cure.
- Unattended, a progressive disease

---

### KEY FACTS

- *E. granulosus* produces cystic disease. Pulmonary cysts are not uncommon (second to liver cysts in adults; more common in children)
- Cysts are round to oval; single or multiple; unilateral (more on the right) or bilateral
- Initially asymptomatic; symptoms are mostly due to compression, erosion, rupture.
- Immunologic reactions with cyst rupture are rare.
- Surgery is the treatment of choice, when possible.

## PULMONARY DISEASE DUE TO E. MULTILOCULARIS (ALVEOLAR FORM)

### Pathogenesis

- The definitive host are wild canids such as foxes and wolves, with rodents, and various deer populations as intermediate hosts.[102]
- Domestic dogs and cats can be infected. Transmission to humans from the latter source occurs due to direct spread of contaminated eggs or with food contamination.
- Pathologic lesions are multicystic with poor differentiation from surrounding tissues.
- Widespread involvement occurs by hematogenous spread with the primary lesion in the liver. Spread is by local extension with tissue destruction also occurs in involved tissues. Pulmonary involvement occurs by transdiaphragmatic spread or hematogenous dissemination.
- As with *E. granulosus*, pulmonary cyst rupture into the mediastinum, pleural cavity, and bronchi can occur.

### Clinical Features

- Commonly asymptomatic for many years
- Hepatic involvement predates pulmonary disease (e.g., abdominal pain, jaundice, and hepatomegaly)
- Nonspecific constitutional symptoms are common.
- Pulmonary symptoms nonspecific and depend on location, size, and complications
- Pulmonary involvement often suggested or investigated because of abnormal radiologic findings

### Diagnostic Workup

- Imaging: Chest x-ray and CT[116]
  - ○ Multiple nodules of varying size and shape; commonly lobulated.
  - ○ Areas of necrosis can be evident.
  - ○ Over time, calcification occurs.
- Serology:
  - ○ ELISA employing specific antigens of *E. multilocularis* (e.g., Em 2 and 18) provides good sensitivity (91% to 100%) and specificity (95% to 100%).

### Treatment

- When possible, radical surgical resection is performed.[102,117]
- With surgery, adjuvant drug therapy with albendazole for a minimum of 2 years is suggested.
- In inoperable cases, long-term pharmacotherapy is employed.

### Natural History/Prognosis

- Has the potential to produce severe fatal disease if untreated (90% 10-year mortality)

---

**KEY FACTS**

- Accounts for a minority of echinococcal disease (< 5%).
- Liver involvement is most common.
- Can produce serious pulmonary morbidity and mortality with lung disease.
- Treatment is radical excision, when possible, and prolonged albendazole therapy.

---

### References

 Interactive references and additional readings for this chapter can be accessed online at *expertconsult.com*.

---

# 17  MASSIVE HEMOPTYSIS

Ciaran McNamee, MD and Allan Conlan, MD

---

Hemoptysis is defined as the expectoration of blood from the lung. This must be differentiated from aspirated blood from the upper respiratory tract or hematemesis from an upper gastrointestinal source.

## DEGREE OF HEMOPTYSIS

- Hemoptysis may be initially classified and triaged as shown in Table 17-1.
- It is often difficult to estimate the amount of blood expectorated by the patient, and pragmatically, it is easier to divide patients into three groups: minor, major (massive), and exsanguinating.
- Minor hemoptysis can change into massive hemoptysis[1,2]; the dilemma is to predict the future severity of an initial episode of minor grade hemoptysis because catastrophic hemorrhage can occur in otherwise stable patients.[3] Rebleeds may have mortality rate as high as 45% if definitive treatment has not been started.[4]

## SURVIVAL FROM MASSIVE HEMOPTYSIS

- Mortality is associated with
  - ○ The severity of bleeding:

- 9% for hemoptysis of < 1000 mL/24 h
- 58% for hemoptysis of >1000 mL/24 h[5]
  - ○ The rate of blood loss
    - 71% mortality for a rate of >600 mL in 4 hours.
    - 45% mortality for a rate of 600 mL in 4 to 16 hours.
    - 5% mortality for a rate of 600 mL in 16 to 48 hours.[6-8]

---

**TABLE 17-1 ▪ CLASSIFICATION OF HEMOPTYSIS**

| Amount of Hemoptysis | Initial Factors Affecting Treatment and Survival |
|---|---|
| Minor—streaking of sputum | Diffuse versus local |
| Moderate—<400 mL | Coagulopathy versus normal |
| Massive—400–1000 mL | Resectable versus nonsurgical |
| Exsanguinating—>1 liter | Medical management versus surgical treatment sentinel |
| | Hemorrhage versus minor hemoptysis |
| | Bronchial artery versus pulmonary artery |
| | Embolization |

○ Hemorrhage that occurs unexpectedly in stable patients may cause death[2,3]; mortality is also associated with rebleeds,[4] and is higher with emergent versus elective surgery[3,9] and neoplasia.[5]

○ The mortality rate for conservative treatment of massive hemoptysis (including later rebleeds) is sufficiently high that in all cases, there should be consideration of other treatment modalities (bronchial artery embolization or surgery, or both) for candidates with localized disease.

## EPIDEMIOLOGY

■ The definition of massive hemoptysis varies widely among authors: in many series, massive hemoptysis has been defined as starting as low as 200 to 400 mL per 24-hour period and may increase to 1000 mL.[1,2,8,10-16] Most authors define massive hemoptysis as expectoration of 400 to 600 mL per 24 hours.[2,12,14,17,18] Others define hemoptysis as one episode of expectoration of at least 200 mL.[19] Massive hemoptysis occurs in only a small percentage of all cases of hemoptysis (1.5%–8%)[11,13,14]; the highest it has ever been in any series of patients with hemoptysis is 14%.[15]

■ Chronic inflammatory nontuberculosis lung disease is one of the leading causes of massive hemoptysis in the Western World.[13-18,20] (See Table 17-1.) However worldwide, tuberculosis is a leading cause of hemoptysis, although the frequency of massive hemoptysis with this infection is low given the wide prevalence of the disease. It is estimated that 2 billion people are infected by the tuberculosis (TB) bacillus and that 5% to 10% of those infected will develop tuberculosis.[14] Regional referral centers for tuberculosis have higher cluster rates of this as the causative agent for massive hemoptysis.[3,4,21,22]

■ The causes for hemoptysis are not only geographic but also seasonal in that in trends in hemoptysis of Western societies follow large population seasonal trends of respiratory infections.[23]

■ Massive hemoptysis is commonly associated with a structural lung abnormality or focus of lung inflammation. Rarely is a hemorrhagic diathesis the primary cause of massive hemoptysis, although it is associated with a higher mortality rate in association with other causes of hemoptysis.[15]

■ There are many causes of hemoptysis, as shown in Table 17-2; however, certain diseases have a higher predilection for massive hemoptysis compared with minor hemoptysis. The common causes of massive hemoptysis in Western societies are as listed in Table 17-2.[2,6,15,17,18,24] Certain disease states (e.g., TB or malignancy) may feature more prominently than others depending on the specialty care and referral pattern for institutional reports.

■ Hemoptysis in children is uncommon, and is disease and center dependent.[25,26] The common causes for childhood hemoptysis are
○ Cystic fibrosis
○ Congenital heart and lung disease
○ Pneumonia and bronchitis
○ Tuberculosis
○ Adenomas
○ Vasculitis

## ANATOMY OF THE PULMONARY CIRCULATION

■ Bronchial artery flow
○ Arise from the aorta or intercostal arteries and form a plexus in the peribronchial space.

---

### TABLE 17-2 ■ COMMON CAUSES OF MASSIVE HEMOPTYSIS

Bronchiectasis (30%–60% of all causes of massive hemoptysis[3,4,17-19,28])
Active tuberculosis[22]
Invasive mycetoma (aspergillus, mucormycosis)
Malignancy (5%–10% of all causes of massive hemoptysis[3,4,17-19] from either endobronchial tumors with bleeding or malignant erosion into major vessels)
Pneumonia/bronchitis
Cystic fibrosis (0.87% incidence and 4% prevalence of patients[30])
Coagulopathies with or without mitral stenosis
Uncommon sources of massive hemoptysis:
  Pulmonary renal syndromes (Goodpasture's syndrome, Wegener's granulomatosis)
  Congenital (arteriovenous malformations, congenital heart disease, unilateral pulmonary artery agenesis)
  Aortic or pulmonary artery fistula to the airway due to trauma or acquired conditions (tracheoinnominate artery fistula, Rasmussen's aneurysm from tuberculosis, lung abscesses, catheter tears of the pulmonary artery)
  Acquired cardiac, large vessel or pulmonary disease (mitral stenosis, pulmonary artery hypertension, Behcet's disease, aortic endo-grafts with erosion into the lung, Dieulafoy's disease of the bronchus)

---

○ Small penetrating arteries then form a submucosal plexus and supply nutrition and oxygen to the airway support structures including the pulmonary artery vessels (vaso vasorum) but play no role in gas exchange.

■ Pulmonary arterial flow
○ Account for 99% of the arterial blood supply to the lungs and are solely responsible for gas exchange.[27]

■ Intersections between the bronchial and arterial blood flow occur as follows:
○ Larger anastomoses between the medium-sized bronchial arteries and the alveolar microvasculature
○ At the level of the vasa vasorum of the pulmonary arteries, which run parallel to the airways
○ There are direct connections (anastomosis) between bronchial and pulmonary arteries at the level of the bronchial submucosa), which is physiologic and accounts for a shunt of 5% of cardiac output.[6]

## PATHOGENESIS

■ Source of hemoptysis:
○ Bronchial artery in 90% of cases
○ Pulmonary artery in 5% of cases
○ Large vessel (aorta or pulmonary artery) fistula to the airway[12]

■ Bronchial artery hemoptysis is usually associated with bronchial artery occlusion due to:
○ Acute or chronic inflammation
○ Acquired
○ Congenital
○ Reduced or occluded pulmonary artery circulation through the pulmonary arterioles secondary to hypoxic vasoconstriction, thrombosis, or vasculitis

■ This induces aberrant bronchial artery vessel proliferation, which leads to hypertrophy of these pulmonary vascular anastomoses. It can also induce collateral flow from extra-bronchial sources, which creates new vessels that are thin walled and fragile. Under inflammatory conditions and exacerbated by systemic arterial pressure, these vessels can rupture to cause hemoptysis of minor or more often major degree.[6,12,16,27,28]

■ Inflammatory vasculitis with vessel wall inflammation and degeneration may also lead to small vessel rupture, leading to alveolar hemorrhage.[29]

## PATHOPHYSIOLOGY

■ Small vessel disease
  ○ Small vessel disease causing hemoptysis is attributable to dilated, aberrant, weak connections in the vaso vasorum between the bronchial arterial system, which, in turn, transmits systemic pressures to the lower pulmonary arterial system. Increased angiogenic factors, such as vascular endothelial growth factor and angiopoietin 1, are induced by the following:
    ● Infection (bronchiectasis, tuberculosis, lung abscesses)
    ● Chronic inflammation[16,28,30,31] may cause enlarged ectatic submucosal arteries from the bronchial arterial system. Degeneration of the vessel walls of these ecstatic vessels may rupture spontaneously to cause hemoptysis.[32]
    ● Neoplasia,[27] primary cancers, metastatic disease, or adenomas with hypervascularity (angiogenesis) or vessel wall fragility
    ● Congenital—Arterovenous malformation, sequestrations (intra- or extralobar, or isolated vascular sequestrations) or isolated pulmonary artery agenesis or stenosis with extrapulmonary aberrant systemic blood supply.[27,33-40]
    ● Immune complex deposition[29,41] due to capillary wall inflammation, and necrosis may produce pulmonary alveolar hemorrhage.
    ● Lung infarction[42]
    ● Diffuse alveolar hemorrhage[29]
  ○ Neoplastic
  ○ Associated with specific disease entities;
    ● Renal failure[43]
    ● Coagulopathies
    ● Blood element dyscrasias: aplasias, or leukemias due to invasive aspergillosis[44] or stem cell trans-plantation[45]
    ● Catamenial hemoptysis with presumed aberrant hypervascularity due to ectopic endometrial tissue in the lung[46]
  ○ Cryptogenic[27,47]
  ○ Iatrogenic—bronchoscopic biopsy of an aberrant submucosal vessel (Dieulafoy's lesion)[39,48]
■ Large vessel disease
  ○ Acquired major vessel disease:
    ● Aortic—fistulas to airways:
      ○ Tracheoinnominate artery fistulas following tracheostomy[49-51]
      ○ Aortic graft fistulas to airways[52,53]
      ○ Aortic false aneurysms with erosion into the bronchus[53a]
      ○ Airway stents with erosions in the aorta[54,55]
  ○ Pulmonary artery aneurysms:
    ○ Pulmonary artery tear by Swan-Ganz catheter[33,56]
    ○ Penetrating trauma to the lungs[33,57]
    ○ Large vessel vasculities, such as Behçet's disease, Takayasu's disease, neoplasia, or chronic inflammation[6,58,59]
    ○ Chronic tuberculous pulmonary infection—Rasmussen's aneurysm[60]
  ○ Malignant invasion with intrapulmonary rupture of either the aorta or the pulmonary artery

## DILEMMAS ON PRESENTATION

■ To emergently deal with massive or exsanguinating hemoptysis

■ To identify those patients whose sentinel bleed may presage a second more massive bleed
■ To identify patients with massive hemoptysis who would not tolerate resectional surgery either as an initial treatment or as an alternative for other failed therapies
  ○ An impaired health status (reduced cardiac, pulmonary or overall performance status)
  ○ Disease progression (locally advanced or disseminated malignancy)
  ○ Siffuse lung bleeds suggesting a systemic problem

## INVESTIGATIONS

■ Urgency of initiation of investigations based on:
  ○ Amount of hemoptysis
  ○ Cardiopulmonary reserve of the patient
  ○ Disease status (large vessel versus small vessel disease)
  ○ Possibility of a massive rebleed following a bleed with a previous lesser grade of hemoptysis[1,3]
■ Initial investigations:
  ○ Complete blood count with platelet count
  ○ Prothrombin time/partial thromboplastin time
  ○ Electrocardiogram
  ○ Chest radiograph
  ○ Urinalysis (rule out [r/o] hematuria for a vasculitis)
    ● Consider:
      ○ Cross match blood for possible transfusion
      ○ Spirometry and arterial blood gas for early assessment of pulmonary function.
      ○ Anti-Gb antibodies for Goodpasture's syndrome
      ○ Erythrocyte sedimentation rate, perinuclear antineutrophil cytoplasmic antibody, or circulating antineutrophil cytoplasmic antibody for vasculitis
■ Subsequent investigations:
  ○ Computed tomography (CT) of the chest
  ○ Multiplanar CT of the chest
  ○ Bronchoscopy (see Table 17-3 for comparison of flexible and rigid bronchoscopy for the evaluation of massive hemoptysis).
  ○ Bronchial artery angiogram (BA)—always consider embolization if BA angiogram is deemed necessary.
  ○ Pulmonary artery (PA) angiogram for specific disease states:
    ● PA aneurysms
    ● Arteriovenous (AV) malformations

## Tips Regarding Investigations

■ Goal of investigations are to
  ○ Regionalize the bleeding focus
  ○ Identify the cause of the bleeding (infection versus cancer versus vasculitis and obtain microbiologic cultures if appropriate)
  ○ Initiate treatment quickly (embolization with angiography or surgical control)
■ *Multiplanar CT* scans are considered better than BA angiograms at detecting bleeding vessels and aberrant vessels. This may be a good first test to help identify aberrant vessels before angiography; this test may also reduce the failure rate of BA embolization by identifying nonbleeding arteries at risk for bleeding before embolization.[27,61]
■ *Bronchoscopy*: rigid versus flexible. Lung soilage without overt endobronchial bleeding requires minimally two different bronchoscopies identifying the same segment for consideration of surgical resection.
■ *Bronchial arteriography versus PA arteriography*

## TABLE 17-3 ■ COMPARISON OF FLEXIBLE AND RIGID BRONCHOSCOPY FOR THE EVALUATION OF MASSIVE HEMOPTYSIS

**Flexible Bronchoscopy**

**Pro:** Performed under local anesthesia
  Ventilation postprocedure not required for poor-risk patients
  May be easier to obtain procedural time
**Goals of:**
  Localization
  Identification of etiology of hemoptysis
  Obtaining culture or pathology specimens
  Cessation of bleeding with vasoactive agents
  Insertion of bronchus blockers if lung isolation is necessary
**Con:** May be aggravated by bleeding, which
  Prevents the identification of lesions
  May overwhelm suction capabilities leading to asphyxiation
  May induce coughing which can aggravate hemoptysis
  Removal of clots difficult with flexible bronchoscope

**Rigid Bronchoscopy**

**Pro:** Performed under general anesthesia, which provides
  Better airway protection for episodes of massive bleeding
  Better airway suctioning for clots or fresh bleeding
  Positive pressure ventilation as counter pressure
  Cessation of coughing as a cause of hemoptysis
  More rapid institution of lung isolation with bronchus blockers or double-lumen endotracheal tubes
  Allows flexible bronchoscopy through the rigid bronchoscope
**Cons:** Requires general anesthesia implying:
  Poor-risk patients may have difficulties with independent pulmonary recovery
  If extubation is not possible due to lung soilage with blood or poor respiratory mechanics, further pulmonary function testing is prevented, which confounds the ability to assess resections of local lesions
  Requires ventilation and care that may not be desired for terminal patients

○ Bronchial artery catherization:
  • Done much more commonly than PA angiograms (90% of bleeding from the bronchial arteries).
  • Need to consider aberrant vessels as sources of hemoptysis:
  • Because contrast extravasation is rarely found at arteriography (3.6%–10.7%), embolization of vessels is commonly based on clinical and radiographic findings.[12,61]
  • Up to 67.5% of patients may have a nonbronchial arterial blood supply in addition to their normal bronchial blood supply.
  • Aberrant bronchial arteries may arise from unusual arterial sites in 8.3% to 35% of patients.[12]
○ PA artery angiograms only for
  • Swan-Ganz catheter tears (sealed) or aneurysms
  • AV malformations
■ Complications of BA angiograms and embolization
  ○ Complications of arterial catheterization: aneurysm of puncture site, arterial wall dissection (0.1%–6%)
  ○ Chest pain (24%–91%)
  ○ Dysphagia (0.7%–18%)
  ○ Embolization causing infarction of other organs (rare)
  ○ Paraplegia rate (1.4%–6.5%) due to occlusion of spinal arteries which originates from or near to a bronchial artery

■ Treatment results of BA:
  ○ Immediate control rate of 73% to 98%.
  ○ Long-term recurrence rate of 10% to 52% due to incomplete embolization, aberrant arteries, recanalization of vessels, or disease progression.[12,22]
  ○ Useful for immediate control of bleeding vessels, stabilizing patients, and converting an emergency situation into a semielective situation.
  ○ Use polyvinyl particles rather then absorbable materials or coils to prevent recanalization or thrombosis of other organs.[12]
  ○ Repeat embolization can be performed; however, its effectiveness is reduced compared with the success rates of initial bronchial artery embolization.[62]

## TREATMENT

### Tips Regarding Treatment

■ Medical management without bronchial artery embolization of massive hemoptysis (>600 mL/24 h) shows a mortality rate of 32% to 85% compared with the mortality rate of 18% to 33% associated with surgical treatment.[2] The high mortality rate associated with conservative management strongly argues for further invasive management with either BA embolization or surgery for patients who have stabilized after an initial episode of massive hemoptysis.
■ BA angiograms with embolization are cost effective compared with surgery; however, they have higher failure rates and rebleeds have a high mortality rate.[22]
○ Factors associated with an increased mortality rate are as follows for:
  ○ Emergency procedures[3,9]
  ○ Pneumonectomy
  ○ Preoperative mechanical ventilation
  ○ Salvage procedures following failed bronchial artery embolization[20]

## MANAGEMENT OF HEMOPTYSIS

■ General supportive:
  ○ Antibiotics
  ○ Correction of coagulopathy
  ○ Antitussives (codeine)
  ○ Consider antifibrinolytics (tranexemic acid, factor VIIa infusion) for diffuse bleeding[45,63]
  ○ Intubation and positive pressure ventilation
■ Treatment for localized massive hemoptysis[8]
  ○ Bronchus irrigation with
    • Iced saline lavage
    • Adrenalin solution
    • Cold probe
    • Topical coagulants
  ○ Laser coagulation
  ○ Radiation therapy (described for hemoptysis with fungal infections)
  ○ Bronchial artery embolization
  ○ Endobronchial blockade or unilateral lung occlusion with a double-lumen tube
  ○ Surgical resection (wedge, lobectomy, pneumonectomy) of diseased lung
  ○ Physiologic exclusion of lung (surgical ligation of the pulmonary artery and the bronchus to a diseased area of the lung without lung resection)[64]
■ Treatment for generalized hemoptysis
  ○ Intubation plus positive pressure ventilation
  ○ Reversal of coagulopathies
  ○ Antibiotics appropriate for organisms

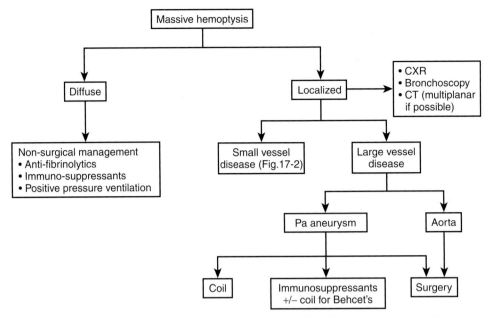

**Figure 17-1:** Algorithm for treatment of massive hemoptysis with diffuse bleeding or large vessel disease.

○ Consider antifibrinolytics (tranexemic acid, factor VIIa infusion) for diffuse bleeding[45,63]
○ Extracorporeal membrane oxygenation[65]
■ Indications for Urgent Surgical Therapy with Massive Hemoptysis:
  ○ Large vessel disease (Fig. 17-1)
    • Tracheoinnominate artery fisutla
    • Benign aortic fistula to the airway
    • Congenital anomalies (sequestrations) with aneurysmal dilation of large vessels
    • Pulmonary artery catheter tears with uncontained hemorrhage[66]
    • Pulmonary artery aneurysms not treatable by coil embolization
  ○ Small vessel disease (patients must have localized and resectable disease and must have the reserve to tolerate surgical resection) (Fig. 17-2):
    • Patients with recurrent hemoptysis after BA embolization
    • Patients who do not respond to conservative management and are not stable enough for BA embolization
    • Patients who are poor candidates for BA embolization (spinal vessels originating from the bronchial arteries, multiple feeder vessels, contrast allergies, patients not able to tolerate the contrast load)
■ Indications for possible surgical resection or exclusion as a semiurgent or elective procedure. (Patients must have localized and resectable disease and must have the reserve to tolerate surgical resection.)
  ○ Cavitary or atrophied lung segments with localized chronic infections or bleeding from multiple feeding vessels[67]
  ○ Patients who have structural or inflammatory lung segments and who live in isolated areas or who live in areas without access to bronchial artery embolization
  ○ Patients who have structural or inflammatory lung segments and who have requirements for anti-coagulation or have ethical or religious concerns about blood transfusions
  ○ Rebleed after initial control with BA embolization
  ○ Patients with a localized inflammatory focus with anticipated poor response to medical therapy (e.g., bronchiectasis with antibiotic resistant bacteria)
  ○ Patients with neoplastic disease that can be resected for cure.

■ Surgical procedure
  ○ Operations almost always require a thoracotomy. The emergent nature of the procedure usually precludes the use of video-assisted thoracoscopic surgery.
  ○ Resection is an anatomic resection (lobectomy or pneumonectomy).
■ Contraindications to surgery
  ○ Diffuse disease (e.g., vasculitis)
  ○ Palliative conditions (neoplasia, poor reserve)
■ Contraindications to BA angiogram and embolization
  ○ Allergy to contrast dye (relative)
  ○ Unable to accept dose of radiation from angiogram (e.g., pregnant patient)
  ○ Spinal arteries arising from bronchial arteries (relative)[68]

## OUTCOMES WITH TREATMENT

■ Table 17-4 illustrates causes and mortality in cases of massive hemoptysis
■ Table 17-5 illustrates success of treatment options for massive hemoptysis

### Brief Illustrative Case

• A 26-year old woman with cystic fibrosis (diagnosed in early childhood) presented to the emergency room (ER) because of significant hemoptysis.
• The volume of hemoptysis in the patient's history and observed in the ER was estimated to be 450 to 500 mL over the last 8 to 12 hours
• The patient was intubated to secure an airway after further coughing up an estimated 150 to 200 mL of blood.
• There were no associated acute events such as an acute infective exacerbation predating the hemoptysis.
• A chest radiograph showed typical bronchiectatic changes bilaterally (tram tracks and ring shadows), together with a vague infiltrate in the right upper lobe
• Her white cell count was elevated (17,000), and the hemoglobin was 9.7. Coagulation studies were within normal limits

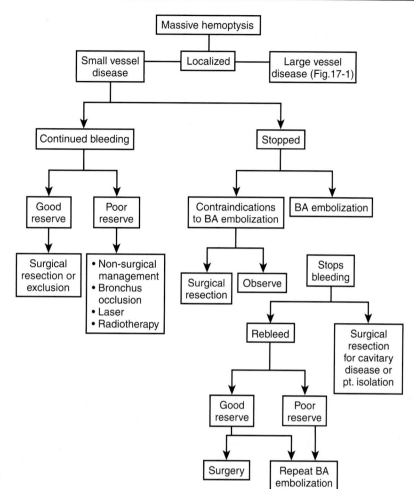

**Figure 17-2:** Algorithm for Treatment of Massive Hemoptysis from small vessel disease.

| | | | ETIOLOGY OF MASSIVE HEMOPTYSIS | | | | |
|---|---|---|---|---|---|---|---|
| Author | Amount of Hemoptysis | n | Bronchiectasis | TB | Malignancy | Abscess/ Pneumonia | Mortality |
| Tuncozgur, 2007[1] | >400 mL/24 h | 20 | 5% | 20% | 15% | 35% (hydatid, fungus) | 15% |
| Reechaipichitkul, 2005[19] | >600 mL/24 h or 200 mL/episode | 101 | 33.70% | 20.80% | 10.90% | 18% | 17.80% |
| Ayed, 2003[28] | >600 mL/24 h | 53 | 58% | | | 19% | 4% |
| Jougon, 2002[16] | >600 mL/24 h | 43 | 28% | 9%, 15% | 28% | 9% | 23% |
| Ong, 2003[17] | >300 mL/24 h | 29 | 61% | 10% | 6% | 13% (mycetoma) | 13% |
| Fidan, 2002[18] | >600 ml/24 h | 20 | 40% | 35% | 10% | 5% | |
| Hirschberg, 1997[15] | >500 mL/24 h | 29 | 21% | | 14% | 31% | 38% |
| Knott-Craig, 1993[4] | >500 mL/24 h in 80% of patients | 120 | 51% | 22.50% | 5% | 7.50% | 10% |
| Conlan, 1983[3] | >600 mL/24 h | 123 | 30.10% | 38% | 5% | 9% | 22.70% |

**TABLE 17-4  ■  CAUSES AND MORTALITY OF MASSIVE HEMOPTYSIS**

TB, tuberculosis.

## TABLE 17-5 ■ SUCCESS OF TREATMENT OPTIONS FOR MASSIVE HEMOPTYSIS

| Author | Amount of Hemoptysis | n | Conservative | BA Embolization | Surgery |
|--------|----------------------|---|--------------|-----------------|---------|
| Tuncozgur, 2007[1] | >400 mL/24 h | 20 | | | 82% |
| Reechaipichitkul, 2005[19] | >600 mL/24 h or 200 mL/episode | 101 | 80.70% | 93% | 85% |
| Jougon, 2002[16] | >600 mL/24 h | 43 | 74% (some BA embolization) | 100% | 81% |
| Ong, 2003[17] | >300 mL/24 h | 29 | | 87.50% | 75% |
| Corr, 2001[22] | >600 mL/24 h | 87 | | 65.50% | ? |
| Lee, 2000[20] | >600 mL/24 h | 54 | 7.40% | 81% | 85% |
| Knott-Craig, 1993[4] | >500 mL/24 h in 80% of patients | 120 | 89% | | 93% |
| Conlan, 1983[3] | >600 mL/24 h | 123 | 36% had recurrent hemoptysis with 45% mortality with conservative management<br><br>12% of patients with conservative management die from massive rebleeds while awaiting a surgical procedure<br><br>69% | | 82% |

BA, bronchial artery angiogram.

## Brief Illustrative Case—cont'd

- She was chronically colonized with *Pseudomonas aeruginosa* and *Staphylococcus aureus*, and an appropriate antibiotic regimen to cover these organisms was instituted
- Bronchoscopy revealed blood oozing from the right upper lobe. The left endobronchial tree was free of blood
- A CT chest ruled out an aspergilloma colonizing an area of cystic bronchiectasis. Figure 17-3 reveals evidence of extensive brochiectasis in both upper lobes.
- It was elected to proceed to bronchial artery embolization.
- Figure 17-4 reveals two large bronchial arteries supplying the right upper lobe, which were embolized.
- Figure 17-5 reveals a tortuous network of 'intercostal' arteries, which appeared to supply the apical segment of the right upper lobe.
- The patient was successfully extubated the following day, with no further episodes of hemoptysis.
- She was evaluated for bilateral lung transplantation.

### Key Points

- The volume and rapidity of hemoptysis in this case qualify for massive hemoptysis, with a high risk of acute asphyxiation from blood clot obstructing the conducting airways (about 140 mL in this patient). Hence, the need for emergent airway control.
- With intubation, appropriate sedation and avoidance of coughing is necessary, because this may aggravate bleeding.

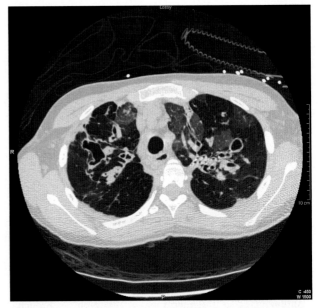

**Figure 17-3:** Computed tomography of the chest showing extensive bronchiectasis in both upper lobes.

- Data from the National CF Patient Registry reported an overall incidence of massive hemoptysis (1990 to 1999) of 4.1%.[69]
- The mean age was 24 +/- 8.7 years; no gender difference.
- Massive hemoptysis was more prevalent in older patients, those with worse pulmonary function and reserve (FEV1 <40% of predicted in 60% of cases) the presence of *S. aureus* in the sputum and associated diabetes.[69]

### Brief Illustrative Case—cont'd

- Massive hemoptysis is associated with increased morbidity, a decline in lung function, and an increased 2-year mortality rate.[69]
- Bronchial artery embolization has proven successful in the management of both adults and children with cystic fibrosis and massive hemoptysis. Re-embolization for relapses is feasible.[70-72]
- The patient was referred for lung transplantation because of limited pulmonary reserve and the episode of massive hemoptysis (given the high risk of death in these circumstances over 2 years).[69]

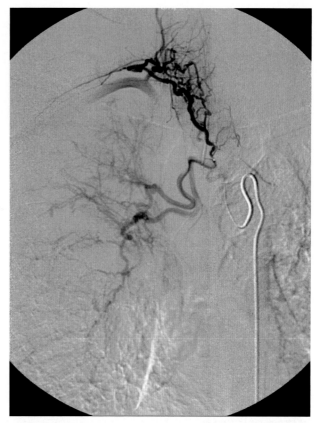

**Figure 17-5:** Tortuous network of 'intercostal' arteries, which supply the apical segment of the right upper lobe (appear black on this image).

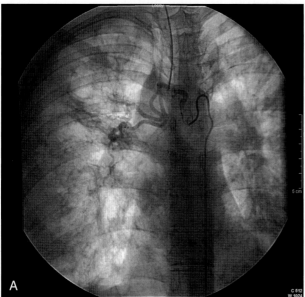

## References

 Interactive references and additional readings for this chapter can be accessed online at *expertconsult.com*.

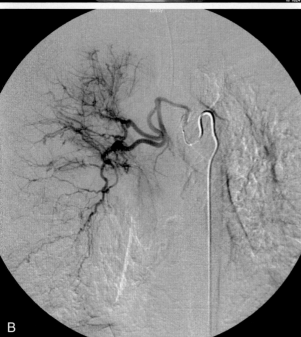

**Figure 17-4: A,** Angiographic depiction of 2 large bronchial arteries supplying the right upper lobe. **B,** Subtraction view.

# 18 ROLE OF LUNG BIOPSY IN DIFFUSE LUNG DISEASE

David Balfe, MBBCh, FCP(SA)

## TERMINOLOGY

- Interstitial lung disease (ILD)
- Idiopathic interstitial lung pneumonia
- Eosinophilic lung diseases

## DEFINITIONS

- Transbronchial biopsy: biopsies taken via the flexible fiberoptic bronchoscopy.
- Surgical lung biopsy: biopsies obtained by surgical mean either by
  - Video-assisted thoracoscopic lung surgery (VATS)—biopsies taken surgically using the VATS approach.
  - Open lung biopsy—biopsies taken surgically using an open thoracotomy.

## INTRODUCTION

- Lung biopsy is frequently required to establish the diagnosis in a number of different lung conditions, including interstitial lung disease, infections, and malignancies.[1,2]
- The indications and methods for obtaining lung tissue, the patterns of pathology encountered, and a number of illustrative cases are presented.
- The term diffuse lung disease covers infiltrative processes that involve the alveolar spaces or the interstitium of the lung.[3]

## INDICATIONS FOR LUNG BIOPSY

Lung biopsy is indicated for the following purposes:

- To provide a specific diagnosis of underlying ILD, malignancy, or infection that may present as diffuse lung diseases. This is important in a patient with atypical features (fever, younger than age 50 years, weight loss, signs of vasculitis, hemoptysis); unexplained extrapulmonary manifestations; a progressive course; a normal, atypical, or rapidly changing chest radiology; or pulmonary vascular disease of unclear origin[4]
- To make a definitive diagnosis and predict prognosis before proceeding with therapies, which may have serious side effects
- To assess disease activity

## DIFFERENT TYPES OF LUNG BIOPSY

Different options are available in obtaining lung tissue specimens.

- Transbronchial biopsy via bronchoscopy
- Lung biopsy via VATS
- Open thoracotomy.

- Transbronchial lung biopsy is more subject to sampling error as a consequence of small sample size.[5] Because processes may be patchy, it is important to take biopsies from multiple sites.[6]

## Transbronchial Lung Biopsy

- Transbronchial lung biopsy via flexible fiberoptic bronchoscopy is often the initial procedure of choice, especially when infection or granulomatous diseases, such as sarcoidosis, are suspected.
- The granulomas of sarcoidosis are often located in the region of the bronchovascular bundles, making them accessible to transbronchial biopsy.[7]
- In addition, it is useful in suspected lymphangitic carcinomatosis, eosinophilic pneumonia, and Goodpasture's syndrome.[4,8-10]
- In patients with sarcoidosis
  - Endobronchial biopsies are frequently positive and may increase the diagnostic yield, compared with transbronchial biopsies alone.[11]
  - The diagnostic yield of transbronchial biopsy exceeds 80%.[7]
- ILD pathology is frequently patchy and difficult to characterize definitively on the basis of small transbronchial biopsies because visualization of whole pulmonary acini is required to fully evaluate disease distribution.
- Bronchoalveolar lavage obtained during bronchoscopy can provide important information, for example, the presence or absence of lymphocytosis in patients with suspected fibrotic diffuse lung disease.[3] If a specific diagnosis is not made by transbronchial biopsy, surgical lung biopsy is often indicated.[4]
- Risks of transbronchial lung biopsies include hemorrhage and pneumothorax, major hemorrhage is rare, and pneumothoraces complicate transbronchial biopsies in 1% to 2% of procedures.[3] Severe pulmonary hypertension and uncontrolled bleeding tendencies are contraindications to performing transbronchial lung biopsies.

## Surgical Lung Biopsy

- Surgical lung biopsy has a very high diagnostic yield (greater than 92%) and low mortality ($\leq$6%)[12-14] and morbidity rates (6% to 19%).[4] Lung tissue can be obtained either by open thoracotomy or by VATS.[12,13] Specimen adequacy and diagnostic accuracy are the same with both procedures.[4,15]
- Increasingly, VATS is the preferred surgical method in part because several retrospective studies have found that morbidity is improved with VATS compared with open thoracotomy[15-17]; however, a small prospective, randomized trial comparing the two procedures found no difference in morbidity or mortality rates (42 patients in the study).[18] The choice of VATS versus open thoracotomy is typically determined by the expertise of the thoracic surgeon.[4]
- Relative contraindications to surgical lung biopsy include[4,12,13]
  - Evidence of diffuse end-stage disease with evidence of honeycombing, without areas of milder disease activity

○ Serious cardiovascular disease, severe pulmonary dysfunction, advanced age, or other major risks for surgery or general anesthesia

○ High likelihood that adequate-sized biopsies from multiple sites (usually from two to three lobes) will not be obtained

○ Mechanical ventilation and immunosuppressive therapy appear to increase the risk of death and other complications of surgical lung biopsy

## SPECIMEN COLLECTION AND HANDLING

■ Optimal handling is essential for the accurate interpretation of biopsies and cytological preparations.[19-28]

■ Transbronchial biopsies
○ Are intended to represent alveolar lung parenchyma beyond the cartilaginous airways[19,26]
○ Crocodile-type forceps (Machida) or cupped forceps are used to obtain the biopsy, ideally at end expiration, with forceps being advanced under fluoroscopic guidance.[5,19] The biopsy appears finely ragged and usually measures between 2 and 3 mm in diameter.[19]
○ The number of biopsies required is at least five to seven adequate samples containing predominantly alveolated tissue.
○ To assess for lung transplant rejection, at least five adequate samples are required.
○ The biopsy is removed from the forceps with a sterile needle, and the specimens are immediately placed into fixative solution (10% neutral buffered formalin) or sterile transport medium.[19]
○ Once processed, the biopsies are serially sectioned for processing.[19]

■ Surgical biopsy
○ The optimal number, size, and location of surgical wedge lung biopsies depend on the suspected diagnosis and the anatomic distribution of the disease process.[4]
○ Before any biopsy is performed, consultation among the radiologist, pulmonologist, and thoracic surgeon is essential to ensure proper sampling and location of ideal biopsy locations.[19] High-resolution CT (HRCT) scanning may further assist in selecting the best location or locations to biopsy.[4]
○ Adequate samples are ideally greater than 30 mm in the greatest dimension and are ideally obtained from more than one lobe of the lung.[28]
○ The surgeon should avoid sampling only subpleural tissue (especially if pleuritis is present) and should avoid the dependent segments of the right middle lobe and lingula, because nonspecific fibrosis may be present at these sites. Areas of severe disease tend to exhibit end-stage fibrosis (i.e., honeycomb lung) without suggesting an etiology and, therefore, are unlikely to yield useful results.[4]
○ Intraoperative pathology consultation with immediate handling of the specimen is ideal, if the lung biopsy is to be divided for microbiologic, electron microscopy, immunofluorescence or molecular studies, these portions can be removed before routine processing.[19]
○ The specimen is injected using a 22- to 25-gauge needle with 10% buffered formalin into the cut edge. Initially the specimen is shaken vigorously within a container of fixative.[19]
○ One biopsy could be taken from an area of lung that appears grossly and radiographically normal and another from an area with mild to moderate disease.[19]
○ Alternatively, both biopsies could be taken from diseased areas of varying severity. This approach provides the pathologist with the data needed to evaluate the extent and distribution of disease. It also increases diagnostic accuracy.[19]
○ The extent and severity of inflammation or fibrosis can provide information regarding the staging of disease. Other histologic parameters (e.g., the extent of fibroblastic foci in usual interstitial pneumonitis) may provide prognostic data.[4,29]

## COMMUNICATION BETWEEN PATHOLOGIST AND CLINICIAN

■ Pathologic abnormalities alone are rarely specific. More often, the findings are characteristic or consistent with a specific diagnosis. They may also be nonspecific reaction patterns common to several diseases that cause inflammation and/or fibrosis in the lungs.[30]

■ Small tissue samples and substantial interobserver variability among pathologists further complicate interpretation.[4,6,31,32]

■ As a result, most cases require careful clinical and pathologic correlation to arrive at a final diagnosis.[33,34] With such an approach, surgical lung biopsy produces a definitive diagnosis in more than 90% of cases of ILD occurring in immunocompetent hosts. The diagnostic yield is lower (35% to 75%) in immunodeficient patients with diffuse parenchymal lung disease.[35,36]

■ Data provided to the pathologist by the clinician at the time of biopsy should include
○ Information regarding the duration of illness, age of patient, and any exposure to occupational or environmental agents
○ Immune status of the patient
○ Any history of medication or illicit drug use
○ Suspected clinical diagnosis, which will often lead to a more targeted search by the pathologist
○ Because a drug reaction is a diagnosis of exclusion, the drug history is more important than the histology in most instances.
○ Similarly, the histology may be diagnostic in several of the pneumoconioses (e.g., silicosis, asbestosis), but lung tissue examination is not commonly required to establish a diagnosis.[4]

## HISTOPATHOLOGIC PATTERNS OF DISEASES

There are six broad histologic lung biopsy patterns.[19]

■ Acute lung injury pattern
○ The lung biopsy is diffusely involved by variable amounts of edema and fibrin accompanied by reactive type 2 pneumocyte hyperplasia.
○ The dominance of noncellular, protein-rich material imparts an overall red or pink appearance to the biopsy at scanning magnification in routine hematoxylin-eosin (H&E) staining.
○ Diseases to be considered include diffuse alveolar damage (DAD) from infection, drug toxicity, collagen vascular diseases, diffuse alveolar hemorrhage, irradiation injury, eosinophilic pneumonia and idiopathic acute interstitial pneumonia (AIP).
○ Other considerations are acute hypersensitivity pneumonitis, acute pneumoconiosis, and acute aspiration pneumonia.

■ Fibrosis pattern
○ The lung biopsy is involved by variable amounts of fibrosis. As in the acute lung injury pattern, the biopsy tends to be more pink than blue at scanning magnification of H&E stained preparations, as a result of collagen deposition.

○ Some fibrosis patterns are accompanied by chronic inflammation that may result in a blue tinge to the process, or dark blue lymphoid aggregates may be present.

○ Diseases to be considered include usual interstitial pneumonia (UIP), nonspecific interstitial pneumonia (NSIP), chronic hypersensitivity pneumonitis (HSP), chronic drug toxicity, collagen vascular diseases, advanced sarcoidosis, chronic eosinophilic pneumonia, and pneumoconiosis.

▪ Chronic cellular infiltrative pattern:

○ The lung biopsy is involved by variable amounts of chronic inflammation and reactive type 2 pneumocyte hyperplasia.

○ The dominance of mononuclear cell infiltrates may impart an overall blue appearance magnification of H&E-stained preparations.

○ Diseases to be considered include HSP, NSIP, collagen vascular diseases, chronic infections, drug toxicities, lymphocytic and lymphoid interstitial pneumonia, lymphomas and leukemias, and lymphangitic carcinomatosis.

▪ Alveolar filling pattern:

○ The dominant finding in alveolar spaces filled with either cellular or noncellular elements.

○ Diseases to be considered include infections, organizing pneumonia, diffuse alveolar hemorrhage, desquamative interstitial pneumonia (DIP), respiratory bronchiolitis-associated interstitial lung disease (RBILD), alveolar proteinosis, alveolar microlithiasis, mucostasis and mucinous tumors, and dendriform calcification.

▪ Nodular pattern

○ Nodules with evidence of an interface between the nodule and more nodule are noted.

○ The nodules can be of various sizes.

○ Diseases to be considered include sacoidosis, Wegener's granulomatosis, berylliosis, aspiration pneumonia, pulmonary Langerhans cell histiocytosis, and primary and metastatic neoplasms.

▪ Near-normal biopsy pattern:

○ The lung biopsy has little or no disease evident at scanning magnification.

○ Diseases to be considered include chronic small airways disease, vasculopathic diseases, lymphangioleiomyomatosis (LAM).[19]

## Idiopathic Interstitial Pneumonias

▪ Patients presenting with clinical and radiological features of interstitial pneumonias without known cause can be grouped into the following seven histologic patterns - UIP, NSIP, DIP, RBILD, organizing pneumonia (OP), lymphocytic interstitial pneumonia (LIP), and AIP with a DAD picture (Table 18-1).[19,37]

▪ UIP (Fig. 18-1)

○ UIP is the histologic pattern typically seen in cases of idiopathic pulmonary fibrosis (IPF), also called cryptogenic fibrosing alveolitis.[38]

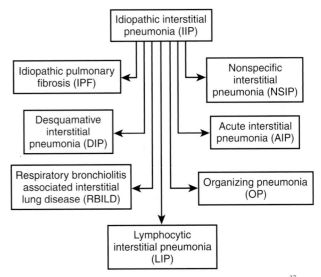

**Figure 18-1:** Classification of idiopathic interstitial pneumonias.[37]

## TABLE 18-1 ▪ FEATURES OF THE IDIOPATHIC INTERSTITIAL PNEUMONIAS

| Features | UIP | NSIP | DIP | AIP | LIP | OP | RBILD |
|---|---|---|---|---|---|---|---|
| Temporal appearance | Variegated | Uniform | Uniform | Uniform | Uniform | Uniform | Uniform |
| Interstitial inflammation | Scant | Prominent | Scant | Scant | Prominent | Scant | Scant |
| Interstitial collagen | Patchy | Variable, diffuse | Variable, diffuse | No | Some cases | No | Mild, focal |
| Interstitial fibroblasts | No | Occasional, diffuse | No | Yes, diffuse | No | No | Mild, focal |
| Organizing pneumonia | Occasional, focal | Occasional, focal | No | Occasional, focal | No | Prominent | No |
| Fibroblastic foci | Typical | Occasional, focal | No | No | No | No | No |
| Honeycomb areas | Typical | Rare | No | No | Sometimes | No | No |
| Intra-alveolar macrophages | Occasional, focal | Occasional, patchy | Yes, diffuse | No | Occasional, patchy | No | Yes, peribronchiolar |
| Hyaline membranes | No | No | No | Yes, focal | No | No | No |
| Granulomas | No | No | No | No | Focal, poorly formed | No | No |
| Terminal airway inflammation | No | No | No | No | No | Sometimes | Prominent |

AIP, acute interstitial pneumonia; DIP, desquamative interstitial pneumonia; LIP, lymphocytic interstitial pneumonia; NSIP, nonspecific interstitial pneumonia; OP, organizing pneumonia; RBILD, respiratory bronchiolitis associated interstitial lung disease; UIP, usual interstitial pneumonia.[19]

○ It is a relatively nonspecific pattern of chronic lung injury with fibrosis, loss of alveolar architecture with a patchy subpleural and paraseptal distribution, with or without honeycombing remodeling.[19]

○ These abnormalities are typically associated with a mild chronic inflammatory cell infiltrate. Varying numbers of fibroblastic foci are another key feature.

○ Additional findings of less diagnostic importance include squamous metaplasia, bony metaplasia, type 2 cell hyperplasia, smooth muscle hypertrophy, and endarteritis obliterans.

○ Rarely, abundant macrophages may be superimposed on the fibrosis, a DIP-like reaction.

○ UIP is a chronic lung disease resulting from repeated subclinical episodes of DAD.[19,21]

○ Episodic deterioration is typical in patients with IPF. In some patients, this deterioration is abrupt and overwhelming.[39] Such exacerbations have mixed histology, with a background of older fibrosis often overshadowed by diffuse acute lung injury, with variable OP and even hyaline membranes.[19]

○ Patients with the histologic pattern of UIP have a worse prognosis than patients with other patterns of interstitial pneumonia, such as DIP, NSIP, RB, bronchiolitis obliterans organizing pneumonia (BOOP), and LIP. As an example, one retrospective series of 104 patients found that the median survival of the UIP group was 2.8 years.[40] This was significantly worse than for other pathologic subgroups of pulmonary fibrosis of unknown etiology.

○ The histologic pattern should always be correlated with clinical findings to ensure that the rare situation in which UIP is associated with a disease other then IPF (e.g., chronic hypersensitivity pneumonia) is not missed.[4,41]

○ See Table 18-2 for a list of potential causes of lung fibrosis with or without honeycombing.[19]

○ IPF usually proves fatal, with a median survival time of about 3 years from the time of diagnosis.[37]

■ NSIP
○ The main histologic feature of NSIP is diffuse and temporally uniform interstitial and chronic inflammation, with or without fibrosis.

---

### TABLE 18-2 ■ POTENTIAL CAUSES OF LUNG FIBROSIS, WITH OR WITHOUT HONEYCOMB REMODELING[19]

Idiopathic pulmonary fibrosis
Desquamative interstitial pneumonia
Lymphocytic interstitial pneumonia
Collagen vascular disease
Drug reactions
Pneumoconioses (asbestosis, berylliosis, silicosis, hard
  metal pneumoconiosis, etc.)
Sarcoidosis
Pulmonary Langerhans cell histiocytosis (histiocytosis X)
Chronic granulomatous infections
Chronic aspiration
Chronic hypersensitivity pneumonitis
Organized chronic eosinophilic pneumonia
Organized, and organizing, diffuse alveolar damage
Chronic interstitial pulmonary edema
Chronic effect of radiation
Sequelae of healed infectious pneumonia/other inflammation
Nonspecific interstitial pneumonia
Hermansky-Pudlak syndrome

---

○ It is characterized by varying degrees of inflammation and fibrosis involving mainly the alveolar walls and variable affecting the bronchovascular sheaths and pleura.[19]

○ Some cases have a primarily chronic inflammatory/cellular pattern (cellular NSIP), but most cases have a fibrotic pattern (fibrotic NSIP).[4,42]

○ Although NSIP may have significant fibrosis, it is usually diffuse in affected lung with a uniform age. Fibroblastic foci and honeycombing, if present, are rare. These features are key in distinguishing NSIP from UIP. Nonetheless, fibrotic NSIP can be difficult to reliably distinguish from UIP and there is significant interobserver variability, even among expert histopathologists.[4,31,32]

○ Compared with patients with UIP, most patients with NSIP have a good prognosis and show improvement after treatment with corticosteroids.[43,44] The 5-year mortality rate is estimated to be 10% to 15%[4]; however, patients with the fibrotic form of NSIP have a worse prognosis.[19]

○ Idiopathic NSIP occurs mostly in middle-aged women who never smoked. The prognosis is very good, with a 5-year mortality rate of less than 18%.[45]

■ DIP
○ DIP is characterized by diffuse filling of alveoli by macrophages that have glassy eosinophilic cytoplasm and fine granular brown pigmentation.

○ Other features that may be seen are mild interstitial chronic inflammation with interstitial thickening by fibrous tissue,[19] type 2 cell hyperplasia, lymphoid follicles, and mild eosinophilic infiltration.[46]

○ DIP was originally thought to be a precursor of UIP. However, it now seems likely that the major cause of DIP is exposure to cigarette smoke.[4]

■ RBILD
○ RBILD is a mononuclear inflammatory process involving the submucosa of the membranous and respiratory bronchioles; these changes may be associated with mild fibrosis that extends into the surrounding alveolar walls.[47]

○ There is also accumulation of macrophages that have glassy eosinophilic cytoplasm and fine granular brown pigmentation with bronchocentric distribution.[47-49] The airway epithelium is abnormal, with goblet cell hyperplasia and metaplastic cuboidal epithelium, which often extends into the nearby alveolar septa and ducts.[4,47]

○ In the appropriate clinical setting, this histologic pattern indicates RBILD. Like DIP, exposure to cigarette smoke is the most common cause.[4]

■ OP
○ OP, also called cryptogenic OP, is the histologic pattern that indicates BOOP in the appropriate clinical setting.

○ More commonly, OP is a nonspecific reaction lung injury or another disorder The distribution of OP is often patchy and peribronchiolar, but the appearance is relatively uniform within involved areas. There are numerous buds of granulation tissue within alveoli, often involving alveolar ducts and small airways.

○ It is sometimes called proliferative bronchiolitis when the granulation tissue is primarily within the airways. Mild chronic inflammation also exists. Foamy macrophages are commonly seen in the alveoli, presumably secondary to bronchiolar occlusion. Eosinophils and neutrophils are usually few in number, and severe fibrotic changes are unusual.[4]

■ LIP
○ In LIP, there is a dense diffuse interstitial lymphoid infiltrate, similar to follicular bronchiolitis.

○ LIP was previously considered to be preneoplastic; however, it is now believed to be a reactive pulmonary lymphoid hyperplasia, similar to that seen in collagen vascular diseases or immunosuppression.[4,50,51]

- AIP
  - ○ In AIP, there is DAD, which is a nonspecific reaction that is most common in patients with acute respiratory distress syndrome (ARDS). AIP is also called the Hamman-Rich syndrome.[4]
  - ○ The characteristic features depend on when the biopsy is taken. During the exudative (acute) phase, there is interstitial edema, acute and chronic inflammation, type II cell hyperplasia, and hyaline membrane formation. Thrombi within small arteries are also common. During the organizing (healing) phase, the features are more similar to those of OP.[4]

## Other Disorders

There are numerous additional causes of ILD that are not classified as interstitial pneumonias. These include eosinophilic pneumonia, pulmonary hemorrhage syndromes, alveolar proteinosis, granulomatous lung diseases, amyloid deposition, smooth muscle proliferation, Langerhans cell granulomatosis (histiocytosis X), honeycomb lung, and unclassifiable interstitial pneumonia.[4]

- Eosinophilic pneumonia
  - ○ The histologic features ILD due to eosinophilic pneumonia are similar to those of OP described earlier, except there is significant eosinophilic infiltration.
  - ○ The eosinophilic infiltration is often accompanied by foci of necrosis and proteinaceous debris, termed eosinophilic microabscesses. Acute and organizing DAD may also be present.[4]
- Pulmonary hemorrhage syndrome:
  - ○ The important finding in these cases is the filling of alveoli with red blood cells and hemosiderin-laden macrophages. The presence of hemosiderin-laden macrophages helps exclude surgical bleeding as the cause of alveolar red blood cells because the quantity of hemosiderin-laden macrophages is proportional to the chronicity of bleeding.[4]
  - ○ Often the underlying lesion is a capillaritis with neutrophilic infiltration of the alveolar septa. This leads to necrosis of these structures, loss of capillary structural integrity, and extravasation of erythrocytes into the alveolar space. Many of the tissue neutrophils are fragmented and eventually become pyknotic; the fragmented neutrophils and nuclear dust fibrin may also enter the alveoli with the red blood cells.[4]
  - ○ True fibrinoid necrosis of the interstitium is sometimes seen, and erythrocytes may also be observed within the interstitial space.
  - ○ Pulmonary hemorrhage without inflammation of the alveolar structures may be seen. DAD can also cause diffuse alveolar hemorrhage.[4]
- Alveolar proteinosis
  - ○ In this entity, the alveoli are filled with acellular pink and finely granular lipoproteinaceous material that stains positively with a periodic acid–Schiff stain for glycogen. Scattered clefts of cholesterol crystals may be seen within the alveolar exudate.[52]
  - ○ The alveolar septa may be slightly thickened, but the normal alveolar architecture tends to be preserved. Typically, there is little or no inflammatory cell infiltration.[4]
- Granulomatous lung disease
  - ○ Granulomas are discrete aggregates of epithelioid histiocytes and T lymphocytes, with varying numbers of Langerhans-type giant cells.[4]

- ○ The differential diagnosis consists largely of sarcoidosis and hypersensitivity pneumonia once fungal and mycobacterial infections have been excluded.[4]
- ○ Sarcoidosis usually has a lymphangitic distribution of granulomas with or without fibrosis and comparatively little lymphocytic inflammation. The granulomas are generally non-necrotizing, but focal central necrosis is occasionally present.[4]
- ○ In hypersensitivity pneumonia, the granulomas are generally bronchocentric, smaller, less discrete, and associated with greater interstitial chronic inflammation.[4]
- Amyloid deposition
  - ○ Deposition of amyloid in the lung can cause diffuse alveolar septal infiltration, single or multiple pulmonary nodules, or diffuse tracheobronchial lesions.[4]
  - ○ Amyloid deposition can be localized to the lung or systemic, with the latter having a worse prognosis.[4]
  - ○ It may be seen in association with multiple myeloma, LIP, or primary pulmonary marginal zone lymphomas of mucosa associated lymphoid tissue (MALT) origin.[4] Also, it is typically of primary light chain (AL)-type of amyloid in symptomatic patients.[4]
- Smooth muscle proliferation
  - ○ Metaplastic smooth muscle proliferation can be seen in several conditions including LAM, benign metastatic leiomyoma, diffuse primary or metastatic spindle cell malignancy, asthma, or other chronic airway diseases.[4]
  - ○ Most cases of LAM are diagnosed without lung biopsy due to the diagnostic accuracy of HRCT. LAM is characterized by multiple cysts whose walls contain bundles of immature smooth muscle cells. These cells typically stain focally for HMB.[45] Areas of proliferation can be sparse.[4]
- Honeycomb lung
  - ○ Honeycomb lung is indicative of end-stage pulmonary fibrosis. Many disorders (e.g., IPF, sarcoidosis, hypersensitivity pneumonia, and eosinophilic granuloma) can progress to end-stage fibrosis but cannot be distinguished reliably by pathologists at this stage of the disease processes.[4]
  - ○ Thus, biopsy of honeycomb lung is not helpful and should be avoided.[4]
- Unclassifiable interstitial pneumonia
  - ○ Unclassifiable interstitial pneumonia exists when histologic features do not allow classification into one of the above-mentioned categories.[4,42]
  - ○ Some of these cases result from sampling error or inadequate specimens. This finding on a transbronchial biopsy should prompt a surgical lung biopsy.[4]
  - ○ Most patients with nonspecific or unclassifiable interstitial pneumonia have a good prognosis and show improvement after treatment with cortico-steroids.[4,43,44]
- ARDS
  - ○ When the cause of ARDS is not apparent, open lung biopsy can be performed with reasonable safety, even in severely hypoxemic patients with ARDS.[4,35,43]
  - ○ This was demonstrated in a retrospective review of 57 patients meeting diagnostic criteria for ARDS with a mean $PaO_2/FiO_2$ ratio of 145 mm Hg. All of the patients successfully underwent open lung biopsy.[4]
  - ○ The rate of major complications was 7%, and no deaths were attributable to the biopsy procedure. Although the overall complication rate was 39%, most of the complications were minor and related to persistent air leaks.[4]
  - ○ The results of the biopsy resulted in the addition of a specific therapy in 60% of patients, and withdrawal of unnecessary therapy in 37%.[4,43]

○ In general, lung biopsy should be reserved for carefully selected patients who have acute respiratory failure of unclear etiology, whose bronchoscopy was nondiagnostic, and who are suspected of having disseminated cancer, vasculitis, alveolar hemorrhage, cryptogenic organizing pneumonitis (COP), or an undiagnosed diffuse lung disease (e.g., sarcoidosis).[4]

- Rheumatoid arthritis (RA)
  ○ HRCT has replaced lung biopsy in many cases.[4,43] However, pathologic diagnosis may be required, especially when atypical features are present on HRCT. A transbronchial biopsy is usually inadequate for diagnosis. Therefore, lung biopsy is typically performed by either VATS or open thoracotomy.
  ○ When deciding whether lung biopsy should be performed, the patient's clinical condition and the impact of the results on the patient's management should be considered. Lung biopsy should not be considered routine.[4]
  ○ A spectrum of findings may be present on lung biopsy including[2-4,9-16,44]:
    - UIP
    - NSIP
    - OP (also called BOOP or COP).
    - Mixed morphology
    - LIP
    - DIP
    - DAD
  ○ The most common pathologic findings among patients with RA-ILD are those of UIP and NSIP, with UIP and NSIP occurring in similar proportions.[4] Men and former smokers are prevalent among patients with RA-ILD who develop the UIP pattern.[4]
- Hypersensitivity pneumonitis (HP)
  ○ Histopathologic confirmation of the diagnosis is required in many instances and should be attempted by transbronchial lung biopsy except in cases of advanced disease, when surgical specimens have a higher yield.[4]
  ○ It is critical that the pathologist be informed when HP is being considered; the findings are often subtle and must be interpreted with knowledge of the clinical setting.[4]
  ○ The histopathologic findings on transbronchial biopsy in HP may include small, poorly formed noncaseating granulomas located near respiratory or terminal bronchioles. These ill-defined aggregates of epithelioid macrophages may be associated with multinucleated giant cells. Well-formed granulomas are not commonly seen, in contrast to their frequent identification in patients with sarcoidosis.[4]
  ○ A patchy mononuclear cell infiltration (predominantly lymphocytes and plasma cells) of the alveolar walls, typically in a bronchocentric distribution.[4]
  ○ Large histiocytes with foamy cytoplasm present in the alveoli and the interstitium.[4]
  ○ With the increased use of surgical lung biopsy in the diagnosis of the idiopathic interstitial pneumonias, it has been recognized that many cases of chronic HP (especially bird fancier's lung), are characterized by varying patterns of organizing pneumonia, NSIP (cellular or fibrotic), and usual interstitial pneumonia-like lesions.[4]
  ○ Often these patterns of injury are seen in the absence of granulomas. Also, the fibrotic changes are commonly located in both centrilobular and perilobular areas, consistent with the pattern suggestive of HP. Multinucleated giant cells with cholesterol clefts are also seen and suggests chronic HP.[4,48,49]

## UTILITY OF OPEN LUNG BIOPSY IN CRITICALLY ILL PATIENTS

### Introduction and Rationale
- Open lung biopsy is considered the "gold standard" for diffuse lung disease in both immunocompromised and immunocompetent critically ill patients.[53-56]
- Clinical workup provides a specific diagnosis in only a third of patients
- Bronchoscopy with bronchoalveolar lavage (BAL) value in many infectious conditions, but sensitivity and specificity is often suboptimal in the critical care arena. For example, organisms isolated may be colonizers or secondary invaders and unrelated to the primary process.
- Provide a specific diagnosis that would effect a change in treatment or withdrawal of unnecessary treatments with their own inherent harmful side effects.
- Improve outcome
- Provide prognostic data

### Patient Population[53-58]
- Commonly immunocompromised (71% in one series)
  ○ Hematologic malignancies
  ○ Blood stem cell transplants
  ○ Solid organ transplants
  ○ Cancer/chemotherapy
  ○ Human immunodeficiency virus/acquired immunodeficiency syndrome
  ○ Corticosteroid therapy
  ○ Immunosuppressive therapies
  ○ Disease-modifying agents (e.g., anti–tumor necrosis factor)
- Immunocompetent
  ○ Atypical pneumonia not responding to usual therapy
  ○ Nonresolving bilateral infiltrate of undetermined etiology
  ○ Comorbid conditions (e.g., diabetes, renal failure)
  ○ Possible drug reactions
  ○ Fulminant idiopathic pneumonias
  ○ Rule out vasculitis

### Open Lung Biopsy Diagnoses in Reported Series[53,57-62]
- Specific
  ○ Fungal infection (e.g., aspergillus)
  ○ Viral infection (e.g., cytomegalovirus [CMV], adeno-virus)
  ○ Miliary tuberculosis
  ○ Chemotherapy toxicity
  ○ Disseminated malignancy
  ○ Pulmonary capillaritis
  ○ Vasculitis
  ○ Acute exacerbation of IPF
  ○ AIP
  ○ Cryptogenic organizing pneumonia
  ○ Panbronchiolitis
- Nonspecific:
  ○ DAD
  ○ NSIP pattern
  ○ Varying elements of an OP pattern

### Surgical Details
- VAT biopsy is the most common approach. In patients who are unable to tolerate single lung ventilation, the classic open approach can be used.
- Biopsy from more than one area, including most and less-involved regions, is recommended. Biopsies from right

middle lobe or lingual did not effect final histopathologic analysis.[62]

- A specimen for culture should always be included
- In adults, most common postoperative complications include air leaks, which are the most common (17%–42%).[53,54] Other complications include bleeding, hypoxemia, arrhythmias, and transient hemodynamic instability.
- Operative mortality rates of 0 to 9% have been reported.

## Issue of Mechanical Ventilation

- The use of mechanical ventilation should not be regarded as a contraindication for surgical biopsy.[53,57,58]
- In this population, however, complications are higher and outcomes worse (in part related to the severity of the underlying disease with or without comorbidities)

## Modification of Therapy and Outcome Data[53,57-61]

- Specific diagnosis:
  - A *specific* diagnosis was made in 46% to 100% (average of series was 70%).
  - In one series,[53] a nonspecific diagnosis was made in 46% (along with a specific diagnosis in another 46%). The nonspecific diagnoses were varying stages of acute lung injury of undetermined etiology.
- Change in therapy
  - Based on the pathology obtained, a change in therapy was instituted in 47% to 81% of recent series (average: 67%)
- Withdrawal of therapy
  - This was reported in 14% to 29% of cases
  - Antibiotics were most frequently withdrawn based on biopsy findings.
- Overall outcome
  - Overall survival rate in patients undergoing open lung biopsy was 30% to 50% in several series (average: 40%)
  - A key issue raised by Soh et al[60] was a survival rate of only 22% of patients in whom specific changes to therapy were made based on pathology findings. This mirrors reports from older series.

## Factors Associated with Poor Outcome[53,57]

- Number of organ dysfunctions (>2 associated with close to 100% mortality)
- Patient age and comorbidity index
- Low $PaO_2/FiO_2$ ratio on day of biopsy
- Longer time to open lung biopsy
- Immunocompromised patients including underlying hematologic malignancy

## Pediatric Population[63]

- Feasible
- Compared with adult patients, higher rate of complications, particularly air leaks. In children in acute respiratory failure, complications were noted in up to 65% compared with a 14% complication rate in those without acute respiratory failure.
- In the latter group, postoperative ventilation was less than 24 hours compared with prolonged ventilation in children with acute respiratory failure
- 24% mortality reported.

## Conclusions

- Can provide a specific diagnosis in a significant number of critically ill patients with undiagnosed diffuse bilateral infiltrates.

- Although pathology results can meaningfully redirect therapy, the overall benefit may be low.
- Careful consideration of risks and benefits needs to be considered in patients with poor prognostic factors, especially those with multiple organ dysfunction.

### Brief Illustrative Case 1

- A 38-year-old woman presented with exertional dyspnea, which has worsened over the last 3 months
- She was a nonsmoker.
- There was minimal dry cough. No fever or constitutional symptoms.
- She had worked for the last 11 years in a "musty" office as a managerial assistant.
- Chest examination revealed late inspiratory crackles at both bases.
- Pulmonary functions revealed a restrictive ventilatory defect (TLC: 4.1 L; 55% of predicted; DLCO: 31%). Blood gases: $PaO_2$: 62 mm Hg; $PaCo_2$: 35 mm Hg. Six-minute walk: 190 m with desaturation to 72%.
- Chest radiograph and chest CT showed prominent honeycombing at the bases, with some interstitial changes noted elsewhere (Fig. 18-2A and B).
- Collagen profile and hypersensitivity pneumonitis panel negative.
- An open lung biopsy via VATS was performed.
- This showed evidence of an "unclassifiable interstitial pneumonia" (Fig. 18-3A to C).

#### Key Points

- Although the honeycombing may suggest UIP and IPF, her young age did not fit such a diagnosis.
- Open lung biopsy was justified to further pursue a diagnosis such as fibrotic NSIP in this young lady.
- The ATS/ERS consensus classification of idiopathic interstitial pneumonia includes a short section on "unclassifiable interstitial pneumonia."[37] Possible reasons for such a diagnosis includes inadequate clinical and investigative data, sampling error (different histopathology can co-exist, e.g., UIP and NSIP in the same or different lobe); previous therapy that modifies pathological features.
- The history of the 11 years in a "musty" office, suggests the possibility of chronic hypersensitivity pneumonitis, which in its late stages, can be indistinguishable from the idiopathic interstitial pneumonias. The presence of fibroblastic foci may be a factor mitigating against such a diagnosis.
- Although a trial of corticosteroids with or without immunosuppressive therapy could be tried, referral for lung transplant evaluation is appropriate.

### Brief Illustrative Case 2

- A 87-year-old man presented with a worsening nonproductive cough and worsening shortness of breath over the last 12 months
- He was an ex-smoker, having a 30-pack year history.
- He previously worked in an office managerial position.

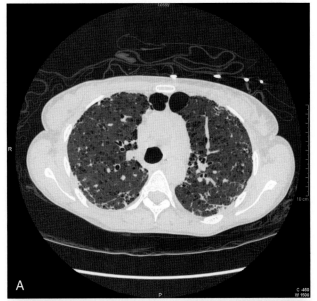

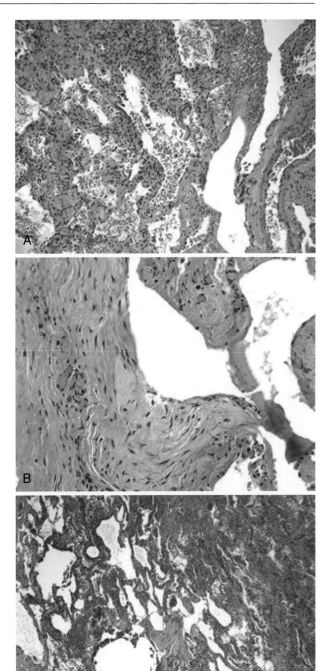

**Figure 18-2: A,** Chest computed tomography (CT) scan of the lung mid zone showing prominent fibrosis with some interstitial changes noted elsewhere. **B,** Chest CT scan showed prominent honeycombing at the bases with some interstitial changes noted elsewhere.

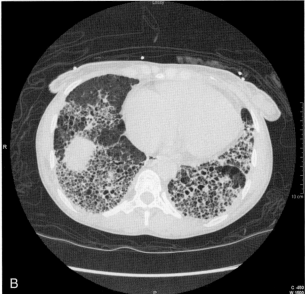

**Figure 18-3:** Pathologic evidence of an "unclassifiable interstitial pneumonia": **A,** Nonspecific interstitial pneumonia pattern. **B,** Fibroblastic focus. **C,** Diffuse interstitial fibrosis.

## Brief Illustrative Case 2—cont'd

- Pulmonary functions revealed a restrictive ventilatory defect (TLC: 3.4 L; 40% of predicted; DLCO: 20%). Blood gases: Room air $PaO_2$: 47 mm Hg; $PaCo_2$: 37 mm Hg.
- Chest radiograph showed bilateral interstitial infiltrates, high-resolution chest CT revealed peripheral honeycomb changes with minimal ground-glass change (Fig. 18-4)
- An open lung biopsy via VATS was performed, which showed evidence of an temporally and spatially heterogeneous interstitial fibrosis with fibroblastic foci and cystic architectural remodeling, consistent with usual interstitial pneumonia pattern of fibrosis (Fig. 18-5)

## Key Points

- The patient's age and peripheral honeycombing suggest the diagnosis of UIP and IPF.
- Obtaining an open lung biopsy could be questioned given the typical clinical and radiologic features.
- The history of smoking is not unusual in patients with IPF.

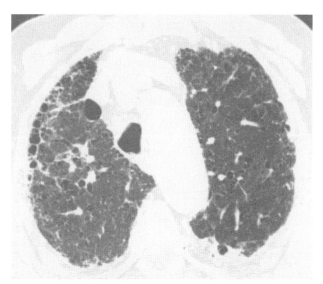

**Figure 18-4:** Usual interstitial pneumonia (UIP) pattern—high-resolution chest computed tomography scan revealed peripheral honeycomb changes with minimal ground-glass change.

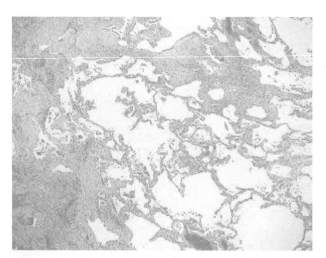

**Figure 18-5:** Evidence of temporally and spatially heterogeneous interstitial fibrosis with fibroblastic foci and cystic architectural remodeling, consistent with usual interstitial pneumonia (UIP) pattern of fibrosis.

## Brief Illustrative Case 3

- A 55-year-old woman presented with a worsening nonproductive cough and fever in addition to some congestion for 2 months. She had been seen for a routine check up 3 months previously and noted to have a normal chest radiograph. She admitted to a viral infection prior to her worsening pulmonary symptoms.
- She is a non smoker and is a homemaker.
- She has no dust exposure or exposure to pet birds
- A rheumatologic workup was negative, and the eosinophil count was normal.
- Pulmonary functions revealed a mild restrictive ventilatory defect
- Chest Xray showed bilateral patchy, high resolution chest CT revealed extensive bilateral patchy infitrates (Fig. 18-6)

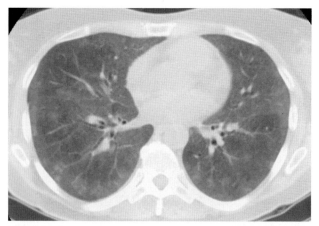

**Figure 18-6:** High-resolution chest computed tomography scan reveals extensive bilateral patchy infiltrates.

- An open lung biopsy via VATS was performed, which showed evidence of lung with organizing pneumonia, no tumor, epithelioid granulomas or viral changes are seen (Fig. 18-7)
- The patient responded to 6 weeks of high-dose oral steroids with complete resolution of the CT changes

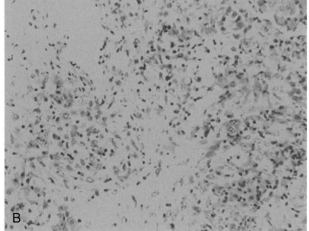

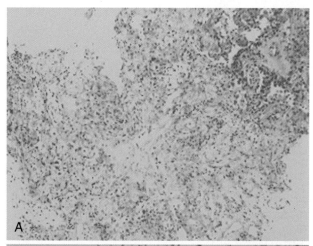

**Figure 18-7:** Evidence of organizing pneumonia. No tumor, epithelioid granulomas, or viral changes are seen on (**A**) low power and (**B**) high power.

• The significant response to steroids is typical for organizing pneumonia, although the condition can recur as the steroids are tapered.

## References

Interactive references and additional readings for this chapter can be accessed online at *expertconsult.com*.

# Neoplastic Disorders

# 19 EVALUATION AND MANAGEMENT OF THE SOLITARY PULMONARY NODULE

Carol C. Wu, MD and Bruce M. Barack, MD

## TERMINOLOGY

■ Solitary pulmonary nodule (SPN)

## DEFINITION

■ An SPN refers to a round lesion smaller than 3 cm in diameter that is completely surrounded by pulmonary parenchyma without other pulmonary abnormalities.[1]

## ETIOLOGY

■ An SPN, which is usually discovered incidentally, is found on 0.09% to 0.02% of all chest radiographs, and approximately 150,000 SPNs are identified each year in the United States.[1]
■ Ten to seventy percent of SPNs are malignant depending on the reported series.[1] However, only 60% to 80% of resected SPNs are malignant.[2]

### Etiology—Key Facts

■ Malignancy
  ○ Bronchogenic carcinoma: accounts for approximately 35% of SPNs.[3]
  ○ The majority of bronchogenic carcinomas in the United States are non–small lung cancer (NSCLC).
    • Adenocarcinomas (including bronchoalveolar cell): most common of the NSCLC, presents as peripheral mass in 49% to 80% of cases.[4,5]
    • Squamous cell carcinomas: now second most common of the NSCLCs, presents as a peripheral mass in 43% to 55% of cases.[4,6]
      ○ Decrease prevalence of squamous cell carcinoma, traditionally presenting as a central tumor, relative to adenocarcinoma, is postulated to be due to the decrease in nicotine and tar levels in cigarettes, which promotes a pattern of deeper inhalation resulting in increased exposure of peripheral lung tissue to smoke and a consequent increase in peripheral origin of lung cancer.[6]

• Large cell carcinoma: a rare cause of an SPN
• Small cell carcinoma: accounts for less than 5% of SPNs
• Proteonomics,[7,8] the study of protein expression, and genomics[9,10] will probably dictate future treatment, deemphasizing the importance of cell type.
  ○ Metastases: accounts for approximately 23% of SPNs.[3]
    • An SPN in patients with lymphoma or leukemia is almost always a primary bronchogenic carcinoma.[11]
    • An SPN in patients with carcinomas of the head and neck, squamous cell carcinoma, carcinoma of the bladder, breast, cervix, bile ducts, esophagus, ovary, prostate, or stomach is more likely to be a primary bronchogenic carcinoma than metastasis.[11]
    • An SPN in patients with carcinoma of the salivary glands, adrenals, colon, kidney, thyroid, thymus, or uterus has an equal probability or being a primary bronchogenic carcinoma and a metastasis.[11]
    • An SPN in patients with melanoma, sarcoma, or testicular cancer is more likely to be a solitary metastasis than primary bronchogenic carcinoma.[11]
    • Colorectal carcinoma accounts for 30% to 40% of all solitary metastatic SPNs to the lung and is the most likely source of a solitary metastatic nodule.[12,13]
    • An SPN in the absence of a known primary is unlikely to be a metastasis, and a persistent diagnostic workup for an extra-thoracic primary is not cost effective.[14]
  ○ Other malignancies
    • Carcinoid, adenosquamous carcinoma, sarcomatoid carcinoma, and salivary gland tumors[15]
■ Benign causes
  ○ Infectious granuloma: about 80% of benign SPNs[1]
    • Histoplasmosis, tuberculosis, are coccidioidomycosis are the etiology of the most commonly resected SPNs[13]
    • The prevalence of coccidioidomycosis or histoplasmosis as the cause of a SPN may be extremely high in a local endemic area.[16]
  ○ Hamartoma: about 10% of benign SPNs[1]
  ○ Vascular:
    • Arteriovenous malformation (AVM)
    • Pulmonary artery aneurysm

- Other:
  - ○ Rheumatoid nodule
  - ○ Wegener's granulomatosis
  - ○ Rounded atelectasis
  - ○ Organizing pneumonia[17]
  - ○ Pulmonary infarct[17]
  - ○ Sarcoidosis[13]
  - ○ Amyloidosis
  - ○ Bronchial atresia[18]

## CLINICAL FEATURES

### Symptoms and Signs
- Frequently asymptomatic
- Cough, fever, hemoptysis

### Pathophysiology
- Cigarette smoking is the overwhelming risk factor for developing a malignant SPN.[19]
- Several clinical models have been developed to estimate the probability of malignancy in an SPN.[14,20-22]
  - ○ In the most recently developed model[22]
    - Current or former cigarette use, older age, increase in nodule diameter are associated with higher risk of malignant SPNs
    - Increase in the number of years since quitting smoking is associated with lower likelihood of malignant SPN
    - Recently diagnosed lung cancer or a history of recent extrathoracic malignancy were not independent predictors of malignancy
    - In contrast to the Mayo Clinic model, this model found that upper lobe SPNs were not more likely to be malignant
  - ○ A history of an extrathoracic malignancy at least 5 years before the time of SPN detection has been reported as an additional predictor of a malignant SPN in the Mayo Clinic model.[14]
  - ○ An additional risk factor is a history of lung cancer in first-degree relatives.[23]
- Evidence for a specific lung cancer susceptible gene has been reported.[24]
- Other risk factors are history of pulmonary fibrosis due to collagen vascular disease, adult respiratory distress syndrome, or radiation, previous exposure to asbestos, uranium and radon.[21,25-28]
- Malignant SPN in usual institial pneumonia develops in periphery of lower lobe in area of fibrosis.[25]
- Lung cancer is uncommon in people younger than age 40 and rare in people younger than age 35.[29]
  - ○ Exceptions are patients with human immunodeficiency virus who have increased risk for developing lung cancer and may develop it at an earlier age.[30]

## DIAGNOSIS

An SPN is most often first identified on a chest radiograph. The first step in the diagnosis is to ascertain that the nodule is indeed solitary and arising from the pulmonary parenchyma, and is not due to etiologies such as a hypertrophied costochondral junction, a pleural nodule, a skin lesion, or other processes extrinsic to the lungs.[31]

### Imaging Studies
- Plain chest radiograph
  - ○ Nineteen percent of SPNs were missed owing to factors such as small size, partial obscuration by superimposing

structures, failure to compare current with prior radiographs, use of a faulty search pattern, poor viewing conditions, and poor technical quality of images.[32,33]
  - ○ An SPN is seldom detected on chest radiography until it is 9 mm in diameter.[34]
  - ○ Approximately 90% of newly discovered SPNs are visible in retrospect on prior chest radiographs.[35]
  - ○ Benign features
    - Size: 90% of SPNs smaller than 2 cm are benign.[14,21]
    - Location: Benign SPNs distributed equally throughout lungs and location cannot be used as an independent predictor of benignity or malignancy.[14]
    - Calcification: Benign patterns of calcifications are laminated (concentric), uniform, central nidus, and popcorn.[36]
      - ○ The first three types are associated with granulomatous disease.
      - ○ Popcorn calcification is seen in one-third of hamartomas.[37]
      - ○ Calcification patterns are more easily demonstrated on CT than chest radiographs.[38]
      - ○ About 45% of benign SPNs demonstrate no calcification.[39]
- Margin characteristics
  - ○ A smooth rounded margin is associated with benign diagnosis.[3]
  - ○ Twenty to thiry-four percent of SPNs with a smooth rounded margin are malignant. Most SPNs are metastatic.[40,41]
- Growth Rate
  - ○ Benign SPNs have doubling time of less than 1 month or more than 16 months.[42]
  - ○ An increase of SPN diameter by 26% is equivalent to doubling of SPN volume.[31]
  - ○ Stability of nodule size over 2 years is no longer considered adequate for diagnosis of benignity, especially with small SPNs.[43]
- Other
  - ○ Unequivocal evidence on previous examinations that the nodule is the end stage of a previous benign process such as infarction or previous granulomatous infection[36]
  - ○ Cavitary wall thickness cannot be used to accurately differentiate between benign and malignant SPNs because of considerable overlap.[44-46] Commonly quoted data is as follows: wall thickness less than 4 mm is generally benign; greater than 16 mm is generally malignant, and a 4- to 16-mm wall thickness is indeterminate.
  - ○ Malignant features
    - Size: SPNs approaching 3 cm are more likely to be malignant.
    - Location
      - ○ Lung cancer is 1.5 times more common in the right lung than the left lung.[47]
      - ○ Seventy percent of lung cancers occur in the upper lobes,[14] but this was not confirmed in one recent series.[22]
    - Calcification
      - ○ An eccentric calcification may represent a malignant lesion with dystrophic calcification or a malignant SPN that has engulfed a benign SPN.[40]
      - ○ Carcinoids, metastatic osteosarcomas, and chondrosarcomas may have dense foci of calcification or be entirely calcified and simulate a benign SPN.[39]
      - ○ Mucin-secreting tumors such as colon or ovarian cancers may have stippled or psammomatous calcification and may also simulate a benign SPN.[39]

- Margin characteristics: spiculated on plain film[14]
- Growth rate
  - Doubling time for most malignant SPNs is between 30 and 400 days[36]
  - Fast-growing metastases[48] and lymphoma[49] can have a shorter doubling time.
- Other: 84% to 95% of cavitary SPNs with irregular-walled cavities thicker than 16 mm tend to be malignant.[44-46]

## Computed Tomography

- Often used to confirm that the nodule seen on chest radiograph is indeed solitary and within the lung parenchyma. Imaging is also useful for further charac-terization.
- Size:
  - Highly accurate at determining nodule size and doubling time.[50]
  - A 6-m nodule incidentally discovered on computed tomography (CT) scan is up to 30 times more likely to be benign than malignant[31]
- Density:
  - Calcification: better than plain radiograph at detecting and characterizing calcification
    - SPN with density above 200 Houndsfield units (HUs) can be considered benign if no other malignant features are present.[51]
  - Fat: can exclude malignancy in most instances by detecting fat density.
    - Fat within an SPN is very specific for hamartoma,[52] and 50% of hamartomas demonstrate focal fat attenuation on high-resolution CT (HRCT).[41]
    - Lipoma is a very rare cause of benign fat-containing SPNs.
    - Metastatic liposarcoma and clear cell renal carcinoma are rare causes of malignant fat-containing SPNs.[53]
  - Pure ground-glass SPN is more likely to be malignant than a solid or partly solid SPN.[54]
- Air bronchograms seen in 30% of malignant and 10% of benign SPNs.[55]
- Enhancement pattern
  - An SPN larger than 5 mm that fail to enhance by more than 15 HU is likely to be benign (negative predictive value greater than 95%).[31,56,57]
  - Tuberculous granulomas show peripheral ring enhancement or curvilinear central enhancement.[58]

## Magnetic Resonance Imaging

- Magnetic resonance imaging is currently not widely used for evaluation of SPNs due to its higher cost and lack of definitive diagnostic advantage relative to CT.

## Positron Emission Tomography (PET) and PET-CT

- SPN is a major indication for $^{18}$F-fluoro-deoxyglucose (FDG) PET imaging. FDG uptake by a nodule is proportional to the metabolic activity of the nodule.[59]
- PDG-PET is less accurate for pulmonary nodules smaller than 1 cm because of the spatial resolution of current PET scanners.[60]
- FDG-PET can be falsely negative in cases of bronchioloalveolar cell carcinoma, carcinoid, and renal cell metastasis.[61-63]
- Inflammatory and granulomatous changes, such as those seen in fungal infection, pneumonia, and sarcoidosis, can give a false-positive result.[62,64]

- Visual or qualitative evaluation by comparing the activity of the SPN relative to the mediastinum may be sufficient for diagnosis. Quantitative analysis with standard uptake value (SUV) may not be necessary in most cases.[65,66] Initially, a lung mass with an SUV greater than 2.5 was thought to be cancer and an SUV smaller than 2.5 was thought to suggest that the lung mass was benign. That is no longer thought to be true. There is no cut points to diagnose cancer in a lung mass. (See chapter 2 on radionuclide imaging for more details.)
- PET/CT has better sensitivity (97%), specificity (85%), and accuracy (93%) in characterizing a nodule as malignant or benign than either CT or PET alone.[65]

## Tissue Diagnosis

- More invasive procedures are undertaken when imaging fails to exclude malignancy.
  - Transthoracic needle biopsy
    - Can sometimes be performed with fluoroscopy or ultrasound guidance, but currently, CT guidance is most commonly used
    - Recent study demonstrates a diagnostic accuracy of 77%, pneumothorax rate of 28%, and chest tube insertion rate of 2.5% for lesions smaller than 20 mm in diameter.[67]
    - Diagnostic accuracy is significantly better for larger (>10 mm) lesions.[67]
    - The accuracy is improved to 97% with the use of multiplanar reconstruction image.[68]
    - The yield for a specific benign diagnosis is improved with core needle biopsy[69] and by having an on-site pathologist to assess the adequacy of biopsy samples at the time of the procedure.[70]
  - Bronchoscopy
    - More useful in lesions that are large, central, or have endobronchial component.[1]
    - However, fiberoptic bronchoscopy has not been shown to be beneficial in most patients with an SPN because diagnostic yield with lesions that are small in size or peripheral in location, is poor.[71,72] Newer techniques such as navigational bronchoscopy have excellent yields (see chapter 4 on diagnostic bronchoscopy).
  - Video-assisted thoracic surgery (VATS)
    - Useful for small indeterminate peripheral pulmonary nodules that are difficult to biopsy or have negative biopsy by transthoracic needle aspiration or bronchoscopy.
    - Preferred over open biopsy due to less pain, shorter hospital stays, and faster recovery.[73,74]
    - Performed under general anesthesia using single lung ventilation via a double-lumen endotracheal tube
    - A recent study demonstrated a 100% success rate in obtaining a tissue diagnosis. Asymptomatic pneumothorax was observed in one case and minor intrapulmonary hemorrhage in 2 cases out of a total of 57 cases.[75]
    - Preoperative CT-guided localization of the pulmonary nodule with hookwire or microcoil is safe, time-saving, and helpful in preventing the need to convert to thoracotomy.[76-78]
  - Open-lung biopsy or excision
    - Overall morbidity is 3% to 7%.[73]
    - For smaller and more central lesions difficult to biopsy by VATS.

## TREATMENT

- Depends on the diagnosis
  - If the lesion is malignant, surgical resection, chemotherapy, or radiation may be used depending on established standard of care for the specific type and stage of the malignancy.

○ If a specific benign diagnosis is obtained, medical therapy may be necessary (i.e., antimicrobials for granulomatous infection)

○ If a non-specific benign diagnosis, such as atypical bronchioloalveolar hyperplasia, inflammation, atypical cells, is obtained, careful clinical and radiographic follow-up is recommended.[72]

## Brief Illustrative Case

- *History:* 55-year-old man with 60-pack-year smoking history and chronic obstructive pulmonary disease (COPD) presents with symptoms of COPD exacerbation.
- *Examination:* Vitals within normal limits except for $O_2$ Saturation of 95%. Diffuse wheezing bilaterally. No other abnormalities.
- *Blood tests:* Complete blood count and electrolytes— normal
- *Imaging:* Chest radiograph demonstrates hyperinflated lungs with an incidental vague nodule in the right lung apex. Contrast CT of the chest (Fig. 19-1): 14 × 15 mm speculated nodule in the apical segment of right upper lobe. Changes of mild centrilobular emphysema are noted. PET demonstrates a hypermetabolic focus in the right upper lobe corresponding to the nodule seen on CT (Fig. 19-2). No other abnormality seen.
- *Diagnosis/Pathology:* CT-guided core needle biopsy (Fig. 19-3) demonstrates a moderately differentiated adenocarcinoma
- *Management:* Surgical right upper lobectomy

### Key Points

- SPNs are often discovered incidentally on chest radiograph.

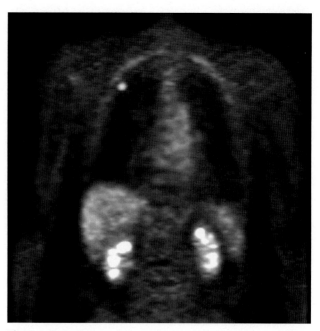

**Figure 19-2:** Fluoro-2-deoxy-D-glucose (FDG) positron emission tomography (PET) whole body scan. The right upper lobe nodule shows high metabolic activity.

- CT of the chest and PET can help further characterize a SPN.
- A spiculated, hypermetabolic SPN in a patient with significant smoking history is highly suspicious for a primary bronchogenic carcinoma.
- CT-guided transthoracic core needle biopsy is the preferred method of obtaining tissue sample if the SPN

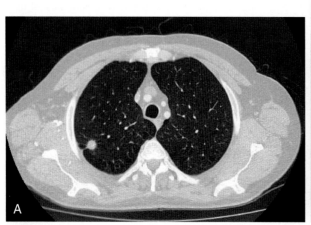

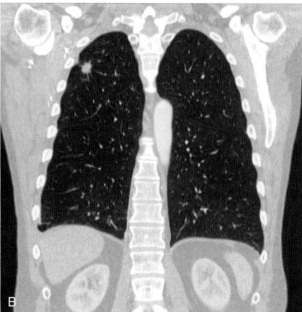

**Figure 19-1: A,** Computed tomography (CT) scan of the chest with contrast, axial view. A spiculated nodule is seen in the right upper lobe. There are also emphysematous changes related to smoking. **B,** CT scan of the chest with contrast, coronal reformation image. The right upper lobe nodule is again demonstrated.

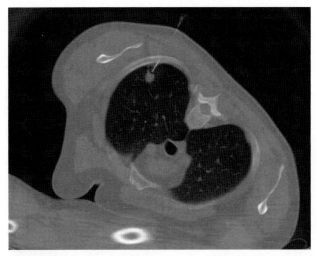

**Figure 19-3:** Transthoracic core needle biopsy. Patient was placed on a left decubitus position for optimal access to the nodule.

## Brief Illustrative Case—cont'd

is suspected to be malignant based on imaging characteristics and is accessible
- Small pneumothorax is a common complication of transthoracic needle biopsy, but most of the time is not clinically significant and does not require chest tube placement
- If a SPN is confirmed to be a primary bronchogenic carcinoma, it is usually surgically resectable.
- Note: A cogent argument could be made to proceed to surgery without CT-guided transthoracic core needle biopsy, in cases with highly suspicious lesions (i.e., based on both clinical risk factors and imaging features) in otherwise operable patients. Rationale: Regardless of the findings on needle biopsy (positive or negative), surgery would be indicated.

*(Continued)*

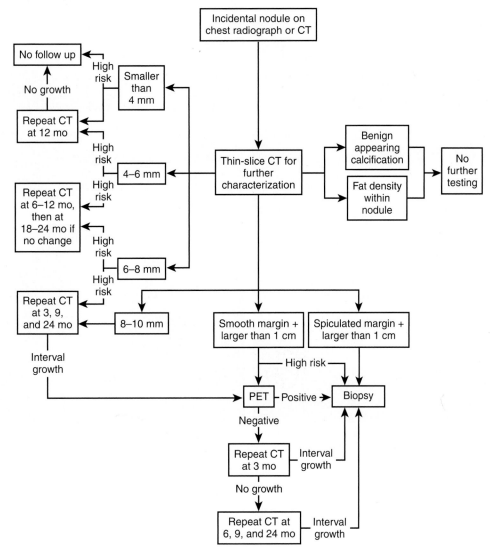

**Figure 19-4:** Algorithm for approach to the incidental finding of a nodule on chest radiograph or computed tomography scan.

## Brief Illustrative Case—cont'd

- An algorithmic approach to the incidental finding of a nodule on chest radiograph or CT is depicted in Figure 19-4.

- Figure 19-5 depicts the natural history of an SPN followed over 18 months in a patient with multiple medical problems. Significant growth was observed over time with the interval development of cavitation. Pathology was non-small cell carcinoma.

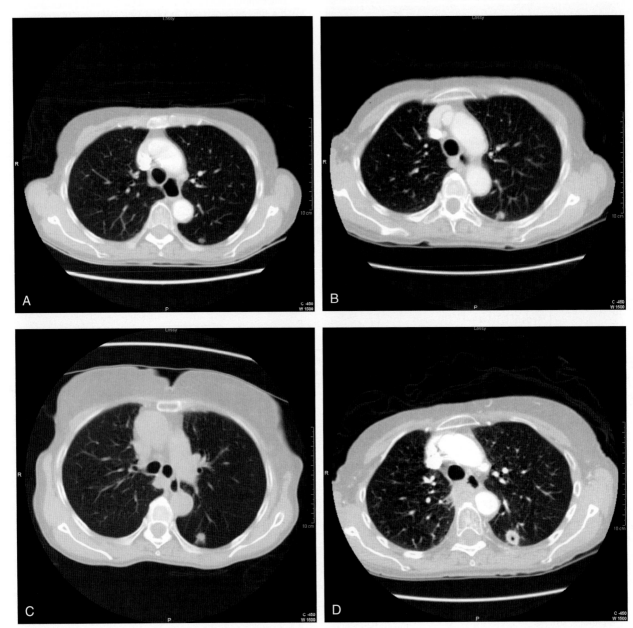

**Figure 19-5:** The natural history of a solitary pulmonary nodule followed over 18 months in a patient with multiple medical problems that rendered the patient inoperable. Pathology was non-small cell carcinoma. **A,** A 5 × 7 mm nodular density noted in the superior segment of the left lower lobe (LLL). **B,** 3-month follow up reveals a slightly larger nodule, which is denser (6 × 8 mm). **C,** Nodule 6 months later was further increased in size (9.9 × 9.3 mm). **D,** Computed tomography scan 9 months later depicts the nodule that demonstrates (1) further increment in size (16 × 12 mm), (2) cavitation, and (3) irregular margins. Note: Although the linear dimensions doubled over the 18-month period, the volumetric increment and doubling times were significantly greater.

## References

 Interactive references and additional readings for this chapter can be accessed online at *expertconsult.com*.

# 20 LUNG CANCER SCREENING

### Brian Tzung, MD and Peter J. Julien, MD

## MAIN POINTS

- Lung cancer is a prevalent disease, and is the leading cause of cancer death in men and women.
- There is a large difference in survival between lung cancer detected at an early stage and lung cancer detected at an advanced stage. Of the four most common cancers, the screening tests have made a big difference in survival for breast, prostate, and colon cancer, but there is no officially approved screening test for lung cancer. A screening test that can detect lung cancer at an early stage would be very desirable because the mortality rate for lung cancer is so high.
- Low-dose computed tomography (LDCT) is sensitive for the detection of early-stage, curable lung cancer
- However, there has been no randomized, prospective screening study to prove that LDCT will reduce the overall mortality for lung cancer. Studies are currently underway to evaluate this more comprehensively.

## SCREENING—DEFINITIONS

- **Screening**: a test used to detect cancer before symptoms develop.
- To be effective, a screening test must be readily available, of low cost, and ultimately influence mortality.

## LUNG CANCER - BACKGROUND INFORMATION / RATIONALE FOR SCREENING

- Epidemiology:
  - Lung cancer is the leading cause of cancer death in men and women.
  - 2007 estimated new cases: 213,380[1]
  - 2007 estimated deaths: 160,390 (compared with 40,910 for breast cancer and 52,180 for colon cancer)[1]
  - Accounts for 15% of cancer diagnoses and 29% of cancer deaths[1]
- Prognosis:
  - Average 5-year survival rate for all patients is very poor, at 16%.[1]
  - Five-year survival rate for localized disease is considerably better, at 67% for stage IA, to 39% for stage IIB.[2]
  - At present, only 16% of lung cancers are diagnosed when still localized.
  - Small cell lung cancer accounts for 13% of all lung cancer cases.[1]
  - Non–small cell lung cancer (NSCLC) constitutes 87%.[1] Screening epidemiology is based on NSCLC data.
- Treatment:
  - For localized cancer, surgery is most often the treatment of choice.
  - Chemotherapy and radiation therapy are used in metastatic disease.
  - For patients with localized (stage I) NSCLC who are not surgical candidates, optimal treatment includes radiofrequency ablation or localized radiation therapy, or both.

## STATISTICAL ANALYSIS

- For a screening test to prove effectiveness, it must ultimately improve mortality, and not just detect cancer and improve 5-year survival.
- Theoretic reasons why a screening test may give a false impression of benefit:
  - Lead time bias—False impression of improved survival in a screened population without affecting mortality, because the cancer is diagnosed earlier in the natural history of the disease but the patient still dies of the cancer (Fig. 20-1).
  - Length time bias—Screened populations are by definition asymptomatic and may therefore be more likely to have less aggressive malignancies.
  - Overdiagnosis bias—A screening program has a tendency to discover cancer that will not affect the life expectancy of the patient.
    - For example, autopsy studies show that up to 22% of men older than 70 dying from unrelated causes still have small kidney cancers.
    - There is also a 1% incidence of lung cancer in the same population, with neither cancer contributing to the patient's demise.

## SCREENING MODALITY: CHEST X-RAY STUDY AND SPUTUM CYTOLOGY

The usefulness of chest x-ray study (CXR) and sputum cytology in lung cancer screening was examined in five randomized control trials in the 1970s and 1980s.[3,4] Screening with CXR (with or without sputum cytology) increased lung cancer diagnosis and an improved survival. However, no definite overall mortality reduction was found. The applicability of these findings is limited by the fact that the American studies used recommended annual CXR as the standard of care for the control group.

- A randomized control trial (RCT) in London evaluated 55,034 men.[5] The experimental group received CXR every 6 months for 3 years, whereas the control group received CXR at the beginning and end of the study. Sixty-two patients died in the semiannual screening group, whereas 59 patients died in the control group. The study was reported as showing no benefit; however, if the data are analyzed differently, interesting results and trends are observed. For example, if the prevalent cases were not included, there was a 60% survival for the incident cases in the screened group and a 0% survival for the incident cases in the control group.
- An RCT in the Czech Republic evaluated 6364 male smokers.[6] Semiannual screening CXR and sputum cytology was compared with a single CXR at the end of 3 years. Lung cancer detection was increased and prognosis improved in the screened group. However, lung cancer mortality was similar. At 15-year follow-up, 247 patients in the semiannual screening group died of lung cancer, compared with 216 in the control group.
- The Mayo Lung Project evaluated 10,933 male smokers older than 45 years of age.[4,7] Initial screening found 51 lung cancers

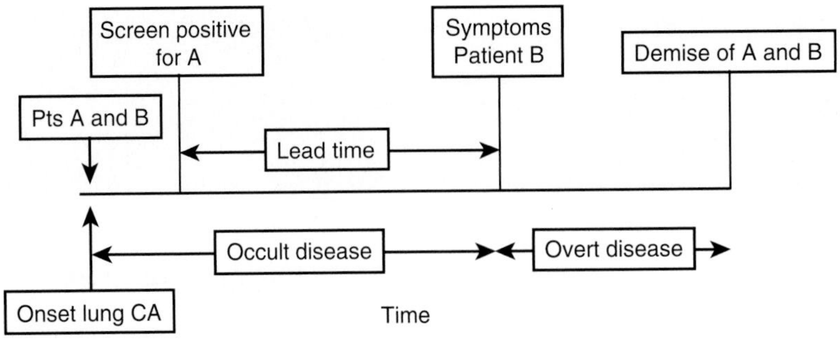

**Figure 20-1:** Schematic showing concept of lead time bias. Hypothetical patients A and B both develop lung cancer (i.e., onset of pathology) at similar times. In A, screening identifies a mass on the chest radiograph that proves to be non–small cell lung cancer. The patient receives appropriate surgical therapy. For patient B, the diagnosis is only made following the development of symptoms, at a much later time compared with patient A. Both patients A and B die from cancer-related causes at similar times. We conclude from this scenario that although the apparent survival of patient A is significantly longer than that of patient B, the mortality and inherent natural history, however, are the same for both patients.

by CXR, 17 by sputum cytology, and 15 by CXR and sputum cytology; these patients were excluded from the study.

- ○ The experimental group (4618 men) received CXR and sputum cytology every 4 months for 6 years
- ○ The control group (4593 men) was less intensively screened. They were recommended to get annual CXR and sputum cytology. At least half of this control group did have at least one CXR in the interim.
- ○ More cancers were diagnosed in the experimental group (206 compared with 160 in the control group).
- ○ More of the detected cancers were resectable in the experimental group (48% versus 32%).
- ○ Overall mortality was similar (3.2 per 1000 person years for the intensively screened group compared with 3.0 per 1000 person years for the less intensively screened group).
- ○ Long-term follow-up of the data from this study discounts the concept of lead time bias for lung cancer.
- ■ Studies performed at the Memorial Sloan-Kettering Cancer Center (MSKCC) in New York and at Johns Hopkins Hospital compared dual screening with CXR and sputum cytology relative to annual CXR. Dual screening did not improve survival.[8,9]

## SCREENING WITH LOW-DOSE COMPUTED TOMOGRAPHY

Because of the early results with LDCT, showing a four-fold increased ability of LDCT to detect lung cancer compared with CXR, and a six-fold increased ability of LDCT to detect Stage I lung cancer (Early Lung Cancer Action Program, 1999),[10] there was renewed interest in the value of imaging to detect early stage lung cancer.

## EXISTING TRIALS

Two prospective, single-arm trials demonstrate the capability of LDCT to detect early-stage lung cancer. The International Early Lung Cancer Action Program (I-ELCAP) study was a multicenter international trial that screened 31,567 patients with LDCT between 1993 and 2005. Another study, combining data from the Mayo Clinic, the Istituto Tumori in Milan, and the Moffitt Center in Tampa, screened 3246 patients, and followed them for an average of 3.9 years.

- ■ I-ELCAP Study[11]
  - ○ 31,567 patients older than 40 years of age with a history of smoking or occupational/second-hand smoke exposure

were screened for lung cancer with LDCT. Of those, 27,546 patients underwent repeat screening 7 to 18 months later.

- ○ The detection rate for lung cancer was 1.3% on baseline examination and 0.3% on follow-up studies. For patients older than 60 years of age who were smokers, the detection rate was 2.7% on baseline examination and 0.6% on follow-up studies.
- ○ Overall, lung cancer was detected in 484 patients. The 10-year survival rate for these patients was projected at 80%. This compares favorably with the 16% 5-year survival rate observed in the average clinically detected lung cancer.
- ○ Most of the patients (412 of 484) were diagnosed as stage I at time of detection.
- ○ In 302 patients with stage I lung cancer who had surgical resection of their tumor within 1 month of cancer detection, there was a 92% 10-year survival for this group.
- ■ Mayo Clinic/Istituto Tumori/Moffitt study[12]
  - ○ Starting in 1998, 3246 current or former smokers were screened with LDCT. Screened patients followed for an average of 3.9 years after screening were compared with expected cancer incidence and mortality based on age- and sex-matched data from the National Cancer Institute's Surveillance, Epidemiology, and End Results (SEER) cancer registry database from 1993 to 1998.
  - ○ One hundred and forty-four lung cancers were diagnosed in the screened population, compared with an expected 44.3 cases of lung cancer.
  - ○ One hundred and nine lung resections were performed, compared with 10.9 expected operations for a nonscreened population.
  - ○ LDCT screening detected lung cancer at an earlier stage than expected. Ninety-six lung cancers (67%) were stage I or stage II.
  - ○ Lung cancer deaths in the screened group:
    - ■ Twelve patients were diagnosed with early-stage lung cancer.
    - ■ Thirteen patients were diagnosed with stage III or stage IV lung cancer.
    - ■ Six patients died of lung cancer who had negative findings on their screening examinations.
  - ○ Only 1 death from lung cancer occurred in screened patients in the first year. The investigators hypothesized that the mortality in the first year was so low because all study patients had to be asymptomatic on enrollment.
  - ○ Overall, 38 screened patients died. This is not statistically different than the expected number of deaths (38.8) in a comparable nonscreened population, as predicted by SEER data.

## Ongoing Trials

- National Lung Screening Trial: 50,000 high-risk smokers have been assigned to annual screening with LDCT or CXR. The study is designed to have a 90% power to detect a mortality reduction of 20% by 2009.
- NELSON trial: In the Netherlands and Belgium, 16,000 smokers have been randomly assigned to LDCT screening or usual care. The study is set to close in 2016.

## Conclusions

- Facts
  - ◦ LDCT detects more lung cancer than CXR (fourfold).
  - ◦ LDCT detects more cases of early-stage lung cancer than CXR (Figs. 20-2 to 20-4).
- Controversy:
  - ◦ Early detection of lung cancer may reduce mortality.

## COST ANALYSIS

- Several models have been proposed estimating the cost effectiveness of CT screening per life year gained.[13] Estimates are extremely variable. Models supporting the use of LDCT screening estimate a cost of $2,500 per life-year gained in a high-prevalence population.[14] Models that do not support the use of LDCT screening estimate a cost of

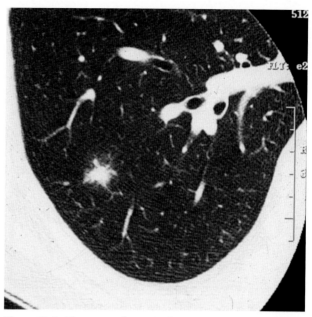

**Figure 20-4:** The computed tomography scan is highly sensitive in the detection of stage I lung cancers, as seen here in the right lower lobe.

$116,300 per quality-adjusted life-year gained, for current smokers.[15]

- Models evaluating cost per life-year gained range from simple to complex.
  - ◦ More simplistic models consider the cost of lung cancer detection to include the cost of limited CT for all screened patients, added to the cost of high-resolution CT and biopsy for patients who have noncalcified nodules.[14]
  - ◦ More complex models augment the costs described earlier with additional costs, including cancer care and surgery performed on detected cancers, complications from biopsy, additional clinical visits, antibiotics, and opportunity costs for travel time.[15]
- Although there are costs associated with lung cancer screening, there are also costs associated with the management of clinically detected lung cancer in unscreened populations.
  - ◦ Surgery for stage I lung cancer is less than half the cost of late-stage treatment.[16,17]
  - ◦ If the assumption is made that LDCT detects lung cancer at an earlier stage, and that early-stage lung cancer is less expensive to manage than late-stage lung cancer, then LDCT screening may actually have significant cost benefits. Comprehensive cost-benefit analyses should weigh the costs of screening against the costs that result from delayed diagnosis in unscreened populations.

## SCREENING CRITERIA

Current guidelines for management of the incidentally detected solitary pulmonary nodule have been outlined by the Fleischner Society. The data reflect the very low incidence of cancer that was observed with small pulmonary nodules in the Early Lung Cancer Action Program. Recommendations are as follows[18]:

- Central, laminar, or dense diffuse calcification patterns are reliable evidence of benignancy
- Fat content suggests a hamartoma, lipid granuloma, or lipoma.
- Solid nodules are likely to grow more rapidly than nonsolid nodules.

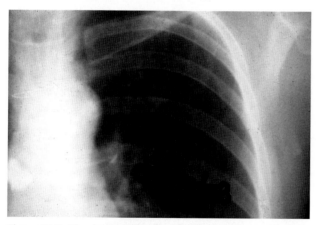

**Figure 20-2:** The chest radiograph often is not sensitive in detecting small lung cancers. The small nodule on this film might easily be interpreted as normal lung markings.

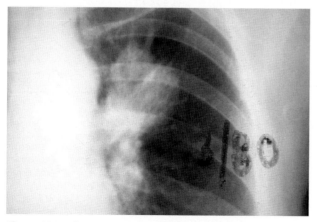

**Figure 20-3:** The same patient (as depicted in Figure 20-2), 3 years later. A large lung mass is now present in the left upper lobe.

| Nodule size | Low-risk patient | High-risk patient |
|---|---|---|
| Less or equal to 4 mm | No follow-up needed | Follow-up at 12 months. If no change, no further follow-up needed |
| >4–6 mm | Follow-up at 12 months If no change, no further follow-up needed. | Initial follow-up at 6–12 months and then at 18–24 months if no change. |
| >6–8 mm | Initial follow-up at 6–12 months and then at 18–24 months if no change. | Initial follow-up at 3–6 months and then at 9–12 months and 24 months if no change |
| >8 mm | Follow-up computed tomography scan (CT) at 3, 9, and 24 months. Dynamic contrast enhanced CT, positron emission tomography scan (PET), or biopsy. | Same as for low-risk patients |

Low-risk patient: Minimal or absent history of smoking and other known risk factors.
High-risk patient: History of smoking or other known risk factors.

## DRAWBACKS OF LUNG CANCER SCREENING WITH LDCT

- Lung cancer screening is associated with costs, both direct and indirect, as discussed earlier.
- Lung cancer screening may lead to overdiagnosis. As a result, unnecessary procedures and surgeries will be performed in some cases, on lung neoplasms that would otherwise never become clinically significant.
- Radiation
  - ○ CT examinations result in larger organ radiation doses compared with other imaging studies. The radiation doses are up to 30 to 90 mSv. Radiation doses for a chest CT range from 7.8 mSv for a reduced-dose CT to 21.4 mSv for a standard-dose CT.[19] An average CXR dose is approximately 0.1 mSv; therefore, a standard dose CT is approximately equivalent to 214 CXRs.
  - ○ The effects of radiation from CT examinations have not been directly studied. A review has suggested that in atomic bomb survivors, low doses of radiation are associated with a small but significant increase in overall risk of cancer. It has also been suggested that radiation workers exposed to an average of 20 mSv have a statistically significant increase in risk of cancer mortality.[20]
    - ■ These conclusions rely on the assumption that certain Hiroshima survivors were exposed to similar doses of radiation as patients undergoing CT examination. Actual radiation exposure experienced by atomic bomb survivors is unclear.
    - ■ The U.S. Food and Drug Administration approves health-care worker exposure up to 50 mSv per year. There is no evidence of increased incidence of cancer in radiologists compared with other physicians.
    - ■ There may be a dose threshhold below which radiation is not significantly carcinogenic. The effects of low doses of radiation are likely to be different than the effects of high doses of radiation.
  - ○ The risk of a CT examination to the individual is low, at less than 1/10th of 1%. The benefits of CT examinations frequently outweigh the possible risks of radiation exposure. At this point, the application of CT scanning must be a balance between the clinical benefit and the potential risks.

## CONCLUSIONS

- The incidence of early stage lung cancer in the United States is 25%, the incidence of early stage lung cancer in CXR screening studies is 40%, and the incidence of early-stage lung cancer in CT screening studies is 80%.
- Nonrandomized screening studies suggest a survival benefit for CT scan screening.
- There is currently no randomized, prospective study to prove that CT scan screening reduces the mortality for lung cancer.

### Brief Illustrative Case

- *History:* A 36-year-old asymptomatic nonsmoking man with an extensive family history of coronary artery disease. He is concerned about his own risk for early coronary disease and decides to have an electron-beam CT (EBCT) performed for calcium scoring.
- *Examination:* Vitals: normal sinus rhythm (62/min); BP 120/65; repirations 13/min; temp: 97.6° F. No apparent distress.
- *Imaging:* Cardiac EBCT demonstrates no significant coronary calcification. However, an irregular noncalcified 9-mm lung nodule is incidentally identified in the right middle lobe. There is no lymphadenopathy. A PET-CT is performed for further evaluation, revealing increased metabolic activity corresponding to the nodule.
- *Diagnosis/Pathology:* Open lung biopsy is performed, and the nodule is removed by limited resection. Pathology is consistent with bronchoalveolar carcinoma.
- *Management:* The patient recovers from the surgical resection. Five years after the procedure, the patient remains asymptomatic, and a CT examination demonstrates no evidence of disease.
- It is possible that "screening" led to a cure. However further follow-up is needed to evaluate possible epidemiological biases, as described above.

## References

 Interactive references and additional readings for this chapter can be accessed online at *expertconsult.com*.

# 21 STAGING OF LUNG CANCER

Clifton F. Mountain,* MD, Kay E. Hermes, BS, and Michael I. Lewis, MD

## TERMINOLOGY

- Stage of disease
- TNM subsets
- Stage grouping
- cStage
- pStage
- rStage

## DEFINITIONS

- The *stage of disease* describes the anatomic extent of the cancer.
- The *TNM subsets* represent description of the primary tumor, the T factor, the status of the regional lymph nodes, the N factor, and the absence or presence of distant metastasis, the M factor.

- *Stage grouping* is the combination of TNM subsets into seven stages of disease that reflect a hierarchy of survival expectations from the best outcome for stage I to the worst in Stage IV: *Stage IA, IB, IIA, IIB, IIIA, IIIB, and IV.*
- All clinical observations and tests performed before the initiation of treatment are the basis for the *clinical* or *cStage.*
- The *postsurgical treatment-pathologic stage, pStage,* is assigned on the basis of pathological examination of resected specimens.
- A *retreatment stage, rStage,* may be assigned following initial or subsequent steps in a multistep treatment program, or at any point in the life history of the cancer.

**Note:** This chapter is divided into two sections: *Section 1* deals with the current staging system in use, and *Section 2* presents the proposed revisions to be incorporated in the seventh edition of the International System for Staging Lung Cancer as published by the International Association for the Study of Lung Cancer (IASLC).

---

## Section 1
# CURRENT STAGING SYSTEM

## INTRODUCTION

- The concept of staging derives from the significant relationship between the anatomic extent of the disease and prognosis in patients with lung cancer.
- The International System for Staging Lung Cancer provides reproducible classification of the anatomic extent of the disease.
- Limitations in treatment strategy are related to:
  - cStage of disease at diagnosis
  - Histologic cell type of the tumor
  - Patient performance status

## INTERNATIONAL SYSTEM FOR STAGING LUNG CANCER

For the past 20 years, the scientific community has been well served by wide application of the International System for Staging Lung Cancer,[1] shown in Tables 21-1 and 21-2. These recommendations were derived and confirmed by analysis of a collected database of the survival experiences of more than 5000 patients with primary lung cancer treated in a contemporary time frame.[2] The present classification was adopted in 1986,[3] and with revisions,[1] has been in place since that time;

it has been included in the past and present published staging manuals of the American Joint Committee on Cancer (AJCC)[4-6] and the International Union Against Cancer (UICC).[7-9] To reduce the inconsistency resulting from the use of multiple systems for classifying regional lymph nodes, recommendations for a lymph node mapping schema[9] were adopted by the AJCC and the UICC that incorporate features of the most frequently used systems.[10]

End results studies according to staging factors provide a benchmark for:

- Estimating prognosis
- Entering patients into clinical trials
- Comparing the effectiveness of differing treatments
- Evaluating new prognostic factors

### Histologic Cell Type

The staging system is applicable for the four major cell types of lung cancer, described in the 2004 World Health Organization Classification of Lung Tumors.[11] This classification emphasizes morphologic aspects of diagnosis using light microscopy and provides a standard nomenclature and criteria for diagnosis that can be used by pathologists worldwide.

- Squamous cell carcinoma
- Adenocarcinoma (including bronchioalveolar carcinoma)
- Large cell carcinoma
- Small cell carcinoma

Specific TNM staging is useful for small cell lung cancer (SCLC), particularly for selecting patients for multimodality programs

---

*\*The editors wish to acknowledge the enormous contributions of Dr. Mountain over many years on the subject of lung cancer staging. Sadly, shortly after submitting this chapter, he passed away. He will be dearly missed.*

## TABLE 21-1 ■ TNM (TUMOR, REGIONAL LYMPH NODES, METASTASIS) DESCRIPTORS

**Primary Tumor (T)**

| | |
|---|---|
| TX | Primary tumor cannot be assessed or tumor proven by the presence of malignant cells in sputum or bronchial washings but not visualized by imaging or bronchoscopy |
| T0 | No evidence of primary tumor |
| Tis | Carcinoma in situ |
| T1 | Tumor 3 cm or less in greatest dimension, surrounded by lung or visceral pleura, without bronchoscopic evidence of invasion more proximal than the lobar bronchus* (i.e., not in the main bronchus) |
| T2 | Tumor with any of the following features of size or extent: |
| | More than 3 cm in greatest dimension |
| | Involves main bronchus, 2 cm or more distal to the carina |
| | Invades the visceral pleura |
| | Associated with atelectasis or obstructive pneumonitis that extends to the hilar region but does not involve the entire lung. |
| T3 | Tumor of any size that directly invades any of the following: chest wall (including superior sulcus tumors), diaphragm, or the mediastinal pleura or pericardium; or tumor in the main bronchus less than 2 cm distal to the carina, but without involvement of the carina; or associated atelectasis or obstructive pneumonitis of the entire lung. |
| T4 | Tumor of any size that invades any of the following: mediastinum, heart, great vessels, trachea, esophagus, vertebral body, carina; or tumor with a malignant pleural or pericardial effusion†, or with satellite tumor nodule(s) within the ipsilateral primary-tumor lobe of the lung. |

**Regional Lymph Nodes (N)**

| | |
|---|---|
| NX | Regional lymph nodes cannot be assessed |
| N0 | No regional lymph node metastasis |
| N1 | Metastasis to ipsilateral peribronchial and/or ipsilateral hilar lymph nodes, and intrapulmonary nodes involved by direct extension of the primary tumor |
| N2 | Metastasis to ipsilateral mediastinal and/or subcarinal lymph node(s) |
| N3 | Metastasis to contralateral mediastinal, contralateral hilar, ipsilateral or contralateral scalene, or supraclavicular lymph node(s) |

**Distant Metastasis (M)**

| | |
|---|---|
| MX | Presence of distant metastasis cannot be assessed |
| M0 | No distant metastasis |
| M1 | Distant metastasis present‡ Specify site(s) |

*T1: The uncommon superficial tumor of any size with its invasive component limited to the main bronchus is classified as T1.
†T4: Most pleural effusions associated with lung cancer are due to tumor. There are, however, some few patients in whom cytopathologic examination of pleural fluid (on more than one specimen) is negative for tumor, the fluid is nonbloody and is not an exudate. In such cases where these elements and clinical judgment dictate that the effusion is not related to the tumor, the patients should be staged T1, T2, or T3, excluding effusion as a staging element.
‡M1: Separate metastatic tumor nodules in the ipsilateral nonprimary tumor lobe(s) of the lung are also classified as M1.
*From Mountain CF. Revisions in the International Staging System for Lung Cancer. Chest 1997;111:1710-1717, with permission.*

## TABLE 21-2 ■ TNM (TUMOR, REGIONAL LYMPH NODES, METASTASIS) BY STAGE

| Stage Subset | TNM |
|---|---|
| Stage 0 | Carcinoma in situ |
| Stage IA | T1 N0 M0 |
| Stage IB | T2 N0 M0 |
| Stage IIA | T1 N1 M0 |
| Stage IIB | T2 N1 M0 |
| | T3 N0 M0 |
| Stage IIIA | T3 N1 M0 |
| | T1 N2 M0 |
| | T2 N2 M0 |
| | T3 N2 M0 |
| Stage IIIB | T4 N0 M0 T4 N1 M0 |
| | T4 N2 M0 |
| | T1 N3 M0 T2 N3 M0 |
| | T3 N3 M0 T4 N3 M0 |
| Stage IV | Any T Any N M1 |

Note: Staging is not relevant for Occult Carcinoma, designated TX N0 M0.
*From Mountain CF. Revisions in the International Staging System for Lung Cancer. Chest 1997;111:1710-1717, with permission.*

involving adjuvant surgery.[12-13] The proportion of patients achieving a complete response to treatment, the duration of the response, and recurrence after a complete response is directly related to the extent of the disease at diagnosis.

### Other Factors and the Present System

- Many factors are reported to have significant influence on the outcome in patients with lung cancer.
- Literature describing prognosis according to the presence or absence of molecular genetic markers, growth factors and receptors, and pathologic factors, such as angiogenesis and cell proliferation, is now available.[14-18]
- In this milieu of evolving knowledge of the molecular biology of lung cancer, its initiation, growth and metastasis, the stage of disease is a standard for evaluating the effect on survival of new factors derived from the research.
- Staging and histologic classifications remain relevant as major indicators of the curative potential and limitations of available therapy for lung cancer.

### TNM Numeric Descriptors

- T—Primary tumor (see Table 21-1)
  - Four distinct levels of tumor progression are classified according to tumor size, location, and extent of invasion, TX, T0, T1, T2, T3, T4.

○ Implications for staging uncommon, limited, superficial tumors and for pleural effusion are addressed in footnotes to Table 21-1.
- N—Regional lymph nodes
  ○ Classification is based on anatomic considerations, that is, the relationship of the nodal drainage to the primary tumor, N0, N1, N2, N3.
- M—Distant metastasis
  ○ Identifies the absence or presence of metastasis to distant organ sites and distant lymph nodes, M0, M1. The implications for staging of separate metastatic nodules in the ipsilateral nonprimary tumor lobe or lobes are addressed in footnotes to Table 21-1.

## Staging in the Life History of the Disease

Identical staging descriptors are useful and applicable at specific points in the life history of the lung cancer.

### cTNM-cStage

- All patients are assigned a clinical stage, which is not changed throughout the course of the disease.
- Importance of clinical staging cannot be overestimated; it is precisely this information that influences treatment selection in most patients.

Sequencing of diagnostic tests usually proceeds from the chest roentgenograms (CXRs) and computed tomographic scans (CTs) and tests to rule out distant metastasis, to examinations for confirming the extent of the primary tumor and the status of regional lymph nodes.[19] The clinical stage includes the results of

- Imaging: CXR; CT; positron emission tomography; magnetic resonance imaging; bone scanning
- Mediastinoscopy, mediastinotomy
- Fine-needle aspiration biopsy
- Diagnostic thoracoscopy
- Transesophageal ultrasound with fine-needle aspiration biopsy may be included; however, it is limited to examination of the posterior mediastinum.[20]

### pTNM-pStage

- For patients assigned to surgical treatment, pathologic examination of resected specimens provides more accurate description of the extent of the primary tumor and regional lymph node metastasis than may be obtained from clinical observations and tests. Except for identifying possible intrapulmonary metastasis, pStage provides no additional information about the cM category.

### rTNM-rStage

- Evaluation of the extent of disease in multimodality therapy programs is useful for assigning subsequent treatment and measuring results of each therapeutic step.

It is useful to specify the evaluations used and the type of staging in end results reports. For example, cStage that includes the results of mediastinoscopy/mediastinotomy provides more accurate evaluation of regional nodes than cStage that does not include the procedure.

## STAGE GROUPING AND SURVIVAL PATTERNS

The TNM subsets, combined in seven stage groups, in addition to a stage 0, are shown in Table 21-2; Figures 21-1 through 21-6

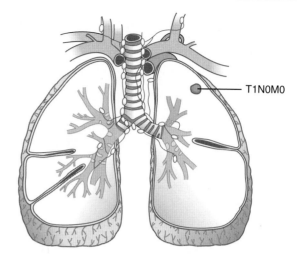

**Figure 21-1:** Diagram—Stage IA includes only patients with T1 tumors and no evidence of metastasis—T1 N0 M0 lung cancer. *(From Mountain CF, Libshitz HI, Hermes KE. Lung cancer: a handbook for staging, imaging and lymph node classification. Houston: Mountain and Libshitz; 1999. p. 28.)*

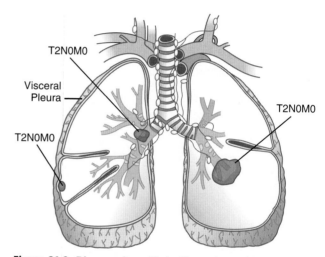

**Figure 21-2:** Diagram—Stage IB classifies patients with T2 primary tumors and no evidence of metastasis, T2 N0 M0 lung cancer. *(From Mountain CF, Libshitz HI, Hermes KE. Lung cancer: a handbook for staging, imaging and lymph node classification. Houston: Mountain and Libshitz; 1999. p. 29.)*

are diagrammatic illustrations of each stage. The implications of the stage classifications for survival rates, according to clinical and surgical pathologic criteria for NSCLC are shown in Figures 21-7 and 21-8, and for SCLC in Figure 21-9. Erosion of prognosis as the lung cancer progresses from stage IA through stage IV reflects the efficacy of treatment, prognosis, and the usefulness of the classification system.

- Stage 0 is assigned to patients with carcinoma in situ.
- Stage IA is reserved for patients with small tumors, less than or equal to 3 cm in greatest dimension, and with no evidence of any metastasis (see Fig. 21-1).[2] The prognosis for these patients is significantly better than that for patients in any other stage, according to both clinical and surgical-pathologic criteria. Figures 21-7 and 21-8 show cumulative 5-year survival rates of 61% for cStage IA patients and 67% for the pStage IA patients with non–small cell lung cancer (NSCLC).[2]

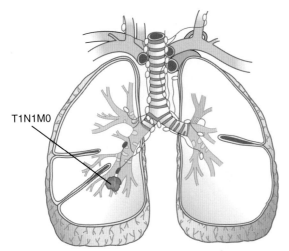

**Figure 21-3:** Diagram—Stage IIA includes patients with T1 primary tumors and evidence of metastasis to hilar, including intrapulmonary lymph nodes, T1 N1 M0 lung cancer. (*From Mountain CF, Libshitz HI, Hermes KE. Lung cancer: a handbook for staging, imaging and lymph node classification. Houston: Mountain and Libshitz; 1999. p. 31.*)

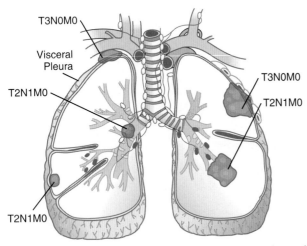

**Figure 21-4:** Diagram—Stage IIB classifies two anatomic subsets of patients, T2 N1 M0 and T3 N0 M0 tumors. The T2 N1 M0 group includes tumors of any size that invade the visceral pleura or the main bronchus more than 2 cm from the carina, or those more than 3 cm in greatest dimension with metastasis involving intrapulmonary, including hilar, lymph nodes T3 N0 M0 includes tumors with limited, circumscribed, extrapulmonary extension and no evidence of metastasis. (*From Mountain CF, Libshitz HI, Hermes KE. Lung cancer: a handbook for staging, imaging and lymph node classification. Houston: Mountain and Libshitz; 1999. p. 33.*)

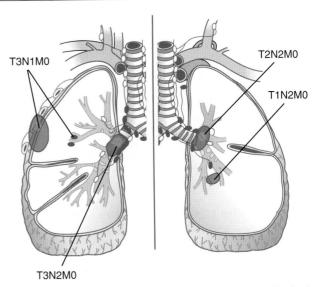

**Figure 21-5:** Diagram—Stage IIIA includes tumors with localized, circumscribed extrapulmonary extension and ipsilateral intrapulmonary, including hilar, lymph node metastasis, the T3 N1 M0 subset. Patients with primary tumor classification of T1, T2, T3 and metastasis to the ipsilateral mediastinal and subcarinal lymph nodes, N2, also are assigned to Stage IIIA - T1 N2 M0, T2 N2 M0 and T3 N0 M0 lung cancer. (*From Mountain CF, Libshitz HI, Hermes KE. Lung cancer: a handbook for staging, imaging and lymph node classification. Houston: Mountain and Libshitz; 1999. p. 35.*)

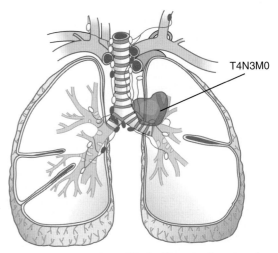

**Figure 21-6:** Diagram—Stage IIIB classifies extensive extrapulmonary tumor invasion of structures such as the trachea, esophagus, heart, and major vessels and metastasis to the contralateral mediastinal and hilar lymph nodes and the ipsilateral and contralateral supraclavicular/scalene lymph nodes, T4 Any N M0 and Any T N3 M0 lung cancer. (*From Mountain CF, Libshitz HI, Hermes KE. Lung cancer: a handbook for staging, imaging and lymph node classification. Houston: Mountain and Libshitz; 1999. p. 38.*)

- Stage IB classifies increasing tumor size and invasiveness, and the presence of associated atelectasis or obstructive pneumonitis; no metastasis is evident, and the proximal extent of disease is at least 2 cm distal to the main carina (see Fig. 21-2).[2] A significant difference between the survival rates for patients with stage IA and those with stage IB NSCLC is documented in Figures 21-7 and 21-8, according to both clinical and surgical pathologic criteria.[2]
- Stage IIA identifies one subset of patients with small primary tumors and limited metastasis to intrapulmonary, including hilar, lymph nodes. These tumors infrequently are

diagnosed clinically; however, in patients undergoing surgical treatment, stage migration to this category is common (see Fig. 21-3)[2] (n = 26, cT1 N1 M0; n = 76, sT1 N1 M0). The survival rates for patients with NSCLC, according to clinical and surgical-pathologic criteria, does not differ significantly from the stage IB groups (see Figs. 21-7 and 21-8); however,

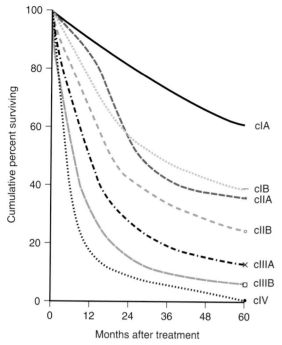

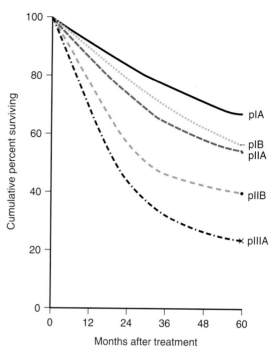

**Figure 21-7:** Cumulative proportion of patients with non–small cell carcinoma expected to survive 5 years according to clinical stage. Number of patients **cIA**, n = 675; **cIB**, n = 1130; **cIIA**, n = 26; **cIIB**, n = 328; **cIIIA**, n = 445; **cIIIB**, n = 836; **cIV**, n = 1166: Overall comparison *P* < .05. Pairwise comparison: **cIA** versus **cIB**, *P* < 0.05; **cIB** vs **cIIA**, *P* > 0.05; **cIIA** vs **cIIB**, *P* < 0.05; **cIIB** versus **cIIIA**, *P* < 0.05; **cIIIA** versus **cIIIB**, *P* < 0.05; **cIIIB** versus **cIV**, *P* < 0.05. (*From Mountain CF, Libshitz HI, Hermes KE. Lung cancer: a handbook for staging, imaging and lymph node classification. Houston: Mountain and Libshitz; 1999. p. 38.*)

**Figure 21-8:** Cumulative proportion of patients with non–small cell lung cancer expected to survive 5 years according to surgical-pathologic stage. **pStage IA**, n = 511; **pIB**, n = 549; **pIIa**, n = 76; **pIIB**, n = 375; **pIIIA**, n = 399. Overall comparison: *P* < 0.05; Pairwise comparisons: **pIA** vs **IB**, *P* < 0.05; **pIB** vs **pIIA**, *P* > 0.05; **pIIA** versus **pIIB**, *P* < 0.05; **pIIB** versus **pIIIA**, *P* < 0.05. (*From Mountain CF, Libshitz HI, Hermes KE. Lung cancer: a handbook for staging, imaging and lymph node classification. Houston: Mountain and Libshitz; 1999. p. 66.*)

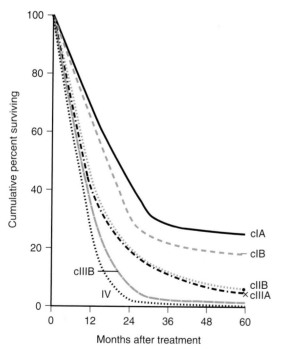

**Figure 21-9:** Cumulative proportion of patients with small cell carcinoma expected to survive 5 years according to clinical stage. Number of patients: **cIA**, n = 12; **cIB**, n = 59; **cIIA**, n = 3; **cIIB**, n = 28; **cIIIa**, n = 66; **cIIIB**, n = 94; **cIV**, n = 261. (*From Mountain CF, Libshitz HI, Hermes KE. Lung cancer: a handbook for staging, imaging and lymph node classification. Houston: Mountain and Libshitz; 1999. p. 67.*)

a specific classification is needed to accumulate data for further study. Radiographic examples of Stage IIA are shown in Figure 21-10A to C.

- Stage IIB includes two anatomic subsets of patients, classified T2 N1 M0 and T3 N0 M0 (see Fig. 21-4).[2] The relationship to survival rates is similar for patients with NSCLC in both of these subgroups: cT2 N1 M0 and cT3 N0 M0, 26% and 21%, respectively, expected to survive 5 years after treatment; pT2 N1 M0 and pT3 N0 M0, 39% and 38% respectively, expected to survive 5 years after treatment.[1] A significant difference in survival rates is shown in Figure 21-7 for patients with cStage IIA NSCLC compared with those with cStage IIB, in which 37% and 24% of patients, respectively, are expected to survive 5 years or more after treatment. In the surgical treatment subset of patients, a significant difference in outcome between pStage IIA and pStage IIB patients also is observed, 55% and 39% respectively expected to survive 5 years after treatment (see Fig. 21-8). Radiographic examples of Stage IIB are shown in Figure 21-11A to B.

- Stage IIIA reflects the implications of ipsilateral, limited extrapulmonary extension of the lung cancer. Classification is provided for four anatomic subsets of patients with extrapulmonary disease and no distant metastasis: Extrapulmonary extension of the primary tumor and metastasis to intrapulmonary, including hilar lymph nodes, is classified as T3 N1 M0, and, T1 N2 M0, T2 N2 M0, and T3 N2 M0 tumors with evidence of metastasis to the ipsilateral mediastinal and subcarinal lymph nodes (see Fig. 21-5).[2] The serious effect on prognosis of clinically detectable lymph node metastasis is shown in the cumulative survival rates for patients with

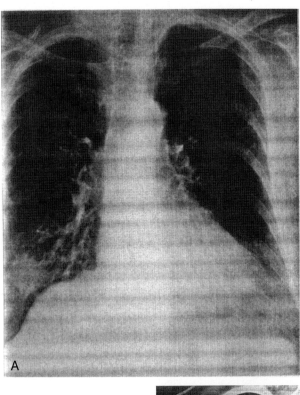

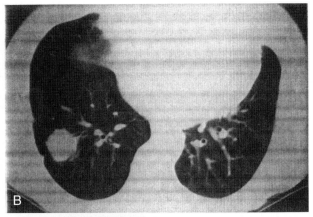

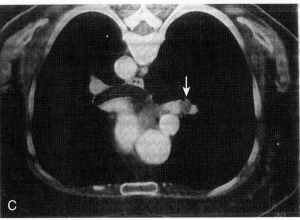

**Figure 21-10: A,** Posteroanterior chest radiogaph shows a speculated bronchogenic carcinoma in the right lower lobe. **B,** Computed tomographic scan (lung windows) through the lesion (**A**) shows the cancer to better advantage and shows tags to the pleura. **C,** Computed tomographic scan (soft tissue windows) shows a right hilar node (*arrow*) that was proven to contain metastatic disease, T1 N1 M0 lung cancer. *(From Mountain CF, Libshitz HI, Hermes KE. Lung cancer: a handbook for staging, imaging and lymph node classification. Houston: Mountain and Libshitz; 1999. p. 31-32.)*

NSCLC in the cT3 N1 M0 and cT1-2-3 N2 M0 subsets, 9% and 13%, respectively, expected to survive 5 years after treatment.[1] Figure 21-7 shows the survival pattern for the cStage IIIA group overall. Selected patients with pStage IIIA NSCLC tumors in whom a complete resection of all known disease is anticipated may have a better prognosis than Stage IIIA patients who are not surgical candidates. Similar cumulative survival rates were observed for patients with NSCLC undergoing surgical treatment in the pT3 N1 M0 and pT1-2-3 N2 M0 groups; 25% and 23% of patients, respectively, expected to survive 5 years after treatment.[1] The survival pattern overall for the pStage IIIA patients is shown in Figure 21-8. Radiographic examples of Stage IIIA are shown in Figure 21-12A to B.

■ Stage IIIB identifies patients with extensive primary tumor invasion of the mediastinum, or with malignant pleural effusion, and metastasis involving contralateral mediastinal, contralateral hilar, and ipsilateral and contralateral scalene/supraclavicular lymph nodes; however, no distant metastasis is present (see Fig. 21-6).[2] Seven TNM subsets include patients with T4 primary tumors and those with N3 disease (see Table 21-1). Only one third of patients with cStage IIIB disease are expected to survive 1 year and 5% for 5 years after treatment. The difference in survival between the Stage IIIB and Stage IV patients is statistically significant, although it may not be clinically relevant (see Fig. 21-7).

■ Stage IV includes only patients with evidence of distant metastatic disease, M1, such as metastases to brain, bone, liver, adrenal

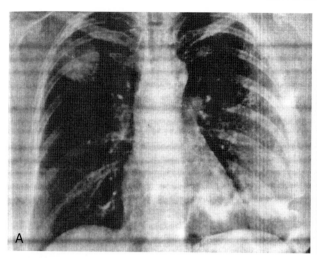
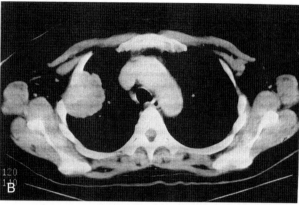

**Figure 21-11: A,** Posteroanterior chest radiograph showing a right upper lobe bronchogenic carcinoma. The chest wall involvement cannot be appreciated. **B,** Computed tomographic scan of the lesion (**A**) shows chest wall invasion (*arrow*). The lymph nodes were free of disease, T3 N0 M0 stage IIB lung cancer. (*From Mountain CF, Libshitz HI, Hermes KE. Lung cancer: a handbook for staging, imaging and lymph node classification. Houston: Mountain and Libshitz; 1999. p. 34.*)

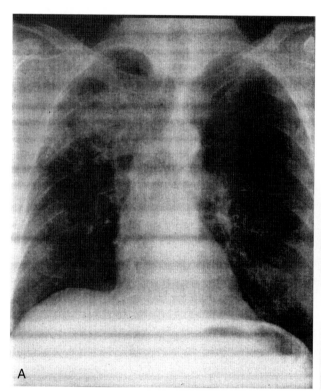
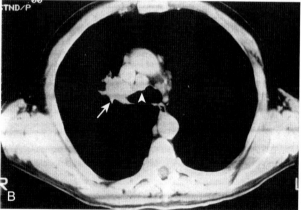

**Figure 21-12: A,** Posteroanterior chest radiograph shows a mass in the right upper lobe and a mass in the right hilum. Mediastinal involvement cannot be excluded. Questionable T2 N2 M0 disease. **B,** Computed tomographic scan of the chest shows the right hilar mass (*arrow*) and right paratracheal adenopathy (*arrowhead*). There is a suggestion of compression of the right main stem bronchus anteriorly. T2 N2 M0-Stage IIIA disease. (*From Mountain CF, Libshitz HI, Hermes KE. Lung cancer: a handbook for staging, imaging and lymph node classification. Houston: Mountain and Libshitz; 1999. p. 36.*)

gland, contralateral lung, pancreas and other distant organs, and metastasis to distant lymph node groups, such as axillary, abdominal, and inguinal. Patients with metastasis in ipsilateral nonprimary tumor lobes also are designated M1. Less than 20% of patients are expected to survive 1 year (see Fig. 21-7).

■ The graphs reflect the erosion of survival expectations as the disease progresses from stage I to stage IV. Differences in outcome for the cStage groups and the pStage patients emphasize the accuracy provided by pathologic evaluation of the extent of disease and the efficacy of surgical treatment.

## IMPLICATIONS FOR TREATMENT SELECTION

The staging process has valid implications for conventional treatment selection; however, it is recognized that no system could be absolute in this regard.

- Surgery is usually the primary treatment option for patient with NSCLC with clinical stages IA, IB, IIA and the T2 N1 M0 subset of Stage IIB. Selected patients with T3 N0 M0—Stage IIB tumors may be referred for surgical treatment, depending on the potential for complete resection of all known disease.
- The proportion of patients expected to survive 5 years after definitive surgical treatment are 67%, pStage IA; 57%, pStage IB; 55%, pStage IIA; 39%, pStage IIB; 23% (see Fig. 21-8).
- Selected patients with cStage IIIA tumors may also undergo surgical treatment, usually in combination with neoadjuvant or adjuvant therapy; 23% are expected to survive 5 years (see Fig. 21-8). The potential for accomplishing an apparent complete resection of all known disease is the key factor in selecting these patients for surgical treatment.
- In patients with stage IIIA and IIIB tumors who are not amenable to a surgical approach, T and N characteristics serve as guidelines for structuring treatment plans, radiotherapy, chemotherapy or combined therapy. Five-year survival rates of 13% and 9% may be expected for cStage IIIA and cStage IIIB, respectively (see Fig. 21-7).
- Stage IV-M1 disease usually indicates only palliative treatment, and the outcome is very poor. Patients with a solitary brain metastasis that are amenable to complete resection are an exception and may have a better prognosis than that of other patients.
- Patients with SCLC are usually treated with chemotherapy. Stage classification for these patients is appropriate and useful because the selection of patients for investigational programs involving adjuvant surgery depends on the initial TNM and stage classifications or the retreatment evaluations following induction therapy.

---

### KEY POINTS

- The International Staging System for Lung Cancer provides a consistent, reproducible method for communicating information and comparing the results of differing treatment approaches for lung cancer.
- The present data support the premise that straightforward indices of the anatomic extent of the cancer permit a simple yet valid classification that best reflects prognosis.
- Patients can be grouped together according to certain measurable common features of their disease so that within each stage group treatment options and survival expectations will be generally similar.
- Survival data according to staging criteria are a measure of the effectiveness of available therapy for lung cancer; thus, the staging information serves as a valuable guide for treatment planning.
- In a given patient, the total tumor burden cannot be precisely quantitated and the balance between host defenses and the heterogeneity of the malignancy is not measurable. These and other complex interacting biologic variables will influence the course of the disease.

---

### Historical Note

The observations of Denoix,[21] who introduced the TNM concept over 60 years ago, remains relevant: "To have a flexible, but reliable (classification) system, it is necessary to agree on the facts of a case. Only then can the cases be grouped in categories in a classification system... The initial descriptions must be definitive, common to all, and based on findings which anyone can confirm with as little margin for personal interpretation among surgeons as possible. It was in concentrating my work on the classification of this common minimum that the TNM system was built up".[22]

---

## Section 2
# PROPOSED REVISIONS TO THE STAGING OF LUNG CANCER (7TH EDITION)

## INTRODUCTION

- Limitations with databases on which prior editions (fifth; 1997, and sixth, 2002) were based, included
  - Small database numbers of cases of NSCLC (n = 5319)
  - Database collected since 1975 (change in modern hospital and other treatment practices)
  - Database drawn mainly from a single institution
  - Database cases most commonly represented a surgical population
  - Very limited internal validation and no external validation
  - Several studies suggested limitations to the current system (e.g., the 3-cm size cutoff)
- In 1998, the IASLC sought to resolve these issues for the seventh edition, by proposed development of a large database drawn globally from multiple geographic regions and which

was to be subjected to intensive validation procedures. The following was achieved[23]:
- Of 100,869 patients submitted, 81,015 passed screening requirements. Of these, 67,725 had NSCLC, with the remainder designated as SCLC. The majority of the cases of NSCLC had pathologic staging (80%)
- The patient cohort was drawn from those treated between 1990 and 2000
- There was wide geographic representation from Europe, North America, Asia, and Australia.
- Treatment modalties were more variable, with only 36% of patients treated with surgery alone.
- High percentage follow-up until death or 2 years (95%) or 5 years (88%), with survivors followed for a median of 5.3 years.
- *Internal validation:* was achieved by analysis and comparison of different types of databases, geographic comparisons and

analysis of survival curves, comparing pTNM and cTNM separately to show consistency. For T validation, a training set of two thirds of the cases used for testing was validated against the remaining third.

- ○ *External validation*: The project database was compared with patients with NSCLC drawn from the 1998–2000 Surveillance, Epidemiology, and End Results (SEER) database.
- ○ Validation procedures demonstrated stability of the data.

## Proposed Revision of T Descriptors

- ■ Revision based on Size: based on clear survival differences (Figs. 21-13 and 21-14), the following changes were proposed (see Table 21-3 for description of all TNM descriptors proposed for the seventh edition[24,25]):
  - ○ T 1 tumors: subclassify as T1a (≤2 cm in greatest dimension) and T1b (>2 cm but = 3 cm)
  - ○ T 2 tumors: subclassify as T2a (>3 cm but ≤5 cm) and T2b (>5 cm but ≤7 cm)
  - ○ T 2 tumors >7 cm: reclassify as T3
- ■ Revision based on Additional Nodule/S: based on better survival in this group compared with other causes of T4 determination (primary lobe) or M1 (ipsilateral different lobe).
  - ○ Additional Nodules in the Primary Lobe: reclassify as T3 (previously T4)

- ○ Additional Nodules in Ipsilateral Lung (i.e., different lobe): reclassify as T4 (previously M)
- ○ With additional nodules, one needs to consider the possibility of synchronous primary tumors, which would have important prognostic implications.

## N Descriptor Proposals

- ■ The large new database provided internal and external validation of clear survival differences with the existing sixth edition staging system for N descriptors. Thus, it was proposed that current N descriptors be maintained in the seventh edition.[26]
- ■ Evaluating survival based on different levels of N1 or N2 disease would require a prospective study with large numbers of patients (e.g., differences between right- or left-sided disease, single versus multiple level involvement, and so on).
- ■ To accomplish meaningful future prospective analyses, comparisons between lymph node zones rather than single lymph node stations were proposed (see Figure 5-1 in Mediastinoscopy chapter for lymph node stations). Six zones were proposed:
  - ○ *Upper zone (R)*: stations 1, 2, 3, and 4 (includes azygous nodes)

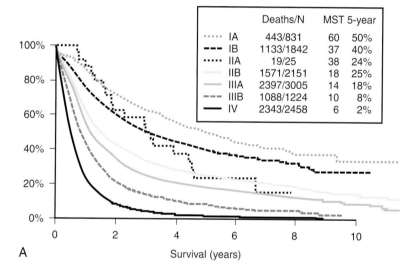

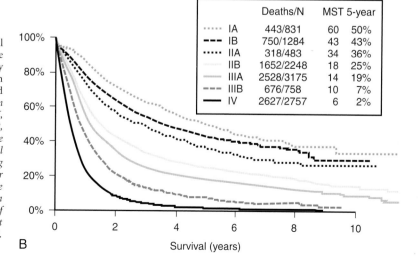

**Figure 21-13:** Overall survival expressed as median survival time (MST) and 5-year survival by clinical stage using the sixth edition of TNM (**A**) and the proposed IASLC recommendations (**B**). *(From Goldstraw P, Crowley J, Chansky K, Giroux DJ, Groome PA, Rami-Porta R, et al; International Association for the Study of Lung Cancer International Staging Committee; Participating Institutions. The IASLC Lung Cancer Staging Project: Proposals for the revision of the TNM stage groupings in the forthcoming [seventh] edition of the TNM classification of malignant tumors. J Thorac Oncol 2007;2:706-714. With permission.)*

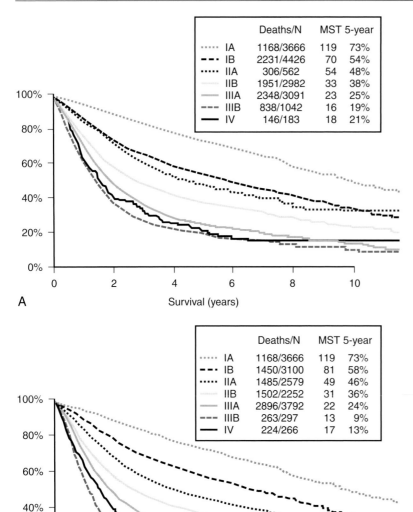

| | Deaths/N | MST | 5-year |
|---|---|---|---|
| ........ IA | 1168/3666 | 119 | 73% |
| --- ▪ IB | 2231/4426 | 70 | 54% |
| ....... IIA | 306/562 | 54 | 48% |
| ——— IIB | 1951/2982 | 33 | 38% |
| ——— IIIA | 2348/3091 | 23 | 25% |
| --- --- IIIB | 838/1042 | 16 | 19% |
| ——— IV | 146/183 | 18 | 21% |

| | Deaths/N | MST | 5-year |
|---|---|---|---|
| ........ IA | 1168/3666 | 119 | 73% |
| --- ▪ IB | 1450/3100 | 81 | 58% |
| ....... IIA | 1485/2579 | 49 | 46% |
| ——— IIB | 1502/2252 | 31 | 36% |
| ——— IIIA | 2896/3792 | 22 | 24% |
| --- --- IIIB | 263/297 | 13 | 9% |
| ——— IV | 224/266 | 17 | 13% |

**Figure 21-14:** Overall survival expressed as median survival time (MST) and 5-year survival by pathologic stage using the sixth edition of TNM (**A**) and the proposed IASLC recommendations (**B**). *(From Goldstraw P, Crowley J, Chansky K, Giroux DJ, Groome PA, Rami-Porta R, et al; International Association for the Study of Lung Cancer International Staging Committee; Participating Institutions. et al. The IASLC Lung Cancer Staging Project: Proposals for the revision of the TNM stage groupings in the forthcoming [seventh] edition of the TNM classification of malignant tumors. J Thorac Oncol 2007;2:706-714. With permission.)*

○ *AP zone (L):* stations 5 and 6
○ *Subcarinal zone:* station 7
○ *Lower zone:* stations 8 and 9
○ *Hilar zone:* stations 10 and 11
○ *Peripheral zone:* stations 12, 13, and 14

### Proposed Revision of M Descriptors

▪ Malignant Pleural Effusion (also Malignant Pericardial Effusion and Pleural Nodules): Survival rates for malignant pleural effusion were worse than for other cT4 tumors (e.g., median survival: 10 versus 13 months; 1-year survival: 36 versus 53%; 5-year survival: 2% versus 15%). Proposal: reclassify as M1a (previously T4)[27]

▪ Additional Nodules in Contalateral Lung: classify as M1a. Note: as above, one still needs to entertain the possibility of synchronous primary lung cancers in this setting.

▪ Extrathoracic Metastases: classify as M1b.

### Proposed New Staging System

▪ Table 21-4: This table depicts the descriptors, proposed T and M categories (with changes from the sixth edition in bold face) and proposed stage groupings.[25]

▪ Table 21-5: This table depicts the proposed TNM stage groupings for the seventh edition.

## LIMITATIONS OF THE SEVENTH EDITION OF THE IASLC LUNG CANCER STAGING PROJECT

▪ A number of geographic regions are not represented (Africa, China, South America and Russia and other States of the former Soviet Union).

▪ Use of multiple existing data sets resulted in missing data in various data fields.

## TABLE 21-3 ▪ PROPOSED DEFINITIONS FOR T, N AND M DESCRIPTORS (7TH EDITION)

**T (Primary Tumor)**

| | |
|---|---|
| X | Primary tumor cannot be assessed, or tumor proven by the presence of malignant cells in sputum or bronchial washings, but not visualized by imaging or bronchoscopy |
| T0 | No evidence of primary tumor |
| Tis | Carcinoma in situ |
| T1 | Tumor ≤3 cm in greatest dimension, surrounded by lung or visceral pleura, without bronchoscopic evidence of invasion more proximal than the lobar bronchus (i.e., not in the mainstem bronchus) |
| T1a | Tumor ≤2 cm in greatest dimension |
| T1b | Tumor >2 cm but ≤3 cm in greatest dimension |
| T2 | Tumor >3 cm but ≤7 cm or tumor with any of the following features (T2 tumors with these features are classified T2a if ≤5 cm) Involves main bronchus, ≥2 cm distal to the carina Invades visceral pleura Associated with atelectasis or obstructive pneumonitis that extends to the hilar region but does not involve the entire lung |
| T2a | Tumor >3 cm but ≤5 cm in greatest dimension |
| T2b | Tumor >5 cm but ≤7 cm in greatest dimension |
| T3 | Tumor >7 cm or one that directly invades any of the following: chest wall (including superior sulcus tumors), diaphragm, phrenic nerve, mediastinal pleura, parietal pericardium; or tumor in the main bronchus <2 cm distal to the carina* but without involvement of the carina; or associated atelectasis or obstructive pneumonitis of the entire lung or separate tumor nodule(s) in the same lobe |
| T4 | Tumor of any size that invades any of the following: mediastinum, heart, great vessels, trachea, recurrent laryngeal nerve, esophagus, vertebral body, carina; separate tumor nodule(s) in a different ipsilateral lobe |

**N (Regional Lymph Nodes)**

| | |
|---|---|
| NX | Regional lymph nodes cannot be assessed |
| N0 | No regional lymph node metastasis |
| N1 | Metastasis in ipsilateral peribronchial and/or ipsilateral hilar lymph nodes and intrapulmonary nodes, including involvement by direct extension |
| N2 | Metastasis in ipsilateral mediastinal and/or subcarinal lymph node(s) |
| N3 | Metastasis in contralateral mediastinal, contralateral hilar, ipsilateral or contralateral scalene, or supraclavicular lymph node(s) |

**M (Distant Metastasis)**

| | |
|---|---|
| MX | Distant metastasis cannot be assessed |
| M0 | No distant metastasis |
| M1 | Distant metastasis |
| M1a | Separate tumor nodule(s) in a contralateral lobe; tumor with pleural nodules or malignant pleural (or pericardial) effusion[†] |
| M1b | Distant metastasis |

*The uncommon superficial spreading tumor of any size with its invasive component limited to the bronchial wall, which may extend proximally to the main bronchus, is also classified as T1.

[†]Most pleural (and pericardial) effusions with lung cancer are due to tumor. In a few patients, however, multiple cytopathologic examinations of pleural (pericardial) fluid are negative for tumor, and the fluid is nonbloody and is not an exudate. Where these elements and clinical judgment dictate that the effusion is not related to the tumor, the effusion should be excluded as a staging element and the patient should be classified as T1, T2, T3, or T4.

*From Goldstraw P, Crowley J, Chansky K, Giroux DJ, Groome PA, Rami-Porta R, et al; International Association for the Study of Lung Cancer International Staging Committee; Participating Institutions. The IASLC Lung Cancer Staging Project: Proposals for the revision of the TNM stage groupings in the forthcoming (seventh) edition of the TNM classification of malignant tumors. J Thorac Oncol 2007;2:706-714. With permission.*

- Inability to control for the precision of clinical and pathologic staging across the large and varied cohort.
- Inability to control for "optimal" treatment measures.
- Lack of prospective data capture
- Lack of nonsize based T2 descriptors such as visceral pleural invasion, hilar atelectasis, obstructive pneumonitis, and main bronchus involvement. For example, in a retrospective analysis of more than 10,000 patients with stage 1B NSCLC, Ou et al[28] reported better survival for patients with visceral pleural invasion, hilar atelectasis, or obstructive pneumonitis when tumor size was smaller than 3 cm compared with 1B patients based on tumor size alone (i.e., >3 cm).
- Challenges to the new staging system include
  ○ New implications for therapy. For example:
  ○ Should T2N0 tumors (moves from stage 1B to IIA) or T3 (size >7 cm) N0 tumors (moves from stage 1B to IIB) require adjuvant chemotherapy post resection?
  ○ What is the correct therapeutic approach to additional ipsilateral tumor nodules?
  ○ What is the optimal approach to malignant pleural effusions? Should systemic chemotherapy become a part of the therapeutic approach?

- Wide-scale education to familiarize treating physicians with a somewhat more complex classification and staging system.

## SMALL CELL LUNG CANCER

- The database contained 12,620 cases of SCLC, with 8088 patients suitable for TNM staging.[29]
- The current staging system separates patients into two groups. Those with limited disease (LD; i.e., confined to the thorax) and those with extensive disease (ED).
- At the time of initial diagnosis, at least two thirds of patients demonstrate evidence of hematogenous spread (i.e., M1 disease)
- Limitations to the current staging system include
  ○ The LD designation does not differentiate size issues.
  ○ The LD designation does not differentiate the presence of ipsilateral or contralateral lymph node involvement (hilar, mediastinal, supraclavicular).
  ○ In the present large series, clinical T1 disease had significantly better survival than those with T2 or other T designations. This group represented only 13.7% of the database.

### TABLE 21-4 ■ DESCRIPTORS, PROPOSED T AND M CATEGORIES, AND PROPOSED STAGE GROUPINGS

| Sixth Edition T/M Descriptor | Proposed T/M | N0 | N1 | N2 | N3 |
|---|---|---|---|---|---|
| T1 (≤2 cm) | T1a | IA | IIA | IIIA | IIIB |
| T1 (>2-3 cm) | T1b | IA | IIA | IIIA | IIIB |
| T2 (≤5 cm) | T2a | IB | **IIA*** | IIIA | IIIB |
| T2 (>5–7 cm) | T2b | **IIA** | IIB | IIIA | IIIB |
| T2 (>7 cm) | T3 | **IIB** | **IIIA** | IIIA | IIIB |
| T3 invasion | | IIB | **IIIA** | IIIA | IIIB |
| T4 (same lobe nodules) | | **IIB** | **IIIA** | **IIIA** | IIIB |
| T4 (extension) | T4 | IIIA | IIIA | IIIB | IIIB |
| M1 (ipsilateral lung) | | **IIIA** | **IIIA** | **IIIB** | **IIIB** |
| T4 (pleural effusion) | M1a | **IV** | **IV** | **IV** | **IV** |
| M1 (contralateral lung) | | IV | IV | IV | IV |
| M1 (distant) | M1b | IV | IV | IV | IV |

*Cells in bold indicate a change from the sixth edition for a particular TNM category.
*From Goldstraw P, Crowley J, Chansky K, Giroux DJ, Groome PA, Rami-Porta R, et al; International Association for the Study of Lung Cancer International Staging Committee; Participating Institutions. The IASLC Lung Cancer Staging Project: Proposals for the revision of the TNM stage groupings in the forthcoming (seventh) edition of the TNM classification of malignant tumors. J Thorac Oncol 2007;2:706-714. With permission.*

### TABLE 21-5 ■ PROPOSED TNM STAGE GROUPINGS (7TH EDITION)

| Occult Carcinoma | TX | N0 | M0 |
|---|---|---|---|
| Stage 0 | Tis | N0 | M0 |
| Stage IA | T1a, b | N0 | M0 |
| Stage IB | T1a, b | N1 | M0 |
| | T2a | N1 | M0 |
| | T2b | N0 | M0 |
| Stage IIB | T2b | N1 | M0 |
| | T3 | N0 | M0 |
| Stage IIIA | T1, T2 | N2 | M0 |
| | T3 | N1, N2 | M0 |
| | T4 | N0, N1 | M0 |
| Stage IIIB | T4 | N2 | M0 |
| | Any T | N3 | M0 |
| Stage IV | Any T | Any N | M1a, b |

*From Goldstraw P, Crowley J, Chansky K, Giroux DJ, Groome PA, Rami-Porta R, et al; International Association for the Study of Lung Cancer International Staging Committee; Participating Institutions. The IASLC Lung Cancer Staging Project: Proposals for the revision of the TNM stage groupings in the forthcoming (seventh) edition of the TNM classification of malignant tumors. J Thorac Oncol 2007;2:706-714. With permission.*

- ○ In the present large series, N0 or N1 disease had better survival than N2 or N3.
- ■ Value of TNM staging in SCLC:
  - ○ It is unclear what impact this would make in LD, because those with good performance status would likely still be offered multi-modality therapy
  - ○ It is unclear if more precise N designation could influence the applied radiation fields with LD (e.g., include supraclavicular regions in the treatment field)
- ■ Recommendations of the IASLC Lung Cancer Staging Project[29]:
  - ○ Incorporate TNM staging for LD, especially in trials of LD (stages I to III)
- ○ Prospective trials should evaluate the impact of nodal disease (especially N3) in LD SCLC
- ○ Prospective trials should evaluate the impact of cytology positive or negative pleural and pericardial effusions in LD SCLC

## References

 Interactive references and additional readings for this chapter can be accessed online at *expertconsult.com*.

# 22 PATHOLOGIC CLASSIFICATION OF LUNG MALIGNANCIES AND SPECIAL PATHOLOGIC PROCEDURES

Alberto M. Marchevsky, MD

## INTRODUCTION

- The lung can be the site of origin of a variety of benign and malignant neoplasms of epithelial, mesenchymal, lymphoid, and other origins.[1-4] These neoplasms are currently classified according to the very comprehensive classification scheme issued by the World Health Organization (WHO) in collaboration with the International Academy of Pathology and the International Association for the Study of Lung Cancer.[5] However, for practical purposes, the majority of lung neoplasms are malignant epithelial neoplasms comprising only four carcinoma cell types: adenocarcinomas, squamous cell carcinomas, large cell carcinomas, and small cell carcinoma (SCLC).[2-4,6] It remains controversial whether the subclassification of pulmonary carcinomas other than SCLC is of current clinical value in terms of their biologic behavior or prognosis. Indeed, squamous cell carcinoma, adenocarcinoma, and large cell carcinoma are usually aggregated together in many clinicopathologic studies under the general category of non–small cell carcinomas (NSCLC).[7-9]

- The WHO classification scheme of neuroendocrine tumors of the lung is somewhat confusing.[5] Although these neoplasms are generally considered as part of a spectrum of neoplasms ranging from low-grade malignancies such as typical carcinoid tumors, intermediate malignancies such as atypical carcinoid tumor, and high-grade neuroendocrine neoplasms such as SCLC and large cell neuroendocrine carcinoma, these neoplasms are categorized in three different subgroups: carcinoid tumor, SCLC, and large cell carcinoma. This problem is compounded by the overlap in the morphologic features of some of these neoplasms, resulting in considerable interobserver variation diagnostic problems.

## GENERAL CONCEPTS ABOUT SPECIAL PATHOLOGIC PROCEDURES FOR THE DIAGNOSIS OF LUNG NEOPLASMS

- Lung neoplasms are generally classified on the basis of their gross pathology and the histopathologic features observed with light microscopy on pathology slides stained with hematoxylin and eosin.[5] The value of histochemistry, immunohistochemistry, and electron microscopy for the diagnosis and subclassification of lung neoplasms is limited in daily clinical practice.[4] The pathologic evaluation of lung neoplasms includes a careful gross description that includes information about the tumor size and location and its relationship to adjacent structures such as the pleura and the airways.

- Microscopic examination of neoplasms requires evaluation of the growth features of the tumor under relatively low-power microscopy (e.g., 4× to 20×) and observation of the cytologic characteristics of the neoplastic cells under higher power light microscopy (e.g., 400× to 1000×). The growth features of a neoplasm are most important for the tumor classification. For example, a squamous cell carcinoma, as it will be discussed below, is diagnosed in the presence of irregular nests of tumor cells that exhibit keratinization, intracellular bridges, and other growth features; adenocarcinomas are diagnosed in the presence of neoplastic cells that grow into acini or papillary structures; and neuroendocrine neoplasms are composed of cells arranged in nests, trabeculae, pseudorosettes, and other structures. The nuclear features of cells under high-power light microscopy are generally useful to distinguish them from non-neoplastic cells. Malignant cells usually exhibit increased cellular size, hyperchromasia, macronucleoli, irregular nuclear membranes, scanty cytoplasm and high nucleo/cytoplasmic ratio (N/C ratio). The cytoplasmic characteristics of tumor cells are generally useful, in addition to the tumor growth features under low-power microscopy for classification of cell type. For example, the cells of squamous cell carcinomas generally exhibit abnormal cytoplasmic keratinization, resulting in a densely eosinophilic cytoplasm, whereas the cytoplasm of the cells of adenocarcinomas can exhibit characteristic intracytoplasmic vacuoles.

- Histochemical stains are of limited value for the diagnosis and classification of lung tumors.[2,5,10,11] Mucicarmine and diastase-PAS stains can be helpful for the distinction between poorly differentiated adenocarcinomas, which exhibit intracytoplasmic red vacuoles with both stains, from large cell carcinomas and squamous cell carcinomas. Other histochemical stains such as Grimelius and other silver stains developed for the detection of intracytoplasmic neuroendocrine granules with light microscopy, are of limited value and have been mostly replaced by modern immunohistochemical techniques.

- Immunohistochemical stains allow for the identification and localization of specific nuclear and cytoplasmic antigens in tissue sections, using detection methods such as peroxidase antiperoxidase, avidin biotin complex, and other chromogenic methods.[11,12] Positive reactivity is interpreted in the presence of brown or red intracytoplasmic or intranuclear staining. These methods are currently used for the diagnosis and subclassification of selected lung neoplasms such as SCLC, and the differential diagnosis from metastatic lesions to the lung from primary lung carcinomas.[13] For example, the cells of metastatic breast carcinomas can exhibit nuclear immunoreactivity for estrogen receptor and progesterone receptor, whereas primary adenocarcinomas of the lung generally exhibit nuclear immunoreactivity for thyroid transcription factor-I (TTF-I). Neuroendocrine lung neoplasms generally exhibit cytoplasmic immunoreactivity for synaptophysin, chromogranin, CD56 and other epitopes.[14,15]

## *PREINVASIVE LESIONS OF THE LUNG*

### Squamous Carcinoma In Situ

- Squamous cell carcinoma of the lung develops through the sequence of squamous metaplasia and dysplasia of the bronchial epithelium (Fig. 22-1).[16,17]
- Squamous dysplasia is characterized by the presence of disorganized growth within the epithelium. Dysplastic cells have altered nuclear polarity, variable nuclear size, and increased mitotic activity above the basal layer (Fig. 22-2).[4]
- The grade of dysplasia is usually classified according to the extent of the dysplastic cells within the bronchial epithelium; mild dysplasia involves only the lower third of the epithelium, moderate dysplasia involves the middle two thirds of the epithelium, and high-grade dysplasia involves the entire thickness of the epithelium.

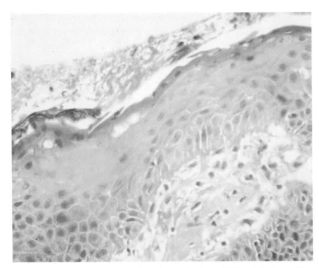

**Figure 22-1:** Squamous metaplasia of the bronchial epithelium. The normal pseudostratified columnar epithelium has been replaced by squamous epithelium with keratinization. Squamous cell carcinoma of the lung is thought to develop through the sequence of squamous cell metaplasia, dysplasia, and squamous cell carcinoma in situ (hematoxylin and eosin, 200×).

### Atypical Adenomatous Hyperplasia

- Atypical adenomatous hyperplasia (AAH) is considered a precursor of adenocarcinoma of the lung.[18-21]
- It is characterized by the presence of atypical pneumocytes with enlarged nuclei showing some hyperchromasia and focal nuclear pseudoinclusions, scanty cytoplasm with high N:C ratio and frequent hobnail features (Fig. 22-3).
- Areas of AAH are frequently small in size, usually smaller than 5 mm in diameter.
- The stroma exhibits no significant fibrosis or inflammation.
- The cells of AAH can exhibit normal genotypic expression, such as immunoreactivity for p53 protein; these immunostains are not helpful for the distinction from bronchioloalveolar carcinoma.[19,21]

### Diffuse Pulmonary Neuroendocrine Cell Hyperplasia

- Diffuse pulmonary neuroendocrine cell hyperplasia (DIPNECH) is an unusual syndrome characterized by the presence of multifocal areas of neuroendocrine cell hyperplasia within the lung. The neuroendocrine cells can present as isolated cells within the bronchiolar epithelium as neuroendocrine bodies or as small pulmonary tumorlets (Fig. 22-4).[22]
- These lesions are thought to be neoplastic precursors of carcinoid tumors and, less likely, high-grade neuroendocrine carcinomas of the lung.[3,5,23]

## *INVASIVE NEOPLASTIC LESIONS OF THE LUNG*

### Squamous Cell Carcinoma
### *Key Pathologic Features*

- Also known as epidermoid carcinoma[4]
- Malignant epithelial cells show cytoplasmic dyskeratosis, keratin pearl formation, and/or intracellular bridges

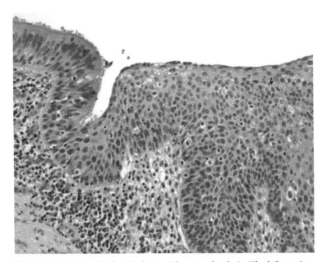

**Figure 22-2:** Bronchial epithelium with severe dysplasia. The left portion of the photomicrograph shows normal ciliated epithelium with abrupt transition to a dysplastic epithelium showing thickening of the bronchial wall and disorganized growth by atypical cells by enlarged hyperchromatic nuclei, loss of polarity and mitotic figures. This lesion is a precursor of squamous cell carcinoma (hematoxylin and eosin, 200×).

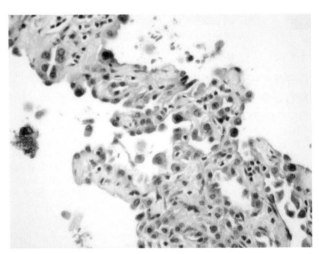

**Figure 22-3:** Atypical adenomatous hyperplasia. The lesion measured approximately 3 mm in size. It shows the presence of hyperplastic pneumocyte type II cells with hyperchromatic, enlarged nuclei with increased nuclear:cytoplasmic ratio. The degree of atypia is less severe than seen in cases with bronchioloalveolar carcinoma (hematoxylin and eosin, 200×).

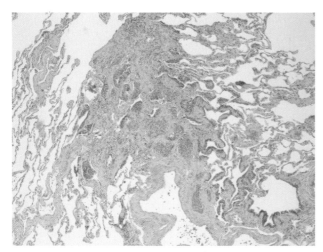

**Figure 22-4:** Carcinoid tumorlet in a patient with diffuse idiopathic neuroendocrine cell hyperplasia (DIPNECH). The lesion is composed of small nests of round cells with minimal nuclear atypia, admixed with a fibrotic stroma (hematoxylin and eosin, 40×).

## Summary of Epidemiology

- Second most common form of carcinoma of the lung.[5]
- More than 90% of squamous cell carcinomas develop in cigarette smokers.[24-29]

## Location

- The majority of squamous cell carcinomas occur as central tumors arising from a major airway (so-called bronchogenic carcinoma).
- Tumors can also develop in subsegmental bronchi or appear as peripheral lung nodules in a minority of patients.

## Gross Features

- Usually located in close proximity to a bronchus with involvement of the bronchial wall (Fig. 22-5)
- The bronchial wall can exhibit a nodular area, a plaque, a polyp, an area of ulceration, or less frequently, diffuse longitudinal involvement of the bronchial wall, resulting in extensive bronchial wall narrowing.

- The lung parenchyma adjacent to the involved bronchus shows a well-circumscribed mass with bosselated borders.
- The surface of the tumor is usually somewhat dry, friable or firm, white or gray with patchy deposition of environmental pigment deposition and variable amounts of necrosis.
- Squamous cell carcinomas can develop extensive central necrosis with cavitation, simulating a lung abscess or other cavitary lesions.

### Histopathological Features

- The tumor cells appear as cohesive sheets with irregular, infiltrating borders associated with an inflamed and fibrotic stroma (Fig. 22-6).[2,5,11]
- The individual tumor cells tend to be polygonal in shape or spindle shaped.
- They characteristically exhibit intracellular bridges that have been shown under electron microscopy to represent tight intracellular junctions (desmosomes) (Fig. 22-7).
- The cytoplasm of the tumor cells is frequently keratinized, appearing as a densely red cytoplasm (Fig. 22-8).

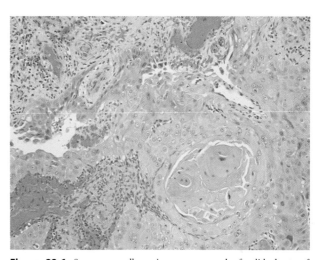

**Figure 22-6:** Squamous cell carcinoma composed of solid sheets of malignant epithelial cells with round nuclei, prominent nucleoli, slightly eosinophilic cytoplasm, and formation of a keratin pearl (hematoxylin and eosin, 100×).

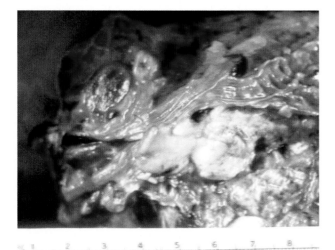

**Figure 22-5:** Squamous cell carcinoma of the lung. The lesion has a small endobronchial component and extends into the adjacent lung parenchyma.

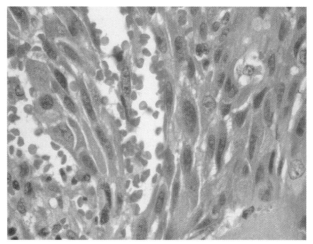

**Figure 22-7:** Squamous cell carcinoma showing the presence of intercellular bridges between the tumor cells (hematoxylin and eosin, 400×).

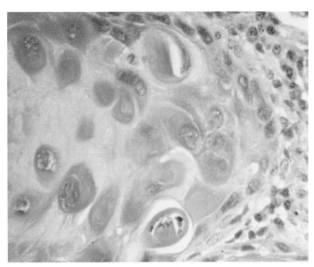

**Figure 22-8:** Squamous cell carcinoma showing the presence of dense eosinophilic cytoplasm in some of the tumor cells, indicative of abnormal keratin formation or dyskeratosis. The presence of intercellular bridges can also be seen (hematoxylin and eosin, 400×).

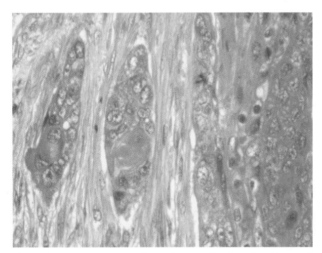

**Figure 22-9:** Squamous cell carcinoma showing keratin pearl formation and stromal invasion (hematoxylin and eosin, 200×).

- Well-differentiated squamous cell carcinomas tend to develop keratin pearls indicative of abnormal keratinization (parakeratosis) and be composed of cells with sharp cytoplasmic membranes and intercellular bridges (Fig. 22-9).
- Squamous cell carcinomas may exhibit lymphatic invasion or vascular invasion; the latter is less frequent than in adenocarcinomas.

## Cytologic Features

- Because squamous cell carcinomas usually present as central lung lesions, the yield of sputum cytology, bronchial brushings and bronchial lavage is higher than for peripheral adenocarcinomas of the lung.[29-36]
- The tumor cells appear in smears as dyscohesive sheets or as individual cells with round to spindled nuclei showing hyperchromasia, occasional prominent nucleoli, and irregular nuclear borders (Fig. 22-10).
- The cytoplasm of the tumor cells tends to have sharp cytoplasmic borders and intracytoplasmic keratinization.
- Pyknotic cells, tadpole cells, and keratin pearls can be found in keratinizing squamous cell carcinoma cases.

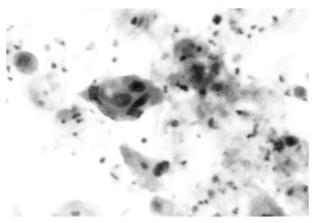

**Figure 22-10:** Sputum cytology showing malignant epithelial cells, consistent with squamous cell carcinoma. The tumor cells exhibit large hyperchromatic nuclei with irregular nuclear membranes and anisocytosis. The cytoplasm is densely red, consistent with dyskeratosis. The tumor cells exhibit increased nuclear:cytoplasmic ratio (Papanicolaou stain, 400×).

## Histochemistry and Immunohistochemistry

- Histochemistry is of limited value for the diagnosis of squamous cell carcinoma.[5,11]
- The lesions stain negative with mucicarmine and d-PAS stains, a useful finding to exclude the possibility of adenocarcinoma in poorly differentiated lesions.
- The tumor cells can exhibit cytoplasmic immunoreactivity for pan-cytokeratin, cytokeratin 5-6, and thrombomodulin and nuclear immunoreactivity for p63.
- Squamous cell carcinomas usually exhibit negative immunoreactivity for TTF-1.[37]

## Variants of Squamous Cell Carcinoma

- Squamous cell carcinomas can present as papillary, clear cell, small cell, or basaloid lesions.[5]
- *Papillary squamous cell carcinomas* usually present as exophytic papillary lesions that tend to grow mostly endobronchially with minimal extension into the peribronchial pulmonary parenchyma; these lesions usually present at a lower stage than other NSCLCs.
- *Clear cell squamous cell carcinomas* are composed mostly of clear cells and exhibit only focal areas diagnostic for squamous cell differentiation. These lesions stain negatively with mucicarmine and d-PAS stain, in contrast to adenocarcinomas with clear cells.
- The *small cell variant of squamous cell carcinoma* is difficult to distinguish from SCLC and /SCLC, combined variant with a squamous cell carcinoma component. The presence of focal nucleoli in some of the tumor cells is a feature that is unusual in small cell neuroendocrine carcinomas of the lung.
- The cells of the small cell variant of squamous cell carcinoma stain negatively with immunostains indicative of neuroendocrine differentiation (e.g., chromogranin, synaptophysin).
- The diagnosis of SCLC, combined variant, is only rendered in the presence of two distinct neoplastic components within a lesion. This diagnosis is particularly difficult to establish in small transbronchial biopsies.
- *Basaloid squamous cell carcinomas* are poorly differentiated lesions that can be difficult to distinguish from basaloid carcinoma, a variant of large cell carcinoma. The presence of keratinization in at least some of the tumor cells and intracellular

bridges is an important diagnostic feature for squamous cell carcinoma and are absent in large cell carcinoma.

## Evaluation of Tumor Grade and Stage

■ Tumor grade
  ○ Squamous cell carcinomas are usually graded as well-differentiated, moderately differentiated, and poorly differentiated lesions (grades I to III).[5,11] It is controversial whether undifferentiated lesions (grade IV) should be classified as poorly differentiated squamous cell carcinomas or simply as undifferentiated large cell carcinomas.
  ○ Grading criteria are not well specified in the WHO publication.[5] Keratinized lesions can be classified on the basis of the percentage of cells that exhibit keratinization (e.g., 0-25%, 25%-50%, 50%-75%, 75%-100%) akin to skin neoplasms, or based on their overall degree of cytologic atypia.
  ○ In our practice, squamous cell carcinomas are graded based on the subjective evaluation of cytologic atypia and relative proportions of keratinized cells within the lesions.
■ Tumor stage[38]
  ○ Important pathologic features that need to be evaluated for the stratification of patients with squamous cell carcinoma into a particular pT category include the tumor size, presence or absence of pleural invasion, and distance to the carina.[7,39,40]
  ○ Measurements of tumor size need to be based on the microscopic edges of the tumor, because squamous cell carcinomas can result in bronchial obstruction with postobstructive endogenous lipoid pneumonia. The latter can inadvertently be included in the measurements of maximum tumor diameter.[39]
  ○ The distance to the carina or the presence of the tumor in the lower bronchus is difficult to evaluate in a lobectomy specimen. This information should be provided by the surgeon at the time of specimen submission.
  ○ The criteria for pleural invasion are somewhat unclear, and some pathologists classify tumors smaller than 3 cm as pT2 in the presence of focal, partial invasion of the pleural elastic tissues as demonstrated by special stains (e.g., elastic von Gieson [EVG] stains). In contrast, other pathologists require the presence of complete involvement of the pleura by a neoplasm that reaches the visceral pleural surface. This issue needs to be clarified in the next edition of the *American Joint Commission on Cancer Staging Manual*.[38]
  ○ The evaluation of intrapulmonary, peribronchial, and mediastinal lymph nodes for the presence of metastasis is important for the classification of the pN status of a patient with squamous cell carcinoma of the lung. According to current American Joint Commission on Cancer (AJCC) guidelines, the presence of a few tumor cells within a lymph node is a result of direct tumor extension or lymphatic invasion and qualifies as a positive node.[38,39,41] According to the location of the node, it would be staged as pN1, pN2, or pN3, as discussed elsewhere in this volume. In contrast, lymph nodes from patients with breast cancer are staged as positive only in the presence of tumor deposits larger than 2 mm in size. In these patients, the presence of a few tumor cells is classified as "isolated tumor cells" and lymph node deposits measuring from 0.2 mm to 2 mm as "micrometastasis"
  ○ In a preliminary study, NSCLC patients with isolated tumor cells or micrometastases had similar prognosis to those with pN0 disease.[41]

## Pathologic Prognostic and Predictive Features

■ To my knowledge, there are no consensus prognostic and predictive features for patients with squamous cell carcinoma of the lung, other than tumor stage.[7-9,42,43]

## Key Pathologic Features for Differential Diagnoses

■ Squamous cell carcinomas need to be distinguished from large cell carcinoma of the lung, adenocarcinoma, and other tumors.[5,11]
■ The presence of individual cell keratinization and/or intracellular bridges are diagnostic features to distinguish squamous cell carcinoma from large cell carcinoma
■ Squamous cell carcinomas frequently exhibit necrosis and artifactual spaces that simulate glandular formation. These spaces are usually not lined by epithelial cells, as malignant glandular lesions are, and lack reactivity with mucicarmine and d-PAS stains.

## Adenocarcinoma
### Key Pathologic Features

■ Peripheral, subpleural tumor.[4,5,11]
■ Glandular formation, papillary formation, lepidic growth feature, mucin production in the tumor cells.

### Summary of Epidemiology

■ Adenocarcinoma is currently the most common histologic subtype of lung cancer.[2,5,11]
■ The majority of cases develop in smokers.[25,26,28]
■ Adenocarcinoma, particularly the bronchioloalveolar variant, more frequently develops in nonsmokers, particularly women, than squamous cell carcinoma and small cell carcinoma.[44-47]

### Histogenesis—Precursor Lesions

■ The histogenesis of pulmonary adenocarcinomas has been the subject of controversy. In the 1970s and 1980s, the lesions were thought to develop from pluripotential basal cells located in the bronchial epithelium.[48] Electron microscopy findings suggested that the basal cells could differentiate into a glandular, squamous, or neuroendocrine phenotype, explaining the frequent heterogeneity seen in lung carcinomas.[48]
■ The more recent literature supports the concept that adenocarcinomas probably develop from a preneoplastic lung lesion, AAH, that develops in small airways or peribronchiolar alveoli through the sequence of AAH, bronchioloalveolar carcinoma, and invasive adenocarcinoma.[18-21,23,44]
■ AAH appears as ill-distinct nodules usually measuring less than 5 mm in diameter, although they can reach a size as large as 10 mm.[5] The nodules of AAH exhibit pneumocyte type II with nuclear enlargement, hyperchromasia, nuclear pseudoinclusions resembling viral changes, focal nucleoli, increased N/C ratio, and nuclear stratification. The degree of cytologic atypia is less severe than that seen in bronchioloalveolar carcinoma.

### Location

■ The majority of pulmonary adenocarcinomas present as peripheral, subpleural lesions (Fig. 22-11).[5,11]
■ Up to 25% of primary adenocarcinomas can present as a peribronchial, more centrally located mass.
■ No consistent predilection for any particular lung lobe has been demonstrated.

### Gross Features

■ Adenocarcinomas of the lung frequently present as peripheral, pigmented lesions with frequent retraction of the overlying pleura (so-called pleural puckering) (Fig. 22-12).[4] This

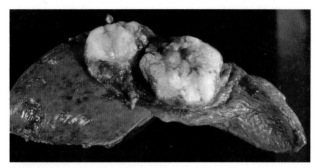

**Figure 22-11:** Peripheral adenocarcinoma of the lung showing focal central necrosis with cavity formation.

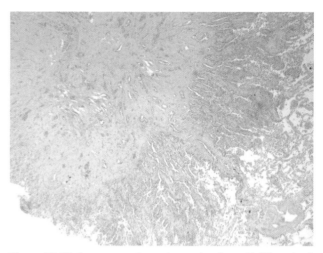

**Figure 22-13:** Low-power photomicrograph of a well-differentiated adenocarcinoma of the lung showing central scarring (hematoxylin and eosin, 20×).

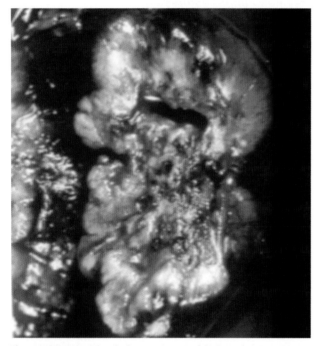

**Figure 22-12:** Peripheral adenocarcinoma of the lung showing pigmentation of the tumor surface and indentation of the pleura (so-called pleural puckering).

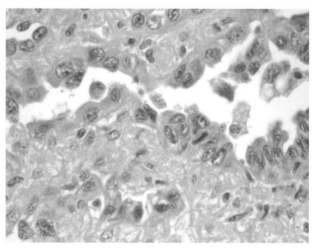

**Figure 22-14:** Adenocarcinoma of the lung showing glandular space (acinar space) lined by malignant epithelial cells with large nuclei showing hypochromasia, prominent nucleoli, irregular nuclear membranes, amphophilic cytoplasm, marked variation in tumor size and shape (anisocytosis), and high nuclear:cytoplasmic ratio (hematoxylin and eosin, 200×).

"triad" can be remembered with the use of the triple "p" acronym (peripheral, pigmented, pleural puckering). Central areas of scarring are frequently present in adenocarcinomas (Fig. 22-13).

■ Adenocarcinomas usually have bosselated, irregular infiltrating margins.

### Histopathologic Features

■ Adenocarcinomas are composed of large polygonal tumor cells with indistinct nuclear membranes and variable N/C ratio.[4]

■ The tumor cells are arranged in acinar (glandular) spaces, papillary fronds, or solid cellular sheets (Figs. 22-14 to 22-16).

■ The nuclei usually show prominent nucleoli and may exhibit nuclear pseudoinclusions that resemble "viral" changes.

■ The cytoplasm is typically vacuolated in well-differentiated adenocarcinoma, although a clear, amphophilic or even eosinophilic cytoplasm can be also noted in selected lesions (Fig. 22-17).

### Cytologic Features

■ The cells of adenocarcinoma typically present in smears and other cytologic preparations as three-dimensional cellular clusters (Fig. 22-18).[31-33,35,36]

■ The tumor cells tend to have large nucleoli and intracytoplasmic vacuoles, features that are useful for the distinction between adenocarcinoma and other forms of NSCLC.

### Histochemistry and Immunohistochemistry

■ The presence of intracytoplasmic mucin detectable with mucicarmine and d-PAS stains can be helpful to confirm the diagnosis of adenocarcinoma, particularly in poorly differentiated neoplasms that are composed mostly of solid sheets of neoplastic cells and exhibit scanty glandular and/or papillary formation.[4]

■ It remains controversial whether a poorly differentiated neoplasm that exhibits only rare cells with intracytoplasmic mucin should be classified as a large cell undifferentiated

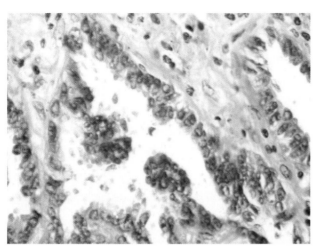

**Figure 22-15:** Adenocarcinoma of the lung showing acinar spaces and finger-like projections (papillary feature) (hematoxylin and eosin, 200×).

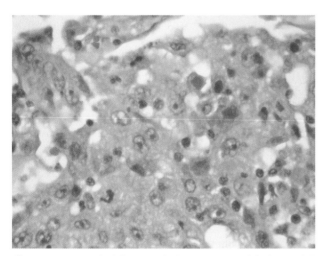

**Figure 22-16:** Poorly differentiated adenocarcinoma of the lung, solid with mucin formation variant. Tumor cells form solid sheets without clear acinar or papillary features. Mucicarmine stain of this lesion showed positive reactivity in many of the tumor cells (hematoxylin and eosin, 400×).

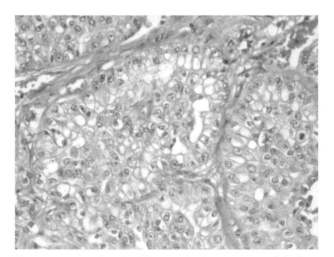

**Figure 22-17:** Moderately differentiated adenocarcinoma of the lung with solid and focal glandular features. Please note the presence of numerous cells with clear cytoplasm (hematoxylin and eosin, 200×).

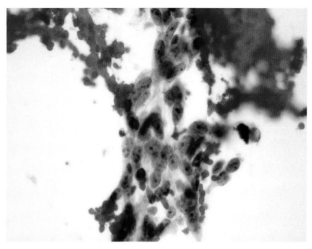

**Figure 22-18:** Fine-needle aspiration of a peripheral lung nodule showing malignant epithelial cells, which is consistent with adenocarcinoma. The tumor cells show nuclear overlap, round nuclei with hypochromasia, and prominent nucleoli, variation in tumor size and shape (anisocytosis), increased nuclear:cytoplasmic ratio, and indistinct cytoplasmic membranes (Papanicolaou stain, 400×).

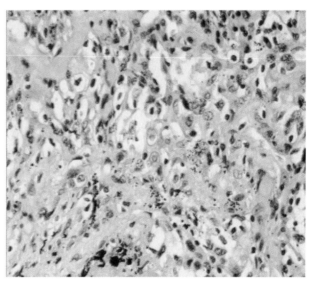

**Figure 22-19:** Large cell carcinoma of the lung showing focal mucin secretion by the tumor cells. Unless this feature is present in a substantial number of the tumor cells, this type of lesion would not be classified as an adenocarcinoma, solid variant with mucin production in our laboratory (mucicarmine stain, 200×).

carcinoma or as a poorly differentiated carcinoma (Fig. 22-19).[11] These lesions are classified in our laboratory as large cell carcinomas unless approximately 10% of the tumor cells exhibit intracytoplasmic mucin.

■ Pulmonary adenocarcinomas usually exhibit the following immunophenotype: cytokeratin 7 (Fig. 22-20), cytoplasmic immunoreactivity, focal or negative cytoplasmic immunoreactivity for cytokeratin 20, and nuclear immunoreactivity for TTF-1 (Fig. 22-21).[49-51] This immunophenotype is seen in approximately 80% of the lesions and can be helpful to confirm the pulmonary origin of an adenocarcinoma and to distinguish it from metastatic lesions (e.g., breast, pancreas, other).[49,50]

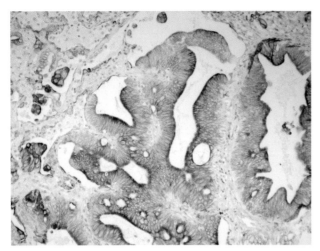

**Figure 22-20:** Adenocarcinoma of the lung showing keratin 7 immunoreactivity of the tumor cells (peroxidase antiperoxidase, 100×).

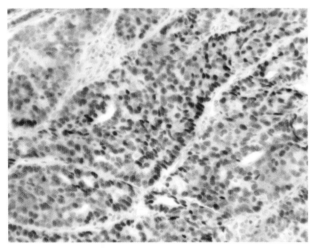

**Figure 22-21:** Adenocarcinoma of the lung showing nuclear immunoreactivity for thyroid transcription factor (TTF-1) (peroxidase antiperoxidase, 400×).

## Variants of Adenocarcinoma

- In addition to adenocarcinomas with acinar, papillary, and mixed features, the following variants of adenocarcinoma are recognized in the WHO classification: bronchioloalveolar carcinoma (BAC), mixed adenocarcinoma-BAC, solid adenocarcinoma with mucin production, fetal adenocarcinoma, mucinous (colloid) carcinoma, mucinous cystadenocarcinoma, signet-ring cell adenocarcinoma, and clear cell adenocarcinoma.[5]
- It is beyond the scope of this chapter to review the pathologic details of all these lesions. Mucinous (colloid) adenocarcinomas and signet-ring cell carcinomas of the lung are composed of cells with abundant intracytoplasmic mucin with or without a signet-ring cell configuration and the presence of abundant extracellular mucin secretion (so-called alveolar mucinosis). They can be difficult to distinguish from metastatic colloid adenocarcinomas of gastrointestinal, ovarian, or other origin; careful clinicopathologic correlation is required because mucinous adenocarcinomas of lung and other sites of origin frequently exhibit negative TTF-1 immunoreactivity and exhibit features seen in colonic adenocarcinomas, such as cytoplasmic immunoreactivity for cytokeratin 20 and nuclear

immunoreactivity for CDX-2.[52,53] The presence of cytoplasmic immunoreactivity for cytokeratin 7 is not seen in colonic adenocarcinomas but can be seen in carcinomas of lung, breast, ovary, pancreas, and other site of origin.[54-56]

## Evaluation of Tumor Grade and Stage

- Adenocarcinomas are classified as well-differentiated, moderately differentiated, and poorly differentiated lesions (grades I to III). To my knowledge, there are no well-recognized criteria for this distinction, which is based on the degree of glandular and papillary formation and cytologic atypia.[2,11]
- Other details about the pathologic staging of NSCLC are discussed in the section on squamous cell carcinoma.

## Pathologic Prognostic and Predictive Features

- It is controversial whether tumor grade predicts the prognosis of patients with lung adenocarcinomas (Figs. 22-22 to 22-24).
- The prognostic significance of lymphatic invasion is controversial (Fig. 22-25).
- Vascular invasion has been associated with a poor prognosis in these lesions.[57-59]
- Immunostains for epithelial growth factor receptor (EGFR) may be a predictor of response to anti-EGFR drugs (Fig. 22-26).[40,60]

## Key Pathologic Features for Differential Diagnoses

- The presence of glandular, papillary formation, or mucin secretion in the cytoplasm of neoplastic cells helps to distinguish pulmonary adenocarcinomas from squamous cell carcinomas, large cell carcinomas, and other NSCLC.[4]
- Immunostains and careful clinicopathologic correlation help to distinguish pulmonary adenocarcinomas from metastases.

## Bronchioloalveolar Carcinoma of the Lung
### Key Pathologic Features

- BAC is currently classified as a variant of lung adenocarcinoma.[42,44-46,61-64]

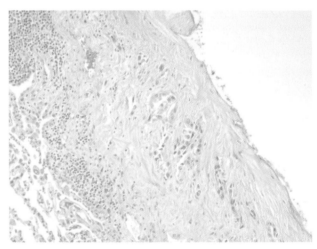

**Figure 22-22:** Evaluation of the presence of pleural invasion is an important step in the pathologic staging of lung neoplasms. Photomicrograph of an adenocarcinoma showing partial pleural invasion without reaching the pleural surface. Partial invasion of the pleura, beyond the pleural elastic lamina, is considered in our laboratory as evidence of pleural invasion. A peripheral neoplasm, smaller than 3 cm in greatest dimension, would be staged as pT2 (hematoxylin and eosin, 100×).

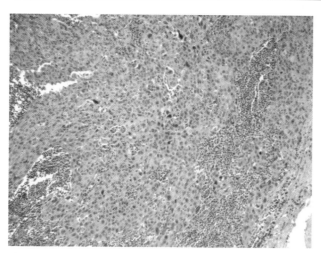

**Figure 22-23:** Evaluation of nodal status is important for the pathologic staging of patients with lung neoplasms. Paratracheal lymph node showing metastatic poorly differentiated adenocarcinoma (pN2) (hematoxylin and eosin, 100×).

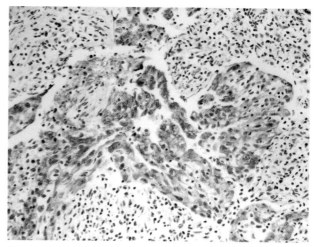

**Figure 22-26:** Adenocarcinoma of the lung showing membrane immunoreactivity of the tumor cells for epidermal growth factor receptor (EGFR) (peroxidase antiperoxidase, 100×).

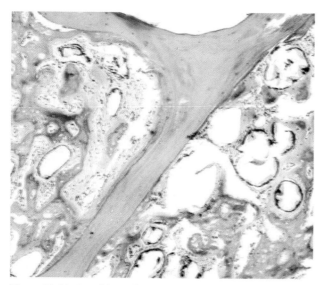

**Figure 22-24:** Bone biopsy showing metastatic adenocarcinoma (pM1) (hematoxylin and eosin, 40×).

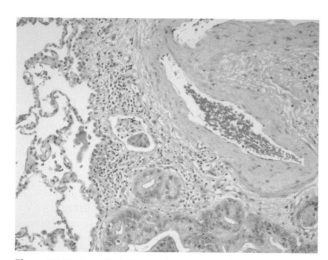

**Figure 22-25:** Lymphatic invasion in a patient with adenocarcinoma of the lung (hematoxylin and eosin, 100×).

- The diagnosis of BAC is established in the presence of lepidic growth of the tumor cells along alveolar septa with no significant alveolar fibrosis and lack of stromal invasion.

### Summary of Epidemiology
- BAC is not significantly associated with cigarette smoking.[63]
- BAC in Asian women appeared to exhibit particular genotypic changes discussed in other chapters of this book.[40,60,65]

### Histogenesis—Precursor Lesions
- BAC develops from areas of AAH.[18-21,23,44]
- The differential diagnosis between AAH and small BAC, nonmucinous type can be difficult.[5] Areas of AAH tend to exhibit smaller size (up to 10 mm in size and frequently less than 5 mm in size) and less cytologic atypia than is seen in small BAC. The interpretation of the degree of cytologic atypia is somewhat subjective and may result in diagnostic problems amongst different pathologists.

### Location
- Similar to other adenocarcinomas of the lung.

### Gross Features
- BAC, nonmucinous type appears as ill-defined gray, nodular, soft areas that blend imperceptively with the adjacent pulmonary parenchyma (Fig. 22-27).[5,11]
- BAC, mucinous type, present as more distinct gray-yellow, glistening, soft nodules that exude mucinous materials. Large BAC mucinous type can simulate pneumonia due to the presence of large areas of gray-yellow consolidation, with indistinct borders (Fig. 22-28).

### Histopathologic Features
- Nonmucinous BAC is characterized by the presence of polygonal cells with round nuclei showing prominent nucleoli and frequent nuclear pseudoinclusions.[4] The cells have increased N/C ratios with frequent hobnail changes. The latter are characterized by the presence of cells with nuclei that protrude into the alveolar lumen and a basally located cytoplasm (Fig. 22-29).
- The cells of BAC tend to show focal nuclear pseudostratification (Fig. 22-30).

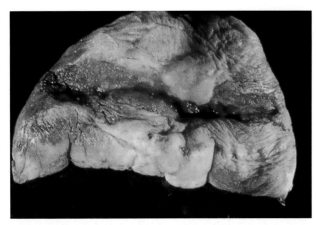

**Figure 22-27:** Small peripheral bronchioloalveolar carcinoma of the lung, nonmucinous type, presenting as an ill-defined, soft subpleural nodule.

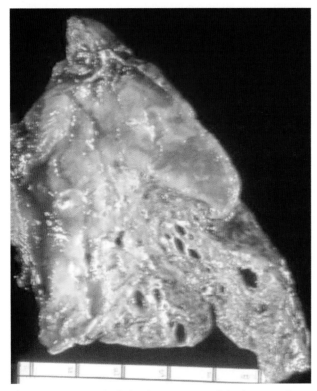

**Figure 22-28:** Bronchioloalveolar carcinoma of the lung, mucinous type presenting as an ill-defined area of gray-yellow consolidation. Please note the presence of interstitial fibrosis in the remainder of the lung. The tumor presents in a patient with usual interstitial pneumonia.

- By definition, no significant interstitial fibrosis or stromal invasion is present in BAC, nonmucinous type.
- Mucinous BAC is characterized by the presence of columnar epithelial cells with basal nuclei and tall columnar cytoplasm growing along alveolar septa in a lepidic growth pattern (Fig. 22-31). The nuclei have frequent nucleoli and occasional nuclear pseudoinclusions. The cytoplasm is abundant, clear, with intracytoplasmic vacuoles, and low N/C ratio (Fig. 22-32). The alveolar spaces adjacent to the tumor are frequently filled with abundant mucin. Mucinous BAC can be particularly difficult to distinguish from metastasis (e.g., gastrointestinal malignancies, pancreatic neoplasms, others).

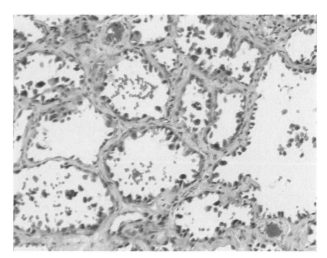

**Figure 22-29:** Bronchioloalveolar carcinoma, non-mucinous type showing the presence of polygonal tumor cells with round nuclei, hobnail features, growing along the inner surface of alveolar spaces (so-called lepidic growth feature) (hematoxylin and eosin, 100×).

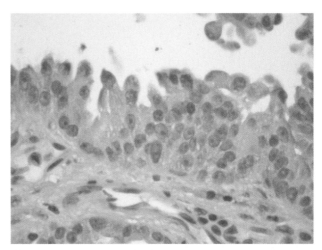

**Figure 22-30:** Bronchioloalveolar carcinoma, nonmucinous type, showing pseudostratification of the tumor cells. The tumor cells exhibit round nuclei with prominent nucleoli and mild anisocytosis (hematoxylin and eosin, 200×).

## Cytological Features

- BAC, nonmucinous type, can be particularly difficult to diagnose in cytologic samples, because the tumor cells frequently exhibit minimal atypia (Fig. 22-33).[36,66,67] The presence in fine-needle aspiration biopsies, bronchoalveolar lavage, or other cytologic samples of many monotonous pneumocytes with mild atypia can be useful to render the correct diagnosis.
- Mucinous BAC can be diagnosed in cytologic samples in the presence of large atypical epithelial cells with large nucleoli and abundant mucin secretion. These lesions cannot be distinguished on cytologic preparations from invasive adenocarcinomas.

## Histochemistry and Immunohistochemistry

- The cells of mucinous BAC exhibit abundant intracytoplasmic mucin detectable with mucicarmine stain and d-PAS stain.[63]
- The cells of nonmucinous BAC stain negative with mucicarmine stain and d-PAS stain, and exhibit the same immunophenotype as other pulmonary adenocarcinomas.

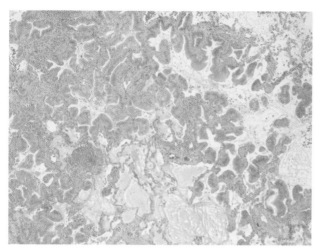

**Figure 22-31:** Bronchioloalveolar carcinoma of the lung, mucinous type, showing tumor cells growing in a lepidic pattern. Please note the presence of abundant intra-alveolar mucin (hematoxylin and eosin, 20×).

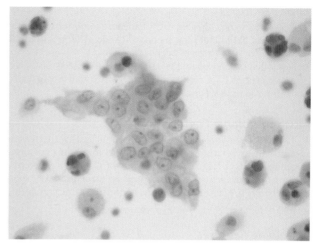

**Figure 22-33:** Fine-needle aspirate biopsy of bronchioloalveolar carcinoma of the lung, nonmucinous type. The tumor cells appear as a flat sheet of epithelial cells with slightly enlarged nuclei, prominent nucleoli, and minimal anisocytosis. These lesions can be difficult to distinguish from reactive pneumocyte hyperplasia (Papanicolaou stain, 400×).

- In contrast, the prognosis of patients with BAC, mucinous type, is usually more guarded because these lesions are frequently multiple and can metastasize.

### Key Pathologic Features for Differential Diagnoses
- BAC is distinguished from invasive adenocarcinomas by the presence of stromal invasion, characterized by the presence of tumor extension into the alveolar septa as individual cells or tumor cords, with reactive fibrosis and local remodeling of the lung architecture.[5] BAC can become secondarily inflamed, for example as a result of infection or other etiologies; in these cases the presence of tumor invasion can be particularly difficult to detect with certainty.
- Lesions with mixed features of BAC and invasive adenocarcinoma are, in our experience, more frequent than pure BAC.

## Adenosquamous Carcinoma
### Key Pathologic Features
- The tumor exhibits the presence of squamous and glandular differentiation. A second cell type needs to be present in at least 10% of the neoplasm for the lesion to be classified as adenosquamous carcinoma.[5,69-71]

### Summary of Epidemiology
- Similar to other forms of NSCLC[69-71]

### Histogenesis—Precursor Lesions
- Dysplasia of the bronchial epithelium is a precursor lesion of squamous cell carcinoma.[3,23] AAH is a precursor lesion of adenocarcinoma.[20,21,44] It is unclear which of these preneoplastic lesions precede an adenosquamous carcinoma of the lung.
- An origin of NSCLC from undifferentiated basal cells or from mucinous cells present in the bronchial epithelium has been proposed. These cells could differentiate into squamous and glandular phenotypes.

### Location
- Adenosquamous carcinomas do not have a predominant location within the lung.

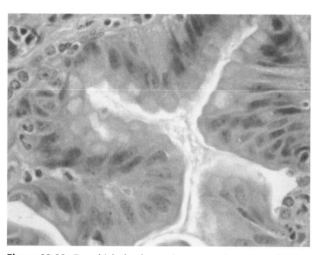

**Figure 22-32:** Bronchioloalveolar carcinoma, mucinous type, showing columnar tumor cells with intracytoplasmic mucin–containing vacuoles. Please note the presence of minimal nuclear anisocytosis (hematoxylin and eosin, 400×).

- The tumor cells of BAC, mucinous type tend to lack TTF-1 immunoreactivity. The tumor cells can exhibit cytoplasmic immunoreactivity for cytokeratin 20 and villin, features usually seen in gastrointestinal adenocarcinomas.[46,63] However, the tumor cells of primary mucinous BAC usually exhibit cytoplasmic immunoreactivity for cytokeratin 7, a feature not seen in colonic adenocarcinomas.

### Evaluation of Tumor Grade and Stage
- BAC usually exhibit low-nuclear grade (grade I) with minimal pleomorphism of the tumor cells.
- They are staged according to the AJCC guidelines for NSCLC; details about pathologic staging are discussed in the section about squamous cell carcinoma.[38,39]

### Pathologic Prognostic and Predictive Features
- BAC, nonmucinous type, is considered as an early lung neoplasm that seldom metastasizes to regional lymph nodes or to extra-pulmonary locations.[42,45,61,63,64,68]

## Gross Features

- In my experience, the majority of adenosquamous carcinomas appear as peripheral lung lesions with identical gross pathologic features to those of adenocarcinoma.[5,11]
- Less often, adenosquamous carcinomas present as bronchogenic, central lung masses that are grossly indistinguishable from a squamous cell carcinoma.

## Histopathologic Features

- The neoplasm is composed of large tumor cells with areas of intracellular keratinization, keratin pearl formation, or intercellular bridges (Fig. 22-34).[5,11] Areas of glandular differentiation exhibit acinar spaces, papillary structures, or solid sheets of neoplastic cells with abundant intracytoplasmic mucin (Fig. 22-35).

## Cytologic Features

- The cells of the squamous cell carcinoma component appear in cytologic samples in flat sheets and as individual tumor cells.[36]

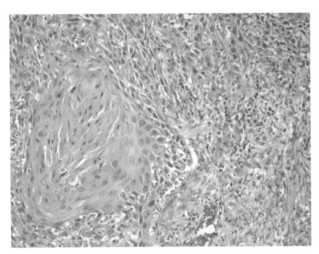

**Figure 22-34:** Adenosquamous carcinoma of the lung. The lesion shows two distinct areas of differentiation. This photomicrograph shows areas of squamous carcinoma with keratinization of the tumor cells (hematoxylin and eosin, 100×).

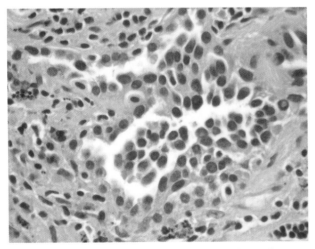

**Figure 22-35:** Adenosquamous carcinoma of the lung. The same neoplasm shown in Figure 22-34 showing areas of adenocarcinoma differentiation (hematoxylin and eosin, 200×).

They exhibit large nuclei with irregular nuclear membranes, focally prominent nucleoli, and hyperchromasia. The cytoplasm is dense, usually with distinct cytoplasmic membranes.

- Cells of the adenocarcinoma component usually present in cytologic samples in three-dimensional clusters with cellular overlap. The nuclei are frequently round, with hypochromasia, irregular chromatin distribution and prominent nucleoli. The cytoplasm frequently has indistinct cytoplasmic membranes and can be vacuolated, a feature useful for the diagnosis of glandular differentiation.

## Histochemistry and Immunohistochemistry

- Mucicarmine and d-PAS stains can be helpful to confirm the presence of adenocarcinoma differentiation in a poorly differentiated lung neoplasm that exhibits histopathologic features suggestive of dual differentiation.[5]
- The immunophenotype of adenosquamous carcinoma is similar to that of adenocarcinomas of the lung.

## Evaluation of Tumor Grade and Stage

- Please refer to the description of pathologic staging in the squamous cell carcinoma section.[39]

## Pathologic Prognostic and Predictive Features

- Tumor stage is the most important prognostic and predictive feature.[38]
- Vascular invasion has been correlated with poor prognosis.[57-59]

## Key Pathologic Features for Differential Diagnoses

- Adenosquamous carcinomas need to be distinguished from squamous cell carcinoma with focal glandular differentiation and adenocarcinomas with focal squamous differentiation.
- According to WHO guidelines, a minimum of 10% of second differentiation is needed to apply this category.[5]
- Adenosquamous carcinomas need to be distinguished from mucoepidermoid carcinomas. The presence of a central tumor with endobronchial component, presence of intermediate cells and lack of keratinization of the tumor cells are histopathologic features that favor the diagnosis of mucoepidermoid carcinoma.

## Large Cell Carcinoma
### Key Pathologic Features

- Large cell carcinoma is an undifferentiated neoplasm composed of malignant epithelial neoplasm that lacks histopathologic features of glandular, squamous, or other differentiation.[5,11]
- The definition of a large cell and distinction from a small cell is somewhat subjective. In general, tumor cells larger than the diameter of three lymphocytes are considered to be large cells.[11]

## Summary of Epidemiology

- Large cell carcinoma accounts for approximately 9% of lung neoplasms.[5]
- It predominates in smokers, and most patients are men.
- Certain variants of large cell carcinoma, such as lymphoepithelioma-like carcinoma, are not related to smoking and tend to affect younger patients. This neoplasm is particularly frequent in Asia.[5]

## Histogenesis—Precursor Lesions

- Unknown

## Location

■ Large cell carcinoma has no particular location within the lung.

## Gross Features

■ The tumor can appear as a subpleural lesion simulating an adenocarcinoma or as a centrally located lung mass more akin to a squamous cell carcinoma (Fig. 22-36). It is unusual, in my experience, for large cell carcinoma to present as an endobronchial mass.

## Histopathologic Features

■ Traditionally, large cell carcinoma of the lung was considered as a "wastebasket" category of lung neoplasms other than small cell carcinomas and was defined by the absence of diagnostic features other than the presence of solid sheets of large malignant epithelial cells.[4]

■ However, the 2004 edition of the WHO Classification of Lung Neoplasms recognizes the presence of several variants of large cell carcinoma: large cell neuroendocrine carcinoma, basaloid carcinoma, lymphoepithelioma-like carcinoma, clear cell carcinoma, and large cell carcinoma with rhabdoid phenotype (Tables 22-1 to 22-4; Fig. 22-37).[5]

■ It is beyond the scope of this chapter to describe these various unusual neoplasms in detail. Large cell neuroendocrine carcinoma are described in the section on neuroendocrine neoplasms of the lung.

## Cytologic Features

■ Large tumor cells with round nuclei exhibiting prominent nucleoli and irregular nuclear membranes, multinucleated giant cells, and high N:C ratio[36]

■ Tumor cells appear in sheets and/or individual tumor cells.

## Histochemistry and Immunohistochemistry

■ The cells of large cell carcinoma of the lung can exhibit occasional intracytoplasmic vacuoles with mucicarmine stain.[4]

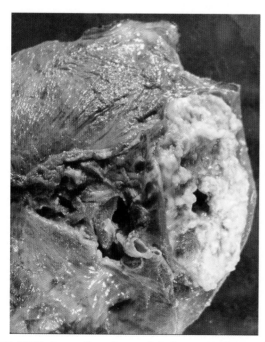

**Figure 22-36:** Large cell carcinoma of the lung presenting as a large gray-yellow lesion with extensive necrosis and central cavitation.

As discussed earlier, it remains controversial where the presence of a small number of these cells would qualify the tumor as a poorly differentiated adenocarcinoma, solid with mucin secretion variant, rather than as a large cell undifferentiated carcinoma.

■ The tumor cells exhibit a similar immunophenotype to adenocarcinomas with cytoplasmic immunoreactivity for cytokeratin 7 and variable nuclear immunoreactivity for TTF-1. Occasional tumor cells can also exhibit focal immunoreactivity for cytokeratin 20.[37,50,72]

## Evaluation of Tumor Grade and Stage

■ Please refer to the description of pathologic staging in the squamous cell carcinoma section.[39]

## Pathologic Prognostic and Predictive Features

■ Tumor stage is the most important prognostic and predictive feature.[38]

■ Vascular invasion has been correlated with poor prognosis.[57-59]

## Key Pathologic Features for Differential Diagnoses

■ Lack of glandular and papillary formation and of significant intracytoplasmic mucin in the cytoplasm of the tumor cells are features that help distinguish large cell carcinoma from adenocarcinoma.

■ Lack of intracellular keratinization, keratin pearls and intercellular bridges are features that allow for the distinction between large cell carcinoma and squamous cell carcinoma.

■ The basaloid variant of large cell carcinoma can be particularly difficult to distinguish from poorly differentiated adenocarcinomas. These neoplasms can have artifactual glandular spaces that can be confused with glandular differentiation.

■ Large cell neuroendocrine carcinomas of the lung can also have focal rosette or glandular formation in combined lesions that can be confused with adenosquamous carcinoma. The latter exhibit the presence of squamous differentiation and lack the expression in the majority of the tumor cells of immunoreactivity for neuroendocrine markers, such as chromogranin, synaptophysin, and others.

## Sarcomatoid Carcinoma
### Key Pathologic Features

■ This is a group of unusual NSCLCs that contain a component of sarcoma or sarcomatoid differentiation.[5,73,74]

■ They have been classified in the past as carcinosarcomas of the lung with homologous or heterologous elements, a terminology that is not currently recommended by the WHO experts.[5]

## Summary of Epidemiology

■ These neoplasms account for less than 1% of all lung malignancies.[74]

■ More frequent in male patients in the seventh decade of life.

■ Sarcomatoid carcinomas have been associated with cigarette smoking and/or asbestos exposure.

## Histogenesis—Precursor Lesions

■ Unknown

## Location

■ Central or peripheral tumors.

■ Some studies have suggested the predominant location to be in the upper lobes.

## TABLE 22-1 ■ MALIGNANT EPITHELIAL TUMORS

**Squamous cell carcinoma**
> Papillary
> Clear cell
> Small cell
> Basaloid

**Small cell carcinoma**
> Combined small cell carcinoma

**Adenocarcinoma**
> Adenocarcinoma, mixed subtype
> Acinar adenocarcinoma
> Papillary adenocarcinoma
> Bronchioloalveolar carcinoma
>> Nonmucinous
>> Mucinous
>> Mixed nonmucinous and mucinous or
>> indeterminate
> Solid adenocarcinoma with mucin production
> Fetal adenocarcinoma
>> Mucinous ("colloid") carcinoma
>> Signet ring adenocarcinoma
>> Clear cell adenocarcinoma

**Large cell carcinoma**
> Large cell neuroendocrine carcinoma
> Combined large cell neuroendocrine
> carcinoma
> Basaloid carcinoma
> Lymphoepithelioma-like carcinoma
> Clear cell carcinoma
> Large cell carcinoma with rhabdoid
> phenotype

**Adenosquamous carcinoma**

**Sarcomatoid carcinoma**
> Pleomorphic carcinoma spindle cell carcinoma
> Giant cell carcinoma
> Carcinosarcoma
> Pulmonary blastoma

**Carcinoid tumor**
> Typical carcinoid
> Atypical carcinoid

**Salivary gland tumors**
> Mucoepidermoid carcinoma
> Adenoid cystic carcinoma
> Epithelial-myoepithelial carcinoma

**Preinvasive lesions**
> Squamous carcinoma in situ
> Atypical adenomatous hyperplasia
> Diffuse idiopathic pulmonary neuroendocrine cell
> hyperplasia

**Mesenchymal tumors**
> Epithelioid hemangioendothelioma
> Angiosarcoma
> Pleuropulmonary blastoma
> Chondroma
> Congenital peribronchial myofibroblastic tumor
> Diffuse pulmonary lymphangiomatosis
> Inflammatory myofibroblastic tumor
> Lymphangioleiomyomatosis
> Synovial sarcoma
>> Monophasic
>> Biphasic
> Pulmonary artery sarcoma
> Pulmonary vein sarcoma

## TABLE 22-2 ■ BENIGN EPITHELIAL TUMORS

**Papillomas**
> Squamous cell papilloma
>> Exophytic
>> Inverted
> Glandular papilloma
> Mixed squamous cell and glandular papilloma

**Adenomas**
> Alveolar adenoma
> Papillary adenoma
> Adenomas of the salivary gland type
>> Mucous gland adenoma
>> Pleomorphic adenoma
>> Others
> Mucinous cystadenoma

## TABLE 22-3 ■ LYMPHOPROLIFERATIVE TUMORS

Marginal zone B-cell lymphoma of the MALT type
Diffuse large B-cell lymphoma
Lymphomatoid granulomatosis
Langerhans cell histiocytosis

### Gross Features

- Sarcomatoid carcinomas tend to present as large neoplasms with similar gross features to other NSCLC (Fig. 22-38).
- Peripheral lesions invade into the pleura and chest wall.

## TABLE 22-4 ■ MISCELLANEOUS TUMORS

Hamartomas
Sclerosing hemangioma
Clear cell tumor
Germ cell tumors
> Teratoma, mature
> Immature
> Other germ cell tumors
Intrapulmonary thymoma
Melanoma

### Histopathologic Features

- Sarcomatoid carcinomas subtypes include pleomorphic carcinoma, spindle cell carcinoma, giant cell carcinoma, carcinosarcoma, and pulmonary blastoma.[5,11,74,75]
- Pleomorphic carcinomas are composed of solid sheets of large pleomorphic tumor cells that grow in a solid, dyscohesive grow pattern. The tumor cells are polygonal, spindled, or multinucleated (Fig. 22-39). They exhibit extreme anaplasia with macronucleoli, irregular nuclear shapes, high N:C ratio, and marked anisocytosis. Necrosis and high mitotic activity are present.
- Spindle cell carcinomas are composed of spindle cells that closely resemble spindle cell sarcoma. Immunohistochemistry is usually required for the diagnosis and to distinguish these lesions from sarcomas.
- Giant cell carcinoma is a variant of sarcomatoid carcinoma characterized by the presence of numerous multinucleated malignant tumor cells (Fig. 22-40). These tumor cells have large nuclei with prominent nucleoli. Their cytoplasm

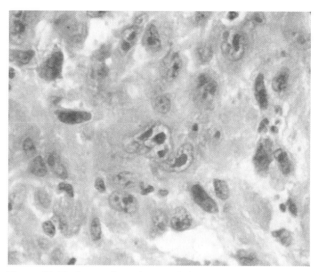

**Figure 22-37:** Large cell carcinoma of the lung composed of solid sheets of very large tumor cells with marked anisocytosis, large nucleoli, irregular nuclear shapes, and high nuclear:cytoplasmic ratio (hematoxylin and eosin, 400×).

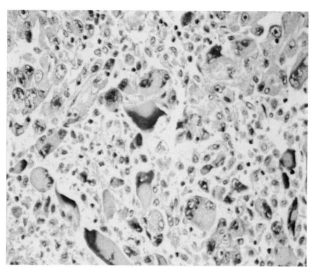

**Figure 22-40:** Giant cell variant of large cell carcinoma of the lung composed of markedly pleomorphic tumor cells with numerous malignant giant cells (hematoxylin and eosin, 100×).

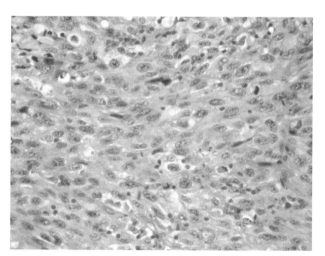

**Figure 22-38:** Sarcomatoid carcinoma of the lung presenting as a cavitary lesion as a result of extensive necrosis.

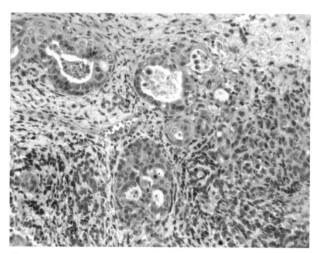

**Figure 22-41:** Carcinosarcoma of the lung composed of an adenocarcinoma with a round cell sarcoma showing rhabdosarcoma differentiation (hematoxylin and eosin, 100×).

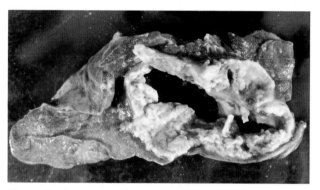

**Figure 22-39:** Sarcomatoid carcinoma of the lung composed of pleomorphic cells with elongated (spindle-shaped) nuclei, growing in solid sheets and simulating a spindle cell sarcoma. This type of lesion can be distinguished from sarcoma only with the aid of immunohistochemical stains for epithelial markers such as keratin AE1/AE3, EMA, MOC31 and others (hematoxylin and eosin, 200×).

exhibits the presence of emperipolesis, with the presence of necrotic nuclei and lymphocytes within their cytoplasm
- Carcinosarcoma and pulmonary blastomas are biphasic malignant lung neoplasms (Fig. 22-41).[75-83] Carcinosarcomas are composed of a carcinoma with squamous cell carcinoma, adenocarcinoma, or large cell carcinoma differentiation associated with a sarcoma that exhibits so-called heterologous elements such as chondrosarcoma, osteogenic sarcoma, rhabdomyosarcoma, and others (Fig. 22-42). The presence of a spindle cell sarcoma component in an undifferentiated lung neoplasm does not qualify the lesion as a true carcinosarcoma under current WHO classifications schema guidelines; such a tumor would be classified as sarcomatoid carcinoma.[5]
- Pulmonary blastomas are malignant biphasic lung neoplasms composed of fetal tissues.[79,83]

## Cytological Features
- Sarcomatoid carcinomas appear in cytologic samples as dyscohesive sheets of large, pleomorphic cells with distinct features of malignancy.[36]

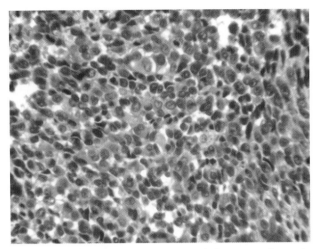

**Figure 22-42:** Rhabdomyosarcoma area of the tumor shown in Figure 22-41. The tumor cells have round hyperchromatic nuclei and eosinophilic cytoplasm with focal gross striations, not visible at this magnification (hematoxylin and eosin, 400×).

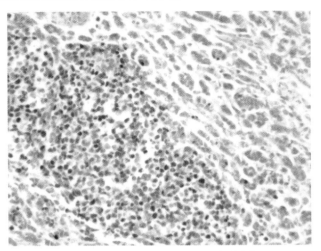

**Figure 22-44:** Carcinosarcoma of the lung with rhabdomyosarcoma features. The sarcoma cells show nuclear immunoreactivity for Myo-D1, a marker of skeletal muscle differentiation (peroxidase antiperoxidase, 200×).

- They are difficult to distinguish from other high-grade NSCLCs, unless a prominent number of malignant giant cells with emperipolesis is present, suggesting the diagnosis of giant cell carcinoma, or sarcomatous elements are present in a cytologic sample.

### Histochemistry and Immunohistochemistry

- Histochemistry is of limited value for the diagnosis of sarcomatoid carcinomas.[73]
- Immunohistochemistry is very important for the distinction between sarcomatoid carcinomas and true sarcomas of the lung.[73-75] The tumor cells of the malignant epithelial lesions usually exhibit immunoreactivity for epithelial markers such as keratin A1/3, CAM 5.2, epithelial membrane antigen (EMA), MOC-31 and other epithelial markers (Fig. 22-43). In the absence of immunoreactivity for an epithelial marker, a pleomorphic lung neoplasm is classified as a sarcoma.

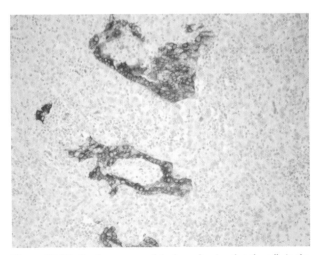

**Figure 22-43:** Carcinosarcoma of the lung showing that the cells in the epithelial area of the neoplasm show strong cytoplasmic immunoreactivity for cytokeratin 7, whereas the sarcoma cells present in between the islands of carcinoma are negative (peroxidase antiperoxidase, 100×).

- Immunostains for S-100 protein, desmin, MyoD1 and others are helpful to characterize the sarcomatous component of carcinosarcomas (Fig. 22-44).

### Evaluation of Tumor Grade and Stage

- Similar to other NSCCCs; please see the discussion in the squamous cell carcinoma section of this chapter.[39]

### Pathologic Prognostic and Predictive Features

- Pleomorphic carcinomas are highly aggressive neoplasms with a poor prognosis.[74,75]
- The neoplasms tend to metastasize via lymphatic and vascular invasion, in a manner similar to sarcomas.
- Stage and vascular invasion are pathologic prognostic and predictive factors.[39]

### Key Pathologic Features for Differential Diagnoses

- Sarcomatoid carcinomas can be difficult to distinguish from large cell carcinoma and pulmonary sarcomas.
- The distinction between a large cell carcinoma and a sarcomatoid carcinoma is based on the perception of epithelial differentiation features. The latter neoplasms usually show these cohesive tumor cells that exhibit extreme cytologic atypia.
- The distinction between sarcomatoid carcinomas and sarcomas is greatly aided by the presence of immunoreactivity for epithelial markers in the carcinomas. The presence of heterologous elements of sarcomatous differentiation such as chondrosarcoma, rhabdomyosarcoma, osteogenic sarcoma, and others would exclude the diagnosis of sarcomatoid carcinoma and favor the possibility of either pulmonary sarcoma or a carcinosarcoma.

## NEUROENDOCRINE TUMORS OF LUNG

Neuroendocrine neoplasms of the lung encompass a spectrum of neoplasms ranging in malignancy grade from low-grade to intermediate malignancy (typical and atypical carcinoid tumors) to high-grade neoplasms (small cell carcinoma, large cell neuroendocrine carcinoma).[2,5,84-88] The current WHO classification of lung neoplasms can be a bit confusing, because these neoplasms are stratified in separate categories within the classification.[5] The WHO scheme includes small cell carcinoma and carcinoid tumors as separate categories from each other and large cell neuroendocrine carcinoma as a variant of yet a third category, large cell carcinoma (see Tables 22-1 and 22-2). However, because these neoplasms are generally considered as a neoplastic spectrum at the time of pathologic diagnosis, they will be described in this chapter as a group of neoplasms ranging in malignancy from carcinoid tumorlet to small cell carcinoma and large cell neuroendocrine carcinoma.

## Carcinoid Tumorlet
### Key Pathologic Features

- Small proliferations of neuroendocrine cells measuring up to 0.5 cm in largest dimension (Fig. 22-45)[5,89]
- They tend to occur in a peribronchial/perivascular location.
- They are composed of small nests and trabeculae of neuroendocrine cells admixed with fibrotic stroma.
- Carcinoid tumorlets can be multiple in patients with DIPNECH.[22]
- Carcinoid tumorlets are generally incidental lesions of no clinical significance. They are generally considered as benign lesions, although a few examples of carcinoid tumorlets metastasizing into hilar lymph nodes have been described.[90-92]

## Carcinoid Tumor
### Key Pathologic Features

- Neuroendocrine tumors of low to intermediate malignancy composed of epithelial cells organized in growth patterns that are characteristic of neuroendocrine differentiation: organoid, trabecular, insular, palisading, ribbon, rosette-like arrangement.[56,84,93,94]
- The tumor cells usually exhibit minimal nuclear anisocytosis and cytologic atypia.
- Typical carcinoid tumors exhibit up to two mitoses in 10 high-power fields (2 mm$^2$) and no necrosis.[5]
- Atypical carcinoid tumors exhibit 2 to 10 mitoses per 10 high-power fields (2 mm$^2$) and focal, punctate areas of necrosis.[5,84,85]
- Carcinoid tumors have been classified in the lung and other locations as neuroendocrine carcinomas (grades I to II), but this terminology is not supported by the current WHO classification schema of lung neoplasms.[5]

### Summary of Epidemiology

- There is no known association between cigarette smoking and the development of carcinoid tumors, although there have been case reports and case series reporting the development of typical or atypical carcinoid tumors in smokers.[5]

### Histogenesis - Precursor Lesions

- Carcinoid tumors arise from pulmonary neuroendocrine cells, first described by Feyrter (Feyrter cells, also known as Kultchitsky's cells).[95-98]
- Normal pulmonary neuroendocrine cells appear as single cells or small cellular groups in the basal portion of the epithelium of small airways.[4] They can also occur as small cellular aggregates located adjacent to respiratory bronchioles, called neuroendocrine bodies.
- Pulmonary neuroendocrine cells can undergo hyperplasia and neoplasia.[97,98]
- Multifocal proliferation of pulmonary neuroendocrine cells has been described in the syndrome of DIPNECH.[22] This lesion is currently considered by the WHO as a precursor lesion of neuroendocrine lung neoplasms.

### Location

- Approximately 75% to 80% of carcinoid tumors are central lesions associated with a bronchus.[5,14,85] The remainder of carcinoid tumors appears as peripheral lung nodules.
- No predilection for any particular lung lobe has been described.

### Gross Features

- Central carcinoid tumors characteristically present as an endobronchial polypoid mass covered by a smooth, hemorrhagic mucosa (Fig. 22-46).[5,11]
- They can also extend into the adjacent pulmonary parenchyma.
- Central carcinoid tumors are highly vascular neoplasms that frequently bleed at the time of endobronchial biopsy.
- Central carcinoid tumors frequently cause postobstructive endogenous lipoid pneumonia that appears as ill-defined areas of yellow-tan consolidation located around the endobronchial mass. The lesions can also completely occlude a major airway resulting in secondary atelectasis.

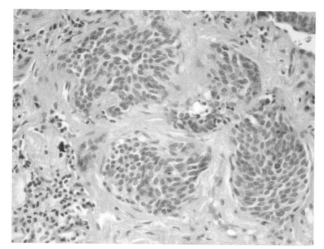

**Figure 22-45:** Carcinoid tumorlet of the lung. The lesion measured 4 mm in size and is composed of small nests of round to oval cells with minimal anisocytosis, no significant hyperchromasia, and amphophilic cytoplasm. The tumorlet nests are admixed with the fibrotic stroma (hematoxylin and eosin, 200×).

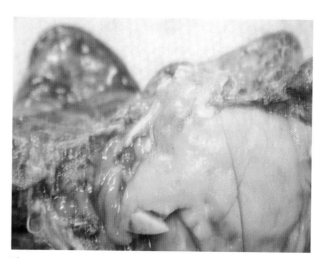

**Figure 22-46:** Central carcinoid tumor of the lung showing an enbronchial mass that is yellow-tan and homogeneous.

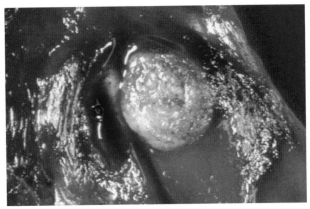

**Figure 22-47:** Peripheral carcinoid tumor of the lung presenting as a well-circumscribed round, red-yellow nodule.

- Peripheral carcinoid tumors appear as well-circumscribed, round, tan-brown nodules that do not tend to infiltrate into the pleura or be associated with pleural puckering as adenocarcinomas (Fig. 22-47).

### Histopathologic Features

- Carcinoid tumors are composed of epithelial cells arranged in various growth patterns that are characteristic for neuroendocrine differentiation (organoid, trabecular, insular, palisading, ribbon, rosette-like arrangements) (Figs. 22-48 and 22-49).[5,11] The tumor cells usually have round to oval nuclei with salt-and-pepper chromatin pattern and inconspicuous nucleoli (Fig. 22-50). The cytoplasm is frequently amphophilic, although carcinoid tumors can be composed of cells with eosinophilic granular cytoplasm resembling Hurthle cells or oncocytes.
- Peripheral carcinoid tumors are frequently composed of spindle cells that tend to be less organized than in the central lesions and can be mistaken for a mesenchymal neoplasm. However, they tend to form solid nests and trabeculae and exhibit at least focal epithelioid features.
- The stroma of carcinoid tumors is highly vascular and can exhibit secondary degenerative changes such as fibrosis, hyalinization, deposition of amyloid material or calcifications, and osseous metaplasia.
- Atypical carcinoid tumors tend to exhibit greater nuclear anisocytosis and more prominent nucleoli than typical carcinoid

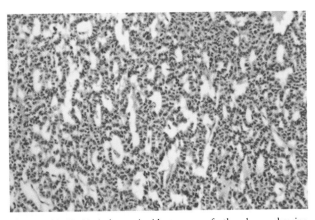

**Figure 22-48:** Typical carcinoid tumor of the lung showing arrangement of the tumor cells in trabeculae and focal solid nests. Please note the absence of nuclear anisocytosis and necrosis (hematoxylin and eosin, 40×).

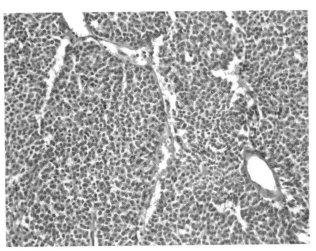

**Figure 22-49:** Typical carcinoid tumor of the lung showing tumor cells in solid nests. Please note the absence of significant nuclear anisocytosis and necrosis. This neoplasm had rare mitoses (hematoxylin and eosin, 100×).

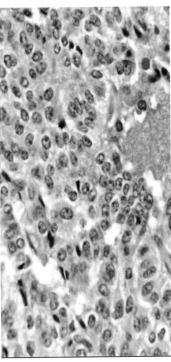

**Figure 22-50:** Typical carcinoid tumor of the lung. The tumor cells have round to slightly oval nuclei with a salt-and-pepper chromatin, inconspicuous nucleolus, and low nuclear:cytoplasmic ratio (hematoxylin and eosin, 400×).

tumors. However, cellular atypia is not a reliable feature to classify these tumors as atypical.[84]
- Typical carcinoid tumors exhibit rare mitoses; mitotic activity of up to two mitoses per 10 high-power fields is consistent with this diagnosis. Mitotic activity of 2 to 10 mitoses/10 high-power fields is consistent with a diagnosis of atypical carcinoid tumor (Fig. 22-51).[5]
- Typical carcinoid tumors lack necrosis, whereas atypical carcinoid tumors can have multifocal areas of punctate necrosis that is considerably less extensive than the necrosis seen in high-grade neuroendocrine carcinomas (Fig. 22-52).

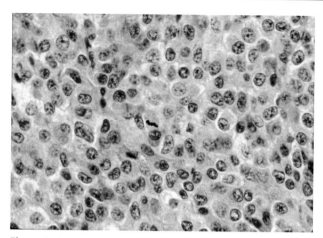

**Figure 22-51:** Typical carcinoid tumor of the lung showing cells with round nuclei and slightly eosinophilic cytoplasm (hematoxylin and eosin, 400×).

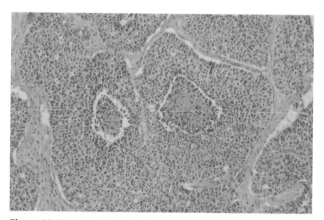

**Figure 22-52:** Atypical carcinoid tumor of the lung showing focal areas of punctate necrosis (hematoxylin and eosin, 100×).

## Cytologic Features

- Cellular samples exhibiting dyscohesive groups of uniform cells with round nuclei, amphophilic or eosinophilic cytoplasm and low N/C ratio. The nuclei are round to oval nuclei with salt-and-pepper chromatin pattern and inconspicuous nucleoli.[36]
- It is probably not reliable to classify typical carcinoid tumors from atypical carcinoid tumors based on cytologic features, because the degree of atypia is not a reliable indicator. The presence of necrosis or of multiple mitoses in a cytologic sample is inconsistent with the diagnosis of typical carcinoid tumor.

## Diagnostic Pitfalls in the Diagnosis of Carcinoid Tumors in Small Biopsies

- Typical and atypical carcinoid tumors can present as neoplasms composed of hyperchromatic small round cells with inconspicuous cytoplasm that can be mistaken for a small cell carcinoma of the lung in a small transbronchial biopsy or needle biopsy.[99,100]
- The presence of necrosis and mitosis is necessary to render a diagnosis of a high-grade neuroendocrine neoplasm such as small cell carcinoma, and in their absence, pathologists should be cautious not to overdiagnose carcinoid tumors as a high-grade neuroendocrine carcinoma.

## Histochemistry and Immunohistochemistry

- Argyrophil and srgentaffin histochemical stains (e.g., Grimelius, Pascal, Fontana, and others) have been used in the past to confirm the diagnosis of carcinoid tumor. These silver stains demonstrate the presence of black granules in the cytoplasm of the tumor cells.[4] They have been currently replaced by more sensitive and specific immunostains.
- Immunohistochemistry can be very valuable to confirm the diagnosis of a neuroendocrine lesion. The tumor cells exhibit cytoplasmic immunoreactivity for synaptophysin, chromogranin, neuron specific enolase, CD56, and other less frequently used neuroendocrine epitopes (Fig. 22-53).[5,54,94]
- Chromogranin and synaptophysin are the most widely used neuroendocrine markers in our laboratory.
- Immunostains for Ki-67, a proliferation marker, are also helpful for the classification of neuroendocrine pulmonary neoplasms. Typical carcinoid tumors exhibit low proliferative activity. Ki-67 stains a minority of the tumor cells of typical carcinoid tumor; atypical carcinoid tumors usually result in nuclear immunoreactivity of 15% to 20% of the tumor cells, whereas high-grade neuroendocrine neoplasms exhibit high proliferative activity in the majority of the tumor cells.[101-104]

## Evaluation of Tumor Grade and Stage

- No current grading system for carcinoid tumors is accepted by the *American Joint Committee on Cancer Staging Manual*.[38]
- Carcinoid tumors are staged in a similar manner to NSCLC. Please refer to the discussion in the squamous cell carcinoma section of this chapter.[39]

## Pathologic Prognostic and Predictive Features

- The classification of carcinoid tumors into typical and atypical has prognostic value.
- Typical carcinoid tumors are low-grade malignancies with approximately 90% 5-year survival rates and 80% 10-year survival rates.[5,84]
- Patients with atypical carcinoid tumors have approximately 60% to 80% 5-year survival rates and 50% 10-year survival rates.

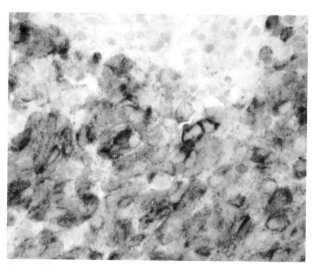

**Figure 22-53:** Carcinoid tumor of the lung showing cells with intense cytoplasmic immunoreactivity for chromogranin (peroxidase antiperoxidase, 400×).

### Key Pathologic Features for Differential Diagnoses

- Carcinoid tumors can be distinguished from high-grade neuroendocrine carcinomas by the presence in the latter group of neoplasms of greater than 10 mitoses/10 high-power fields and extensive areas of necrosis.
- Nuclear immunoreactivity in the majority of the tumor cells with antibodies to Ki-67 excludes the diagnosis of a carcinoid tumor.
- Metastatic breast carcinomas to the lung can closely simulate a carcinoid tumor.[13,91] The cells of these metastatic lesions exhibit greater nuclear pleomorphism and lack the characteristic salt-and-pepper features of the neuroendocrine lesions. Metastatic breast lesions also may have greater numbers of mitoses than expected in a carcinoid tumor. Immunohistochemistry can be helpful for this differential diagnosis; for example, carcinoid tumors would be expected to exhibit cytoplasmic immunoreactivity for chromogranin and synaptophysin, whereas metastatic breast cancers may exhibit nuclear immunoreactivity for estrogen receptor and cytoplasmic immunoreactivity for gross cystic disease protein 15.

## HIGH-GRADE NEUROENDOCRINE CARCINOMAS OF THE LUNG

- This group of neoplasms includes small cell carcinoma and large cell neuroendocrine carcinoma.[5] As explained earlier, these two neoplasms are categorized as separate neoplasms in the WHO scheme (see Table 22-1), although they are components of a spectrum of neoplasms that frequently exhibit overlapping histopathologic features. Indeed, studies of high-grade neuroendocrine carcinomas of the lung with morphometry and by multiple experts analyzing the frequency of interobserver variability have shown that approximately one third of these neoplasms can be classified as either small cell carcinoma or large cell carcinomas by different pathologists.[85,87]

### Small Cell Carcinoma
#### Key Pathologic Features

- Malignant epithelial cells have small round to oval nuclei which are markedly hyperchromatic and lack nucleoli. The cells have scanty cytoplasm with high N:C ratio.[4,88] As suggested in The Armed Forces Institute of Pathology textbook entitled *Tumors of the Lower Respiratory Tract*, the use of an arbitrary size of three lymphocytes diameters to distinguish small from large cells.[11]

### Summary of Epidemiology

- Small cell carcinoma encompass approximately 10% to 15% of lung neoplasms.[86,88,105,106]
- The majority of these neoplasms develop in cigarette smokers.[107]

### Location

- The majority of small cell carcinomas occur as central tumors arising from a major airway (bronchogenic carcinoma)
- The neoplasms can be difficult to identify on imaging studies because the primary lesions can be small in patients, with widespread metastasis at the time of initial diagnosis

### Gross Features

- Usually located in close proximity to a bronchus with involvement of the bronchial wall

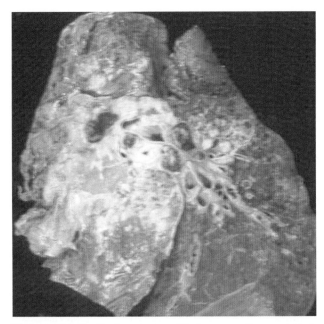

**Figure 22-54:** Small cell carcinoma of the lung presenting as a central, wide, soft peribronchial lesion extending to peribronchial lymph nodes. Please note the presence of tumor in different lobes (pM1 lesions).

- The bronchial wall characteristically exhibits diffuse thickening with narrowing of the bronchial lumen (Fig. 22-54).
- The tumors appear grossly as ill-circumscribed gray friable neoplasms with extensive necrosis
- They frequently involve multiple peribronchial and mediastinal lymph nodes at diagnosis.

### Histopathologic Features

- The tumor cells appear in cohesive sheets forming nests, trabeculae, festoons, pseudorosettes and other features of neuroendocrine differentiation.[88,105]
- The tumor cells have small round to oval hyperchromatic nuclei with a salt-and-pepper chromatin pattern (Fig. 22-55).

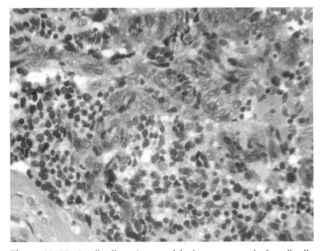

**Figure 22-55:** Small cell carcinoma of the lung composed of small cells arranged in trabeculae. The tumor cells have hyperchromatic nuclei with salt-and-pepper chromatin pattern. Please note that the tumor cells are 2 to 3 times the size of adjacent lymphocytes, seen in the lower portion of the photomicrograph (hematoxylin and eosin, 200×).

- The cytoplasm is inconspicuous, resulting in a very high N:C ratio.
- The tumor cells are usually twice or three times the size of mature lymphocytes.
- The tumor cells frequently exhibit a spectrum of nuclear sizes, with some cells larger than three lymphocytes in diameter; these tumors with intermediate morphology can be particularly difficult to categorize with certainty.
- The cells of small cell carcinomas usually lack prominent nucleoli. The presence of this feature should raise concern about this diagnosis.
- The tumor cells are friable and the tumors frequently exhibit crush artifact on biopsy materials, because they easily crumble under the pressure of biopsy instruments (Fig. 22-56).
- Mitoses are frequent, usually more than 20 to 30 mitoses/10 high-power fields.
- Necrosis is usually extensive in small cell carcinomas.

## Cytologic Features

- The tumor cells appear in cohesive sheets with frequent crush artifact.[36]
- Necrosis and dyscohesive cells are frequently present.
- Individual tumor cells show the cytologic features described earlier.

## Histochemistry and Immunohistochemistry

- Cells of small cell carcinoma seldom stain with argyrophilic (e.g., Grimelius stain) and argentaffinic (e.g., Fontana) stains used in the past for the diagnosis of neuroendocrine carcinomas.
- Immunohistochemistry is very useful for the diagnosis of small cell carcinoma.[49,86,108,109] Although the WHO classification schema does not require the use of immunohistochemistry for the diagnosis of small cell carcinoma, it is our practice to confirm this diagnosis routinely with the use of immunostains for keratin to confirm the epithelial nature of the tumor (e.g., keratin AE1/AE3, CAM 5.2), leukocyte common antigen (CD45) to exclude the possibility of a malignant lymphoma, and synaptophysin and chromogranin to confirm the neuroendocrine nature of the tumor (Fig. 22-57).[5]
- Immunostains for TTF-1 are very often positive.
- Rarely small cell carcinomas can stain negatively with all these antibodies, and epithelial markers such as MOC-31 can be helpful to confirm the epithelial nature of the neoplasm.

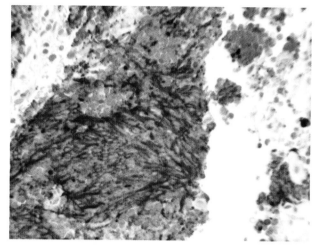

**Figure 22-57:** Small cell carcinoma of the lung showing strong immunoreactivity of the tumor cells for synaptophysin (peroxidase antiperoxidase, 200×).

- In small biopsies, small cell carcinomas can be difficult to distinguish from carcinoid tumors, particularly in lesions that lack necrosis or visible necrotic figures. The use of proliferation markers such as Ki-67 (MIB-1) can be helpful, because almost 100% of the cells of small cell carcinomas exhibit nuclear immunoreactivity with this marker (Fig. 22-58).[109]

## Variants of Small Cell Carcinoma

- Small cell carcinomas can present with areas of squamous cell carcinoma, large cell carcinoma, or adenocarcinoma differentiation. These lesions are currently classified as small cell carcinoma, combined variant.[5]
- Rare tumors exhibit all areas of differentiation (small cell, squamous, adenocarcinoma) and have been classified in the past as lesions with tripartite differentiation.[110,111]
- It has been suggested that patients with small cell carcinoma, combined variant, have a worse prognosis than those with pure small cell carcinoma.[86]

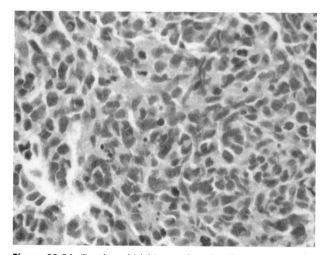

**Figure 22-56:** Transbronchial biopsy of small cell carcinoma of the lung. The tumor cells show marked crush artifact. Please note the presence of some viable tumor cells and mitoses (hematoxylin and eosin, 400×).

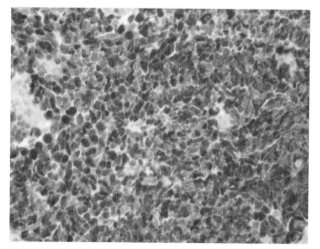

**Figure 22-58:** Small cell carcinoma of the lung showing that almost all tumor cells exhibit nuclear immunoreactivity for Ki-67 (Mib-1). This feature is seen in high-grade neuroendocrine carcinomas of the lung and can be helpful to differentiate these neoplasms from carcinoid tumors in small biopsy samples (peroxidase antiperoxidase, 400×).

### Evaluation of Tumor Grade and Stage

- There is no current grading system for small cell carcinomas.
- The distinction in the past between oat cell carcinoma and carcinomas of intermediate differentiation is no longer in use. Older literature has suggested that patients with small cell carcinomas of the intermediate variant had a slightly worse prognosis than those with oat cell carcinoma, but these differences have not been validated.
- Patients with small cell carcinomas can be staged using the same AJCC criteria developed for non-small cell carcinoma of the lung.[38]
- However, the classification of patients with small cell carcinoma into localized and diffuse disease is more widely used in clinical practice.[112] Patients with localized small cell carcinomas have the disease confined to the chest, whereas those with diffuse small cell carcinomas present with multiple extrathoracic metastases.

### Pathologic Prognostic and Predictive Features

- There are no consensus pathologic prognostic and predictive features for patients with small cell carcinoma of the lung other than tumor stage.[5]

### Key Pathologic Features for Differential Diagnoses

- Small carcinoma of the lung needs to be distinguished from the small cell variant of squamous cell carcinoma, malignant lymphoma, Ewing's sarcoma/peripheral neuroendocrine tumor (PNET), and, less frequently, from other neoplasms composed of small cells with hyperchromatic nuclei and scanty cytoplasm.[5,11]
- Squamous cell carcinoma, small cell variant, usually includes the presence of cells with cytoplasmic keratinization and focal areas with epithelial cell exhibiting intercellular bridges, keratin pearls, or other features of squamous differentiation. The presence of nucleoli in the tumor cells is also seen more frequently in squamous cell carcinomas than in small cell carcinomas. Squamous cell carcinoma, small cell variant, can be particularly difficult to distinguish from small cell carcinomas, combined variant. The latter neoplasms exhibit two distinct areas of differentiation and the neuroendocrine component, as confirmed by immunohistochemistry.
- Malignant lymphomas are usually composed of cells that are more dyscohesive than seen in small cell carcinoma. The chromatin pattern of the cells of malignant lymphomas tend to be more granular than that of small cell carcinomas, and the lymphoid cells usually present more irregular nuclear membranes than seen in epithelial malignancy. The use of lymphoid markers such as CD45, light chains, and markers for B-cell and T-cell differentiation can be helpful to distinguish these lesions.
- Relatively infrequent cases of Ewing's sarcoma/PNET can be confused for small cell carcinomas. Both neoplasms are high-grade malignancies with necrosis and high mitotic activity. Ewing's sarcoma/PNET tends to occur in younger patients than those with small cell carcinoma. Immunohistochemistry is also helpful as the lesions of the sarcoma usually lack keratin immunoreactivity and exhibit immunoreactivity for CD99.

### Large Cell Neuroendocrine Carcinoma
#### Key Pathologic Features

- Tumor can present in any location within the lung and is composed of solid sheets of large cells with histopathologic features of neuroendocrine differentiation.[113]

- Tumor cells are usually larger than three lymphocytes in diameter.[5,85] The tumor cells exhibit focal nucleoli and slightly more abundant cytoplasm than seen in cases of small cell carcinoma.

### Summary of Epidemiology

- Large cell neuroendocrine carcinoma of the lung is an unusual neoplasm that represents less than 1% of lung neoplasms.[5]
- The majority of cases have been described in cigarette smokers.

### Histogenesis—Precursor Lesions

- It is unclear whether large cell neuroendocrine carcinoma arises from Kulchitsky's cells or from undifferentiated basal cells in the bronchial epithelium, as other NSCLCs.[5]

### Location

- Large cell neuroendocrine carcinomas of the lung have no particular predilection for any area of the lung.

### Gross Features

- Ill-circumscribed gray, soft tumors with extensive necrosis.

### Histopathologic Features

- Large cell neuroendocrine carcinomas are composed of large cells with round to oval hyperchromatic nuclei with salt-and-pepper chromatin pattern and small to prominent nucleoli (Fig. 22-59).[88]
- The tumor cells have scanty to moderate amount of cytoplasm with high N:C ratio.
- The tumor cells are arranged, at least in focal areas, in nests, trabeculae or pseudorosettes, features indicative of neuroendocrine differentiation.

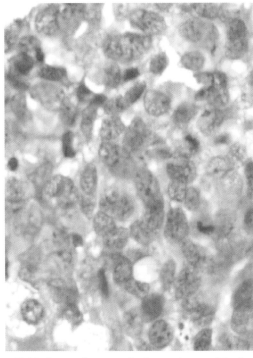

**Figure 22-59:** Large cell neuroendocrine carcinoma of the lung. The tumor cells are large, hyperchromatic with salt-and-pepper chromatin pattern and high nuclear:cytoplasmic ratio. Please note the presence of several mitotic figures, characteristic of high-grade neuroendocrine carcinomas (hematoxylin and eosin, 600×).

### Cytologic Features

- The tumor cells present in cytologic preparations as flat sheets of large cells with the features described earlier.[36]
- Frequent necrosis and high mitotic activity are present.

### Histochemistry and Immunohistochemistry

- Large cell neuroendocrine carcinomas have similar phenotypes with histochemical stains and immunostains as described for small cell carcinoma.
- Immunostains are not helpful to distinguish small cell carcinomas from large cell neuroendocrine carcinomas.
- Large cell neuroendocrine carcinomas exhibit high proliferative activity with immunostains for Ki-67.[104]

### Variants of Large Cell Neuroendocrine Carcinoma

- Large cell carcinomas can be combined with squamous cell carcinoma and adenocarcinoma components.[5]

### Evaluation of Tumor Grade and Stage

- No grading system is available for large cell neuroendocrine carcinoma, and these neoplasms are considered as high grade lesions.
- Patients with large cell neuroendocrine carcinoma are staged according to AJCC guidelines.[38]

### Pathologic Prognostic and Predictive Features

- It is controversial whether patients with large cell neuroendocrine carcinoma have a worse prognosis than patients with other forms of non–small cell carcinomas of the lung.[113-115]
- Several publications have suggested that these neoplasms have an aggressive biologic behavior, even when detected at stage I.[114]

### Key Pathologic Features for Differential Diagnoses

- Large cell neuroendocrine carcinomas need to be distinguished from small cell carcinomas by the presence of larger cells with occasional nucleoli and lower N:C ratio.
- These neoplasms also need to be distinguished from undifferentiated large cell carcinomas of the lung with focal cells exhibiting immunoreactivity for chromogranin, synaptophysin, or other neuroendocrine markers (so-called non–small cell carcinoma-neuroendocrine). The presence of histopathologic features of neuroendocrine differentiation, seen on hematoxylin and eosin-stained sections is needed for the diagnosis of large cell neuroendocrine carcinoma in addition to immunostains.[5]

## SALIVARY GLAND TUMORS

Salivary gland tumors comprise less than 5% of all lung neoplasms.[5,11] They include mucoepidermoid carcinoma, adenocystic carcinoma, and other less frequent neoplasms such as acinic cell tumor, epithelial-myoepithelial carcinoma, oncocytoma, and others. It is beyond the scope of this chapter to describe these neoplasms in detail.

## Mucoepidermoid Carcinoma
### Key Pathologic Features

- Central (bronchogenic) neoplasms[116,117]
- Usually present with a polypoid bronchial mass (Fig. 22-60)
- Tumors are composed of glandular cells, intermediate cells, and cells with squamous differentiation.
- Neoplasms lack the presence of frank keratinization and/or keratin pearls.

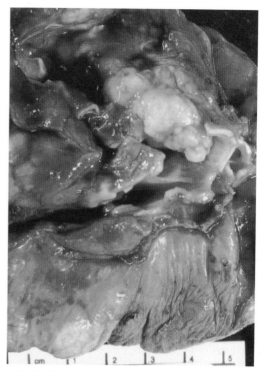

**Figure 22-60:** Mucoepidermoid carcinoma of the lung presenting as a yellow, soft endobronchial lesion.

### Summary of Epidemiology

- Mucoepidermoid carcinomas are not associated with cigarette smoking.[5,11]
- They occur in patients in their fourth to eight decades, with no sex prevalence.

### Histogenesis—Precursor Lesions

- They arise from bronchial glands.
- No precursor lesion has been described.

### Gross Features

- Endobronchial polypoid tumors (see Fig. 22-60)

### Histopathologic Features

- The tumors can be divided into low-grade and high-grade neoplasms.[11]
- Low-grade mucoepidermoid carcinomas frequently have cystic changes with focal solid areas
- The cystic changes are lined by mucin-secreting cells forming small glands and tubules admixed with intermediate cells and squamoid cells (Fig. 22-61)
- The tumor cells exhibit minimal cytologic atypia and have abundant eosinophilic, mucin-rich cytoplasm and round to oval nuclei with inconspicuous nucleoli.
- Admixed with mucinous epithelium are non-keratinizing epithelial cells with squamous differentiation, forming solid sheets.
- Focal intercellular bridges are present.
- The stroma has foci of dense fibrosis and hyalinization that may simulate amyloid deposition.
- High-grade mucoepidermoid carcinomas are unusual neoplasms that can be difficult to distinguish from adenosquamous carcinomas.
- They exhibit a combination of mucinous cells, squamoid cells with marked nuclear atypia.

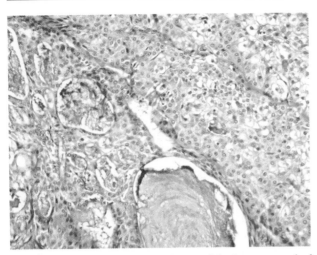

**Figure 22-61:** Mucoepidermoid carcinoma of the lung composed of mucin-secreting cells and intermediate cells. Please note the absence of significant nuclear pleomorphism (hematoxylin and eosin, 100×).

### Histochemistry and Immunohistochemistry

- Mucicarmine stain and d-PAS stains are helpful to confirm the presence of cells with glandular features in high-grade mucoepidermoid carcinomas.
- Immunostains are not helpful in the diagnosis of these neoplasms.
- The tumor cells exhibit negative immunoreactivity for TTF-1.

### Evaluation of Tumor Grade and Stage

- Mucoepidermoid carcinomas are staged according to the AJCC staging rules for non–small cell carcinomas of the lung.[38]
- The evaluation of tumor grade has been controversial, with some studies proposing the subclassification of mucoepidermoid carcinomas into low-grade, intermediate grade, and high-grade lesions, whereas others favor a two-grade system.[5]
- The WHO favors the separation of these tumors into only two categories: low-grade and high-grade neoplasms.

### Key Pathologic Features for Differential Diagnoses

- Low-grade mucoepidermoid carcinomas need to be distinguished from bronchial adenomas. Bronchial adenomas are rare benign bronchial neoplasms composed of glandular elements. They lack the presence of intermediate cells with squamous differentiation, characteristic of low-grade mucoepidermoid carcinoma.
- High-grade mucoepidermoid carcinomas can be difficult to distinguish from adenosquamous carcinoma.[5,11] The presence of a central lesion with an endobronchial component and the lack of keratinization in the tumor cells are features that favor the diagnosis of mucoepidermoid carcinoma.

## Adenoid Cystic Carcinoma
### Key Pathologic Features

- Malignant epithelial neoplasm with characteristic histologic growth patterns of the tumor cells including cribriform, tubular and glandular arrays associated with hyalinized basement membrane-rich extracellular matrix[5,11,118]

### Summary of Epidemiology

- Adenoid cystic carcinomas comprise less than 1% of lung neoplasms.[118]
- Equal sex distribution

- More frequent in the fourth and fifth decades of life
- No association with cigarette smoking or other risk factors

### Histogenesis - Precursor Lesions
- No preneoplastic lesions
- Origin in bronchial glands

### Location
- Adenoid cystic carcinomas of the lower respiratory tract are more frequent in the trachea than in the lungs
- Intrapulmonary lesions usually involve major bronchi

### Gross Features
- Tumors grow along the bronchial submucosal area, producing a cylindrical narrowing of the bronchial lumen.[11]
- Polypoid component of the tumor can be present.

### Histopathologic Features
- Adenoid cystic carcinomas grow along the bronchial wall, frequently without disturbing the overlying bronchial epithelium.[5,11]
- The latter feature can be misleading to thoracic surgeons, who may not be able to visualize the tumor grossly at the time of resection.
- The tumor cells are organized in characteristic cribriform patterns or cylindromatous pattern forming cellular trabeculae surrounded by hyalinized stroma, tubules and solid nests (Fig. 22-62).
- The tumor cells are small with scant cytoplasm and dark hyperchromatic nuclei.
- Mitotic figures are infrequent.
- Cribriform areas frequently contain central basophilic material that simulates glandular contents; however, this material has been recognized by electron microscopy to represent basement membrane material.
- The epithelial cells are associated with myoepithelial cells.

### Histochemistry and Immunohistochemistry
- Histochemistry is of limited value for the diagnosis of adenoid cystic carcinoma.
- Epithelial cells exhibit cytoplasmic immunoreactivity for keratin.
- Myoepithelial cells can also exhibit vimentin, smooth muscle actin, S100 protein, and calponin immunoreactivity.[5]

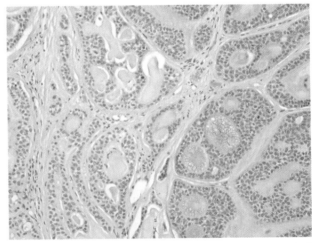

**Figure 22-62:** Adenocystic carcinoma of the lung showing the typical arrangement of the tumor cells in a cribriform pattern (hematoxylin and eosin, 100×).

### Evaluation of Tumor Grade and Stage

- Adenoid cystic carcinomas are staged according to the AJCC guidelines for non–small cell lung neoplasms.[38]
- No grading system has been developed for adenoid cystic carcinomas.
- The lesions tend to behave in an aggressive manner with frequent local recurrences, in spite of their bland cytologic features.[118]

### Key Pathologic Features for Differential Diagnoses

- Adenoid cystic carcinomas can be mistaken for mucoepidermoid carcinomas, the latter contain mucin-secreting cells that are not characteristic of adenoid cystic carcinoma.

- Adenoid cystic carcinomas can be mistaken in small biopsies for small cell carcinomas.[5] The cells of the salivary gland tumor lack neuroendocrine differentiation, necrosis, and high mitotic activity, all features characteristic of small cell carcinoma.

## References

 Interactive references and additional readings for this chapter can be accessed online at *expertconsult.com*.

# 23 SURGICAL MANAGEMENT OF NON–SMALL CELL LUNG CANCER

Robert J. McKenna Jr., MD and Ali Mahtabifard, MD

Although there have been great strides in the biologic understanding of lung cancer, new chemotherapy agents, and new radiation modalities, such as Cyberknife, surgery remains the mainstay of treatment for non–small cell lung cancer (NSCLC). Current major issues for thoracic surgery include minimally invasive surgery for the lung and surgery after multimodality treatment.

## TERMINOLOGY

- **VATS** (video-assisted thoracoscopic surgery): thoracic surgery through small incisions without spreading the ribs.
- **Thoracotomy:** thoracic surgery through a larger incision with rib spreading.
- **Muscle-sparing thoracotomy:** thoracic surgery with rib spreading but without cutting major chest wall muscles (latissimus dorsi or serratus anterior).
- **Wedge resection:** nonanatomic resection of lung tissue (less than a lobectomy)
- **Lobectomy:** anatomic resection of a lobe of the lung
- **Sleeve resection:** anatomic resection of a segment, lobe, or lung with transection and reconstruction of the bronchus or artery, or both.

## EPIDEMIOLOGY

- In the United States, lung cancer is the leading cause of cancer death in both men and women. The rise and, more recently, the decline in the incidence and mortality rate of lung cancer have paralleled the increase and decrease in smoking.[1]
- Tobacco is the world's leading cause of preventable death.[2]
- Lung cancer mortality rates among Hispanics, Native Americans, and Asians/Pacific Islanders are significantly lower than the rates among blacks and non-Hispanic whites.[3]
- Worldwide, lung cancer is the most commonly diagnosed cancer, but there is a wide geographic variation.[3] It is most common in North America and Europe, whereas it is much less common in South America and Africa.

- Women appear to have a higher risk of developing lung cancer and a greater susceptibility to the effects of smoking.
- The National Research Council reports that approximately 15,000 to 20,000 lung cancer deaths per year in the United States are caused by radon.[4]
- Doll and Peto,[5] in their 1981 review of the causes of cancer, estimated that perhaps 1% to 2% of lung cancer cases were related to air pollution.

## Pathogenesis

- In the United States, smoking roughly accounts for 87% of lung cancer cases (90% in men and 79% in women). The remaining cases are due to occupational exposures, radon causes,[6] and outdoor air pollution (perhaps 1% to 2% of lung cancer cases).[7] The impact of nutritional factors is undetermined, but dietary factors have been hypothesized to account for approximately 20% (range, 10% to 30%) of lung cancer cases.[8]
- The United States Environmental Protection Agency estimates that one in 15 homes in the United States has **radon** levels above the recommended guideline of 4 picoCuries per liter (pCi/L).[9]

### Smoking

- Smoking causes a 20-fold increase in lung cancer risk. The incidence of lung cancer follows patterns of smoking, with a 20-year lag.[10]
- A threefold increase of the number of cigarettes smoked per day triples the risk of lung cancer, whereas tripling the duration of smoking leads to a 100-fold increase in lung cancer.[11]
- The longer a former smoker abstains from smoking cigarettes, the lower the risk of lung cancer (Table 23-1). However, even for periods of abstinence of more than 40 years, the risk of lung cancer among former smokers remains elevated compared with that of people who never smoked.[12]

| TABLE 23-1 ▪ RELATIVE RISK OF SMOKING AND ASBESTOS AS RISK FACTORS FOR LUNG CANCER | | |
|---|---|---|
| | No Asbestos | Asbestos |
| No smoking | 1 | 5.17 |
| Smoking | 10/85 | 53.24 |

- **Passive smoking:** The National Research Council concluded that nonsmoking spouses married to smokers were about 30% more likely to develop lung cancer than nonsmoking spouses married to nonsmokers.[12]
- In the United States, passive smoking accounts for approximately 3000 lung cancer deaths per year.[13]
- A 1997 meta-analysis[14] showed a 20% increased risk associated with marriage to a smoker.

### Nontobacco Causes of Lung Cancer
- **Occupational agents** are known to act as lung cancer carcinogens. Arsenic, asbestos, and chromium have the highest risk. An estimated 2% to 9% of lung cancers are related to occupational exposures.
- **Dietary factors** can modify risks. Higher consumption of fruits and vegetables is associated with a reduced lung cancer risk, and an increased dietary fat intake may lead to a higher risk. Supplementation with vitamins A, E, or beta-carotene has not positively influenced risk.[7]
- Theoretically, **antioxidants** may prevent oxidative DNA damage and thereby protect against cancer[15]; however, because cigarette smoking is associated with less healthful lifestyles, such as poor diets,[16] it is difficult to separate dietary factors from cigarette smoking as a cause of lung cancer.
- The studies with **retinols** are also equivocal.
- The case controlled studies for **carotenoids**, beta-carotene, and vitamin C suggest a reduction in lung cancer risk. However, three randomized, double-blind, placebo-controlled chemoprevention trials showed no benefit.[17]
- The studies about silica dust are equivocal,[18] but asbestos is clearly associated with lung cancer.[19] A sevenfold excess of lung cancer was subsequently observed among insulation workers in the United States.[20] The peak incidence occurred 30 to 35 years after the initial exposure to asbestos.

## PATHOLOGY
- NSCLC comprises 80% of lung cancer cases. Adenocarcinoma has surpassed squamous cell carcinoma as the most common histologic type of lung cancer.[1] (See Chapter 22 on pathology of lung malignancies.)
- Staging for NSCLC: See Chapter 21 on lung cancer staging–current and new proposed systems.

## CLINICAL FEATURES
- In the United States in 2004, approximately 173,770 new cases of lung cancer were diagnosed. Lung cancer accounts for approximately 28% of all cancer deaths.

### Male-to-Female Ratio
- In the United States, the male-to-female ratio is 60:40.
- In 1984, the incidence was 86.5 per 100,000 men, and it has subsequently been declining (69.1 per 100,000 in 1997).

- The incidence of lung cancer in women increased during the 1990s, with a leveling off toward the end of the decade (43.1 per 100,000 women).

### Symptoms
- From 85% to 95% of patients with lung cancer will be symptomatic at presentation.
- Symptoms may include cough, hemoptysis, dyspnea, chest pain, hoarseness, headaches, weight loss, bone symptoms, or neurologic symptoms.

## DIAGNOSTIC WORKUP

### Imaging Studies (also see Chapters 1 and 2 on Imaging)
#### Chest Computed Tomography Scan
- The computed tomography (CT) scan is a critical part of the workup because it helps stage the tumor and gives the surgeon anatomic information that allows the surgeon to determine technical details about what procedure will be required. Reports of CT scans rarely give the surgeon all the information needed, so the surgeon needs to view the actual images.
- Radiographic features suggestive of malignancy include the absence of a benign pattern of calcification in the detected lesion, a nodule or mass that is growing, a nodule with a spiculated or lobulated border, a larger lesion (larger than 3 cm is malignant unless proven otherwise), and a cavitary lesion that is thick walled (larger than 16 mm).
- The appearances of lung cancers on CT scan are quite varied. Figure 23-1 shows a large cavitary cancer in the right upper lobe. This appearance is most commonly seen with squamous cell carcinoma. Figure 23-2 shows a lobe with three synchronous primary tumors, each of which exhibited a different histological type. Figure 23-3 shows extensive nodal metastases in a patient with Stage IIIB disease. In evaluating a lung mass, chest CT scans should extend down to include the liver and adrenal glands. Figure 23-4 shows adrenal metastases in a patient with an incidental discovery of a lung mass on chest radiograph.

### Positron Emission Tomography Scan
- The positron emission tomography scan (PET) uses [18F] fluorodeoxyglucose.
- It has a sensitivity of 97% and a specificity of 78%, as used in clinical practice.[21] PET scan is commonly used for evaluation of a lung mass and staging.

### Assessment and Follow-Up of Solitary Lung Masses
- If a mass is PET positive, there is an 80% chance that it is cancer. False-negative findings occur in masses smaller than 1 cm and in bronchioalveolar cancer (BAC). Note: PET standard uptake value (SUV) thresholds commonly cited, such as larger than or smaller than 2.5 SUV have come under critical review and appear not to as robust as previously stated (see Chapter 2 on Radionuclear Imaging by Waxman for more details); therefore, SUV greater than 2.5 is not to be used as a cutoff point for the diagnosis of lung cancer on PET scan
- If the mass is PET negative, there is a 5% chance of cancer so those masses are often watched. If the mass is suspicious, such as a ground-glass opacity or a spiculated mass, then it should be resected if the follow-up CT scan shows that the mass is stable or enlarged. If the appearance of the mass is less suspicious, then it can be watched if it is smaller or stable.
- Our experience with the PET scan evaluation of the mediastinum has been that the false-positive rate for mediastinal nodes

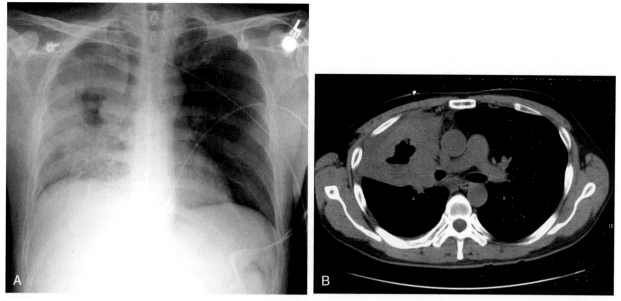

**Figure 23-1:** Chest x-ray study (**A**) and CT scan (**B**) of a large cavitary squamous cell carcinoma of the right upper lobe (stage 2B, T3N0) tumor that invaded the chest wall.

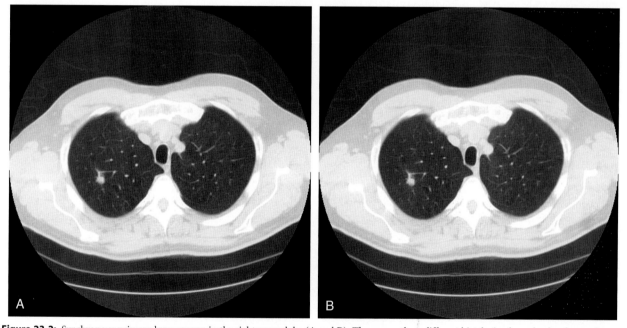

**Figure 23-2:** Synchronous primary lung cancers in the right upper lobe (**A** and **B**). There were three different histologies: bronchoalveolar carcinoma, adenocarcinoma, and squamous cell carcinoma.

is about 30% so positive nodes on CT scan should be biopsied to properly stage the cancer.

- **Nuclear** scans are used much less frequently since the advent of the PET scan, although a PET scan may not rule out bony metastasis and a bone scan may be indicated if bony metastases are suspected.
- **Brain magnetic resonance imaging (MRI) or CT scans:** Although some physicians obtain brain imaging for all patients suspected to have lung cancer, most surgeons use brain imaging selectively because the incidence of brain metastases is very low for clinical stage 1 lung cancer. Indications for brain imaging are seen in Table 23-2.

| TABLE 23-2  ■  **INDICATION FOR BRAIN IMAGING (BRAIN MR OR CT SCAN) IN A PATIENT WITH KNOWN OR SUSPECTED LUNG CANCER** |
|---|
| New onset headaches |
| New onset neurologic symptoms |
| Weight loss |
| Stage 3 cancer by CT or PET scans |

CT, computed tomography; PET, positron emission tomography.

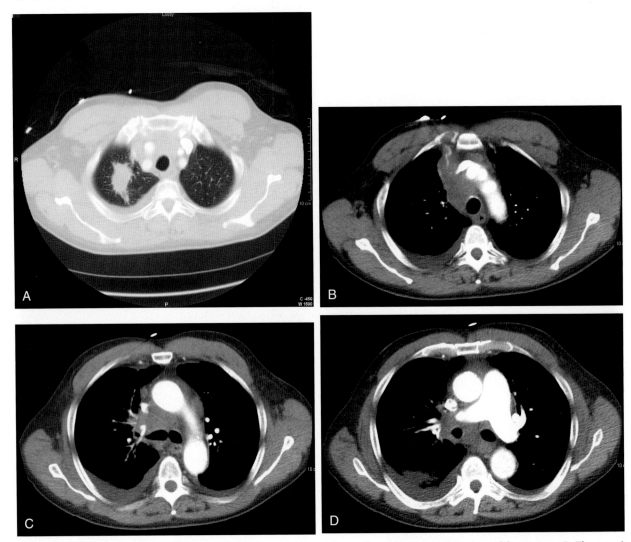

**Figure 23-3:** **A** and **B**, Stage 3B (T2N3) right upper lobe tumor with extensive mediastinal and supraclavicular nodal metastases. **B**, The extensive nodal metastases on the mediastinal windows. **C**, Extensive mediastinal adenopathy plus contralateral subaortic nodes plus (R) malignant pleural effusion. **D**, shows subcarinal nodal metastases.

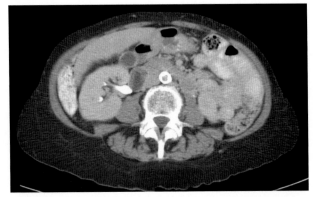

**Figure 23-4:** Computed tomography scan depicting adrenal metastases from lung cancer.

---

### KEY POINTS

- Resect a mass if it looks suspicious and is PET positive.
- Follow a mass if it does not look suspicious and is PET negative.
- Continue follow-up if a mass decreases in size.
- Resect a mass that remains stable on follow-up but has a suspicious appearance (spiculated or ground glass appearance).
- Resect a mass that has increased in size on follow-up.

### *Pulmonary Function Tests*

- The pulmonary function test should be performed before lung resection in order to assess the postoperative predicted $FEV_1$. **A postoperative predicted $FEV_1$ of greater than or equal to** at least 40% of predicted after any resection is associated with a lower incidence of respiratory failure postoperatively.
- In the past, the recommendation was that the postoperative $FEV_1$ would equal 800 to 1000 mL, but % predicted is a better approach because 800 mL may be adequate for a small person but inadequate for a large person.

- If the $FEV_1$ is predicted to be marginal, a quantitative lung perfusion scan will demonstrate if the part of the lung to be resected is functional. If it is not functional, then an operation should be tolerable.
- **Diffusion capacity** should be greater than 40% predicted. If it is less than 40% predicted, an operation has a significantly greater risk.
- For marginal patients, **exercise studies** are helpful. If the $VO_2$ **max** is greater than 20, the patient should tolerate the operation; if it is less than 10, an operation carries a very high risk.[22]

### Diagnostic Studies

- The use of the **needle biopsy** is slightly controversial. Some centers perform needle biopsies on any suspicious mass. Others do not because the biopsy rarely can prove that a mass is benign so both a positive biopsy and a nondiagnostic biopsy lead to a resection of the mass. Needle biopsy of a suspicious mass rarely changes the decision to operate. A suspicious mass needs to be resected if the biopsy shows cancer and if the biopsy is nondiagnostic.
- Preoperative needle biopsy is cost effective if wedge resection of a mass and frozen section takes longer than 30 minutes.
- **Bronchoscopy** has a high diagnostic yield for centrally located tumors but a diagnostic yield well below 50% for peripherally located masses.
- **Bronchoscopy** is routinely performed at the beginning of a VATS procedure to position the double-lumen tube to look for any endobronchial pathology and to assess the extent of resection for a centrally located tumor (standard lobectomy versus sleeve lobectomy versus pneumonectomy).
- **Wedge resection** is the definitive diagnostic test for a lung mass. Centrally located masses may not be amenable to a wedge resection. In such cases, a lobectomy may be needed, and is perfectly reasonable for suspicious masses. We prefer to not perform a pneumonectomy without a specific diagnosis.

## SURGERY

- Surgery is the mainstay for treatment of lung cancer and has the best chance for cure of lung cancer. Unfortunately, an operation is most effective for stage 1 cancer and less than 25% of patients are found to have lung cancer at an early stage. Table 23-3 shows the standard treatment for lung cancer by stage.

### Indications

- For stage 1A, 1B, 2A, and 2B NSCLC, an operation is the treatment of choice. Adjuvant treatment should be considered for patients after resection for stage 2 lung cancer. For incidental finding of mediastinal lymph node involvement from surgical specimens (unexpected), adjuvant therapy can be considered.
- Selected patients with stage 3A and 3B may be candidates after neoadjuvant treatment. The 6-year survival rate for both stage 3A and 3B patients treated with preoperative cis-platin, VP-16, and 4500 rads of radiotherapy was 22%.[23]

### TABLE 23-3 ■ STANDARD TREATMENT FOR LUNG CANCER BY STAGE

| Stage | Treatment |
| --- | --- |
| 1A and 1B | Surgery |
| 2A and 2B | Surgery and postoperative chemotherapy |
| 3A | Neoadjuvant Treatment and Surgery |
| 3B | Usually Palliative |
| 4 | Palliative |

### Contraindications

- Stage 3 patients are generally not surgical candidates, although patients with technically resectable stage 3A (N2 disease) can be surgical candidates after neoadjuvant treatment.
- Stage 4 patients are rarely candidates for resection. If a patient has a solitary brain met or solitary adrenal met and otherwise a stage 1 lung cancer, then both sites can be resected.
- Medically inoperable patients.

### Extent of the Pulmonary Resection for Lung Cancer

- Many factors that determine the extent of the pulmonary resection. Careful review of the preoperative CT scan and a thorough understanding of thoracic anatomy show the relationship of the tumor to vessels, bronchi, chest wall and the pericardium.
- A randomized, prospective study by the Lung Cancer Study Group showed a lower local recurrence rate for a lobectomy compared with wedge resection or segmentectomy.[24] Therefore, for patients with adequate pulmonary function, a lobectomy is the most common type of resection for lung cancer.

### Wedge Resections

- Occasionally, the size of the tumor and the cell type may lead to a wedge resection as the definitive treatment for lung cancer. Although a lobectomy is considered the standard of practice, lesser resections are again being considered in special circumstances. The increasing use of screening CT scans has led to the finding of tiny pulmonary masses for which a wedge resection might be appropriate. For small peripheral BACs, a wedge resection is adequate.[25,26]

### Wedge Resections with Brachytherapy

- To reduce the chances of local recurrence after a wedge resection in a patient who cannot physiologically tolerate a lobectomy, local radiation can be used.
- External beam radiation can compromise pulmonary function as much as a lobectomy, so localized radiation (brachytherapy) can be used with wedge resection.
- Brachytherapy technique can be either via placement of a mesh embedded with low-dose radioactive seeds on the pulmonary resection site or suturing afterload catheters on the lung.[27] If afterload catheters are used, patients go to the radiation department for temporary placement of high-dose radioactive seeds. The potential advantages of the afterload catheter approach include the following: it minimizes radiation exposure to hospital personnel and contacts of the patients, and there is no need for an isolation room for the patient.

### Video-Assisted Thoracic Surgery Lobectomy

- A VATS lobectomy should have the same anatomic dissection and the same individual ligation of vessels and bronchi that is used with a lobectomy by thoracotomy. Although some surgeons have compromised the standard anatomic dissection in order to perform a minimally invasive pulmonary resection, this technique is to be avoided. An operation should not be compromised in order to make it a minimally invasive operation. Therefore, a VATS lobectomy should be an anatomic dissection of the vessels and bronchus with individual ligation of these structures.
- The intent of a minimally invasive procedure is that the same procedure is performed safely with less pain and earlier recovery for the patient, but this remains controversial in the minds of many thoracic surgeons. Although we first performed a VATS

lobectomy in February 1992, the acceptance of the procedure was slow for many years; however, the momentum for that approach has been steadily growing in the last few years.[28-30]

- The relative contraindications for VATS lobectomy are shown in Tables 23-4 and 23-5. The contraindications include larger tumors that cannot be removed without spreading ribs, conditions that compromise the safety of the dissection (preop treatment with chemotherapy, radiation therapy, or both), the invasion of extrapulmonary structures (chest wall or pericardium), and pathologic lymph nodes. The assessment for and performance of a sleeve resection may require a thoracotomy, although we have performed sleeve lobectomies by VATS.

---

**KEY POINTS**

- VATS lobectomy must use a standard anatomic resection with removal of lymph nodes.

---

### Open Versus Video-Assisted Thoracic Surgery Lobectomy

- Since 1990, the trend in thoracic surgery has been toward less invasive approaches, with a switch from traditional posterolateral thoracotomy incision to the muscle-sparing thoracotomy and now to VATS procedures. In the United States at the present time, 10% of the lobectomies are performed via VATS. In 2005, we performed 94% of our lobectomies, including sleeve resections, with VATS.[28] The majority of lobectomies could likely be performed by VATS.

- Although some thoracic surgeons are still concerned that a VATS lobectomy is unsafe, an incomplete cancer operation, and offers no advantage over a thoracotomy for lobectomy, current data show those concerns to be unfounded. Proponents believe that VATS lobectomy is a safe and effective treatment for lung cancer.

---

**TABLE 23-4 ▪ GENERAL INDICATIONS FOR A VATS LOBECTOMY**

Clinical stage 1 or 2 lung cancer
Tumor less than 6 cm
Elderly patients
Patients with compromised performance status
Inflammatory disease (destroyed lobe)

VATS, video-assisted thoracic surgery.

---

**TABLE 23-5 ▪ RELATIVE CONTRAINDICATIONS FOR A VATS LOBECTOMY**

Tumors larger than 6 cm
T3 tumors
Preoperative chemotherapy
Preoperative radiation
Centrally located tumors
Abnormal lymph nodes

VATS, video-assisted thoracic surgery.

---

- The evidence is mounting that a VATS lobectomy may have advantages over a lobectomy by thoracotomy, although there are very little data from randomized, prospective studies to compare the two approaches.

- Demmy[31] showed **shorter hospitalizations** (5.3 + 3.7 versus 12.2 + 11.1 days, $P = 0.02$) and chest tube durations (4.0 + 2.8 versus 8.3 + 8.9 days, $P = 0.06$) for VATS lobectomy.

- A randomized trial from Germany showed **fewer complications** after the VATS approach (14.2%) than for thoracotomy (50%).[32]

- A Japanese study showed that **financial costs** (anesthesia charges, laboratory charges, and hospital charges) were lower for the VATS approach than those for thoracotomy.[33] Postoperative pain (visual pain scale, total dose of narcotic, need for additional narcotic, need for intercostal blocks, and sleep disturbances) is less after VATS than for thoracotomy.[34]

- There appears to be an **earlier postoperative recovery** for the VATS approach than a thoracotomy. Demmy[31] reported earlier returns to full preoperative activities ($P < 0.01$). less postop pain ($P = 0.014$), and less shoulder dysfunction than with thoracotomy.[35,36]

- Suguira reported **better short-term and long-term quality of life**.[37]

- There is **less impact on the immune system** after VATS than with thoracotomy. In this study, patients who underwent VATS also had reduced postoperative release of both proinflammatory and antiinflammatory cytokines. Although the postop release of tumor necrosis factor-α and interleukin-1β (IL-1β) were minimal for both groups, the levels of IL-6, IL-8, and IL-10 were higher in the open group.[38] The clinical significance of these findings remains to be fully elucidated.

### Concerns Unique to Video-Assisted Thoracic Surgery Lobectomy

- The biggest concerns regarding VATS lobectomy center on three issues: risk and management of intraoperative bleeding, tumor recurrence in the incision, and the adequacy of the cancer operation, but the incidence of these complications is low.

- The incidence of **bleeding** is less than 1%.[28-30]

- Cancer **recurrence at an incision** happens in only 3/1321 (0.2%) cases.[28-30] We have not experienced a trocar site recurrence in our VATS procedures for lung cancer since we switched to the Lapsack for removal of the tumors.

- The **adequacy of a cancer operation** is measured by survival. In a nonrandomized series of VATS lobectomy for stage 1A (T1N0) lung cancer, the 5-year survival has been 72% to 94.4%.[26-27,39] Others have reported a survival rate that is the same as that reported with thoracotomy-treated lung cancer (McKenna and colleagues[28] [72% at 5 years] and Walker and associates[41] [77.9% at 5 years]). It certainly appears that a VATS approach does not compromise the survival for lung cancer patients.

---

**KEY POINTS**

- Bleeding can occur with VATS lobectomy, but this appears to be rare and manageable.
- Recurrence in an incision can occur with VATS lobectomy, but this appears to be rare.
- Cure rates for a lobectomy by VATS and a thoracotomy appears to be the same.

---

## Sleeve Lobectomy

- The goal of resection for lung cancer is to obtain clear margins with preservation of as much pulmonary tissue as possible. Pneumonectomy is required in approximately 10% of resections for lung cancer. At times, pneumonectomy can be avoided if a sleeve resection is performed.
- For example, if a tumor is at the origin of the right middle lobe bronchus, clear surgical margins could be obtained with resection of the right middle lobe and the right lower lobe (seven pulmonary segments). Alternatively, a sleeve resection of the right middle lobe and the superior resection of the right lower lobe can be performed with reimplantation of the basilar bronchus into the intermediate bronchus (resection of three segments). This sleeve resection can provide clear margins with resection of only 30% of the right lung, rather than resection of 70% of the right lung with a bilobectomy.
- The CT scan in Figure 23-5 shows a tumor at the origin of the right upper lobe and the main stem bronchus. A right upper lobe sleeve resection can be performed with transection of the main stem bronchus and the intermediate bronchus. The intermediate bronchus and the main stem bronchi are then anastamosed.
- Sleeve resection has been shown to provide the same cure rate as a pneumonectomy for selected patients while providing significantly better quality of life.[42]

## Pneumonectomy

- Usually, about 10% of resections for lung cancer require a pneumonectomy, but that increases to 30% when the resection is after neoadjuvant treatment for stage 3 lung cancer. The operation should provide clear margins and save as much lung tissue as possible. Pneumonectomy can be performed with VATS or a thoracotomy.
- The overall mortality rate is 5% to 10% but 2 to 3 times higher for a right pneumonectomy. The mortality rate for a right pneumonectomy for stage 3 lung cancer after chemotherapy and radiation approaches 25%.

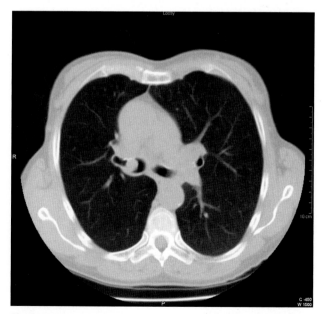

**Figure 23-5:** Computed tomography scan showing a tumor at the origin of the right upper lobe bronchus in a patient who subsequently underwent sleeve lobectomy.

- The risk for atrial fibrillation after lung surgery increases with the patient's age and the amount of lung resected. After a pneumonectomy, the risk for atrial fibrillation is 25% so prophylaxis (calcium channel blocker or beta blocker) is indicated.
- If the expected postoperative $FEV_1$ is not at least 40%, then a quantitative lung perfusion scan should be performed to determine if a pneumonectomy would be tolerated.
- Indications include
- Central tumors involving the main pulmonary artery or the bronchus, if they are not amenable to a sleeve resection
- Tumors crossing the fissures

---

**KEY POINTS REGARDING SURGERY FOR LUNG CANCER**

- For selected patients, sleeve resection can provide the same cure rate and better quality of life compared to pneumonectomy.
- Sleeve lobectomy has now been performed by VATS.
- Lobectomy is the standard of practice for most lung cancers.
- Wedge resection and brachytherapy are reasonable treatments for patients with poor pulmonary function that precludes lobectomy for lung cancer.

---

## Conversion to Thoracotomy

- There is no shame in converting from VATS to thoracotomy. This is necessary in 2% to 20% of VATS cases.[28-30] Many surgeons perform a VATS wedge resection and then a thoracotomy for a lobectomy. In the United States, about 10% of lobectomies are now performed by VATS. There is a strong trend toward more cases being performed by VATS.
- Reasons for conversion include the following: patient disease (tumor invading the chest wall, need for sleeve lobectomy), surgeon skills (lack of training or skills to perform a VATS lobectomy), and intraoperative complications (bleeding).

## Postoperative Management

- See chapter 6 on VATS surgery.

## SPECIAL SITUATIONS

### Bronchioloalveolar Carcinoma
#### Definitions

- A subtype of adenocarcinoma that is characterized by a well-differentiated histology in which tumor cells grow in a lepidic fashion (i.e., grow along intact alveolar septae) without distortion of the lung architecture. There is a tendency for aerogenous and lymphatic spread but no stromal, vascular, or pleural invasion.[44-46] This lesion is referred to as pure BAC.
- More commonly, a mixed histology consisting of invasive elements of adenocarcinoma and BAC coexist and is referred to as a mixed subtype. This can range from BAC predominance to minimal focal elements of BAC.
- BAC subtypes include: mucinous, nonmucinous, and a mixed/intermediate form (both mucinous and nonmucinous). The mucinous form accounts for up to a quarter of cases, whereas the nonmucinous form accounts for up to two thirds. The cell of origin for the mucinous variety is thought to be the goblet cell, whereas nonmucinous BAC likely arises from type II pneumocytes and Clara cells.

- Possible progression: atypical adenomatous hyperplasia; premalignant (AAH), to BAC (generally low grade malignancy), to BAC with adenocarcimoma (more malignant) to adenocarcinoma.[47]
- The above-mentioned definitions are important because the varying histopathologies affect both clinical presentation and prognosis.

### Epidemiology and Prevalence

- The incidence of BAC has been reported to be on the rise, with a reported prevalence as high as 20% to 24%. However, this likely reflects data on mixed tumors because the incidence of pure BAC has been reported to be less than 5% of NSCLC.[48]
- There is a higher proportion of women affected than in other types of NSCLC, with the male-to-female ratio about equal.
- Not associated with smoking as much as other types of lung cancer. About a third are life-long nonsmokers.[49]

### Clinical Subtypes and Presentation

- Different patterns of BAC:
  - *Solitary nodule* (most common). Peripheral in location. Tends to be nonmucinous in type.
  - *Segmental or lobar consolidation.* More likely mucinous variety. Diffuse infiltrative (much less common than 20 years ago)
  - *Multifocal nodule (multiple pulmonary nodules)*
- Symptoms and signs
  - Frequently asymptomatic and an incidental finding (solitary nodule or nodules)
  - Cough, sputum, hemoptysis, dyspnea, weight loss (all in <35%)[50]
  - Bronchorrhea: copious (>100 mL/d) watery sputum. True incidence lower than in early studies (likely 5%). Described with consolidative subtype
  - Extensive consolidation associated with dyspnea and hypoxemia
- Radiologic CT appearances[50,51]
  - Localized ground-glass attenuation noted in 94% of pure BACs.
    - Small, pure ground-glass opacity (<1 cm) likely AAH and may be removed with a wedge resection with nearly 100% cure rate
    - Larger (>1 cm) masses, especially with punctuate white areas, usually contain areas of adenocarcinoma and are treated like adenocarcinoma
    - May have associated consolidation producing "open bronchus sign."
    - Nodules can display pseudocavitation (bubble-like areas of low attenuation), spiculated margins, cavitation, pleural tags.
      - *Consolidation* (segmental, lobar, multilobar) with heterogeneous attenuation
      - *Multiple nodules:* often a mix of well and poorly defined nodules and area of ground-glass attenuation.
- PET scans[44]
  - Significant proportion of false-negative scans (up to 60%)
  - Most false-negative findings with focal BAC

### Treatment

- Early stage disease[44]
  - Surgery:
    - As in other forms of NSCLC, surgery is the gold standard approach.[44,52]

- Primary treatment is resection (usually lobectomy, depending on size and location)
- Sublobar resection may be appropriate in the following circumstances: pure ground-glass appearance on CT; small size: 1 to 2 cm; intraoperative pathologic confirmation of pure BAC; no evidence of invasion; free surgical margins (see the Appendix: ACCP evidence-based practice guidelines, 2007). Small peripheral lesions may also factor in (e.g., 1 cm peripheral ground glass opacities)
- This approach is also supported by the fact that pure BAC rarely involves lymph nodes.
- Koike and associates[53] offered all stage 1 patients with BAC limited resection. One hundred and fifty-nine patients underwent lobectomy, whereas 74 had segmentectomy or wedge resection. No survival differences between the groups were observed at 3 and 5 years or in the incidence of recurrence.
- In patients with mutifocal disease or with metachronous lesions evident over time, limited resection may be necessary to preserve lung parenchyma and function
- Thus, follow-up is very important because patients with solitary BAC may develop metachronous tumors. If solitary and peripheral, they may be removed with a wedge resection.
- **Radiation:** rarely needed. Similar efficacy as in other forms of NSCLC.
- Systemic disease and systemic therapies
  - Chemotherapy
    - No good data on adjuvant treatment exists
    - BAC has traditionally been believed to be not as sensitive to chemotherapy as other adenocarcinomas. The first International Association for the Study of Lung Cancer (IASLC)/American Society of Clinical Oncology (ASCO) consensus conference on BAC[54] concluded that there was insufficient evidence to answer this question.
    - Epidermal growth factor receptor (EGFR) mutations have been found in up to a quarter of patients with BAC[55] and are limited to nonmucinous forms of BAC.
    - EGFR blockers (e.g., erlotinib or gefitinib) are more effective for BAC than other types of adenocarcinoma.
    - The 2007 American College of Chest Physicians (ACCP) evidence-based practice guidelines recommend standard chemotherapy for unresectable BAC patients with good performance status (see the Appendix).
    - EGFR inhibitors can be considered in patients with advanced disease and poor performance status or who have failed standard chemotherapy regimens.

### Prognosis

- Stage for stage, BAC has a better survival rates than other forms of NSCLC.[46,56-58]
- Stage I BAC 1-year survival is 81% to 83% versus 63% to 65% for other NSCLCs.

### Synchronous and Metachronous Lung Primary Tumors

- Definitions[59-63]
  - *Synchronous:* primary tumors occurring at the same time
  - *Metachronous:* primary tumors occurring at different times

- Synchronous primaries are much more common than appreciated. Two to four synchronous primary tumors can coexist (see Fig. 23-2).
- In one series, synchronous and metachronous primary tumors were observed in 8.4% of 369 patients with adenocarcinoma.[61]
- Criteria for synchronous primary tumors:
  ○ Different cell types (e.g., squamous cell and adenocarcinoma)
  ○ Different Immunostains
  ○ Different degree of differentiation
  ○ Solitary, bilateral upper lobe spiculated masses
  ○ Both have radiologic appearance of primary lung cancers
- Satellite tumors currently make the tumor T4 (stage 3B), but the new staging system will make satellite tumors resectable stage 2B.
- Patients should be given the benefit of the doubt in presence of what appears as two separate primary masses, because the cure rate for resection is reasonable and the long-term survival for palliative chemotherapy is poor.
- Workup generally includes PET/CT scan, brain MRI, and mediastinoscopy.
- When possible, usual surgical principles pertain.

## Association with Other Malignancies
- Patients with aerodigestive cancers, especially laryngeal cancers, have a 40% incidence of developing a primary lung cancer, so they require careful follow-up.[64-66]
- Patients with leukemia and lymphoma have a 50% increased incidence of developing a primary lung cancer
- Patients treated with radiation (for lung cancer, lymphoma, etc.) have a 50% increased incidence of developing a primary lung cancer

## Adrenal Masses
- The adrenal glands need to be evaluated in patients suspected of having lung cancer.
- Four percent of patients with lung cancer have benign adrenal adenomas.
- MRI can be used to detect fat in an adrenal mass that may suggest the diagnosis of a benign adenoma.
- Patients with adrenal masses that are irregular or larger than 2 cm in size are likely to have metastatic disease (see Fig. 23-4).
- If the diagnosis is uncertain, CT-guided biopsy may be required
- Patients with adrenal metastases usually exhibited clinical or biochemical evidence of advanced disease.[67]

## Brief Illustrative Case 1

- A 74-year-old, asymptomatic physician underwent a screening CT scan that showed a spiculated 3-cm mass in the right upper lobe (Fig. 23-6).
- The mass lit up on PET scan, and there was no evidence of nodal or distant metastases.
- Pulmonary function was good. FEV₁: 3.26 (84%); FVC: 4.42 (90%)
- Because the workup suggested that he had a stage 1A lung cancer, he underwent a VATS wedge resection.
- The frozen section showed non–small lung cancer. He then underwent a VATS lobectomy and node dissection.
- Final pathology showed a stage 1A adenocarcinoma.
- He was discharged from the hospital on postoperative day 1.

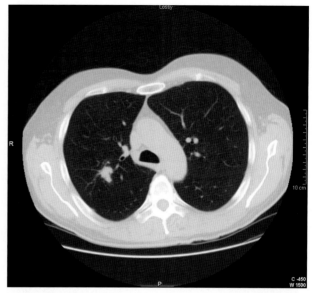

**Figure 23-6:** Spiculated mass in the posterior segment of the right upper lobe (stage 1A, T1N0 adenocarcinoma).

- On the seventh postoperative day, he returned to his office to see patients.

## Key Points

- VATS lobectomy certainly does not always produce such remarkable results but does allow some patients to return to regular activities much more quickly than patients who undergo a thoracotomy for a lobectomy.

## Brief Illustrative Case 2

- A 60-year-old man went for his routine check up for his emphysema. A chest x-ray study showed the emphysema and a new left upper lobe mass.
- His pulmonary function was terrible (FEV₁ = 38% predicted, TLC = 135% predicted, and RV = 287% predicted)
- The CT scan showed a speculated mass at the left apex and a very heterogeneous pattern of emphysema, with severe emphysematous destruction in the upper lobes and much better parenchyma at the bases (Fig. 23-7).
- Needle biopsy showed an adenocarcinoma
- PET scan staged it as a stage 1A (T2N0) lung cancer.
- He underwent a VATS left upper lobe with preservation of the lingula and a node dissection. There was no need for resection of the lingula for a tumor in this location and his pulmonary function was poor.
- Final pathology showed a stage 1B (T2N0M0) BAC with areas of adenocarcinoma.
- No adjuvant treatment is needed.

## Key Points

- Some patients can have combined operation for severe emphysema (lung volume reduction surgery [LVRS]) and a lung cancer lobectomy if the cancer and the emphysema are in the same location (preferably upper

*(Continued)*

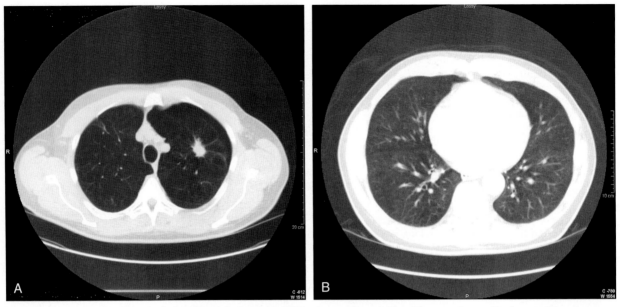

**Figure 23-7: A,** A spiculated mass in the left upper lobe (stage 1A, T1N0, adenocarcinoma). Note: The parenchyma of both upper lobes shows severe emphysematous changes, whereas in **B,** much better lung parenchyma is noted at the bases of both lungs. The patient thus has a very heterogeneous pattern of emphysema.

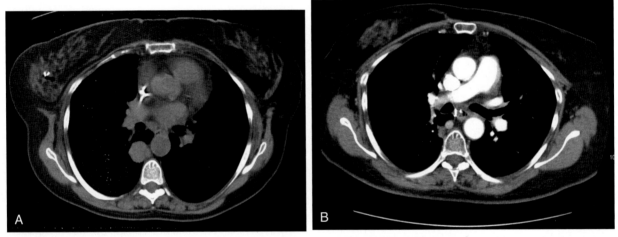

**Figure 23-8: A,** Initial computed tomography scan with a carcinoma in the apex of the superior segment of the right lower lobe. **B,** The tumor after preoperative treatment with radiation and chemotherapy. There has been a dramatic response to the treatment.

### Brief Illustrative Case 2—cont'd

lobe). If the cancer is not in the area of the severe emphysema, then a wedge resection can be performed in the better area of lung and the LVRS in the worse areas.

### Brief Illustrative Case 3

- A 62-year-old woman with a history of breast cancer went for routine follow-up that included a PET scan. No symptoms of metastases.
- CT showed a right lower lobe 4-cm mass (Fig. 23-8).
- Mediastinoscopy showed subcarinal nodal metastases (pathologic stage 3A, T2N2).
- She received preoperative carboplatin, taxol, and 45cG.

- Follow-up CT/PET showed no distant metastases and a good response on the CT.
- She underwent a thoracotomy, right lower lobectomy, node dissection, and intercostal muscle flap on the bronchial stump.
- Final pathology showed a complete remission.

### References

Interactive references and additional readings for this chapter can be accessed online at *expertconsult.com*.

### Appendix

Appendices for this chapter can be accessed online at *expertconsult.com*.

# 24 ADJUVANT AND NEOADJUVANT CHEMOTHERAPY IN NON–SMALL CELL LUNG CANCER

Ronald Natale, MD

## INTRODUCTION

Worldwide, nearly 1 million people die annually from non–small cell lung cancer (NSCLC).[1] Traditionally, complete surgical resection has been considered the only treatment with a curative potential in the 35% or so of these patients with early-stage disease (i.e., stages IA–IIIA). However, more than one half ultimately die from recurrent disease resulting from micrometastases not apparent at the time of surgery. Hence, there is a clear need for systemic treatment in the form of chemotherapy and perhaps newer biologically targeted agents to compliment the critical local role of surgery.

## SURVIVAL FOLLOWING COMPLETE SURGICAL RESECTION IS RELATED TO STAGE AND RISK OF MICROMETASTASES

- Five-year survival rates in completely resected NSCLC ranges from 70% in patients with stage I disease to about 10% in patients with stage IIIA disease.[2]
- In most cases, the failure of surgery to cure localized NSCLC results from the growth and progression of micrometastatic cancer not detected at the time of surgery.[3,4]

## POST-OPERATIVE RADIATION THERAPY MAY HAVE A DELETERIOUS EFFECT ON SURVIVAL

- The Post-Operative Radiation Therapy (PORT) Meta-Analysis Trialists Group first published a meta-analysis based on individual data on 2128 patients from nine randomized clinical trials comparing postoperative observation with postoperative radiotherapy in NSCLC in 1998.[5] In 2005, the PORT group updated their meta-analysis with the addition of individual patient data from a 10th clinical trial, bringing the patient total to 2232.[6] The results indicated a deleterious effect of radiotherapy on survival in patients with stage I or II lung cancer (18% increased risk of death over 5 years and an absolute decrease in 5-year survival of 6%). No definite adverse effect of PORT could be identified in patients with stage III (N2) NSCLC.

## CHEMOTHERAPY AFTER SURGERY (ADJUVANT) OR BEFORE SURGERY (NEOADJUVANT)

- **Risks versus benefits:** If the primary goal of adding chemotherapy to surgery is to eradicate micrometastatic disease, biologically there should be no major difference in whether the chemotherapy is given after or before the surgery. However, because surgery provides the only curative potential for patients with clinically localized lung cancer, the risks of delaying surgery, increasing surgical morbidity or mortality, or, worse, making surgery impossible because of a severe chemotherapy-related adverse event, most chemotherapy studies over the past 15 years have been in the postoperative (adjuvant) setting. As postoperative chemotherapy becomes better established and more effective, it is rational for chemotherapy to be more commonly administered in the preoperative setting when patients are better able to tolerate it and when it might enhance the feasibility and limit the extent of surgery by tumor downstaging.

## POSTOPERATIVE (ADJUVANT) CHEMOTHERAPY

- **Goal:** Improve survival following complete surgical resection of early stage NSCLC by administration of systemic therapy that eradicates microscopic residual or metastatic disease.
- **Early efforts with first-generation platinum-based chemotherapy regimens:** Clinical trials before 1985 were generally small, poorly designed, and used chemotherapy regimens with minimal efficacy. After 1985, cisplatin-based chemotherapy regimens that appeared to improve survival in patients with stage IV NSCLC began to be used in the adjuvant setting.
  - **Lung Cancer Study Group (LCSG) trial 772:** 141 patients with completely resected stage II or III adenocarcinoma or large cell undifferentiated carcinoma were randomized to receive six cycles of cyclophosphamide, doxorubicin, and cisplatin (CAP) chemotherapy or putative immunotherapy (intrapleural BCG and levamisole). Patients in the adjuvant chemotherapy arm achieved significant delay in time to recurrence of lung cancer and improved cancer-free survival at 1 year (77% versus 62%) but no statistically significant long-term or overall survival advantage.[7]
  - **LCSG trial 791:** Patients with positive surgical margins or metastases to high paratracheal lymph nodes (level 2) randomized to post-operative radiation therapy alone or radiation therapy followed by adjuvant CAP chemotherapy. One-year survival rates favored chemotherapy arm, but survival at 2 years and overall survival were not different between the two arms of the trial.[8]
  - **LCSG trial 801:** Patients with completely resected T2N0 or T2N1 NSCLC were randomized postoperatively to observation or four cycles of CAP chemotherapy. There was no difference in survival, but nearly half of the patients in the adjuvant chemotherapy arm failed to receive the planned four cycles of treatment. Subset analysis suggested that patients receiving more than 80% of planned treatment may have a survival advantage. There is uncertainty whether this represents an effect of chemotherapy or an

effect of a better patient subset. This clinical trial demonstrated the difficulty patients have in tolerating the toxic side effects of some chemotherapy regimens.[9]

○ **A Finnish** trial demonstrated an 11% improvement in 5-year survival in patients with completely resected T1-3N0 NSCLC receiving adjuvant CAP chemotherapy compared with observation. More than 60% of patients received less than the planned four cycles of CAP because of severe hematologic or gastrointestinal side effects.[10]

○ **The Non–Small Cell Lung Cancer Collaborative Group** conducted a **meta-analysis** of 52 randomized clinical trials performed between 1965 and 1991 with a total of 9387 patients with completely resected NSCLC.[11] Overall, adjuvant chemotherapy improved the 5-year survival rate by 5%, representing a 13% reduction in the relative risk of death. Chemotherapy regimens that used primarily alkylating agents worsened 5-year survival (15% relative increase risk of death), whereas platinum-based chemotherapy regimens produced a 13% relative decrease in the risk of death.[11]

■ **More successful results with second- and third-generation platinum-based regimens:** In the 1980s, new agents such as etoposide, vinblastine, and vindesine demonstrated improved outcomes combined with a platinum in patients with advanced or metastatic NSCLC (second-generation platinum-based regimens). In the 1990s, newer agents such as gemcitabine, paclitaxel, docetaxel, and vinorelbine (third-generation platinum-based regimens) appeared to improve survival in the advanced disease setting further still. These new regimens set the stage for more promising randomized clinical trials in the adjuvant disease setting.

○ The **International Adjuvant Lung Trial (IALT)** randomized 1867 patients with completely resected stage I, II, or IIIA NSCLC to observation or adjuvant chemotherapy with cisplatin combined with etoposide or vinblastine or vindesine or vinorelbine. The chemotherapy arms resulted in an absolute 4.1% improvement in the proportion of patients surviving 5 years (44.5% versus 40.4%), translating to a 14% decrease in the relative risk of dying.[12]

○ The **National Cancer Institue of Canada (NCI-C) JBR-10 trial** randomized 482 completely resected patients with stage IB-II NSCLC patients to observation versus four cycles of adjuvant cisplatin and vinorelbine.[13] Although only 58% of patients were able to tolerate three or more of the planned cycles of treatment, there was a 15% absolute improvement in 5-year survival favoring the chemotherapy arm (69% versus 54%, $P = 0.03$) representing a 40% reduction in the relative risk of dying.

○ The **Cancer and Leukemia Group B (CALGB) trial 9633** evaluated the role of adjuvant carboplatin and paclitaxel in 344 patients with surgically staged IB NSCLC randomized to observation versus chemotherapy.[14] Unfortunately, an 8% improvement in survival at 3 and 4 years (79% versus 71% and 69% versus 61%, respectively) narrowed to only a 2% advantage at 5 years (59% versus 57%). The overall hazard ratio for survival of 0.8, suggesting a 20% decreased risk of death, was not statistically significant ($P = 0.10$).

○ The **Adjuvant Navelbine International Trialist Association (ANITA) trial** randomized 840 patients with completely resected stage IB-IIIA NSCLC to postoperative observation versus four cycles of cisplatin and vinorelbine (identical to NCI-C JBR-10 trial).[15] Again only 61% of patients completed three or more cycles of the planned chemotherapy regimen because of the severity of treatment-related side effects. However, the adjuvant chemotherapy arm was associated with an absolute 8.6% improvement in 5-year survival and an improvement in median survival from 43.7 months to 65.7 months ($P = 0.017$).

■ Uracil/Tegafur-Based Adjuvant Trials in Japan

○ **Uracil/Tegafur (UFT)** is an oral prodrug of 5-fluorouracil that has been studied in six randomized clinical trials in Japan.[16-21]

○ A **meta-analysis** of 2003 Japanese patients with stage I NSCLC randomized to postoperative observation versus UFT demonstrated a 26% decreased risk of death with UFT taken orally for 2 years.[22] UFT was associated with an absolute 5% improvement in survival at 5 years (81.5% versus 76.5%, $P = .011$) and 7.7% at 7 years (77.2% versus 69.5%, $P = .01$).

○ These results have not been confirmed in randomized clinical trials outside Japan.

■ Current standard of care for adjuvant chemotherapy in NSCLC

○ Patients with completely resected stage IIA, IIB, or IIIA NSCLC should be offered platinum-based adjuvant chemotherapy

■ The data support the preferential use of cisplatin in most patients.

■ Carboplatin is acceptable in patients who are intolerant of cisplatin and who are unable to tolerate or accept risks of nephrotoxicity (e.g., creatinine clearance below 60 mL/min, congestive heart failure, or cardiovascular condition intolerant of copious normal saline hydration and mannitol-forced diuresis, or diabetes), ototoxicity (e.g., pre-existing hearing loss or tinnitus) or peripheral neuropathy (e.g., pre-existing peripheral neuropathy, diabetic neuropathy, or trade or activity dependent on fine manual motor skills), and the elderly.

■ The data most strongly support the use of vinorelbine added to cisplatin. Based on the results of randomized trials in patients with advanced stage IIIB or IV NSCLC, other third-generation agents, such as gemcitabine, paclitaxel, or docetaxel are probably at least equally efficacious, but direct data in the adjuvant setting are limited.

○ Subset analyses suggest that improvement in survival is greatest in patients with the most advanced stage of localized disease (stage IIIA) and decreases proportionately with earlier stage. For example, no survival benefit can be convincingly demonstrated in patients with stage IB disease except in the T2N0 subgroup with tumor diameter greater than 4 cm.

■ Future directions

○ **Patient selection:** Use of genomic analyses of resected tumor specimens to identify patients at highest risk of disease recurrence thus sparing chemotherapy toxicities in patients more likely to be cured with surgery alone.[23]

○ **Chemotherapy selection:** Use of biochemical, biologic or genomic analyses of resected tumor specimens to identify drug sensitivity or resistance features (e.g., high ERCC-1 tumor expression predicts unfavorable response to platinum).[24-27]

○ **Biologically targeted therapy:** The addition of biologically targeted agents to chemotherapy. Current studies exploring the use of the epidermal growth factor receptor–targeted agent, erlotinib, or the vascular endothelial growth factor–targeted agent, bevacizumab.[28-31]

## PREOPERATIVE (NEOADJUVANT) CHEMOTHERAPY

■ **Goal:** Reduce locoregional disease to improve surgical resectability and eradicate micrometastatic disease to improve survival.

○ Patients with pathologic N2 NSCLC have a survival rate of 5% to 15% following complete surgical resection, depending on the extent of mediastinal nodal involvement and less than 5% following incomplete surgical resection.[32,33]

○ The fact that two thirds of first recurrences following complete surgical resection occur at distant sites reflects the micrometastatic nature of NSCLC and the potential benefit from effective systemic therapy.[34]

○ Stage IIIA (N2) NSCLC is a heterogeneous disease and can be divided into three general groups[35,36]:

■ Patients with minimal N2 involvement found incidentally during or after surgery

■ Patients with limited N2 disease (one or two nodal stations) diagnosed preoperatively with imaging or surgical procedures (mediastinoscopy or transbronchial/transesophageal biopsy)

■ Patients with multistation or bulky mediastinal nodal involvement

○ The potential benefit of preoperative chemotherapy intended to improve the rate of complete surgical resection and reduce micrometastatic disease must be weighed against the potential growth of tumor that may occur by delaying surgery and the potential adverse effects of cytotoxic therapy on perioperative morbidity and mortality

■ **Early feasibility studies:** Several small phase II studies of preoperative chemotherapy performed in the early 1990s.

○ Established the safety of this approach (no apparent increase in surgical morbidity or mortality)

○ Suggested that chemotherapy effectiveness, as measured by objective response rates, was significantly better in this earlier disease setting than in stage IIIB/IV disease (response rates of 50% to 70% versus 20% to 30%, respectively)

○ Answered valid concerns regarding the frequency of chemotherapy-resistant tumors progressing to an unresectable stage by delaying surgery (less than 10%)

○ Demonstrated that 5% to 15% of patients with pathologically documented N2 involvement could be downstaged to pN0 with possible improved survival outcomes[37-40]

■ **Initial phase III randomized trials:** Several pioneering phase III randomized trials were conducted in the early to mid 1990s. Although some of the results were promising, these first efforts suffered from several problems including trial size, variable pretreatment assessment of mediastinal nodal involvement, or variable stages of disease, the noncontrolled use of postoperative chemotherapy or radiation therapy and the use of older second-generation, platinum-based regimens.

○ A randomized trial conducted in **Spain** selected patients with stage IIIA (not all N2 documented) disease to undergo surgery alone or preoperative chemotherapy with mitomycin, ifosfamide, and cisplatin. All patients received postoperative radiotherapy. The study was closed early, with only 60 total patients (30 per arm) because of a striking survival benefit from chemotherapy. The median survival time was 22 months in the neoadjuvant chemotherapy group versus 10 months in the surgery only group.[41] Survival at 3 years was 20% versus 10%, respectively.[42]

○ A randomized trial conducted at the **MD Anderson Cancer Center** selected patients with stage IIIA (not all N2 documented) disease for randomization to surgery alone versus preoperative chemotherapy with etoposide, cyclophosphamide, and cisplatin. Patients with incompletely resected disease received postoperative radiation therapy and patients evaluated to have responded to the induction chemotherapy received three additional cycles of chemotherapy postoperatively. This study was also closed early with only 60 patients because of an impressive survival benefit from neoadjuvant chemotherapy. The median survival time was 21 months in the neoadjuvant chemotherapy group (28 patients) versus 14 months in the surgery only group

(32 patients).[43] Survival at 3 years was 43% versus 19%, respectively.[44]

○ A larger phase III trial in **France** randomized 355 patients with resectable stage IB to IIIA NSCLC to two cycles of mitomycin, ifosfamide, and cisplatin before surgery (and two additional cycles following surgery) or to surgery alone. Despite a striking difference in median survival between the two arms of the study (37 months versus 26 months, respectively), the difference was not statistically significant ($P = 0.15$). The percent of patients surviving 3 years was 52% and 41%, respectively.[45]

○ A fourth trial conducted in **Japan** was closed early because of slow accrual and no apparent differences in survival. In this study, 62 patients with documented mediastinal nodal involvement (N2) were randomized to preoperative treatment with vindesine and cisplatin or to surgery alone. The median survival times were 17 months and 16 months, respectively, and the percent of patients surviving 3 years was 23% and 26%, respectively.[46]

■ **Neoadjuvant trials with newer platinum-based regimens:** As was the case in adjuvant chemotherapy trials, the newer and more effective platinum-based regimens that incorporated gemcitabine or one of the taxanes, paclitaxel or docetaxel, began to be tested in the preoperative setting in the late 1990s and early 2000s. Furthermore, lessons learned from the pioneering neoadjuvant trials mentioned earlier led to more standardized patient selection and mediastinal nodal staging.

○ At least four phase II trials tested cisplatin and gemcitabine in the preoperative setting in patients with resectable N2 disease or more advanced and unresectable stage IIIB disease.[47-50] The treatment was well tolerated, and the radiographic objective responses ranged from 57% to 70%, which is considerably higher than what generally occurs in patients with stage IV disease. Furthermore, complete resection rates appeared to be increased and complete pathologic downstaging of mediastinal nodal involvement to pN0 occurred in about 10% of patients overall. Median survival times generally ranged from 19 to 20 months.

○ The **Lung Cancer Project Group of the Swiss Group for Clinical Cancer Research (SAKK)** treated 90 patients with stage IIIA (pN2) NSCLC with three consecutive cycles of cisplatin and docetaxel before surgical resection.[51] Overall, 66% of patients achieved a radiographic clinical response (greater than 50% tumor regression). Surgery was performed in 78 of the 90 patients (12 nonsurgical patients included one ineligible, nine progressive disease during or after chemotherapy, one deteriorated lung function, and one refusal); 75 were able to undergo resection (three were found to be unresectable). Radiographic clinical response was associated with a higher complete resection rate (93% versus 57%) and higher rate of nodal downstaging (73% versus 40%). Fourteen of the 75 patients (19%) completing surgical resection achieved pathologic complete response (pCR) with complete tumor necrosis or necrosis plus fibrosis. Multivariate analysis identified mediastinal nodal clearance and complete resection as strongly prognostic for increased survival.

○ The **European Organization for Research and Treatment of Cancer (EORTC)** studied carboplatin and paclitaxel in 90 patients with biopsy-proven N2 disease.[52] The objective radiographic response rate was 66%. Patients responding to the neoadjuvant chemotherapy were subsequently randomized to receive either surgery or radiotherapy; therefore, there are limitations in assessing the effects on resectability and survival. The efficacy of the carboplatin and paclitaxel regimen was further investigated in a multicenter phase II study in the **United States** in 94 patients with stage IB-II NSCLC and negative mediastinoscopy.[53] Patients received two cycles of chemotherapy, followed by surgery, followed by three cycles of chemotherapy. This study demonstrated that patients better tolerate preoperative chemotherapy than postoperative chemotherapy and that relatively high radiographic response rates and complete resection rates could be achieved (60% and 81%, respectively).

- Randomized phase III neoadjuvant trials in early stage lung cancer
  ○ Because the trials summarized above appeared to demonstrate that preoperative chemotherapy could be given safely and effectively to patients with N2 disease or early-stage disease, several randomized trials in patients with stage IB-IIIA NSCLC were initiated.
    - The **Southwest Oncology Group (SWOG) 9900** selected patients with clinical stage IB-IIIA (N1) disease for randomization to neoadjuvant carboplatin and paclitaxel, followed by surgery or to surgery alone.[54] Mediastinoscopy was required in all patients with mediastinal adenopathy. However, this study was closed early with 354 patients because of the emerging positive results of adjuvant chemotherapy trials and the ethical problems of not giving adjuvant chemotherapy to the surgery-only group. Despite the early closure, it was the largest randomized trial comparing preoperative chemotherapy to surgery alone. Nearly half of the patients in the neoadjuvant chemotherapy arm achieved greater than 50% radiographic reduction in cancer preoperatively and an improvement in median progression free survival (35 months versus 20 months, $P = 0.07$).
    - Several other neoadjuvant trials are either ongoing or recently closed, including trials in which neoadjuvant chemotherapy is compared directly with adjuvant chemotherapy.
- Role of radiation therapy in the neoadjuvant (preoperative) setting
  ○ Although radiation therapy and concurrent chemotherapy are the standard of care for patients with unresectable stage IIIA or IIIB NSCLC, the role of radiation therapy combined with neoadjuvant chemotherapy in resectable stage IIIA-N2 NSCLC is more controversial.
    - In a trial headed by the **SWOG** and participated in by other cooperative groups in the United States (**Intergroup Study 0139**), 429 patients with documented N2 disease were treated with concurrent chemotherapy (cisplatin and etoposide) and radiation therapy (45 Gy) and then randomized to surgery or to an additional 18 Gy of radiation therapy (63 Gy total).[55,56] Both groups were eligible to receive an additional two cycles of cisplatin and etoposide following surgery or radiation therapy. There were no statistically significant differences in survival between the two treatment arms except in subset analyses based on the type of surgery performed (pneumonectomy versus lobectomy). Patients undergoing pneumonectomy demonstrated a significantly inferior survival compared with matched patients undergoing chemotherapy and radiation therapy only in part related to a postoperative mortality rate of 26% in patients undergoing pneumonectomy. Many of the postoperative deaths were due to severe acute respiratory distress syndrome in the remaining lung. On the other hand, patients undergoing lobectomies appeared to have a survival advantage compared with matched patients undergoing chemotherapy and radiation therapy only (median survival 34 months versus 22 months, respectively, and 5-year overall survival of 36% versus 18%, respectively, $P = 0.002$). Most interestingly, the 5-year survival of the 42% of patients achieving pathologic downstaging of mediastinal nodes to N0 was greater than 40%. These provocative results are currently being pursued in further studies.

- Current standard of care regarding treatment of patients with stage IIIA (N2) NSCLC
  ○ Patients with N2 NSCLC represent a relatively heterogeneous group of patients. Therefore, no one treatment plan fits all.
    - Patients with multistation nodal involvement or bulky nodal metastases are probably best treated with concurrent chemotherapy and radiation therapy. Surgery in this subset is best limited to patients who achieve an excellent radiographic response and in whom all disease can be resected without the need for a pneumonectomy. But this requires that radiation therapy be limited to not more than 45 Gy because of the great difficulty in performing complete surgical resections safely following higher doses of radiation that usually result in considerable fibrosis of soft tissue and lung. Most patients in this category are probably best treated with chemotherapy and concurrent definitive (>60 Gy) radiation therapy.
    - Patients with minimal single nodal station N2 disease can be treated either with preoperative (neoadjuvant) or postoperative (adjuvant) chemotherapy, although emerging data make the former a very attractive consideration.
    - Patients with intermediate volume N2 metastases involving one or two nodal stations can be treated with either neoadjuvant chemotherapy alone or with concurrent radiation therapy (45 Gy). As noted earlier, radiation therapy should not be performed in patients requiring a pneumonectomy for complete surgical resections.

## Brief Illustrative Case

- The patient is a 62-year-old man with a 50-pack year history of cigarette smoking who was evaluated for a cough.
- A chest x-ray study revealed a 3- to 4-cm right lower lobe mass.
- A subsequent chest computed tomography (CT) scan confirmed a 3.6-cm mass in the right lower lobe and a 2-cm diameter lymph node in the right pretracheal region, which is consistent with a primary lung neoplasm and mediastinal nodal (N2) metastasis (Fig. 24-1).
- A positron emission tomography scan demonstrated intense hypermetabolic activity confined to the right lower lobe mass, hilum, and right pretracheal nodal regions only.
- Mediastinoscopy with biopsies of R level 2, 4, and 7 lymph node regions confirmed a moderate to poorly differentiated adenocarcinoma involving a right pretracheal lymph node without extranodal spread.
- The patient received three cycles of carboplatin (AUC 5) and paclitaxel (200 mg/m²) administered at 3-week intervals for three successive cycles.
- He tolerated treatment well, with no serious adverse effects.
- A follow-up chest CT scan demonstrated significant interval decrease in the size of the right lower lobe mass that now measured 1.8 cm in maximum diameter with extensive central cavitation. The right pretracheal lymph node that now measured 0.8 cm in diameter with central heterogeneity (Fig. 24-2).
- Four weeks following the third cycle of chemotherapy, the patient underwent a right lower lobectomy and mediastinal lymph node dissection.

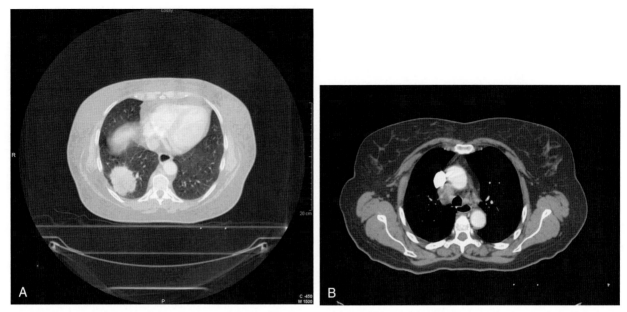

**Figure 24-1:** Preneoadjuvant chemotherapy. **A,** Chest computed tomography scan showing a 3.6 cm mass in the right lower lobe consistent with a primary lung neoplasm and mediastinal nodal (N2) metastasis. **B,** Mediastinal window demonstates a lymph node 2 cm in diameter in the right pretracheal region. (Mediastinoscopy confirms N2 disease.)

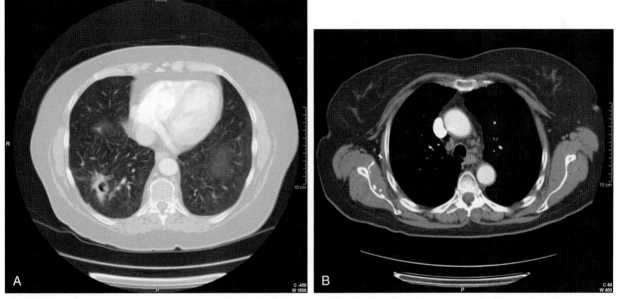

**Figure 24-2:** Postneoadjuvant chemotherapy. **A,** A follow-up chest computed tomography scan demonstrated significant interval decrease in the size of the right lower lobe mass, which now measured 1.8 cm in maximum diameter, with extensive central cavitation. **B,** A follow-up chest CT scan with mediastinal windows demonstates that the right pretracheal lymph node now measured 0.8 cm in diameter with central heterogeneity.

- All hilar and mediastinal lymph nodes were negative for evidence of metastatic disease and the previously involved right pretracheal lymph node demonstrated extensive necrosis (N0).
- The right lower lobe pulmonary mass also demonstrated greater than 90% necrosis with less than 10% viable malignant cells and a maximum tumor diameter of 0.8 cm.

- Neoadjuvant chemotherapy was thus an appropriate modality.
- Significant radiologic and pathologic response to N0 disease and very low residual tumor (<10%) were observed.
- Following appropriate surgical resection, predicted survival would be considerably improved (up to or greater than 40%).

### Key Points

- This patient illustrates a typical patient with N2 disease involving 1 to 2 stations 9 (intermediate volume N2 disease).

### References

Interactive references and additional readings for this chapter can be accessed online at *expertconsult.com*.

# 25 OVERVIEW OF RADIATION THERAPY TERMS AND PROCEDURES IN THE MANAGEMENT OF THORACIC MALIGNANCIES

Amin J. Mirhadi, MD

## INTRODUCTION

### Terminology

- Radiation therapy

### Definition

- Radiation therapy (or radiotherapy [RT]) is the medical use of ionizing radiation as part of cancer treatment to control malignant cells (not to be confused with radiology, the use of radiation in medical imaging and diagnosis).
- RT may be used for curative or adjuvant cancer treatment. It is used as palliative treatment when cure is not possible and the aim is for local disease control or symptomatic relief, or as therapeutic treatment when the therapy has survival benefit and it can be curative.
- RT is commonly used for the treatment of malignant tumors, and may be used as the primary therapy. It is also common to combine RT with surgery, chemotherapy, hormone therapy, or some mixture of the three.
- Most common cancer types can be treated with RT in some way. The precise treatment intent (curative, adjuvant, neoadjuvant, therapeutic, or palliative) will depend on the tumor type, location, and stage, as well as the general health of the patient.
- The radiation fields may also include the draining lymph nodes if they are clinically or radiologically involved with tumor, or if there is thought to be a risk of subclinical malignant spread. It is necessary to include a margin of normal tissue around the tumor to allow for uncertainties in daily set-up and internal tumor motion. These uncertainties can be caused by internal movement (for example, respiration and bladder filling) and movement of external skin marks relative to the tumor position.
- To spare normal tissues (such as skin or organs which radiation must pass through in order to treat the tumor), shaped radiation beams are aimed from several angles of exposure to intersect at the tumor, providing a much larger absorbed dose there than in the surrounding, healthy tissue.

## HISTORICAL PERSPECTIVE

- On November 8, 1895, while passing electricity through a high-vacuum tube, Wilhelm Conrad Roentgen noted the fluorescence of a nearby piece of paper painted with barium cyanide. Because he had wrapped the Crookes tube in heavy opaque paper before beginning the experiment, he realized that this fluorescence of the paper could have been caused by a new, invisible type of ray that the tube was now emitting that was affecting both the shielded walls of the tube and the nearby piece of paper. This is the first known record of the x-ray.[1]
- Roentgen studied the attenuation and the intensity of these x-rays and noted the inverse square law, which describes the loss of intensity of the x-rays with the inverse square of the distance between the tube and the plate.[2]
  - He also noted that he could see the shadow of the bones in his hand when it was placed between the Crookes tube and the fluorescent paper. This led to the first human x-ray film on December 22, 1895, when he placed his wife's hand between the x-ray tube and a photographic plate.
- Roentgen first presented his findings on December 28, 1895 and sent the details of his experiments to physicists throughout the world.[3] Because the x-ray tube was a simple apparatus to replicate, many experiments on x-rays took place within a very short time.
  - This quick, widespread experimentation rapidly produced advances in the new field. Within months of the discovery of x-rays, they were being used diagnostically in hospitals throughout the world. For example, the first medical x-rays at the University of Pennsylvania were taken in February of 1896 (within 3 months of the discovery of the x-ray).
- Almost immediately, the biologic effects of ionizing radiation were recognized. Scientists and workers performing early experiments experienced significant radiation effects. Soon after learning of these, physicians at St. Louis Hospital in Paris began treating patients with radiation. They found that tumors could be eradicated by radium exposure, thus beginning the use of ionizing radiation in the treatment of cancer.
  - The first cure with radiation, involving a patient with basal cell epithelioma, was reported in 1899.[4]
- External beam radiation therapy took longer to develop and might have been abandoned had it not been for the work of Claude Regaud and Henri Coutard. They used smaller doses of radiation in several treatments delivered over several weeks.
  - This eventually gave birth to the concept of fractionated RT, which is the most common form of treatment today.[5]
- With time, ionizing radiation became more precise, and higher energy machines capable of depositing dose at depth were invented. High-energy photons and electrons in the megavoltage range are now available, with accurate treatment planning and delivery. As the technology has progressed, radiation therapy has become increasingly sophisticated, with computer controls to deliver exact and modulated doses to depths and specific areas within the treatment field.
  - Heavy particles—most notably neutrons and protons—are now being used, with even greater accuracy using greatly increased therapeutic ratios.

## THE PHYSICS BEHIND RADIATION ONCOLOGY

To understand radiation oncology, an understanding of the particles and processes involved in the production and delivery of radiation must be attained. The following is an introduction to the physical properties of radiation that are fundamental to the clinical application of radiation to patients.

## Types of Radiation

- Electromagnetic radiation is energy that is transmitted at the speed of light through oscillating electric and magnetic fields. A photon has a wavelength $\lambda$, frequency $v$, and energy $E = hv$, where h is Planck's constant ($6.6 \times 10^{-34}$ Joule seconds).
- The electromagnetic spectrum ranges from wavelengths of $10^5$ m for AM radio waves to $10^{-12}$ m for gamma rays and cosmic rays (Fig. 25-1).
- Although electromagnetic radiation is conventionally described as waves, it is also valid to describe radiation in terms of photons, or particles with packets of energy.
- Because energy varies inversely with wavelength, x-rays have a much greater energy than do radio waves. This high energy gives x-rays the property of being deeply penetrating, and hence, they are able to be used therapeutically to treat deep-seated tumors.[6]
- Radiation used clinically consists of teletherapy, external beam radiation (from an outside source), and brachytherapy (using a source of radiation inserted or implanted into the patient).
- The electromagnetic radiation used in external beam radiation therapy consists of x-rays and gamma rays. They differ only in terms of their production, as gamma rays are produced within the nucleus from natural radioactive decay, and x-rays are produced outside of the nucleus.
- In practice, almost all x-rays are produced by machines (linear accelerators), and gamma rays used in radiation therapy are produced by the decay of radioactive substances. The vast majority of forms of radiation used in the clinic today, whether external beam radiation or brachytherapy, are from x-rays, gamma rays, or electrons.[6]

## Radiation Production by Radioactive Decay

- The nucleus contains protons and neutrons that usually have stable configurations. When these configurations are not stable, they undergo spontaneous transformations to attempt to reach a more stable state.
- These disintegrations of isotopes into a more stable state are called radioactive decay, and the species that undergo these transformations are called radioactive. With these disintegrations, energy is released as a photon (gamma ray), which can be used for radiation therapy.
- The type of radioactive decay and type of particle emitted depend on the nuclear composition of the radioactive species.
- Regardless, the energy released as these decays occur is in the form of gamma rays, and it is these that are (usually) used clinically to deliver radiation dose.[6]
- Cobalt-60 is a very important radioisotope that is used in external beam RT (teletherapy). Cobalt machines were the first practical megavoltage machines and were pioneered by the Canadian physicist, Herbert Johns.[7]
    - The radioactive decay of Cobalt-60 releases 1.2-megavolt (MeV) gamma rays, which represents a major advance in external beam radiation treatment.
- The depth of penetration in tissue increases with increasing x-ray energy, but with x-ray energies up to 250 kilovolts (keV), the maximal dose is always deposited at the skin surface, and thus x-ray doses have always been limited by skin tolerance.
    - This follows from the physics of x-ray interaction with matter, which is discussed in more detail in subsequent sections.
- At energies up to 250 keV, x-rays interact with matter via the photoelectric effect, whereby they interact with the tightly bound electrons close to the nucleus of an atom to cause ionization.
    - This process begins to occur as soon as the photon interacts with matter (i.e., at the skin surface).
- Cobalt-60 machines were simple in design and mechanically highly reliable, and they revolutionized the practice of RT. By their skin-sparing effect, doses of radiation required for treatment could be given safely for the first time without the desquamating skin toxicity that was the hallmark of kilovoltage radiotherapy.
- In time, Cobalt machines in the United States were largely replaced by linear accelerators, which have the advantage of producing more sharply defined beams of a variety of different energies and which can produce both electrons and x-rays.
- Linear accelerators can also be used with devices such as computer-controlled multileaf collimators, allowing much more precise dose delivery. Cobalt machines remain the workhorses of cancer treatment in much of the less developed world, however.

THE ELECTROMAGNETIC SPECTRUM

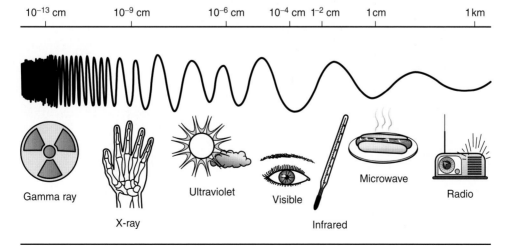

**Figure 25-1:** Electromagnetic spectrum.

## Radiation Production from Linear Accelerators

- Most radiotherapy is delivered with beams of x-rays that were produced by directing highly accelerated electrons into a target.
- Two processes can produce x-rays when electrons are directed onto target atoms.
  ○ The electrons can ionize these atoms by depositing sufficient energy so that an inner shell electron is ejected. The vacancy in the inner shell is filled by an outer shell electron with the release of a photon called a characteristic x-ray. Characteristic x-rays are of low energy and of little utility in therapy.
  ○ Another way of producing x-rays involves the interaction of an electron with the electromagnetic field of a nucleus. This interaction decelerates the electron, with the conservation of energy leading to the production of bremsstrahlung (braking energy) x-rays.
- Before 1950, external beam radiation therapy was accomplished by accelerating electrons in a vacuum tube to hit a target, producing bremsstrahlung x-rays, with a maximum energy of about 300 keV. As just stated, these x-rays are low in energy compared with what is used today, with disadvantages of poor penetration and the deposition of dose maximally at the skin.
- The modern radiation therapy treatment machine is called a linear accelerator.
  ○ These machines use microwaves (with a frequency of 3000 MHz) to accelerate electrons to very high energies.
  ○ These electrons strike an x-ray target (usually tungsten) to produce a beam of (mainly bremsstrahlung) x-rays.
  ○ This x-ray beam is flattened with a flattening filter, so that the beam is uniform throughout, and collimated by the collimator, so that the size of the beam can be selected.
  ○ This high-energy beam is directed at the target volume within the patient, which is made up of the tumor and surrounding tissue that is to be treated (Fig. 25-2).[6]

## Deposition of Dose

- The absorbed dose from an x-ray beam is the measure of the energy deposited by the beam and absorbed by the target.
- The unit of absorbed dose is the Gray (Gy), named after the British radiobiologist L.H. Gray.
  ○ It is defined as the Joules of energy absorbed in a kilogram of tissue (J/kg). Clinical doses are often communicated as centiGray (cGy), equal to the older term of rad.
- Because the amount of radiation absorbed by the target is assumed to be closely related to the observed biologic effects, how and where the dose is deposited is obviously very important.
- As stated previously, x-rays in the megavoltage energy range, such as those used in radiation therapy, exhibit the phenomenon of skin sparing, whereby the dose deposited in tissue is relatively low at the surface but increases rapidly over the first few millimeters. The region of rapidly increasing dose is known as the build-up region. This rapid increase occurs because of the forward-moving photons interacting with electrons of the target tissue via the interactions described previously.
- Linear accelerators typically produce beam energies ranging from 6 to 18 MeV, and the dose at depth increases with beam energy.
- Therefore, an 18 MeV photon beam would deliver more dose to a given depth in a patient than would a 6 MeV photon beam.
  ○ An 18 MeV beam would also show more skin sparing (i.e., it would have a greater $D_{max}$).
- Another aspect that affects the depth dose is the size of the field of radiation used to treat the patient. With a larger field size, there is greater scattering of photons within the field during the interactions with electrons.
- This scatter effect leads to more interactions, which translates into a higher deposition of dose at depth.
  ○ In other words, the dose at 10 cm depth within a patient from a photon beam that has a field size of 20 cm × 20 cm

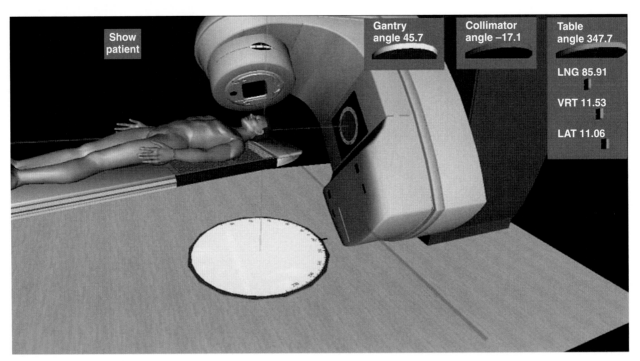

**Figure 25-2:** Linear accelerator.

would be higher than the same photon beam with a field size of 5 cm × 5 cm.

- Many other factors go into the calculation of dose delivered at varying depths in a patient, including scatter from the collimators in the machine, blocks to shield normal tissue, and wedges and compensators (which are used to shape the photon beam).
- Another main modifier in the target tissue that affects dose at depth is the density of the tissue being treated.
  - ○ Lung, for example, being less dense than soft tissue, allows more photon transmission.[6]

## THE BIOLOGIC BASIS OF RADIATION ONCOLOGY

- The basic understanding of the physical properties of a radiation beam must be coupled with an understanding of how radiation interacts with biologic tissues to cause damage. Through interactions with biologic tissue, radiation deposits energy as it travels through the patient. These interactions set secondary electrons in motion that go on to produce further ionizations. This ultimately results in the breaking of chemical bonds and damage to molecules and structures within the cell. If these broken bonds and subsequent damage occur to cells' critical structures, the most significant effect of the accumulation of radiation damage will be cell killing.
- This process is obviously not as simple as just described. The deposition of radiation dose and the damage it induces is random and complex, and depends on many aspects of both the radiation and the biologic tissue.

### Interactions with Biologic Materials

- Cell killing occurs when critical targets within the cell are damaged by radiation. Therefore, radiation that deposits dose near critical structures is more likely to incur a biologic effect.
- A number of biologic molecules or structures are potential targets for radiation damage, and there is still lively debate within the field as to whether there are multiple targets within the cell.
- Many circumstantial data indicate that DNA is the critical target for the biologic effects of radiation, although this speculation remains without definitive proof. Measurement of DNA damage after radiation closely correlates with cell lethality.[8]
- Cells that are inhibited from repairing DNA damage or that are naturally deficient in DNA repair enzymes show a distinct radiosensitivity
- Also, experiments in which the nucleus was irradiated selectively show that radiation caused cell death at a higher rate than did radiation of the cytoplasm.[9-10]
- DNA damage can be termed direct or indirect. If radiation is absorbed by the DNA itself, the atoms of the DNA can become ionized and damaged.
- This is termed the direct effect of radiation. Because the width of DNA is 1 to 4 nm and there is relatively little DNA in the cell, direct damage must be a relatively infrequent event.
- More commonly, water molecules surrounding the DNA are ionized by the radiation. The ionization of water creates hydroxyl radicals, peroxide, hydrated electrons, and oxygen radicals. All of these species are highly reactive free radicals. These radicals, in turn, interact with the DNA and cause damage. This is termed indirect damage.
- Eighty percent of a cell is composed of water, making indirect damage a much more common event.[11]

- ○ Direct and indirect damage work to cause broken bonds in the DNA backbone.
- ○ These broken bonds can result in the loss of a base or of the entire nucleotide, or in complete breaking of one or both of the strands of DNA. Single-strand breaks are easily repaired using the opposite strand as a template.
- ○ Therefore, single-strand breaks show little relation to cell killing, although they might result in mutation if the repair is incorrect.
  - ○ Double-strand breaks, on the other hand, are thought to be the most important lesion in DNA produced by radiation. Double-strand breaks, as the name implies, results in the chromatin being snapped into two pieces.
  - ○ These double-strand breaks can result in mutations or, most important, in cell killing. Because x-rays are sparsely ionizing, there can be random stochastic processes in regions within the cell where ionization events are much more densely clustered than in other areas.
  - ○ The free radicals produced are also thought to be clustered in discrete areas.
  - ○ Therefore, the multiple broken bonds and resultant DNA damage that occurs could be highly localized. The term *locally multiply damaged site*, coined by John Ward, or the cluster hypothesis described by Goodhead refers to this phenomenon, and Ward suggests that it is these clustered regions of DNA damage that lead to clinically significant effects.[12-13]
- Most investigators believe that the dominant form of lethal radiation-induced DNA damage is the double-strand break, which ultimately results in mitotic death. In surviving irradiated cells, chromosomal aberrations such as nondisjunctions and micronuclei are detectable.
- Radiation controls cancer cells through at least three main effects:
  - ○ Inducing apoptosis.
  - ○ Causing permanent cell cycle arrest or terminal differentiation.
  - ○ Inducing cells to die of mitotic catastrophe.
    1. Apoptosis is also known as "programmed cell death." The triggering of cell death is a process frequently seen in normal development, differentiation, immune responses, menstruation, neuronal development, and tissue turnover, and it also can be triggered by several noxious stimuli, including ionizing radiation. In this case, radiation damage triggers signaling cascades that invoke pre-existing mechanisms by which the cell self-destructs. Cells undergoing apoptosis show very characteristic features as they die, including dramatic blebbing and fragmentation of the nucleus. Radiation with doses typically used in the clinic often induces apoptosis in lymphomas and other malignancies of hematopoetic origin. In contrast, apoptosis is far less commonly seen in tumors of epithelial origin, such as head and neck squamous cell cancers. Tumors that commonly undergo apoptosis often have a brisk clinical response to radiation therapy.[14-15]
    2. All of these factors must be taken into consideration when a fractionation scheme is being designed. Although the "standard" fractionation schedule differs in many parts of the world, 1.8 to 2.0 Gy per day is considered the conventional fractionation schedule in the United States. Most regimens that deviate from this norm use more than one fraction in a day. This reduces both the size of the fraction and the total treatment time, to take advantage of the radiobiologic principles as they apply to early-responding tissues (and tumors) and to late-responding tissues as described previously.

## Altered Fractionation Schemes

- The standard of five fractions per week and 9 to 10 Gy of dose per week has evolved not as a biologically designed, optimal method of administration of radiation but rather from considerations such as the convenience of patients and staff, the availability of equipment, and financial concerns.
- Outside of the United States, the same nonmedical constraints have often dictated other fractionation regimens that usually employ fewer fractions over a shorter time period because of limited availability of high-energy treatment machines or trained radiation oncologists.
- In the 1990s, more attention was paid to attempts to alter the customary fractionation protocols toward schemes that would improve the biologic outcome from treatment, either through increased tumor sterilization or decreased normal tissue toxicity, or both.
- These attempts were undertaken because of the knowledge that the effects of radiation on acutely reacting tissues (e.g., skin and mucosa) are different from those on late-reacting tissues. Early-reacting tissues, which determine the patient's tolerance to treatment, are time dependent in their reactions.
- Because these tissues proliferate rapidly, prolonging the total time of therapy allows proliferation to take place and thus lessens the severity of the overall reaction. This is especially true about breaks (days off) from treatment, during which a mucosal or skin reaction can heal substantially in just a few days. Late-reacting tissues do not proliferate during a 6- to 7-week course of treatment, and their reaction is thus not sensitive to overall treatment time.
- Late-reacting tissues are very sensitive to fraction size, however. It is now clear from a number of clinical studies that for the same total dose, late reactions are worse when large fractions are used compared with smaller ones. This is understandable from the shape of the cell survival curves for early- and late-reacting tissue. Late-reacting tissues have low $\alpha/\beta$ ratios, and their survival curves bend at higher doses, causing a substantial difference in cell kill with large rather than small fractions.
- With little proliferation to make up the difference, the tissues become fraction-size dependent. If large fractions are used, the total dose must be lowered to achieve the same effect on long-term toxicity.
- Clinical examples of this effect are found most often in palliative regimens, in which 20 Gy in five fractions or 30 Gy in 10 fractions are given to spinal metastases and equate with 50 Gy in 25 fractions for spinal cord tolerance.
- Many Canadian and European centers give fewer numbers of larger fractions for curative treatment as well, reducing total dose for the sake of not amplifying late toxicity. It becomes clear that a few large fractions preferentially damage late-reacting tissues, whereas larger numbers of smaller fractions preferentially spare them.
- The other side of this coin is tumor proliferation. If many small fractions are used and the time it takes to deliver a course of radiation is protracted, tumor proliferation could negate any gains. When the aims are to both take advantage of the sparing of late tissue damage and avoid having treatment last for too many days, treatment has been given with multiple fractions per days.[16-18]

## *THE EFFECTS OF RADIATION ON NORMAL TISSUES*

- The goal of all investigations into the physical aspects and biologic principles behind radiation therapy is to attempt to increase the therapeutic index, which is defined as the tumor response for a fixed level of normal tissue damage. Or to restate it another way, the goal is to increase tumor cell kill and hence tumor control while maintaining normal tissue toxicity within a tolerable range.
- Obviously, acute toxicity (encountered during treatment) is a concern and must be managed aggressively to ensure that the patient is able to complete the course of radiation therapy. When discussing normal tissue toxicity, however, late effects, which translate into end-organ damage, are usually considered the dose-limiting toxicity.
- All organs have a threshold for normal tissue toxicity. These thresholds, though, often lack rigidity and are poorly defined, as they depend on the interaction of many factors. The most important factors in terms of normal tissue tolerance and toxicity are total dose delivered and the volume of the organ exposed to this dose. Calculating this relationship for normal tissue is not as simple as it is for tumors, however.
- When speaking in terms of tumor cure, the fraction of cells surviving determines the success of treatment, because a single surviving cell might suffice for regrowth of the tumor.
- For normal tissues, the tolerance is greatly dependent on the ability of stem cells to maintain a sufficient number of mature cells for proper organ function. This statement is an oversimplification, however, because the tolerance of an organ also depends on the structural organization of the organ, which some have termed functional subunits. For example, consider the kidney and the spinal cord. If radiation permanently damages a number of nephrons, the end-organ function might not be affected as long as enough nephrons remain to maintain function.
- The functional subunits of the kidney, then, are said to be arranged in parallel. On the other hand, if one section of the spinal cord is damaged, the entire cord distal to the lesion will be disrupted. Organs such as the spinal cord, in which damage to one portion of the organ affects the function of the entire organ, have what is called serial functional subunits.
- Functional subunits have yet to be identified for many organs, and the use of functional subunits to describe radiation tolerance of many organs remains a hypothesis. We can say, however, that as the irradiated volume of an organ increases, the complications increase.
- Although the volume of the organ that is exposed to radiation is important, this might not be observed as toxicity if the total dose delivered remains below the dose that would damage the normal tissue in question. The concept of a threshold for total dose exposure becomes an important concept as we attempt to escalate dose to increase tumor control. Clinical and in vitro data are consistent with the view that increased dose kills more cells, although few clinical trials have demonstrated this directly. Retrospective data, however, have confirmed a dose response in many clinical sites, including head and neck, Hodgkin's disease, high-grade glioma, non–small cell lung cancer (NSCLC), prostate cancer, breast cancer, and cervical cancer.
- Therefore, the total dose to the tumor and the volume of normal tissue treated must be considered when designing a radiation treatment course. Success might be possible in any tumor, regardless of size and histology, if sufficiently high doses are used. Clinically, however, this consideration must be balanced against the toxicity that would result to normal tissue. To increase the therapeutic ratio, many of the radiobiologic and physical principles of radiation have been used. These include all that have been described, such as tumor localization, choosing the optimal energy and radiation modality, manipulating the dose rate, fractionation schemes, and the use of radiosensitizers and radioprotectors or targeted therapies. All are dependent on the accurate localization of the tumor and the accurate delivery of the radiation.[19-22]

## Acute Effects on Normal Tissues

- The acute effects of radiation result from direct damage to parenchymal cells of organs that are sensitive to radiation. For purposes of discussion, an acute effect is defined as an effect seen during treatment and up to 3 months after the conclusion of therapy. A detailed discussion of this subject is beyond the scope of this chapter, but it has been reviewed elsewhere.[23]

## Late Effects on Normal Tissues

- Late effects are those that occur 3 months or longer after the end of therapy. Virtually any organ or tissue that is treated can express a syndrome of late radiation damage. The etiology of late damage is debated. Some believe that it is due to slow dropout of small vasculature, leading to organ cell loss, fibrosis, and eventual late organ failure. Evidence for this viewpoint is supplied by morphologic studies of irradiated tissues where decreased vascularity can be observed in virtually every tissue type. Others believe that late damage is due in large part to direct damage to parenchymal cells. This theory is plausible, because organs have widely differing sensitivities to radiation, but there is little evidence to suggest that blood vessels in one part of the body are more or less radiosensitive than in any other part. Thus, if vascular damage were a final common pathway, then most organs should share similar radiation tolerance doses, and they do not. In all likelihood, late damage represents a combination of vascular damage and direct organ cell depletion.[24-25]

## THE CLINICAL APPLICATION OF RADIATION THERAPY

- After evaluation of the patient has been done and the decision to use radiation has been made, perhaps the most important step in a radiation treatment course is the design of the radiation treatment itself. Advances are constantly being investigated, with the aim of increasing the therapeutic ratio in radiation therapy. Many of the largest advances have been in the technology used to deliver radiation. The concept is that if a higher dose of radiation can be delivered to the tumor volume with respect to the surrounding normal tissues, radiation can be delivered with less toxicity or a greater dose can be delivered to the target volume with the same toxicity. These goals constitute the basis for these investigations.

## Treatment Planning and Set-Up

- Successful treatment planning is imperative to the success of a radiation treatment course. The goal is to identify the full extent of the tumor and areas of possible spread. Several considerations must be taken into account when considering this volume. These include the tumor histology, the extent of the gross disease, regions of microscopic spread but no gross disease, whether the treatment is being given postoperatively or in an undisturbed tumor bed, and the tolerances of adjacent structures. A plan must then be devised to treat this entire region to the dose desired for each region while keeping the volume of each normal tissue below its tolerance dose.
- At one time, radiation treatment was performed by placing the patient directly on the treatment machine and setting up the fields for radiation treatment using surface anatomic landmarks. Although some radiation oncologists became highly skillful at this process and it is still occasionally used in emergency situations, it is obviously an uncertain process with

many possibilities for error. In the modern era, the process of designing a radiation field starts with the simulation. In simulation, the treatment fields are designed for the patient before treatment is initiated. Simulation is used to determine the extent of disease and its relationship to other organs. The earliest simulators were fluoroscopy units designed to mimic the geometry of the treatment machines. The oncologist could thus obtain a "beam's eye view" of what would be included in the treatment field. Fluoroscopy was used to outline the boundaries of the field, with plain film x-rays being taken to include the general outline of the area to be treated. Although fluoroscopic simulators are still in use and efficacious, many three-dimensional (3D) treatment planning systems to design conformal radiation treatment plans are now available to radiation oncologists. 3D treatment planning systems use computed tomography (CT) (or in some cases magnetic resonance imaging [MRI] or even positron emission tomography [PET]) data to assist in setting up the radiation fields. This can be accomplished generally by three different methods:
- ○ The field can be set up by transferring CT data onto conventional simulation films.
- ○ CT images can be transferred to a computer-based treatment planning system. The fields are designed using the CT-based planning system, with verification done by taking films on a conventional simulator.
- ○ The third and most efficient method is to use a CT simulator to set up the radiation fields. The CT simulator combines the processes of obtaining CT images and field design into a single process. CT images of the patient are transferred directly to a computer system that allows the physician to outline the tumor volume and critical structures on individual CT slices. This, in effect, creates an accurate 3D recreation of both the patient's tumor that is to be treated and of normal tissues that are to be avoided during the delivery of radiation.

## Established Techniques
### Three-Dimensional Conformal Radiotherapy

- After the image data sets are obtained in any type of simulation, careful review of the clinical data must be done to delineate the tissue in need of treatment. This volume to be treated is defined as the target volume and is created by adding three components together. First, the gross tumor volume is noted. This volume is expanded to create the clinical tumor volume by accounting for the areas at risk for spread, such as adjacent tissues or draining lymphatic regions. The planning tumor volume (PTV) is reached by adding margin to correct for possible variability in daily positioning and patient motion during treatment.
- The remainder of the planning process involves choosing the number of radiation beams required, the energy of these beams, and the angles and weighting of these beams needed to deliver the required radiation dose to the tumor with optimal sparing of normal tissues. After these beams are designed, digitally reconstructed radiographs are produced to reflect the designed treatment fields. The availability of 3D treatment planning has allowed for greatly increased complexity of plans in the attempt to increase the therapeutic ratio via the designing of radiation fields, because the doses to the tumor and normal organs can be evaluated accurately and three-dimensionally. This evaluation process allows assessment of the possible toxicity that could result from the radiation treatment via the evaluation of a dose volume histogram, which shows the dose delivered throughout the volume of the organ. Although it is never acceptable to treat an entire organ beyond its tolerance, there are circumstances when portions of an

organ may be treated to close to or even beyond its tolerance. A consideration here is whether the organ in question is considered to have a serial or parallel structure. In an organ with a serial structure, failure of any component of the organ will cause failure of the entire organ. An example of this might be the spinal cord, where taking any segment of the cord beyond cord tolerance will cause failure of everything downstream. In a parallel organ, such as the lung or kidney, the patient might be able to tolerate loss of part of the organ's function, provided certain volume considerations are not exceeded.

■ Normal tissues are shielded from the radiation beams in various ways. The first shields or blocks were simply handplaced pieces of lead or depleted uranium that were inserted in the radiation field to shield the structures below them. When Powers invented a low-melting-point alloy of lead with similar beam-attenuating properties, it became possible to create complex blocks that followed the divergent properties of the beam to more accurately shield organs defined on the simulation films. Blocks were then custom made for each patient. A newer method of shielding is with the use of a multileaf collimator. The multileaf collimator system uses 1-cm or 0.5-cm "leaves" that are actually partitioned jaws of the collimator of the treatment machine. These leaves can be moved to block the radiation field to effectively shape the field as desired.

■ Once treatment planning is completed, the patient begins the course of radiation therapy. The first step is to set up the patient to verify the simulation fields on the actual treatment machine. Each day, the patient is repositioned into the exact position in which the simulation and subsequent treatment planning were done. To aid in the repositioning, immobilization devices are often used, consisting of foam body casts or plastic head masks. These are made before simulation and are kept for use throughout the entire radiation course. Laser lights that converge on the exact isocenter (the point around which the treatment machine rotates) of the treatment machine are available within the treatment room and are used to assist in this repositioning. Because 3D techniques allow for greater refinement of treatment volumes and of the increasing complexity of plans, exact daily repositioning is absolutely imperative. A course of radiation can be any number of fractions, although in palliative cases, it is usually between five and 15 fractions, with curative treatments often being between 25 and 40 fractions. Treatment is almost always delivered with five daily fractions per week, but accelerating treatment beyond this has shown some efficacy, although in some cases, it has resulted in increased toxicity (Fig. 25-3).[6,26-28]

### Modulated Radiotherapy

■ Radiation oncology has striven to deliver the dose to the tumor ever more precisely and to diminish the dose to adjacent normal structures. The linear accelerator offered the ability to deliver shaped uniform beams from multiple angles as it rotated about the patient and represented a major step forward toward reaching this goal. The introduction of the multileaf collimator, whereby the machine itself (rather than an added beam-shaping device) shapes the beams, increased the efficiency of this process. Now, radiation oncologists and physicists are attempting to push this technology one step further. Because the leaves in a multileaf collimator are computer driven, it becomes possible to move the leaves continuously during treatment. Treatment thus becomes four-dimensional (in both time and space) rather than 3D and allows for the selection of beams that are deliberately nonuniform, to deliver

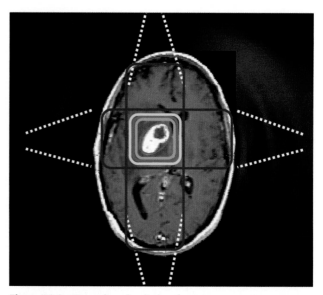

**Figure 25-3:** 3D conformal radiation therapy.

varying doses to varying parts of the treatment field. The CT simulator allows the patient to be simulated for treatment in virtual time rather than in real time, allowing the physician or a computer program under the physician's control to evaluate dozens (if not hundreds) of treatment plans to optimize the dose to the tumor. The beams chosen need no longer be coplanar in such a system. This technology forms the basis for what has become known as intensity-modulated radiation therapy. Intensity-modulated radiotherapy (IMRT) is based on the use of several noncoplanar radiation beam intensities incident on the patient to achieve a shaped, irregular dose distribution. It represents the state of the art in technologic advancements in the field of radiation oncology in manipulation of dose distributions and represents an advance on 3D conformal radiation treatments.

■ Many authors have completed treatment planning comparisons between IMRT plans and conventional treatment plans. These have been followed by publications that have emphasized clinical endpoints in patients treated with IMRT. The entire goal of IMRT is to increase the therapeutic ratio, delivering a higher tumor dose relative to normal tissues. Keeping this in mind, IMRT can be used to escalate the tumor volume to a higher dose while maintaining normal tissue toxicity at the same level. Among the sites and cancers investigated using IMRT to escalate total dose are NSCLC, intracranial tumors, and prostate cancer. Alternatively, IMRT can be used to deliver conventional doses to the tumor bed, resulting in lower dose to normal tissues, with hopes of reducing toxicity. This strategy has been reported on in patients with breast cancer, head and neck cancer, mesothelioma, pancreatic cancer, and gynecologic cancers. Many of these studies report favorable outcomes or dose distributions that conceivably would result in decreased toxicity, although no definitive study has conclusively demonstrated the clinical impact of IMRT. The dose distributions made possible by IMRT's planning and treatment delivery, however, show a significant potential for improvement in clinical outcomes.

■ IMRT is very much an evolving technique at this time and carries with it a number of potentially difficult problems that still need to be addressed. With IMRT, it is much more difficult than with 3D conformal therapy to verify that treatment has been delivered correctly to the patient. If there is organ motion, and virtually every organ below the calvarium is in motion, then there is a possibility that the dose delivered differs significantly from the dose planned, because planning was done on static images. Finally, as more beams are added to the treatment and the daily treatment time increases, then although less normal tissue will be treated to tolerance doses, the volume of normal tissue that receives some dose of radiation in fact increases, as does the total-body dose of radiation. It remains to be seen how significant these problems will be to the development of this new technology (Fig. 25-4).[29-32]

### Proton Therapy

- Although protons have a slightly higher linear energy transfer than x-rays, they are not generally considered as high linear energy transfer particles. They achieve most of their advantage over x-rays in their physical dose distribution. When a heavy, charged particle, such as a proton, passes through tissue, the dose it deposits increases slowly with depth, then reaches a sharp increase at its maximum depth of penetration. This is called the Bragg peak. The maximum depth of penetration can be adjusted by varying the energy of the proton beam or by adding or removing compensating material placed in the path of the beam. Frequently, in clinical use, the Bragg peak is spread out in depth using specialized filters to achieve the dose deposition pattern desired, but still with the sharp dose fall-off at the deep edge of the beam. Using multiple beams or varying compensators, it is possible to design a 3D dose deposition that is precisely confined to the tumor volume with minimal dose to the surrounding normal tissue.
- The majority of patients treated with proton therapy have been patients whose tumors are in close proximity to critical structures. The precise dose deposition patterns made it possible to treat these tumors without crossing the threshold of toxicity of the normal structures.
- Proton therapy is one of the most promising modalities that have resulted from technologic advances in the field of radiation oncology. It represents the optimal therapeutic ratio available in terms of dose delivery. Therefore, although neutron therapy

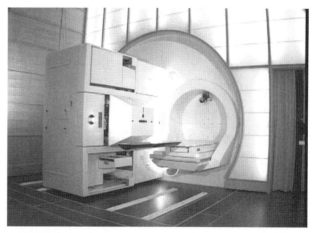

**Figure 25-5:** Proton therapy unit.

is falling out of favor in the radiation community, research into proton therapy dose planning and delivery continues to grow (Fig. 25-5).[33]

## Newer Techniques
### Image-Guided Radiation Therapy

- Image-guided radiation therapy (IGRT) is the process of frequent 2D and 3D imaging, during a course of radiation treatment, used to direct radiation therapy utilizing the imaging coordinates of the actual radiation treatment plan. The patient is localized in the treatment room in the same position as planned from the reference imaging dataset. 3D IGRT would include localization of a *cone-beam computed tomography* (CBCT) dataset with the planning CT dataset from planning for example. -2D IGRT would include matching planar kilovoltage (kV) radiographs *fluoroscopy* or megavoltage (MV) images with digital reconstructed radiographs from the planning CT.
- This process is distinct from the use of imaging to delineate targets and organs in the planning process of radiation therapy. However, there is clearly a connection between the imaging processes because IGRT relies directly on the imaging modalities from planning as the reference coordinates for localizing the patient. The variety of image gathering hardware used in planning includes CT, MRI, and PET, among others. Through advancements in imaging technology, combined with a further understanding of human biology at the molecular level, the impact of IGRT on radiotherapy treatment continues to evolve (Fig. 25-6).[34]
- Goals and clinical benefits
  - The goal of the IGRT process is to improve the accuracy of the radiation field placement, and to reduce the exposure of healthy tissue during radiation treatments. In years past, larger PTV margins were used to compensate for localization errors during treatment. This resulted in healthy human tissues receiving unnecessary doses of radiation during treatment. PTV margins are the most widely used method to correct geometric uncertainties. By improving precision and accuracy through IGRT, radiation is decreased to surrounding healthy tissues, allowing for increased radiation to the tumor for control.
  - At present, certain radiation therapy techniques employ the process of IMRT. This form of radiation treatment uses computers and linear accelerators to sculpt a 3D radiation dose map specific to the target's location, shape, and motion characteristics. Because of the level of precision required for IMRT, detailed data must be gathered about

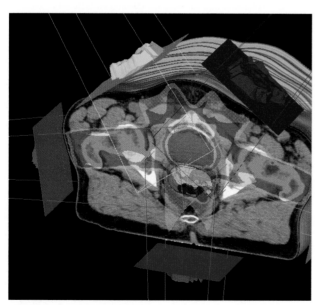

**Figure 25-4:** An intensity-modulated radiotherapy plan.

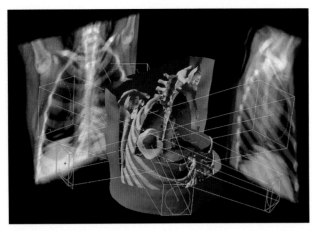

**Figure 25-6:** Using imaging during treatment (image-guided radiation therapy).

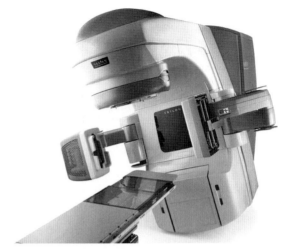

**Figure 25-7:** The Trilogy system.

tumor locations. The single most important area of innovation in clinical practice is the reduction of the PVT margins around the location. The ability to avoid more normal tissue or employ dose escalation strategies is a direct byproduct of the ability to execute therapy with the most accurate geometric precision.

○ IGRT will continue to increase the amount of data collected throughout the course of therapy. Over the course of time, whether for an individual or a population of patients, this information will allow for the continued assessment and further refinement of treatment techniques. The clinical benefit for the patient is the ability to monitor and adapt to changes that may occur during the course of radiation treatment. Such changes can include tumor shrinkage or expansion, or changes in shape of the tumor and surrounding anatomy.[35]

■ Rationale for IGRT
  ○ There are many factors that may contribute to differences between the planned dose distribution and the delivered dose distribution. One such factor is uncertainty of patient position on the treatment unit. IGRT is a component of the radiation therapy process that incorporates imaging coordinates from the treatment plan to be delivered in order to ensure the patient is properly aligned in the treatment room.[36]
    ■ Trilogy System: The system (Fig. 25-7) is an advanced linear accelerator with IGRT capabilities. It also has the capacity to integrate many other features that enhance target localization and allow for more aggressive treatment approaches. The following features are noteworthy:
      ○ Cone beam CT: CBCT-based image-guided systems have been integrated with medical linear accelerators to great success. With improvements in flat-panel technology, CBCT has been able to provide volumetric imaging and allows for radiographic or fluoroscopic monitoring throughout the treatment process. CBCT acquires many projections over the entire volume of interest in each projection. Using reconstruction strategies pioneered by Feldkamp, the 2D projections are reconstructed into a 3D volume analogous to the CT planning dataset.
      ○ Optical tracking: The use of a camera to relay positional information of objects within its inherent coordinate system by means of a subset of the electromagnetic spectrum of wavelengths spanning ultraviolet, visible, and infrared light. Optical

navigation has been in use for the last 10 years within image-guided surgery (neurosurgery, ear, nose, and throat, and orthopaedic) and has increased in prevalence within radiotherapy to provide real-time feedback through visual cues on graphical user interfaces. For the latter, a method of calibration is used to align the camera's native coordinate system with that of the isocentric reference frame of the radiation treatment delivery room. Optically tracked tools are then used to identify the positions of patient reference set-up points and these are compared with their location within the planning CT coordinate system. A computation based on least-squares methodology is performed using these two sets of coordinates to determine a treatment couch translation that will result in the alignment of the patient's planned isocenter with that of the treatment room. These tools can also be used for intrafraction monitoring of patient position by placing an optically tracked tool on a region of interest to either initiate radiation delivery (i.e., gating regimes) or action (i.e., repositioning).[37]

■ Cyberknife: CyberKnife (Fig. 25-8) is the name of a frameless robotic *radiosurgery* system invented by John R. Adler, a Stanford University Professor of Neurosurgery and Radiation Oncology. Numerous CyberKnife systems have been installed around the world, for example in China, Japan, Italy, and the United States. Many of the prestigious American University Medical Centers operate a CyberKnife system. Examples are the Stanford Blake Wilbur CyberKnife Center and at the Comprehensive Cancer Center at Stanford University, Georgetown University Hospital, University of California-San Francisco Medical Center, and the University of Pittsburgh. Stanford University has treated more than 2500 patients using the CyberKnife system, and worldwide, more than 15,000 patients have been treated.

■ Several generations of the CyberKnife system have been developed since its initial inception in 1990. There are two essential features of the CyberKnife system that set it apart from other stereotactic methods.
  ○ Robotic mounting: The first is the fact that the radiation source is mounted on a precisely controlled industrial robot. The original CyberKnife used a Fanuc robot; however, the more modern systems use a Kuka

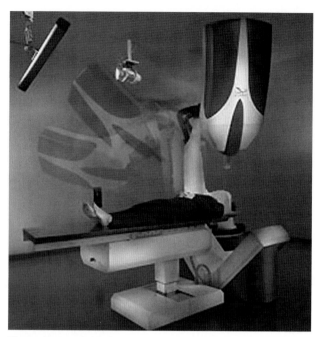

**Figure 25-8:** CyberKnife.

240. Mounted on the robot is a compact X-band linac that produces 6MV x-ray radiation. The linac is capable of delivering approximately 600 cGy of radiation each minute. The radiation is collimated using tungsten collimators (also referred to as cones), which produce circular radiation fields. At present, the radiation field sizes are 5 mm, 7.5 mm, 10 mm, 12.5 mm, 15 mm, 20 mm, 25 mm, 30 mm, 35 mm, 40 mm, 50 mm, and 60 mm. Mounting the radiation source on the robot allows complete freedom to position the radiation within a sphere about the patient. The robotic mounting allows very fast repositioning of the source, which allows the system to deliver radiation from many different directions, which is impossible using a conventional gantry-based linear accelerator system due to the mechanical limitations of the gantry.

○ Synchrony: The second technology of image guidance that the CyberKnife system can use is called the Synchrony System. The Synchrony System is used primarily for tumors that are in motion while being treated, such as lung tumors and pancreatic tumors. The Synchrony System uses a combination of surgically placed internal fiducials and light-emitting optical fibers (markers) mounted on the patient skin. Because the tumor is moving continuously, to continuously image its location using x-ray cameras would require prohibitive amounts of radiation to be delivered to the patient's skin. The Synchrony System overcomes this by periodically taking images of the internal fiducials, and predicting their location at a future time using the motion of the markers that are located on the patient's skin. The light from the markers can be tracked continuously using a camera, and the markers are placed so that their motion is correlated with the motion of the tumor. A computer algorithm creates a correlation model that represents how the internal fiducial markers are moving compared with the

external markers. Therefore, the Synchrony System is continuously predicting the motion of the internal fiducials, and therefore, the tumor, based on the motion of the markers. The correlation model can be updated at any time if the patient's breathing becomes irregular in any way. The advantage of the Synchrony System is that no assumptions about the regularity or reproducibility of the patient's breathing have to be made. To function properly, the Synchrony System requires that for any given correlation model, there is a functional relationship between the markers and the internal fiducials. The external marker placement is also important, and the markers are usually placed on the patient's abdomen, so that the motion will reflect the internal motion of the diaphragm and the lungs.[38-40]

### Brachytherapy

- Some patients with cancer in the lung need an alternative treatment to a lobectomy when pulmonary function is poor. A lobectomy is preferred over a wedge resection for a stage I lung cancer because the latter has a higher local recurrence rate and a lower survival.[41-44] For patients with pulmonary function that precludes a lobectomy, alternative treatment options include radiofrequency ablation, external beam radiation, stereotactic radiation, and wedge resection with brachytherapy.

- Brachytherapy is the direct placement of a decaying radioactive source directly against a tumor using catheters that house the source (Fig. 25-9). Depending on the source, the radiation can be delivered at a rapid rate (high-dose rate brachytherapy) or at a reduced rate (low-dose rate brachytherapy). Both techniques have wide-ranging clinical applications, but high-dose rate brachytherapy is rapidly becoming the application of choice in lung cancer.

- Brachytherapy after wedge resection has been shown to reduce the rate of local recurrence after wedge resection alone.[45-47] One approach for the brachytherapy has been to sew radioactive seeds in a mesh that is then placed on the lung at the resection margin.[45,47] As an alternative, afterload catheters can be sewn on the resection margin and the radioactive seeds are passed into the catheters for short time intervals for a few days, and then the catheters are removed.

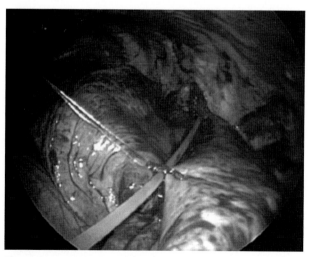

**Figure 25-9:** Brachytherapy.

■ McKenna and colleagues evaluated the efficacy of high-dose rate brachytherapy in 48 patients who underwent wedge resection.[48] They concluded that, in the short term, wedge resection and brachytherapy with afterload catheters appears to be a safe treatment for lung cancer in patients in whom a lobectomy is not advisable because of poor pulmonary function. Long-term follow-up is needed to determine the cure rate for wedge resection and brachytherapy, however.

### Stereotactic Lung Radiosurgery

■ Although surgical resection is the preferred approach for patients with early stage primary NSCLC, radiotherapy (RT) is used in patients who are not candidates for surgery. Previous experience with conventional external beam RT showed that control of the primary lesion is directly related to the dose of radiation, suggesting that higher doses might offer better local control.

■ Lung radiosurgery has been extensively evaluated in patients with early stage primary NSCLC.[49-51] Stereotactic body RT (SBRT) dosing is influenced by a number of parameters, including the size of the tumor and the number of fractions, and the optimal dose and fractionation schedule is not yet known.

■ In the largest reported experience, 300 patients with stage I NSCLC were treated at multiple institutions with varying doses and schedules, ranging from 18 to 75 Gy in 1 to 22 fractions.[49] The rate of local recurrence was 15%, and a dose-response relationship was found for a biologic equivalent dose (BED) 100 Gy versus less than 100 Gy (recurrence rate, 14% versus 33%). Among medically operable patients, the 5-year survival rate was significantly higher in those treated with BED 100 Gy (74 versus 37 percent, compared to a BED <100 Gy).

  ○ Toxicity

    ■ Although direct comparisons are not possible, use of detailed modeling suggests that the doses used with SBRT are biologically equal to or greater than those used with conventional fractionated RT, and SBRT has generally been associated with an acceptable toxicity profile.[52]

    ■ The lung parenchyma generally tolerates the high fractional and total doses used in SBRT. Although radiographic evidence of asymptomatic radiation pneumonitis and radiation fibrosis have been identified in more than 60% of cases in most series, symptomatic or disabling pneumonitis is rare. Despite this, pulmonary function studies have not found a decline in $FEV_1$ or carbon monoxide diffusing capacity (DLCO) values following therapy. Total lung capacity, vital capacity, and forced expiratory volume were unchanged 1 year after SBRT, whereas DLCO improved in patients who had been heavy smokers before treatment.[53-55]

    ■ Other thoracic tissues may be more sensitive than lung parenchyma. Reported complications have included bronchial stenosis, rib fracture or chest wall pain, esophageal ulceration, and perforation and pulmonary artery bleeding.[56,57]

■ Treatment of lesions in the perihilar and mediastinal region has been associated with an increased risk of serious toxicity compared to peripheral lesions. In a series of 70 patients with stage I NSCLC treated with a total of 60 to 66 Gy in three fractions, the 2-year incidence of severe toxicity was higher in patients with central lesions (46% versus 17% in those with peripheral lesions).[58]

## Brief Illustrative Case

- A 75-year-old smoker presented with a 2.5-cm spiculated mass in his right upper lobe on a screening computed tomography scan (CT) for coronary calcification analysis.
- This was shown to be a NSCLC on needle aspiration cytology. Bronchoscopy revealed no endobronchial lesions.
- Comprehensive workup culminated in the tumor being clinical staged as stage 1a (i.e., T1N0).
- Chest CT revealed extensive homogeneously distributed emphysema.
- Pulmonary function studies revealed an $FEV_1$ of 0.62 L.
- Thus, although he was potentially resectable for cure, his poor pulmonary reserve and underlying coronary artery disease made him inoperable (i.e., serious comorbidities precluded resectional surgery).
- He was thus managed with stereotactic lung radiosurgery using IGRT. This delivers three very large fractions of radition to the tumor only, with a very sharp fall off of radiation immediately around the tumor. Without IGRT, it would be difficult to accomplish this because the targeting would be imprecise.

### Key Points

- This approach is unlikely to be curative. However in the presence of the patient's serious comorbidites, the patient may well succumb "with the cancer," as opposed to "from the malignancy."
- The absence of a distinctly heterogeneous pattern of emphysema affecting the upper lobes precluded lung volume reduction surgery, with the tumor included in the resected lung specimens.[59]
- Radiofrequency ablation may also have been an option.

## References

 Interactive references and additional readings for this chapter can be accessed online at *expertconsult.com*.

# ADJUVANT AND NEOADJUVANT RADIATION THERAPY FOR LUNG CANCER

Richard D. Pezner, MD

## INDICATIONS FOR RADIATION THERAPY IN LUNG CANCER

### Historical

- External beam radiation therapy (EBRT) has been used for several decades for definitive and palliative treatment of non-small cell lung cancer (NSCLC) patients.[1]
- A dose of 60 Gy (1 Gray = 100 centiGray = 100 rad) in daily treatments over 6 to 6 1/2 weeks has been a standard dose for inoperable locally advanced cases based on a major randomized study in the 1970's showing that dose to be superior to lower doses.[2]
- More recently, numerous studies have shown that combined radiochemotherapy regimens are superior to EBRT alone in local control and survival for inoperable locally advanced NSCLC patients.[3-5]
- EBRT is routinely used in patients with limited-stage small cell lung cancer.
- EBRT is highly effective in palliating lung cancer, which produces superior vena cava syndrome, obstruction of major airways, hemoptysis from endobronchial tumor involvement, and severe tumor pain. Palliative EBRT doses may range from 30 to 45 Gy in 2 to 5 weeks.

### Adjuvant Radiation Therapy

- Postoperative radiation therapy (PORT) to hilar and mediastinal nodes can significantly reduce the frequency locoregional recurrence, but has not improved overall survival rates in stages I to III.[6,7]
- PORT fell out of favor with publication of a major meta-analysis that revealed poorer survival rates with PORT due to cardiopulmonary complications.[8]
- Modern EBRT techniques that use well-fractionated dose-schedules and better limit dose to heart and lungs do not appear to increase the risk of treatment-related mortality.[9]
- PORT may have future indications in early-stage lung cancer if adjuvant chemotherapy decreases the frequency of distant metastases but not the frequency of locoregional recurrences.

### Neoadjuvant Radiochemotherapy

- Preoperative EBRT alone has not been shown to be of benefit for NSCLC in downstaging, improved local control, or higher survival rates. In the past, the exception to this was for superior sulcus lung cancers (Pancoast tumors), in which preoperative RT and surgery appeared to produce superior results to either modality alone.[10]
- Preoperative chemotherapy alone has demonstrated downstaging and improved survival in some studies.
- Preoperative radiochemotherapy using platinum-based regimens has also demonstrated downstaging, improved locoregional control, and in some studies, improved survival.
  - The typical EBRT dose is 45 to 50 Gy over 5 weeks.[11-13]
  - Small studies have used EBRT doses of 59 to 66 Gy, particularly for patients with bulky primary or nodal disease.[14,15]
  - Treatment fields encompass the primary tumor and involved nodes.
  - Major acute toxicities are myelosuppression and radiation esophagitis, both of which may be severe.
  - Postoperative complications and mortality are mainly due to pulmonary toxicities, including pneumonia, pulmonary embolism, acute respiratory distress syndrome (ARDS), and bronchopleural fistula, particularly in patients who underwent pneumonectomy.[11-13] Fatal pulmonary complications have been reported in 13% to 26% of patients who undergo pneumonectomy but only 1% to 3% who undergo lobectomy.[11,13] Placement of an intercostal muscle flap to cover the bronchial stump has significantly reduced the frequency of bronchopleural fistulas.[11,15]
  - Pathologic complete responses occurred in 7% to 45% of cases.[11-15]
  - Overall survival has been reported to be 22% to 46% at 3 to 5 years.[11-15]
  - Preoperative radiochemotherapy combined with surgical resection is considered the standard optimal approach for superior sulcus tumors.[16,17] The intergroup trial had a 2-year survival rate of 55% for eligible patients entered in the study.[17] Of 111 patients entered in the study, there were only three (2.7%) treatment-related deaths. Complete pathologic responses were found in 28 (25%) of patients.

## ACUTE AND LATE TOXICITIES OF THORACIC RADIATION THERAPY

### Acute Side Effects During Course of Thoracic Radiotherapy

- Radiation esophagitis is the most common acute toxicity and occurs to some degree in a large majority of patients. With concurrent chemotherapy, grade 3 or greater dysphagia may occur in 3% to 13% of patients.[11,12,15,17] Treatment includes oral xylocaine-based medications, narcotics, intravenous fluids, and/or breaks from treatment. Radiation esophagitis quickly resolves, typically within 7 to 14 days, following discontinuation of EBRT to the esophagus. In some cases, esophageal candidiasis may aggravate the severity of the dysphagia.
- Myelosuppression is more frequent and more likely to be severe in patients who receive concurrent chemotherapy.
- Skin reaction is typically a mild erythema on chest or back.
- Acute pericarditis is extremely rare (<0.1%).

### Acute Radiation Pneumonitis

- Acute radiation pneumonitis (ARP) is an inflammatory reaction that appears in the high-dose irradiated portion of the lungs after the completion of EBRT. Pathophysiology is incompletely understood but appears to involve a cascade of inflammatory cells and cytokine production.[18-20]

- Symptomatic ARP may develop in up to 20% of lung cancer patients, with 5% to 10% of all lung cancer patients having moderate to severe symptoms.[3,4,18-21] It is not understood why only a small minority of irradiated patients develop ARP.

- The relative risk or frequency of ARP can be estimated before the start of EBRT based on any of several EBRT treatment planning parameters. The $V_{20}$, the percentage of total lung volume receiving at least 20 Gy, has been shown to be a very useful predictive parameter.[21] It has been incorporated into many intergroup studies to put an upper limit to the volume of lung that may be irradiatied. The $V_{20}$ can be determined before the start of EBRT when CT simulation and computerized treatment planning are used by the radiation oncologist.

- Symptoms include any combination of dyspnea, dry hacking cough, low-grade fever up to 101.5°F, or ipsilateral chest aching discomfort. High-grade fevers or productive cough are more likely due to other etiologies such as infections.

- Symptoms may arise 3 weeks to 3 months after the last day of EBRT but may also arise up to a year after treatment. Typically symptoms gradually progress in severity. However, unrecognized cases may progress to respiratory failure requiring intubation.

- There are no laboratory tests or pathologic findings that are specific for ARP. Lung biopsies show inflammatory alveolar changes consistent with ARDS. Bronchoscopy with bronchoalveolar lavage shows nonspecific inflammatory findings.

- Chest computed tomography (CT) scans show a restricted zone of fluffy infiltrates, often with air bronchograms. The infiltrate does not have a lobar distribution.

- The diagnosis is established by the determination that the region of infiltrate corresponds to the zone of irradiated lung.[19,22] This often requires the radiation oncologist to compare the diagnostic CT scan with the radiation therapy simulation or port films or the EBRT dosimetry planning CT scans (Fig. 26-1).

- If the zone of infiltrate does not closely correspond to the irradiated volume, other diagnoses should be entertained, such as infection or lymphangetic metastases. In some cases, pulmonary infiltrates may be due to multiple diagnoses (e.g., pneumocystis in a patient with simultaneous ARP). In such cases, bronchoscopy may be helpful to search for diagnoses other than ARP.

- The ARP infiltrate may be different when newer methods of EBRT are used.[23] When multiple small EBRT fields are aimed from several directions toward a lung tumor, the high-dose volume will surround the tumor in a very restricted and irregular shape. In addition, intensity-modulated radiation therapy (IMRT) uses sophisticated computer-controlled delivery to each EBRT field so that the portion of a particular field that passes through the tumor receives a higher dose and the portion of the field that passes through a critical structure receives a lower dose. Compared with standard EBRT fields, this results in a very conformal treatment region in which a much smaller lung volume receives a high EBRT dose. This, in turn, can reduce the frequency and severity of ARP. However, when ARP does develop, its appearance will be a vague irregular cloud-like region surrounding the treated tumor (Fig. 26-2).

- Prednisone 30 to 100 mg per day in divided doses (or its equivalent if other corticosteroids are used) is highly effective. Symptoms may dramatically improve within 24 to 48 hours. Rapid significant relief confirms the diagnosis of ARP.

- Patients with ARP who are either asymptomatic or minimally symptomatic do not necessarily need to be placed on steroids. Often, mild cases will resolve without medication. Prednisone can always be started if symptoms worsen.

- Pulse oximetry at rest and after a 5-minute walk may be of value in estimating the severity of ARP and in making decisions about how much steroid, if any, to prescribe for an individual case. Although pulse oximetry cannot establish a diagnosis of ARP, subsequent determinations after the start of steroids can confirm clinical improvement.

- Once started, gradual tapering of the steroid should begin within several days of symptom relief. Tapering needs to be gradual so as

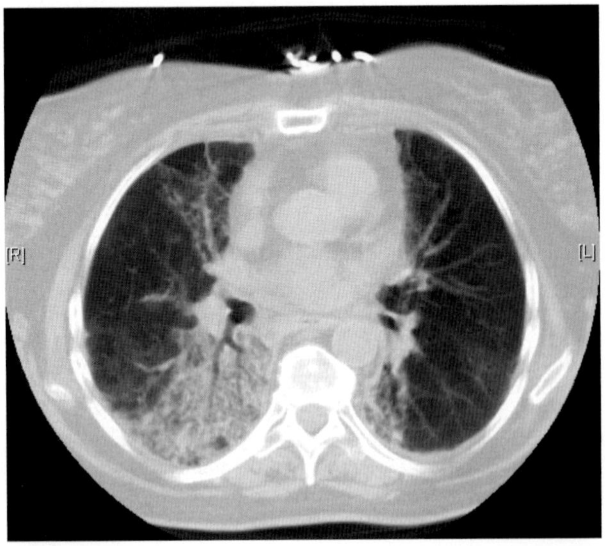

**Figure 26-1:** Acute radiation pneumonitis (ARP) in a patient with right-sided lung cancer who underwent radiotherapy with standard anterior and posterior opposed fields encompassing the primary tumor and mediastinum. The interstitial infiltrate closely matched the irradiated region of the right lung and left paramediastinal lung tissue. Symptoms were promptly relieved with prednisone.

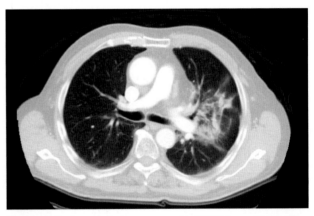

**Figure 26-2:** Acute radiation pneumonitis (ARP) in a patient with a small medically inoperable left lung cancer who was treated with intensity-modulated radiation therapy (IMRT). IMRT involves the use of multiple computer-controlled radiation beams centered on the tumor. The ARP infiltrate from IMRT formed a cloud-like pattern around the tumor. The patient was asymptomatic and did not require steroids. The infiltrate gradually condensed over several months into a smaller zone of radiation pulmonary fibrosis.

not to trigger steroid-withdrawal radiation pneumonitis (see later). Typically, the total daily prednisone dose can be tapered by 5 mg, with stepdowns taking place once or twice a week. A detailed written schedule helps most patients. Any worsening of symptoms should lead to a return to the previous steroid level at which the patient's symptoms were under control. Serial chest x-ray studies or CT scans are not particularly helpful, because resolution of the ARP infiltrates significantly lags behind clinical improvement.

- After completion of steroid tapering, ARP rarely returns.
- Follow-up chest x-ray studies and CT scans often show development of chronic radiation pulmonary fibrosis in the portion of lung involved by ARP.
- Surgery following acute radiation pneumonitis and vice versa:
  - There are no reports of acute radiation pneumonitis developing in patients receiving neoadjuvant radiochemotherapy precluding surgery.
  - Perhaps this is because surgery is performed about 5 to 7 weeks after the end of radiation therapy and the window for majority of cases of acute radiation pneumonitis occur 3 weeks to 3 months after the end of treatment in those 10% to 20% of treated patients who develop it.
  - In the setting of this rare possibility, a prudent approach might be to resume prednisone perioperatively and delay surgery a week or two with cautious tailing postoperatively.
  - As for the possibility of acute radiation pneumonitis arising in the postoperative period, the risk is considered to be low for pneumonectomy patients. For these patients, the only unresected potentially irradiated lung tissue may be a small strip of contralateral lung immediately adjacent to irradiated mediastinal lymph nodes.
  - In the setting of acute radiation pneumonitis developing after surgery, clinicians would have a tough time teasing out this complication from ARDS including chemotherapy-related lung toxicity, hospital-acquired pneumonia, and other post-operative complications.
  - Radiographic diagnosis would also be difficult because part but not all of the irradiated lung would have been resected. What remains would expand through the hemithorax and no longer have the shape of the irradiated fields.

## Steroid-withdrawal Radiation Pneumonitis

- Rapid tapering or discontinuation of a corticosteroid in the months after EBRT of the chest may trigger ARP in a patient who never had symptoms or radiographic evidence of ARP.[24]
- This can occur when steroids were prescribed for a completely unrelated problem (e.g., dexamethasone prescribed for brain metastases that develop several months after the end of thoracic EBRT for a lung cancer, dexamethasone given before administration of a taxane chemotherapy drug, or steroids prescribed for exacerbation of chronic obstructive pulmonary disease or arthritis).
- Steroid-withdrawal radiation pneumonitis is diagnosed and managed the same as a de novo case of ARP.

## Late Radiation Toxicities

- Chronic radiation pulmonary fibrosis will develop to some degree in a large majority of patients but will be symptomatic in only a small minority.[18-20,23]
- Esophageal stricture is infrequent. It may require esophageal dilatation.
- Osteoporotic vertebral collapse of the irradiated thoracic spine may infrequently occur. MRI spine scan may be needed to differentiate from a vertebral metastasis.
- Rib fracture in the irradiated rib cage (rare).
- Pericardial effusion/constrictive pericarditis (rare)
- An increased risk for coronary artery disease has been extensively described for young adults with lymphomas who receive mediastinal EBRT and for breast cancer patients who received adjuvant EBRT. A complete discussion is beyond the scope of this chapter. More recent studies have demonstrated that the risk is highly dependent on total radiation doses, daily radiation dose, and EBRT field technique.[25-27] Most lung cancer patients have a long smoking history and other factors that already put them at risk of coronary artery disease.
- An increased risk for cardiac valvular disease has been described in young lymphoma patients decades after receiving mediastinal irradiation.[27] An increased risk has not been described for lung cancer and breast cancer patients.
- Spontaneous pneumothorax is an uncommon complication in lymphoma patients.[28] Rarely, it may occur in lung cancer patients.
- Hypothyroidism may occur when the thyroid gland is irradiated. For lung cancer patients, this would be a rare complication. It would only occur if the EBRT fields extended superiorly to include the supraclavicular nodes and incidentally encompass the thyroid gland.
- EBRT delivered as a few extremely large radiation dose fractions (up to 22 Gy per fraction) by extremely well-targeted and conformal radiation techniques, termed stereotactic body radiation therapy, may lead to fibrotic obstruction of major airways, fatal hemorrhage from major blood vessels, and other late complications not typically encountered with standard well-fractionated EBRT.[29]
- Although there is an extensive literature about patients treated for childhood neoplasms, benign disease, breast cancer, and Hodgkin's disease,[30,31] the chance of a radiation-related second malignant neoplasm as a *consequence* of treatment of NSCLC is extremely unlikely. This is due to poor overall survival, comorbidities, and long lead time to develop radiation-induced tumors, such as chest wall sarcoma (10–30 years).

## References

 Interactive references and additional readings for this chapter can be accessed online at *expertconsult.com*.

# 27 RADIOFREQUENCY ABLATION OF LUNG TUMORS

Fereidoun Abtin, MD and Robert D. Suh, MD

## INTRODUCTION

Radiofrequency (RF) ablation is an alternative technique to surgical resection of lung tumors, either primary or secondary, through delivery of high-frequency alternating current using electrodes precisely placed at the target sites. Although not absolutely necessary, the vast majority of radiofrequency ablation is performed under image guidance.

## DEMOGRAPHICS OF LUNG CANCER

- Lung cancer is most common cause of cancer death in both men and women, accounting for 29% of all cancer deaths in the United States.[1-3]
- In the United States, 170,000 new cases of primary lung cancer are diagnosed annually.[1]
- Despite advances in treatment technology, the overall 5-year survival rate for newly diagnosed lung cancer remains at only 15%.[1] Survival differs with pathology, staging, and treatment.
  - Non–small cell lung cancer (NSCLC)
    - Stage 1(T1 N0 M0 and T2 N0 M0):
      - Surgery is the treatment of choice.
      - 5-year survival rate at approximately 75%.
    - Stage 2 (T1 N1 M0, T2 N1 M0 and T3 N0 M0):
      - Surgery is the treatment of choice.
      - 5-year survival rate at approximately 50%.
    - Stage 3 A (T1 N2 M0, T2 N2 M0, T3 N1 M0 and T3 N2 M0):
      - Radiotherapy, chemotherapy, surgery, and combinations of these modalities are used for treatment.
      - Overall 5-year survival does not exceed 10% to 15%.
    - Stage 3 B (Any T, N3, M0 and T4, any N, M0):
      - Surgery is of no benefit. Combination of chemotherapy and radiotherapy is used.
      - 5-year survival rate is less than 5%.
    - Stage 4 (Any T, Any N, M1):
      - Palliative chemotherapy is used.
      - Median survival at time of diagnosis is 7.9 months.[4]
  - Small cell lung cancer (SCLC)
    - Limited-stage disease: Combination chemotherapy is the cornerstone of treatment, combined with radiotherapy. Median survival of 18 to 24 months and 40% to 50% 2-year survival rate.[2,5]
    - Extensive-stage disease: Combination chemotherapy is the cornerstone of treatment. Radiotherapy alone is not beneficial.
- Lung Cancer:
  - For early-stage (1 and 2) NSCLC, (15% of cases at diagnosis) surgical resection is standard therapy because it confers the best opportunity for long-term disease-free survival.[6]
  - However, only one third of these patients meet pulmonary physiologic guidelines for lobar or sublobar resection ($FEV_1 > 60\%$ predicted and carbon monoxide diffusing capacity > 60% predicted).[7]
  - For medically inoperable surgical candidates, sublobar resection, specifically wedge resection and segmentectomy, has been proposed; however, these approaches have shown high local recurrence rates of up to 50% and, therefore, are considered less favorable.[5]
  - According to the Surveillance, Epidemiology and End-Results database, 14,555 patients, or 15.7%, present with stage 1 and 2 lung cancer but are medically inoperable.[8]
  - Despite comorbid medical illness, patients who receive therapy for early-stage lung cancer enjoy better outcomes than those who do not receive therapy.[9]
  - Therefore, a sizeable proportion of patients with stage 1 and 2 lung cancer are medically inoperable and can benefit from less invasive and nonsurgical techniques, such as radiofrequency ablation.
- Metastasis:
  - The lungs are the second most common organ involved by solid tumor metastases, following the lymphatic system and virtually tied with the liver.[10,11]
  - Hematogenous metastasis from nongastrointestinal tumors to the lungs is common, because the lung acts as the first capillary bed for blood-borne and lymphatic system–borne dissemination.[12]
  - Approximately 20% of patients with lung metastases and resected primary soft tissue tumors have a limited number of metastases located only in the lung. Therefore, they are potential candidates for surgical resection or metastasectomy.[11]
  - Surgical metastasectomy may result in improved disease-free survival in properly selected patients.[13-15] However, with multiple surgical resections, pulmonary capacity compromise may become an important issue. A lung-sparing technique, such as radiofrequency ablation, may be an attractive option in those candidates who have limited disease, those who have controllable disease but are medically inoperable, and those who have limited recurrent or residual disease, following prior surgical resection, chemotherapy, or radiotherapy.

## PHYSICS OF RADIOFREQUENCY ABLATION

- RF ablation is a technique that requires precise placement of an electrode or electrodes into a specific location to cause local tissue destruction by controlled heating. The mechanism involves
  - Application of rapid alternating electrical current with a frequency of 460 to 500 kHz in the range of radio waves. Applied electric power ranges from 10 W to 200 W with maximum current from 500 mA to 2000 mA.
  - The RF electrical current is concentrated near the noninsulated tips of the electrode, and the circuit is completed by returning either to electrical grounding pads usually located on the patient's thighs (monopolar system) or to a nearby grounding electrode (bipolar system).
  - The alternating electrical current causes agitation of ionic dipolar molecules in surrounding tissue and fluids, resulting

in frictional heating that is greatest adjacent to the noninsulated portion of the electrode.[16]

○ When living tissue is heated to more than 50° C for at least 5 minutes, cells undergo coagulation necrosis that results in denaturation of proteins. The heat energy is then distributed radially to surrounding tissues. For ablation of tumors, tissue temperatures typically range between 60° C and 100° C, which results in rapid coagulation necrosis, enzymatic deactivation, and subsequent nearly instantaneous cell death.[13,16]

■ Control of the ablation zone and area of cell death are of utmost importance. For ablation of tumors within the lung and liver, the goal is homogeneous necrosis of the entire tumor, as well as an acceptable surrounding margin of noncancerous tissue, generally at least 1 cm.[17,18] Preservation of surrounding vital structures and organs is an additional key consideration.

○ RF thermal distribution in tissue has been described by the bioheat transfer equation. The dimensions of tissue undergoing necrosis are dependent on

  ■ Length and thickness of noninsulated active portion of the electrode.
   ○ The longer the length of the active portion, the larger the area of ablation.
   ○ The larger the diameter of the electrode, the larger the area of ablation.

○ The ablation zone is usually elliptical, its width measuring approximately 2 to 3 cm in diameter. In order to accomplish therapeutic goal of complete tumor kill in tumors larger than 2 to 3 cm diameter, multiple overlapping spheres or cylinders of ablation are required.[19,20] As the number of overlapping ablations increase, so do the overall duration of the procedure, the likelihood of leaving islands of viable tumor, and the probability of complications.

  ■ The highest rates of complete tumor ablation and lowest rates of complications are achieved in tumors less than 2 to 3 cm diameter.

○ Power and duration of applied RF current.
  ■ 10 W to 200 W, with maximum current from 500 mA to 2000 mA.
  ■ A minimum of 5 minutes is required to obtain cell death. Twelve minutes is optimal and usually repeated.
  ■ Multiple electrodes and switch boxes can be used to increase the ablation zone.

○ Surface temperature of RF electrode.
  ■ Temperatures ranging from 60° C to 100° C result in rapid coagulation necrosis, enzymatic deactivation, and subsequent cell death nearly instantaneously.[13,16]
  ■ At temperatures in excess of 105° C to 115° C, tissue charring and carbonization, gas formation, and cavitation may occur, insulating the surrounding tissue from the effects of RF current and interfering with heat diffusion.

○ Composition of surrounding tissue.
  ■ "Heat sink" is a phenomenon of heat removal by rapidly flowing blood within an adjacent artery or vein, thereby preserving the blood vessel and an adjacent cuff of malignant perivascular tissue. Heat sink can also occur with larger bronchi.

## PATIENT SELECTION CRITERIA

■ Proper patient selection is highly dependent on the anticipated goal to be achieved. Although no solid or strict criteria exist, emerging goals for ablation thus far established within the current medical literature include

○ Potential for cure.
  ■ In stage 1 and 2 NSCLC.
  ■ In medically inoperable surgical candidates or in those with stage 1 and 2 NSCLC who refuse surgical resection.
  ■ Limited metastases.

○ Prolongation of survival.
  ■ Pulmonary malignancy with limited disease outside the lung that can be treated with systemic therapy or locoregional methods.
  ■ Slowly growing pulmonary malignancy, with the main bulk of tumor within the lung.
  ■ Cytoreduction of large tumors to potentially alter the susceptibility of viable tumor tissue to chemotherapy or radiotherapy.

○ Relief of symptoms.
  ■ Pain commonly present with peripheral tumors invading the parietal pleura or chest wall, for example, mesothelioma
  ■ Ablation of tumors adjacent to vital structures as a preemptive strike before invasion
  ■ Cytoreduction of tumor volume, resulting in reduction of symptoms and significant improvement in the quality of life

## PROCEDURE

### Preprocedure Evaluation

Once the patient is selected, evaluation before ablation includes:

■ Directed patient history
■ Directed physical examination with special attention to cardiopulmonary compromise
■ Electrocardiogram and pulmonary function tests (PFTs), the latter particularly with lung disease and/or resection. Many patients with lung cancer are or have been smokers. PFTs are required to establish:
  ○ Adequacy of oxygenation
  ○ Pulmonary reserve
  ○ Flow volume spirometry
■ Medication history
  ○ Anticoagulant and antiplatelet medications need to be tapered or stopped before the anticipated procedure.
  ○ Before the procedure, conversion to subcutaneous or low-molecular-weight heparin can be considered, which is stopped at least 24 hours before the procedure.
■ Current computed tomography (CT) scan should be available that is not older than 4 weeks. In case of primary lung cancer, current staging with positron emission tomography (PET) or mediastinoscopy is required. CT scan is used
  ○ To ensure amenability of tumor size and number to ablation.
  ○ Evaluate a safe access route
  ○ Comorbid disease in the lung
  ○ Location and relationship of tumor to vital structures
■ Presence of pacemaker or implantable cardioverter defibrillator
  ○ RF current can cause potential device malfunction.
  ○ Possibility of coagulation necrosis at myocardial implantation site seems invalid, likely from massive heat sink effect of cardiac ventricular blood flow.
  ○ Patients dependent on pacemaker for small percentage of time can have temporary deactivation with temporary cardiac passing available on standby.
  ○ Patients with constant dependence on pacemaker may benefit from alternative modalities, like cryoablation, microwave and laser thermal ablation.

■ Histopathologic diagnosis of the lesions should be obtained before the ablation. Biopsy can be performed before the ablation as a separate session or immediately before the ablation as a concurrent session. The latter is less preferred because
  ○ Procedure time may be prolonged.
  ○ Presence of complications from biopsy procedure can delay or postpone the ablation.
  ○ Postbiopsy hemorrhage along the needle tract may obscure the tumor margins and detection of post ablation zone of ground-glass opacity (GGO) less accurate.

## Anesthesia

RF ablation can be painful, especially in close proximity to the parietal pleura, and controlled breathing with a stationary targeted tumor is desirable. The procedure can be performed under general anesthesia or deep or moderate conscious sedation. No consensus exists among authors, and each operator's decision is dependent on many variables including comorbid disease, tumor location, and risk for potential complications.[21-24]

■ General anesthesia
  ○ Advantages
    ■ Greater degree of patient comfort
    ■ Better control of the airways
    ■ Presence of an expert in pulmonary and cardiac management in case of complications
  ○ Disadvantages
    ■ Higher cost
    ■ Logistical challenges requiring second participating service
    ■ Longer procedure times related to anesthesia setup and availability
    ■ Increased risk for pneumothorax owing to positive pressure ventilation
    ■ Risks specific to general anesthesia
■ Deep conscious sedation
  ○ Advantages
    ■ Lower cost than general anesthesia
    ■ Shorter procedure times than with anesthesia
  ○ Disadvantages
    ■ Potential for less patient comfort and procedural pain

## Preparation for Procedure

■ Consent for the procedure and other interventions, if needed, should be obtained.
■ Coagulation cascade, including prothrombin time, partial thromboplastin time, International Normalized Ratio, and bleeding time, needs to be checked on the day of procedure, especially if the patient is on anticoagulation, or within 7 days.
■ Prophylactic antibiotics are given routinely by some interventionists 1 hour before the procedure and in postprocedural period, the argument being that devitalized tissue at the end of ablation is a potential nidus for superinfection. However, the benefits have yet to be proven.
■ For the lung, CT is the most widely used modality for directed and precise electrode placement. Volumetric acquisition of imaging data allows for computer reconstruction of three-dimensional volume data sets for pre-, intra-, and postprocedure analysis. Multiplanar reformatted display of images both parallel to (long axis views) and perpendicular to (short axis views) the axis of the RF electrodes can provide valuable

information regarding depth of device penetration, position of an electrode shaft or tines within or adjacent to tumor, the configuration of multiple devices, and the relationship to essential, nontargeted structures.[25] The principal limitation of CT is the lack of real-time imaging feedback for interactive advancement of devices into the targeted tumor. Some operators have found CT fluoroscopy to be a useful adjunct for device placement (Fig. 27-1A and B).
■ Patient positioning on the CT table warrants attention.
  ○ In general, the shortest distance from skin to the tumor is optimal.
  ○ When equivocal, posterior approach with the patient in prone position is favorable to supine patient position, because posterior ribs are less subject to respiratory variation.

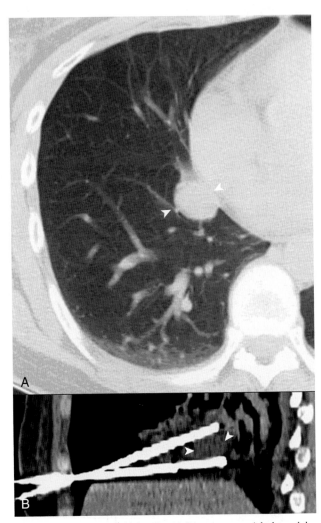

**Figure 27-1:** A 60-year-old female with biopsy-proven right lower lobe metastatic uterine sarcoma. **A,** Axial noncontrast computed tomography image at the level of the right atrium shows the soft tissue metastasis adjacent to the right atrium (*arrowheads*). Owing to its firm consistency, multiple attempts to place an electrode through its center were unsuccessful. **B,** Multiplanar reformat (MPR) with sagittal reconstruction demonstrates two electrodes placed at the superior and inferior surface of the target lesion, pinching the lesion in between (*arrowheads*). The conferred ablation zone geometry is certain to encompass the tumor and provide an acceptable margin.

○ In general, access should pass over the superior margin of the rib to minimize the probability of intercostal artery injury, should avoid traversing bullae or interlobar fissures, and should avoid injury of essential non-target structures.

○ Care should be taken when positioning the upper extremities to avoid injury to the brachial plexus.

○ Off-center position of the patient on the CT table may be required to provide sufficient clearance between the chest wall and the inner surface of the CT gantry in order to accommodate the RF electrode. The CT table should be as low as possible to maximize gantry clearance.

■ Dispersive grounding pads with large surface areas must be applied to the patient's body, preferably perpendicular to the RF electrode path and not located over bony prominences. The grounding pads should be in good contact with the skin, and if necessary, the skin must be shaved. Grounding pads are usually placed over thighs. When more than one electrode is used, more than two grounding pads and usually at least two pads can be placed to prevent cutaneous pad burns.

## Intraprocedural Technique

■ The Initial CT is performed, and the site of entry is marked using radiopaque grid or radiopaque marker like a lead ball.

■ Once the skin entry site is confirmed, it is prepared with antiseptic solution and draped with sterile towels.

■ After cutaneous anesthesia is achieved, a coaxial or Chiba needle is directed to the pleural surface, where liberal local anesthetic is deposited to achieve pleural anesthesia.

■ Several techniques have been used to successfully place the RF electrode into the targeted tumor:

○ One option initially places a 21- or 22-gauge, 10- to 15-cm length localizing needle into the tumor. The thinner localizing needle is believed to be associated with a lower risk of pneumothorax and hemorrhage than the larger bore electrode should multiple passes be necessary to obtain optimal device position. Once the small-gauge localizing needle is situated satisfactorily within the tumor, it can be used as a guide for advancement of RF electrode. Because the localizing needle is not electrically insulated, it must be removed before switching on the RF current.[21]

○ Alternatively, some operators advance a coaxial cannula or RF electrode directly, with or without CT fluoroscopy guidance.

■ Electrode selection depends on operator preference. Three electrodes have been most widely used, each electrode unique in its design and ablation zone geometry

○ The LeVeen electrode (Boston Scientific; Watertown, MA) employs tines within the shaft of the electrode. Once in position, the tines are deployed laterally, then arching backward, forming an umbrella-like array (Fig. 27-2A). The LeVeen electrode is optimally deployed when its tines arise from the center of the target tumor and extend immediately beyond the peripheral edges of the tumor. The resultant ablation zone appears as a horizontal oval.

○ The tines of the Starburst and Side-Deployment (SDE and Talon) type electrodes (Angiodynamics; Queensbury, NY) course forward from either the tip (Starburst) or the side of the electrode (SDE) and laterally, similar to the stems in a bouquet of flowers (see Fig. 27-2B). With this design, the tines are deployed from the electrode shaft at the near aspect of the tumor and then advanced until they reach the far aspect of the tumor. The ablation zone achieved is a vertical oval, oriented to the shaft of the electrode.

○ The straight internally cooled single-electrode or triple-cluster electrodes (Covidien; Boulder, CO) are placed such

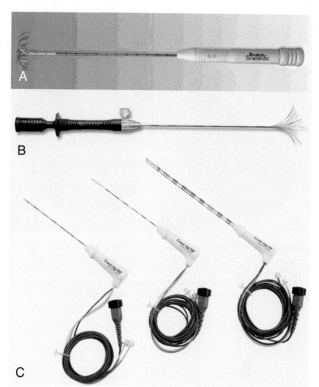

**Figure 27-2:** The most commonly used radiofrequency ablation electrodes. **A,** The LeVeen electrode (Boston Scientific; Watertown, MA) employs an expandable multiarray, in which all tines are initially contained within the electrode shaft. Once the tip of the shaft is in position, the tines are deployed, arcing horizontally and backward, forming its umbrella-like array. **B,** The Starburst XL electrode (Angiodynamics; Queensbury, NY) also employs an expandable multiarray, in which its tines course forward from the shaft tip. Once deployed, the completed array is reminiscent of the stems in a bouquet of flowers. **C,** The internally cooled single-needle electrode or triple-cluster electrode (Covidien; Boulder, CO) uses an active tip of varying length that determines the size of the ablation zone.

that the active exposed tip is situated in the deep portion of the tumor and extends 0.5 to 1.0 cm into nontumorous lung (see Fig. 27-2C). The resultant ablation zone is a vertical oval.

■ Once the electrode or electrodes are in position, RF ablation is started. The goal is to achieve homogenous coagulation necrosis of the entire tumor, as well as an adjacent 0.5- to 1.0-cm margin of nontumorous lung.

■ End point parameters.

○ Each device vendor has provided end point parameters that presume adequate ablation. Repeat ablations can be performed, if these endpoints are not achieved.

■ The LeVeen system increases the electrical power (Watts) delivered in a stepwise fashion at prescribed intervals until the impedance (Ohms) rises precipitously, a phenomenon frequently termed roll-off.[26]

■ The angiodynamics generator provides full power at 250 W. When tissue temperature exceeds target temperature, usually 90°C, as detected by thermocouples located in alternate tines, the tines are advanced until the desired array diameter is achieved. Following manufacturer recommendations, ablation is continued at target temperature until specified ablation end times are achieved.

■ The Cool-tip system gradually increases electrical power until an impedance rise of 20 O over baseline is detected,

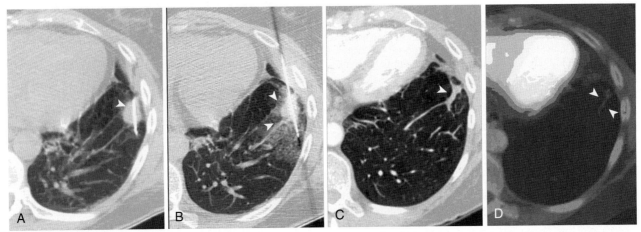

**Figure 27-3:** Metastatic colon carcinoma to the left lower lobe in a 62-year-old woman. **A,** Axial noncontrast computed tomography (CT) image demonstrates a single-needle electrode placed through the center of the targeted metastasis (*arrowhead*). **B,** Immediate postablation image demonstrates ground-glass envelopment (*arrowheads*) of the newly ablated tumor. **C,** A single-axial CT image from the CT-positron emission tomography (PET) at 12 months shows that the original tumor has been replaced by an irregular band of density, which is consistent with postablation pleuroparenchymal scar (*arrowhead*). **D,** Axial fused CT-PET image at the same level confirms no metabolic activity within the scar (*arrowheads*).

at which time power delivery is reduced. The heating cycle is terminated after an ablation time of 12 minutes. The tissue temperature, as measured by an embedded thermocouple, should exceed 70° C immediately after power termination and remain above 60° C for at least 3 minutes.

○ Irrespective of the electrode used, imaging end points can be helpful to determine adequate ablation, specifically the appearance of GGO on CT encompassing the treated tumor in its entirety, measuring at least 0.5 to 1.0 cm in width (Fig. 27-3A and B).

○ After completion of ablation, many, but not all, operators practice tract cauterization of the lung parenchyma with low-power application (e.g., 10 W) while withdrawing the RF electrode. Theoretically, this maneuver may lower the probability of parenchymal hemorrhage, pneumothorax, and tumor tract seeding.

■ After removal of the RF electrode, a limited set of CT images should be obtained in the area of ablation to screen for procedural complications.

## Precautions

■ During the course of RF ablation, ensure that perspiration has not caused the pads to peel away from the skin, because skin burns can occur.

■ Palpate the skin adjacent to the leading edge of grounding pads to ensure that excessive heating is not occurring. If so, dry the edges regularly.

■ Electrical burns can occur when current passes between the pads and RF electrodes through alternate routes, typically from arm and fingers. Ensure adequate insulation by placing a blanket or other insulators between arms and body.

■ After placement of the electrodes and immediately before starting the ablation, an extra dose of analgesic is given. It is believed that initiation of RF ablation may stimulate nerves, particularly intercostal, and induce pain even before onset of significant tissue necrosis.

■ Oxygen should be administered by nasal prong or mask, especially in patients with chest tightness and dyspnea.

## RECOVERY

Following RF ablation, patients need to be observed for recovery and for potential complications from anesthesia and the procedure.

■ Patients need to be observed in a postanesthesia care unit, and vital signs and pulse oximetry must be checked frequently.

■ Chest radiographs should be obtained and reviewed between 1 and 4 hours to exclude complications, including pneumothorax, pleural effusion or hemorrhage, and pulmonary infiltrates.

■ Hemoglobin and hematocrit levels can be obtained approximately 3 to 4 hours postprocedure to screen for occult hemorrhage.

■ Postprocedural pain management can include either oral analgesics or patient-controlled analgesia pumps for parenteral administration of narcotics.

■ Use of anti-inflammatory agents, like ibuprofen, is recommended. Suppression of inflammation postablation for at least 5 days may decrease the degree of pleural reaction, pleural pain and pleural effusion, and systemic inflammatory response.

■ Low-grade fever for 2 to 3 days is common.

■ Typically, patients can be discharged to home within 1 to 2 days after RF ablation, unless a thoracostomy drain was required. Many operators discharge patients home on the same day but closely follow-up the patient from home.

■ Patients should generally be instructed not to travel by air for at least 3 weeks. Airplane cabins are not fully pressurized to sea level, and exposure to this environment could potentially result in a pneumothorax. However, at our institute, we allow air travel within 3 days after a repeat chest radiograph and evaluation.

## COMPLICATIONS

■ Society of Interventional Radiology clinical practice guidelines define major complications and minor complications as with the following guidelines[27]:

○ Minor complications.
  ■ No therapy, no consequence.
  ■ Nominal therapy, no consequence, including overnight admission for observation only.
○ Major complications
  ■ Require therapy, minor hospitalization (<48 h)
  ■ Require major therapy, unplanned increased level of care, prolonged hospitalization (>48 h)
  ■ Permanent adverse sequelae
  ■ Death

■ For many years, as a general indication, the US Food and Drug Administration (FDA) has allowed the use of RF ablation for the cutting and coagulation of soft tissues. However, more recently through a number of statements, the FDA clarified that although RF ablation is not cleared specifically for lung tumor ablation, RF ablation for lung tumor ablation is still considered on-label and covered under the general indication.

■ Review of the medical literature on reported complications for RF ablation performed between 2000 and 2006 on 824 patients in 1081 sessions is shown in Table 27-1.

■ A review of the medical literature by Rosen and colleagues[22] showed a similar pattern of complications, with pneumothorax topping the list. The higher incidence of pneumothorax among this group was most likely affected by a group of patients receiving RF ablation through open thoracotomy.

■ Pneumothorax
  ○ Most common complication, and seen to some degree in almost all patients
  ○ The incidence of minor or major pneumothorax ranges between 25% and 35%. However, only a small portion of this group requires intervention. The majority are managed conservatively, needing only observation.[22,28]
  ○ The incidence of pneumothorax requiring chest tube placement or aspiration is approximately 10% to 20%.[22,28]
  ○ The incidence of RF ablation–related pneumothorax can be affected by
    ■ The degree of intraparenchymal manipulation of the electrode. The less the electrode is repositioned, the less the rate of air leak.
    ■ Traversal of the emphysematous lung or bullae, obviously associated with more serious pneumothoraces
    ■ Traversal of interlobar fissures, each fissure crossed associated with a linear rate of pneumothorax

■ Postprocedural incentive spirometry
■ Number of lesions ablated. The higher number of lesions treated per session generally accounting for a higher rate of air leak complications
■ Tract ablation on retraction and removal of the electrode.
■ Use of conscious sedation versus general anesthesia with intubation. Pneumothorax rates are higher with regard to general anesthesia with intubation due to positive pressure ventilation.

■ Postablation syndrome:
  ○ Described as a complex of symptoms thought to arise secondary to increased circulating cytokines.
  ○ The typical presentation includes mild fever, cough occasionally productive with rust-colored sputum, chills, pain, nausea, and malaise. These symptoms can be seen in up to 36% of patients and vary in severity.
  ○ The effects of postablation syndrome can be expected to last from 1 to 7 days, occasionally up to 14 days.
  ○ Treatment is largely symptomatic with antipyretics, pain control, and anti-tussives, as needed.

■ Pleural effusion and hemorrhage:
  ○ Usually sympathetic and very common, but only 4% of patients require drainage for symptomatic relief with thoracocentesis or chest tube placement.
  ○ Hemothorax is a more serious complication and is usually caused by mechanical injury to the intercostal or other chest wall arteries. Hemorrhage into the pleural space can be rapidly fatal due its large potential volume and the negative pressure that occurs with each inspiration.[29]
  ○ Rapidly accumulating pleural fluid on intraprocedural CT scans or follow-up chest radiographs or signs of intra- or postprocedural hypotension or tachycardia are suggestive evidence for massive, potentially lethal hemothorax and should stimulate prompt intervention, including either transcatheter arterial embolization or operative ligation.
  ○ Empyema occurs infrequently and is likely related to pulmonary infections.

■ Bronchopleural fistula
  ○ Peripheral juxtapleural lesions, particularly in patients with emphysema, squamous cell cancers, and bronchiectasis, may cavitate and breech the viscera pleura, which communicates with the pleural space.[30]
  ○ Bronchopleural fistulas are hard to manage and require frequent treatments, including pleurodesis, endobronchial management, and surgical repair.
  ○ In one series, 0.6% of patients developed this complication.[30]

■ Mediastinal and neural injury
  ○ Care must be taken with ablation of apical lung and superior sulcus tumors. Ablation of these tumors can cause injury to brachial plexus.
  ○ Recurrent laryngeal nerve injury and Horner's syndrome have been reported with mediastinal mass or lymph node ablations.[31]
  ○ Ablation of tumors abutting the mediastinum can cause phrenic nerve injury and resultant diaphragmatic palsy.

■ Microembolization
  ○ Gas microembolization detected by intraprocedural carotid duplex ultrasonography has been studied by many authors. From the ablation bed, these gas microemboli pass into and through the pulmonary veins and enter the systemic circulation. These microemboli are believed to arise from the water vapor during ablation.[32-35]
  ○ Overall no CT, magnetic resonance imaging (MRI), or clinical evidence of neurologic deficit has been reported in any of these studies.

---

**TABLE 27-1 ■ REPORTED COMPLICATIONS FOLLOWING COMPREHENSIVE REVIEW OF MORE THAN 1000 ABLATION SESSIONS***

| Complications | Major (%) | Minor (%) | Total (%) |
|---|---|---|---|
| Pneumothorax | 111 (10.3) | 285 (26.4) | 396 (36.6) |
| Effusion | 8 (0.7) | 155 (14.3) | 163 (15.1) |
| Hemorrhage related | 4 (0.4) | 66 (6.1) | 70 (6.5) |
| Pain | 0 | 86 (8) | 86 (8) |
| Fever | 0 | 34 (3.1) | 34 (3.1) |
| Infections | 24 (2.2) | 0 | 24 (2.2) |
| CNS related | 1 (0.1) | 7 (0.6) | 8 (0.7) |
| Tumor reeding | 1 (0.1) | 0 | 1 (0.1) |
| Excessive recrosis | 1 (0.1) | 0 | 1 (0.1) |
| Pulmonary embolus | 1 (0.1) | 0 | 1 (0.1) |
| Death | 4 (0.37) | 0 | 4 (0.37) |

CNS, central nervous system.
*Pneumothorax is the most common major and minor complication.

○ However, one case of massive cerebral infarction immediately following lung RF ablation has been reported,[35] but this event may have been as a result of air emboli as opposed to gas emboli.

- Death
  ○ The procedure-specific 30-day mortality rate in one large series was 2.6%, and the overall 30-day mortality rate was 3.9%.[28] Despite this one published series, cumulative review of articles between 2000 and 2006 showed a mortality rate of only 0.4%.
  ○ The reported causes of death include massive hemoptysis and hemorrhage, acute respiratory distress syndrome (ARDS), pulmonary sepsis, pulmonary embolism, heart failure, exacerbation of underlying disease and the combination of above-mentioned disorders.

## HISTOPATHOLOGY RESPONSE AND IMAGING CORRELATION FOLLOWING RADIOFREQUENCY ABLATION

- Animal studies
  ○ Postmortem histologic evaluation of the lung following RFA in animal models shows a relatively large central zone of coagulation necrosis surrounded by a relatively thin rim of hyperemia and edema, which on CT scan corresponds to an area of GGO.[36-42]
  ○ Within 1 week, these zones develop a sharp demarcation from surrounding viable lung. The ground glass opacities seen on CT after RF ablation correlate histologically with thermally injured lung.
  ○ After 1 week, the entire ablated region appears as a well-demarcated homogeneous dense opacity on CT that corresponds to necrotic tissue and its surrounding rim of granulation tissue on histopathologic examination. The enclosing extensive area of GGO on the initial CT scan represents an ongoing necrosis.[42]
  ○ Within 2 to 3 weeks, the ablated region gradually contracts on CT, representing a tissue-repairing process in which the granulation tissue encroaches on the inner necrotic tissue.
  ○ Cavity formation was associated with injury to nearby bronchi.
  ○ In a significant minority of cases, microscopic islands of residual viable tumor was found.
- Human subjects: Assessment of adequate RF ablation and annihilation of tumor can be challenging as the ablated tumor remains in situ.
  ○ In general, Response Evaluation Criteria in Solid Tumors (RECIST),[43] based on lesional diameter changes on CT or MRI, is a widely accepted system that is used to objectively measure tumor response to chemotherapy.
  ○ Adequate ablation during the procedure can be assumed when a zone of GGO of 0.5 to 1.0 cm encompasses the tumor in its entirety. This zone corresponds to ongoing necrosis demonstrated in animal models.[42]
  ○ Measurement of the ablation zone alone does not distinguish viable from nonviable tumor or adjacent devitalized tissue, or an adequate treatment response. Steinke and associates[44] showed that following RF ablation, lesion diameters were larger than baseline in 100%, 95%, 76%, and 46% of patients on follow-up CT scans at 1 week, 1 month, 3 months, and 6 months, respectively.
  ○ Postcontrast CT scan, nodule (or ablation zone) CT densitometry, and fluorine-18-fluorodeoxyglucose PET to evaluate for viable tissue appear more accurate than RECIST criteria alone.[10,21,40,45,46]

- Akeboshi and colleagues[40] used a combination of contrast-enhanced CT and PET imaging to evaluate the presence of residual tumor. In a group of patients in whom a discrepancy existed between contrast CT and PET, percutaneous biopsy of the lesions was performed. Histologic assessment found PET imaging to be both more sensitive and specific than contrast-enhanced CT with regard to detection of residual viable tumor.
- Lee and colleagues[45] employed contrast-enhanced CT to assess the extent of tumor necrosis. Viable tumor was defined as intralesional tissue that increased by at least 10 HU compared with its appearance on the noncontrast CT. The mean survival of patients with complete RF-induced necrosis was 19.7 months ± 2.0, compared with only 8.7 months ± 1.8 ($P < 0.01$) for those patients with partial necrosis.
- Suh and colleagues[21] used CT nodule densitometry before tumor treatment and CT ablation zone densitometry after tumor ablation. Contrast enhancement less than 15 HU[46] and an uptake profile of less than 50% of baseline enhancement (the latter at 6 months follow-up) may be a good predictor of outcome and recurrence.

## FOLLOW-UP

- After discharge, periodic imaging is required to follow the disease response to RF ablation and to screen for disease progression. The CT scan is the most widely used modality, with CT-PET and MRI used as supplementary imaging modalities. PET imaging appears to be more sensitive and specific than CT for the detection of residual viable tumor.[40,47,48]
- Typical imaging intervals for CT are at 1, 3, 6, 9 and 12 months, followed by 3- to 4-month intervals thereafter (see Fig. 27-3C). Generally, PET is incorporated at 6-month intervals or at times when CT findings are equivocal for tumor progression. With the advent of newer multidetector CT-PET platforms, operators have liberally substituted CT-PET at time points when CT alone was used, allowing for improved incorporation and integration of both contrast enhancement and metabolic data.
- In some reports, the adequacy of RF ablation can be foretold from a PET scan at 1 to 2 months. However, PET without CT is limited by its lack of anatomic rendering. With CT-PET, however, anatomic detail is restored and can be fused with metabolic information, providing improved insight into the ablation zone.
  ○ Metabolic activity on PET appears to mirror contrast enhancement patterns on CT.
  ○ Expected PET findings at 1 to 2 months include absence of metabolic activity at tumor focus and the presence of a surrounding moderately photointense larger diameter ring. The latter represents inflammatory granulation tissue at the interface of necrotic and viable tissue.[49]
  ○ By adding CT, the 1-month CT-PET scan allows anatomic evaluation for any complications, measurement of baseline postablation tumor size, and any obvious residual tumor.
  ○ In most cases, because treated tumor size will be larger than the baseline tumor, a CT scan alone may not be helpful in the evaluation of treatment response. Therefore, many authors advocate the use of CT-PET.[40,48]
  ○ The 1-month CT-PET can carry a high rate of false-positive findings because the area of inflammation within the ablated mass has not settled and may show high metabolic activity. For this reason, some authors prefer deferring the first CT-PET to 2 or 3 months after ablation, and instead,

obtaining a contrast CT scan or contrast nodule densitometry at 1 month.
- Less well-studied, post gadolinium-enhanced MRI has been used to evaluate response to RF ablation. In general, the ablated tumor appears as a cystic lesion with thin rim-like enhancement. Irregular and thickened rim enhancement or the presence of solid tumor suggests residual tumor tissue.[50]
- For those patients with pulmonary metastases and elevated serologic tumor markers, serial assay of these same markers can be useful nonimaging parameters to record the adequacy and durability of treatment response following RF ablation.
- At our institute, the recommended form of follow-up imaging is contrast-enhanced CT with contrast densitometry at 1, 3, 6, 9, and 12 months. PET is included in the 6- and 12-month follow-up studies as a CT-PET (see Fig. 27-3D).

## RESULTS

- Survival following RF ablation is affected by and dependent on many factors.
- For patients with NSCLC, survival is strongly correlated with clinical tumor stage. A potential cure can be achieved in patients with stage IA or IB NSCLC.
  - ○ Baseline tumor size and attainment of complete necrosis with RF ablation are strongly correlated with and influence survival in patients with inoperable early stage NSCLC.
  - ○ Many authors have shown lower local tumor progression rates following RF ablation for NSCLC measuring less than 3.0 to 3.5 cm compared with those tumors larger than 3.0 to 3.5 cm.[28,45,51-55]
  - ○ Long-term results for RF ablation for lung tumors are surfacing.
    - Simon and coworkers[28] reported the median survival for stage I NSCLC as 29 months. In their study, survival rates at 1, 2, 3, 4, and 5 years were 78%, 57%, 36%, 27%, and 27%, respectively. Median time to death was 30 months (95% confidence interval [CI], 22–38) and 28 months (95% CI, 14–36) for stage IA and IB, respectively, although statistical significance was not achieved ($P = 0.578$).
    - In this same study, in the subset of 21 patients with large or advanced stage tumors that RF ablation was performed for symptom palliation, median survival was 6 months. Survival rates at 1 and 2 years were 27.8% and 5.8%, respectively.[28]
    - When stratified for tumor size, statistically significant lower local tumor progression-free rates occurred with tumors smaller than 3 cm, as compared with larger tumors. The 1-, 2-, 3-, 4-, and 5-year local tumor progression-free rates, respectively, were 83%, 64%, 57%, 47%, and 47% for tumors 3 cm or smaller, and 45%, 25%, 25%, 25% and 25% for tumors larger than 3 cm.[28]
- For metastatic disease, factors that influence survival include baseline tumor size, tumor cell type and grade, whether the primary tumor has been resected, the presence of extrapulmonary metastases, the number of pulmonary metastases, and the use of and response to chemotherapy.
  - ○ In a recent study evaluating response following ablation in a mixed population of metastatic tumor types, the median time to local tumor progression was 45 months for those with tumors 3 cm in diameter or smaller and 12 months for tumors larger than 3 cm.[28]
  - ○ In another study, local tumor progression in metastatic disease following ablation was seen in 11% of patients with tumors no greater than 3 cm in diameter compared with 50% in patients with tumors 3 to 6 cm in diameter.[55]

- ○ The most extensive follow-up after RF ablation for metastatic tumors has been with colorectal carcinomas.
  - In recent reports by Yamakado and associates[55] and Yan colleagues,[56] relatively similar median survival following therapy has been shown at 31 and 33 months, respectively.
  - The 1-, 2-, and 3-year survival rates are also comparable, with the largest of these studies by Yamakado and associates showing 84%, 64%, and 46% survival, respectively.[55] Although many factors were implicated, risk ratios for poorer outcome were statistically significant for tumors larger than 3 cm, the presence of extrapulmonary metastases, or both.
- In patients with NSCLC, RF ablation and radiotherapy can be synergistic.
  - ○ Proposed mechanism: RF ablation causes central coagulation necrosis, including areas of least oxygenation (presumably these areas are least responsive to radiotherapy), with a surrounding zone of nonlethal heat injury that increases sensitivity to external beam irradiation or brachytherapy.[57]
  - ○ With synergism, the acceptable tumor diameter for potential cure may be larger for combined therapy than with RF ablation alone.
  - ○ Grieco and colleagues[57] reported results for patients after thermal ablation (either RF ablation or microwave ablation), followed by radiation therapy (either external beam irradiation or interstitial brachytherapy) for stage I or II NSCLC.
    - Overall survival rates were 86.8%, 70.4%, and 57.1% for 1, 2, and 3 years, respectively. Similar to their earlier experience and others, the reported survival rates for combination therapy were higher than for RF ablation alone.[28,45,57]
    - The survival rates were similar in stage IA and IB, suggesting that radiotherapy may improve the efficacy of thermal ablation for the treatment of larger tumors.
    - However, local recurrence remained higher in tumors larger than 3 cm.[57]
  - ○ The survival rates in patients with stage I and IIA tumors receiving combination RF ablation followed by radiotherapy are higher than in those receiving either treatment alone.[28,45,57,59] Overall survival rates in patients with stage I and IIA receiving radiotherapy alone is 57% at 1 year, 36% at 2 years, and 21% at 3 years after treatment[59] versus 86.8% at 1 year, 70.4% at 2 years, and 57.1% at 3 years for a similar group receiving combination therapy.[57]

## ADVANCES IN THERMAL ABLATION

Since the first published report by Dupuy and associates[58] in 2000 on RF ablation of lung malignancies, new thermal energies have been introduced and developed for tumor ablation. Of these, microwave ablation and cryoablation[60-62] appear the most promising, and each with its advantages and disadvantages is briefly discussed below.

- Microwave (MW) ablation
  - ○ Principles
    - MW used for tissue ablation works on a principle similar to an MW oven.
    - MW ablation is performed by induction of greater than 900 MHz frequency. The MW energy induces dipole excitation, which, in turn, causes the water molecules to spin, transferring some of their kinetic energy and creating friction, resulting in heat generation and tissue hyperthermia.[60]

○ Advantages
  ■ Ability to obtain higher intratumoral temperatures and to ablate larger tumors
  ■ The generator allows multiple applicators to be connected and simultaneously enacted, thereby decreasing ablation times and enabling larger ablation volumes.
  ■ Less "heat sink" effect
  ■ Shorter procedure and room times due to faster ablation times
  ■ No pads or grounding is necessary with MW energy, lessening the chance of skin burns or short circuiting between pads and body parts.
  ■ Less pain on initiation of the procedure, due to absence of current travelling through the intercostal nerves.
  ■ Improved convection profile
  ■ Less pain associated with MW for treatment of subpleural and juxtapleural and chest wall lesions in close proximity to the somatically innervated parietal pleura and chest wall.
○ Disadvantages:
  ■ The presence of surgical clips or staples may affect the area of ablation with larger or unpredictable patterns.
  ■ The antennae and the generator are more expensive.
  ■ Implantable cardiac devices, including pacemakers and cardiac defibrillators, may be susceptible to interference from electromagnetic energy in the MW frequency range. It is recommended to reprogram pacemakers to automatic pacing modes and temporarily disable implanted defibrillators during the procedure. External pacemakers can be used during temporary deactivation.
  ■ MW antennae should preferably be positioned more than 5 cm from cardiac device leads, which can limit the area of ablation.
■ Cryoablation:
○ Principles
  ■ Cryoablation uses the principles of cold temperature dissipation to induce thermal injury in target tissues. The applicators allow conduction of compressed argon gas

in their interior hollow chambers, which, in turn, lead to subzero temperatures in the applicator and surrounding tissue.[61,62]
  ■ Based on the duration of ablation and the diameter of the applicator, the size of ice ball formation varies.
  ■ The ice ball consists of an innermost isotherm with temperatures of -40°C, an inner isotherm of -20°C, and an outer isotherm rim with temperatures ranging from -20°C to 0°C.
  ■ Cell death occurs at subzero temperatures by immediate post-thaw-freeze rupture, followed by long-term coagulation necrosis.
○ Advantages
  ■ No need for electric current.
  ■ The formed ice ball can be seen on CT, and thus, the margins of ablation clearly demarcated.
  ■ Less conferred pain, when compared with heat-induced thermal ablation. This is particularly beneficial when treating subpleural and juxtapleural and chest wall tumors.
  ■ Multiple applicators can be used simultaneously, creating a larger zone of ablation in shorter time.
  ■ Cryoablation can be used with pacemakers and implantable cardiac devices.
○ Disadvantages
  ■ The ice ball formed in the lung is not visible because of the air surrounding the targeted tumor.
  ■ Tissue hemorrhage has been reported. Parenchymal hemorrhage in the lung can be troublesome, and therefore, performance of ablation under general anesthesia is suggested.
  ■ The gas containers are cumbersome and need to be checked for adequate pressure before every procedure.

## References

 Interactive references and additional readings for this chapter can be accessed online at *expertconsult.com.*

# Special Circumstances: Neoplastic Disorders

# 28 SUPERIOR VENA CAVA SYNDROME

Isabel Pedraza, MD, Clark Fuller, MD, and Michael I. Lewis, MD

## TERMINOLOGY

■ Superior vena cava (SVC) syndrome
■ Superior vena cava obstruction
■ Superior mediastinal syndrome

## DEFINITION

The SVC syndrome refers to a constellation of symptoms and signs secondary to obstruction of blood flow through the SVC, producing severe reduction in venous return from the head and neck, upper trunk and extremities. The obstruction is due either from invasion or external compression of the SVC, thrombosis within the SVC, or both.

## ETIOLOGY

The epidemiology of underlying causes of SVC obstruction, continues to evolve, with recent new trends[1-5]:

■ Before the discovery of antibiotics, the most common etiologies were syphilitic aortic aneurysms (original description by William Hunter in 1757), fibrosing mediastinitis from untreated histoplasmosis, and compression from tuberculous lymphadenitis.
■ In the present day, the most common etiology is malignancy (60%–85%), followed by benign causes (15%–40%).
■ There is an increasing incidence of benign causes due to increased use of intravascular devices. This distinct trend is well illustrated in the most recently published series (Table 28-1).

## TABLE 28-1 ■ ETIOLOGY UNDERLYING SUPERIOR VENA CAVA SYNDROME

| Condition | Rice, et al[4] 1996–2001 n = 78 (%) | Yellin, et al[3] 1972–1987 n = 63 (%) |
|---|---|---|
| **Malignant/Tumor** | | |
| Small cell lung cancer | 22 | 6 |
| Non–small cell lung cancer | 24 | 41 |
| Lymphoma | 8 | 21 |
| Germ cell tumors | 3 | 2 |
| Thymoma | – | 3 |
| Esophageal cancer | – | 2 |
| Metastatic tumors (e.g., breast) | | 6 |
| **Benign/Nontumor** | | |
| Portacath/Hickman | 22 | – |
| Dialysis catheter | 5 | 2 |
| Fibrosing mediastinitis | 8 | 5 |
| SVC thrombosis | – | |

SVC, superior vena cava.

Note: ≤2%: Pacer wire, aortic dissection, pseudotumor, S/P Mustard operation, Behcet's syndrome, retrosternal goiter, idiopathic.

## Etiology—Key Facts

### Malignancy

- Bronchogenic carcinoma[3-7] is the most common cause of SVC syndrome, occurring in 2% to 4% of patients overall during the disease course:
  - Small cell carcinoma:
    - Higher prevalence of SVC obstruction compared with non–small cell lung cancer (6%–20% of patients; central location)
    - SVC obstruction has been associated with a higher incidence of brain metastases.
  - Non–small cell carcinoma:
    - Large cell and other centrally located tumors are the most common types associated with SVC obstruction.
    - SVC obstruction is a poor prognostic indicator.
- Lymphoma[3-9]
  - Non-Hodgkin's lymphoma:
    - Most common group of lymphomas causing SVC obstruction, primarily due to lymph node compression
    - Diffuse large cell and lymphoblastic most commonly associated subtypes
    - Primary mediastinal B-cell lymphoma has been associated with SVC obstruction as a presenting feature, in 57% of cases
  - Hodgkin's lymphoma:
    - Much rarer (7 times), despite bulky mediastinal and hilar adenopathy in some subtypes[1,7]
- Germ cell tumors[10]
  - 2% to 3%
  - Primary mediastinal germ cell tumors: all types except mature teratoma; SVC syndrome in 20% of a series cohort
- Thymus tumors
  - Includes thymoma, invasive thymoma, thymic carcinoma
- Other malignancies
  - Solid tumors with mediastinal nodal metastases (breast cancer most common; thyroid, renal, rectal)
  - Esophageal cancer
  - Granulocytic sarcoma associated with acute or chronic myeloid leukemia[11]

## Benign Causes

- Intravascular devices[12-14]
  - Increasing incidence; 25%
  - Indwelling venous catheters: SVC obstruction has been linked to Port-a-Cath, dialysis catheters, and Hickman and other central venous catheters.
  - Development of SVC obstruction with indwelling catheters has been associated with suboptimal extension of catheters to the SVC/RA junction.
  - Pacemaker/implantable cardioverter defibrillator wires—proposed risk factors include:
    - Presence of prior temporary pacing lead, more than one pacer lead, retention of a severed lead, previous lead infection, and dual coil leads
    - Trauma to the vessel wall during insertion
    - Prior venous thrombosis; hormonal therapy
- Fibrosing mediastinitis[15,16]
  - 2% to 10% of several series
  - Excessive host response to infectious or noninfectious agent that involves mediastinal lymph nodes and that culminates in an excessive sclerosing process, with compressive of regional structures (SVC, pulmonary arteries and veins, airways, esophagus).
  - Most commonly due to *Histoplasma capsulatum* infection.
  - Can also be caused by tuberculosis, actinomycosis, blastomycosis, aspergillosis, nocardiosis, and bancroftian filiariasis.
- Other
  - Postradiation[17]
  - Primary SVC thrombosis
  - Sarcoidosis
  - Behcet's disease[18]
  - Coronary artery bypass[19]
  - Sclerosing cholangitis
  - See Table 28-1

## CLINICAL FEATURES

### Symptoms and Signs

- May occur as presenting manifestations of the underlying disorder, at any time during its course, and occasionally following surgical or other manipulation that disturbs adaptive collateral flow.
- With SVC obstruction, venous collaterals form to promote venous return to the right atrium (Fig. 28-1).
- With SVC syndrome, proximal venous pressures remain high despite collateral formation in the azygos, internal mammary, lateral thoracic, paraspinous, hemiazygous, intercostal, and esophageal venous systems.
- With high obstruction, collaterals drain into the azygos vein (most efficient decompressor). Obstruction below the azygos confluence drains to the inferior vena cava via hemiazygous or chest wall veins (less efficient).
- The rapidity with which SVC obstruction occurs affects the severity of the syndrome. Rapid development allows less time for adaptive collaterals to form, and thus greater severity.
- The duration of symptoms before diagnosis depends on the underlying cause or condition. In one series, 43% presented in less than 1 month and 50% after 1 to 6 months.[3,4]
- Presenting symptoms and signs are outlined in Table 28-2.

### Pathophysiology

- Symptoms are milder when the azygos vein is patent and recruitable, because it can accommodate more than 35% of the venous return.
- Changes in posture can exacerbate symptoms (bending forward; supine posture).

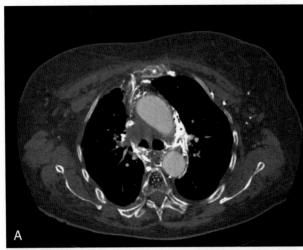

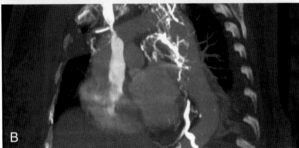

**Figure 28-1: A,** Transaxial computed tomography (CT) section showing compression of superior vena cava (SVC) by tumor together with a profusion of collaterals. **B,** CT reconstructed oblique view showing focal narrowing of SVC and prominent collateral vessels.

■ Clinical features of malignant and benign causes are similar, except for less weight loss, cough, hoarseness (trend), and hyponatremia with malignant etiologies.[4]
■ Facial, neck, upper trunk plethora and swelling: venous stasis
■ Dilated vessels: visible collaterals
■ Headache, head fullness, and other neurologic manifestations: reduced cerebral venous drainage, cerebral edema
■ Hoarseness: laryngeal edema
■ Hypoxemia: multifactorial; systemic to pulmonary venous shunts also described.[20]
■ Cough: variable mechanisms/multifactorial.

## DIAGNOSIS

Diagnosis and cause should be established, because management, at least in part, depends on etiology. For standard workup of specific malignant and benign conditions, see specific chapters on those topics. The diagnostic approaches presented in the next section refer specifically to the workup of patients with SVC syndrome.[3-5,21]

### Imaging Studies
■ Plain chest radiograph
  ○ Abnormal in majority (>85%)
  ○ Clues: superior mediastinal widening, dilated azygos, mediastinal hilar mass
■ Computed tomography (CT) scan
  ○ Most useful imaging modality.
  ○ Contrast imaging demonstrates narrowed or obstructed SVC, level of obstruction, and presence of collaterals (see Fig. 28-1).
  ○ May suggest etiology
  ○ Multidetector row CT with three-dimensional volume rendering provides the most accurate depiction of collateral circulations.[6]
■ Magnetic resonance imaging scan
  ○ Similar to CT
  ○ Useful with dye allergy or limited venous access.
■ Upper extremity venography
  ○ Reliably demonstrates obstruction; less informative than CT

### Establishing a Tissue Diagnosis in the Presence of Superior Vena Cava Obstruction

More invasive procedures are undertaken when less invasive approaches fail to make a diagnosis (e.g., bronchoscopy, peripheral lymph node biopsy)

■ Invasive techniques:
  ○ Prior concerns regarding the safety of invasive diagnostic procedures have been recently clarified.[7]
  ○ Cervical mediastinoscopy and anterior mediastinotomy have the potential for complications because of the possibility of bleeding from dilated veins.
  ○ Cervical mediastinoscopy and anterior mediastinotomy have been associated with increased morbidity in patients with SVC obstruction compared with those without (12.8% versus 2.8%), with major bleeding accounting for 40% of the morbidity.[22] In another series, major bleeding occurred in 4.3% with cervical mediastinoscopy but not with anterior mediastinotomy.[7] No increased mortality was observed in either reports. Diagnostic accuracy was 97.4%
  ○ Ultrasonography-assisted videomediastinoscopy can help minimize complications and increase diagnostic yield.[23]

### TABLE 28-2 ■ PRESENTING SIGNS AND SYMPTOMS OF SUPERIOR VENA CAVA SYNDROME

| Sign/Symptom | Rice, et al[4] 1996–2001 n = 78 (%) | Yellin, et al[3] 1972–1987 n = 63 (%) |
|---|---|---|
| Venous congestion head/neck | 82 | 86 |
| Upper extremity/trunk swelling | 62 | 32 |
| Dyspnea at rest | 53 | 30 |
| Cough | 50 | 21 |
| Dilated chest veins | 38 | NS |
| Chest/shoulder pain | 19 | 6 |
| Facial plethora | 18 | NS |
| Syncope/ pre-syncope/dizziness | 13 | NS |
| Headache | 12 | NS |
| Hoarseness | 12 | NS |
| Hemoptysis | 9 | 8 |
| Dysphagia | 6 | 6 |

NS, not stated.
Note: ≤5%: Confusion, epistaxis, tinnitus, proptosis, ischemic stroke, no signs or symptoms.

○ Video-assisted thoracic surgery and thoracotomy are rarely reported in published series. High yield; no report of increased major complications attributable to presence of SVC obstruction.

▪ Anesthesia in patients with SVC obstruction[24,25]:

○ Anesthesia generally can be performed safely. However, depending on the size, location, pathology and potential for compression of airways and great vessels, life-threatening cardiorespiratory complications can occur upon induction, or at any time during the procedure.

○ Acute airway obstruction occurred in 5% of 39 patients undergoing cervical mediastinoscopy or anterior mediastinotomy

○ Preventative measures: preanesthesia planning; airway evaluation and planning; Fowler position with induction/intubation; alternative approaches, if risk is too high.

## TREATMENT

Endovascular therapies including percutaneous stenting of the SVC are rapidly emerging as the initial primary therapeutic modality in many cases because of rapid and effective symptom relief.[26] This does not preclude the use of other treatment measures, depending on the underlying etiology and circumstance.[27,28]

▪ Endovascular approaches[29-35]

○ *General procedures with stent deployment:* predilatation of the stenosis by angioplasty generally needed to overcome radial forces and optimize stent deployment (Fig. 28-2). With extensive clot, local thrombolyic therapy (e.g., tPA) can be used. The final diameter of self-expanding stents should be 1.2 to 1.5 times the vessel diameter, with appropriate length, to account for up to 30% shortening in situ (Fig. 28-3). Most often, one stent is used but multiple devices can be employed.

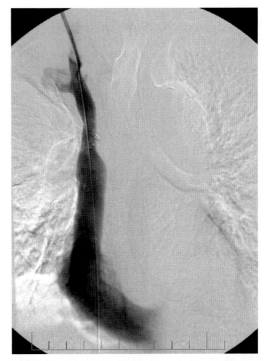

**Figure 28-3:** Contrast study following stent deployment. Note improved superior vena cava flow across stent.

○ *Types of stents:* most commonly used are self-expanding Smart Control Stent (Cordis) and other self-expanding nitinol or balloon expandable stents (allows size adjustment). The Wallstent (stainless steel mesh; Meditech-Boston Scientific) is now not commonly used.

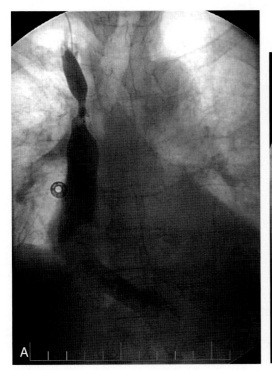

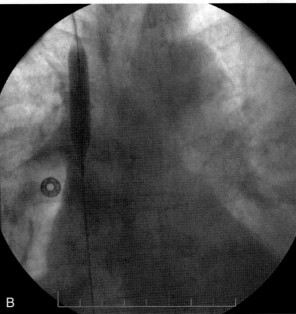

**Figure 28-2: A,** Superior vena cava obstruction before angioplasty and stent placement. **B,** Figure depicting angioplasty procedure.

○ *Indications:*
  - Primary modality with moderate to severe symptoms for rapid relief
  - In combination with chemoradiation therapy
  - Rapid progression
  - Failure of chemoradiation therapy
  - Reached dose limitation for chemoradiation therapy
  - Benign etiologies
○ Complications:
  - Thrombosis (can use anticoagulation or antiplatelet drugs to prevent; can treat with endovascular approaches)
  - Stent migration (can reposition or remove from RV or pulmonary arteries percutaneously)
  - Infection (rare; remove; antibiotics)
  - Rupture and pericardial tamponade (rare)
  - Transient hemidiaphragm paralysis (rare), pleuritic chest pain
  - Pulmonary edema (rapid increase in venous return)
○ Efficacy and long-term outlook:
  - Rapid relief in 95%; long-term patency rate 92%
  - Recurrent SVC obstruction in 11% (amenable to endovascular therapy in majority).
- Chemotherapy and radiation therapy[9,26-28,36]
  ○ May be indicated for definitive treatment of the underlying condition
  ○ May induce rapid response in some conditions (e.g., non-Hodgkin's lymphoma).
  ○ May reduce tumor bulk and prolong survival
  ○ Can be combined with endovascular therapy
  ○ With small cell lung cancer, chemoradiation relieved SVC obstruction in 77%, with recurrence in 17%
  ○ With non–small cell lung cancer, chemoradiation relieved SVC obstruction in 60%, with recurrence in 19%
- Corticosteroids
  ○ No defined role established on systematic review[28]
- Surgical bypass[37-40]
  ○ Mostly performed for benign causes, such as extensive mediastinal fibrosis with complete obstruction not amenable to endovascular approaches.
  ○ Successful bypass with prolonged graft patency has been reported
  ○ Internal jugular–SVC bypass, using autologous superficial femoral vein graft; can also use saphenous veins to bypass
  ○ Internal jugular-femoral vein bypass (using synthetic graft via subcutaneous tunnel)

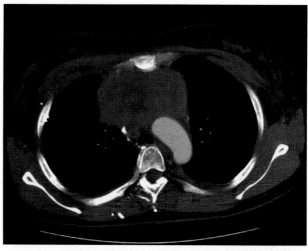

**Figure 28-4:** Transaxial computed tomography section showing marked compression of the superior vena cava by lymphoma (9 × 11 cm anterior mediastinal mass). Note no evident collateral vessels present.

vein. Only few collaterals evident. Small pericardial and pleural effusions.
- *Echocardiogram:* Pericardial effusion with features of tamponade (right atrial [RA] collapse; right ventricular [RV] invagination). Pericardiocentesis removed 300 mL, with temporary catheter left in situ. (cytology-negative)
- *Diagnosis/Pathology:* Right anterior mediastinotomy with biopsies. Pathology: Diffuse large B-cell lymphoma.
- *Management of SVC syndrome:* Anticoagulation and chemotherapy. Rapid reduction in size of anterior mediastinal mass and sustained resolution of SVC syndrome, clinically and on serial CT scans.

### Key Points

- Typical presentation of SVC syndrome.
- Rapid course suggests rapid tumor growth with little chance for adaptation (few collaterals on CT).
- Absence of plethora not unusual (present in a fifth of patients).
- Pleural and pericardial effusions can complicate lymphoma. Pleural effusions reported in 70% of malignant and 58% of benign cause of SVC syndrome.[41]
- Respiratory symptoms suggest potential for airway problems with anesthesia (special precautions with high-risk anesthesiologist required; may need to ventilate in lateral decubitus or other postures in extreme unanticipated cases).
- Pathology illustrates most common lymphoma type associated with SVC syndrome.
- Stenting could have been performed with slow or poor response to chemotherapy, which was not the case in this patient.

---

### Brief Illustrative Case

- *History:* A 32-year-old woman with 10-day history of progressive facial and bilateral arm swelling. Also, new headaches, cough, and mild dyspnea on effort and orthopnea. Low-grade night fever and sweats.
- *Examination:* Vitals: tachycardia (100–114/min); BP 120/68; respirations 16/min; temp: 99.8° F, $SPO_2$ 99% (2 L/min NC $O_2$). Obvious facial swelling. No plethora. Distended veins neck and upper chest.
- *Blood tests:* Complete blood count and electrolytes—normal; LDH 628; beta HCG and alpha fetoprotein: normal.
- *Imaging:* Contrast CT scan of chest (Fig. 28-4): 9 × 11 cm anterior mediasinal mass with marked compression of SVC and thrombosis in proximal left brachiocephalic

### References

Interactive references and additional readings for this chapter can be accessed online at *expertconsult.com*.

# SUPERIOR SULCUS TUMORS

Peter Smethurst, MD, Clark Fuller, MD, and Michael I. Lewis, MD

## TERMINOLOGY

- Superior sulcus tumor
- Superior pulmonary sulcus tumor
- Pancoast tumor
- Pancoast's syndrome

## DEFINITION

A superior sulcus (or Pancoast) tumor is a neoplasm of pulmonary origin that is located in the most apical recess of the pulmonary sulcus (i.e., the thoracic costovertebral gutter) and that arises from the lung apex. Pancoast's syndrome is classically associated with pain in the arm and shoulder, weakness and atrophy of small muscles of the hand, and Horner's syndrome (ipsilateral ptosis, miosis and anhidrosis).

## EPIDEMIOLOGY

- Superior sulcus tumors account for less than 5% of all non–small cell lung cancers (NSCLC).[1-3]

## PATHOLOGY

- The majority of superior sulcus tumors are NSCLC.[3-9]
  - Most commonly squamous cell, followed by adenocarcinoma and large cell. Some series cite adenocarcinoma as the most common.
- Small cell lung cancer accounts for approximately 5% of cases.[1,2,10-13]
- Rarely other masses or tumors may simulate Pancoast's syndrome.[1,14-38] These include
  - Neoplastic: adenoid cystic carcinoma, metastatic disease, lymphoma, plasmacytoma, other primary thoracic tumors
  - Aneurysms, cervical rib syndrome, amyloid nodules
  - Pulmonary infections (including fungal, bacterial, mycobacterial, and parasitic)

## ANATOMIC CONSIDERATIONS

- Knowledge of the thoracic inlet anatomy is important because superior sulcus tumors can invade important anatomic structures contained therein (Fig. 29-1).[39]
- The thoracic inlet can be divided into anterior, middle, and posterior compartments.[39]
- *Anterior compartment*: ventral to the anterior scalene muscle (subclavian vein, internal jugular vein, sternomastoid, omohyoid muscle)
- *Middle compartment*: between middle and anterior scalene muscles (subclavian artery, trunks of brachial plexus, phrenic nerve)
- *Posterior compartment*: posterior to middle scalene muscle (brachial plexus nerve roots, stellate ganglion, vertebral bodies)
- Although posterior involvement is the classic more common presentation, anterior, middle, or combined involvement

may occur, which complicates the optimal surgical approach (see later).
- Figure 29-2 depicts the anatomy of the brachial plexus.

## CLINICAL FEATURES

### Clinical Presentation

- The most common initial presenting symptom in most superior sulcus tumors is arm and shoulder pain (90%, but wide range).[1,2,5,10,40-43]
  - Mechanism of pain: tumor invasion of brachial plexus, parietal pleura, ribs (first and second) or vertebral bodies.[40]
  - Pain may radiate to the ipsilateral head and neck, axilla, anterior chest, scapula, or arm. (The latter often in an ulnar distribution, that is, half of fourth and fifth digit ipsilateral to the tumor.)
  - Pain is often initially misdiagnosed as nonspecific musculoskeletal pain or bursitis.
- Pancoast's syndrome is seen later in the course of disease.
  - Pancoast described superior vena cava (SVC) syndrome as part of this syndrome
  - Shoulder and arm pain in the C8, T1, and T2 dermatomes, as described earlier (axilla, medial aspect of the arm, forearm and medial portion of fourth finger and the fifth finger)
  - Hand small muscle weakness, atrophy, and paresthesias occur with involvement of the C8 and T1 nerve roots.
  - Horner's syndrome (ipsilateral ptosis, miosis and anhidrosis) is seen in 25% to 50% of patients (83% in one study).[40,44,45]
    - Caused by involvement of the paravertebral sympathetic chain and the stellate ganglion (see Fig. 29-2).
- Supraclavicular lymph nodes are noted in 25% to 35% of patients.[1,40]
- Extension of the tumor through the intervertebral foramen may result in spinal cord compression, with variable neurologic sequelae, including paraplegia.[1] Intervertebral foramen invasion is noted in about 5% earlier in the course of the disease and as high as 25% in patients presenting late.
- Occasionally a SVC syndrome may develop (see Chapter 28 on Superior Vena Cava Syndrome).[1]
- Phrenic nerve involvement can occur.
- Typical "pulmonary" symptoms including cough, hemoptysis, and dyspnea are uncommon presenting symptoms, likely as a result of the peripheral location of the tumor.[1,40]

### Staging Classification

- Staging is done as per the International System for Staging Lung Cancer (TNM staging system) as adopted by American Joint Committee for Cancer (see Chapter 21 on Staging of Lung Cancer).[46]
  - Owing to the location, most superior sulcus tumors are T3 (chest wall involvement) or T4 (invasion of vertebrae, great vessels, esophagus, or trachea).
  - Depending on the nodal status, nonmetastatic tumors are stage IIB (N0), IIIA (N1, N2) or IIIB (N3).
  - Metastatic tumors are by definition stage IV.

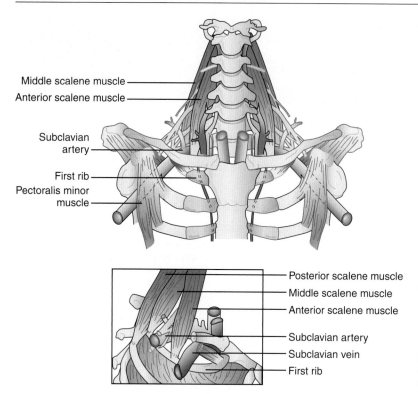

Middle scalene muscle

Anterior scalene muscle

Subclavian artery

First rib

Pectoralis minor muscle

Posterior scalene muscle
Middle scalene muscle
Anterior scalene muscle
Subclavian artery
Subclavian vein
First rib

**Figure 29-1:** Anatomy of the thoracic inlet. *(From Rusch VW. Management of pancoast tumours. Lancet Oncol 2006;7:997-1005, with permission.)*

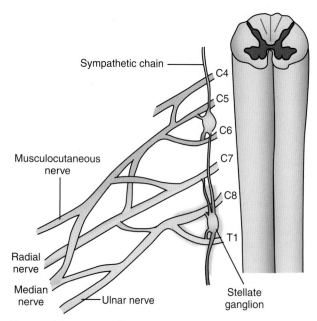

Sympathetic chain

C4

C5

C6

C7

C8

T1

Musculocutaneous nerve

Radial nerve

Median nerve

Ulnar nerve

Stellate ganglion

**Figure 29-2:** Anatomy of the brachial plexus. *(From Arcasoy SM, Jett JR. Superior pulmonary sulcus tumors and Pancoast's syndrome. N Engl J Med 1997;337:1370-1376, with permission.)*

## *DIAGNOSITIC WORKUP*

### **Laboratory Studies**

- Serum chemistries and cell counts, including a complete blood count, liver function tests, and electrolytes, are indicated as part of the routine workup of lung cancer patients.[47]

## **Imaging Studies**
### *Chest X-ray Study*

- Findings include an apical cap greater than 5 mm, a discrepancy between the apical caps greater than 5 mm, an apical mass, and first- or second-rib or thoracic vertebrae destruction (Fig. 29-3).[5,42,48]

### *Computed Tomography*

- Contrast-enhanced computed tomography (CT) is more useful than a chest x-ray study (CXR) in tumor staging and in further delineating the tumor.
- Sensitivity of mediastinal lymph node involvement is about 65%. If the CT scan shows normal nodes, there is an 18% chance of N2 disease (Fig. 29-4).
- Limited ability to identify vessel, nerve, and chest wall invasion[48-51]
- Can demonstrate obvious rib and vertebral destruction
- Inferences for chest wall involvement: no visible fat plane; significant apposition of tumor with pleural surface (>3 cm) but specificity low.
- Can demonstrate vessel compression or encasement

### *Magnetic Resonance Imaging*

- Superior to CT for evaluation of brachial plexus, vertebral body destruction, extension into spinal canal through intervertebral foramina, vascular, and chest wall involvement (Fig. 29-5).[49,52-58]

### *Positron Emission Tomography*

- Positron emission tomography (PET), while not well studied in this subset of patients, is generally accepted as part of the workup of patients with NSCLC.[47] This method may be helpful in the evaluation of mediastinal nodal involvement and distant metastases.

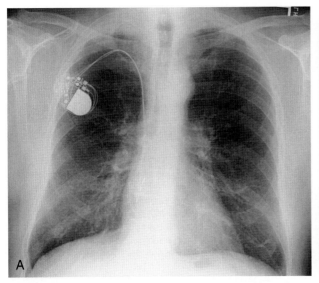 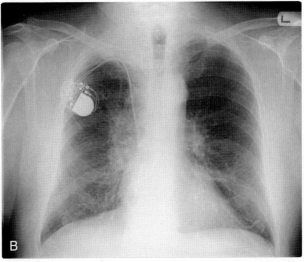

**Figure 29-3:** Chest radiographs in a patient with right superior sulcus tumor. **A,** Note: in the upper film, an apical density larger than 5 mm is just discernable and the patient was asymptomatic. **B,** Seventeen months later, the patient presented with typical symptoms, and the superior sulcus tumor has grown in size and is now clearly present.

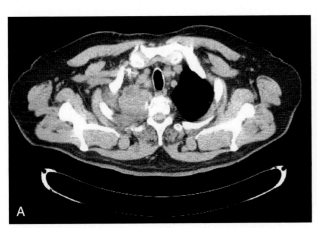 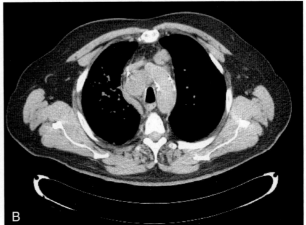

**Figure 29-4:** **A,** Chest computed tomography scan showing large superior sulcus tumor on the right. **B,** Significant mediastinal adenopathy is evident in this patient.

## Tissue Diagnosis

- Because the differential is broad (benign apical cap, infection such as tuberculosis or aspergillus-associated pleural reaction, lymphoma, primary chest wall tumors, neural tumors, lipoma, metastatic pleural disease, radiation fibrosis, cervical rib), tissue is required for diagnosis.
  - ○ Guided transthoracic needle biopsy is diagnostic in up to 95% of cases.[6,11,59-61]
  - ○ Sputum cytology has a yield between 11% and 20%.[6,62]
  - ○ Bronchoscopy is typically low yield due to the peripheral location of the tumor (diagnosis in 10% to 40% of cases).[5,47,59,62,63]
  - ○ Video-assisted thoracic surgery or thoracotomy will be diagnostic if other modalities fail.

## Further Workup/Special Studies
### Mediastinoscopy

- Pathologic staging of mediastinum is necessary before treatment.

- Thus, it is generally recommended as part of the surgical staging before final treatment decisions, especially as this study affects treatment approaches and prognosis.[64-66]

### Imaging for Metastatic Disease

- The CT scan of the chest generally includes cuts of the upper abdomen including the liver and adrenals, and thus, may be useful in the evaluation of metastasis to these sites.
- Superior sulcus tumors commonly metastasize to the brain; therefore, routine brain imaging (CT or MRI) is generally recommended.[1,67]
- PET scans, as noted earlier, are generally useful in the evaluation of patients with NSCLC.[47]
- A bone scan is indicated in patients with appropriate symptoms.[1]

### Pulmonary Functions Testing

- Indicated in all patients in whom surgical resection is considered

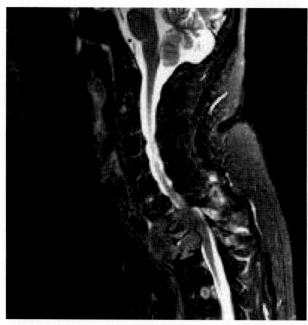

**Figure 29-5:** Magnetic resonance imaging scan depicting superior sulcus tumor with vertebral involvement and cord compression by the tumor mass. *(Reprinted with permission from eMedicine.com, 2007. Available at: http://www.emedicine.com/radio/topic515.htm.)*

## PROGNOSIS

- Poor prognostic factors include the presence of Horner's syndrome, advanced stage, invasion of the great vessels or vertebral bodies, and longer duration of symptoms.[2,64,65,68-71]
- Good prognostic factors include early stage, complete respectability, less than 5% total body weight loss, and good preoperative performance status.[13,40]

## TREATMENT

- The treatment of superior sulcus tumors continues to evolve but typically involves multimodality therapy
- An outstanding historical perspective has been provided by Valerie Rusch, in which four eras of management were described.[39] These eras can be summarized as follows:
  - ○ **First Era:** early treatment approaches by Chardack and MacCallum (1956; radical resection and postoperative radiation[72]), and Shaw, Paulson, and Kee (1961; preoperative radiation followed by radical resection[73]).
  - ○ **Second Era:**
    - 30 Gy preoperative radiation over 2 weeks, followed by an en bloc resection of the lobe and chest wall nerve roots via an extended posterolateral thoracotomy. This became the standard approach for the next 3 decades.[4,12,68,69,74-78]
    - Studies over this time highlighted issues with limited ability to perform curative resection and poor outcome with mediastinal node involvement, vertebral, or vascular involvement. This was confirmed in a study of 225 patients treated between 1974 and 1988.[68]
    - Survival in that study highlighted the need for new treatment strategies.[68] Five-year survival after treatment was 46% for T3N0, 13% for T4N0 and 0% for N2 disease.[68]
  - ○ **Third Era:** This was characterized by several new surgical approaches to deal with tumors in which subclavian vessels or the spine was involved. This included

- Anterior transcervical-thoracic approach for tumor invasion of subclavian vessels[79]
- Transmanubrial osteomuscular sparing approach (spares clavicle)[80,81]
- Approaches to facilitate lung and spine exposure, including hemiclamshell anterior thoracotomy and partial median sternotomy[82,83]
- Approaches to deal with spinal involvement to include vertebrectomy and spine stabilization[45,58,84-86]
  - ○ **Fourth Era:** This relates to induction chemoradiation, followed by en bloc resection. Key trials and data summary:
    - 4th era treatment applies to patients in whom mediastinoscopy is negative.
    - Southwest Oncology Group (SWOG 9416-1060) phase II trial. N = 110 (T3-4; N0-1)[87]
    - Two cycles of etoposide and cisplatin plus 45 Gy concurrent radiation, then resection (if stable or tumor regression), then 2 additional cycles of etoposide and cisplatin
    - Main results[87,88]:
      - ○ Seventy-five percent of patients underwent resection (most lobectomy and chest wall resection)
      - ○ Of these, a third had a complete pathologic response (CR) and a third showed minimal residual disease.
      - ○ Complete resection in 91% of T3 lesions and 87% for T4 lesions.
      - ○ Only 42% could complete post operative chemotherapy.
      - ○ Survival data[88]: The 5-year survival rate was 54% in patients with complete resection and 44% overall. In patients with CR at surgery, the estimated 5-year survival rate was about 70% versus about 40% in those with residual disease. Note: these are impressive data compared with studies over the last 30 years, in which the 5-year survival rate was 30% and complete resection possible in less than 50% of patients.
      - ○ Disease progression was mainly due to metastatic disease (e.g., brain).
      - ○ Similar survival data were reported in single institution study.[89]
- Summary details of posterior and anterior surgical approaches, including management of spine/neurologic involvement
  - ○ Posterior
    - The posterior approach for Pancoast's tumors is the optimal approach for lesions attached to the ribs posteriorly or to the vertebral bodies. It begins with an extended posterolateral incision. This usually involves transection of the latissimus dorsi and serratus anterior muscles. Posteriorly, the incision is extended to the top of the scapula with transection of the teres and rhomboid muscles.
    - Resection of ribs is part of the procedure, and it is the reason that this is not a minimally invasive procedure. An adequate margin around the tumor is imperative, so at least one rib above and one rib below the ribs to which the tumor is attached are resected.
    - The rib resection is performed first, and then a standard lobectomy and node dissection are performed. Visualization of the tumors attachment to the ribs can be very helpful to determine which intercostal space is entered for the resection.
    - The pulmonary resection should be a lobectomy, not a wedge resection because a wedge resection has a higher local recurrence rate. The margins of resection must be clean because local radiation does not then prevent local recurrence.

○ Anterior
■ The anterior approach is the procedure of choice for a Pancoast tumor attached anteriorly to the ribs of the anterior chest or subclavian vessels.
■ The incision is made just superior to the clavicle, then in the midline of the chest over the sternum, and then laterally into (usually) the fourth intercostal space. This provides excellent exposure to the subclavian vessels and the brachial plexus. This is not seen well through a posterior incision.
○ Spine/neurologic involvement:
■ Spinal involvement is not a contraindication to resection if all disease can be resected. This requires a spine surgeon as part of the team. The operation should include an en bloc resection of the ribs, the lobe, and the spine.
■ Neurologic involvement is also not an absolute contraindication to resection.
■ The posterior cord of the brachial plexus can be resected. However, more extensive involvement of the brachial plexus is a contraindication to resection.
■ The phrenic nerve is adjacent to the brachiocephalic vein and SVC. This means that clear margins will not be obtained with the resection, so phrenic nerve involvement precludes a resection with *curative intent.*
■ Treatment complications[47]:
○ Surgical mortality rates range from 0 to 14%.[47,70,88-90]
○ *Post-thorocotomy complications* include
■ Pneumonia (chest wall instability and pain limit effective bronchial toilet)
■ Wound infection
■ Bronchopleural fistula
■ Chylothorax and hemothorax
■ Ulnar nerve paralysis (damage to C8 +/- T1)
■ Horner's syndrome (high dorsal root sympathectomy)
■ Pulmonary embolism
■ Subclavian vein injury or thrombosis
○ *Radiation* may result in skin irritation, esophagitis, pneumonitis, and pulmonary fibrosis
○ *Chemotherapy-related complications* specific to the therapy or regimen chosen
■ Primary stand-alone radiation therapy and other issues:
○ Indication: patients with unresectable or metastatic disease,[2,10] serious comorbidities that render them inoperable, poor performance status
○ Provides good palliation for pain
○ 60 to 65 Gy given with unresectable disease
○ In unresectable disease, concurrent chemotherapy and radiation can be considered depending on patient factors
○ Some studies have shown up to 40% 5-year survival rates using radical radiation alone in localized tumors.[2,10,70,91]
○ Postoperative radiation therapy may be considered in unresectable or incompletely resected tumors.[3,43,69,92]

## *KEY FACTS*

■ Most (>95%) of superior sulcus tumors are NSCLC.
■ The most common initial presenting symptom is shoulder pain.
■ Owing to their location, most superior sulcus tumors are T3 or T4.
■ MRI is better than CT for the evaluation of nerve and vascular involvement.
■ Percutaneous/transthoracic needle biopsy is diagnostic in up to 95% of cases.

■ Radiation plus chemotherapy before complete surgical resection is the treatment of choice for resectable superior sulcus tumors (Fourth Era of treatment), provided that the mediastinum has negative findings for affected nodes.
■ Prophylactic cranial irradiation has been recommended by some groups.[10,67,78,93]
■ With complete resection, 5-year survival may now surpass 50%.

### Brief Illustrative Case

- A 62-year-old woman with a heavy smoking history
- In her usual state of health until she developed left shoulder and anterior chest wall pain, which became progressively worse, requiring codeine analgesics
- She was initially misdiagnosed as having musculoskeletal pain.
- She had no headaches, neurologic symptoms, or bone pain.
- Dry cough, with no sputum or hemoptysis
- Anorexia and a 10-pound weight loss were noted over several months.
- Examination revealed no signs of a Horner's or SVC syndrome. No supraclavicular adenopathy
- Auscultation revealed diminished breath sounds in the region of the left upper lobe (LUL)
- Some wasting of the small muscles of the left hand was evident
- CXR and subsequent CT revealed a 6.6-cm mass in the LUL compatible with a superior sulcus tumor (Fig. 29-6).
- PET scan was strongly positive for the tumor. Lymph nodes were negative, and no distant metastatic disease was found.
- Cervical mediastinoscopy was negative.

*(Continued)*

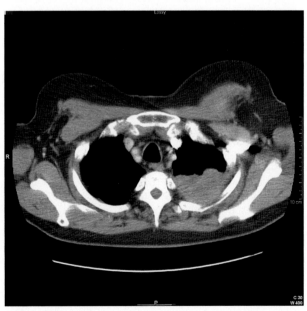

**Figure 29-6:** Computed tomography (CT) scan showing 6.6-cm lobulated superior sulcus tumor (*left upper lobe*). The tumor abuts the pleura posteriorly. There are however no distinct CT signs of invasion of pleura and no invasion of bone or muscle.

## Brief Illustrative Case—cont'd

- The patient underwent neoadjuvant chemoradiation therapy. (Two cycles of chemotherapy with concurrent 45 Gy radiation therapy.)
- Subsequent CT scans showed tumor regression. Surgery was undertaken about 3 months after start of neoadjuvant therapies.
- At surgery, the tumor (now 3.5 cm) was found to be attached to the chest wall, requiring ribs 2 to 4 to be resected en bloc with the left upper lobe.
- Tumor pathology revealed 50% of the tumor mass to be necrotic, 20% fibrotic, with the remainder showing poorly differentiated adenocarcinoma. No pleural involvement was evident. No muscle or bone invasion was noted. Lymph nodes negative.
- Lessons to be learned from this case are
  - Patient symptoms are often misdiagnosed as nonspecific musculoskeletal complaints, as in this case.

- Shoulder pain with radiation is a common presenting symptom in up to 90% of cases.
- Pancoast's tumors should be staged with a PET scan, brain MRI, and a cervical mediastinoscopy.
- Treatment for Pancoast's tumors has evolved from surgery alone to preoperative radiation (3000 Rads in 2 weeks), to the current standard of chemotherapy plus radiation followed by resection with or without chemotherapy (Fourth Era)
- In this case, the response to neoadjuvant therapy, while significant, was not greater than 90% on surgical pathology.
- Postoperative chemotherapy should be considered.

## References

 Interactive references and additional readings for this chapter can be accessed online at *expertconsult.com*.

# 30 CHEST WALL INVASION IN LUNG CANCER

Ashraf Elsayegh, MD, Michael I. Lewis, MD, and Robert J. McKenna Jr., MD

## DEFINITIONS

- **Chest wall invasion:** In the context of non–small cell lung cancer (NSCLC), chest wall invasion refers to invasion of the parietal pleura with or without invasion beyond the endothoracic fascia.[1] This may include invasion of soft tissues including muscle with or without invasion of ribs. In most series of chest wall invasion by NSCLC, superior sulcus tumors are excluded from the analyses. (See Chapter 29 on Superior Sulcus Tumors.)
- **R0 resection:** Refers to complete resection of the tumor with adequate margins that are tumor free.

## EPIDEMIOLOGY

### Prevalence

- Approximately 5% to 8% of NSCLC extends beyond the lung to invade chest wall structures.[1,2]
- Prevalence numbers refer to those cases with chest wall invasion that were pathologic Stage IIB (T3N0M0) or IIIA (T3N1M0; T3N2M0).
- In series published over the last 10 years, the breakdown of stages in patients undergoing surgical therapy was as follows[1-8]:
  - *T3N0M0:* 54-75% (65+/-7%)
  - *T3N1M0:* 10-26% (16+/-6%)
  - *T3N2M0:* 9-23% (16+/-6%)

### Demographics

- In several recent series, 66% to 90% of patients were male.[3,6,7,9]
- The average age in more recent series was 63 years (range: 32-93).[1,3,6-8]

## PATHOLOGIC CONSIDERATIONS

### Tumor Histology

- Squamous cell carcinoma: 42% to 60% (50+/-8%)[1,3,5,6,9]
- Adenocarcinoma: 27% to 57% (39+/-11%)
- Large cell carcinoma/other: 12% to 22% (16+/-6%)

### Chest Wall Invasion

- Chest wall invasion may be limited to the parietal pleura only, or it may be more expansive to encompass soft tissues, including intercostals muscles and ribs. Rarely, extrathoracic muscle invasion can occur.[3,5,8-12]
  - Parietal pleura only: 18% to 69% (37+/-18%)
  - Soft tissue invasion: 13% to 67% (38+/-22%)
  - Bony invasion: 24% to 46% (36+/-9%)
  - Very rarely, NSCLC can present as a palpable, chest wall mass.

## CLINICAL FEATURES

### Symptoms

- *Chest Pain:* Although intuitively one might expect a high incidence of chest pain with chest wall involvement, a sizeable number of patients were pain free. For example, Burkhart and colleagues[6] reported chest pain as a presenting symptom in only 45% of patients. Similarly, other series reported chest pain in 47% and 51% of their patients.[3,7] Chest pain ranges from a vague ache to a discrete localized pain.
- **Other symptoms:** *Hemoptysis* was reported in 6% in one series,[3] whereas *cough* was a presenting symptom in 18% in another.[6] In both series, 17% to 21% of patients were asymptomatic on presentation.

## DIAGNOSIS

The diagnosis of chest wall involvement may be made based on several clinical and imaging studies. However, it should be emphasized that these studies, either singly or in combination, are not totally sensitive or specific. Finite diagnosis thus often rests with direct visual examination and exploration at the time of surgery and should be confirmed as such in all cases. In some cases, frozen section or permanent histologic sections may confirm early invasion.

### Plain Chest Radiograph

- This is the least sensitive modality.
- Pleural-based masses do not confirm invasion and should not be relied on for diagnosis.
- In some cases, clear rib destruction by a contiguous mass may be evident.

### Computed Tomography of the Chest

- As with other imaging modalities, one needs to distinguish between tumor invasion and tumor impression, in which the tumor abuts the pleura but there is no actual pleural invasion. The latter may be the case in the often reported pleural-based mass.[13-16]
- Pleural thickening adjacent to the mass, lengthy contact, and angulation of the mass interface are neither sensitive nor specific.
- Loss of the normal extrapleural fat plane is suggestive, whereas obvious rib destruction is highly specific.
- In a recent prospective study by Bandi and coworkers[16] in 136 patients with lung cancer and possible chest wall invasion, the sensitivity of thoracic computed tomography (CT) was reported as only 42%, with the specificity at 100%. In another study, standard CT had a sensitivity of 50% and a specificity of 71%.[17]
- Improved sensitivity (70%) was reported for thin section cuts with multiplanar CT reformatting.[18] Likewise, much improved sensitivity was reported for high-resolution CT using an algorithm for soft tissue.[17]
- Usually in patients with a tumor abutting the chest wall on CT scan, the presence of chest wall pain is a better predictor of chest wall invasion than the appearance of the scan.

### Magnetic Resonance Imaging of the Chest

- Several studies have suggested that magnetic resonance imaging (MRI) may have several advantages over CT in the diagnosis of chest wall invasion.[13,19-22]
- This stems from the fact that the extrapleural fat plane can be more readily determined on MRI because of high signal intensity on T1-weighted images. Differences in signal intensity due to tumor invasion of the chest wall musculature can be appreciated on T2-weighted images.
- Improved accuracy over conventional CT or MRI was recently reported using respiratory dynamic MRI in 98 patients with suspicious CT scans.[23] Cine images assessed tumor movement along the chest wall to note the presence or absence of free movement. Following surgical and pathologic correlation, sensitivity was 100% and specificity was 83%.
- A case can be made that more sophisticated testing is not usually warranted, because a localized tumor should be resected, whether or not the chest wall is invaded.

### Ultrasound

- Ultrasound, using high frequency linear probes (5–7.5 MHz), may also be a useful modality, employing several of the principles reported above for other imaging modalities.[16]

- Two or more of the following criteria suggested chest wall invasion: (1) impairment of movement along the chest wall (as in the dynamic MR study above); (2) interruption of the pleural reflection; (3) tumor growth into the chest wall; and (4) invasion of the ribs.
- In 136 patients who were evaluated, ultrasound had a sensitivity of 89% and a specificity of 95%.
- The false-positive rate was attributed to benign adhesions noted at surgery, which limited movement with respiration.
- **Other:** The utility of positron emission tomography (PET), PET/CT, and other modalities needs further investigation. At present, the PET scan would not appear a good test to determine chest wall invasion.

## TREATMENT

### Surgical Approaches

- When chest wall invasion is suspected, a preoperative CT-guided needle biopsy is preferred to alternative biopsy approaches. This is because it is not desirable to cut into the tumor for diagnosis, or to cut across a tumor to separate it from the chest wall for a wedge resection.[1-12,24-28]
- The operation should start with video-assisted thoracic surgery for the following reasons:
  - To make sure that there is no evidence of pleural seeding
  - To determine if the tumor is indeed attached to the chest wall
  - To determine what interspace should be used to enter the chest, with an adequate margin around the tumor
  - To determine where to cut the ribs for an adequate margin around the tumor.

### Principles of Complete Resection

- When the attachment between the lung and the chest wall is minimal, an **extrapleural dissection** or an **en bloc chest wall resection** can be performed. An en block chest wall resection is generally recommended because it provides a lower local recurrence rate and a better survival rate.[3] If the adhesions are inflammatory, such as those due to adhesions caused by a central tumor resulting in distal atelectasis, then chest wall resection is not needed if the frozen section shows that the tumor does not go to the pleural surface.
- Tumors invading the chest wall should be resected, with removal of the involved ribs and one additional rib inferior and superior to the involved ribs and a 3- to 5-cm margin anteriorly and posteriorly. In a large recently reported series, one rib was resected in 12.9%, whereas two, three, four, and five ribs were resected in 31.5%, 38.3%, 15.8%, and 1.4% of cases, respectively.[3]
- An en bloc resection should be performed with removal of the chest wall and the lung tissue.
- Even if the amount of lung involved by tumor is small, the recommended pulmonary resection is a lobectomy, not a wedge resection, because the latter has a greater local recurrence rate. Adjuvant radiation therapy after a wedge resection has an inferior survival rate compared with lobectomy.

### Chest Reconstruction

- When to consider[29-33]:
  - Chest wall reconstruction is generally indicated for cases in which more than one rib has been resected.
  - Chest wall reconstruction is not necessary for the following situations:
    - If the resection involves ribs 1 through 4 posteriorly under the scapula. If the resection includes rib 5, then

reconstruction is needed because the tip of the scapula goes inside the remaining ribs.

- If the chest wall is ulcerated or infected over the tumor, reconstruction of the chest wall with a prosthetic is not usually performed because the prosthetic material may become infected.

- Types of reconstruction: prostheses and muscle/myocutaneous flaps.
  - Chest wall reconstruction can be performed using a variety of prosthetic materials or a myocutaneous flap.[29-32] Use of a stabilizing prosthesis has been reported as important in decreasing the need for prolonged postoperative mechanical ventilation.[31] However, use of only a myocutaneous flap has not resulted in respiratory compromise in our experience (i.e., the presence of a persistent flail segment postoperatively did not significantly affect rapid weaning from mechanical ventilation or produce respiratory compromise).
  - A sandwich of Marlex (a plastic mesh) and methyl methacrylate is most commonly used to reconstruct the chest wall. The combination makes a solid prosthesis for reconstruction. The methyl methacrylate comes in the form of a liquid and powder that are mixed to make a solid prosthesis in the shape of the chest wall defect. The mesh is sutured to the surrounding ribs. This sandwich is used for chest wall resections that involve the curved part of the chest or the sternum.
  - An alternative is to reconstruct without the methyl methacrylate. For this method, the following variety of materials is available: plastic mesh, absorbable polyglactin mesh, and biologic xenografts. These are used primarily when the resection involves a flat area of the chest wall, such as the anterior surface between the sternum and the anterior axillary line.
  - A myocutaneous flap is used when the chest wall resection involves a significant amount of soft tissue and especially if skin is resected.
  - A muscle flap is used if the resection includes ribs and the overlying muscle so that there is no muscle to separate the marlex/methyl methacrylate mesh from the overlying subcutaneous tissue. Usually, a single muscle is used. The choice depends on several factors including proximity, technical and anatomic feasibility of rotating it in place, and the size of defect that needs to be covered.[30] If the sandwich is too close to the skin, an erythematous reaction in the skin commonly ensues.
  - Muscle and myocutaneous flaps may decrease the risk of infection while covering the defect and mesh.[30]

## Perioperative Management and Highlight of Potential Complications and Management

- Perioperative management is basically the same as the postoperative care for all lung resections (see Chapter 23 on Surgical Management of Lung Cancer). The keys are pain relief, early ambulation, and good pulmonary toilet.
- Pain control is usually administered by an epidural or a pain pump. If an epidural is too high in the chest, respiratory depression may occur, so if the resection involves the first three ribs, a pain pump is preferable.
- Complications after pulmonary resection plus chest wall resection are basically the same as for other pulmonary resections. Rib resection includes resection of the intercostal nerves, so patients experience permanent paresthesias in the distribution of those nerves.

## Factors Negatively Influencing Outcome

- In all series[1,3-12]:
  - Mediastinal and hilar lymph node involvement
  - Incomplete resection

- In some series:
  - Depth of invasion
  - Male gender
  - Poor tumor differentiation
  - Tumor size
  - Extent of resection
  - Older age
  - Type of surgical approach

## Resection in Patients with Limited Pulmonary Function

- The same general principles employed in other potentially resectable cases should be used. Because of the added morbidity of a chest wall resection however, a more conservative approach is prudent and is advised for patients with limited pulmonary function. (See Chapters 3 and 31 on resection in patients with limited reserve and perioperative assessment.)
- A case series of en bloc resection and limited lung resection in 10 patients with poor pulmonary function ($FEV_1$ <1.3 L) was reported.[34] There was no perioperative mortality, and long term follow-up results were acceptable.

## Adjuvant Therapies

- Radiation:
  - Adjuvant radiotherapy may be employed even in R0 resections. When resection margins are positive or narrow, radiation may be given in an effort to reduce local recurrence. The discovery of hilar or mediastinal adenopathy in surgical specimens will likely also prompt adjuvant chemotherapy with or without radiation therapy.
  - In 209 patients who underwent en bloc chest wall resections, adjuvant radiation therapy did not impact on the rate of local recurrence or overall survival in patients with stage IIB (T3N0) disease. In contrast, adjuvant radiation therapy did increase survival in those patients with stage IIIA disease.[3]
  - Radiation therapy improved outcome in some series,[12,35] but not in another.[4]
- Chemotherapy
  - The role of chemotherapy in patients with chest wall invasion who are pStage IIB is unclear. The number of patients with lung cancer involving the chest wall is small, so there are no randomized, prospective trials to assess the value of adjuvant chemotherapy. However, the studies do show a small benefit for adjuvant chemotherapy for stage 2 and 3 lung cancer (see Chapter 24 on Adjuvant and Neoadjuvant Chemotherapy of NSCLC). Therefore, patients with lung cancer invading the chest wall generally receive adjuvant chemotherapy.
  - There is no proven benefit for preoperative chemotherapy in patients with lung cancer invading the chest wall.

## SURVIVAL DATA

For many years, prognosis was believed to be dismal with chest wall invasion. However, with surgical advancements, survival has improved tremendously. In fact, in patients without nodal involvement, survival has improved by nearly 50% with the performance of surgery.

Many studies have evaluated different prognostic factors for these patients using univariate and multivariate statistical analyses. We summarize this data in order to better understand prognosis. Unless otherwise stated, survival relates to 5-year data/estimates.

## Overall (5-Year Survival)

- Doddoli and associates[3] reported a median survival of 19 months and a 5-year survival rate of 31%. Similarly, Burkhart and coworkers[6] reported a 38% 5-year survival rate, while

Chapelier and colleagues[9] had a slightly higher 5-year survival rate of 41%. In one study by Facciola and coworkers,[12] the 5-year survival rate was as high as 61%.

## Stage

- Now that surgical approaches and techniques have become more standardized, the most important prognosticating factor has become stage. The main issue appears to be nodal involvement (N0 vs N1 or N2 disease).
- Survival in patients with N0 disease ranged from 22%, 25%[4,9] to 40%, to 44%.[3,6,10]
- The survival rate in patients with N1 disease was not as high. Chaplier and associates[9] reported a 9% survival rate. Doddoli and associates[3] and Magdlienat and coworkers[4] reported survival rates of 24% and 20%, respectively. At least two studies had much higher survival rates. Matsuoka and colleagues[10] and Burkhart and associates[6] reported survival rates of 40% and 44%, respectively.
- N2 involvement was associated with very poor survival rates, that is, 8%,[3] 6%,[10] and 0%[9] in several studies.
- Aside from nodal involvement, several studies have evaluated other prognostic factors.

## R0 Versus non-R0 resections (i.e., Incomplete Resection)

- Downey and coworkers[11] showed a 5-year survival difference of 32% in patients with R0 resection vs. 4% in those who did not have R0 resection.
- Magdeleinat and associates[4] had 24% with R0 resections versus 13% with incomplete resection.
- Matsuoka and colleagues[10] had similar results, with 34% with R0 versus 14% with incomplete resection.

## Tumor Size

- Doddoli and associates[3] showed that there was worse survival in patients with a tumor size larger than 6 cm.

## Gender

- Doddoli and associates[3] showed a worse rate of survival in men than in women.
- Similarly, Burkhart and colleagues[6] reported an overall 5-year survival rate of 53% in women, whereas men had a 31% survival rate.

## Depth of Invasion

- Several studies reported a worse prognosis if the tumor invades deeper into the chest wall (beyond the parietal pleura).[4,9]
- Facciola and coworkers[12] showed a survival rate of 79% if the tumor was solely limited to the parietal pleura versus 54% if invasion included the soft tissue and the ribs.

## Other Factors

- Both Doddoli and coworkers[3] and Chapelier and associates[9] reported a worse prognosis if patients had more than two ribs resected.
- Megdeleinat and colleagues[4] noticed a worse prognosis in older patients.

### Brief Illustrative Case

- A 47-year-old man complained of left shoulder pain.
- He had a 40-pack year smoking history.
- He denied having headaches, neurologic symptoms, bone pain, or weight loss.

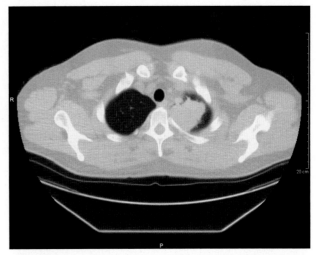

**Figure 30-1:** Computed tomography scan of chest showing a 6-cm mass in the left upper lobe. The mass abuts the posterior chest wall.

- Chest x-ray study suggested the presence of a mass in the apex of the left chest.
- CT scan confirmed the presence of a 6-cm mass in the apex of the left lung. The mass abutted the chest wall posteriorly (Fig. 30-1).
- Needle biopsy revealed the presence of a NSCLC.
- He received chemotherapy (carboplatin and taxol), together with 50 cGy radiation.
- The chest wall pain completely resolved.
- Restaging with a PET/CT and a brain MRI showed a good response to the neoadjuvant treatment and no evidence of distant or nodal metastases.
- Five weeks after the last radiation and chemotherapy treatments, he underwent a left-sided thoracotomy, left upper lobectomy, node dissection, and en bloc resection of ribs 1 through 4.
- Final pathology showed a residual tumor with 90% necrosis as a result of the neoadjuvant treatment. Furthermore, there were clear margins and no nodal metastases.

### Key Points

- This case was treated as a superior sulcus tumor, with an appropriate treatment regimen.
- This case differs from the case scenarios outlined earlier
- Superior sulcus tumors are often reported in case series, along with chest wall invasion at other sites. This complicates matters in view of different approaches, with only high grade evidence available in the literature for management of superior sulcus tumors. (See Chapter 29.)
- In cases of chest wall invasion (apart from the superior sulcus region), treatment approaches should follow the general considerations outlined earlier.
- For further details on chest wall resection in a variety of other situations (e.g., other chest wall tumors, chest wall and sternal infections, chest wall reconstruction and thoracoplasty), see Chapter 50 on the Chest Wall by Francis C. Nichols.

## References

 Interactive references and additional readings for this chapter can be accessed online at *expertconsult.com*.

# 31

# PREOPERATIVE ASSESSMENT OF HIGH-RISK PATIENTS FOR LUNG CANCER RESECTION

Heather D. Jones, MD and Zab Mosenifar, MD

## INTRODUCTION

Patients who develop pulmonary lesions requiring resection often have underlying parenchymal lung abnormalities. Pulmonary function tests may reveal clinically significant obstruction or gas diffusion abnormalities, which require careful consideration; a patient's immediate operative risks and possible long-term disability related to loss of lung function must be weighed against the benefit of a potentially curative surgery for lung cancer. Numerous studies have examined methods of preoperative risk Zassessment for these patients, and although individual findings vary, a general consensus for risk stratification has begun to emerge, as recently outlined in an algorithm by the American College of Chest Physicians (ACCP) (Fig. 31-1).[1] In this chapter, we provide a background for understanding the current guidelines, discuss high-risk patient groups who do not meet usual criteria for surgery, and describe the application of these guidelines in practice.

## LUNG CANCER RESECTION: STRATIFICATION OF RISK

- Who does not need further workup?
  - There is general consensus that those with an $FEV_1$ of greater than 80% predicted have an average perioperative risk.[1,2]
  - If a patient has a preserved $FEV_1$, but unexplained dyspnea or diffuse parenchymal disease on chest computed tomography (CT) scan, ACCP 2007 guidelines recommend measuring carbon dioxide diffusing capacity (DLCO).[1]
  - Patients with a DLCO of less than 80% predicted may have increased pulmonary complications (Table 31-1); those with less than 60% predicted may have increased mortality.[3]
  - *Patients with an $FEV_1$ greater than 80% predicted and DLCO greater than 80% predicted do not have increased risk for lobectomy or pneumonectomy, and do not require further preoperative testing.*[1,2]
- Next step in evaluation: split-function determinations
  - Patients with $FEV_1$ or DLCO less than 80% predicted require further evaluation
  - The ACCP 2007 algorithm and other sources suggest split-function evaluation for determination of predicted postoperative (ppo) $FEV_1$ and DLCO values as next step (see Figs. 31-1 and 31-2).[1,4,5]
    - Split-function evaluation can be done by using CT scan data or by a nucleotide lung perfusion scan (see Fig. 31-2).
    - Nucleotide lung perfusion scan is best for patients with marginal lung function and/or for patients requiring pneumonectomy.[6]
  - Risk stratification based on ppo lung functions
    - For $ppoFEV_1$ less than 40% predicted, the perioperative mortality rate is approximately 50%.[7-9]

- ppoDLCO of less than 40% predicted is also associated with high mortality and morbidity.[3,7]
- When the product of the ppoDLCO and $ppoFEV_1$ is less than 1650, this number predicts increased surgical mortality.[10]
- ppoDLCO as % predicted closely correlated with operative mortality: odds of death increased 3.5-fold for every 20-point decrease in ppoDLCO%.[11]
- DLCO can be decreased by induction (preoperative) chemotherapy, and this decrease in DLCO is an additional risk factor for postoperative complications[12-14]; therefore, repeating pulmonary function tests after induction treatment should be considered.
- In some studies, even patients with ppoDLCO or $ppoFEV_1$ of less than 40% can have uncomplicated postoperative courses, but mortality risk is higher and physician discretion is important in these patients.[2,5,15,16]
- Next step in evaluation: cardiopulmonary exercise testing (CPET):
  - CPET is recommended for further evaluation of patients with $ppoFEV_1$ or ppoDLCO of less than 40%.
  - Determination of $VO_2$ max via CPET can be the next step instead of a split-function test in some algorithms.[2,17]
  - Incremental exercise testing—Most widely used and studied type of exercise test for assessing preoperative risk in high-risk patients.
    - Patient exercises on a cycle ergometer or treadmill, with continuous (ramp) or incremental increase each minute in work rate; continuous exhaled $O_2$ and $CO_2$ measurements, electrocardiogram (ECG) and $O_2$ saturation, and intermittent blood pressure readings are measured.[18]
    - Work rate increments targeted based on patient's predicted $VO_2$ max to reach maximal exercise within 6 to 12 minutes.[18]
    - Risks of complications during exercise testing are low, with overall rate of death of 2 to 5 per 100,000 clinical exercise tests; risks are related to underlying comorbid conditions.[19]
    - Absolute contraindications are few and include syncope, unstable angina, uncontrolled systemic hypertension, and the presence of serious dysrhythmias on resting ECG.[19]
    - In patients with multiple or no medical conditions, the many variables measured allow detailed analysis and determination of etiology of impaired exercise tolerance or unexplained dyspnea
    - For patients with lung cancer, the most frequently used parameter for preoperative assessment and risk stratification is $VO_2$ max.
      - $VO_2$ = cardiac output × oxygen extraction.
      - Maximal $VO_2$ can be reduced for many reasons (Fig. 31-3).
      - This multifactorial variable is most often the best predictor of perioperative risk (see below).

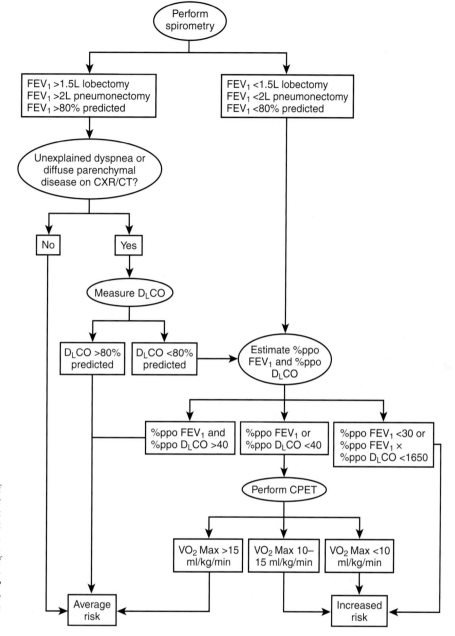

**Figure 31-1:** American College of Chest Physicians algorithm for preoperative physiologic assessment of perioperative risk. CXR, chest radiograph. (*From Colice GL, Shafazand S, Griffin JP, Keenan R, Bolliger CT. Physiologic evaluation of the patient with lung cancer being considered for resectional surgery: ACCP Evidenced-Based Clinical Practice Guidelines. 2nd ed. Chest 2007;132: 161-177. Reprinted with permission.*)

---

### TABLE 31-1 ■ PERIOPERATIVE COMPLICATIONS*

Need for prolonged (more than 48 h) mechanical ventilation or reintubation
Myocardial infarction
Cardiac arrhythmias requiring treatment
Pneumonia
Atelectasis—on radiologic studies or lobar requiring bronchoscopy
Pulmonary embolism
Acute $CO_2$ retention
Death

---

*Complications included in most studies examining predictive value of pulmonary function tests and cardiopulmonary exercise tests in estimating perioperative risks for lung cancer resection surgery.[2,5,7,8,16,23]

○ Risk assessment based on CPET
  ■ Patients with a preoperative $VO_2$ max of greater than 15 to 20 mL/kg/min, or greater than 75% predicted have acceptably low perioperative mortality rates.[2,4,16,20-24]
  ■ Patients with a $VO_2$ max between 10 and 15 mL/kg/min are at an increased risk for perioperative complications (see Fig. 31-1)[1,5,20,21,24]
  ■ Percent predicted $VO_2$ max may be a better discriminator than absolute $VO_2$ max,[21] and patients with a $VO_2$ max of less than 60% predicted are at increased risk for perioperative complications.[5,21,23]
  ■ A low anaerobic threshold (<11 mL/min/kg), especially in conjunction with cardiac ischemia, is associated with a high mortality rate.[25]
  ■ Patients with a ppo$VO_2$ max of less than 10 mL/kg/min have a very high perioperative mortality rate and are generally considered to be inoperable.[1,2,20,21]

CALCULATING THE PREDICTED POST-OPERATIVE LUNG FUNCTIONS

**Functional segments for lobectomy:**

ppo F = preoperative F × (1 − y/z)

where F = the lung function being evaluated (FEV1, DLCO, VO2max), y is the number of *functional segments* (determined by CT) to be removed and z is the total number of functional segments (**6**), as estimated by CT scan.

**Quantitative CT scans for pneumonectomy:**

For *pneumonectomy*, functional segment evaluation is not accurate (**6**), and underestimates the actual post-operative values. CT scans can be used to evaluate the functionally relevant lung parenchyma, as identified by falling within a defined range of attenuation values. A radiologist can identify the tissue to be resected and the tissue remaining by outlining them using a drag ball, and standard CT software can provide the areas of functionally relevant tissue. By this method, the quantitative CT scan calculation would be:

ppo F = preoperative F × (1 − [RFLV/TFLV])

where RFLV = regional functional lung volume to be resected, and TFLV = total functional lung volume (**6**).

**Perfusion scans:**

Perfusion scans remain the gold standard and should be used for patients with severe impairment for whom highest accuracy is needed; many studies using ppo values to predict risk are based on perfusion scan-derived numbers (**2,5,7,8,17**). Technetium-99m ($^{99m}$Tc)-labeled macroaggregates are used to quantify the contribution of different areas of lung parenchyma to lung function. Ppo values are calculated by fractional contributions of each lung or lobe (**7,33**):

ppo F = preoperative F × (1 − fractional contribution of resected lung or lobe)

**Figure 31-2:** Calculation of predicted postoperative pulmonary functions. Formula used is determined by degree of impairment and degree of resection required (see text).

■ Even patients who are deemed inoperable by the above-mentioned criteria can successfully undergo surgery, and median survival for these patients is twice as long as for patients who do not undergo surgery (30 vs 15 months).[5]
■ Presurgical exercise training can increase VO$_2$ max by 2 or more mL/kg/min in borderline patients within 4 to 6 weeks.[26]
○ Fixed challenge exercise testing: assessment of ability to perform a fixed amount of work; that is, climbing stairs or walking a fixed distance[4]:
■ Stair climbing:
○ Classic test for estimating perioperative risk—usually involves physician accompanying patient to climb stairs in a hospital or office building at patient's own pace with monitoring pre-exercise vital signs, continuous pulse, and O$_2$ saturation during climb, and postexercise vital signs; some studies include calculation of VO$_2$ max by estimation of work done (step height × steps/min × wt in kg × conversion factor).[27,28]
○ Inability to climb 12 meters, or 75 steps, predicts a high rate of complications (>50%).[27-29]
○ Ability to climb three flights, or 90 steps, predicts a lower rate of perioperative complications (6–20%).[28-31]
■ 6-minute walk test:
○ Patient is instructed to walk at a brisk pace in a hallway for 6 minutes and is allowed to rest as needed during the interval; total distance walked is recorded.
○ Data are limited in this test in preoperative assessment of lung cancer patients.[32]

○ One study demonstrated that a 6-minute walk distance of greater than 1000 feet predicted successful surgical outcome.[31]

## PREDICTING LONG-TERM EFFECTS OF LUNG RESECTION: PNEUMONECTOMY VERSUS LOBECTOMY

■ ppo formulas generally underestimate postoperative lung function at 1 year, especially for pneumonectomies.[33,34]
■ Patients have an initial decrease in exercise tolerance at 3 months after surgery, but this factor recovers at 6 months for lobectomy patients.[35-38]
■ Pneumonectomy patients often do not recover exercise tolerance, which postoperatively becomes limited by dyspnea.[35-37]
■ Postoperative pulmonary function and exercise tests correlate poorly with quality of life measures, which are reduced in lung cancer patients, but which return to preoperative levels at 3 months after surgery.[39]

## LUNG VOLUME REDUCTION SURGERY COMBINED WITH LUNG CANCER RESECTION

■ Several studies describe combined operations for lung volume reduction surgery and lung cancer resection.[40-43]
■ Patients in these studies had ppoFEV$_1$ values less than 40%, with average ppoFEV$_1$ values of 21% and 26% of predicted in two series,[40,41] and would have been considered inoperable

VO2 PEAK = CARDIAC OUTPUT × (CAO2 − CVO2) = [SV × HR]

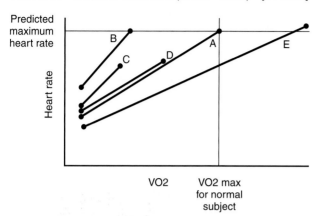

**Figure 31-3:** Peak VO$_2$ (maximum delivery to and extraction of oxygen from tissues) can be limited by multiple factors:
**A,** Normal: VO$_2$ max is limited by reaching maximum cardiac output via maximum heart rate (stroke volume reaches plateau earlier)
**B,** Maximum heart rate reached at lower level of exercise (and O$_2$ extraction from tissues):
  ▪ Heart disease: maximum cardiac output impaired, usually due to impaired stroke volume (reach maximum heart rate early)
  ▪ Deconditioning: decreased stroke volume and extraction of oxygen from tissues leads to maximum heart rate and fatigue early.
**C,** Limited by factors other than heart rate (with increased heart rate as compensatory mechanism):
  ▪ Respiratory disease: oxygenation impaired, arterial oxygen decreased and limits oxygen delivery, causing lactic acidosis and fatigue, exercise terminated.
  ▪ Pulmonary vascular disease: oxygenation and stroke volume impaired, both limiting oxygen delivery, causing lactic acidosis and fatigue, exercise terminated.
  ▪ Anemia: impaired oxygen content/delivery to tissues, causing lactic acidosis and fatigue, exercise terminated.
  ▪ Peripheral vascular disease: impaired delivery of blood/oxygen to tissues, causing lactic acidosis and fatigue, exercise terminated.
  ▪ Mitochondrial disease: oxygen extraction impaired, causing lactic acidosis and fatigue, exercise terminated.
**D,** Limited by factors not related to oxygen delivery:
  ▪ Respiratory disease: ventilation impaired, CO$_2$ rise causes dyspnea and exercise terminated.
  ▪ Anxiety, poor motivation.
**E,** Elite endurance athlete: Stroke volume and oxygen extraction supraphysiologic, with resultant VO$_2$ much higher at maximum heart rate.

for lung cancer resection by usual criteria, although CPET data were not collected for further risk stratification.
■ Results of these studies[40,41,43] showed:
  ○ Perioperative mortality and complications were low (0-14%)
  ○ FEV$_1$ improved and dyspnea was improved or unchanged.
■ These findings suggest that different criteria should be used for assessing lung cancer patients who also meet criteria for lung volume reduction surgery
■ Risks of mortality from surgery must be weighed against mortality from lung cancer in these patients

## Brief Illustrative Cases

### Case 1

- A 54-year-old man with a 30 pack-year smoking history referred for preoperative risk assessment before right upper lobectomy for a solitary pulmonary nodule.
- FEV$_1$ is 82% predicted; however, patient reports dyspnea with moderate exertion.

- DLCO = 73% predicted.
- An incremental exercise test is performed, and patient's VO$_2$ max is 17 mL/kg/min.

### Key Points

- This patient's DLCO was appropriately measured, because although the FEV$_1$ was greater than 80%, he reported dyspnea that would not be expected with normal spirometry. Because the DLCO was less than 80% predicted, further evaluation was required; an exercise test *or* determination of patient's predicted postoperative FEV$_1$ and DLCO would be an acceptable next step.
- ACCP 2007 guidelines would suggest calculation of predicted postoperative pulmonary function tests (PFTs), which could be done based on functional segments (because a lobectomy is planned) as demonstrated on CT scan, and requires no further studies. These values could be calculated as follows:
- ppo Function = preoperative Function × (1–3 right upper lobe [RUL] segments)
- 18 total segments
  - ppo Function = preop Function × (.83)
  - ppoFEV$_1$ = 82% × (.83) = 68% predicted
  - ppo DLCO = 73% × (.83) = 61% predicted
- Values for ppoFEV$_1$ and DLCO greater than 40% predict an average risk for surgery, and this estimation would have been sufficient.
- In this case, a CPET was performed, and this patient's VO$_2$ max of greater than 15 mL/kg/min confirms the perioperative risk to be average.
- Because this patient is to undergo a lobectomy, he is unlikely to be more limited by dyspnea postoperatively than preoperatively.
- One advantage to a CPET in this patient would be to further investigate the etiology of the preoperative dyspnea and to rule out cardiac ischemia.

### Case 2

- A 73-year-old woman with long-standing COPD has a lung mass involving the left lower lobe bronchus with distal atelectasis
- A left lower lobectomy is planned.
- FEV$_1$ is 59% predicted, and DLCO is 48% predicted.
- A perfusion scan is performed, which shows 22% fractional contribution from the left lower lobe.

### Key Points

- This patient required further evaluation based on FEV$_1$ and DLCO of less than 80%.
- Because her preoperative pulmonary function is marginal, a perfusion scan is better than functional segment calculations for estimation of predicted postoperative values.
- Alternatively, an exercise test to measure VO$_2$ max could have been performed as the next step.
  - ppoFunction = preoperative function × (1–.22)
  - ppoFEV$_1$ = 59% × (.78) = 46% predicted
  - ppoDLCO = 48% × (.78) = 37% predicted
- Because the ppoDLCO is less than 40% predicted, this patient is at increased risk for post-operative complications and required a CPET to determine whether her operative mortality was prohibitive.
- A CPET demonstrated a VO$_2$ max of 11 mL/kg/min.
- ppoVO$_2$max = 11 mL/kg/min × (.78) = 8.58 mL/kg/min

*(Continued)*

## Brief Illustrative Cases—cont'd

- Patients with ppoVO$_2$ max values of less than 10 mL/kg/min are at very high risk for complications.
- However, the perioperative morbidity and mortality must be balanced against the morbidity of an unresected lung cancer. In these cases, physician discretion is particularly important for determining which patients are candidates for surgery.
- Alternative therapies, such as radiofrequency ablation or Cyberknife, may be considered.[44]

### Case 3

- A 65-year-old woman with a right upper lobe mass abutting the right pulmonary artery requires a right pneumonectomy.
- Her FEV$_1$ is 78% predicted, and DLCO is 85% predicted.
- A perfusion scan reveals 62% fractional contribution of the right lung.

### Key Points

- A perfusion scan was appropriate in this patient, because the FEV$_1$ was less than 80%, requiring further evaluation, and functional segment analysis is not accurate for predicting postoperative function after pneumonectomy.
    - ppoFunction = preoperative function × (1−.62)
    - ppoFEV$_1$ = 78% × (.38) = 30%
    - ppoDLCO = 85% × (.38) = 32%
- This patient is at increased risk for perioperative complications because her predicted postoperative FEV$_1$ and DLCO are less than 40%, and further evaluation with an exercise test is indicated.
- A stair climbing test was performed, and the patient was able to climb four flights of stairs, or 100 steps, suggesting that the patient will be able to tolerate the operation.
- The predicted postoperative calculations underestimate postoperative pulmonary function with pneumonectomy, and this patient is likely to have better postoperative values than calculated. However, this patient may have her postoperative exercise capacity limited by dyspnea, as has been found in patients after pneumonectomy.

### Case 4

- A 68-year-old man with severe upper lobe bullous emphysema has a left upper lobe mass in an area of nonfunctional lung.
- FEV$_1$ is 32% predicted, and DLCO is 41% predicted.
- A stair climbing test was performed, and the patient was unable to climb more than two flights secondary to dyspnea.

### Key Points

- This patient should be referred to a thoracic surgeon experienced in lung volume reduction surgery (LVRS) for consideration of a combined lung volume reduction surgery with resection of the lung mass.
- By all established criteria, this patient's perioperative mortality risk would be considered prohibitive.

- However, patients with heterogeneous upper lobe emphysema and low exercise capacity have a mortality benefit from LVRS,[45] the survival benefit to resection of the lung cancer is significant, and these patients have been shown to tolerate such combined procedures well. Hence, they must be considered differently from other patients being evaluated for lung cancer resection.

### Case 5

- A 58-year-old man with a right middle lobe nodule found on an "executive physical" CT scan is being evaluated for surgery.
- As part of his physical, PFTs showed an FEV$_1$ of 82% predicted.
- A CPET was also performed, which showed a VO$_2$ max of 16 mL/kg/min, which was 58% of predicted for his age and height.
- The anaerobic threshold was reached at 11 mL/kg/min, and there was evidence of 1 mm ST segment depressions in the inferior leads.

### Key Points

- A VO$_2$ max of less than 60% predicted indicates an increased risk of complications in this patient, despite an absolute VO$_2$ max value of greater than 15 mL/kg/min.
- Moreover, patients with an early anaerobic threshold and suggestion of cardiac ischemia on the ECG during the exercise test have significantly increased perioperative mortality for lung resection.
- This patient requires further evaluation, probably with cardiac catheterization, due to his increased risks.

## SUMMARY AND PRACTICAL PEARLS

- Patients with preoperative FEV$_1$ and DLCO greater than 80% of predicted do not need further evaluation for lung resection.
- Patients with an absolute VO$_2$ max of less than 15 mL/kg/min[20,24] or a VO$_2$ max of less than 60% of predicted[5,21,23] have a significantly increased risk of postoperative complications.
- Patients with a ppoFEV$_1$ or DLCO less than 40%[7] or a ppoVO$_2$ max of less than 10 mL/kg/min[8,20] have very high perioperative risk of mortality or mortality with lung cancer resection.
- Even patients at very high risk who undergo surgery at their physician's discretion have higher 5-year survival than those who do not undergo surgery.[5]
- Pneumonectomy, but not lobectomy, results in significant decreases in exercise tolerance and increased dyspnea.[35-37]
- Patients who meet criteria for lung volume reduction surgery and have lung cancer in a nonfunctional area targeted for resection may not fall within the above-mentioned criteria; tumor resection in these patients, even with very poor preoperative function, may improve status as well as increasing survival.[40-43]

## References

 Interactive references and additional readings for this chapter can be accessed online at *expertconsult.com*.

# 32

# SMALL CELL LUNG CANCER

Leland Green, MD

## INTRODUCTION

- Accounts for 15% of all cases of lung cancer.[1]
- Decreasing incidence in the United States, Europe, and Japan.[2]
- Unique clinical aspects, response to treatment, and therapeutic strategies.

## PATHOLOGY

- Characteristic ovoid, small cells with scant cytoplasm. Crush artifact commonly seen (Fig. 32-1).
- Histologic subtypes include small cell (90%) and combined small and non–small cell components, including large cell neuroendocrine.[3]
- Neuroendocrine markers of differentiation help make the diagnosis (chromagranin, synaptophysin, and CD 56 Neural Cell Adhesion Molecule [NCAM]).[4]
- Electron microscopy shows dense-core neurosecretory granules.

## INCIDENCE

- Decreasing incidence and mortality rate over the last few decades. Possibly due to decreasing smoking incidence and increasing use of low tar filters.
- Rising incidence of women who present with small cell lung cancer (SCLC), approaching 50%. This is attributed to rising smoking incidence in women.
- SCLC has the strongest association with smoking of all lung cancers.[5]

## PATHOGENESIS

- Strong linkage to tobacco. Ninety-five percent of patients have a prior smoking history.[6]
- Interplay of environmental factors with genome of respiratory epithelium:
  - Autocrine growth loops with peptides that perpetuate cell growth.[7]
  - Oncogene overexpression (myc oncogene, tumor suppressor gene underexpression-p53, Rb gene inactivation)
  - Apoptosis (programmed cell death) inhibited by BCL-2 overexpression in over 90% of patients.[8]

## PRESENTATION

- Historically male predominant; now equal (Tables 32-1 and 32-2)[9]
- Typical patient is older than 50 years of age.
- Respiratory symptoms are the most common (see Table 32-1).
- Majority present with advanced disease (66%).
- Higher incidence of paraneoplastic syndromes, mainly neurologic and endocrinologic.[10]
- Endocrine entities parallel disease activity, whereas neurologic complications progress independently of illness.

## CLINICAL FEATURES

- "Central disease" with hilar, mediastinal, large volume, bulky radiographic features.[11]
- Most common malignant etiology of superior vena caval syndrome, with facial and neck swelling, jugular and anterior chest venous engorgement.
- Ten percent present with peripheral, solitary pulmonary nodule.[12]
- The majority present with metastatic disease, most commonly to liver, bone, adrenals, brain, and bone marrow.
- Paraneoplastic syndromes (Tables 32-3 and 32-4)[13]

### Endocrine (Protein Mediated)

- Inappropriate antidiuretic hormone (ADH)—hyponatremia (15%)
- Cushing's syndrome—hypertension, hypokalemia related to increased adrenocorticotropic hormone production.
- Acromegaly—secondary to increased growth hormone–related protein production.
- Hypercalcemia—related to increased parahormone-related protein (much more common in non–small cell cancer).

### Neurologic (Antibody Mediated)

- Definition of neurologic paraneoplastic syndromes[14]:
  - A classic neurologic syndrome associated with SCLC, developing within 5 years of neurologic presentation
  - Nonclassic syndrome that significantly improves or resolves after cancer treatment
  - The presence of "paraneoplastic antibodies"
- Syndromes:
  - Eaton-Lambert syndrome:
    - Occurs in about 3% of patients with SCLC
    - Tumor-associated antigens cross-react with voltage-gated calcium channels on presynaptic nerve terminals, with generation of antibodies directed against these channels in 95% of patients.
    - Ptosis is common, but diplopia is rare.
    - Muscle weakness in the pelvic girdle exceeds that of muscle groups around the shoulder girdle
    - Respiratory muscle involvement and respiratory failure can occur.
    - Repetitive nerve stimulation studies typically produces augmentation of the amplitude of compound action potentials initially (opposite with myasthenia gravis)
    - Can coexist with either cerebellar degeneration or encephalomyelitis
    - Successful therapy results in improvement in 50% of cases.
    - Plasma exchange, intravenous immunoglobulin and 3,4, diaminopyridine (enhances acetylcholine release from nerve terminals) has been used to treat the disorder per se.

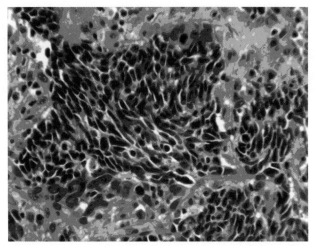

**Figure 32-1:** High-power photomicrograph showing clusters of small round to ovoid cells with scant cytoplasm, typical for small cell lung cancer.

### TABLE 32-1 ■ SYMPTOMS OF SMALL CELL LUNG CANCER

| Symptom | Percent of Patients |
| --- | --- |
| Cough | 50 |
| Weakness | 40 |
| Dyspnea | 40 |
| Chest pain | 35 |
| Anorexia | 30 |
| Hemoptysis | 20 |

### TABLE 32-2 ■ SIGNS OF SMALL CELL LUNG CANCER

| Sign | Percent of Patients |
| --- | --- |
| Weight loss | 50 |
| Paraneoplastic process | 1–15 |
| Fever | 10 |

### TABLE 32-3 ■ ENDOCRINE PARANEOPLASTIC SYNDROMES IN SMALL CELL LUNG CANCER

| Syndrome | Clinical Presentation | Protein |
| --- | --- | --- |
| Inappropriate secretion of antidiuretic hormone (SIADH) | Hyponatremia | ADH |
| Cushing's syndrome | Hypokalemia, hypertension | ACTH |
| Acromegaly | Acromegaly, Hypertension, Glucose Intolerance | Growth hormone release hormone (GHRH) |

ACTH, adrenocorticotropic hormone; ADH, antidiuretic hormone.

## STAGING

- The concept of limited and extensive disease is the currently employed staging system in patients with SCLC (Table 32-5).
- Limited disease is disease confined to one hemithorax, with the tumor encompassing one radiation port. Disease that is beyond those confines is defined as extensive disease.
- The International Association for the Study of Lung Cancer Lung Cancer Staging Project has published proposals regarding the clinical staging of SCLC in the forthcoming (Seventh)

○ Other syndromes:
  ■ See Table 32-4.
  ■ Neurologic syndromes are generally progressive and run a course independent of the therapeutic response of the tumor.

### TABLE 32-4 ■ NEUROLOGIC PARANEOPLASTIC SYNDROMES IN SMALL CELL LUNG CANCER

| Syndrome | Clinical | Pathophysiology |
| --- | --- | --- |
| Lambert-Eaton | Proximal limb muscle weakness, Initial increase in strength with activity (i.e., transient postrecruitment augmentation) | Antibody directed against voltage gated calcium channel antigens |
| Encephalomyelitis (includes cortical, limbic, and brainstem, as well as cerebellar, cord, and peripheral nervous system involvement) | Lethargy, sensory neuropathy, autonomic neuropathy | Antineuronal antibody, (Hu) (also anti-Ri with brainstem encephalitis) |
| Cerebellar degeneration | Ataxia, poor coordination, nystagmus. | Purkinje cell antibody mediated; Anti-Tr |
| Stiff man syndrome* | Progressive muscle rigidity; superimposed painful muscle spasms and gait impairment due to continuous motor activity | Antiamphiphysin |
| Subacute pandysautonomia | Cholinergic and/or adrenergic dysfunction | Antineuronal acetylcholine receptor antibody |

*Benzodiazepines (for muscle relaxation) and immune modulators such as intravenous immunoglobulin, plasmapheresis, and prednisone may provide effective treatment.

| TABLE 32-5 ■ CLINICAL AND INVESTIGATIVE STAGING OF SMALL CELL LUNG CANCER |
| --- |
| History and physical<br>CT scan of chest, abdomen and pelvis<br>Brain imaging (CT scan or MRI)<br>PET/CT scan (acceptable)<br>Bone scan<br>Chemistry panel, CBC, LDH, CEA<br>Bone marrow (only if abnormal CBC, high LDH and potential to change treatment plan) |
| CBC, complete blood count; CEA, carcinoembryonic antigen; CT, computed tomography; LDH, lactate dehydrogenase; MRI, magnetic resonance imaging scan; PET, positron emission tomography. |

| TABLE 32-6 ■ ACTIVE DRUGS FOR TREATMENT OF SMALL CELL LUNG CANCER |
| --- |
| Cisplatin/carboplatin<br>Etoposide<br>Vincristine<br>Doxorubicin<br>Irinotecan<br>Cyclophosphamide/ifosfamide<br>Topotecan/taxanes<br>Methotrexate |

Edition of the Tumor, Node, Metastasis Classification for Lung Cancer[15] (see Chapter 21 on Lung Cancer Staging). Use of TNM staging for early stage SCLC was recommended in future trials.

## STAGING WORKUP

- The staging workup and studies described below classify the patient into either category and determine therapeutic goals, treatment strategy and prognosis.
  - History and physical with attention to lymph nodes, upper body venous distension (superior vena cava syndrome), and organomegaly.[16]
  - Complete blood count (CBC), chemistry panel, lactate dehydrogenase (LDH), and carcinoembryonic antigen (CEA).
  - Computed tomography (CT) scan of chest, abdomen, and pelvis.
  - Brain imaging (CT scan or magnetic resonance imaging [MRI]).
  - Positron emission tomography (PET)/CT scan is an acceptable modality for staging, complementing the anatomic focus of CT scanning with the enhanced metabolic uptake of malignant cells of PET technology.[17]
  - Bone scan.
  - Bone marrow is rarely needed, unless an abnormal CBC on presentation, and the likelihood of changing treatment decisions. In addition, increased LHD levels often correlate with bone marrow involvement.

## THERAPY

- The natural history of untreated SCLC is a 6- to 12-week survival.

### Limited Disease (30% of Patients)

- Concurrent chemoradiotherapy is treatment of choice.[18]
- Radiation adds to overall survival (about 5% at 3 years). No role for surgery except in rare circumstances (see later).[19]
- Chemotherapy: Cisplatin/etoposide is the chemotherapy regimen of choice, but numerous drug combinations show similar activity (Table 32-6). The usual course of treatment is four cycles.
- With initial treatment of SCLC, chemotherapy results in significant treatment responses in the majority of cases (70%

to 90%). The problem is that for the majority of cases, relapse and progressive disease ensues.
- Combination chemotherapy including more than two active drugs has not been shown to improve survival.
- There is no current proven role for maintainance therapy, stem cell transplant, biologic therapy, or consolidation chemotherapy at this time.
- Chemotherapy side effects include nausea, vomiting, myelosuppression, sepsis, hair loss, and renal insufficiency.
- Etoposide has been reported to rarely cause lung toxicity (acute pneumonitis, diffuse alveolar damage, hypersensitivity reactions and bronchospasm). It may also potentiate the risk of radiation pneumonitis.
- Relapse occurs in up to 80% (within 2 years) despite an initial response to chemoradiation, due to the development of tumor cells that are chemoresistant
- Thoracic radiotherapy, in daily or twice-daily dosing, is initiated within the first two cycles of chemotherapy, concurrently, in limited disease.[20] If the patient has a reasonably poor functional status, or is not tolerating the treatment-related mucositis, then the treatment modalities can be given sequentially. (However, the latter approach has been shown to produce less optimal survival.)
  - Daily: 54 to 60 Gray in 25 to 30 fractions once a day.
  - Twice daily: If the patient has an excellent performance status and is younger than 60 years of age, hyperfractionation can be used.
  - With hyperfractionation, mucositis is typically much higher, but local control is better compared with conventional regimens. A trial is ongoing to evaluate if a high-dose daily regimen is equivalent (with regard to survival) compared with twice-daily regimens.
  - With hyperfractionation, 1.5 Gray is given twice a day to a total dose of 45 to 50 Gray.
  - The treatment field included in the radiation portal (both conventional and hyperfractionation) includes the prechemotherapy tumor volume (including any positive lymph nodes), as delineated by CT, PET, or both, plus a 2-cm margin around this area. In contrast to management of NSCLC, high-risk lymph node–bearing regions are not included.
  - Radiation side effects include esophagitis, pneumonitis during or after therapy, and weakness.
- Continued smoking has been shown to worsen survival.
- Combined modality therapy for early-stage limited disease produces a 5-year survival rate of 20% to 25%.[21]

### Extensive Disease (70% of Patients)

- Chemotherapy is the mainstay of treatment. Drugs are the same as in limited disease.
- Median survival is 8 to 10 months, with a 60% to 80% response rate.
- Usually patients receive four to six cycles of therapy.

- Radiation is useful for palliation of local symptoms. For example, lung masses causing postobstructive pneumonia and symptomatic atelectasis.
- The radiation dose is usually 30 Gray in 10 fractions.

## Relapsed Disease

- Definitions[22]
  - Relapse: Disease that recurs more than 3 months after completion of initial first-line treatment.
  - Refractory disease: No response (or indeed disease progression) with first-line treatment or if the disease recurs less than 3 months after completion of initial first-line treatment.
  - General comment: In reported studies, relapsed and refractory disease are often grouped together, despite the fact that the latter likely represents more chemoresistant tumors, and the response to salvage therapy and prognosis is worse.
- Median survival in this setting is 4 to 6 months, once there is progression of disease or relapse on therapy.
- Results are better if the disease-free interval is 6 months or more, but median survival is still less than 1 year. The longer the duration between initial treatment and relapse, the better the response rate to salvage chemotherapy.
- Salvage chemotherapy has been shown to improve survival and quality of life compared to best supportive care approaches.[23]
- Enrolling relapsed patients into clinical trials is appropriate when feasible.
- In patients with good performance status, combination chemotherapy regimens using non cross-resistant agents to those employed previously is suggested.
- In patients with poor performance status, single agents with fewer side effects are suggested (e.g., topotecan).
- Alternative agents include topotecan, taxanes, adriamycin, and vincristine.
- Newer agents include antiangiogenesis agents, e.g., bevacizumab (Avastin) and epidermal growth factor inhibitors (EGFR-Tarceva).[24]

## SPECIAL CIRCUMSTANCES

### Role of Surgery

- Rationale not to consider surgery:
  - SCLC is considered a systemic disease (i.e., early dissemination at the time of diagnosis), even in those designated to have apparent limited stage disease.
  - Early reports on surgery found no benefit as a primary treatment modality.[12]
- Rationale to consider surgery in select circumstances:
  - Despite optimal chemoradiation measures in patients with limited disease, the local recurrence is still high (35% to 50%).[19]
  - Solitary pulmonary nodules are reported in 4% to 12% of patients with SCLC. Often the diagnosis is confirmed following surgical resection. Survival rates in stage 1 solitary pulmonary nodules treated with surgery as part of therapy is higher than that generally reported for limited stage disease (40% to 53% 5-year survival rate).[25]
  - The new proposed IASLC staging for SCLC, recommends TNM staging for limited disease SCLC, in view of data showing improved outcomes in early TMN staged in a large database. (See Chapter 21 on Lung Cancer Staging.)
  - The above-mentioned changes, together with the results of more recent trials, suggest that the role of surgery in patients with early stage SCLC should be reconsidered and

further studied (as part of a multimodality approach in selected cases).
  - The following are recently reported survival data for surgery in SCLC:
    - Brock and associates[26] reported the experience at Johns Hopkins, in which 82 of 145 patients with SCLC (from 1976-2002) underwent surgical resection. Mixed histology was present in 14 of the 82 patients. The majority of patients also received chemotherapy, with about a quarter given prophylactic cranial irradiation. The overall 5-year survival rate was 42%. In patients with stage 1 disease receiving platinum-based chemotherapy (n = 24), the 5-year survival was 86%.
    - A Spanish study reported prospective data for 47 patients with SCLC (T1-2 N0). The overall survival rate at 5 years was 26% and 36% (n = 15) with pathologic stage 1 disease.[27]
    - A recent Japanese study reported a 68% 3-year survival rate for clinical stage 1 SCLC patients treated with complete surgical resection and adjuvant cisplatin and etoposide therapy.[28]
  - As stated earlier, surgery is rarely performed in patients with SCLC with the current state of the art but may be considered in the following circumstances[29]:
    - In selected cases with a peripheral, solitary pulmonary lesion and no nodal involvement or metastases. In these cases, postoperative adjuvant chemoradiotherapy is recommended.
    - Mixed tumor histology (i.e., combined SCLC with non-SCLC elements). Rationale: the non-SCLC elements are less responsive to chemotherapy; thus, with early stage lesions a combined approach including surgery may offer the potential of cure.
    - Localized disease unresponsive to chemotherapy (resistant tumor may have mixed histology)

## Prophylactic Cranial Irradiation

- The brain is a sanctuary for metastases, and it is poorly permeated by chemotherapy. Thirty to sixty percent of patients with SCLC develop brain metastases in the first 2 years of their illness. This has led to the strategy of prophylactic brain irradiation (PCI).[30]
- Initially, the treatment was given only to patients with limited disease and complete response to therapy. However, it has been shown to be effective in patients with metastatic disease with good systemic response. It has reduced the incidence of brain metastases by 50% to 60% with a small survival benefit as well.
- It is now recommended for use in all patients, with both limited and extensive disease, with an excellent systemic response.[31]
- The PCI dose is either 25 Gray in 10 fractions, or 30 Gray in 15 fractions.
- Complications of PCI include neuropsychiatric impairment (memory loss, cognitive impairment, dementia).

## DELAYED COMPLICATIONS OF THERAPY

- Second malignancies[32,33]
  - Lung cancer (non–small cell) is the most common
  - Head and neck cancer
  - Acute leukemia

## CONCLUSIONS

- SCLC has unique, characteristic clinicopathologic features.
- It is a chemosensitive and radiosensitive disease.

■ Despite typical rapid response to therapy, cure in limited disease patients remains elusive, with an overall 10% 5-year survival.

■ Treatment is dictated by the extent of disease at presentation, and response to initial therapy.

## Brief Illustrative Cases

### Case 1

• A 52-year-old woman presented with a cough, substernal pain, and shortness of breath.

• A chest x-ray study revealed a left upper lobe density and left hilar mass.

• A chest CT revealed a mass of enlarged lymph nodes in the aortopulmonary window and a mass-like area in the left upper lobe, with consolidation (Fig. 32-2A).

• Mediastinoscopy revealed a small cell carcinoma.

• The patient has a 60 pack-year tobacco history.

• Staging including PET/CT scan bone scan, brain MRI, and chemistry panel were all negative for extrapulmonary disease.

• She underwent chemoradiation with four cycles of cisplatin/etoposide and concurrent thoracic radiation therapy, and obtained a complete response (see Fig. 32-2B).

• She then completed a course of prophylactic cranial irradiation (PCI).

• She remains free of disease and symptom free 2 years post therapy.

### Key Points

• This patient had limited disease.

• She was a smoker, as noted in 98% of patients with SCLC.

• The location of the tumor was central, which is typical for SCLC.

• Appropriate workup was needed to prove limited disease staging.

• This is important because it has implications for therapeutic approaches.

• A standard approach was taken, as described earlier.

• In view of good performance status, a concurrent hyperfractionated radiation regimen was employed.

• PCI was appropriate in view of her significant response to multimodality therapy.

• This approach has a 20% to 25% chance of 5-year survival and cure.

• Her disease-free status 2 years after completion of therapy is encouraging. However careful follow-up is needed to evaluate for relapse.

### Case 2

• A 63-year-old woman presented with progressive abdominal pain.

• The patient also complained of back pain, anorexia, and nausea.

• Her physicians ordered an abdominal CT scan (Fig. 32-3), which revealed multiple hepatic lesions and a 3-cm left lower lobe lung mass.

• PET/CT imaging confirmed the left lower lobe mass, and mediastinal and hilar adenopathy.

• There is a 40 pack-year tobacco history.

• Physical examination revealed a chronically ill woman with temporal wasting and no adenopathy or organomegaly.

• Laboratory studies were notable for a serum sodium of 116 (normal 135–142), Calcium of 9 (normal) and elevated LDH of 653 (<300).

• A CT-guided biopsy of the lung mass revealed a small cell carcinoma.

• Further staging confirmed extensive bony metastases in the spine, with normal brain imaging.

• The patient was begun on cisplatin/etoposide chemotherapy, and bisphosphonate for bony metastases.

• She required narcotic analgesia.

• Demeclocycline was used to treat her syndrome of inappropriate ADH (SIADH) and hyponatremia.

• After two cycles of therapy, her hyponatremia has resolved, and she is pain free and no longer on narcotics.

*(Continued)*

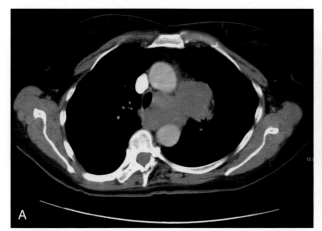
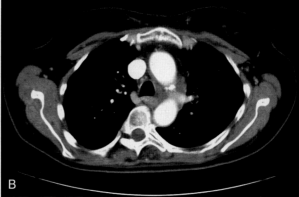

**Figure 32-2: A,** Computed tomography scan of the chest showing a large mass lesion in the aortopulmonary window. The mass extends posterior to the trachea deviating the airway slightly to the right. The mass significantly narrowed the left pulmonary artery (not shown). **B,** Following chemoradiation, a complete response (resolution of tumor mass) is noted, with trachea assuming a normal position.

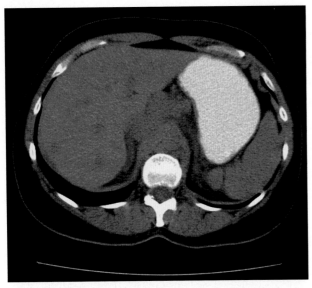

**Figure 32-3:** Computed tomography scan on presentation showing multiple hypodense liver metastases.

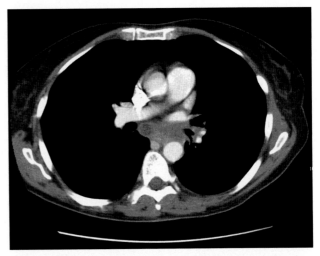

**Figure 32-4:** A repeat computed tomography scan of the chest following chemotherapy showing distinct improvement in her primary lung lesion and necrosis of hilar/mediastinal adenopathy.

### Brief Illustrative Cases—cont'd

- A repeat CT scan has shown distinct improvement in her primary lung lesion and necrosis of her hilar/mediastinal adenopathy (Fig. 32-4).

#### Key Points

- This patient had extensive disease.
- Extensive disease SCLC occurs in the majority of cases (70%).
- Widespread metastatic disease was evident on presentation, in keeping with the systemic nature of the disease.
- Nonpulmonary symptoms dominated her presentation.
- SCLC is an important cause of SIADH. The significantly low level of serum sodium clearly occurred over some time (absence of major neurologic symptoms) and should not be rapidly corrected.
- The high LDH level in this patient is one of several markers that correlates with a poor outcome.

- Standard chemotherapy regimens were appropriate in this patient and clearly resulted in symptomatic and radiologic improvement (short-term response rates with extensive disease reported as 60% to 80%).
- PCI could be considered.[34]
- Despite her initial reponse to chemotherapy, the outcome in this patient would be expected to be poor and the treatments palliative. Indeed relapse or progression would be expected in 98% to 99% of such cases.
- The median survival of patients with extensive disease treated with etoposide and cisplatin was reported as 8 to 10 months.[34]

### References

 Interactive references and additional readings for this chapter can be accessed online at *expertconsult.com*.

# 33    OTHER NEOPLASTIC LESIONS: BENIGN AND MALIGNANT

Francis C. Nichols, MD and Daniel L. Fortes, MD

## *OTHER NEOPLASTIC LESIONS*

### Introduction

- Histologically most cases of lung cancer are adenocarcinoma, squamous cell carcinoma, large cell undifferentiated carcinoma, and small cell carcinoma.
- If carcinoid and atypical carcinoid tumors are added to the above-mentioned histopathologic types, 99% of all primary lung neoplasms are accounted for.[1]

- In addition to carcinoid tumors, this chapter will focus on benign lung tumors, as well as a variety of nonbronchogenic primary pulmonary malignancies.
  - Classification of these neoplasms is problematic because of disagreement regarding the histogenesis of these varied tumors.
  - It is easiest to just discuss these neoplasms individually.

## BENIGN NEOPLASMS OF THE LUNG

### Hamartoma

- Most common benign lung neoplasm
- Arrigoni and colleagues[2] reported on 130 benign lung tumors from Mayo Clinic and found that 100 (76.9%) were hamartomas (Table 33-1).
- Pathology: These tumors are derived from peribronchial mesenchyme and are composed mostly of cartilage, connective tissue, fat, smooth muscle, and respiratory epithelium (Fig. 33-1).
- Clinical presentation: Most are asymptomatic and account for 7% to 14% of pulmonary coin lesions.[3]
  - In a review of 215 patients with hamartomas, Gjevre and associates[4] found only 3% were symptomatic.
  - Commonly occur between the ages of 40 and 70 years, with a 2:1 to 4:1 male-to-female ratio.
- Radiology: often solitary and can occur in any part of the lung but are more common in the periphery
  - The tumors measure from 1 to 7 cm (average 2 cm) in diameter.

**TABLE 33-1 ■ BENIGN LUNG TUMORS AND THEIR INCIDENCE***

| Tumor | Number (%) |
|---|---|
| Hamartoma | 100 (76.9) |
| Benign mesothelioma | 16 (12.3) |
| Xanthomatous and inflammatory pseudotumors | 7 (5.4) |
| Lipoma | 2 (1.5) |
| Leiomyoma | 2 (1.5) |
| Hemangioma | 1 (0.8) |
| Mucous gland adenoma | 1 (0.8) |
| Mixed tumor | 1 (0.8) |

*Adapted from Arrigoni MG, Woolner LB, Bernatz PE, Miller WE, Fontana WS. Benign tumors of the lung. A ten-year experience. J Thorac Cardiovasc Surg 1970;60:589-599.

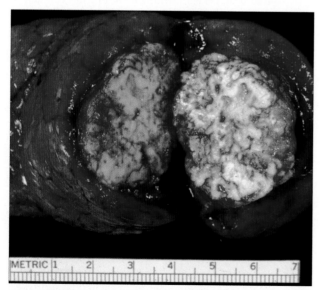

**Figure 33-1:** Hamartoma. It is well demarcated from the surrounding lung. Note the variegated white and yellow appearance which corresponds to the cartilage and fat.

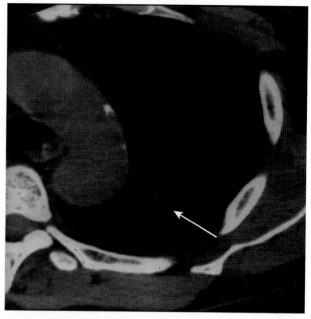

**Figure 33-2:** Computed tomography scan showing a 1-cm pulmonary nodule with a central fat density (*arrow*). This lesion has an appearance consistent with a hamartoma.

  - A characteristic popcorn pattern of calcification may be present on computed tomography (CT) scan in up to 30% of cases, but some authors report a much lower incidence of calcification.
  - CT may also demonstrate fat within the lesion. Siegelman and colleagues[5] reported fat in 50% of hamartomas (Fig. 33-2).
    - The presence of fat density by high-resolution CT in a peripheral solitary lesion is strong presumptive evidence for a benign hamartoma.
- Pathology: Malignant transformation is rare.
  - Growth is slow.
  - Needle biopsy may be diagnostic.
  - This may be useful after CT studies when the diagnosis of hamartoma is still in doubt and the patient is poor risk for surgical intervention.
- Treatment
  - Excision should be considered if the diagnosis is in doubt.
  - Small (<2 cm) hamartomas can be observed.
  - Hamartomas larger than 2.5 cm should be considered for excision.[6]
  - Video-assisted thoracoscopic wedge resection is the preferred treatment.
    - Segmentectomy or lobectomy may be required, and pneumonectomy should be avoided.
  - Recurrence is highly unlikely.

### Inflammatory Pseudotumor

- Numerous synonyms: histiocytoma, plasma cell granuloma, plasmacytoma, xanthoma, xanthogranuloma, xanthofibroma, and inflammatory myofibroblastic tumor.
- Pathology: Classically considered a non-neoplastic process characterized by unregulated growth of inflammatory cells.
  - Historically, cause was unknown but thought to represent an exaggerated tissue response to injury.
  - Now thought to be of neoplastic origin with evidence of rearrangement of the anaplastic lymphoma kinase gene on chromosome 2p23.[7]

- Presentation: The true incidence is unknown; however, in 56,400 general thoracic surgical procedures performed at Mayo Clinic between 1946 and 1993, 23 patients (0.04%) had resection of inflammatory pseudotumors.[8]
  - Median age 47 years (range, 5 to 77 years).
  - They are the most common benign lung tumor in children.
  - Presentation is usually with symptoms: cough, weight loss, fever, fatigue.
- Radiology: usually appear as well-defined solitary parenchymal masses 0.5 to 36 cm in diameter; the most common size is 1 cm to 6 cm.[9,10]
- Pathology: Grossly they consist of multilobular or bosselated tumor with a rubbery surface. They commonly have a white shiny appearance due to the large amount of fibrous tissue present; however, as the number of histiocytes or xanthomatous cells increase, their color becomes more yellow due to lipid accumulation (Fig. 33-3).
- Treatment is complete resection to avoid local recurrence.
  - In the Mayo Clinic series, complete resection was accomplished in 18 (78%) patients. Resection required pneumonectomy in six patients, bilobectomy in one, lobectomy in six, segmentectomy in one, wedge resection in seven, and chest wall resection in two.[8]
    - Two patients with positive margins underwent re-resection, and two have been observed without evidence of tumor growth.
    - The 5-, 8-, and 10-year survival rates were 91.3%, 91.3%, and 77.7% respectively.

## Lipoma

- Presentation: Rare, with only two found out of 130 benign lung tumors in the Mayo Clinic series.[2]
  - Most are endobronchial and cause obstruction.
- Radiology: Because of their fatty composition, CT may strongly suggest the diagnosis of endobronchial lipoma.
- Treatment: Use bronchoscopic removal whenever possible.
  - Muraoka and associates[11] reported on 64 cases with surgical procedures including pneumonectomy in four patients,

lobectomy in 24, bilobectomy in eight, bronchotomy in four, bronchoscopic removal with Nd:YAG laser in 17, cautery in five, and a combination of laser and cautery in five.
  - Reasons for surgical resection include
    - Difficulty in obtaining a definitive diagnosis and the existence of a possible complicated malignant tumor
    - Peripheral destruction of the lung secondary to longstanding atelectasis or pneumonia
    - Extrabronchial growth or the existence of subpleural lipomatous disease
    - Technical difficulties encountered during the bronchoscopic procedure

## Leiomyoma

- Presentation:
  - Account for 1.5% to 2% of benign lung neoplasms
  - Most common in young and middle-aged women
  - Location split almost evenly between lung parenchyma and tracheobronchial[12]
  - Peripheral lung parenchymal leiomyoma are often asymptomatic while tracheobronchial leiomyoma may cause pulmonary obstruction.
- Radiology: On CT, there are no distinguishing features from other pulmonary nodules.
- Pathology: Grossly, they resemble smooth muscle tumors (Fig. 33-4).
- Treatment
  - Endobronchial leiomyoma without destroyed distal lung parenchyma may be treated with endobronchial resection with or without the use of Nd:YAG laser.
  - Surgical resection is the treatment of choice for peripheral leiomyoma and those endobronchial leiomyoma with destroyed distal lung tissue.
- Benign metastasizing leiomyoma
  - Term used for multiple (occasionally single) well-differentiated pulmonary smooth muscle nodules found almost exclusively in women, many of whom have a history of uterine leiomyoma.
  - Pathology: very bland cytologic appearance, with minimal mitosis or necrosis very similar to uterine leiomyomas.
    - Controversial term because they have hematogenously spread from benign uterine leiomyoma; this contradicts their "benign" designation.

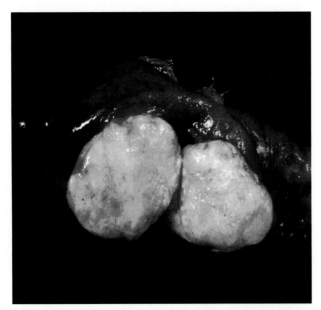

**Figure 33-3:** Inflammatory pseudotumor. Note the sharp demarcation from the surrounding lung. The presence of xanthoma cells imparts a yellow color, plasma cells and lymphocytes a tan color, and fibrous connective tissue a white color.

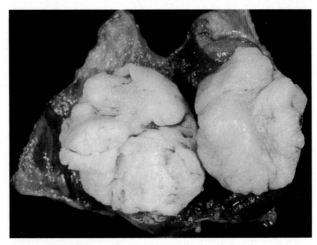

**Figure 33-4:** Benign pulmonary leiomyoma. The nodule is lobulated with a typical pale white smooth muscle appearance.

- Kayser and colleagues[13] compared benign metastasizing leiomyomas with uterine leiomyomas using a variety of markers such as estrogen receptor (ER) and progesterone receptor (PR) receptors and Ki-67. They concluded that benign metastasizing leiomyomas are in reality slow-growing uterine leiomyosarcomas.
    - Takemura and colleagues[14] believe that benign metastasizing leiomyomas could be due to multicentric benign leiomyomatous growths instead of actual metastases.
- Treatment
    - Pulmonary resection can be considered when feasible and for establishment of diagnosis.
    - These tumors can regress following oophorectomy.
    - Because these tumors are ER- and PR-receptor positive, they may respond favorably to hormonal therapy.

## Hemangioma

- Sclerosing hemangioma
    - Presentation: Sugio and colleagues[15] reported sclerosing hemangioma as the 2nd most common benign lung neoplasm following hamartoma.
        - Eighty percent occur in women.
        - Most are asymptomatic.
    - Radiology: they appear as a solitary, circumscribed, homogeneous mass that occasionally is calcified.
        - They range in size from 0.4 cm to 8.0 cm, with an average of 2.8 cm.[16]
    - Pathology: Four major histologic patterns exist: solid, papillary, sclerotic, and hemorrhagic. Most of these neoplasms exhibit combinations of these patterns.
    - Treatment: Surgical resection is the procedure of choice.
        - Miyagawa-Hayashino and colleagues[17] have reported on 4 patients with sclerosing hemangioma and lymph node metastases.
            - Lymph node metastases were described as peribronchial, regional, and hilar.
            - Despite the presence of lymph node metastases, these authors still consider sclerosing hemangiomas to be benign.[17]
            - Because of the possibility of lymph node metastases, a regional and hilar lymph node dissection should be done in addition to surgical resection of the sclerosing hemangioma.
    - Prognosis is excellent, and prognosis did not appear to be affected by the presence of lymph node metastases.[17]
- Cavernous hemangioma
    - Presentation: Extremely rare, occurring in all age groups
        - Shields and Robinson[18] consider these to be pulmonary arteriovenous malformations (AVMs).
        - May occur in the tracheobronchial tree or in the peripheral lung parenchyma
        - Presentation may be asymptomatic or include hemoptysis, respiratory distress, or congestive heart failure.
    - Treatment
        - Endobronchial lesions are managed by Nd:YAG laser.
        - Parenchymal AVMs can be embolized with metal coils and occasionally require surgical excision.

## Mucous Gland Adenoma

- Synonyms: mucous gland cystadenoma, adenomatous polyp, and adenomas of mucous gland type
- Presentation: Rare neoplasm that occurs in both children and adults, and is more common in women.[19]
    - Arises in the bronchus and derived from bronchial mucus glands
    - Because of their bronchial location, patients often have symptoms secondary to obstruction or hemorrhage: cough, fever, hemoptysis, recurrent pneumonia.
- Pathology: Grossly the tumors are soft, spherical, polypoid endobronchial nodules that are usually smaller than 2 cm in diameter but may range up to 7 cm.
    - They are more common lower or middle lobe lobar or segmental bronchi.[19]
    - The differential diagnosis includes low-grade mucoepidermoid carcinoma.
    - Distinguishing between the two types may be difficult with small biopsies. The lack of cytologic atypia, mitoses, and necrosis aids in differentiation.
- Treatment
    - Endobronchial resection with or without the use of Nd:YAG laser or cryotherapy if there is no distal lung destruction
    - Surgical resection is the treatment of choice for these neoplasms if there is destroyed distal lung parenchyma or there are contraindications to endoscopic resection
- Prognosis: excellent.

## Chondroma

- Benign tumors composed of hyaline cartilage, which may be parenchymal or involve the cartilaginous airways.
- Presentation:
    - Endobronchial chondromas are often associated with obstructive symptoms, are more common in men, and may be treated by endobronchial removal or surgical resection.[18]
    - Although parenchymal chondromas are frequently asymptomatic, they are more common in women and may be associated with Carney's triad.[20,21] In fact, the presence of a pulmonary chondroma in a young woman should lead to consideration of this triad, which includes
    - Chondroma of the lung single or multiple
    - Gastrointestinal stromal tumor
    - Extra-adrenal paraganglioma
- Treatment: repeated surgical resections of the respective tumors
    - Lung parenchymal–sparing resections are adequate for pulmonary chondromas.
- Prognosis
    - For a single pulmonary chondroma, overall survival is excellent.
    - For patients with Carney's triad, despite repeated resections, the development of recurrent neoplasms is common. Neoplasms that grow or cause symptoms should be resected. Carney's triad is a chronic, persistent, indolent disease extending over a long period of follow-up. Sixteen percent of patients eventually die of the disease.[21]

## Atypical Adenomatous Hyperplasia

- Atypical adenomatous hyperplasia (AAH) is of increasing interest because of its association with bronchoalveolar carcinoma (BAC).
- Pathology: AAH is a focal lesion smaller than 5 mm in diameter due to proliferation of atypical bronchoalveolar cells lining centriacinar alveoli.[22]
    - Autopsy studies have demonstrated AAH in 2% to 4% of cases.
- Presentation: Demographic data are conflicting.
    - May be more common in women
    - May be more frequent in Japanese individuals

- Radiology:
  - Most AAH is completely invisible; however, when visible, it may present on thin-section high-resolution CT as tiny foci of ground-glass opacification within the lung parenchyma.
  - These ground-glass features, however, are not specific to AAH.
- Differential diagnosis is primarily with BAC.[22]
  - Grossly, AAH is typically smaller than 5 mm in diameter and BAC is larger than 10 mm; however, size alone cannot reliably make the distinction between the two.
  - Pathology: cell population of AAH may be more heterogenous and BAC more monomorphic. Of the following histologic features, AAH rarely demonstrates more than one, whereas BAC exhibits three or more.
    - Marked cell stratification
    - High cell density, with marked overlapping of nuclei
    - Coarse nuclear chromatin and prominent nucleoli
    - True papillae or an obvious picket-fence growth pattern
    - Increase in columnar cell height in excess of those lining terminal bronchioles
  - BAC
    - There are little data on the appropriate treatment of AAH.
    - In most cases, treatment is determined by the associated lesions that may be present.
      - If a ground-glass opacity is resected and AAH is identified, then only a wedge resection with free margins is required.
      - Even for BAC, there is a growing consensus that sublobar resection may be adequate therapy.[23]

## MALIGNANT NEOPLASMS OF THE LUNG

### Bronchial Adenomas
- Describe a group of slow-growing neoplasms, most of which arise from the bronchial glands
- Three histologic types of tumors
  - Bronchial carcinoids
  - Adenoid cystic carcinoma
  - Mucoepidermoid carcinoma
- The term bronchial adenoma is a misnomer because these tumors are usually low-grade malignancies and not benign neoplasms as the term adenoma implies.
- The term bronchial adenoma should be avoided whenever possible.

### Carcinoid Tumors
- History: First described by Otto Lubarsch in 1888 who identified multiple tumors in the distal ileum of two patients at autopsy.[24]
- Sigfried Oberndorfer in 1907 coined the term *karzinoide* to describe tumors with carcinoma-like features but a much more indolent behavior.[24]
- Pathology
- Pulmonary carcinoids are malignant neuroendocrine tumors comprising 1% to 2% of all primary lung tumors[25] and 85% of bronchial gland tumors.
  - Carcinoid tumors are part of the spectrum of malignant neuroendocrine tumors, which range from low-grade typical carcinoid tumors to intermediate-grade atypical carcinoid tumors to high-grade tumors, including large cell neuroendocrine carcinoma and small cell lung carcinoma.
  - Most pulmonary carcinoid tumors arise in major bronchi.[26]
    - Ten percent in mainstem bronchi
    - Seventy-five percent in lobar bronchi

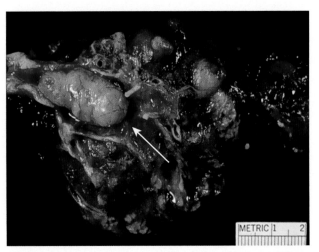

**Figure 33-5:** Carcinoid tumor. Note the large endobronchial tumor mass (*arrow*). The bronchial wall is largely intact and does not appear replaced by tumor as seen with either large cell neuroendocrine or small cell lung carcinomas.

    - Fifteen percent in the lung periphery that is segmental bronchi and distal
  - Frequently have a large endobronchial component with a fleshy smooth polypoid mass protruding into the bronchial lumen (Fig. 33-5). The cut surface may appear tan-yellow or red depending on the extent of vascularity.
  - Arrigoni and colleagues[27] proposed that bronchial carcinoids be divided into the categories of typical and atypical.
    - Typical carcinoid tumors
      - Constitute approximately 90%
      - Tend to be central in location
      - Characterized by an orderly, often acinar-like, grouping of small polygonal cells with abundant clear to eosinophilic cytoplasm and oval nuclei with fine granular chromatin. Pleomorphism, mitoses, necrosis, and disorganization of architecture are rare.
      - The 1999 WHO classification of this group of neoplasms is based on the absence of necrosis and less than two mitoses per high power field (HPF).[28]
      - Approximately 10% to 15% metastasize to lymph nodes.[25,26,29]
    - Atypical carcinoid tumors
      - Constitute approximately 10% of bronchial carcinoids
      - Are usually larger at presentation and more likely located in the lung periphery[25]
      - Are characterized by maintenance of a recognizable carcinoid pattern; however, degrees of cellularity with architectural disorganization, increased mitotic activity, pleomorphism, and irregularity of nuclei with prominent nucleoli, hyperchromatism, abnormal nuclear-cytoplasmic ratio, and areas of tumor necrosis.
      - Presence of 5 to 10 mitoses per HPF is a characteristic finding; however, the 1999 WHO classification includes the presence of necrosis or two to 10 mitoses per HPF[28]
      - Twenty to seventy-five percent have regional lymph node involvement.[25]
- Clinical findings
  - Occur in the 5th and 6th decades of life. Atypical carcinoid tumors reach their peak incidence approximately 1 decade later than typical carcinoids.[26]
  - Equal female-to-male distribution

○ Signs and symptoms
- Spectrum of symptoms dependent on tumor size, location, and growth pattern
  ○ Peripheral tumors are often asymptomatic.
  ○ Central tumors because of bronchial compression often present with cough, hemoptysis, wheezing, and recurrent infection
- No clear difference exists in the clinical manifestations in most patients with typical versus atypical carcinoid tumors
- Average interval from symptom development to diagnosis has been estimated to be 29 to 37 months ranging up to 14 years.[25]
- Carcinoid syndrome occurs in less than 5% of cases.[24]
  ○ May occur with very large carcinoid tumors or when liver metastases are present.
- Carcinoid crisis has been reported following endobronchial manipulation or biopsy of these tumors.[30]
  ○ Manifestations include bronchoconstriction, hypotension, hypertension, prolonged cutaneous flushing, confusion, and coma.
- One percent of cases of Cushing's syndrome is due to bronchial carcinoid tumors.[31]
- Five to fifteen percent of bronchial carcinoid tumors result in Cushing's syndrome.[32,33]
  ○ Bronchial carcinoid tumors are the most frequent cause of Cushing's syndrome resulting from ectopic ACTH secretion.
  ○ Adrenocorticotropic hormone (ACTH)–secreting bronchial carcinoids are most commonly typical carcinoid tumors and are not a more aggressive variant of typical carcinoids.[31]
- Other paraneoplastic syndromes, such as acromegaly, may rarely occur.
■ Diagnosis
○ In asymptomatic patients, conventional chest radiography (CXR) may provide the earliest indication of a bronchial carcinoid tumor.
- Conventional CXRs show abnormal findings in 75% of patients with bronchial carcinoids.[26,27,34]
  ○ Fifteen percent of peripheral solitary pulmonary nodule
  ○ Sixty percent show evidence of a central mass, obstructive pneumonitis, or lung volume loss
- CT has superseded other standard radiographic views and is capable of delineating the endobronchial and parenchymal aspects of the tumor in most patients.
○ Nuclear scanning
- OctreoScan: somatostatin analogue octreotide may be useful but is not widely used unless a pulmonary carcinoid tumor is suspected.
- Positron emission tomography (PET): PET with $^{18}$F-fluorodeoxyglucose has become useful in the evaluation of indeterminate pulmonary nodules and screening for metastatic disease. Its utility in bronchial carcinoid tumors is still uncertain given the low mitotic activity of the majority of these tumors. More promising results may be forthcoming with different radiolabeled precursors. Approximately 60% of carcinoid tumors light up on the PET scan.
○ Bronchoscopy remains a reliable means of diagnosing bronchial carcinoids. Because many of these tumors are central, an endobronchial lesion is commonly visible.
- The typical lesion is smooth and pink or slightly red in color.
- Biopsy reveals the diagnosis in 85% of patients.[26,27]

○ Normal biopsy findings do not exclude the diagnosis because an intact mucus membrane may preclude biopsy of the actual tumor.
- Because bronchial carcinoids are vascular, care must be exercised when obtaining biopsies as significant bleeding has occurred.
- Bronchoscopy provides valuable information about the tumor's location, which may be critical in planning for surgery.
■ Treatment
○ Pulmonary resection is the treatment of choice.[26,27,35-37]
- Primary goals
  ○ Complete tumor removal
  ○ Relief of airway obstruction
  ○ Preservation of as much normal lung as possible
- Unlike bronchogenic carcinoma, carcinoid tumors infrequently invade adjacent tissue and more limited resection margins are acceptable. Lobectomy with or without removal of a sleeve of bronchus, segmental resection, or sleeve resection alone are the most commonly performed procedures. Occasionally, pneumonectomy is required because of the tumor's location (Table 33-2).
- Thorough lymph node sampling or resection of all mediastinal, hilar, and pulmonary level lymph nodes is essential.
  ○ Our preference is for formal mediastinal lymphadenectomy
○ Endobronchial therapy
- Endoscopic resection is not recommended as primary therapy because it is almost always incomplete with recurrence likely.
- Useful in
  ○ Patients with central obstructing endobronchial lesions who are poor risk for surgical resection.
  ○ Patients symptomatic from postobstructive pneumonia in which bronchoscopic debulking may allow resolution of the infectious process before surgical resection.
○ Adjuvant chemotherapy or radiation therapy remains controversial.
- In general, chemotherapeutic agents have been largely ineffective.
○ Somatostatin analogue (octreotide) may effectively treat the carcinoid syndrome due to metastases, but does not make the tumors shrink.
○ Prognosis
- Bronchial carcinoids are extremely slow growing, and in general, the long-term prognosis is excellent.

### TABLE 33-2 ■ TYPES OF RESECTION FOR TYPICAL BRONCHIAL CARCINOID TUMORS IN 203 PATIENTS*

| Type of Resection | Number (%) |
| --- | --- |
| Pneumonectomy | 54 (26.7) |
| Lobectomy including bilobectomy | 131 (64.5) |
| Segmental resection | 9 (4.4) |
| Sleeve resection & lobectomy | 5 (2.5) |
| Sleeve resection alone | 4 (2.0) |

*Adapted from Okike N, Bernatz PE, Woolner LB: Carcinoid tumors of the lung. Ann Thorac Surg 1976;22:270-277.

- Overall typical carcinoid tumors have an 87% to 100% 5-year survival rate and an 82% to 100% 10-year survival.[24,25]
  - Patients with typical bronchial carcinoids without lymph node involvement (T1-2, N0, M0) have a 5-year survival rate of 94% and 25-year survival of 66%.[26]
  - Patients with typical carcinoid tumors with metastatically involved lymph nodes (T1-2, N1-2, M0) have a 5-year survival rate of 71%.[27]
  - Overall, patients wtih atypical carcinoid tumors have a 40% to 83% 5-year survival rate and a 31% to 83% 10-year survival rate.[24,25]

## Carcinoid Tumorlets

- A nodular proliferation of neuroendocrine cells forming a nodule smaller than 5 mm in size.[38]
- Typically are an incidental pathologic finding
  - Reported incidence of 0.22% in one autopsy series[39]
- Often occur in conditions of chronic lung damage such as bronchiectasis, chronic or granulomatous inflammation, or pulmonary fibrosis.
- Histologically, they are well differentiated and lack atypia, mitoses, and necrosis.
- Carcinoid tumorlets must be distinguished from metastatic carcinoma.

## Adenoid Cystic Carcinoma

- Synonym: cylindroma
- Presentation:
  - Less common than bronchial carcinoids, comprising only 10% of bronchial gland tumors
  - Very slow growing with propensity for submucosal and perineural spread as well as metastasizing.
  - Central tumors that exhibit both tracheal and bronchial involvement
  - Can be seen at all ages but most common in the 5th decade of life.
  - Eighty percent of patients are symptomatic.[40]
  - Commonly cough, hemoptysis, wheezing, stridor, respiratory distress, fevers, recurrent pneumonias
- Radiology:
  - May be a central mass
  - CT scans give details about the intraluminal and extraluminal extent of tumor, as well as assessment of the mediastinal lymph nodes.
- Bronchoscopy
  - Often diagnostic showing localized polypoid masses or sessile lesions with diffuse submucosal involvement.[41]
- Treatment
  - Surgical resection is preferred.[42]
    - Frozen section pathology should be used to ascertain free margins.
    - On occasion, a positive surgical margin remains, which is acceptable if further tracheal resection would result in tension on the anastomosis.
  - Radiation therapy
    - These are radiosensitive tumors, and radiation can be used when the resection margins are positive or in patients at too high risk for surgical resection.
    - With postoperative radiation therapy, the recurrence rate is low.
  - Endobronchial therapy with Nd:YAG laser may be beneficial for tumor debulking in patients with recurrent or unresectable disease.

- Prognosis
  - Grillo found 12% of their resected patients died of their tumors during a 26-year period of follow-up.[42]
  - Even patients with incomplete resection can survive for a long time.

## Mucoepidermoid Carcinoma

- Presentation:
  - Accounts for 1% to 5% of all primary bronchial gland tumors.[43,44]
  - In contrast to adenoid cystic carcinoma, tracheal involvement is rare, and these tumors most commonly arise distal to the carina in mainstem bronchi.
  - Because these tumors are usually located in a major airway, patients are commonly symptomatic.
    - Cough, dyspnea, hemoptysis, wheezing, and pneumonia
- Pathology
  - Classified as high-grade or low-grade tumors
- Radiology: the appearance is similar to adenoid cystic carcinoma.
- Diagnosis:
  - Transbronchial biopsies are needed for diagnosis.
- Treatment
  - Surgical resection is preferred along with hilar and mediastinal lymph node dissection.
  - Radiation therapy is ineffective.[44]
  - Endobronchial therapy should be considered only for palliation of obstructive symptoms.
- Prognosis
  - Patients with low-grade tumors who undergo resection enjoy long-term survival with high cure rates.
  - Heitmiller and colleagues reported a 100% mortality rate for high-grade tumors within 16 months.[44] Vadasz and colleagues reported a 31% 5-year survival rate in 29 patients with high-grade tumors, but there were no survivors if there was mediastinal lymph node involvement.

## Pulmonary Sarcomas

- Presentation:
  - Primary soft tissue sarcomas of the lung are extremely rare with a frequency of one case per 500 primary lung cancers (Table 33-3).
  - Soft tissue sarcomas in the lung are most commonly metastatic.
    - A careful search for a nonpulmonary sarcoma should be undertaken before classifying a sarcoma of the lung as primary.

| TABLE 33-3 ▪ PRIMARY SARCOMAS OF THE LUNG |
| --- |
| Angiosarcoma |
| Chondrosarcoma |
| Fibrosarcoma |
| Kaposi's sarcoma |
| Leiomyosarcoma |
| Liposarcoma |
| Malignant fibrous histiocytoma |
| Malignant hemangiopericytoma |
| Neurogenic sarcoma |
| Osteosarcoma |
| Pulmonary artery sarcoma |
| Rhabdomyosarcoma |
| Spindle cell sarcoma |
| Synovial sarcoma |

○ The mean age at presentation is 53 years (range: 1.5 years to 78 years).[47,48]

○ Twenty-five to fifty percent of patients are asymptomatic, with the sarcoma discovered coincidentally on a CXR performed for unrelated reasons.[47,48]

○ Symptoms when present include cough, dyspnea, chest pain, hemoptysis, fatigue, malaise, fever, and weight loss.

▪ Pathology:

○ Median tumor diameter was approximately 6 cm (range: 1 to 17 cm).[47,48]

○ In order of decreasing frequency, the most common histologic sarcoma subtypes were leiomyosarcoma, rhabdomyosarcoma, spindle cell sarcoma, angiosarcoma, malignant fibrous histiocytoma, fibrosarcoma, hemangiopericytoma, and blastoma.[48]

▪ Treatment is surgical resection when feasible.

○ Lobectomy and wedge resection are most common.

○ Mediastinal lymphadenectomy should also be performed

▪ Prognosis

○ High cure rates for chondrosarcoma and low cure rates for osteosarcoma[7]

○ In one of the largest series, overall 1-, 3-, 5-year survival rates were 55%, 31%, and 25% respectively.[48]

▪ Survival varies with different series and seems to correlate best with complete surgical resection, tumor grade, and tumor stage.

○ Pulmonary sarcomas smaller than 5 cm correlated with improved survival.[7,47]

## Pulmonary Lymphomas

▪ Presentation:

○ Although it may involve the lung in 25% to 40% of cases of generalized lymphoma, primary pulmonary lymphoma is rare.

○ Primary pulmonary lymphoma accounts for only 3.6% of extranodal lymphoma and less than 1% of all primary pulmonary malignancies.[48-50]

▪ Pathology:

○ Primary pulmonary lymphoma is not a single disease but rather a histologic spectrum of malignant lymphomas including Hodgkin's disease and non-Hodgkin's lymphoma.

○ Most primary lymphomas of the lung arise from the mucosa-associated lymphoid tissue of the bronchus also called bronchus-associated lymphoid tissue (BALT).

▪ The peak incidence is in the 6th decade of life (range: 15–87 years).

○ Most BALT lymphomas are low-grade small B-cell lymphomas; however, high-grade large B-cell lymphoma and non-BALT lymphomas are also seen.[1,49,51]

▪ Half of patients can be asymptomatic.[51]

▪ Radiographic findings can vary: nodule, mass (single or multiple), ill-defined infiltrates or consolidation without any dominant features.[51]

▪ They usually pursue an indolent course and can remain localized to the lung for prolonged time periods before disseminating.[51]

▪ Treatment:

○ No consensus on the best treatment.

○ There are several treatment options: surgical resection, chemotherapy alone, radiation therapy, and surgery followed by adjuvant therapy.

○ The role of surgery in primary pulmonary lymphoma is twofold: to obtain diagnostic tissue and in appropriate patients to obtain a therapeutic resection.

▪ Tumors that appear to be resectable should be approached with intent to cure by performing

complete surgical resection and a staging lymph node dissection.

▪ When presented with large, unresectable tumor or bilateral disease, obtaining adequate tissue to establish a diagnosis of lymphoma is the goal.

▪ When dealing with an indeterminate, resectable lung mass at thoracotomy, the surgeon's primary concern is bronchogenic carcinoma. In an otherwise healthy patient, the goal is complete resection and obtaining negative margins.

○ In the series by Ferraro and colleagues,[49] surgery entailed pulmonary biopsy in seven patients, wedge resection in 21, lobectomy in 11, segmentectomy and pneumonectomy in two each.

▪ For BALT lymphoma, survival rates at 1, 5, and 10 years were 91%, 68%, and 53%, respectively.

▪ For non-BALT lymphoma 1-, 5-, and 10-year survival rates were 85%, 65%, and 64%, respectively.

▪ None of the prognostic factors studied (histology, postoperative stage, complete resection, adjuvant chemotherapy) was found to influence overall survival.

○ Owing to the rarity of this disease, there are insufficient data, to make a clear recommendation on the proper surgical management of these patients. Survival in patients with low-grade lymphoma is good despite the resection type. If the patient can tolerate a complete resection, then that would seem to be a reasonable approach. In the case of low-grade lymphoma adjuvant therapy is probably unnecessary.

○ The 5-year survival rate for patients with high-grade lymphoma is only 44% to 60%, much less than that of those patients with low-grade lymphoma. Standard treatment for high-grade lymphoma is surgical resection, followed by radiation therapy with or without chemotherapy.[48]

## Primary Pulmonary Hodgkin's Disease

▪ Presentation:

○ Hodgkin's disease commonly involves the lung as a reflection of disseminated disease or by direct extension from the mediastinum.

○ The incidence of primary pulmonary Hodgkin's disease is very low, with none being reported in Miller and colleagues' rare pulmonary neoplasms series.[1]

○ Many patients with primary Hodgkin's disease of the lung have the diagnosis established during biopsy of the lung for a solitary lesion.

○ In such a situation, if all evident disease can be removed, it is reasonable to perform formal surgical resection with mediastinal lymph node dissection.

○ If all disease cannot be removed, then biopsy to obtain adequate tissue for diagnosis is sufficient.

▪ Treatment:

○ The standard treatment for primary pulmonary Hodgkin's disease includes combination chemotherapy and radiation therapy.

## Brief Illustrative Case

• A 46-year-old woman presented with hemoptysis (<50 mL)

• There was a history of "walking pneumonia" 6 months prior, which responded to oral antibiotics. No imaging was obtained at that time.

*(Continued)*

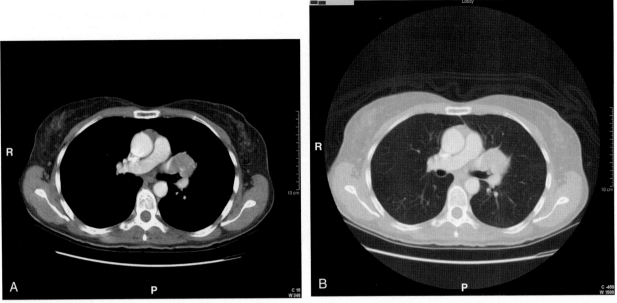

**Figure 33-6:** Mediastinal (**A**) and lung (**B**) views on computed tomography chest showing large left hilar mass, calcification in mass, and endobronchial component (**B**).

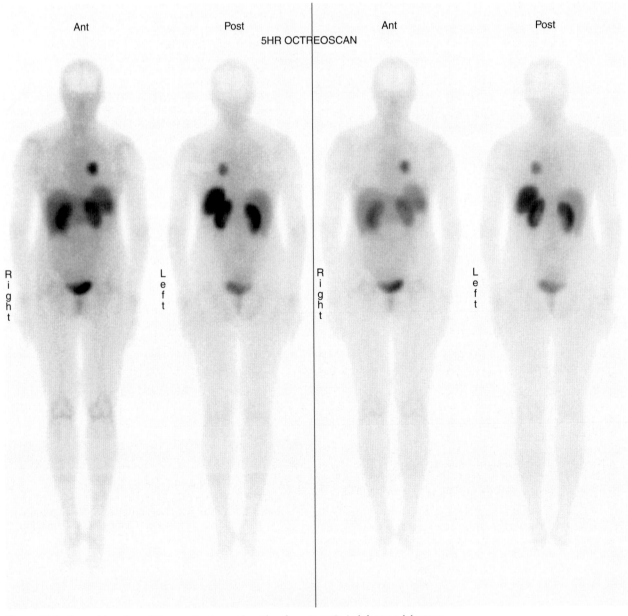

**Figure 33-7:** Octreotide radionuclide scan showing avid uptake of somatostatin in left upper lobe mass.

## Brief Illustrative Case—cont'd

- There were no current symptoms of fever, sweats, chills, weight loss, diarrhea or flushing.
- A chest x-ray study and CT scan (Fig. 33-6) showed a large left hilar mass that appeared to extend into the lumen of the left upper lobe bronchus. Calcifications were noted in the mass.
- Bronchoscopy revealed a glistening smooth surface tumor extending into the left upper lobe bronchus and close to its origin (Fig. 33-7). There was no active bleeding.
- An octreoside scan avid somatostatin uptake in the left perihilar mass (Fig. 33-8).
- A left upper lobectomy with sleeve resection was performed.
- Pathology revealed features of a typical carcinoid with rare mitoses, trabecular and nesting patterns, oncocytic differentiation and no evidence of lymphatic or vascular invasion. All lymph nodes from the comprehensive lymph node dissection were negative for tumor (Fig. 33-9).

### Key Points

- Common presentation of a typical carcinoid tumor.
- There was likely a long period in which she was completely asymptomatic.
- A biopsy was not obtained at the time of bronchoscopy because it was clear that surgery would be necessary; CT and endoscopy findings suggested a carcinoid tumor and her presentation with hemoptysis, albeit not massive.
- However, bronchoscopic biopsy is not contraindicated. Significant bleeding after biopsy is very rare, but if undertaken, all precautions to deal with such an event should be in place.
- On CT, the tumor appeared to be closely abutting the pulmonary artery and to be close to the origin of the left upper lobe origin. Thus, decisions are to be made

at surgery to determine if pneumonectomy, vascular sleeve resection, or bronchial sleeve resection is the best operative procedure.
- At surgery, the tumor was close to, but did not involve, the pulmonary artery. Left upper lobectomy with bronchial wedge resection was necessary (i.e., wedge resection of a portion of the left main bronchus [LMB] with suture of the LMB to the lower lobe bronchus).

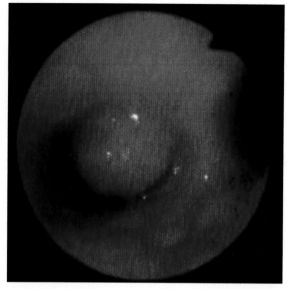

**Figure 33-8:** Bronchoscopic view of left upper lobe tumor with features compatible with carcinoid tumor (smooth, rounded, glistening surface, pink/red hue).

## References

 Interactive references and additional readings for this chapter can be accessed online at *expertconsult.com*.

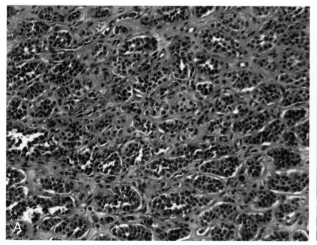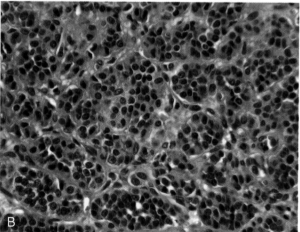

**Figure 33-9:** Low (**A**) and high (**B**) power views of histopathology showing features of a typical carcinoid. **A,** The tumor is composed of small nests of cells in an organoid pattern (hematoxylin and eosin stain; original magnification 200×). **B,** Tumor cells have regular, monomorphic nuclei with fine chromatin and inconspicuous nucleoli (hematoxylin and eosin stain; original magnification 400×).

# 34 | RESECTION FOR PULMONARY METASTASES

Reza J. Mehran, MD

## INTRODUCTION

- The lungs are one of the most common sites of involvement for metastatic neoplasms. About 30% of patients with malignant disease will eventually develop pulmonary metastases. For melanomas and sarcomas, the incidence may be as high as 80%.[1-3]
- Therapeutic success depends on early diagnosis, appropriate selection of patients for surgery, complete resection, and a favorable tumor-host relationship.
- The tumor-host relationship includes factors such as the histology of the primary tumor, disease free interval and the doubling time of the tumor.
- Other important factors in determining the operability include the number, size, and location of the metastasis.
- Survival benefits from surgery depend on a careful selection of the patient and stratifying the risk factors associated with the tumor-host relationship.

## SELECTION CRITERIA FOR RESECTION

- The primary site must be controlled locally with no evidence of active disease.
- There must be no evidence of extrathoracic metastatic disease. However, involvement of other extrathoracic sites may not be a contraindication to the resection of the pulmonary disease as long as all disease sites can be resected completely before the lung resection.
- All pulmonary metastases must be resectable.
- The patient must have an adequate pulmonary reserve to tolerate the pulmonary resection.

## INVESTIGATION OF PATIENTS WITH PULMONARY METASTASES

- Most patients are asymptomatic (85%), and the diagnosis of pulmonary metastases is usually made in the context of staging and follow-up of a primary extrathoracic malignancy.[4-8]
- The computed tomography (CT) scan is the gold standard for the evaluation of pulmonary metastases.
- With standard CT techniques using collimations of 1 cm, the risk of underestimating the number of metastases is 35% to 40%. The risk of overestimating the lesions is 25% to 30%. Therefore, accurate information is only obtained in about 70% to 75% of patients. When CT is used to look for metastatic disease, collimations of 5 mm or less should be used because this increases the accuracy of the preoperative evaluation.
- A single pulmonary lesion in a patient with a previous history of malignancy cannot be assumed to be metastasis unless properly investigated. This requires getting a tissue diagnosis.

A solitary pulmonary nodule is likely to be a metastasis in 60% to 80% of patients with a prior history of sarcoma or melanoma, in 50% of patients with prior adenocarcinoma, and in less than 20% of patients with prior squamous cell or prostatic carcinoma.

- Some primary tumors when metastatic to the lung can also spread to local and regional lymph nodes. Typical examples are colon and renal cell carcinoma. In these patients, the preoperative evaluation should also include a search for such nodes in the hilum or the mediastinum.
- The indication for surgery in patients with the suspicion of lymph node involvement is not clear. Enlarged lymph nodes can be biopsied by mediastinoscopy or by endobronchial ultrasound–guided biopsy. If the patient suffers from a single metastatic disease with lymph nodes in one station only, a case can be done to resect all visible disease.
- All patients with pulmonary metastases should also have a careful search for any occult extrathoracic metastases, particularly to the liver, brain, and the retroperitoneum.

## ASSESSMENT OF OTHER RISK FACTORS OF RECURRENCE AFTER SURGERY

- Tumor doubling time and disease-free interval must be long enough (>40 days, >2 years) to suggest slow-growing disease. However, surgery should not be denied to patients based on these criteria alone, but the prognosis will be negatively affected in those with rapid-growing tumors.[9]
- Some tumor histologies do better than others after complete resection. These tumors tend to metastasize only to the lung and include such tumors as bone and soft tissue sarcomas, as well as germ cell tumors. On the other hand melanoma and breast carcinoma tend to metastasize not only to the lung but also to other extrathoracic sites and the prognosis after lung resection is more guarded.
- The extent of the disease includes the number of metastases, their size, whether they are unilateral or bilateral, and whether or not the metastases have spread to the locoregional lymph nodes. The more extensive the disease, the less is the chance to be able to obtain a complete surgical resection.
- The number of metastases is usually not a limiting factor for surgery, as long as all metastases can be removed leaving the patient sufficient pulmonary function.

## THE ROLE OF CHEMOTHERAPY PRIOR TO SURGERY

- A trial of chemotherapy before surgery is recommended if the tumor is sensitive to the medication.[10]
- Osteosarcomas and germ cell tumors are typically treated by chemotherapy before consideration for pulmonary metastatectomy.

- If effective chemotherapy is not available, visible pulmonary metastases can be used to assess the efficacy of new or experimental treatments. Alternatively, in the absence of good chemotherapy, the patient can be offered surgery. This is often the case of metastases from renal cell carcinoma.
- The role of chemotherapy after surgery is not clear. Many factors are used to weigh the benefits of more chemotherapy after surgery, such as the amount of residual viable tumor in the resected metastases and the completeness of resection.

## PLANNING OF SURGERY

- Oligometastases (<4) located in the periphery of the lung can be resected by multiple wedges by video-assisted thoracoscopic surgery (VATS). The issue with VATS is that complete palpation of the lung is more difficult with this technique. In patients with numerous small metastases, there is a strong possibility that a metastasis could be missed.[11-13]
- Metastatectomy should not be attempted for lesions less than 1 cm in size unless the tumor is on the surface of the lung, or tissue is needed for diagnostic or therapeutic reasons such as the determination of genetic targets. Small lesions of indeterminate etiology can be followed by serial CT scans.
- Patients with initial bilateral disease can be approached by staged thoracotomies or by median or transverse sternotomy.
- Larger and centrally located metastases may require a segmentectomy or a lobectomy.
- Pneumonectomy is rarely indicated in the management of pulmonary metastases unless the patient can obtain an excellent prognosis after the resection or a single central lesion is causing significant problems such as pulmonary collapse or hemoptysis and the resection is done for cure. Pneumonectomy can be considered in the care of patients with central endobronchial metastases.
- In patients who are not candidates for curative resection, single lesions can be treated by stereotactic radiation therapy or radio-frequency ablation.

## POSTOPERATIVE CARE AFTER SURGICAL RESECTION

- The immediate postoperative care of patients after metastatectomy is similar to those having had any type of pulmonary resection. Chest tubes are used to drain fluid and air under suction until they are ready to be removed.
- In patients with a small residual lung left after resection, airway mucus mobilization should be encouraged aggressively. In patients with continuous leak of air beyond 3 days who have lung that does not re-expand to the chest wall, pneumoperitoneum, blood patch or talc sclerotherapy should be entertained.
- Serum tumor markers when appropriate should be repeated immediately after the surgery. The usual markers are β-human chorionic gonadotropin (βhCG), a fetoprotein, and carcinoembryonic antigen (CEA).
- All patients treated surgically for metastatic disease need a careful follow-up after the resection to detect recurrence. Patients should have a baseline CT scan repeated once the lung has healed at about 3 months after the resection and then every 6 months thereafter. The disease will eventually recur in about 50% of patients after an initial resection, and the patient will require more surgery, which is an argument for using pulmonary sparing maneuvers at the time of each resection.

## RESULTS OF SURGICAL RESECTION

- Results of pulmonary metastatectomy are mainly histology dependent. Soft tissue sarcomas have a 5-year survival rate of 30% to 60%; colorectal carcinoma, 25% to 30%; renal cell carcinoma, 20% to 50%, testicular carcinoma, 60% to 80%; head and neck carcinoma, 20% to 30%; and the prognosis for patients with melanoma and breast carcinoma metastatic to the lung is poor.[14,15]
- There has never been a comparative evaluation of the actual usefulness of pulmonary metastatectomy compared with nonoperative maneuvers. Furthermore, the effect of lung resection in the quality of life of patients has not been determined either.

## FUTURE APPLICATIONS

- Recent advances in understanding the biology of tumors which become metastatatic may able the identification of subgroups of patients who can do better after resection.[16]
- Genetic mapping and proteomics will lead to better targeted therapies in which certain types of drugs can be given with better results for specific tumors or other drugs can be used to deliver missing or mutated genes to prevent recurrence or spread of the disease.
- Numerous centers anticipating such advances are already banking serum and tumor samples for research purposes but also for clinical applications in their patients.

### Brief Illustrative Case

- A 74-year-old woman with a past history of rectal cancer, presents with a biopsy-proven single metastatic deposit in the right lower lobe (Fig. 34-1). She was treated after the resection of the rectal carcinoma with 5

*(Continued)*

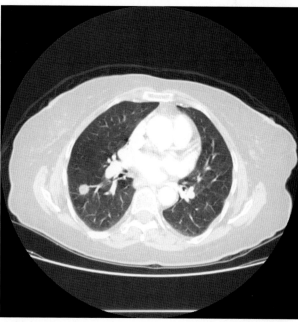

**Figure 34-1:** Single metastasis from a rectal carcinoma in a 74-year-old woman.

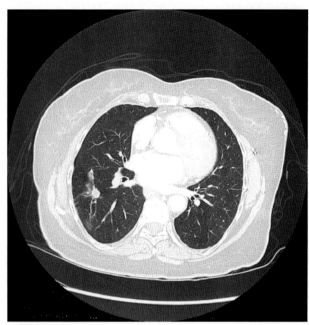

**Figure 34-2:** First recurrence 16 months later.

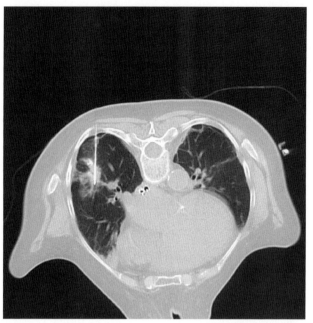

**Figure 34-3:** Recurrence treated with radiofrequency ablation.

### Brief Illustrative Case—cont'd

fluoro-uracil (5-FU) and leucovorin. On treatment, she developed neurocognitive changes. It was decided to not treat her with more systemic therapy and to refer her for surgery. There is no mediastinal involvement. She sustained a single-wedge resection to clear margins by VATS.

- Sixteen months later, her tumor recurred in the same position. Because of chronic obstructive pulmonary disease (COPD), she was treated with radiofrequency ablation (Figs. 34-2 and 34-3).
- The lesion recurred again 1 year later (Fig. 34-4). Her COPD treatment was optimized, and she was able to tolerate a lobectomy. She remains disease free.

## References

 Interactive references and additional readings for this chapter can be accessed online at *expertconsult.com*.

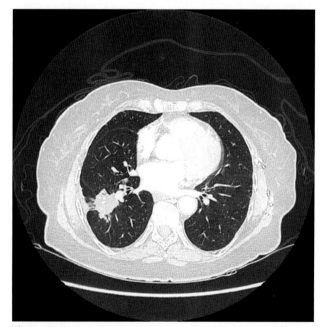

**Figure 34-4:** Second recurrence 1 year after radiofrequency ablation. This time, the tumor was resected with a right lower lobe lobectomy.

# LUNG TRANSPLANTATION

## 35 PATIENT EVALUATION AND SELECTION

Sara Ghandehari, MD, Jeremy A. Falk, MD, and George E. Chaux, MD

### GOAL OF LUNG TRANSPLANTATION

- Provide survival benefit for patients with advanced lung disease
- Improve quality of life for patients with advanced lung disease[1]

### GENERAL INDICATIONS

- Advanced lung disease with[2]
  - Chronic progressive respiratory failure refractory to maximal available medical treatment
  - Absence of effective medical therapy for patients with advanced lung disease and poor prognosis
- Poor prognosis with estimated life expectancy of approximately 2 years

### ABSOLUTE CONTRAINDICATIONS

- Malignancy in the last 2 years[1,2]
  - With the exception of cutaneous squamous and basal cell tumors, at least 2-year disease-free survival after definitive therapy for a malignancy is recommended but a 5-year disease-free interval is prudent, especially in the case of malignant melanoma and breast cancer.
- Advanced dysfunction of another major organ, although combined organ transplantation can be considered on an individual basis
- Systemic inflammatory disease such as sarcoidosis, amyloidosis, or progressive systemic sclerosis with primary lung involvement but also with extensive extrathoracic involvement
- Chronic extrapulmonary infection that cannot be treated and resolved
- Human immunodeficiency virus infection and disease have traditionally been considered to be an absolute contraindication to lung transplantation. However, increasing experience with transplantation of other solid organs in this patient population may render this a relative contraindication.
- Significant chest wall/spinal deformity
- Medical noncompliance
- Uncontrolled psychiatric condition that cannot be treated and resolved
- Lack of stable social support system
- Substance abuse within the last 6 months, including smoking and alcohol abuse

### RELATIVE CONTRAINDICATIONS[1,2]

- Age older than 65 years for single lung transplantation, 60 years of age for bilateral lung transplantation, and 55 years of age for heart-lung transplantation
- Acute critical clinical condition
- Poor functional status without potential for rehabilitation
- Colonization or active infection with resistant or highly virulent microorganisms including *Burkholderia cepatia,* molds, and atypical mycobacteria
- Obesity, with body mass index (BMI) greater than 30 kg/m$^2$.[3]
- Advanced malnutrition with BMI less than 20 kg/m$^2$
- Severe or symptomatic osteoporosis.
- Mechanical ventilation for acute respiratory failure, although patients have successfully undergone transplantation surgery who have relatively stable chronic respiratory failure on non-invasive mechanical ventilation or on mechanical ventilation via tracheotomy
- Comorbidities that have not yet resulted in advanced organ dysfunction
- Chronic high-dose steroid therapy usually defined as the equivalent of more than 20 mg of prednisone a day
- Lack of adequate medical insurance coverage

### REFERRAL FOR LUNG TRANSPLANTATION

In general, evaluation for lung transplantation is recommended for patients with advanced lung disease when

- 2- to 3-year predicted survival is less than 50%
- Level of function at New York Heart Association (NYHA) class III or IV
- There is refractory hypoxemia
- There is development of cor pulmonale

### DISEASE-SPECIFIC GUIDELINES

#### Chronic Obstructive Pulmonary Disease

- Chronic obstructive pulmonary disease (COPD) is currently the most common indication for lung transplantation.[4]
- Very symptomatic COPD patients may have a relatively good prognosis, which makes identifying the appropriate timing for transplantation rather challenging.[5]

- An acute exacerbation with hypercapnia and requiring hospitalization carries a poor prognosis of 49% 2-year survival.[6]
- In general, the goal of thoracic organ transplantation in this patient population is improvement in quality of life rather than prolongation of survival and life expectancy.

### When to Refer

- Continued deterioration despite optimal medical and surgical therapy including
  - Smoking cessation
  - Maximal bronchodilating treatment
  - Pulmonary rehabilitation
  - Long-term oxygen therapy
  - Lung volume reduction, if indicated
- Decline in measures of health-related quality of life: BODE Index–the components include:
  - **B**MI
  - Degree of airflow **o**bstruction (percent predicted $FEV_1$)
  - Degree of **d**yspnea (based on modified Medical Research Council dyspnea scale)
  - **E**xercise capacity (based on 6-minute walk test [6-MWT])
- In a prospective study of 625 patients with COPD, a BODE index of 7 to 10 was associated with a median survival of about 3 years, which is less than would be expected after transplantation.[7]
- Patients with a BODE score of 5 to 6 would less likely derive a survival benefit from transplantation but may be candidates for early referral.

### When to Transplant

- Patients with a BODE index of 7 to 10 or at least 1 of the following:
  - Hospitalization for exacerbation associated with acute hypercapnia ($Pco_2$ exceeding 50 mm Hg), which suggests a 49% 2-year survival
  - Pulmonary hypertension or cor pulmonale, or both, despite oxygen therapy
  - $FEV_1$ of less than 20% and either carbon monoxide diffusing capacity (DLCO) of less than 20% or homogenous distribution of emphysema

## Idiopathic Interstitial Pneumonia

- Idiopathic pulmonary fibrosis (IPF) is the most common of idiopathic interstitial pneumonia and carries the worst prognosis.[8]
- IPF is the second most frequent indication for lung transplantation.[4]
- Median survival time from diagnosis of IPF is 2.5 to 3.5 years.
- Patients with IPF have the highest mortality on the transplant waiting list.[4]
- A subset of patients with fibrotic nonspecific interstitial pneumonia (NSIP) with severe functional impairment at diagnosis or a rapid decline in their functional indices over 6 to 12 months follow-up have a similar poor prognosis to IPF with a dismal 2-year survival, regardless of treatment.[9,10]

### When to Refer

- Histologic or radiographic evidence of usual interstitial pneumonia (UIP)
- Histologic evidence of fibrotic NSIP
- Other forms of interstitial lung disease such as desquamative interstitial pneumonia (DIP), chronic hypersensitivity pneumonitis or eosinophilic granulomatosis refractory to medical therapy

### When to Transplant

- Histologic or radiographic evidence of UIP and any of the following:
  - DLCO less than 39% predicted
  - Decline in forced vital capacity (FVC) of 10% or greater during 6 months of follow-up
  - Oxygen desaturations to less than 88% during 6-MWT
  - Honeycombing on high-resolution computed tomography (HRCT) scan (fibrosis score of >2)
  - Development of secondary pulmonary hypertension
  - Development of hypercapnia
- Histologic evidence of fibrotic NSIP and any of the following:
  - DLCO less than 35% predicted
  - Decline in FVC of 10% or greater during 6 months of follow-up
  - Decline in DLCO of 15% or greater during 6 months of follow-up
  - Development of secondary pulmonary hypertension
  - Development of hypercapnia

## Collagen Vascular Disease

- Introduction
  - There has been limited experience with collagen vascular disease (CVD)[2]
  - By 2004, The International Society for Heart and Lung Transplantation registry had documented only 65 cases.
  - Reluctance centered around the concern for an active systemic disease and extrapulmonary involvement that could complicate the post-transplant course.
  - General considerations in such cases now include
    - Quiescent status of systemic disease
    - Failure of state-of-the-art medical therapeutic approaches
    - Each candidate needs to be evaluated on an individual basis.
- Scleroderma
  - Interstitial lung disease and pulmonary arterial hypertension are the major thoracic complications of scleroderma
  - Severe lung disease with or without pulmonary arterial hypertension is a leading cause of death in scleroderma
  - Previously, patients with scleroderma have been regarded as suboptimal candidates for lung transplantation.
  - More recent data, however, are more encouraging.[11-13]
  - Data on 29 patients with scleroderma who underwent transplantation in the Johns Hopkins and University of Pittsburgh lung transplant programs were reported[11]:
    - The 2-year mortality rate for scleroderma patients was 38%, which is similar to that for IPF (33%) and idiopathic pulmonary arterial hypertension (IPAH; 37%)
    - Early survival was less in scleroderma patients (69% at 6 months versus 80% and 79% for IPF and IPAH, respectively)
    - Early deaths with scleroderma occurred in those with single lung transplants and PAH who developed primary graft dysfunction. Bacterial pneumonia was also a contributor
    - In another analysis of 47 patients from 23 US centers, 1- and 3-year survival rates were 68% and 46%, respectively.[12]
  - Lung transplantation should be considered a viable option in appropriate candidates with scleroderma
  - Pre- and post-transplant challenges include enhanced likelihood of renal dysfunction, hypertension (with risk of crisis), and aspiration from esophageal dysmotility

## Pulmonary Langerhans Cell Histiocytosis (Eosinophilic Granuloma)

- There is a variable natural history with 10% to 15% mortality rate from progressive pulmonary disease and respiratory failure.[2,14] Median survival overall is 13 years.
- In addition, pulmonary arterial hypertension, which is often severe and disproportionate to the degree of lung disease or hypoxemia can complicate the disease. The latter is thought to be due to a small vessel vasculopathy
- In patients referred for lung transplantation, mean pulmonary artery pressure was 59 mmHg.[15]
- In a 2005 report, pulmonary Langerhans cell histiocytosis (PLCH) has accounted for only 0.2% of lung transplants.[4]
- Considerations for lung transplantation include[2]
  - Progressive respiratory dysfunction: $FEV_1$ less than 40%; FVC less than 55%, and DLCO less than 40% of predicted.
  - Significant PAH
  - NYHA functional class III or IV
  - Progressive decline in quality of life measures

## Lymphangioleiomyomatosis

- This is a rare disease affecting women in which proliferation of atypical smooth muscle produces thin-walled lung cysts. Angiomyolipomas of the kidney and other intra-abdominal and retroperitoneal structures also occur in 30% to 70% of patients.[16]
- In a 2005 report, lymphangioleiomyomatosis (LAM) has accounted for only 1.1% of lung transplants.[4]
- Considerations for lung transplantation include[2]
  - Progressive respiratory dysfunction despite optimal antiestrogen therapy: $FEV_1$ less than 30%; FVC less than 50%, and total lung capacity (TLC) less than 130% of predicted.
  - Severe cystic lung disease and complications
  - NYHA functional class III or IV
- Transplant and post-transplant considerations
  - Double lung transplant suggested to avoid native lung complications (e.g., pneumothorax, chylothorax)
  - Postoperative bleeding from lung explantation in the face of extensive pleural adhesions can pose a serious problem.
  - Postoperative chylothorax, which may require thoracic duct ligation, can occur.
  - LAM recurrence in transplant allografts reported but rare.

## Cystic Fibrosis

- Cystic fibrosis (CF) is the third most common indication for lung transplantation.[4]
- CF patients are often chronically infected with multidrug-resistant organisms, increasing their potential risks for infection with post-transplant immune suppression.
- Despite increased risk of infection and comorbidities associated with CF, post-transplant survival of patients with CF is similar to or greater than in others undergoing lung transplantation.[17-19]
- Bilateral lung transplantation is mandatory in patients with CF and others with chronic suppurative lung disease.

### When to Refer

- $FEV_1$ greater than 30% predicted or a rapid decline in $FEV_1$
- Acute exacerbation requiring stay in intensive care unit
- Increasing frequency of exacerbations and requirement for antibiotic therapy
- Recurrent or refractory pneumothorax
- Recurrent hemoptysis despite embolization treatment
- Development of colonization or infection with increasingly resistant microorganisms

### When to Transplant

- Oxygen-dependent respiratory failure
- Hypercapnia

- Pulmonary hypertension
- Decreasing exercise tolerance

## Pulmonary Arterial Hypertension

- PAH is a disorder with varying etiologies, induced by increase in pulmonary vascular resistance that progressively worsens, leading to right-sided heart failure.
- Untreated idiopathic PAH carries a reported median survival rate of 2.8 years.[20]
- In general, these patients are managed with bilateral lung transplantation, although successful unilateral lung transplantation has been reported by several centers. Heart-lung transplantation is reserved for those individuals who have very severe right ventricular dysfunction.[21]

### When to Refer

- Rapidly progressive disease refractory to medical therapy
- Intolerance to or severe adverse reaction attributed to available medical therapy
- NYHA functional class III or IV

### When to Transplant

- NYHA class III or IV despite maximal medical therapy, including IV epoprostenol or its analogues
- 6-MWT of less than 380 meters
- Declining 6-MWT
- Cardiac index of less than 2 L/min/m$^2$

## Sarcoidosis

- Sarcoidosis currently accounts for 2.6% of indications for adult lung transplantation.[4]
- Patient with sarcoidosis on lung transplant waiting list have a reported 30% to 50% mortality rate.[22,23]
- Sarcoidosis has a variable course that makes finding the appropriate time for transplantation referral relatively difficult.

### When to Refer

- NYHA functional class III or IV
- Failure to respond to medical therapy
- Progressive restriction on pulmonary function tests
- Stage III and IV disease, which is less likely to respond to steroid therapy

### When to Transplant

- NYHA functional class III or IV and any of the following:
  - Hypoxemia at rest
  - Pulmonary hypertension
  - Right atrial pressure greater than 15 mm Hg.

## References

 Interactive references and additional readings for this chapter can be accessed online at *expertconsult.com*.

## Appendix 1

 Appendices for this chapter can be accessed online at *expertconsult.com*.

## Appendix 2

 Appendices for this chapter can be accessed online at *expertconsult.com*.

# LUNG TRANSPLANT DONOR SELECTION AND MANAGEMENT

Jeremy A. Falk, MD, Sinan Simsir, MD, and George E. Chaux, MD

## INTRODUCTION

The number of lung transplants performed worldwide has increased exponentially over the past 20 years.[1] The availability of suitable organs has limited the number of patients who can undergo transplantation surgery as increasing numbers of patients are placed on waitlists for lung transplantation. Strategies to increase the donor pool have been diverse and have included increasing public awareness, use of extended donors, active donor management, and use of donation after cardiac death (DCD) donors.

## SHORTAGE OF ORGANS

- Improved outcomes have led to an increased demand for lung transplantation surgery (Fig. 36-1).
- Trend toward bilateral rather than single lung transplants, among other factors, has led to a need for increased numbers of donors.[1]
- In May of 2005, the lung allocation score (LAS) was developed by the United Network for Organ Sharing (UNOS) and Organ Procurement and Transplant Network (OPTN) networks to decrease the mortality rate of patients on the lung transplant waiting list. The high death rate of these patients is primarily a result of limited organ availability.[2]
  - ○ LAS altered allocation of organs to recipients with the greatest need rather than to those with the longest time on the transplant list.

- Despite measures to increase rates of transplantation, significant numbers of patients die while on the waiting list.[3]
- Very few lungs (15%–20%) are procured or used from potential donors,[4] particularly when compared with procurement rates of other solid organs (Figs. 36-2 and 36-3).
- Reasons for low use of lung allografts (Fig. 36-4)[5]:
  - ○ Perceived poor lung function in donor
  - ○ Medical or social history of donor
  - ○ No suitable recipient found
  - ○ Organ unsatisfactory
  - ○ Donor positive for human immunodeficiency virus/hepatitis/HTLV-1
  - ○ Cardiac arrest
  - ○ Abnormal findings of allograft biopsy

## PHYSIOLOGY OF BRAIN DEATH

- The vast majority of lung allografts are from brain-dead donors.
- The process of brain death is referred to as coning.
- Central nervous system ischemia typically occurs in a stepwise fashion, progressing from the cerebrum and pons to hypothalamus and pituitary (Fig. 36-5)[6]:
- Autonomic and hypothalamic dysfunction results in a predictable fashion with direct implications for the lung.
  - ○ Hypernatremia
  - ○ Hypotension

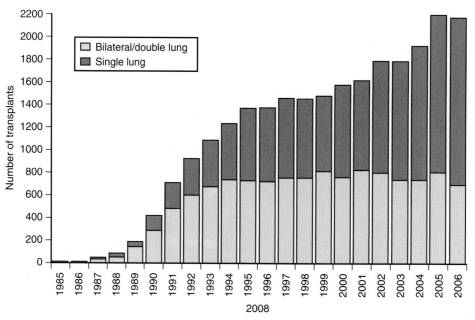

**Figure 36-1:** Number of lung transplants reported by year and procedure type. (*Adapted from Hertz MI, Aurora P, Christie JD, Dobbels F, Edwards LB, Kirk R, et al. Registry of the International Society for Heart and Lung Transplantation: a quarter century of thoracic transplantation. J Heart Lung Transplant 2008;27:937-983.*)

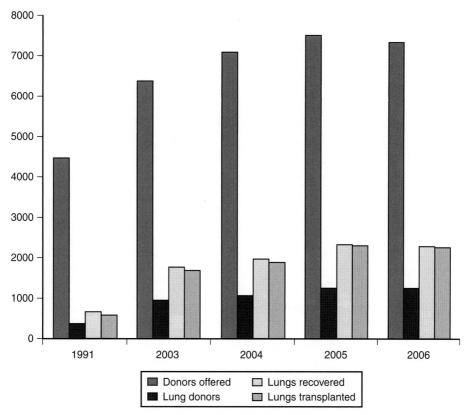

**Figure 36-2:** Lung offers translate to few transplants. *(Based on OPTN data as of February 2, 2007.)*

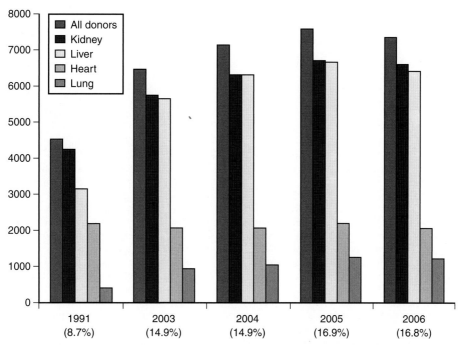

**Figure 36-3:** Cadaveric donors by organ type. *(Based on OPTN data as of February 2, 2007.)*

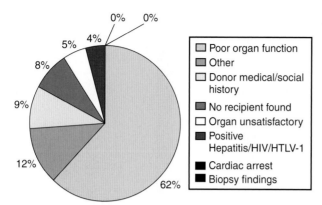

**Figure 36-4:** Reasons for non-recovery of consented organs, 2004. (*Based on OPTN/SRTR data as of May 2, 2005.*)

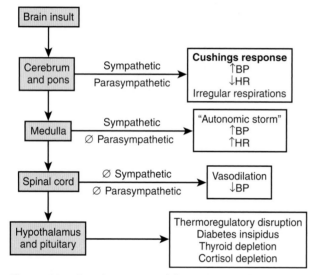

**Figure 36-5:** Stepwise process of brain death and physiologic consequences.

○ Pulmonary edema
○ Systemic inflammation
▪ Procedures aimed at reversing these changes have been shown to increase rates of procurement.[7]

## DONOR MANAGEMENT

▪ On identification of a potential donor, management must often be done to maximize not only lung but other organs that may potentially be used for transplant surgery.
▪ Different organs often have very different, sometimes conflicting, management strategies.[6]
▪ Use of a protocol published by the UNOS, entitled "Critical Pathway for the Organ Donor," has provided general guidelines for management of organ donors, which take into account the specific needs of each potential organ and has been shown to improve procurement and transplantation rate (see the chapter appendix).[7]
▪ General management principles[6]
○ Invasive monitoring including arterial line and a pulmonary artery (PA) catheter or central venous catheter
○ Central venous pressure (CVP) 6 to 8 mm Hg, or lowest CVP needed to maintain blood pressure (BP) and urine

output, pulmonary capillary wedge pressure (PCWP) 8 to 12 mm Hg (if PA catheter placed)
○ Appropriate use of antibiotics
○ Vasopressor use to maintain BP greater than 90 mm Hg systolic
○ Endocrine replacement
  ▪ Insulin drip, if needed
  ▪ Arginine vasopressin—1 unit bolus: 0.5 to 4.0 unit/h drip (titrate systemic vascular resistance [SVR] 800–1200)
  ▪ Methylprednisolone—15 mg/kg bolus (Repeat q 24 h PRN)
    ○ Improves gas exchange
    ○ Increases rate of procurement[8,9]
  ▪ Tri-iodothyroxine ($T_3$)—4 μg bolus: 3 μg/h continuous infusion
    ○ Little data suggest that thyroid replacement is beneficial in lung recipients
○ Ventilator management, not validated[6]
  ▪ Tidal volume suggested 8 to 10 mL/kg
  ▪ Positive end-expiratory pressure (PEEP) is 5; ideally, it should be less than 10 cm $H_2O$
  ▪ Maximize lung compliance (plateau pressure < 30 cm $H_2O$)

## THE IDEAL LUNG DONOR

▪ Traditional criteria[10,11]
○ Age younger than 55 years
○ ABO compatibility
○ Clear chest radiograph
○ Adequate oxygenation ($PaO_2$ > 300 mm Hg at $FiO_2$ = 1.0, or $PaO_2/FiO_2$ > 250–300)
○ No chest trauma
○ No evidence of aspiration/sepsis
○ Normal sputum gram stain
○ Normal bronchoscopy
○ No history of significant lung disease
○ Limited smoking history (<20 pack-years)
▪ Very little data to support traditional criteria because extensive data now exists challenging their usefulness.
○ Despite registry data suggesting worse early and late outcomes using lungs from older donors (>50 years), advanced donor age, in the absence of prolonged ischemic time (>6 hours) is associated with acceptable outcomes.[1,12,13]
○ Several studies have shown equivalent outcomes in donors with normal and abnormal chest x-ray studies (atelectasis or infiltrate).[14-19]
○ One published report suggested that as many as 41% of lungs rejected based on clinical criteria, including chest x-ray study, were actually suitable organs when examined pathologically.[20]
○ No data available linking donor smoking history with transplant outcomes.[15-19]
○ Markedly abnormal bronchoscopic evaluation of the potential lung donor is common despite normal radiographs and arterial blood gases.[21]
▪ No strong evidence exists that has shown that the presence of significant airway secretions leads to unacceptably performing lung allografts, although this is frequently cited as a reason for lungs not being used.
○ $PaO_2/FiO_2$ ratio greater than 300 appears to be most important single factor in predicting outcomes after transplantation surgery.[22,23]
  ▪ Little is known about the minimal acceptable $PaO_2/FiO_2$ ratio as a modality to improve gas exchange (aspiration of secretions, diuresis, and use of corticosteroids can transform unacceptable organs to acceptable ones).[8,11,17]

| Study | N | Infiltrate | Secretions | Age | Smokers | Low PF | Other |
|---|---|---|---|---|---|---|---|
| *Kron, et al., 1993* | 10 | • | • | | | | Aspiration |
| *Shumway, et al., 1994* | 52 | • | | • | • | • | |
| *Sundaresan, et al., 1995* | 44 | • | | • | • | • | |
| *Gabbay, et al., 1999* | 64 | • | • | • | • | • | |
| *Bhorade, et al., 2000* | 52 | • | | • | • | | Vent > 5 days Inhaled drugs |
| *Whiting, et al., 2003* | 42 | • | • | | • | • | |

**Figure 36-6:** Use of "extended" donors. Common conclusion: No effect on short- or long-term survival.

- There have been several reports of the successful use of lungs from donors with a $PaO_2/FiO_2$ ratio of less than 300.[15,16,24] This factor may affect outcomes only when accompanied by significant purulent secretions.[25]
- Several published studies have challenged the notion of "ideal donor" as the use of "extended donors" has not been shown to impact significantly on early or late outcomes (Fig. 36-6)
- Poor correlation between traditional criteria and clinical outcomes has led to a clinical scoring system of donors.[26]
  - Five components include $PaO_2/FiO_2$ ratio, donor age, appearance on chest x-ray study (CXR), smoking history, and secretions observed during bronchoscopy.
  - Although preliminary results have suggested utility in predicting early clinical outcomes in bilateral lung transplants, routine use of the scoring system is still in question.

## STRATEGIES TO INCREASE THE NUMBER OF AVAILABLE ORGANS

- Increase rates of donation
  - Public awareness increased after the Uniform Anatomic Gift Act of 1968, which allowed patients and family the right to donate organs.[11]
  - In 1998, the Health Care Financing Administration mandated that all US hospitals contact their local organ procurement organization (OPO) to notify them of patients likely to die in order to increase the number of potential donors.
  - Community outreach programs
- Increased organ procurement and transplantation rates
  - "Active" management
    - Aggressive management, including diuresis, electrolyte correction, recruitment maneuvers, and endocrine replacement, has increased procurement rates.[7,17,27,28]
    - Close involvement by a member of the transplant team, including ventilator adjustment, antibiotic choices, fluid management, interpretation of x-ray studies, physiotherapy, and bronchoscopy, has increased the number of viable organs and helped convert poor organs to acceptable ones.[29]
  - Prolonged ischemic times
    - Often limits the geographic procurement area
    - A traditional ischemic time of 4 to 6 hours has been typically used because longer durations are associated with increased risk of early graft dysfunction, chronic rejection, and worse survival rates.[11,30,31]

- Several studies examining lungs with ischemic times longer than 6 hours from donors younger than 55 years of age have shown more favorable results.[32,33]
  - Procurement protocols
    - Protocolized management of potential donors including active involvement by members of the transplant team within an OPO has not only been very successful in significantly increasing lung donors but also in converting poor donors to acceptable ones.[29]
    - One such management protocol included[29]
      - Alveolar recruitment if $PaO_2/FiO_2$ is less than 300, pulmonary infiltrates are present, or both: (1) pressure control ventilation with $\Delta P$ 25 cm $H_2O$ and PEEP 15 cm $H_2O$ for 2 hours, followed with assist control 10 mL/kg, PEEP 5 cm $H_2O$; (2) successful if $PaO_2/FiO_2$ are greater than 300 and CXR improved
      - Restriction of fluids
      - Diuretics to maintain negative fluid balance
      - Minimize aspiration risk: (1) elevate head of bed to 30 degrees; (2) set endotracheal cuff pressure to 25 cm $H_2O$
  - Ex vivo lung conditioning
    - Lungs ventilated and perfused ex vivo before implantation in recipient[34,35]
    - Allows for more aggressive and "lung specific" management to maximize potential performance once patient has undergone transplantation surgery
    - Primary role likely to be in nonliving donors (donation after cardiac death—see later)
    - Only one reported use in humans[35]
- Alternative sources of organs
  - Living lobar donors
    - Left lower lobe and right lower lobes from two healthy living donors[36-38]
    - Recipients typically children or small adults
    - Unclear what role LAS will play in the future of living donor lobar transplantation
    - Outcomes similar to cadaveric transplantation
    - More common in countries such as Japan, where the concept of brain death is generally not recognized and where as many as two thirds of lung transplants performed nationally are from living lobar donors.[39,40]
  - DCD
    - Organs procured from non–brain-dead donors, with impending cardiac death scheduled for withdrawal of support
    - Donors categorized according to Maastricht criteria[41]
      - Category I: dead on arrival
      - Category II: unsuccessful resuscitation

- ○ Category III: awaiting cardiac death
- ○ Category IV: cardiac death in a brain-dead donor
- ■ DCD done exclusively in Maastricht Category III donors under controlled conditions
  - ○ Death occurs on withdrawal of life support in the intensive care unit or operating room as opposed to occurring spontaneously.
- ■ Ongoing ethical debates regarding the appropriateness of this approach[42]
- ■ Several small case series show outcomes similar to those of traditional brain-dead donors[43,44]
- ■ UNOS has established a protocol for DCD procurement (see appendix)
- ○ Xenotransplantation[45]
  - ■ Although no human experience yet exists in procuring nonhuman lungs for use in lung transplantation, interest remains high.

- ■ Great potential to increase supply of organs
- ■ Bulk of research has been done using porcine to primate transplant

## References

Interactive references and additional readings for this chapter can be accessed online at *expertconsult.com*.

## Appendix

Appendices for this chapter can be accessed online at *expertconsult.com*.

---

# 37  SURGICAL TECHNIQUES AND OPTIONS

### Wen Cheng, MD, Robert M. Kass, MD, and Ross Bremner, MD, PhD

## TERMINOLOGY

- ■ Donor
- ■ Lung preservation
- ■ Single lung transplantation
- ■ Sequential bilateral lung transplantation
- ■ Living donor (lobar) transplantation
- ■ Heart-lung transplantation

## DONOR

- ■ Twenty percent of otherwise suitable organ donors have lungs that meet standard donor lung criteria (Table 37-1).[1-3]
- ■ Many brain-dead donors have significant lung parenchymal issues such as contusion, infection, aspiration, or neurogenic pulmonary edema.
  - ○ Size matching between donor and recipient lung volumes is important.
  - ○ Lung volumes are calculated using standard nomograms based on age, sex, and height.[4]
- ■ In patients with obstructive lung disease, allografts up to 20% larger than the predicted lung volume can be placed due to the increased size of recipient's pleural space.
- ■ In patients with restrictive lung disease or pulmonary vascular disease, pleural space is reduced in size; therefore allograft should not be oversized.
- ■ In sequential bilateral lung transplant, do not oversize.
- ■ "Marginal" donors refer to organs that are transplanted despite not meeting all of the standard donor selection criteria.
- ■ "Marginal" donors can provide postoperative function that is nearly equivalent to the standard donors.[5-8]
- ■ Other strategies to increase donor pool include living donor lobar transplantation.[9]

## LUNG PRESERVATION

### Basic Principles

- ■ Systemic donor heparinization and administration of pulmonary vasodilator prostaglandin $E_1$ (PGE$_1$) 500 μg into the main pulmonary artery (PA).
- ■ Pulmonary artery flush in a state of moderate inflation/ventilation with an $FiO_2$ greater than room air.
- ■ Extracellular low potassium dextran solution used (Perfadex at temperature of 4° C). Perfadex (Vitrolife, Sweden), a low-potassium Dextran solution has been shown by several groups to produce better results than Euro-Collins solution.[10-12] This has not been reproduced in all centers.[13] Despite this, most programs have switched to Perfadex as their flush solutions.[14]
- ■ Ideally, ischemic time should be less than 6 hours.[15]

| TABLE 37-1 ■ STANDARD LUNG DONOR SELECTION CRITERIA |
|---|
| Age younger than 55 years |
| No history of pulmonary disease |
| Normal serial chest radiographs |
| Adequate gas exchange (PaO$_2$ 300 mmHg on FiO$_2$ and PEEP 5 CM [H$_2$O]) |
| Normal bronchoscopic examination |
| Negative serologic screening for hepatitis B and human immunodeficiency virus (HIV) |
| Recipient matching for ABO blood group |
| Size matching |
| |
| PEEP, peak end-expiratory pressure. |

## Donor Extraction

- Chest x-ray study assessed for infiltrates, and fiberoptic bronchoscopy performed at donor hospital by harvesting team.
- Final assessment by gross inspection of lungs after median sternotomy.
- Trachea, vena cavae, and aorta encircled in chest.
- Donor heparinized, then the cardioplegia cannula is placed in the ascending aorta if the heart is being harvested, and a large-bore pulmonary artery flush cannula is placed in main pulmonary artery (MPA) proximal to bifurcation.
- $PGE_1$ may be given into the MPA, producing immediate drop in systemic blood pressure.
- The superior vena cava is ligated, and inferior vena cava (IVC) is clamped. (Note: IVC drain placed by liver team to drain liver flush.)
- IVC—right atrial junction is incised to allow cardioplegia to vent from coronary sinus to pericardium.
- The aorta is cross-clamped, and cardioplegia and PA flush initiated (Fig. 37-1).
- Left atrial appendage is incised to vent pulmonary artery flush solution.
- The lungs are ventilated as 3 to 4 L of Perfadex solution are delivered at low pressure (<30 mm Hg).
- Topical iced slush is applied.
  - ○ Donor heart is removed in situ.
  - ○ After the superior vena cava, aorta, and MPA are divided, the heart is retracted to the right, and the left atrium is opened between the coronary sinus and the inferior pulmonary vein.
  - ○ The left atrial wall is divided leaving a rim of muscle on the pulmonary vein side (Fig. 37-2).

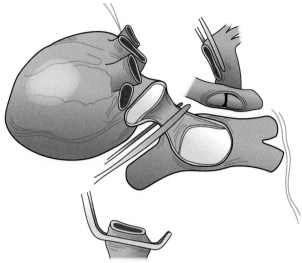

**Figure 37-2:** The ascending aorta is divided. The main pulmonary artery has been transsected at its bifurcation. The heart is retracted upward and to the right to enable safe division of the left atrium leaving suitable cuffs on both cardiac and lung allografts. *(From Sundaresen S, Trachiotis GD, Aoe M, Patterson GA, Cooper JD. Donor lung procurement: Assessment and operative technique. Ann Thorac Surg 1993; 546:1409-1413.)*

- Optional retrograde flush of pulmonary veins is performed with balloon tipped catheter.
- The trachea divided with stapler above the carina with the lungs inflated, then the lungs are removed.
- If the individual lungs are going to recipients at different hospitals, the donor left main stem bronchus is divided with a cutting stapler, leaving both lungs inflated (Fig. 37-3). Otherwise

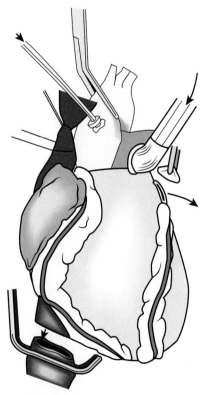

**Figure 37-1:** Cardioplegia is administered proximal to an aortic cross clamp and vented through the transsected inferior vena cava (*open arrow*). Pulmonary flush solution is administered through the main pulmonary artery and vented through the amputated tip of the left atrial appendage (*solid arrow*). *(From Sundaresen S, Trachiotis GD, Aoe M, Patterson GA, Cooper JD. Donor lung procurement: Assessment and operative technique. Ann Thorac Surg 1993;56:1409-1413.)*

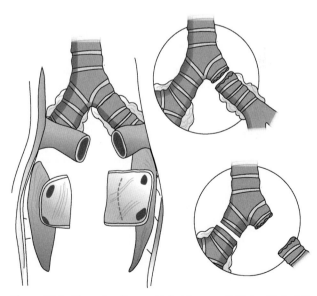

**Figure 37-3:** The pericardium and left atrium are divided, with the left atrium further trimmed (*dotted lines*). The airway is transsected and kept sealed with the use of a gastrointestinal anastomosis stapling device across the proximal left main stem bronchus. The donor airway is further revised for implantation, as shown in the bottom right. *(From Sundaresen S, Trachiotis GD, Aoe M, Patterson GA, Cooper JD. Donor lung procurement: Assessment and operative technique. Ann Thorac Surg 1993; 546:1409-1413.)*

both lungs should be transported en bloc to be separated at the recipients hospital.

- The lung allografts are immersed in cold flush solution for transport.
- Before implantation, the pulmonary venous cuffs are trimmed.
- Hint: The donor pericardium can be used to augment the size of the pulmonary venous cuff.
- The pulmonary artery is separated from its pericardial attachments out to its upper lobe branch.
- The main stem bronchus is divided 1 to 2 rings proximal to upper lobe origin.
- Hint: Minimize dissection at site of bronchus transection to preserve bronchial collateral blood flow to donor bronchus after implantation.

## Recipient Anesthesia

- Full hemodynamic monitoring is performed with a Foley catheter, PA Swan-Ganz catheter, and radial artery catheter.
- A transesophageal echo probe is useful in patients with pulmonary hypertension to monitor right and left ventricular function.
- Left-sided double-lumen endotracheal tube for separate ventilation of left and right lung.
- A single-lumen tube may be necessary in patients with suppurative lung disease such as cystic fibrosis because thick purulent secretions may need to be suctioned frequently from the tube.

## Cardiopulmonary Bypass

- Cardiopulmonary bypass (CPB) is used for patients who do not tolerate single-lung ventilation.
- For patients of small stature when a single-lumen tube is used
- For patients with significant pulmonary hypertension who do not tolerate pulmonary artery occlusion
- For double-lung transplants after implantation of the first lung, to prevent the development of primary graft dysfunction in the first lung due to the entire cardiac output perfusing this lung while implanting the second lung ("first lung syndrome")
- For patients who do not tolerate left atrial clamping for construction of the pulmonary venous anastomosis

## Technique

- Right thoracotomy, ascending aortic cannulation for arterial return and right atrium for venous drainage.
- Left thoracotomy, proximal left pulmonary artery or main pulmonary artery cannulation for venous drainage and descending aorta for arterial return.
- Median sternotomy, or bilateral thoracosternotomy (clamshell), ascending aorta for arterial return and right atrium for venous drainage. MPA vent catheter.
- Femoral artery and vein can be used for peripheral cannulation.

## SINGLE-LUNG TRANSPLANTATION

### Choice of Side

- Transplant side with least pulmonary function as determined by preoperative quantitative nuclear perfusion scan.
- Right side preferred if CPB needed as in pulmonary fibrosis patients with associated pulmonary hypertension.

## Exposure

- Posterolateral thoracotomy through fifth interspace is the preferred incision.
- A median sternotomy can be used for a right-sided single-lung transplant, especially if concomitant coronary bypass surgery or intracardiac repair is performed.

## RECIPIENT PNEUMONECTOMY

- Pleural adhesions are divided.
- PA and vein are encircled.
- Care is taken to avoid the phrenic and recurrent laryngeal nerve.
- Need to use CPB assessed by occluding the pulmonary artery and assessing gas exchange and hemodynamic stability.
- Intraoperative transesophageal echocardiogram (TEE) useful to assess left and right ventricular function.
- Upper lobe PA branches are ligated and divided.
- Distal PA is stapled and divided.
- Pulmonary vein branches are divided with silk ligatures or stapler.
- Pericardium around vein stumps is widely opened, and the interatrial groove is dissected.
- The bronchus is divided proximal to upper lobe origin (Fig. 37-4).

## IMPLANTATION

- Bronchial anastomosis is performed first. The membranous posterior wall is closed with a continuous #4-0 absorbable monofilament suture (PDS or Maxon). The anterior cartilaginous airway is reapproximated with interrupted simple or figure-of-eight absorbable suture (Vicryl, PDS, or Maxon) (Fig. 37-5).
- No attempt is made to intussuscept the smaller bronchus to avoid future bronchial stenosis.
- The pulmonary artery anastomosis is similarly fashioned with a vascular clamp placed proximally to control the recipient branch pulmonary artery. Excess length is trimmed from the donor and recipient branch PAs before creating an anastomosis with #5-0 polypropylene suture (Fig. 37-6).
- After an atrial clamp is placed controlling the pulmonary vein stumps and part of the recipient left atrial wall, the pulmonary vein stumps are amputated and the bridge of tissue is divided to create a left atrial cuff.
- The pulmonary veins are anastomosed with a #5-0 monofilament suture (Fig. 37-7).

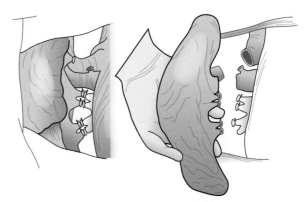

**Figure 37-4:** Excision of the native right lung is depicted. The pulmonary artery is stapled beyond its first upper lobe branch. Pulmonary veins are divided between ligatures, and the bronchus is transsected just proximal to the upper lobe orifice. *(From Shields TW: General Thoracic Surgery. Philadelphia: Lea & Febiger; 1994.)*

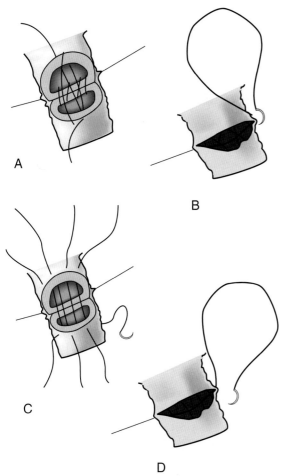

**Figure 37-5:** A bronchial anastomosis is depicted. The membranous wall is approximated (**A** and **C**). If the airways are large, a figure-eight cartilaginous suture technique can be seen (**A**). Smaller airways require simple, interrupted sutures (**C**). Peribronchial mediastinal tissue covers the anastomosis (**B** and **D**). *(From Meyers BF, Patterson GA. Bilateral lung transplantation. Op Tech Thorac Cardiovasc Surg 1999;4:169.)*

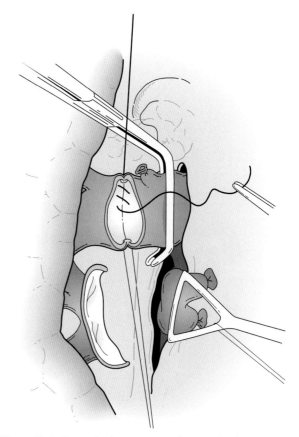

**Figure 37-6:** A central pulmonary artery clamp is placed, the staple line is excised, and an end-to-end anastomosis is constructed with 5-0 polypropylene. *(From Meyers BF: Technical aspects of adult lung transplantation. Semin Thorac Cardiovasc Surg 1998;10:213.)*

## Allograft Reperfusion

- One gram of methylprednisone (Solu-Medrol, Pfizer, New York, NY) is given before reperfusion.
- The lung is gently inflated while the PA clamp partially removed to flush the perfusate and air through the open left atrial anastomosis before tying the sutures and removing both the PA and left atrial clamp.
- Two chest drains are left in pleural space, with an optional drain left in the pericardium.

## *SEQUENTIAL BILATERAL LUNG TRANSPLANTATION*

### Exposure

- Through the bilateral anterolateral fourth or fifth interspace, thoracotomies are performed with or without a transverse sternotomy "clamshell incision" (Figs. 37-8 and 37-9).
- CPB is created by ascending aorta and right atrial cannulation if the sternum divided. Femoral artery cannulation if sternum intact.
- Omitting the transverse sternotomy leads to better and less painful sternal healing.

- Through a median sternotomy for recipients with "midline" hearts, that is, patients with COPD. Left lung exposure facilitated by CPB support.

## Pneumonectomy and Implantation

- Identical to single-lung transplantation
- CPB instituted for patients who do not tolerate double-lumen endotracheal tubes or develop gas exchange or hemodynamic instability during removal or replacement of the recipient lung.
- Following implantation of first lung, CPB is initiated to protect this lung from the effects of excessive perfusion in a newly transplanted lung, which is called first-lung syndrome.

## *LIVING DONOR LUNG TRANSPLANTATION*

### Background

- First Living Donor Lung Transplant performed by Vaughn Starnes at the University of Southern California in 1992.[16]
- Derived from the need for dying patients to undergo transplantation surgery while waiting for a cadaveric organ.
- Initially, donors were considered only if they were related to the recipient. With the success of the procedure, unrelated individuals who can demonstrate an emotional attachment to the recipient are also considered.

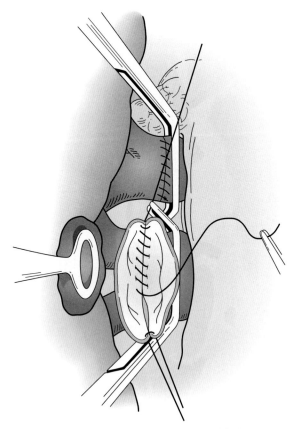

**Figure 37-7:** A central left atrial clamp is in place while the vein stumps are amputated and the bridge of atrial muscle is divided. The 4-0 polypropylene suture is used to complete the anastomosis. *(From Meyers BF: Technical aspects of adult lung transplantation. Semin Thorac Cardiovasc Surg 1998;10:213.)*

- Donors are healthy, and they donate a single lobe from one side of the chest.
- Recipients receive two healthy lobes from two donors, and each lobe acts as an entire lung.

## RECIPIENT SELECTION

- Must meet criteria for cadaveric transplantation
- Cystic fibrosis is most common indication
  - Patients with cystic fibrosis are often children and young adults and are small, that is, the donor lobe is more often of adequate size for the chest cavity in these patients and provides adequate pulmonary tissue
  - Indications for transplantation include:
    - Increase in number and severity of infections
    - Increasing antibiotic resistance
    - Progressive weight loss
    - Deteriorating pulmonary function tests
    - Increasing hypercapnia
  - Contraindications:
    - Panresistant respiratory flora or active viral infections
    - Major organ dysfunction
    - Lack of social support or non-compliance
    - Other indications have included fibrosis, pulmonary hypertension, bronchopulmonary dysplasia, and bronchiolitis obliterans[17]

## DONOR SELECTION[18]

- The recipient provides the names of potential donors, who must be in excellent health.
- Donors are evaluated initially for height, weight, age, relationship to the recipient, comorbidities, previous lung problems or chest procedures, and smoking history

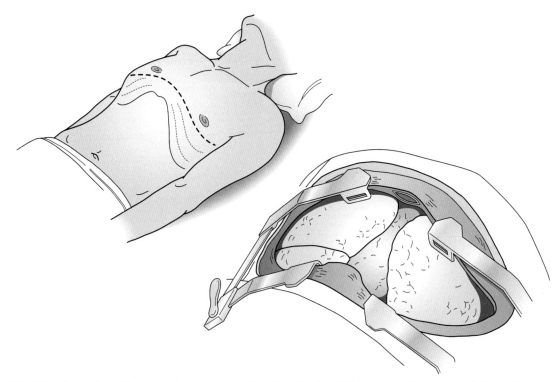

**Figure 37-8:** Bilateral anterolateral thoracotomies are performed through the fourth or fifth interspace with transverse division of the sternum. *(From Shields TW: General thoracic surgery. Philadelphia: Lea & Febiger; 1994.)*

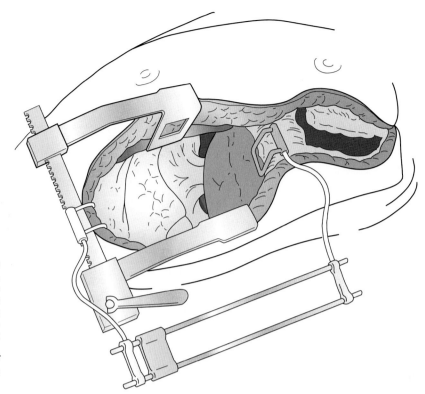

**Figure 37-9:** A chest retractor is used to spread the ribs vertically, while a Balfour retractor is used to open the muscle and skin of the lateral chest wall laterally. The combined use of these two retractors results in excellent exposure without sternal division. *(From Meyers BF: Technical aspects of adult lung transplantation. Semin Thorac Cardiovasc Surg 1998;10:213.)*

- Must be 18 to 55 years old.
- Tall donors are preferred (taller donors have larger lobes than shorter donors).
- Donors undergo intensive psychosocial evaluation to understand the motivation for donating. Donors who are construed to be under pressure to donate for whatever reason are excluded.
- Preliminary screening:
  ○ Spirometry
  ○ Chest x-ray study
  ○ Blood typing (human leukocyte antigen matching not required)
- Further testing is then performed:
  ○ Transplant serologies
  ○ Electrocardiogram and stress testing is performed for donors older than 40 years of age
  ○ V/Q scan
  ○ High-resolution computed tomography scan

## DONOR OPERATION

- A major difference between living donor and cadaveric procedures is that cold ischemic time is minimized.[9,19]
- Three operating rooms are needed concurrently: one for each of the donors, and one for the recipient. The recipient operation starts at the same time that the donor lobes are harvested.
- The taller donor is used for the right lobe.
- Lower lobes are used because these provide the best anatomy for implantation.
- After anesthesia is administered, the donor airway is evaluated bronchoscopically.
- PGE$_2$ is used until explantation to dilate the pulmonary vascular bed.
- Use of a posterolateral 5th interspace incision is optimal.

- Key to the procedure: The lobe must be removed with an adequate cuff on bronchial and vascular margins to enable implantation in the recipient and closure in the donor without compromise to the remaining lung.
- Similarly, fissure dissection should be performed sharply as much as possible so that parenchymal compression with stapling is avoided.
- Right lobectomy:
  ○ Fissure dissection is done sharply, vessels and bronchus are dissected free, and then heparin and steroids are administered parenterally.
  ○ Division of the artery and veins is illustrated in Figures 37-10 and 37-11. Division of the lower lobe bronchus should be done so as not to compromise the orifice of the middle lobe when closing the stump (Fig. 37-12). Closure of the bronchus is done with simple figure-of-eight 4-0 PDS suture.
  ○ If a second middle lobe artery is compromising the vascular margins, this may be ligated because the first branch is usually larger. A single middle lobe artery must obviously be preserved.
  ○ If the middle lobe vein drains into the lower lobe vein, this should be reimplanted to the upper lobe vein, or transection of the lower lobe vein should be done in the parenchyma in such a way to preserve drainage of the middle lobe vein.
  ○ Closure of the vessels is done with 4-0 or 5-0 prolene.
  ○ Liberal use of fine suture and lung sealants, such as Co-seal or Tisseal, is recommended to eliminate any obvious air-leaks in the remaining lobe before closing the chest.
- Left lobectomy
  ○ Dissection and heparinization, as above.
  ○ Division of the artery and bronchus are illustrated in Figures 37-13 and 37-14. An angled transection of the artery is necessary to preserve both the superior segment

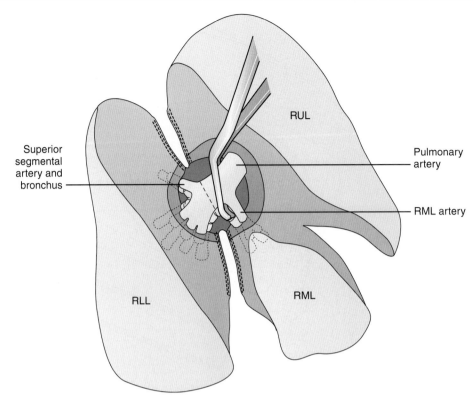

**Figure 37-10:** Placement of the pulmonary artery clamp following dissection for the donor right lower lobectomy. *(Reprinted with permission from Cohen RG, Barr ML, Schenkel FA, DeMeester TR, Wells WG, Starnes VA. Living-related donor lobectomy for bilateral lobar transplantation in patients with cystic fibrosis. Ann Thorac Surg 1994;57:1423-1428.)*

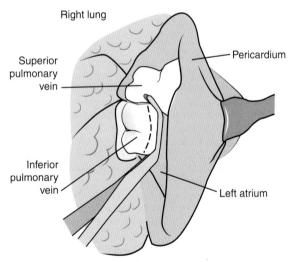

**Figure 37-11:** Placement of the vascular clamp after dissection of the intrapericardial inferior pulmonary vein and right atrium. *(Reprinted with permission from Cohen RG, Barr ML, Schenkel FA, DeMeester TR, Wells WG, Starnes VA. Living-related donor lobectomy for bilateral lobar transplantation in patients with cystic fibrosis. Ann Thorac Surg 1994;57: 1423-1428.)*

vessel (to go to the recipient), and the lingular vessel (to remain functional in the donor).

○ Occasionally, the lingular artery takes off some distance distal to the superior segment vessel. If the lingular artery is small, it can be ligated. However, if it is large, it may have to be reimplanted proximally.

- Preparation of the donor organ
  ○ A separate team prepares the preservation solutions on the back table.
  ○ Once the lobe is explanted, it is perfused with approximately 2 L of Perfadex (see above) in both the antegrade and retrograde manner while the lobe is gently ventilated. Care should be taken to keep the open airway clear of pneumoplegic solution.
  ○ The bronchus is gently clamped when the lobe is partly inflated, and the lobe is placed on ice and taken to the next room for implantation.
- Postoperative donor management.
  ○ Postoperative management is similar to that for the "usual" lobectomy patient; however, the sharp fissural dissection and the normal nonhyperinflated remaining lobe may result in a space or a prolonged air leak. This is managed with chest tube drainage and rarely requires further surgical intervention.

## THE RECIPIENT OPERATION

- The diseased recipient lungs are removed through a bilateral thoracosternotomy (clamshell incision). Because most of these patients have cystic fibrosis, intrathoracic adhesions and collateral bronchial vessels can make explantation challenging.[16]
- CPB is used because of the critical condition of these patients and to allow controlled reperfusion to both lobes. This helps avoid pulmonary edema from reperfusing a single lobe with the entire cardiac output.

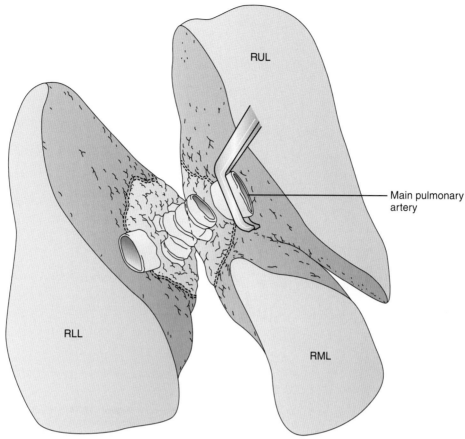

**Figure 37-12:** Dissection and division of the bronchus to the right lower lobe. *(Reprinted with permission from Cohen RG, Barr ML, Schenkel FA, DeMeester TR, Wells WG, Starnes VA. Living-related donor lobectomy for bilateral lobar transplantation in patients with cystic fibrosis. Ann Thorac Surg 1994;57:1423-1428.)*

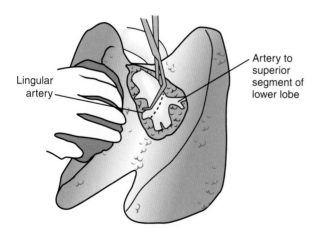

**Figure 37-13:** Dissection and division of the pulmonary artery for donor left lower lobectomy. *(Reprinted with permission from Cohen RG, Barr ML, Schenkel FA, DeMeester TR, Wells WG, Starnes VA. Living-related donor lobectomy for bilateral lobar transplantation in patients with cystic fibrosis. Ann Thorac Surg 1994;57:1423-1428.)*

- The pleural cavity of patients with cystic fibrosis is irrigated copiously with an aminoglycoside and amphotericin B solution before implantation.
- Dissection of pulmonary vessels and bronchus is performed as in a cadaveric transplant (Fig. 37-15).

- The bronchial anastomosis is performed using 4-0 PDS suture in a continuous fashion, taking care to avoid narrowing the superior segment orifice, which is close to the anastomosis (Fig. 37-16).
- The venous and arterial anastomoses are performed with 5-0 polypropylene suture, again using a continuous technique (Figs. 37-17 and 37-18).
- After completing the anastomoses, the arterial clamp is slowly removed and the preservation perfusate is allowed to egress from the venous anastomosis before tying the venous suture.
- Nitric oxide is started at 20 ppm, and ventilation is begun.
- Slow reperfusion of the lobes is performed by allowing increased cardiac ejection fraction and subsequent weaning from cardiopulmonary bypass.
- TEE and bronchoscopy are performed to evaluate anastomotic patency.

## POSTOPERATIVE MANAGEMENT

- Because the entire cardiac output is passing through only two lobes, there are unique challenges to postoperative management compared with cadaveric transplantation.
- The recipient is kept heavily sedated and intubated for 48 to 72 hours to minimize atelectasis- and agitation-induced pulmonary hypertension, and to allow continuous nitric oxide administration.

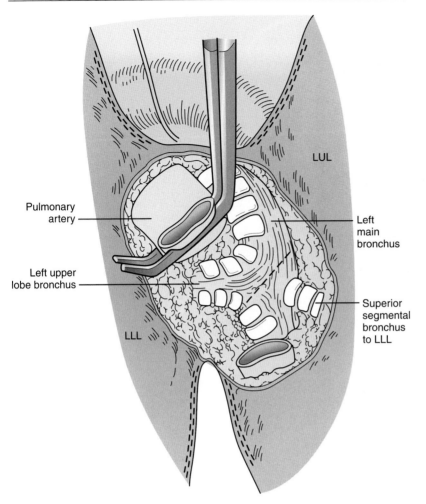

Pulmonary
artery

Left upper
lobe bronchus

LUL

LLL

Left
main
bronchus

Superior
segmental
bronchus
to LLL

**Figure 37-14:** Dissection and division of the bronchus to the left lower lobe. *(Reprinted with permission from Cohen RG, Barr ML, Schenkel FA, DeMeester TR, Wells WG, Starnes VA. Living-related donor lobectomy for bilateral lobar transplantation in patients with cystic fibrosis. Ann Thorac Surg 1994;57:1423-1428.)*

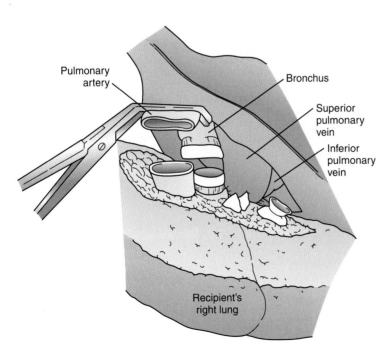

Pulmonary
artery

Bronchus

Superior
pulmonary
vein

Inferior
pulmonary
vein

Recipient's
right lung

**Figure 37-15:** Recipient right pneumonectomy. *(Reprinted with permission from Starnes VA, Barr ML, Cohen RG. Lobar transplantation: Indications, technique, and outcome. J Thorac Cardiovasc Surg 1994; 108:403-411.)*

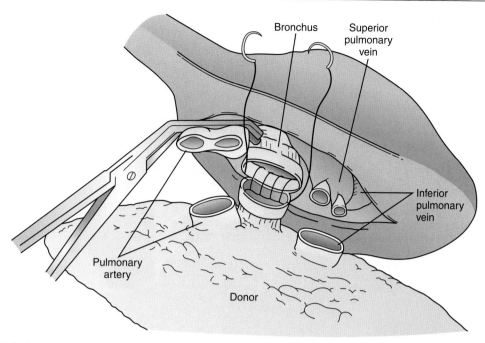

**Figure 37-16:** Right lower lobe implantation: bronchial anastomosis. *(Reprinted with permission from Starnes VA, Barr ML, Cohen RG. Lobar transplantation: Indications, technique, and outcome. J Thorac Cardiovasc Surg 1994;108:403-411.)*

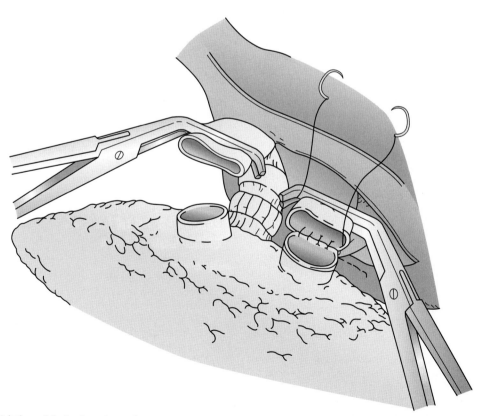

**Figure 37-17:** Right lower lobe implantation: pulmonary venous anastomosis. *(Reprinted with permission from Starnes VA, Barr ML, Cohen RG. Lobar transplantation: Indications, technique, and outcome. J Thorac Cardiovasc Surg 1994;108:403-411.)*

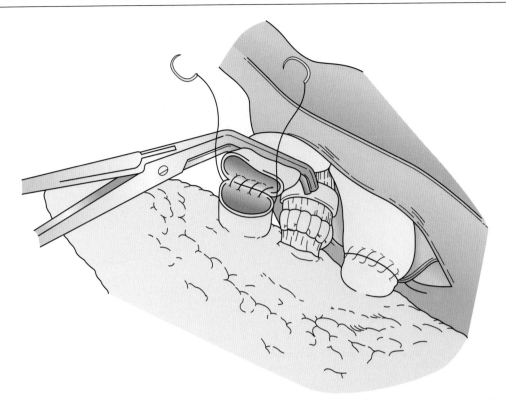

**Figure 37-18:** Right lower lobe implantation: pulmonary arterial anastomosis. *(Reprinted with permission from Starnes VA, Barr ML, Cohen RG. Lobar transplantation: Indications, technique, and outcome. J Thorac Cardiovasc Surg 1994;108:403-411.)*

- Chest tubes are not placed on conventional -20 cm water suction because this can result in impaired deflation mechanics. This is because the lobe does not conform entirely to the intrathoracic cavity. We have initially applied -10 cm suction in a rotational fashion to each chest tube to evacuate blood and minimize suction hyperinflation.[20]
- Patients are kept on nitric oxide in a relatively hypovolemic state with continuous nitroglycerine drip to keep pulmonary arterial pressures as low as possible.
- After 48 to 72 hours, patients are weaned of their drips and ventilatory support.
- Chest tubes are kept in situ for longer periods than in cadaveric transplantation surgery because of increased output resulting from topographic mismatch of the lobes, and for fear of fluid collections becoming infected from the contaminated space in patients with cystic fibrosis. Empyema is subsequently a very uncommon event.[21,22]

## RESULTS

### Recipients

- More than 130 recipients have now undergone transplantation surgery at the University of Southern California, and many other centers throughout the world are now performing the procedure.
- Results for children and adult recipients are similar to those for cadaveric transplantation surgery despite the recipients being critically ill at the time of implantation.[23,24]
- Infection is the major cause of 1-year mortality and is reflective of the cystic fibrosis population. Pseudomonas and Aspergillus are the most common causative organisms.

### Donors

- One of the major concerns with living lobar transplantation is the potential morbidity and mortality of the healthy donors.[25]
- To date, there have been no cases of donor mortality, and a low incidence of morbidity.
- One- and two-year postoperative pulmonary function testing has shown an average of 15% decrease in forced expiratory volume in one second ($FEV_1$).
- Using a RAND 36-item survey, no donors had regrets about donating and 85% said their health was no different from before donation.

## COMBINED HEART-LUNG TRANSPLANTATION

### Indications

- Eisenmenger's syndrome
  - A recent analysis to determine possible survival benefits for heart-lung transplantation (HLT) versus lung transplantion (LT) was conducted on data from the United Network for Organ Sharing and International Society for Heart and Lung Transplantation.[26]
  - Multivariate analysis on 605 patients with Eisenmenger's syndrome subjected to HLT or LT was performed.
- Multivariate analysis showed significantly better survival for patients subjected to HLT with Eisenmenger's syndrome due to ventricular septal defect or multiple congenital abnormalities compared with LT at 1 year.[26]

- Uncorrectable congenital heart disease with pulmonary artery atresia or hypoplasia and progressive heart failure.
- Severe cardiac and pulmonary disease with end stage heart or lung failure.

## Contraindications (Relative)

- Age older than 60 years
- Prior intrathoracic surgery where bleeding is anticipated to be significantly greater than usual

## Donor

- Same criteria as for lung transplantation and heart transplantation
- HLT recipients must have normal thoracic volumes, and size matching is important.
- Heart and lung preservation is currently used for each organ individually.

## Recipient

- The basic technique of HLT, as described by Reitz, is generally unchanged, except for changes in preservation.[27-29]
- Because mediastinal bleeding is common and can be difficult to control, meticulous hemostasis while excising the recipient heart and lungs is essential.
- Special care to avoid injury to the phrenic nerves is essential (carefully isolated on sizable pedicles of pericardium).[28]
- The donor heart-lung block is placed in the recipients's thorax, with the airway connection being a tracheal anastomosis. In

pediatric cases, interrupted polypropylene sutures are used to allow for growth at the anastomotic region.[28]

## Postoperative Care

- Generally, the same immunosuppression protocol as used in heart transplantation is followed.
- Rejection is most often discordant, more frequent, and more severe in the lung than in the heart.

## Survival

- The 1-, 3-, and 5-year survival rates for 372 adult patients for the period from 2000 to June 2004 were approximately 74%, 60% and 49%, respectively.[30]
- Complex congenital heart disease survival was significantly less than for patients with Eisenmenger's syndrome.[30]
- For pediatric patients over the time period from 1999 to June 2004 (n = 68), the overall survival data was somewhat lower (1-, 3-, and 5-year survival rates were approximately 67%, 51%, and 40% respectively).[30]

## References

 Interactive references and additional readings for this chapter can be accessed online at *expertconsult.com*.

# 38 | LUNG TRANSPLANTATION: PERIOPERATIVE MANAGEMENT AND EARLY COMPLICATIONS

Kamyar Afshar, DO, Jeremy A. Falk, MD, and George E. Chaux, MD

## INTRODUCTION

Lung transplantation has gained increased success over the past 20 years owing to improved surgical techniques, refinements in donor and recipient selection, and overall improved postoperative care of the recipients. The perioperative management for lung transplantation has expanded to a global focus of various organ systems. In this chapter, we discuss issues regarding mechanical ventilation, hemodynamic monitoring, the prevention and treatment of infectious pathogens, and the institution of immunosuppressive therapy. These matters are balanced with the prevention of various complications; such as those involving the vascular and airway anastomosis, acute cellular and humoral allograft rejection, primary graft failure, and impairment in the function of other end-organs. For the purposes of this chapter, we will primarily focus the discussion on the first 30 days following lung transplantation.[1]

## AIRWAY MANAGEMENT/VENTILATORY SUPPORT

- Standard mechanical ventilation techniques are used to maintain adequate gas exchange while minimizing risk of barotrauma and ventilator-induced lung injury. Some centers use pressure control or pressure-regulated volume control modes to decrease airway pressures. At present, there are no trials to determine the optimal mode of ventilation, but data in literature that focuses on patients with adult respiratory distress syndrome (ARDS) are extrapolated for the lung transplant patients.
- Tidal volume adjusted to 6 to 8 mL/kg and respiratory rate to 10 to 16 breaths per minute are recommended to decrease the risk of stretch and tidal trauma, and to decrease the risk of ventilator-induced lung injury.[2]
- Administer the least $FiO_2$ to maintain adequate oxygenation; the goal $FiO_2$ is 30% to 40% immediately postoperatively.

■ Mode of ventilation and airway pressures should also take into account the physiology of the native lung in single lung transplants; i.e., overly aggressive ventilation of a single lung transplant patient may lead to overdistension of the more compliant native lung in patients with emphysema. This overdistension of a single native lung may lead to development of mediastinal shift towards the allograft in addition to hemodynamic derangements resulting from the development of "auto-peep."

■ Migration of the endotracheal tube into one of the airways can result in barotrauma to the ipsilateral lung, which is due to high airway pressures to a single lung, as well as lung collapse of the contralateral lung.

■ Postoperatively, airway secretion clearance becomes ineffective owing to incision pain, decreased cough reflex from lung denervation, and reduced mucociliary function. Bronchoscopy before extubation is generally used for airway clearance; once the patient is extubated, postural drainage with chest percussion therapy is performed. Early patient mobility is also very important in this regard.

■ Standard weaning parameters and modes of ventilation are used to allow for early extubation, ideally 24 to 48 hours postoperatively.

## CARDIOVASCULAR MANAGEMENT

■ With the exception of those transplanted for pulmonary arterial hypertension or for parenchymal lung disease with secondary pulmonary hypertension, most patients are on minimal vasopressors, if any, during the immediate postoperative phase. Theses agents are generally weaned off in the first few hours of admission to the intensive care unit (ICU). Optimization of the preload and afterload is vital for spontaneous hemodynamic compensation. The pulmonary artery (PA) catheter waveforms and values are used to achieve optimization.

■ Continued need for or escalation of the vasopressor agents should prompt further investigation into possible sepsis, bleeding, or myocardial dysfunction. If a single lung transplant is performed for emphysema, then dynamic hyperinflation of the native lung may be a contributing factor.

■ Although anticoagulation is used during cardiopulmonary bypass, patients are still at risk of developing a thromboembolic event. Owing to the loss of the bronchial circulation, there is a greater degree of hypoxemia if pulmonary emboli occur. In two retrospective single-center studies, 8.6% to 29% of patients developed thromboembolic complications, with 20% occuring in the first month of transplantation.[3,4]

■ Arrhythmias are generally supraventricular in origin owing to the location of the anastomosis in the right or left atrium. Atrial flutter and atrial fibrillation are the most common arrhythmias. They are more likely to occur within 6 weeks of the operation. Some centers provide prophylactic beta-blockers, calcium channel blockers, or amiodarone.

■ Pulmonary hypertension can complicate the postoperative course. Although little data exist to support its use, inhaled nitric oxide (iNO), 10 to 40 parts per million, is often used to reduce elevated pulmonary artery pressure (PAP) and to minimize the occurrence of primary graft dysfunction. The goal is to maintain a systolic PAP less than 40 mm Hg with iNO. Most patients tolerate discontinuation of iNO within the first 24 hours. Methemoglobinemia and paradoxical pulmonary hypertension are known adverse events of continued iNO use and during weaning, respectively.

## COMMON EARLY COMPLICATIONS IN THE POSTOPERATIVE PERIOD

### Primary Graft Dysfunction

■ Previously referred to as the reimplantation respose, this is a non-alloimmune process with noncardiogenic pulmonary edema characterized by diffuse parenchymal infiltrates associated with various degrees of hypoxemia (Fig. 38-1)

■ Overall incidence has been reported between 10.2% and 25%, with a 30-day mortality rate of up to 42%.[5-8]
  ○ Chronic obstructive pulmonary disease (COPD) 3% to 9%
  ○ Suppurative lung diseases 10% to 35%
  ○ Restrictive lung diseases 10% to 40%
  ○ Primary pulmonary arterial hypertension 33% to 59%

■ Risk factors: lower donor $PaO_2/FiO_2$ (P/F) ratio, higher donor age, high inotrope requirement in the allograft recipient, pulmonary arterial hypertension as the underlying disease, and cardiopulmonary bypass requirement.[9,10] The pathophysiology of pulmonary graft dysfunction (PGD) is thought to be related to

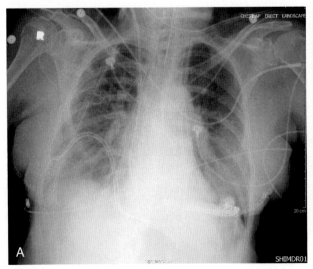
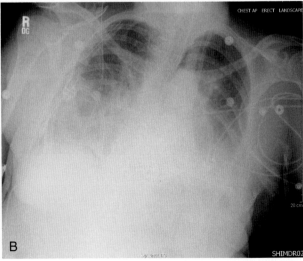

**Figure 38-1: A,** Chest radiograph shortly after surgery. **B,** Marked progression several hours later (bilateral consolidation and effusions), which is compatible with primary graft dysfunction.

cold ischemia time of the allograft, reperfusion lung injury, and other factors leading to an acute lung injury characterized by neutrophyllic infiltration of the lung allograft leading to a capillary leak syndrome.

■ Monitor for PGD from 0 to 72 hours after surgery. A low P/F ratio at 6 hours found to correlate with mechanical ventilation need, length of ICU admission and 30-day mortality

■ Grades (mild to severe)
  ○ Grade 0: No chest x-ray study (CXR) abnormality and P/F ratio greater than 300
  ○ Grade 1: CXR abnormality and P/F of 200 to 300
  ○ Grade 2: CXR abnormality and P/F between 100 and 200
  ○ Grade 3: CXR abnormality and P/F < 100

■ Treatment options include supportive care, judicious administration of intravenous fluids balanced with adequate perfusion of end organs, and diuresis. Inhaled nitric oxide improves oxygenation for up to 72 hours, but it has not been shown to positively effect the duration of mechanical ventilation requirement or mortality. In severe cases, extracorporeal membrane oxygenation (ECMO) is used. When clinically indicated, early use shows a survival benefit. Late initiation (greater than 7 days after severe PGD) has a 100% mortality rate associated with it.[11] In cases refractory to ECMO support, retransplantation can also be considered in select cases.

## Pleural Space Complications

■ Exudative, serosanguinous pleural effusions are very common in the early postoperative course. This is due to interruption of the lungs' lymphatic drainage. Chest tube drainage catheters should remain in place until the output is less than 100 to 150 mL/day. A persistent pleural effusion with high output should prompt the treating physician to consider a pathologic process such as an acute cellular rejection, primary graft failure, infectious process, bleeding, or injury to the thoracic duct.

■ Complicated pleural effusions and empyema are not very common, but when they occur, they are associated with a high rate of morbidity and mortality.

■ Chylothorax is rare but should be considered in the differential diagnosis of persistent pleural effusions early in the postoperative period.

■ Postoperative hemorrhage is more common in patients requiring cardiopulmonary bypass because anticoagulation is required. A re-exploration of the chest may be required to evaluate for a source of bleeding and to evacuate a potential hemothorax.

■ Small intermittent air leaks are common early after surgery. A persistent air leak is reported in approximately 10% of patients. It may be due to a donor-recipient size mismatch, but the possibility for the development of a bronchial anastomotic dehiscence should be evaluated via bronchoscope. Bronchial anastomotic dehiscence is rare, but when it is present, it usually occurs within the first month of transplantation because of impaired wound healing. Earlier studies attributed this to high dose corticosteroid use, but subsequent studies have refuted this.[12] The single most effective way to prevent this complication from developing is to place the bronchial anastomosis as distal as possible, thereby preserving as much of the native bronchus and its bronchial circulation. Sirolimus utilization within the first 3 months is associated with a high risk of developing bronchial anastomotic dehiscence and should be avoided in the early postoperative period.[13,14]

■ In double-lung transplantations, the anterior pleural reflection is taken down and there is communication between both hemithoraces. It is not uncommon that if a particular pathology occurs on one side that output or air leaks may be visualized on the contralateral side.

## IMMUNOSUPPRESSANT THERAPY

■ Immunosuppressive therapy is initiated just before transplantation to prevent rejection of the allograft. Similar to other solid organ transplantation therapy is aimed as a two-phase process: induction and maintenance.

■ Induction therapy
  ○ Induction therapy is used in order to prevent the activation and proliferation of alloreactive T cells. Up to 49% of the transplant centers have induction therapy as part of their protocol, but not all centers use induction as part of their immunosuppressive protocol due to lack of data demonstrating efficacy against development of chronic rejection and improved survival.[15,16] Alloreactive T cells are activated by the interleukin-2 (IL-2) receptor activation with the presence of the T cell–antigen complex. A number of different agents are available that can be used for induction immunosuppression.
  ○ Induction therapy with thymoglobulin antibodies (monoclonal versus polyclonal) (anti-lymphocyte or anti-thymocyte globulins) is used for induction through a complement-dependent cytotoxic methodology. They inhibit alloreactive T cells but also promote regulatory T cells. These agents reduced the rate of acute rejection in the first year compared to no induction or induction with IL-2 antibodies.[17,18] Major adverse drug effects include hypotension, systemic inflammatory response syndrome, capillary leak syndromes, and an increased risk of post-transplant lymphoproliferative disorder.
  ○ Mouse-human or rabbit-human IL-2 receptor antibodies (daclizumab or basiliximab) have been found to decrease incidence of acute cellular rejection compared with no induction, without an increased risk of CMV infection or malignancy and therefore have gained some favor among centers that do have induction protocols.[15,19]
  ○ The anti-CD52 monoclonal antibody alemtuzumab has recently been introduced but has not been compared in head-to-head studies with other agents used for induction in lung transplantation.[20]
  ○ Induction therapy does not alter risk of bronchiolitis obliterans syndrome and has not been shown to improve long-term survival outcomes after lung transplantation.[15,16]

■ Maintenance immunosuppressant therapy
  ○ Maintenance therapy may be administered by nasogastric tube, sublingually, or through intravenous routes.
  ○ A high-dose corticosteroid bolus is administered intraoperatively and can then be continued at 125 mg intravenously every 8 hours in the first 24 hours as part of the induction protocol. Prednisone is then administered orally starting at 0.5 to 1 mg/kg daily and tapered on a weekly basis to a maintenance dose of 0.2 to 0.3 mg/kg daily by 6 months if no induction immunosuppression is used. In cases in which induction immunosuppression is used, prednisone therapy can be initiated at the maintenance dose immediately after surgery.
  ○ Approximately 75% of lung allograft recipients are currently receiving a tacrolimus, prednisone, and mycophenolate mofetil combination as a standard triple-drug immunosuppression regimen. Other immunosuppressive agents used include cyclosporine, azathioprine, sirolimus, and on occasion, methotrexate. Sirolimus, however, is not used in the first 3 months owing to the risk of bronchial anastomotic dehiscence and chest wound complications.

## INFECTIONS IN THE EARLY POST–LUNG TRANSPLANTATION PERIOD

- Infections are a significant cause of morbidity and mortality.
- Exposure to infectious agents occurs from four potential sources: donor transmission, recipient derived, nosocomial infection, and community-acquired infection.
- Early in the course of lung transplantation, nosocomial bacterial infections are primary causes of infectious complications; particularly bacterial pneumonia.[21,22]
- The etiology of bacterial pneumonia may be due to retained secretions, ventilator-associated pneumonia or an infectious transmission from donor to recipients.
- Prophylactic antibiotics are primarily tailored to cover for gram negative (*Pseudomonas sp, Haemophilus influenza and Klebsiella sp*) and gram-positive organisms (*Staphylococcus aureus*). In patients with cystic fibrosis, the most recent culture results and sensitivities dictate the choice of antibiotic administered.
- Prophylactic intravenous antibiotics are given for approximately 7 to 14 days.
- Additional nosocomial infections to monitor include *C. difficile* colitis, donor-derived viremia, or candidemia.
- The use of prophylactic medications for cytomegalovirus, pneumocystis, and fungal infections has markedly reduced the incidence for these infections.

## PAIN MANAGEMENT

- Patients undergoing a thoracotomy or clamshell incision experience severe pain, thereby impairing optimal respiration.
- A thoracic epidural is generally placed postoperatively in addition to intravenous opioid administration. Epidural infusion of analgesics has been shown to allow for earlier extubation.[23] This needs to be balanced with the risk of gastrointestinal complications, increased incidence of hypotension, and complications related to the catheter itself, including bleeding and infection.

## Complications
### Anastomotic Complication

- Bronchial anastomosis—A bronchoscope is used after lung transplantation to evaluate for evidence of ischemia, anastomotic dehiscence, fixed or dynamic bronchial narrowing, and purulent airway secretions.
- Hypotension, hypoxemia, and unilateral lung opacification on chest radiograph may be due to a pulmonary vein occlusion or pulmonary artery occlusion. Both of these complications are rare and can be easily detected by a transesophageal echocardiogram. Immediate revision is imperative to prevent graft ischemia and loss of the allograft.

### Acute Cellular Rejection

- Acute rejection is a cell-mediated immune response against the allograft. It has been detected as early as 2 weeks postoperatively; the highest risk for this adverse event is within the first 6 weeks.
- Chest radiographic appearance includes opacification, interlobular septal thickening, and pleural effusions. The chest radiograph may also be unrevealing. Computed tomography can also feature a ground-glass opacification, although this is not specific, as well as a mosaic pattern (Fig. 38-2).
- Acute rejection grades
  - A1 (minimal rejection): rare mononuclear cells cuffing small pulmonary vessels
  - A2 (mild rejection): mononuclear invasion restricted to perivascular adventitia
  - A3 (moderate rejection): perivascular and septal mononuclear infiltration
  - A4 (severe rejection): alveolar airspace involvement containing mononuclear and neutrophilic infiltration.
- Lymphocytic bronchiolitis grade
  - BX: upgradeable
  - B0: none
  - B1
  - B2

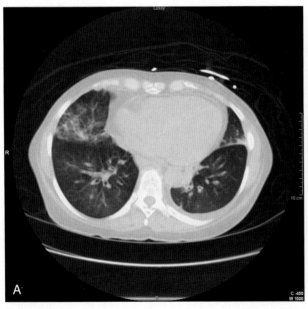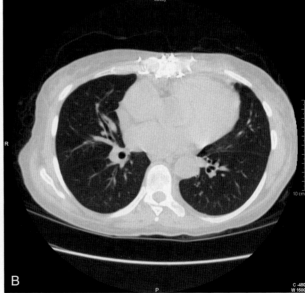

**Figure 38-2: A,** Acute cellular rejection on chest computed tomography (CT) scan (infiltrates, ground-glass, mosaic pattern). On biopsy, A2 rejection documented. **B,** Follow-up CT scan showing complete resolution after treatment for rejection.

- Repeated episodes of acute cellular rejection are a major risk factor for the development of bronchiolitis obliterans syndrome.[24,25]
- Treatment includes pulse corticosteroid therapy with a tapering of oral prednisone. Rapid resolution of radiographic features is noted within 24 to 48 hours of therapy. Although most experts agree that grade A2 or greater acute rejection should be treated, there is controversy as to treatment of acute grade A1 cellular rejection, which is often asymptomatic and may resolve spontaneously.[26]

### Antibody-Mediated or Humoral Rejection

- Preformed donor specific antibodies to human leukocyte antigens (HLAs) can cause a fulminant clinical syndrome quickly after transplantation known as hyperacute rejection.
- The diagnosis is based on early lung allograft dysfunction, the pre-existence of donor-specific antibodies, and the presence of subendothelial antibody and complement deposition in the biopsy specimen, which is examined by immunofluorescence or immunohistochemistry.
- Therapy includes high-dose corticosteroids, plasmapheresis, intravenous immune globulin, and rituximab.

### Native Lung Complications in Single-Lung Transplantation

- Early complications developed from the native lung, regardless of the underlying disease, have been reported in up to 60% of lung transplant recipients and can affect the outcome of transplantation.
  - ○ Infectious etiology: bacterial pneumonia, invasive aspergillus, tuberculosis
  - ○ Native lung emphysema hyperinflation
  - ○ Hemothorax/pneumothorax
  - ○ Retention of secretions causing bronchial obstruction and atelectasis

### Renal Failure

- Up to 56% of recipients develop acute renal failure within the first 2 weeks of transplantation. 8% of these patients require hemodialysis.[27]
- This is generally a multifactorial etiology with hemodynamic changes, intravascular volume shifts, and the use of nephrotoxic agents.
- Predictors for the need of hemodialysis include baseline renal function, use of parenteral amphotericin B (and other nephrotoxic agents), and mechanical ventilation requirement for longer than 1 day.[27]

### Gastrointestinal Complications

- Gastrointestinal (GI) complications are more frequent with the lung transplantation compared with other solid organ transplants. Up to 49% of recipients have one or more GI problems.[28]
- GI complications include nausea and vomiting, adynamic ileus, gastroesophageal reflux, ischemic bowel, colonic perforation, CMV colitis, gastroparesis, and diaphragmatic hernia. The etiology may be from the lingering effects of anesthesia, postoperative effects, and narcotic use for pain relief.
- Gastroparesis is particularly common and related in part to vagus nerve injury that is sustained during the transplant operation.[29,30]
- Patients with cystic fibrosis are at particular risk due to higher incidence of small bowel obstruction.

### Phrenic Nerve Injury

- Results from hypothermia from the cold ice slush, mechanical retraction of local structures, or electrocaudery for dissection of tissue, leading to loss of diaphragmatic function.
- Phrenic nerve injury has contributed to longer days on mechanical ventilation, a higher likelihood of tracheostomy, and prolonged ICU stays.[31]
- Phrenic nerve conduction studies and diaphragmatic electromyography (EMG) are the most reliable ways to evaluate phrenic nerve and diaphragmatic dysfunction. The sniff test is less invasive but also less sensitive and specific for diagnosing these disorders of diaphragmatic function.

### Post-Transplant Diabetes Mellitus

- It is a common complication in patients receiving tacrolimus-based triple-drug immunosuppression, particularly in older lung transplant recipients, obese individuals, and those experiencing more episodes of acute cellular rejection. Half of the patients develop post-transplant diabetes mellitus (PTDM) within the first 3 months of transplantation.[32,33]
- Associated complications include the loss of allografts, cardiovascular disease, infections, and even death.[34]

## Brief Illustrative Case

- A 67-year-old man with idiopathic pulmonary fibrosis was admitted for bilateral sequential lung transplantation.
- The diagnosis was confirmed on open lung biopsy.
- He had shown a progressive decline in pulmonary function studies and exercise tolerance in the 9 months before admission.
- There had been no response to a regimen of prednisone, azathiprine, and mucomyst and subsequent experimental therapy, since he was diagnosed more than 2 years ago.
- He was known to be colonized with a pan-sensitive pseudomonas over the last 3 months (intermittent on serial sputum cultures).
- He fulfilled criteria for transplant consideration:
- Progressive decline in FVC (>10%) and DLCO (>15%) in the last 6 months. DLCO: 33% of predicted.
- Marked desaturation with 6-minute walk test (180 m).
- Associated pulmonary hypertension (mean pulmonary artery pressure of 48 mm Hg).
- Failure of medical therapy
- WHO functional class III
- At the time of his preoperative evaluation, he was in a stable state with no active issues.
- On call to the operating room, 1g of mycophenolate and daclizumab (Zenapax, Roche Pharmaceuticals, Nutley, NJ) (1 mg/kg IV over 15 minutes) were given.
- The following is a sample of postoperative orders in such a patient (Fig. 38-3)

### Key Points

- The approach to orders as noted in Figure 38-3 is only an example. Although the general principles of management are relatively common across different transplant programs, specific approaches to induction, immunosupression, and other issues may vary widely.

*(Continued)*

**Panel A**

Time: _____ Date: _____ ALLERGIES/REACTIONS: _____ ☒ NKA

1. Admit to: _Lung Transplant_ Service
2. Notify Pulmonary Fellow on call of patient's arrival and location.
3. Diagnosis: _IPF with Pulm. Htn._
4. Procedure: _Bilateral sequential lung transplant (on pump)_
5. Warming blankets on bed
6. Follow strict isolation precautions, per Lung Transplant protocol, including:
   ☒ Strict handwashing, wear mask and gloves, No labcoats
7. Monitoring Procedures:
   ☒ Vital signs every 15 minutes until stable, then every 30 - 60 minutes.
   ☒ Temperature on admission & every hour until normothermic or if > 101ºF
      A. Temp < 96ºF - use warming blanket
      B. Temp > 101ºF - Notify MD, obtain pan cultures, and use cooling measures.
   ☒ Hemodynamic profile on admission and every _3 hours_
      A. Document PAP, CI, SVR, PVR, RVSWI, LVSWI
      B. Do not wedge PA line unless ordered by MD
   ☒ Daily weight and record.
   ☒ Continuous pulse oximetry
      A. Notify MD for O₂ saturation < _92 %_
8. Intake and Output:
   ☒ Strict Intake & Output every hour
   ☒ NPO
   ☒ NG tube to straight drainage; check patency and position every 2 hours
   ☒ Chest tubes to -20 cm water seal drainage, strip tubes prn
      A. Record hourly and cumulative drainage
      B. Notify MD if output > _200 cc_ and obtain spun hematocrit, TBT, and coagulation profile
      C. Notify MD of leak or if subcutaneous emphysema develops
   ☒ Urine output every hour
   A. Notify MD if < _0.5 mL/Kg/hr_

A

**Panel B**

9. Respiratory Procedures:
   ☒ _Assist Control_ Ventilator settings:
      A. FiO₂ _40%_
      B. Tidal volume _500cc_
      C. Rate _12_
      D. PEEP _5_
      E. Other _____
   ☒ Chest physiotherapy: _None_
   Start: _____

10. Medications:
   ☐ Epinephrine 4 mg / 250 ml D5W (16 mcg / ml) at _None_
   ☐ Dopamine 400 mg / 250 ml D5W (1600 mcg / ml) at _____
   ☐ Dobutamine 250 mg / 250 ml D5W (1000 mcg / ml) at _____
   ☐ Nitroprusside 50 mg / 250 ml D5W (200 mcg / ml) at _____
   ☐ Other: _____

11. Immunosuppression & immunological agents:
   ☒ Tacrolimus (0.1 mg / kg) _3_ mg PO at 06:00 and 18:00
   ☒ Mycophenolate mofetil 1 / 1.5 gm PO / NGT at 08:00 and 20:00; start _1gm BID_
   ☒ Prednisone _10_ mg PO / NGT daily

12. Antimicrobial agents: _Piperacillin/Tazobactam 3.375mg IV Q6°_
   ☒ Bactrim DS (for non-Sulfa allergic patients), 1 tablet PO every Monday, Wednesday, Friday
   ☒ Valcyte 450 mg PO daily to start after extubation

B

**Panel C**

13. Other Medications:
   ☒ Follow potassium replacement protocol as follows:
      A. Notify MD if K < 3.6 or > 5.2
      B. K < 3.8  Give 10 meq KCl in 50 cc / h over 1 hour x3
      C. K 3.9 - 4.2 Give 10 meq KCl in 50 cc / h over 1 hour x2
      D. K 4.3 - 4.6 Give 10 meq KCl in 50 cc / h over 1 hour x1
   ☒ Esomeprazole (Nexium®) 40 mg PO / NG daily
   ☒ Vitamin C 1 gm PO / NG daily
   ☒ Vitamin A 25,000 units PO / NG daily
   ☐ Other: _____

14. VTE Prophylaxis (choose at least one of the following)
   ☒ Heparin 5000 units SQ BID. Start AM after surgery.  ☐ Heparin 5000 units SQ TID. Start AM after surgery.
   Additional VTE Prophylaxis (combine with above): ☐ SCD's  ☐ TED's
   ☐ Patient at High Risk for Bleeding:  No Heparin  ☐ SCD's  ☐ TED's

15. Pain Management: (for pain exceeding patient's comfort goal)
   ☒ Intubated patient give: hydromorphone (Dilaudid) _0.2_ mg (usual dose 0.2 - 0.4 mg) IV every 15 min PRN
   Post extubation
      ☒ Severe pain (pain scale score 7 - 10), give: hydromorphone (Dilaudid) 0.4 mg IV every hour
      ☒ Moderate pain (pain scale score 3 - 6), give: hydromorphone (Dilaudid) 0.2 mg IV every hour
      Schedule for analgesia: ☐ around the clock (ATC) ☐ ATC for ___ hours, then PRN ☒ PRN
   ＊ _Anesthesia/pain Consult for epidural catheter placement._
16. IV fluids and blood products (Leukocyte depleted blood only to be used)
   ☒ To keep central lines open, infuse _10cc/° NS_
   ☐ _____
   ☐ _____

17. Diagnostic Procedures:
   ☒ Stamp all requisitions with "Lung Transplant Patient" stamp
   ☒ STAT on admission to CSICU
      A. ABG, CBC with manual differential, tacrolimus level, CMP, PT / PTT, TBT, Ionized Calcium, Magnesium, Amylase
      B. 12 lead EKG
   C. Portable chest X-ray: _Supine_ (position)

C

**Panel D**

18. Daily:
   ☒ ABG, CBC with manual differential, platelet count, CMP, Tacrolimus level (to be drawn before morning dose is given), Magnesium, Amylase (x _1_ days), PT / PTT (x _3_ days)
   ☒ Portable chest X-ray
      A. X-ray tech to maintain flowsheet for recording techniques used each time Chest X-ray is obtained
      B. Must be done no later than 0600 each day
   ☒ Sputum for gram stain, Culture & Sensitivity, Fungal culture x _1_ days

19. Frequent Studies:
   ☒ ABG every _4° x 1 day_
   ☒ CBC, CMP every _6°_
   ☒ BS accucheck every 6 hours: call MD for _<60 or >200_
   ☐ Other _____

20. Wound Care:
   ☒ Wound care to incision site, as per protocol

D

**Figure 38-3:** A to D, Example of postoperative orders for the patient outlined in the brief illustrative case.

## Brief Illustrative Case—cont'd

- Induction immunosuppression not universally done at all centers and several different agents are available. (See Chapter 40 on Transplant Pharmacology.)
- Because this patient had significant pulmonary hypertension, a decision a priori to go on cardiopulmonary bypass was made.
- In such cases, or if cardiopulmonary bypass is a possibility, calcineurin inhibitors are withheld until after the surgery in order not to aggravate renal function.
- Because the patient was known to colonize *Pseudomonas aeruginosa* in sputum cultures, appropriate antibiotic cover was given perioperatively.

- An epidural catheter for pain control was not inserted before transplant surgery in anticipation of coagulation issues related to cardiopulmonary bypass procedures.
- Low-dose prednisone was given. Note: large-dose methylprednisolone is administered in the operating room with cross-clamp release.
- Other orders and management issues need to be tailored to the patients's perioperative serial status.

## References

Interactive references and additional readings for this chapter can be accessed online at *expertconsult.com*.

# 39 INTERMEDIATE AND LATE COMPLICATIONS OF LUNG TRANSPLANTATION

Jeremy A. Falk, MD, Scott Oh, DO, C. Joyce Lee, MD, Hari Reddy, MD, George E. Chaux, MD, and Michael I. Lewis, MD

## LUNG TRANSPLANT REJECTION

### Definitions

- Acute rejection: a rapid onset of worsening lung function, typically in the first year after transplant, often accompanied by radiographic deterioration with histologic appearance of lymphocytic vascular invasion on biopsy.[1]
- Chronic rejection: a clinical symptom referred to as bronchiolitis obliterans syndrome (BOS) clinically manifested by a persistent drop in lung function in the absence of potentially reversible etiologies typically occurring more than 6 months after transplant sugery.[2,3]

### Acute Rejection

- Incidence
  - Very common with estimates of one or more episodes in first year after transplant between 27-85%[4-7]
  - True incidence rates not well described because nonuniformity in definition of acute rejection is common.[1]
- Clinical presentation[8]
  - Symptoms include
    - Malaise
    - Dyspnea
    - Low-grade fever
  - Signs
    - Drop in lung function, typically $FEV_1$ or FVC
    - Abnormal findings on chest x-ray study
      - Infiltrates
      - Pleural effusions
    - Hypoxia
    - Elevation in white blood cell count, often with peripheral eosinophilia
- Risk factors
  - HLA mismatching[9-11]
    - Owing to time constraints at time of surgery, human leukocyte antigen (HLA) matching is often not possible.
    - Associated with episodes of acute rejection as well as worse long-term survival.
    - "Virtual" cross-matching in which potential donors' HLA profiles are known and can be compared against recipients' HLA antibodies may improve short and long-term outcomes by minimizing HLA mismatches; however, data on this technology are evolving.[12]
  - High levels of recipient anti-HLA antibodies
    - Measured by panel reactive antibodies associated with increased rates of acute rejection and decreased survival[13]
    - Development of anti-HLA antibodies after transplant also reported to increase risk for acute rejection[14]
  - Cytomegalovirus (CMV) mismatch/infection
    - Relationship not clear at this point[15,16]
  - Community-acquired viral infections[16,17]
  - Gastroesophageal reflux disease (GERD)[18-21]
- Diagnosis
  - Transbronchial biopsies via flexible fiberoptic bronchoscope
    - Gold standard
    - Generally minimum of six biopsies taken from single side
    - Use of surveillance bronchoscopy (SB) controversial[22-25]
      - Approximately two thirds of lung transplant programs perform SB.[1]
      - Biopsies are performed at fixed intervals in first year in asymptomatic individuals looking for occult rejection and infection.
      - Recent finding of low-grade rejection linked to the development of BOS infers benefit to early diagnosis and treatment; however, data showing this are scant.[26]
      - A recent study showed that 31.5% of biopsies taken as part of SB were "clinically useful," and argued for the use of SB universally.[27]
  - Clinical symptoms
    - Not sensitive or specific[28]
  - Pulmonary function
    - Not sensitive or specific[29,30]
  - Radiographic abnormalities
    - Neither chest x-ray study (CXR) or computed tomography (CT) scanning is adequately sensitive or specific and cannot differentiate rejection from infection.[31-33]
  - Exhaled breath condensate
    - Essentially not helpful[34]
  - Hepatocyte growth factor
    - Serum marker recently shown to be elevated in both infection and acute rejection, although this still must be validated.[35,36]
- Pathology[37]
  - Hallmarked by presence of perivascular and mononuclear cell infiltrates.
  - Acute rejection has traditionally been considered a T-cell mediated event, however, humoral rejection has gained interest recently.[38]
  - Lymphocytic airway infiltration and lymphocytic bronchiolitis have long been recognized in lung transplant; however, clinical importance in both acute and chronic rejection is evolving.[39]
- Grading
  - Grading scheme updated in 2007.[37]
  - ABCD grading scheme (Table 39-1 and Figs. 39-1 through 39-8)
    - A: acute vascular mononuclear cell infiltration
      - A0: no evidence of rejection
      - A1: scattered, infrequent perivascular mononuclear infiltrates in alveolated lung parenchyma

## TABLE 39-1 ■ REVISED WORKING FORMULATION FOR CLASSIFICATION AND GRADING OF PULMONARY ALLOGRAFT REJECTION

| A | Acute rejection | |
|---|---|---|
| | Grade 0 | None |
| | Grade 1 | Minimal |
| | Grade 2 | Mild |
| | Grade 3 | Moderate |
| | Grade 4 | Severe |
| B | Airway inflammation | |
| | Grade 0 | None |
| | Grade 1R | Low grade |
| | Grade 2R | High grade |
| | Grade X | Ungradable |
| C | Chronic airway rejection – Obliterative Bronchiolitis | |
| | 0 | Absent |
| | 1 | Present |
| D | Chronic vascular rejection | Accelerated graft vascular sclerosis |

*From Stewart S, Fishbein MC, Snell GI, Berry GJ, Boehler A, Burke MM, et al. Revision of the 1996 working formulation for the standardization of nomenclature in the diagnosis of lung rejection. J Heart Lung Transplant 2007;26:1229-1242.*

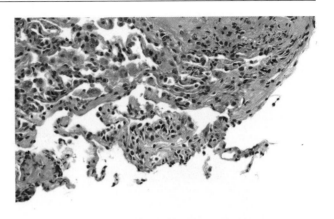

**Figure 39-2:** Rejection grade A1—minimal infiltration of mononuclear cells around small vessel (hematoxylin and eosin; original magnification 200×).

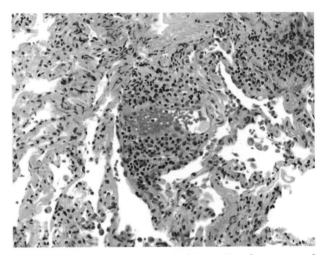

**Figure 39-3:** Rejection grade A2—prominent perivascular aggregate of mononuclear cells observable at scanning power (hematoxylin and eosin; original magnification 200×).

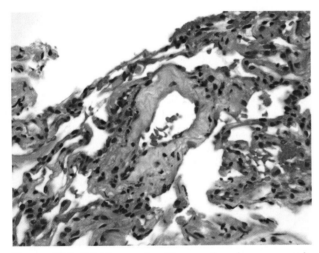

**Figure 39-1:** Rejection grade A0—normal pulmonary venule (hematoxylin and eosin; original magnification 400×).

- ○ A2: more frequent perivascular mononuclear infiltrates are seen surrounding venules and arterioles and are readily recognizable at low magnification, often with presence of perivascular eosinophils
- ○ A3: easily recognizable cuffing of venules and arterioles by dense perivascular mononuclear cell infiltrates, which are commonly associated with endothelialitis and frequent eosinophilic and neutrophilic involvement
- ○ A4: diffuse perivascular, interstitial and air-space infiltrates of mononuclear cells with prominent alveolar pneumocyte damage and endothelialitis
- ■ B: acute bronchiolar mononuclear cell infiltration
  - ○ B0: no bronchiolar inflammation
  - ○ B1R: mononuclear cells within submucosa of the bronchioles (R: "revised" from 1996 scheme)

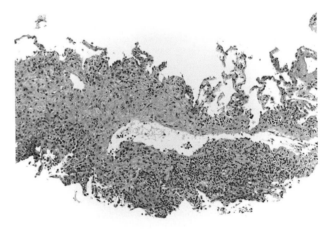

**Figure 39-4:** A3—prominent aggregate of mononuclear cells with infiltration into surrounding interstitium (hematoxylin and eosin; original magnification 100×).

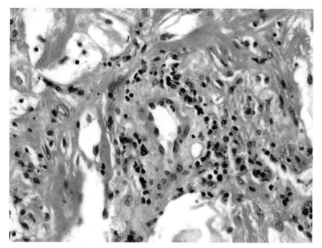

**Figure 39-5:** Rejection grade A4—infiltrate of mononuclear cells around vessel with adjacent hyaline membranes of diffuse alveolar damage (hematoxylin and eosin; original magnification 400×).

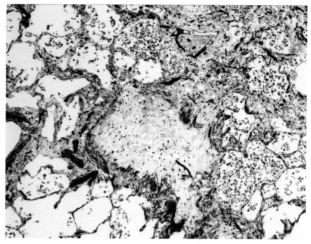

**Figure 39-8:** Rejection grade C1 (obliterative bronchiolitis)—terminal bronchiole obliterated by intraluminal fibrosis (Masson Trichrome; original magnification 40×).

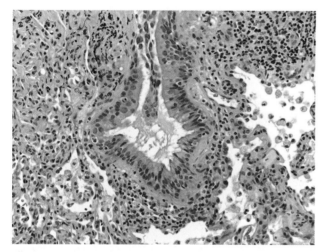

**Figure 39-6:** Rejection grade B1R (low-grade) lymphocytic bronchiolitis—mild peribronchiolar infiltrate of mononuclear cells (hematoxylin and eosin; original magnification 200×).

- ○ B2R: larger and more numerous mononuclear cells within the submucosa with evidence of epithelial damage
- ○ BX: ungradeable due primarily to technical problems not allowing adequate inspection of bronchioles
- ■ C: presence of chronic airway rejection (obliterative bronchiolitis)
  - ○ C0: not present
  - ○ C1: dense eosinophilic hyaline fibrosis in the submucosa of membranous and respiratory bronchioles, resulting in partial or complete luminal occlusion
- ■ D: presence of chronic vascular rejection
  - ○ Fibrointimal thickening of arteries and veins seen only on open lung biopsy, not transbronchial biopsy
  - ○ May represent progressive humoral rejection
- ■ Prevention
  - ○ Optimization of immunosuppression
  - ○ Use of induction therapy at time of transplant (anti-interleukin-2 [IL-2] receptor monoclonal antibodies, antilymphocyte/anti-thymocyte globulin, or anti-CD3 monoclonal antibodies)
    - ■ Limited data suggest that rates of acute rejection are decreased with induction.[39-43]
  - ○ Choice of calcineurin inhibitor - cyclosporine (CsA) versus tacrolimus (Tac)
    - ■ Mixed data favoring the use of Tac over CsA in several studies have shown superior rates of acute rejection or with conversion from CsA to Tac, but with no overall changes in survival.[44-47]
  - ○ Use of mycophenolate mofetil (MMF) over azathioprine[6,48]
    - ■ No convincing evidence MMF decreased rate of acute rejection
- ■ Treatment
  - ○ Mainstay of treatment is a short course of high-dose systemic steroids, typically 500 mg to 1000 mg intravenous (IV) methylprednisolone (Solu-Medrol, Pfizer, New York, NY) for 3 days
  - ○ Many centers also increase dosing of other immunosuppressive medications after an episode of acute rejection

## Chronic Rejection

- ■ Incidence
  - ○ Very common, in fact nearly 50% of patients have evidence of chronic rejection (BOS) at 5 years.[7]

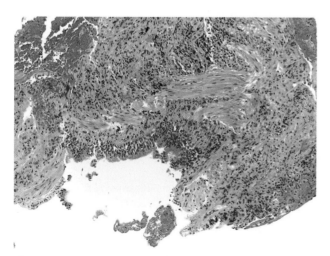

**Figure 39-7:** Rejection grade B2R (high-grade) lymphocytic bronchiolitis—extensive infiltrate of mononuclear cells through bronchiolar wall (hematoxylin and eosin; original magnification 100×).

- Clinical presentation
  - ○ Characteristic decline in lung function in BOS.
  - ○ Biopsy is not needed to establish diagnosis.
  - ○ Defined as a drop in $FEV_1$ to less than 20% from baseline, where the baseline is the average of two measurements separated by a minimum of 3 weeks in the absence of another potential cause of loss of lung function, that is, airway stenosis or infection.[49]
  - ○ Graded stages 0 to 3 with a new classification developed in 2002 called 0-p (Table 39-2), which refers to "potential" BOS.
- Risk factors
  - ○ Episodes of severe rejection[50]
  - ○ Episodes of persistent mild acute rejection[51]
  - ○ CMV pneumonitis[26,52]
  - ○ Lymphocytic bronchiolitis[53,54]
  - ○ GERD[21]
- Diagnosis
  - ○ Transbronchial biopsy
    - Obliterative bronchiolitis (OB), the pathologic correlate of BOS, is missed frequently by transbronchial as OB tends to be a patchy process with significant portion of the allograft unaffected.[55]
  - ○ Pulmonary function testing
    - Alterations in $FEV_1$ and $FEF_{25-75}$ are expected, as are implicit in definition of BOS.
    - May be lowered in many clinical scenarios not related to transplant
  - ○ Single-breath washout tests
    - Changes in the slope of the alveolar plateaus using nitrogen and helium have been shown to be predictive of declines in lung function attributable to BOS.[1]
  - ○ Other tests including measurements of exhaled nitric oxide, exhaled breath condensate, induced sputum, bronchoalveolar lavage (BAL) cellular concentration, and CT scanning.[56]
- Pathology
  - ○ "Obliterative bronchiolitis describes dense eosinophilic hyaline fibrosis in the sub-mucosa of membranous and respiratory bronchioles, resulting in partial or complete luminal occlusion"[37] (see Fig. 39-8)
- Grading
  - ○ See earlier text (see Table 39-2).
- Treatment
  - ○ No intervention has conclusively shown benefit for patients with established BOS.
  - ○ Most interventions aim to stabilize or decrease rate of decline of lung function rather than reversing decline

---

### TABLE 39-2 ■ 2002 CLASSIFICATION OF BRONCHIOLITIS OBLITERANS SYNDROME

| Class | Features |
|---|---|
| BOS 0 | $FEV_1 > 90\%$ of baseline and $FEF_{25-75} > 75\%$ of baseline |
| BOS 0-p | $FEV_1$ 81% to 90% of baseline and/or $FEF_{25-75} \leq 75\%$ of baseline |
| BOS 1 | 66% to 80% of baseline |
| BOS 2 | 51% to 65% of baseline |
| BOS 3 | 50% or less of baseline |

*From Estenne M, Maurer JR, Boehler A, Egan JJ, Frost A, Hertz M, et al. Bronchiolitis obliterans syndrome 2001: an update of the diagnostic criteria. J Heart Lung Transplant 2002;21:297-310.*

- ○ Avoidance, when possible, of known risk factors
- ○ Alteration of immunosuppression
  - Change cyclosporine A (CsA) to tacrolimus (Tac)
    - ○ May help for early BOS; no benefit over the long term[57,58]
- ○ Inhaled CsA
  - Not approved by the U.S. Food and Drug Administration. Large prospective placebo-controlled trial looking at rate of acute rejection showed no benefit. However, improved survival and BOS-free survival were observed with use of inhaled CsA.[59]
- ○ Statins
  - Limited studies have shown benefit in reducing the incidence of BOS in patients started on a statin during the first postoperative year, presumably from its anti-inflammatory effects.[60]
- ○ Azithromycin
  - Pooled data have shown a reverse decline in pulmonary function in a subset of patients, suggesting a diverse pathogenesis of BOS[61]
- ○ Retransplantation
  - Although initial data suggested significantly worse outcomes for retransplantation surgery, more recent data suggest that 5-year survival rates are approaching those of first-time transplants.[62]
  - Given the shortage of transplantable organs, some centers have argued this practice given poorer outcomes.

## *INFECTIONS FOLLOWING LUNG TRANSPLANTATION*

### Introduction

- Infections are the leading cause of morbidity and attributable mortality following lung transplantation, in both single and double lung transplants.[63-65]
- Infections account for up to 50% of deaths, with chronic rejection the second leading cause. Infections can also complicate patients with chronic rejection.[64]
- Two thirds of infections involve the respiratory system.[66-68]
- Infections can complicate both the early and late stages, although the risk is highest in the first 100 days following lung transplant.[66]

### General Factors Predisposing to Infection

- Immunosuppression[69,70]:
  - ○ Impaired cell-mediated immunity
  - ○ Neutropenia (e.g., adverse side effect of medications)
  - ○ Cytolytic therapy
  - ○ Augmented immunosuppression for rejection episodes
  - ○ Posttransplant hypogammaglobulinemia[71]
- Impaired lung defenses:
  - ○ Denervation:
    - Depressed cough reflex
    - Impaired mucociliary clearance
  - ○ Impaired lymphatic drainage
  - ○ Primary graft dysfunction
- Environment:
  - ○ Transplant lungs are continuously exposed to external environment and conditions.
- Donor Transmission:
  - ○ Prolonged ventilation
  - ○ Aspiration
  - ○ Latent infections (e.g., tuberculosis [TB], endemic fungi)
  - ○ Increased use of extended criteria lung donors

- Recipient conditions
  - Harboring resistant organisms (e.g., in sinuses in patients with cystic fibrosis)
  - Latent infection in native lung with single-lung transplant
  - Reflux and silent aspiration
  - Inadequate prophylaxis (e.g., perioperative, pneumocystis, CMV, fungal)
- Airway
  - Anastomotic stenosis with impaired clearance of secretions
  - Anastomotic stenosis with enhanced colonization
  - Airway dehiscence
  - Anastomotic infection (e.g., aspergillosis)
- Presence of chronic rejection (bronchiolitis obliterans)
  - Bronchiectasis
  - Chronic colonization
  - Augmented immunosuppression
  - Impaired clearance
- Comorbid conditions
  - Diabetes
  - Renal dysfunction
  - Nutritional depletion and cachexia
  - Breakdown of skin and mucosal barriers

## Post-Lung Transplantation Infection Timeline

- Period 1: first month post-transplant[70,72]
  - Usual bacterial postoperative infections are the most common (90%)
    - Pneumonia
    - Urinary tract infections
    - Wound infection
    - Line-associated blood stream infection
  - Donor-colonizing organisms, active or latent infection
  - Recipient-colonizing organisms, active or latent infection
  - Infection related to surgical complications:
    - Bleeding with retained hemothorax, leading to empyema
    - Anastomotic issues associated with infectious complications
  - Herpes simplex
  - Note: Notable absence of opportunistic infections
  - Also see Chapter 38 on Peri-operative Management and Early Complications
- Period 2: 1 to 6 months after transplant surgery
  - Opportunistic infections:
    - Fungal (e.g., Aspergillus, Cryptococcus and so on)
    - Viral (e.g., CMV, Epstein-Barr virus [EBV])
    - Pneumocystis
    - Mycobacterial
    - Nocardia
    - Listeria
  - Immunomodulating viruses can in conjunction with standard immunosuppressive therapy, enhance the predilection to opportunistic infection
  - Infection in this period may be modified by prophylactic therapies
  - Prophylaxis can prevent or delay the onset of opportunistic infections to period 3 (e.g., CMV).
- Period 3: greater than 6 months after transplant surgery
  - Absence of BOS and receiving low-level immunosuppression:
    - Significantly reduced incidence of opportunistic infections
    - Community-acquired pneumonia
    - Respiratory viruses
  - Presence of BOS:
    - Owing to high-level immunosuppression, continue to see opportunistic infections.

- Chronic colonization with resistant bacteria and other organisms, often refractory to clear
- Multiple recurrent infections
- Chronic viral infections

## Specific Pathogens
### Bacterial Infections

- Bacterial pathogens are responsible for the largest proportion of infections.[70,72]
- During the first year, up to 70% of patients have experienced a bacterial infection, mostly resulting in pneumonia.[69,73]
- Other sites of bacterial infection include urinary tract; blood stream (line), pleural space wound, airway, mediastinum.[74]
- The cumulative incidence after the first year remains high (30%–40%)[69,73]
- Common bacterial pathogens: These depend on timeline, level of immunosuppression, and presence or absence of BOS
  - A large prospective analysis of pneumonia in lung transplant recipients was recently reported.[76]
    - Early and intermediate periods accounted for the largest number of infections.
    - In patients in whom a cause of pneumonia was determined, bacteria accounted for 82.7% of cases. Of these, gram-negative bacilli accounted for 77%, gram-positive cocci accounted for 18%, and nocardia for 5%.
    - In this series, the most common gram-negative organisms in descending order were *Pseudomonas aeruginosa, Acinetobacter baumanii, Escherichia coli, Klebsiella pneumoniae,* and *Stenotrophomonas maltophilia. Staphylococcus aureus* was responsible for all gram-positive infections.
    - These prospective data mirror retrospective analyses.[66]
  - *Resistant bacteria:* MRSA, extended spectrum β lactamase organisms (*E. coli,* Klebsiella) and multidrug-resistant organisms (Pseudomonas, Acinetobacter) are increasingly being encountered, particularly in the hospital setting.[70]
  - Colonization with multidrug resistant organisms is common in patients with cystic fibrosis (upper airway, sinuses) and in patients with BOS, predisposing to infection. Azithromycin may be of value in these settings because the drug has anti-inflammatory properties and also impairs synthesis of Pseudomonas virulence factors.[76,77]
  - Community acquired pneumonia pathogens:
    - Pneumococcal pneumonia has been reported late after transplant (median 1.3 years) in 6.4% of transplant patients.[78] Most of the serotypes were resistant to trimethoprim-sulfamethoxazole and were accounted for in the 23-valent pneumococcal vaccine.
    - *Chlamydia pneumoniae* and *Mycoplasma pneumoniae* can produce severe pneumonia in the lung transplant patient, particularly with concomitant hypogammaglobulinemia in the case of Mycoplasma. Chlamydial infection has been associated with acute and chronic rejection.
    - *Legionella pneumophila* can produce severe disease in the transplant patient. Acquisition occurs both in the community setting as well as in the hospital environment, through contamination of water systems.
  - *Clostridium difficile:* use of multiple courses of broad-spectrum antibiotics is a major contributing factor. Severe colitis can also result in bacterial gut translocation and sepsis.
- Uncommon bacterial pathogens
  - Nocardia
    - Nocardia species are gram-positive filamentous bacteria that are partially acid fast. At least two thirds of infections occur in immunocompromised hosts.

- The incidence of infection following lung transplantation is low (1.85, 2.1 and 3.5% in three large series).[79-81]
- Nocardia species included: *Nocardia nova* (30%–49% of nocardial infections), *Nocardia farcinica* (28%–30%), *Nocardia asteroides* (23%–30%), and *Nocardia brasiliensis* (3%–10%).[80,81] This is important because of treatment implications (see later).
- Infection occurred late in reported series (i.e., mean of 13 to 34 months after transplant surgery and a median of 34.1 months in a third series).[79-81]
- Of note, 30% to 69% were receiving trimethoprim-sulfamethoxazole prophylaxis, suggesting that this should be relied on to prevent nocardiosis.
- Overall, 77% to 100% of patients had pulmonary disease only. In single-lung transplant patients, the majority occurred in the native lung.[79-81]
- Pulmonary involvement includes single or multiple nodules, cavitation, interstitial infiltrates, lobar consolidation, and pleural effusions.[82]
- Extrapulmonary involvement: Neurologic (brain abscess most important; epidural abscess; meningitis), bone, joints, skin, kidney, and multiple other sites (rare but reported)
- Risk factors with lung transplantation: high-dose steroids, CMV in preceding 6 months, high calcineurin inhibitor levels in the preceding month.[81]
- Diagnosis: compatible clinical and radiologic findings, stain (Gram and acid fast) and culture of appropriate specimens (may need tissue). Note, routine cultures require 5 to 21 days. Polymerase chain reaction (PCR) is not generally available.
- Treatment
  - Effective antibiotics include: trimethoprim-sulfamethoxazole, amikacin, imipenem, and third-generation cephalosporins.
  - Variable resistance noted in different species: imipenem (*N. asteroides*; *N. brasiliensis*); *N. farcinica* (third-generation cephalosporins). Note: *N. nova* is generally sensitive to all of the above-mentioned antibiotics.
  - Principles of therapy: (1) Two- to three-drug coverage for severe infection. Susceptibility testing is key. (2) IV trimethoprim-sulfamethoxazole is used as part of first-line therapy in conjuction with amikacin and imipenem. With central nervous system (CNS) disease, include a third-generation cephalosporin. Aim for sulfonamide level of 100 to 150 μg/mL 2 hours after dose. With sulfur allergy, use alternate combinations. (3) Duration of initial therapy: 6 weeks. (4) Oral maintenance: two drugs for 12 months or life long because of relapse potential (agents: trimethoprim-sulfamethoxazole, minocycline, amoxicillin/clavulanic acid, extended spectrum fluoroquinolone). (5) Reduce level of immunosuppression, as feasible. (6) Potential surgical indications: empyema, mediastinitis, pericarditis, brain abscess
  - Outcome: Mortality rate can be high (40%) in one series.[80]
- Listeria:
  - *Listeria monocytogenes* is an aerobic or facultative anaerobic intracellular gram-positive rod. It may be found in soil and decaying vegetable matter, and can contaminate a variety of processed foods including soft cheeses.
  - Impaired cell-mediated immunity/corticosteroids are an important predisposing factor.
  - Clinical features include sepsis, meningoencephalitis, febrile gastroenteritis, pneumonia, endocarditis, and so

on. It has rarely been described after lung transplantation (usually renal and liver).[83]
- There is a single report of pleural infection following lung transplantation.[84]
- Treatment principles
  - Ampicillin plus gentamicin. Imipemen or meropenem are alternatives.
  - In penicillin allergic patients, trimethoprim-sulfamethoxazole can be used. Meropenem is another possibility, although some cross-reactivity exists with penicillin. There is limited experience with linezolid.
  - Duration of therapy is 6 to 8 weeks.
  - Reduce level of immunosuppression, as feasible.
- Burkholdaria:
  - Microbiology: Formally named *Pseudomonas cepacia*, the *Burkholdaria cepacia* complex comprises nine different genomovars or species. Genomovars I through IX have recently been given species names.[85,86]
  - Consideration of Burkholdaria infections predominate in patients with cystic fibrosis, particularly those being considered for lung transplant.
  - In the United States, the majority of isolates are *B. cenocepacia* (genomovar III; 50%) and *Burkoldaria multivorans* (genomovar II; 38%). Similar trends for *B. cenocepacia* were reported for the United Kingdom, Canada, and Italy.[86]
  - The clinical significance of the different genomovars in lung transplantation stems from reports of poor short-term survival following transplant surgery in patients colonized with Burkholdaria.[87] These patients died of "cepacia syndrome" (i.e., necrotizing pneumonia and severe sepsis).
  - More recent data reports that *B. cenocepacia* (genomovar III) is most often associated with the cepacia syndrome and poor outcomes, with excellent outcomes in patients with non–*B. cenocepacia* infections.[88]
  - Thus, genomovar testing should be performed and isolation of non–*B. cenocepacia* should not preclude transplantation.
  - In patients with *B. cenocepacia* isolates before transplant surgery, the decision to transplant or not rests with each center and is likely not an absolute contraindication. In such patients, the Toronto group had excellent 1-year survival rate using a protocol of multiple antibiotics perioperatively (inhaled and IV tobramycin, chloramphenicol, ceftazidime) and reduced goals of immunosuppression.[89]

## Mycobacterial Infections

- Introduction[90]
  - Incidence: In lung transplant cases, the reported incidence of *Mycobacterium tuberculosis* varies from less than 1% to 6.5%.[90,91] For nontuberculous mycobacteria, only selected case reports and one series have been reported (see Saggar and colleagues for a comprehensive review[90,92])
  - Risk factors for mycobacterial disease
    - Residence or origin in high-prevalence endemic areas
    - Environmental factors (prevalence of a particular organism, contact, poor ventilation, etc.)
    - Latent disease in recipient (or donor)
    - High-intensity immunosuppression
    - CMV infection
    - BOS
    - Comorbid conditions (e.g., diabetes mellitus)
  - Risk reduction[91]
    - Screen potential recipients (PPD, interferon release assays)

- INH prophylaxis for PPD greater than 5 mm induration or significantly positive interferon release assays
- Imaging showing old granulomatous disease
- History positive PPD or treated TB in donor
- Close TB contacts
- Test for TB in donor and recipient BAL fluid specimens (stain and culture)
- *M. tuberculosis* (TB)
  ○ Usually due to reactivation. Transmission of TB from a donor to recipient has been reported.[93]
  ○ Usually manifests within the first year and most commonly in the intermediate period (1–6 months).
  ○ Although pulmonary involvement is most common, disseminated disease can manifest in up to a third of cases.[92] In solid organ transplants, imaging revealed focal infiltrates (40%), military features (22%), nodules (15%), pleural effusion (13%), and interstitial changes (5%). Of note: cavitation was distinctly rare (4%).[91] Usual diagnostic approaches apply. The key to diagnosis is a high index of suspicion.
  ○ Treatment considerations
    - Usual guidelines as proposed by the American Thoracic Society (ATS), The Centers for Disease Control and Prevention (CDC) and Infectious Diseases Society of America (IDSA) are followed.[95] Treatment should likely be continued for 1 year.[95] High mortality rates were reported for treatment courses of 6 and 9 months.[96]
    - Susceptibility testing is essential.
    - For further details on the approach to multiple drug resistant isolates and surgical considerations, see Chapter 16 by Reece and colleagues, earlier in this text.
    - An important consideration in management is that rifampin and other rifamycins significantly reduce the serum levels of calcineurin inhibitors and sirolimus, thus increasing the risk of rejection.[97]
    - Fluoroquinolones have been suggested as part of multidrug regimens in transplant recipients with TB.[95]
- Nontuberculous mycobacteria (NTB)
  ○ NTB can occur following lung transplantation. However, there is only one series reported together with several case reports.[90,92]
  ○ In a series of 23 patients of a cohort of 261 lung transplant patients, NTB included *Mycobacterium avium* complex (13 patients), *Mycobacteium abscessus* (two patients), *Mycobacterium kansasii* (one patient), *Mycobacterium asiaticum* (one patient) causing lung disease. Skin infections due to *Mycobacterium haemophilum* occurred in five patients. Rapid growers (*Mycobacterium chelonae* and *Mycobacterium fortuitum*) have been reported causing pulmonary disease and wound infection, respectively. Empyema due to *M. abscessus* has been noted.[98] Colonization with *Mycobacterium gordonae* and *Mycobacterium scrofulaceum* has also been reported.[90]
  ○ Infections due to NTM usually occur late (i.e., >1 year) but can present in the intermediate period.[90,92]
  ○ Treatment considerations
    - Regimens commonly use rifampin (especially important for *M. kansasii*), which reduces serum levels of calcineurin inhibitors and sirolimus, thus increasing the risk of rejection, and macrolides such as clarithromycin (important for *M. avium* complex), which increase levels of calcineurin inhibitors, thus increasing the risk of toxicity.
    - For further details, treatment of NTB and surgical considerations, see Chapter 16 by Reece and colleagues, earlier in this text.

## *Fungal Infections*

Note: For further details on mycology, clinical presentation, diagnosis, and treatment of specific fungal infections, including possible surgical considerations, see Chapter 16 by Reece and colleagues, earlier in this text.

- Introduction
  ○ Incidence: Invasive fungal infections were reported in 2.7% of a large cohort of thoracic organ transplant recipients, most of whom were heart transplant recipients. In lung transplant recipients, the incidence was higher (9%).[99] In a recent analysis of pneumonia following lung transplantation, fungi were the cause in 14%.[75]
  ○ Candida and Aspergillus species are the most common fungal offenders.
  ○ Risk factors[100]
    - Most of the overall risk factors described earlier pertain to
    - Broad-spectrum antibiotics
    - Corticosteroids
    - Neutropenia
    - Impaired alveolar macrophage function
    - IV catheters
    - Parenteral nutrition
    - Pretransplant colonization
    - Latent endemic fungal disease in recipient
    - Donor-related fungal transmission (rare)
    - Airway problems
    - BOS
    - Comorbid conditions (e.g., diabetes, malnutrition)
    - Environmental and recreational exposures (e.g., construction, gardening, endemic fungi)
  ○ Colonization versus infection: Distinction can be difficult after transplant surgery. Clinical disease criteria include combinations of
    - Compatible disease process
    - Pathologic demonstration and/or culture of a mold or yeast in fluid or tissue normally sterile
    - Specimens showing inflammation with or without necrotizing granulomas
    - Ancillary serologic and other tests (e.g., cryptococcal antigen)
  ○ Timeline for fungal infections:
    - Early: Candida, aspergillus (in recipients with pretransplant colonization).
    - Intermediate: Opportunistic fungal infections. Aspergillus (most prominent 1–4 months); Cryptococcus (most prominent 4–6 months); endemic fungi (most prominent >4 months).
    - Late: Cryptococcus; endemic fungi; new fungal pathogens (see later); late-onset aspergillus.
  ○ Fungal prophylaxis:
    - Recommendations by the American Society of Transplantation in 2004 were based on limited prospective uncontrolled studies.[100] Nevertheless, important principles still apply. These include
      ○ Prophylaxis is essential in all high-risk patients, such as those with preoperative fungal isolates or donor bronchus–culture positive for Candida spp or other fungi.
      ○ Risk factors for Aspergillus include primary graft dysfunction, ischemic bronchial segments (particularly with mucosal sloughing/necrosis), anastomotic dehiscence, early recovery of aspergillus or CMV infection.[101]
      ○ Because Aspergillus is responsible for a significant proportion of post lung transplant fungal infections, agents

without Aspergillus cover are suboptimal, unless the subject is a low-risk patient.

○ Traditional agents used are fluconazole, inhaled amphotericin, and itraconazole.

○ In high-risk patients, newer azoles may be used. A recent study compared use of voriconazole with itraconazole with or without inhaled amphotericin, in lung transplant recipients.[102] At 1 year, the rate of invasive aspergillosis was 1.5% in the voriconazole group compared with 23% in the comparator group.

○ With use of voriconazole, regular assay of liver enzymes is necessary, as well as serum levels of calcineurin inhibitors and renal dysfunction to avoid toxic levels. Posaconazole is another promising azole. However, it requires multiple daily dosing and intake of fatty foods to facilitate absorption.

○ Duration of prophylaxis is also not well defined. Low risk: 4 months. High risk: 1 year or indefinite.

### Specific Fungal Pathogens

■ Candida
  ○ Colonization frequent
  ○ With prophylaxis or preemptive treatment, invasive complications now rare (e.g., invasive pneumonia)
  ○ Candidal infections now most commonly seen in association with airway anastomotic problems.[103] Treatment includes inhaled and systemic antifungal drugs.
  ○ Other clinical sequelae include mucocutaneous infection, esophagitis, wound infection, line infection, pneumonia (very rare), empyema, abdominal infection, and sepsis.
  ○ There has been a noticeable increase in the emergence of non–*Candida albicans* species. This is important as some of these (e.g., *Candida glabrata*) are generally resistant to fluconazole and even new azoles.[104] In a large cohort of thoracic transplant patients in whom invasive fungal infection was reported, one third of candidal infections were non–*C. albicans* (e.g., *C. glabrata, Candida kruzei, Candida parapsilopsis*).[99]
  ○ Treatment with fluconazole is appropriate for infection with *C. albicans*. In non–*C. albicans* infections, especially *C. glabrata* infection, an echinocandin such as caspofungin should be used.

■ Aspergillus
  ○ Aspergillus airway colonization is high in lung transplant recipients (20%–46%). This is a risk factor for invasive disease. For example, about a quarter of colonizers went on to develop invasive disease and the risk was 11-fold higher in the first 6 months compared with those who were not colonized.[105] Hence, the importance of preventive therapies. There are several aspergillus species: *Aspergillus fumigatus* (most common), *Aspergillus flavus*, and *Aspergillus niger*.
  ○ Aspergillus syndromes following lung transplantation
    ■ Invasive pulmonary aspergillosis (in some series, accounts for 9% of deaths). Primary site is lung allograft in single-lung recipients but can occur in the native lung.
    ■ Tracheobronchitis (ulcerative or pseudomembranous)[70,106]
    ■ Aspergilloma
    ■ Bronchial impaction and stent infection
    ■ Empyema
    ■ Disseminated disease
    ■ Rhinosinusitis, CNS infection, endophthalmitis, and so on
  ○ Diagnosis:
    ■ For more details, see Chapter 16.
    ■ While serum galactomannin in lung transplant patients has low sensitivity as an adjunctive test, BAL

galactomannin plus compatible clinical picture has good predictive value.[107]

○ Treatment:
  ■ For more details, including ISDA guidelines, see Chapter 16.
  ■ For invasive pulmonary aspergillosis, voriconazole is the treatment of choice. Combination therapies are currently being evaluated.

■ Cryptococcus
  ○ Third most common fungal infection[108]
  ○ Acquisition: primary acquisition after transplant surgery or reactivation of latent disease.
  ○ In patients with solid organ transplants, a third were limited to the lungs, and 53% to 72% were disseminated or involved the CNS (meningitis; brain parenchymal lesions in a third).
  ○ In patients with pulmonary disease, pleural effusions are not uncommon.
  ○ An immune reconstitution inflammatory syndrome, resembling worsening disease or relapse, has recently been described in transplant patients.[109]
  ○ Diagnosis
    ■ For more details, see Chapter 16.
    ■ In patients with single pulmonary nodules, cryptococcal antigen was commonly negative compared with patients with infiltrates and effusions.[110]
    ■ With meningitis in transplant recipients, serum cryptococcal antigen was positive in 88% to 91%.
  ○ Treatment
    ■ For more details, including ISDA guidelines, see Chapter 16.
    ■ Severe disease/meningitis: induction—liposomal amphotericin plus flucytosine for 2 weeks; consolidation with fluconazole (400–800 mg/d) for 8 weeks; maintenance: fluconazole (200–400 mg/d) for 6 to 12 months
    ■ Isolated pulmonary disease: fluconazole (400 mg/d) for 6 to 12 months

■ Geographically limited fungi (Note: For more details on coccidioidomycosis, histoplasmosis, and blastomycosis, see Chapter 16)
  ○ The reported incidence in lung and other solid organ transplants ranges from 0.3% to 3%.[100]
  ○ Acquisition: primary infection in endemic areas or reactivation of latent disease. Donor transmission has been described with lung transplantation.[111,112]
  ○ Coccidioidomycosis[113]
    ■ The incidence varies year by year in relation to local geographic conditions.
    ■ Disease often severe. Patients present with isolated pulmonary disease or disseminated disease plus pneumonia.
    ■ Diagnosis
      ○ For more details, see Chapter 16.
    ■ Treatment
      ○ For more details, including ISDA guidelines, see Chapter 16.
      ○ With lung transplantation, drug interactions need to be considered (all azoles increase levels of calcineurin inhibitors and sirolimus).
      ○ Initial therapy is with liposomal amphotericin, which has good tissue penetration, followed by lifelong suppressive therapy with fluconazole (200–400 mg/d). Newer azoles are also active, but clinical experience is limited.
  ○ Histoplasmosis:
    ■ Reactivation can produce disseminated disease
    ■ Can also present with fever of unknown origin and pancytopenia
    ■ Diagnosis:
      ○ For more details, see Chapter 16.

- Treatment;
  - ○ For more details, including ISDA guidelines, see Chapter 16.
- Rare and emerging new fungal pathogens[100,104]
  - ○ Zygomycosis[104]
    - Species include Mucor spp; Rhizopus; Cunninghamella, Absidia
    - Most commonly seen in diabetic allograft recipients
    - Previous exposure to voriconazole may be a risk factor.
    - Rhinocerebral disease, pulmonary, gastrointestinal, genitourinary, skin, and bone disease have been reported in transplant patients.
    - Treatment with lipid amphotericin plus surgery as indicated is the primary approach. Posaconazole has activity, but there is limited experience with this drug
    - For more details, see Chapter 16.
  - ○ Scedosporium[104,114]
    - *Scedosporium apiospermum* (a form of *Pseudoallescheria boydii*) and *Scedosporium prolificans* (mold)
    - Invasive pneumonia or nodular disease; empyema; mycetoma; sinusitis; fungemia; isolated organ involvement or disseminated disease
    - Resistant to amphotericin
    - Treatment: voriconazole
    - High mortality rate, especially with disseminated disease (>50%)
  - ○ Fusarium[104]
    - Mold
    - Neutropenia a risk factor
    - Clinical presentation includes sinopulmonary infection, disseminated disease, skin/soft tissue bone
    - Treatment: lipid amphotericin B; voriconazole
  - ○ Paecilomyces:
    - Produce hyphae in tissue
    - Skin and sinus disease
    - Treatment: voriconazole (posaconazole and ravuconazole have good activity in vitro)
  - ○ *Pneumocystis jiroveci* (formally carinii)[115]
    - Thought to be more closely related to fungal organisms
    - Risk greatest between 1 and 6 months
    - Universal prophylaxis has virtually eliminated pneumocystis pneumonia in lung transplant recipients, provided compliance is exercised.
    - Life-long prophylaxis is recommended in lung transplant recipients, because the incidence in these patients did not decrease after the first year.[116]
    - Prophylactic agent of choice is trimethoprim-sulfamethoxazole (one single- or double-strength tablet three times a week). In sulfur-allergic patients, inhaled pentamidine, dapsone, or atovaquone are options. Atovaquone failures have been reported.[117]

## Viral Infections

- CMV
  - ○ Introduction
    - CMV is a member of the herpes family of viruses
    - Responsible for significant morbidity after transplant surgery
    - Prophylactic and preemptive treatment strategies have significantly reduced mortality rates due to CMV
    - The incidence of CMV infection and disease is greatest in lung transplant recipients compared with that of other solid organ transplants
    - Without prophylaxis, the combined rate of infection and disease has been reported as high as 54% to 92%.[118]
    - CMV may be associated with augmented immunosuppressive properties, predisposing to opportunistic infections.
  - Definitions:
    - ○ *Latent infection*: primary latent infection that persists for life. In the United States, more than 50% of adults have positive serologic evidence of prior exposure
    - ○ *CMV infection*: refers to evidence of active replication and shedding of the virus (positive culture from BAL and other fluids, positive PCR). Patient asymptomatic without clinical evidence of a disease process.
    - ○ *CMV disease*: Evidence of CMV inclusion bodies in tissue. Usually patients are symptomatic with clinical localization. Viral copies on PCR rises sharply and progressively if the condition is left untreated.
  - Acquisition of CMV infection after transplant surgery
    - ○ Donor transmission
    - ○ CMV-positive blood products
    - ○ Reactivation of latent disease
  - ○ Risk factors[118]
    - The lung is regarded as a primary site for CMV latency and recurrence.
    - Risk has been reported in relation to baseline CMV serologic data on donor (D) and recipient (R):
      - ○ D+/R−: Considered high risk[119]
      - ○ D+/R+: Moderate risk
      - ○ D−/R−: Low risk, particularly if seronegative blood products used[119]
    - Enhanced immunosuppression and cytolytic therapy
  - ○ Clinical disease
    - Timeline for infection and disease: mean of 40 and 55 days, respectively[120]
    - Pneumonitis (need to distinguish from acute rejection because the two conditions clinically share common features; Note: acute rejection can present earlier than the CMV timeline)
    - Chest imaging: infiltrates, focal consolidation, interstitial changes, pleural effusion
    - Rare: endobronchial polyps
    - Flu-like syndrome
    - Extrapulmonary sites of disease
      - ○ Hepatitis
      - ○ Gastrointestinal: colitis, gastroenteritis (inflammation, ulceration, hemorrhage)
      - ○ Bone marrow suppression: leukopenia, thrombocytopenia
      - ○ Retinitis
      - ○ Neurologic: meningoencephalitis; Gullian-Barré (rare)
  - ○ Diagnosis
    - Compatible clinical picture
    - CMV PCR
    - Culture (blood, BAL, urine); rapid shell vial culture
    - Bronchoscopy (detection of typical viral inclusions in biopsy specimens). Positive BAL provides only presumptive evidence.
  - ○ CMV prophylaxis[118]
    - Definitions:
      - ○ *Prophylaxis*: antiviral therapy to prevent infection and disease, particularly in high-risk patients.
      - ○ *Preemptive therapy*: antiviral treatment of infection to prevent the progression of disease.
    - Antiviral therapy:
      - ○ Gancyclovir inhibits replication of CMV but does not treat latent infection. Thus, prophylactic regimens can delay the onset of infection.
      - ○ The most common oral agent used for prophylaxis is valgancyclovir, a gancyclovir prodrug with an oral

bioavailability of about 60% (10× greater than oral gancyclovir).[121]

○ For prophylaxis, the generally recommended dose of valgancyclovir is 900 mg/d (dose adjustment for renal dysfunction is required).[118] However, encouraging experience with 450 mg daily has recently been reported.[122]

○ CMV—Intravenous immunoglobulin (IVIG) in conjunction with valgancyclovir could be considered in high-risk patients.

○ Ensure all blood products are treated to be free of CMV.

○ Duration of prophylaxis: (1) There is no consistent consensus in the literature. (2) At least 100 days (or 180 days) has been recommended.[118] (3) Our practice is as follows: (a) D+/R−: valgancyclovir for 12 months. (b) D+/R+: valgancyclovir for 6 months. (c) D−/R+: valgancyclovir for 6 months. (d) D−/R−: acyclovir for 3 months.

○ Treatment of disease and preemptive therapy.[118]
  ■ Preemptive therapy: if viremia occurs after completion of prophylaxis.
  ■ For preemptive therapy and treatment of disease:
    ○ IV gancyclovir (5 mg/kg twice a day) for 3 weeks
    ○ Oral valgancyclovir (900 mg twice a day) for 3 weeks.[121]
  ■ CMV-resistant strains
    ○ Suggested by poor clinical or virologic response, recurrent infection, and so on.
    ○ Gancyclovir susceptibility testing is possible.[123]
    ○ Treatment considerations include the use of foscarnet alone or in combination with CMV-IVIG or gancyclovir.[118] The down side of foscarnet is enhanced renal toxicity in combination with calcineurin inhibitors. Treatment end point in such cases is reduction in viral load below assay detection.

■ Community respiratory viruses
  ○ Introduction:
    ■ Can cause significant morbidity and mortality in lung transplant recipients.[124,125]
    ■ *Incidence:* Community respiratory viruses have been reported in 3% to 21% of lung transplant recipients.[125,126]
    ■ *Variability:* owing to varying awareness, robustness, and stringency of detection methodologies, geographic and climatic variation, contact with susceptible population groups.
    ■ *Seasonal variation:* Respiratory syncytial virus (RSV), influenza, parainfluenza 1 and 2, and rhinovirus occur mainly in winter. Adenovirus and parainfluenza 3 occur year round.
    ■ *Acquisition:* contagious contact, reactivation of latent infection, nosocomial transmission, donor transmission (e.g., adenovirus)
  ○ Parainfluenza[126]
    ■ Time of diagnosis: range 0.6 to 5 years, with a median of 2.1 years[126] Serotype 3 is most common.
    ■ Clinical
      ○ Tracheobronchitis
      ○ Pneumonia
      ○ Respiratory failure in a fifth of cases (n = 24) in one series.
      ○ Can be associated with rejection
    ■ Diagnosis: BAL fluorescent antibody (FA), culture
    ■ Treatment: anecdotal reports of aerosolized ribavirin; mainly supportive

○ RSV
  ■ Onset: 2 weeks to 2 years
  ■ Clinical
    ○ Tracheobronchitis
    ○ Pneumonia
    ○ Respiratory failure in a fifth of cases (n = 24) in one series.[124]
    ○ Secondary bacterial infection
  ■ Diagnosis:
    ○ BAL FA, culture, shell vial assays
  ■ Treatment:
    ○ aerosolized ribavirin in severe cases
    ○ RSV immune globulin
○ Adenovirus[127]
  ■ DNA virus with six subgroups
  ■ Presentation can be early (intermediate phase) or late
  ■ Clinical
    ○ Upper respiratory tract infection
    ○ Pneumonia (mild to severe)
    ○ Coinfection with bacteria or other opportunistic infections
    ○ Hepatitis
    ○ Hemorrhagic colitis; enterocolitis
    ○ Hemorrhagic cystitis, nephritis
    ○ Disseminated disease
  ■ Diagnosis:
    ○ Culture (routine, shell vial)
    ○ Fluorescent antibody (FA) and electron microscopy (EM) of tissue or secretions
    ○ Enzyme immunoassay (EIA) of respiratory specimens
    ○ PCR
  ■ Treatment:
    ○ Cidofovir (has renal, hematologic, and ocular side effects). Treatment of choice with severe infection or disseminated disease.
    ○ Limited data for zalcitabine and gancyclovir
○ Influenza
  ■ Rarely reported in the lung transplant literature
  ■ Annual influenza vaccine advisable (efficacy not well established)
  ■ Oseltamivir can be used in prevention in special circumstances
  ■ Oseltamivir can also be used in treatment (avoid amantadine/rimantidine because of resistance issues)
○ Human metapneumovirus[128]
  ■ Member of the Paramyxoviridae family (first isolated in 2001)
  ■ Can produce disease resembling RSV
○ Herpes simplex
  ■ Clinical
    ○ Can present early after transplant surgery
    ○ Tracheobronchitis
    ○ Pneumonitis
  ■ Prophylaxis and treatment
    ○ Acyclovir for both
    ○ Gancyclovir prophylaxis for CMV covers *Herpes simplex*
○ Parvovirus B19[129]
  ■ Single-stranded DNA virus
  ■ Sixty to ninety percent of adults have antibodies against parvovirus B19
  ■ Median time to onset after solid organ transplant reported as 7 weeks
  ■ Clinical findings in series of 98 cases post transplant[129]
    ○ Anemia (99%), leucopenia (36%), thrombocytopenia (21%)

○ Pneumonitis
○ Myocarditis
○ Hepatitis
■ Diagnosis
○ Serology for immunoglobulin M (IgM) antibodies (a third negative with disease onset)
○ PCR (96%)
■ Treatment
○ IVIG

# AIRWAY COMPLICATIONS FOLLOWING LUNG TRANSPLANTATION

■ Introduction:
○ Airway complications at the bronchial anastomosis was a major cause of mortality in the early lung transplantation experience, occurring in 16 of the first 20 patients who had survived for more than 7 days after lung transplantation.[130,131]
○ At present, airway complications after lung transplantation still contribute to significant morbidity and mortality rates but now occur later and with reduced incidence.
○ In the modern era of lung transplantation, airway complications occur in approximately 7% to 15% of patients, with a mortality rate of 2% to 3%, a reduction that reflects improved surgical techniques.
■ Airway complications
○ Airway complications range from bronchomalacia, anastomotic stenosis, and partial or complete bronchial dehiscence.
○ Patients with anastomotic stenosis may present with focal wheezing, recurrent lower respiratory tract infections, and decreased spirometric indices.
○ Patients with bronchial dehiscence may present with pneumomediastinum, pneumothorax, and the associated complications such as respiratory compromise and cardiovascular collapse. Infections and sepsis leading to multiorgan failure may also occur.
■ Tracheal airway complications
○ In the early lung transplantation experience, the most common airway complication was dehiscence at the tracheal anastomosis.[130]
○ En bloc double-lung transplantation was the routine surgical approach in the early lung transplantation experience. Poor circulation due to prolonged re-establishment of bronchial arterial supply at the tracheal anastomosis is thought to be the major contributing factor.[132-134]
○ Immunosuppressive medications used during the early lung transplantation experience, such as high-dose steroids and azathioprine, were also thought to contribute to poor healing at the anastomosis site.
○ Various technical measures, such as bronchial circulation reconstruction and omental wrap, have been tried to improve healing of the donor bronchus, but as en bloc double-lung transplantation with tracheal anastomosis became replaced by bilateral sequential lung transplantation with bilateral bronchial anastomosis, tracheal airway complications are now rarely seen.
■ Bronchial airway complications:
○ The complications of bronchial anastomoses may be divided into early (<3 months) and late (>3 months).
○ These complications include bronchial necrosis, dehiscence, excessive granulation tissue, bronchomalacia, and stricture.
○ The risk factors for bronchial anastomosis airway complications traditionally were thought to include
■ Ischemic time
■ Rejection

■ Immunosuppresion
■ Infection
■ Inadequate organ preservation.
○ One recent retrospective study from Belgium, consisting of 232 lung transplants over 13 years, suggests that the duration of mechanical ventilation in the donor, height of recipient, and telescoping technique are also risk factors for developing airway complications within the first year after transplantation.[135]
○ A retrospective study from Spain, consisting of 255 patients over 14 years, suggested however, that the technique of bronchial anastomosis does not increase the risk of airway complications. They identified double lung transplantation, postoperative airway colonizations, and post-transplant mechanical ventilation for more than 72 hours as risk factors for airway complications.[136]
■ Treatment options
○ Surgical repair is indicated in complete dehiscence. Transplantectomy and retransplantation have sometimes been performed due to complete dehiscence of anastomosis site.[136]
○ Partial dehiscence can be managed conservatively, with evacuation of the associated pneumothorax, but stent insertion may or may not be required to allow anastomosis healing.[135,136]
○ Bronchomalacia is usually treated with tracheobronchial prostheses (stent insertion).
○ Treatment options for anastomosis stenosis include
■ Rigid bronchoscopy with bougie dilatation
○ Requires general anesthesia and its use has been decreasing over time.
■ Flexible bronchoscopy and balloon dilation:
○ A mean gain in $FEV_1$ of 24% after balloon dilatation has been reported.[137]
○ Up to 80% recurrence requiring further intervention such as stent placement.
■ Silicone and metal tracheobronchial prostheses or stents
○ Increase in $FEV_1$ ranging from 56% to 117% after stent insertion has been reported.[137-139]
■ Silicone stents often require rigid bronchoscopy and general anesthesia for deployment, but insertion with flexible bronchoscopy has been described. Silicone stents migrate more commonly than other stents, and therefore may require repeated bronchoscopies for repositioning.
■ Obstruction can also occur due to accumulation secretions, and the presence of granulation tissue at either end of the stent may then require laser therapy for removal.
○ Metal stents can be inserted using fiberoptic bronchoscopy and rarely migrates within the tracheobronchial tree.
■ Neodymium: yttrium-aluminum-garnet laser (Nd: YAG Laser) therapy
○ For thermoablation of granulation tissue
○ Has been used since 1990s but only small series published (Fig. 39-9)[136,140]
■ High-dose-rate brachytherapy with iridium-192.
○ Some small studies have shown efficacy in managing recurrent stenoses caused by hyperplastic granulation tissue at the bronchial anas-tomosis.[141,142]

# CARDIOVASCULAR COMPLICATIONS

■ Hypertension
○ Patients with poorly controlled hypertension generally excluded from lung transplant consideration

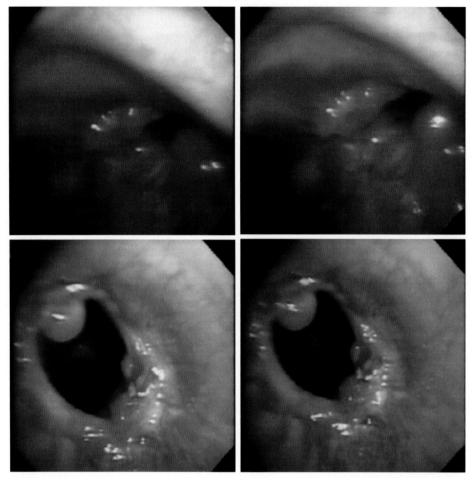

**Figure 39-9:** Bronchoscopic view of stenotic right mainstem (*upper panels*) bronchus secondary to granulation tissue. This patient is 8 weeks out from a bilateral lung transplant secondary to idiopathic pulmonary fibrosis. The lower panels reveal the stenotic bronchus after débridement of granulation tissue using YAG laser. The patient had a significant improvement in lung function after the procedure.

○ New-onset hypertension is common and is usually a consequence of drug toxicity.[143] Its prevalence increases with time

○ Pre-existing elevation in diastolic blood pressure (BP) only predictor for development of hypertension after transplant surgery.[143]

○ Treatment regimens generally avoid the use of angiotensin-converting enzyme (ACE) inhibitors secondary to nephrotoxicity.

○ Non-nephrotoxic agents such as diltiazem are used frequently as diltiazem has an advantageous effect on calcineurin inhibitor levels (elevates them)

■ Hyperlipidemia

○ This develops commonly in patients after lung transplant with the prevalence reaching nearly 50% at 5 years.[143]

○ Hyperlipidemia has been recently shown to be associated with accelerated chronic kidney disease after lung transplant.[144]

■ Coronary artery disease

○ Most patients undergo rigorous cardiovascular screening including coronary angiogram before listing for lung transplant (See Chapter 35 on Evaluation of the Lung Transplant Recipient)

○ Select patients who are candidates for revascularization by percutaneous procedures or surgical bypass have shown good outcomes when combined with lung transplantation.[145-147]

○ Little longitudinal data exists on the development of coronary artery disease after transplantation.

## RENAL COMPLICATIONS AFTER LUNG TRANSPLANTATION

■ Introduction

○ Chronic kidney disease is a frequently recognized complication of lung transplantation

○ 2008 International Society for Heart & Lung Transplantation (ISHLT) registry data showed a 25.3% prevalence of renal insufficiency at 1 year and 37% at 5 years, with approximately 3% going on to require hemodialysis[7]

■ Factors contributing to chronic kidney disease[144,148]

○ Calcineurin inhibitors

○ Chronic effective volume contraction

○ Perioperative acute renal failure

○ Increasing incipient age

○ Diabetes mellitus

○ Hypertension

○ Dyslipidemia

○ Chronic infection

- ○ Hepatitis C
- ○ Hepatitis B
- ▪ Treatment modalities for chronic kidney disease associated with lung transplantation have included
  - ○ Lowering Tac or CsA levels
  - ○ Using sirolimus to lower or replace calcineurin inhibitors[149]
  - ○ Chronic dialysis
  - ○ Renal transplant

## GASTROINTESTINAL COMPLICATIONS OF LUNG TRANSPLANTATION

### Gastroparesis[150-153]

- ▪ Incidence:
  - ○ The incidence of gastroparesis posttransplant has been reported to be up to 24%.
- ▪ Clinical
  - ○ Symptoms include nonspecific gastrointestinal symptoms such as early satiety, epigastric fullness, anorexia, nausea, or vomiting. Undigested food found in the stomach after an overnight fast on endoscopy is also suggestive of significant gastroparesis.
- ▪ Pathophysiology
  - ○ The etiology of increased gastroparesis after transplant surgery is thought to be secondary to surgical vagal nerve injury as well as medication side effects of calcineurin inhibitors.
- ▪ Diagnosis
  - ○ Diagnosis is typically confirmed with a nuclear medicine gastric emptying study. Esophagogastroduodenoscopy is also useful to identify associated findings such as erosive esophagitis and undigested gastric contents after an overnight fast, as well as to exclude other pathology.
- ▪ Treatment
  - ○ Treatment includes typical dietary and lifestyle modifications, along with promotility agents such as metoclopramide and erythromycin.
  - ○ Conversion to medications with less gastroparesis such as cyclosporine to tacrolimus should also be considered.
  - ○ Invasive treatment options include transcutaneous electrical nerve stimulation, gastric pacing, and jejunal feeding tubes.
  - ○ Successful management of refractory gastroparesis with Roux-en-Y esophagojejunostomy gastric bypass surgery has also been reported.
- ▪ Sequelae
  - ○ Severe gastroparesis may lead to malnutrition, erosive esophagitis, transfusion-dependent upper gastrointestinal hemorrhage, and recurrent aspiration pneumonia.
  - ○ A growing body of literature has also linked gastroparesis to an increased risk of BOS. One study reported a 44% incidence of BOS in patients with gastroparesis in comparison with 21% in those without gastroparesis. Food particles detected in the BAL suggest microaspiration as the underlying mechanism.

### GERD[19,20,154-161]

- ▪ Incidence
  - ○ There is a high incidence of GERD in lung transplant patients, which has been reported to increase substantially after transplant surgery.
  - ○ One study noted an increase in the incidence from 35% pretransplant to 65% posttransplant.
- ▪ Clinical
  - ○ Usual clinical symptoms, however, are frequently asymptomatic.

- ▪ Pathophysiology
  - ○ The etiology of the increased incidence of GERD after transplant surgery has been attributed to vagal nerve dysfunction due to surgical injury.
  - ○ Medication side effects on gastric motility and lower esophageal sphincter function may also play a role.
- ▪ Diagnosis
  - ○ Confirmation of clinical suspicion is typically done with ambulatory pH monitoring, along with endoscopic evaluation for associated changes such as esophagitis as well as to exclude other pathology.
- ▪ Treatment
  - ○ Treatment includes usual dietary and lifestyle modifications along with pharmacologic antacid therapy.
  - ○ Surgical interventions including gastric fundoplication has also been reported to be an effective treatment for refractory cases (Fig. 39-10).
- ▪ Sequelae
  - ○ There is now a growing body of literature linking GERD and BOS possibly from aspiration-induced airway injury and inflammation in combination with altered pulmonary defense mechanisms such as impaired mucociliary clearance leading to airway fibrosis.

### Peptic Ulcer Disease[162]

- ▪ Incidence
  - ○ The incidence of giant gastric ulcers defined as greater than 3 cm has been reported to be 40 times greater in bilateral orthotopic lung transplant patients.
- ▪ Risk factors
  - ○ All patients found to have giant gastric ulcers were noted to be on nonsteroidal anti-inflammatory drug therapy.
  - ○ Corticosteroids
- ▪ Diagnosis
  - ○ Usual diagnostic workup including endoscopy.
  - ○ Rule out *H. pylori*
- ▪ Treatment
  - ○ Usual treatment approaches including medical, endoscopic and surgical.

### Acute Abdomen[163-170]

- ▪ An increased risk has been associated with lung transplantation. Etiologies include:
  - ○ Bowel perforation
  - ○ Appendicitis
  - ○ Colitis including *Clostridium difficile*
  - ○ Diverticulitis

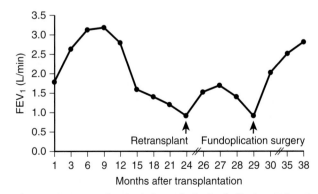

**Figure 39-10:** Lung function before and after fundoplication. *(Adapted from Palmer SM, Miralles AP, Howell DN, Brazer SR, Tapson VF, Davis RD. Gastroesophageal reflux as a reversible cause of allograft dysfunction after lung transplantation. Chest 2000;118:1215.)*

- ○ Cholecystitis (cholelithiasis, sludge)
- ○ Pneumoperitoneum
- ○ Ischemic bowel and hemorrhage
- ▪ A high index of suspicion is critical because the use of high-dose immunosuppressants and corticosteroids can mask clinical symptoms and contribute to delayed diagnosis with poorer outcomes.

## OSTEOPOROSIS[171-175]

- ▪ Incidence
  - ○ The incidence of osteoporosis is high in lung transplant patients.
  - ○ The prevalence has been reported to be 29% to 61% in the patients awaiting lung transplant and up to 73% in post-tranplant patients.
- ▪ Risk factors in lung transplant
  - ○ Hypercapnia
  - ○ Tobacco use
  - ○ Glucocorticoids
  - ○ Pancreatic insufficiency in patients with cystic fibrosis
  - ○ Hypogonadism in patients with cystic fibrosis
  - ○ Inactivity
  - ○ Failure to achieve peak bone mass in patients with cystic fibrosis
  - ○ Calcineurin inhibitor therapy
- ▪ Diagnosis
  - ○ Bone density scan
  - ○ Plain films for fractures
- ▪ Sequelae
  - ○ The fracture rate in the first year posttransplant has been reported to be 18% to 37%
- ▪ Treatment
  - ○ Initiate therapy even with normal bone mineral density (BMD) after transplant surgery given high risk.
  - ○ Bisphosphonate therapy has been shown to prevent bone loss in lung transplant patients, but the optimal dosing regimen and route of administration are unclear.
  - ○ Resistance training has been shown to improve BMD after transplant surgery alone or in combination with a bisphosphonate.
  - ○ Hormone replacement therapy has been shown to protect BMD after transplant surgery in women who are also postmenopausal.
  - ○ Given high side effect profile of testosterone including prostatic hypertrophy, dyslipidemia and abnormal liver function enzymes, its use is recommended to be limited to men who are truly hypogonadal.
  - ○ Vitamin D and analogues have limited efficacy and a narrow therapeutic window with a relatively high side effect profile including hypercalcemia and hypercalciuria. Thus, they are not ideal first-line agents.

## RESPIRATORY AND LIMB MUSCLE DYSFUNCTION AFTER LUNG TRANSPLANTATION

- ▪ Pretransplant factors:
  - ○ Pretransplant respiratory and/or limb skeletal muscle dysfunction can persist, partially recover, fully recover, or develop de novo following lung transplantation or be aggravated by various factors post-transplantation.[176]
  - ○ Mechanisms for respiratory and limb skeletal muscle dysfunction in pretransplant candidates include[177,178]
    - ▪ Nutritional depletion (affects all skeletal muscles, including respiratory)
    - ▪ Comorbid states associated with loss of fat-free mass (e.g., chronic obstructive pulmonary disease [COPD], chronic heart failure, cystic fibrosis, and so on)
    - ▪ Mechanical inefficiency of the diaphragm with hyperinflation
    - ▪ Chronic hypoxemia
    - ▪ Deconditioned state
    - ▪ Prolonged immobilization
    - ▪ Corticosteroids and other agents (e.g., statins)
    - ▪ Inflammatory states (e.g., cystic fibrosis, COPD)
    - ▪ Repeated infections (promotes proteolysis of muscle with each episode; recovery inadequate or prolonged)
    - ▪ Critical illness neuropathy and myopathy with inadequate recovery
    - ▪ Prior episodes of mechanical ventilation (impaired diaphragm contractility and muscle atrophy)
- ▪ Post-Transplant Respiratory or Limb Muscle Dysfunction
  - ○ Exercise capacity
    - ▪ Despite significant improvement in lung function with single- (60%) and double- (can be near normal) lung transplants, maximal work rates and maximal oxygen uptake, remain significantly reduced (40%–60%)[179-182]
    - ▪ The reduced exercise capacity occurs despite clinical improvement, an active nonsedentary lifestyle, and rehabilitation/exercise training.
    - ▪ Potential mechanisms
      - ○ Deconditioning as suggested by reduced lactate threshold on cardiopulmonary exercise testing[181] and P31 MR spectroscopy of quadriceps muscle[182]
      - ○ Impaired muscle oxygen utilization at a mitochondrial or microcirculatory level. This is supported by dynamic findings on magnetic resonance spectroscopy (MRS).
      - ○ Calcineurin inhibitors: Studies in rats given cyclosporine reported significantly reduced oxidative capacity (succinate dehydrogenase [SDH], a mitochondrial enzyme) in all fiber types of a limb muscle as well as reduced capillarity (limb muscle and diaphragm).[183] Impaired mitochondrial respiration has also been reported.[184]
      - ○ Ventilatory and cardiac factors do not appear to be the limiting factors.[185,186]
- ▪ Respiratory muscles and diaphragm
  - ○ *Inspiratory and expiratory muscle strength:* in stable patients 5 to 102 months after transplant surgery, maximum inspiratory mouth pressures were similar to control values.[187,188] However, maximum expiratory mouth pressures were reduced by 30%.[187] Poor expiratory muscle function could impair cough efficiency.
  - ○ *Diaphragm strength:* in patients who have undergone transplant surgery for COPD, sniff transdiaphragmatic pressure (Pdi) was significantly increased, because the reduced lung volumes optimized diaphragm force generating capacity.[189]
  - ○ *Diaphragm paralysis:*
    - ▪ See section on diaphragm paralysis in Chapter 51 on "Diaphragm Disorders."
    - ▪ Diaphragm paralysis after lung transplant surgery is likely the result of phrenic nerve injury (e.g., cold-induced or mechanical traction)
    - ▪ Incidence: 5% to 9% in several series.[190-192] One prospective series reported an incidence of 30% (similar to that reported in heart-lung transplants).[196] It is postulated that if more sensitive measures are employed (e.g., twitch Pdi), some diaphragm weakness may be common early after transplant surgery.

- Diaphragm dysfunction results in prolonged mechanical ventilation and ICU time.[191]
  - ○ Other factors responsible for respiratory muscle dysfunction after transplant surgery.
    - Infection[194]
    - Rejection
    - Drugs (corticosteroids, especially large pulse dosing with rejection[195]; calcineurin inhibitors)
    - Mechanical ventilation[196,197]
    - Metabolic disorders[177]
    - Critical illness neuropathy and myopathy
    - Poor nutrition
    - Renal dysfunction
- Limb muscles
  - ○ In stable post-transplant patients, maximal volitional isometric forces of ankle dorsiflexors were significantly reduced.[187] Reduction in quadriceps force generation has also been reported.[198] Improvement following rehabilitation was less in female patients.
  - ○ After pulse steroids, reduced limb muscle strength has been reported in 45% of patients. Recovery took about 2 months.[195]
  - ○ *Other factors responsible for limb muscle dysfunction:* see those listed for respiratory muscles earlier.

## POST-TRANSPLANT LYMPHOPROLIFERATIVE DISORDER (PTLD)

- Definition[199]
  - ○ A heterogeneous spectrum of lymphoproliferative disorders that occurs following solid-organ transplantation, including lung and heart/lung transplants (as well as blood stem cell transplantation).
  - ○ A close association with Epstein-Barr virus (EBV) infection is reported.
- Pathology:
  - ○ Histology varies from benign polyclonal lymphoid proliferation, as might be seen in infectious mononucleosis to frank high-grade lymphoma. Most cases stain immunohistochemically for B cells (e.g., CD 20)
  - ○ Three major forms described[200]
    - "Reactive-like" lesion with polyclonal B lymphocyte proliferation and normal cytogenetic features.
    - Polyclonal (occasionally monoclonal) B lymphocyte proliferation, with early features of malignant lymphomatous transformation
    - Monoclonal B lymphocyte proliferation with features of high-grade lymphoma
- Risk factors for post-transplant lymphoproliferative disorder (PTLD)
  - ○ EBV
    - EBV can colonize B lymphocytes to produce asymptomatic infection.
    - EBV can disrupt signaling pathways that regulate antigen-dependent activation, differentiation and proliferation of B cells. In addition, immunosuppressive therapy may impair the regulatory role of T cells on B cell proliferation.
    - EBV-seronegative patients before transplant surgery with seroconversion after transplant surgery are considered a major risk factor.[201-205]
    - Immunohistochemical staining of PTLD tissue reveals positive staining for EBV nuclear antigen and latent membrane protein in the majority of cases.[199]

- Elevated EBV DNA levels in serum and especially BAL fluid may highlight high-risk patients.[206,207]
    - EBV-negative cases of PTLD have been described.[208]
  - ○ Immunosuppression
    - Aggressive immunosuppression, particularly use of induction agents, has been reported but is controversial.[209,210]
    - No correlation with standard immunosuppression regimens.[210]
  - ○ Rejection
    - Increased rejection frequency has been reported but is controversial.[210]
  - ○ HLA-A3 expression
    - Expression of HLA-A3 in the recipient or donor has recently been reported to confer an added risk in seronegative recipients.[206]
- Clinical demographics
  - ○ Incidence:
    - 1.8% to 20% range reported.[199,201,211-213]
    - In three studies of more than 1000 lung transplant recipients, the incidence was 1.8%, 2.5%, and 6.1%, respectively.[199,211,214]
    - A higher incidence has been reported in children following lung transplantation (16%).[219]
  - ○ Temporal relationships
    - Early presentation (<1 year) is most common.
    - In adults, the diagnosis is made on average 339 days after transplant (range: 113–800 days)
    - In children, the range for time to diagnosis was 2 months to 11 years, with 77% presenting less than 1 year.[215]
- Diagnosis
  - ○ Imaging studies
    - CXR and CT[199,215]
      - ○ Single nodule (can be large)
      - ○ Multiple nodules (mostly well defined; ill-defined borders with or without halo can be noted). Most common feature.
      - ○ Patchy alveolar infiltrates
      - ○ Mediastinal with or without hilar adenopathy
      - ○ Pleural effusion and thickening (effusions occasionally chylous)
      - ○ Combined features can be seen
    - Positron emission tomography scan: can reflect increased metabolic activity; may be useful to follow response to treatment[199]
  - ○ Serology
    - EBV PCR and full PCR panel to detect EBV markers[216]
  - ○ Pathology
    - Histologic and immunohistochemical assay of biopsy tissue
    - Flow cytometry
  - ○ High clinical index of suspicion
    - Rule out other causes such as infection
- Clinical features
  - ○ PTLD most commonly presents in the lung allografts in single- or double-lung transplants (70% in one adult series, with the remainder presenting with disseminated disease).[199] Localized disease may progress to a disseminated state.
  - ○ A similar breakdown was reported in pediatric patients.[215]
  - ○ Clinical features are relatively nonspecific.
    - Incidental finding on imaging study
    - Constitutional: fever, weight loss
    - Intrathoracic: depend on thoracic findings and extent of pathology. Often progressive. See section on imaging earlier.[199,215,217]

■ Extrathoracic
  ○ Head and neck: cervical adenopathy, tonsils, adenoids
  ○ Gastric, small and large bowel involvement
  ○ Intra-abdominal and retroperitoneal adenopathy
  ○ Solitary or multiple liver masses
  ○ Kidney involvement
  ○ CNS: brain mass or masses; meningeal
■ Treatment[199,215]
  ○ Optimal treatment approaches have not been well defined, with high mortality rates using traditional approaches.
  ○ *Reduced immunosuppression:*
    ■ May be of value in earlier type reactive lesions
    ■ Risk is an increased rate of rejection
  ○ *Surgical excision:* Presumes localized disease
  ○ *Radiation:* Presumes localized disease
  ○ *Chemotherapy:*
    ■ Single-agent chemotherapy inferior to combination regimens, such as CHOP with or without E, ProMACE-CytaBOM (prednisone, adriamycin, cyclophosphamide, etoposide, cytarabine, bleomycin, oncovorin, and methotrexate).[218]
    ■ Side effects, such as infection and cardiotoxicity, are limiting factors.
  ○ Rituximab
    ■ A chimeric human/murine monoclonal antibody targeted against the CD20 antigen of normal and malignant B lymphocytes.
    ■ Encouraging results have been reported, with the infusion well tolerated.[219]
    ■ Complete response (CR): 54% to 66%, with progressive disease or death despite therapy, in about a third
    ■ Anecdotal reports of failure with rituximab, yet CR following combination chemotherapy[220]
    ■ Can be given in conjunction with reduced immunosuppression as a first-line treatment.
  ○ *Other:* Antiviral therapy, Interferon alpha, LAK cells, and re-transplant controversial.
■ Outcomes
  ○ Survival still poor despite CR to rituximab or chemotherapy
  ○ Despite an overall response rate of 64% to rituximab, the median survival was only 14.5 months.[219]
  ○ With intrathoracic disease, nodules have a better 1-year survival compared with involvement of mediastinal/hilar lymph nodes (89% versus 35%).[221]
  ○ Apart from the aggressive behavior of many forms of PTLD, side effects of treatment, including infection, and increased propensity to rejection with reduction in immunosuppression, add to attributable mortality rate.
■ Other malignancies: increased risk in lung transplant patients[222]
  ○ Lip cancer
  ○ Skin cancer
  ○ Perineal cancer
  ○ Cervical cancer

# DEPRESSION[223]

■ Depressive symptoms remain low in the period soon after surgery with associated increase in quality of life.
■ Depressive symptoms and quality of life dramatically increase with decline in functional status.
■ Serotonin reuptake inhibitors and new generation antidepressants such as mirtazapine are thought to be first-line agents, but drug interactions need to be carefully monitored including QT prolongation.
■ Adjuvant and complementary therapies such as psychoeducational interventions may strengthen coping strategies.

# RECURRENCE OF PRIMARY DISEASE FOLLOWING LUNG TRANSPLANTATION[224-250]

■ The overall recurrence rate of the primary lung disease post-transplant has been reported to be about 1%.
■ The diseases that have been reported to recur include
  ○ Sarcoidosis
  ○ Lymphangioleiomyomatosis
  ○ Pulmonary Langerhans' cell histiocytosis
  ○ Bronchoalveolar carcinoma
  ○ Diffuse panbronchiolitis
  ○ Desquamative interstitial pneumonia
  ○ Giant cell interstitial pneumonia
  ○ Pulmonary alveolar hemosiderosis
  ○ Pulmonary alveolar proteinosis
  ○ Talc granulomatosis, bronchiectasis secondary to aspiration
  ○ Emphysema due to alpha 1 antitrypsin deficiency.
■ The highest incidence of recurrence includes bronchoalveolar carcinoma (50%), sarcoidosis (35%), and Langerhans' cell histiocytosis (20.5%).
■ Although pathologic recurrence of sarcoidosis is high, 3- and 5-year outcomes are similar to patients transplanted for other diagnosis.

## Brief Illustrative Case

• A 63-year-old male patient received a single lung transplant for emphysema 2 years before his present presentation
• While on vacation at a lake resort, he presented to the local emergency room (ER) because of right-sided chest discomfort. He was told he had pneumonia and was placed on a course of antibiotics.
• Over the next 3 weeks, he still had mild chest discomfort and intermittent headache. His temperature over this period was not significantly elevated (maximum: 99° F).
• On presentation to the emergency room, he now complained of severe unrelenting headache and fever of 102° F over the prior day.
• Vital signs were stable. Temperature: 100° F. Chest: dull at both bases R>L. Markedly diminished breath sounds at right base with bronchial character. No neck stiffness. Normal fundi
• Laboratory
  • White blood cell count: 2900; Metabolic: normal electrolytes; glucose: 124
  • LP: opening pressure was 43 and CSF: clear; 5 white cells/UL; protein: 37 mg/dL; glucose: 65 mg/dL; rare "yeast-like" organisms
  • Pleural tap: exudate; glucose: 19 mg/dL; 110 white cells (68% lymphocytes)
• Imaging:
  • CT brain: normal
  • Chest x-ray study and CT chest: Extensive volume loss and consolidation of right middle and lower lobes;

emphysema of native left lung with patchy infiltrates in left lower lobe. Large complex effusion on right. Smaller left pleural effusion (Fig. 39-11).

- The patient was started on fluconazole in the ER pending results of the LP. He was then switched to liposomal amphotericin B once CSF results are available. The level of immunosupression was reduced as feasible.
- Soon thereafter, serum cryptococcal antigen was reported positive (1024; normal <4). Cryptococcal antigen was also positive in the CSF (1:16) and blood cultures were positive for cryptococcus.
- Because of the complex right loculated pleural effusion with compressive atelectasis, video-assisted thoracic surgery pleural fluid evacuation and decortication was performed on hospital day 7, to permit full lung expansion.
- Pathology: chronic granulomatous pleuritis with foamy histiocytes containing intra- and extracellular fungal spores compatible with Cryptococcus (Gomori methenamine silver [GMS] positive with mucicarmine staining of capsule) (Figs. 39-12 and 39-13).
- Liposomal amphotericin B was continued for 4 weeks and converted thereafter with oral fluconazole for 1 year.
- The patient improved progressively and on follow-up exhibited no clinical signs of relapse with serum cryptococcal antigen remaining negative.

## Key Issues

- Patient presented in the late transplant phase likely associated with significant immunosuppression.
- This patient had disseminated cryptococcosis.
- Diagnosis was delayed, which was a likely contributing factor.
- Despite clear evidence of meningitis, classic signs such as neck stiffness were absent, which is common, particularly in immunocompromised patients.

- This case highlights pleural involvement with cryptococcal infection.
- The addition of flucytosine to liposomal amphotericin B was considered but not given in view of marrow suppressive side effects of flucytosine in the face of leukopenia on admission.

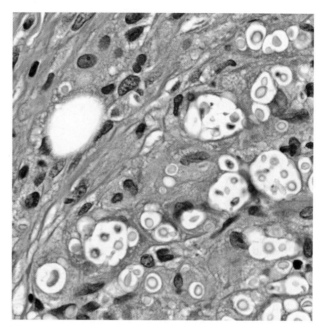

**Figure 39-12:** Numerous variably sized yeast with narrow based budding and clear halos compatible with cryptococcus (hematoxylin and eosin stain; original magnification 600×).

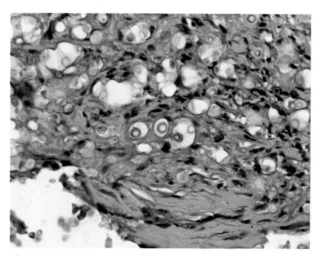

**Figure 39-13:** Mucin stain highlights mucinous capsules confirming cryptococcus (red; mucicarmine stain; original magnification 600×).

## References

 Interactive references and additional readings for this chapter can be accessed online at *expertconsult.com*.

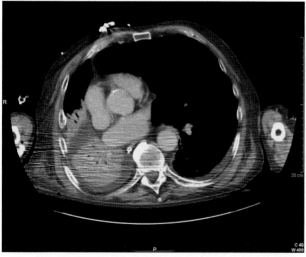

**Figure 39-11:** Computed tomography scan of the chest showing extensive volume loss and consolidation of right middle and lower lobes. Note large complex effusion on right and smaller left pleural effusion.

## TRANSPLANT IMMUNOSUPPRESSION

### Immunosuppressive Agents

Immunosuppressive agents are the mainstream therapies used to overcome immunologic barriers to transplantation[1] and to prevent allograft rejection. Immunosuppressive agents are divided into different categories depending on when they are given in relation to time of transplant (Fig. 40-1).

### Categories of Agents

- Induction agents
  - Antibody induction
  - Monoclonal antibodies: basiliximab, daclizumab, alemtuzumab, OKT3
  - Polyclonal antibodies: antithymocyte globulin (rabbit), antithymocyte globulin (equine)
  - Administered intravenously in the perioperative period
  - Induce acute, powerful, short-lived immunosuppression
- Primary Immunosuppressant[2,3]
  - Calcineurin inhibitors (CNIs) are the cornerstones of immunosuppressive therapy. These drugs include tacrolimus and cyclosporine A (CsA) and can be administered by the oral, intravenous, or inhalational route.
- Adjuvant agents
  - One or more medications prescribed in addition to a CNI
  - Antiproliferative agents
    - Azathioprine, mycophenolate mofetil, mycophenolate sodium, sirolimus, and everolimus
  - Corticosteriods
    - Methylprednisolone and prednisone

### Induction Agents

- Interleukin-2 (IL-2) receptor blockers
  - Basiliximab (Simulect)
    - Mechanism of action
      - Binds to activated lymphocyte IL-2 receptor alpha chains (Fig. 40-2)
    - Dosing
      - 20 mg intravenous piggyback (IVPB) given on POD #0 and #4; total of two doses
    - Diluent: normal saline only
    - Chimeric (70%/30%)
    - Administration time: 15 minutes
    - Line access: either peripheral or central line
    - Side effects
      - Hypotension, hypersensitive reaction, tachycardia, bronchospasm, pulmonary edema, and infection
  - Daclizumab (Zenapax)
    - Mechanism of Action
      - Same as basiliximab
    - Dosing
      - 1 mg/kg (maximum 100 mg) IVPB Q14 days for total of up to five doses
    - Diluent: normal saline only
    - Ninety percent humanized
    - Administration time: 15 minutes

- Line access: either peripheral or central line
- Side effects: same as basiliximab
- Humanized anti-CD52 monoclonal antibody
  - Alemtuzumab (Campath)
    - Mechanism of action[4]
      - Proposed antibody dependent lysis of lymphocytes after binding
      - Unconjugated; therefore, it relies on the Ab itself to kill cells directly or through activation of complement T cells
      - Causes transient but profound depletion of mature T cells and some depletion of B cells and monocytes but not bone marrow
    - Dosing
      - Alemtuzumab is administered one time as 30-mg subcutaneous injection (2 ×15-mg syringes) in either the buttocks or thighs.[5]
      - Premedications: methylprednisolone, acetaminophen, and diphenhydramine
    - Side effects
      - Anemia, neutropenia, thrombocytopenia, autoimmune hemolytic anemia (rare), infusion site reactions (rigors, fever, nausea and vomiting [N/V], rash, itching), infections
    - Monitoring
      - Complete blood count, absolute lymphocyte account Anti-CD3 murine monoclonal antibody
  - Muromonab CD3 (Orthoclone OKT3)
    - Mechanism of action
      - Reacts with T-3 antigen, recognizing structure
      - Blocks T-cell effector function
    - Dose:
      - 5 mg intravenous piggyback (IVP) in less than 1 minute for 7 to 14 days
    - Premedications: methylprednisolone, acetaminophen, and diphenhydramine
    - Side effects
      - Flulike syndrome
      - Pulmonary edema
      - Aseptic meningitis
      - Hypotension
      - Serious infection (including cytomegalovirus, posttransplant lymphoproliferative disease)
      - Seizure
    - Monitoring parameters
      - Fluid status: chest x-ray study, body weight (BW)
      - Frequent vital signs
      - First dose reactions
      - Efficacy: CD3 level
      - Tolerance: OKT-3 antibody
    - Note: Owing to severe adverse reactions (e.g., anaphylactic and cytokine release syndrome), which may occur with any dose or course, use of OKT3 is less desirable in the current era.
- Antithymocyte globulin (ATG)
  - Equine polyclonal immunoglobulin G (IgG) antibody (Atgam)
    - Mechanism of action

MECHANISMS OF ACTION

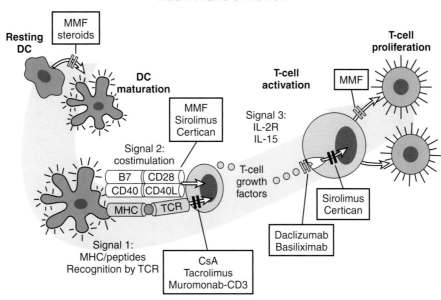

**Figure 40-1:** Sites of action of various immunosuppressive medications commonly used in solid organ transplantation.

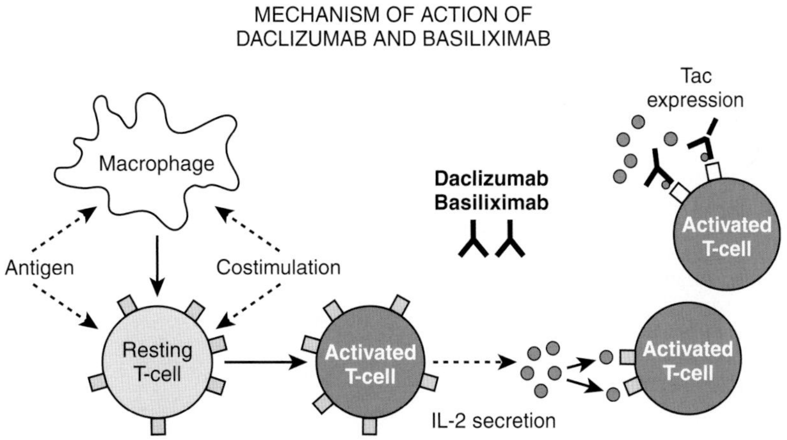

MECHANISM OF ACTION OF
DACLIZUMAB AND BASILIXIMAB

**Figure 40-2:** Mechanism of action of daclizumab and basiliximab. Daclizumab is a selective, modified human IgG1 monoclonal antibody specific for alpha subunit (CD25) of interleukin-2 receptor; inhibits interleukin-2–dependent human T-lymphocyte activation. Basiliximab is a chimeric interleukin-2 receptor antagonist. It is directed against the interleukin-2R-alpha chain (CD25) on activated T lymphocytes, and is a potent inhibitor of interleukin-2–mediated activation of lymphocytes, a critical pathway in the cellular immune response involved in allograft rejection.

○ Reduces number and alters function of circulating T lymphocytes
▪ Dose
  ○ 10 to 20 mg/kg/d intravenous (IV) over 6 to 8 h for 7 to 14 days via central line
▪ Premedications: methylprednisolone, acetaminophen, and diphenhydramine
▪ Skin testing is required
▪ Side effects[6]
  ○ Fever, chills, leukopenia, pain, headache, abdominal pain, diarrhea, hypertension, nausea, and thrombocytopenia
▪ Monitoring parameters
  ○ ATG/thymoglobulin protocol
  ○ Platelets higher than 100,000 or white blood cell count (WBC) higher than 3000: Full dose
  ○ Platelets between 50,000 and 100,000 or WBC between 2000 and 3000: Half dose

  ○ Platelets less than 50,000 or WBC less than 2000: Hold dose
    1. Rabbit polyclonal IgG antibody (thymoglo-bulin)
▪ Mechanism of action
  ○ Same as equine polyclonal IgG antibody
▪ Dose
  ○ 1.25 to 1.5 mg/kg/d for 7 to 14 days
▪ Pharmacokinetic (PK) profile: t 1/2 30 days (14–45 days)
▪ Infusion rate: First dose over 6 to 8 hours; subsequent doses over 4 to 6 hours
▪ Central line preferred
▪ No skin testing required
▪ Premedications methylprednisolone, acetaminophen, and diphenhydramine
▪ Side effects and monitoring
  ○ Same as equine polyclonal IgG antibody

## Summary of Antibody Therapy Prior to Anti-CD25 (IL-2 Blockers) mAbs

- Polyclonal antibodies (e.g., ATG, antilymphocyte globulin [ALG]) and monoclonal antibody (OKT3) used for reversal of acute rejection and prophylactic induction
- When used in prophylactic setting:
  - Reduce incidence of early calcineurin-associated nephrotoxicity
  - Decrease incidence and duration of graft dysfunction
  - Delays the time of first rejection
  - Antigen nonspecific, increasing the risk of over immunosuppression

## Primary Immunosuppressants

- CNIs
  - CsA (Neoral)
    - Mechanism of action[7]
      - CsA binds to cyclophylin. This action inhibits the antigenic response of helper T lymphocytes and suppresses the production of IL-2 and interferon-gamma. In addition, production of the receptor site for IL-2 on T lymphocytes is inhibited.
    - Dose
      - PO: 4 to 6 mg/kg/day, given in divided doses, every 12 hours
      - IV: 1/3 of PO dose BID over 4 hours
    - Target CsA levels
      - First 3 months, 250 to 300 ng/mL
      - 3 to 6 months, 200 to 250 ng/mL
      - 6 to 12 months, 150 to 200 ng/mL
      - More than 12 months, 100 to 150 ng/mL
  - Tacrolimus (Prograf)
    - Mechanism of action[8]
      - Tacrolimus binds to an intracellular protein, called FKBP-12. A complex is formed that inhibits the phosphatase activity of calcineurin. This may prevent dephosphorylation and translocation of nuclear factor of activated T cells, which is believed to initiate gene transcription for lymphokines.
    - Dose
      - PO: 0.1 to 0.2 mg/kg/d given in divided doses, every 12 hours
      - IV: 1/3 of PO dose via continuous infusion.
      - IV should be avoided unless absolutely necessary. Switch to oral or nasogastric tube feeding as soon as possible to avoid nephrotoxicity.
    - Target tacrolimus levels
      - First 3 months, 15 to 20 ng/mL
      - 3 to 6 months, 12 to 15 ng/mL
      - 6 months and beyond, 10-12 ng/mL
- CNI side effects (Table 40-1)[9-11]
- Metabolic interactions that increase CNI levels
  - Calcium channel blockers
    - Verapamil, diltiazem, nicardipine
  - Antifungal agents
    - Ketoconazole, fluconazole, itraconazole, voriconazole (typically decrease tacrolimus level by two thirds)
  - Immunosuppressants
    - Sirolimus
  - Antibiotics
    - Erythromycin, clarithromycin, josamycin, ponsino-mycin
  - Protease inhibitors
    - Saquinavir, indinavir, nelfinavir, ritonavir
  - Foods
    - Grapefruit, grapefruit juice
- Metabolic interactions that decrease CNI levels

| TABLE 40-1 ■ COMMON TOXICITIES OF CALCINEURIN INHIBITORS | |
|---|---|
| **Event[9]** | **Comments** |
| Hepatotoxicity | Liver function should be monitored at regular intervals |
| Cardiovascular | Fewer TAC-treated patients require antihypertensive medications |
| Hypertension | |
| Hypercholesterolemia | TAC impacts lipid levels less than CsA |
| Glucose intolerance | Recent studies indicate little difference between TAC and CsA with regard to diabetes[10,11] |
| Neurotoxicity | Seen more often with TAC and generally improve with dose reduction |
| Tremor | |
| Headache | |
| Insomnia | |
| Paresthesia | |
| Physical | |
| Gingival hypertrophy | Use of corticosteroids may exaggerate development |
| Hirsutism | Gingival hypertrophy and hirsutism are associated with CsA |
| Alopecia | Alopecia can occur with TAC |
| Malignancy | Incidence appears to be a function of overall amount and duration of immunosuppression rather than any specific agent |
| Skin cancers | |
| Cervical cancer | |
| Lymphoproliferative disorders | |

CsA, cyclosporine A; TAC, tacrolimus.

- Antituberculosis drugs
  - Rifampin, rifabutin
- Anticonvulsants
  - Barbiturates, phenytoin, carbamazepine
- Herbal preparations
  - St John's wort
- Antibiotics
  - Nafcillin, IV trimethoprim, IV sulfadimidine, imipenem, cephalosporins, terbinafine, ciprofloxacin
- Other drugs
  - Ticlopidine, octreotide, nefazodone
- Agents that potentiate toxic effects of CNIs (Table 40-2)

## Adjuvant Agents[9]

- Antiproliferative agents
  - Azathioprine (Imuran)
    - Mechanism of action
      - A purine analogue; affects purine nucleotide synthesis and metabolism, and alters the synthesis and function of RNA and DNA.
    - Dose
      - 1 to 3 mg/kg/d PO or IV
    - Side Effects[12]
      - Leukopenia, anemia, thrombocytopenia, hepatitis, cholestasis, pancreatitis
    - Monitoring
      - Complete blood counts should be performed regularly to monitor for hematologic side effects.
  - Mycophenolate mofetil (Cellcept)
    - Mechanism of action[13]
      - A prodrug, rapidly hydrolyzed to the biologically active mycophenolic acid after oral administration.
      - Produces potent, noncompetitive inhibition of inosine monophosphate dehydrogenase, thus blocking de novo synthesis of guanosine nucleotides.

<br>

**TABLE 40-2 ■ AGENTS KNOWN TO POTENTIATE TOXIC EFFECTS OF CALCINEURIN INHIBITORS**

| Drug Type | Comments |
|---|---|
| Nephrotoxic agents<br>NSAIDs<br>Aminoglycosides<br>Amphotericin | Monitor kidney function<br>NSAIDs may have increased nephrotoxicity with hepatic impairment<br>Liposomal preparations of amphotericin are generally well tolerated |
| Potassium-sparing diuretics | Hyperkalemia has been reported |
| Antacids | Magnesium and aluminum antacids may inhibit CNI absorption<br>If necessary, should be taken 2 hours after CNI dose |
| HMG-CoA reductase inhibitors (statins) | Increased risk of rhabdomyolysis, bone marrow suppression |

CNI, calcineurin inhibitors; HMG-CoA, 3-hydroxy-3-methyl-glutaryl coenzyme A; NSAIDs, nonsteroidal anti-inflammatory drugs.

- Dose
  - 750 to 1500 mg BID (typical dose is 1 g BID)
  - Doses used with tacrolimus are typically lower
- Pharmacokinetic
  - Immediate release; release in stomach
  - Exposure in patients taking tacrolimus is substantially higher than in those taking CsA
- Side effects[13]
  - Leukopenia, anemia, thrombocytopenia, diarrhea, nausea, bloating/dyspepsia, vomiting, esophagitis, gastritis
- Monitoring
  - Complete blood counts should be performed.
  - Gastrointestinal side effects are more common when dose exceeds 1 g BID, and they respond to dose reduction or more frequent administration of smaller doses.
○ Mycophenolate sodium (Myfortic)
  - Mechanism of Action
    - Same as mycophenolate mofetil
  - Dose
    - 360 to 720 mg BID (720 mg = 1 g mycophenolate mofetil)
  - Pharmacokinetic
    - Release in small intestine, enteric coated
  - Side effects and monitoring
    - Same as Mycophenolate Mofetil
○ Sirolimus (Rapamune)
  - Mechanism of action
    - Acts on the molecular target of rapamycin (mTOR) and blocks the ability of cells to enter the cell cycle.
    - Inhibits IL-12- and IL-15-driven proliferation, and thus inhibits T-lymphocyte activation and antibody production.
  - Dose
    - 2 to 5 mg daily (target whole blood trough level is 5 to 15 ng/mL)
  - Pharmacokinetic
    - T1/2: 60 hours
    - Time to reach steady state: 6 days
    - Trough levels do not reach steady state for several days after dose adjustment
  - Side effects[14]
    - Hypercholesterolemia, edema, hypertriglyceridemia, hypertension, rash, leukopenia, anemia, thrombocytopenia, interstitial pneumonitis, delayed wound healing, mouth ulcers, myalgia/weakness, proteinuria
    - Bronchial dehiscence associated with use of sirolimus within first 3 months after lung transplant; black box warning[15]
  - Monitoring-lipid panel, urine protein
    - 5-mg dose was not associated with better efficacy but was less well tolerated than 2-mg dose
    - Pneumonitis occasionally resolved with discontinuation of sirolimus
    - Sirolimus rescue in children has been associated with heavy proteinuria; patients should be monitored closely for this side effect[16]
○ Everolimus (Certican); not yet approved
  - Mechanism of action
    - Same as sirolimus
  - Dose
    - Range, 0.5 to 1.5 mg BID
  - Pharmacokinetic
    - T1/2: 23 hours
    - Time to reach steady state: 4 days
  - Side effects, drug interactions, and monitoring
    - Same as sirolimus
○ Corticosteroids
  - Mechanism of action[2,17]
    - Corticosteroids have multiple actions that produce anti-inflammatory effects and result in their widespread use.
    - Corticosteroids block T cell–derived and antigen-presenting cell–derived cytokine and cytokine-receptor expression.
  - Dose
    - 5 to 10 mg QD tapered per center protocol
  - Side effects[9]
    - Acne, cushingoid facial appearance, hirsutism, mood disorders, hypertension, glucose intolerance, cataracts, osteoporosis, growth retardation in children
  - Monitoring
    - May potentiate adverse events of CNIs

## Possible Drug Interactions with Adjuvant Agents

- Azathioprine[12]
  - Coadministration with ganciclovir, angiotensin-converting enzyme (ACE) inhibitors, carbamazepine, clozapine, or cotrimoxazole can lead to the exacerbation of hematologic toxicity.
  - Allopurinol is contraindicated, because concomitant administration can lead to life-threatening myelosuppression; reduce the dose of azathioprine by 75%.
- Mycophenolate mofetil/mycophenolate sodium[13]
  - Coadministration with ganciclovir, ACE inhibitors, carbamazepine, clozapine, or cotrimoxazole can lead to the exacerbation of hematologic toxicity.
- Sirolimus/everolimus[14]
  - Because sirolimus is metabolized by the same pathway as the CNIs (P-450 3A4), interactions are the same.
  - Sirolimus has been shown to raise blood levels of CsA.
  - CsA has been shown to raise blood levels of sirolimus.
  - Limited reports of coadministration of sirolimus and voriconazole have shown no adverse outcomes.
    - Close monitoring of sirolimus levels after reduction in dosage by 50% to 90% is suggested.[18,19]
- Corticosteroids[17]
  - No significant drug interactions

## Immunomodulation

- Rituximab-anti-CD20 monoclonal antibody[20]
  - Mechanism of action[21-26]
    - Chimeric murine/human monoclonal antibody selectively depletes B cells bearing the CD20 surface marker via
      - Antibody-dependent cellular cytotoxicity
      - Complement-dependent cytotoxicity
      - Apoptosis
  - Dose
    - $375$ mg/m$^2$ IVPB for one dose or 1000 mg IVPB (in one to two doses)[27]
    - Pre-medications 30 minutes before infusion
      - Acetaminophen 650 mg PO
      - Diphenhydramine 50 mg PO
      - Methylprednisolone 40 mg IVP
  - Pharmacokinetic
    - Long serum half-life ($375$ mg/m$^2$)
    - Single dose t1/2 = 76 hours
    - Multidose t1/2 = 206 hours
  - Side effects
    - Headache, nausea, vomiting, rash
  - Monitoring
    - Complete blood count
- Intravenous Immunoglobulin
  - Mechanism of action[28]
    - Regulation of B-cell repertoire and antibody production
    - Induction of B-cell apoptosis through FcgR-mediated signals
    - Inhibition of dendritic cell maturation and function through FcgR-mediated signals/T-reg induction
    - Inhibition of macrophage maturation and function through FcgR-mediated inhibition of FN-g receptor
    - Inhibition of complement-mediated inflammation inhibition of C5b-9 MAC
    - Induction of anti-inflammatory cytokines (IL-10, tumor growth factor-β [TGF-β])/Increased T-reg activity
    - Inhibition of cytokines IL-1b, interferon-γ, IL-2, IL-6
    - Anti-human leukocyte antigen (HLA)
    - Neutralization of anti-HLA antibodies by anti-idiotypic antibodies
  - Dose
    - High dose: 2 g/kg monthly; range two to four doses (max 140 g for patient weighing more than 70 kg)[27,29]
  - Side effects
    - Headache, nausea, vomiting, rash
    - Acute renal failure, thrombotic complications, hemolysis (brand specific)[30]
  - Monitoring
    - Complete blood count, basic metabolic panel (BMP)

## CONCLUSION

- Proper immunosuppression is critical to allograft survival.
- Understanding proper dosing and monitoring is especially critical in the presence of comorbid conditions.
- Some side effects are associated with immunosuppression; others are associated with specific agents.
- Patient education on adherence should continue throughout the life of the transplant.
- Awareness of important drug-drug interactions is critical in avoiding toxicity and potential over- and under-immunosuppression.

## References

 Interactive references and additional readings for this chapter can be accessed online at *expertconsult.com*.

# 41  TRANSPLANT IMMUNOLOGY

### Stanley C. Jordan, MD and Mieko Toyoda, PhD

## INTRODUCTION

- The optimal treatment for patients with end-stage organ failure is transplantation.[1,2] This is especially true for patients who are candidates for lung, heart, and heart-lung transplantation because no long-term life support system such as dialysis is available.
- The study of transplantation has played a critical role in advancements in our understanding of immunology.
- Organ donors and recipients are genetically distinct. This factor results in a genetically encoded immunologic barrier to transplantation that was first recognized in experiments performed in the early 20th century.
- The first successful kidney transplant was performed in 1954 between identical twins.[3] However, the true implementation of transplantation as a reasonable therapy for end-stage organ failure awaited advancements in understanding the immunologic basis of allograft rejection and advancements in immunosuppressive therapy.[4,5]
- The surgical techniques for kidney transplantation and heart transplantation were developed in the 1950s and 1960s, but the success of these organ transplants were dismal due to the severe rejection that often accompanied these procedures.
- For heart transplant especially, the ultimate graft failure and death of most patients led to a feeling that the fledgling transplant enterprise was a failure and could offer little hope for anyone. This was best depicted in a feature article that appeared in the September 17, 1971 issue of *LIFE*. The article describes "The Tragic Record of Heart Transplants: A New Report on an Era of Medical Failure" (Fig. 41-1).
- Clearly, the rapid advancements in surgery could not compensate for the poor and incomplete understanding of the allograft-directed immune responses and how to deal with them. Fortunately, a few years later Dr. Borel, a biochemist working at Sandoz in Switzerland, discovered a novel fungal derivative drug with immunosuppressive properties (cyclosporine A [CsA]) that would eventually revolutionize the field of transplantation.[5]
- The field of clinical transplantation developed alongside clinical immunology.
- The rejection of allograft tissue was found to be a result of an active immunologic process in which antigens of the allograft are processed and an acquired immune response developed with multiple effectors that evolve to destroy the transplant.[4,6,7]

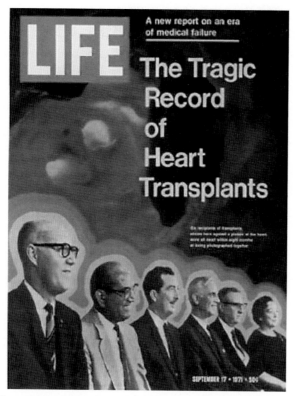

**Figure 41-1:** A feature article that appeared in the September 17, 1971 issue of *LIFE*. The article describes "The Tragic Record of Heart Transplants: A new report on an era of medical failure."

- This knowledge was augmented by the finding that the primary target for the allograft-directed immune response was the major histocompatibility complex (MHC). Genes in this region encode dominant transplant antigens that were first identified serologically and defined as human leukocyte antigens (HLA).[6,7]
- These HLA antigens were not created as transplant antigens by nature and were ultimately found to be responsible for self-restriction of immunologic responses.[1,4] These fundamental observations represent the cornerstone of the scientific basis for the practice of transplantation.
- Further developments in immunology have revealed a high degree of complexity of the immune response to allografts and cellular events that lead to the loss or acceptance of an organ transplant. These events are shown in Figure 41-2A and B.

## HISTOCOMPATIBILITY AND ALLORECOGNITION

- Humans and all higher animals evolved histocompatibility molecules (HLA system in humans) with matching receptors to allow them to distinguish their cells and tissues as "self."
- These molecules represent a system of diversification and amplification that allows different organisms among the same species to preserve individual immunologic integrity.[8]
- Clearly, allotypic differences between donor and recipients of transplanted tissues can simulate immune responses that are characterized as rejection. This arises, in large part, because of the extreme polymorphism of the HLA system and the role of these molecules in antigen recognition.

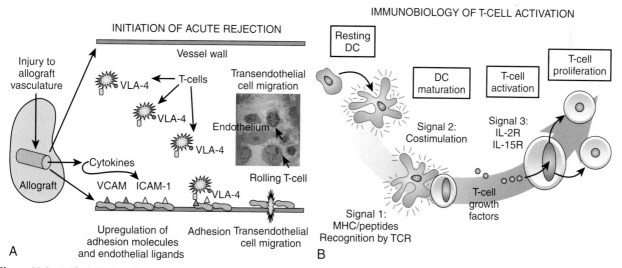

**Figure 41-2: A,** The initiation of acute rejection in an unmodified allograft lies in events related to procurement and surgery. Once the organ is removed, perfused, and transplanted, cytokines such as TNF-α, IL-1a and IL-6 are generated and activate the endothelium of the allograft. This allows infiltrating T-cells to bind and migrate from the endothelium to the interstitium of the allograft (*inset photo*). These migrating T cells move into the host lymphoid tissues and process alloantigens that result in T cell activation and allograft rejection, as shown in **B. B** shows that resting dendritic cells (DC) or antigen presenting cells (APCs) become activated in the cytokine-rich environment of an ischemic-reperfused organ. This activates the DC and allows it to interact directly with the activated T cells that have migrated through the endothelium. This allows interaction of the T-cell receptor (TCR) with the MHC class II antigen presenting machinery on the DC/APC. This is called Signal 1. With signal 1 only, the T cell would receive incomplete activation and die. However, the DC contains other molecules called costimulatory molecules (CD80/86, CD40/CD40L) that are responsible for delivering a full activation signal to the T cell (Signal 2). Once activated, T cells produce cytokines such as interleukin-2 (IL-2), IL-15, and interferon-γ (IFN-γ) that drive T-cell proliferation and cytotoxic effector functions (Signal 3).

■ Although other minor histocompatibility differences have been identified in humans, the MHC is the major target for allotypic responses in transplant rejecton.[9]

## T-CELL ACTIVATION AND ALLOGRAFT REJECTION

■ The structure of the human MHC class I and class II molecules is shown in Figure 41-3.
■ MHC class I proteins
  ○ Cell-surface glycoproteins that are highly polymorphic and composed of a heavy chain and a less variable light chain (b2 microglobulin).
  ○ MHC class 1 proteins are expressed on most nucleated cells and interact exclusively with CD8+ T-cells through the T-cell receptor (TCR) complex.
  ○ The interaction of CD8+ T cells with the MHC class I peptide complex is "self-restricted," meaning that CD8+ T cells from another individual would not recognize this individual's MHC class I peptide complex. When CD8+ T cells interact with sel-MHC class I/peptide complex, the CD8+ T cell becomes activated and generates effector CD8+ T cells directed at this target (see Fig. 41-3).
■ MHC class II proteins
  ○ Consist of two membrane anchored glycoproteins (a chain approximately 35 kD; b-chain, approximately 28 kD). The tissue distribution of MHC class II molecules is much more restricted than that of MHC class I.
  ○ MHC class II is constitutively expressed on B-lymphocytes and dendritic cells, which have very specialized functions as antigen-presenting cells (APCs). MHC class II/peptide-bearing cells generally interact with CD4+ T cells only.
  ○ Again, these interactions are self-restricted and result in the activation of the CD4+ T cell with designated effector functions aimed at the presented peptide (see Fig. 41-3).[1,4]

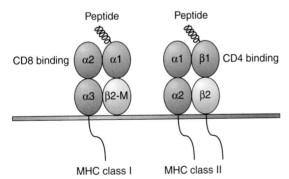

**Figure 41-3:** This figure is a schematic diagram of the human MHC class I and class II molecules. MHC class I consist of three a chains bound to β2 microglobulin (not membrane bound). Foreign peptides are bound in the peptide groove. This APC then interacts with CD8+ T cells from the host to allow activation of peptide-specific CD8 response (cytotoxicity). The major histocompatibility complex (MHC) class II consists of two alpha chains and two beta chains both tethered to the cell membrane. Peptides bound to the MHC class II interact with the individual CD4 cells only. Activation of CD4 T cells interacting with this peptide results in helper CD4 T-cell functions (regulation of T-cell effectors, activation of B cells and initiation of antibody production by B cells).

## ALLOANTIGEN RECOGNITION AND EFFECTOR FUNCTIONS

■ Because the graft is infiltrated by T cells, alloantigen recognition can occur in one of two ways: direct allorecognition and indirect allorecognition.
■ Direct allorecognition:
  ○ Is of particular importance for lung and heart lung allografts because this is the direct interaction of infiltrating T cells with allogenic MHC molecules present on the dendritic cells present in the allograft and adjacent lymphoid tissue.
  ○ The frequency of alloreactive lymphocytes stimulated through this process is high and likely accounts for most cases of early allograft rejection.
  ○ Although direct allorecognition would appear to violate the "self-restriction" principle of T-cell activation, it is likely that the TCR of infiltrating lymphocytes can discriminate between subtle differences in MHC structure and peptides binding in their grooves. Because the infiltrating lymphocytes are not from naïve animals, there is likely a large repertoire of T-cell memory that constitutes infiltrating cells that have the capacity to become activated more easily and can result in allograft directed T-cell responses. This is shown in Figure 41-4.[1,4,10]
  ○ This is why the achievement of tolerance in humans is much more difficult than in inbred mouse strains that have limited pathogen exposure and T-cell repertoires.
■ Indirect allorecognition:
  ○ Is a more traditional process of T-cell activation.
  ○ In allogenic transplantation, alloantigens of the graft are processed by self-MHC–bearing APCs and presented to self T cells. Thus effector T cells are generated and respond to the allograft in a more chronic manner.
  ○ The importance of indirect presentation is underscored by the intense immune responses generated by skin grafts from MHC class II–deficient mice transplanted into normal mice.[10] Rejection occurs as a result of indirect presentation only and results in long term memory.
  ○ In human transplantation, the indirect pathway is likely responsible for chronic allograft rejection and stimulation of antibody responses to the allograft. Established immune responses initiated via the indirect pathway are long lasting and difficult to suppress.[1,11] This is summarized in Figure 41-4.

## COSTIMULATION IN T-CELL ACTIVATION

■ The fate of T cells after engagement of the TCR with cognate MHC/peptide complex varies widely. Outcomes include activation, proliferation, effector functions, apoptosis, anergy and evolution to memory cells.
■ Clearly, the various outcomes of T-cell activation depend on costimulation and soluble cytokines.[1,12] This has been an area of great interest in transplantation because manipulation of costimulatory molecule interaction with T cells has the potential to delete alloreactive T-cell clones and mute alloreactive T-cell responses.
■ Many experiments have detailed the importance of costimulation. If T cells engage antigen through the TCR/MHC peptide complex alone (Signal 1), T cells either die or become anergic (Fig. 41-5).
■ Costimulation occurs through numerous molecules and cognate receptors on T cells and APCs. However, of considerable importance is the CD40/CD40L(CD154) and CD28/CD80/86 molecules.

DIRECT ANTIGEN PRESENTATION

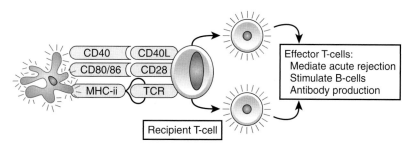

INDIRECT ANTIGEN PRESENTATION

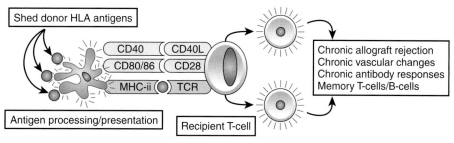

**Figure 41-4:** Allorecognition pathways for allograft infiltrating lymphocytes. T cells infiltrating the allograft can be activated by direct antigen recognition (interaction of host T cells with alloantigen present on antigen-presenting cells [APCs] present in the allograft). This is likely to be associated with early acute rejection (AR). Second, long-term indirect allorecognition can occur (interaction of self APCs processing donor antigens and presenting to self–T cells). This is a more traditional form of immune activation and results in more chronic immune responses to the allograft.

T-CELL ENGAGEMENT PARTNERS PREDICTS T-CELL FATE

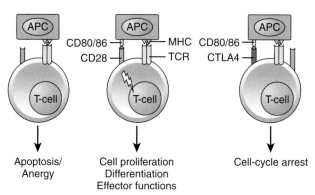

**Figure 41-5:** T cells interacting with cognate receptors on APCs can result in different "fates" for the T cell. Signal 1 only (TCR/MHC) results in apoptosis/anergy of the T cell. A full "immunizing" signal of the T-cell is seen when Signal 1 (TCR/MHC) and Signal 2 (CD80/86-CD28) occur together. This process results in cell proliferation, differentiation and effector functions. Finally, when T cells express CTLA4 as a costimulatory molecule with TCR/MHC interactions, cell cycle arrest and apoptosis can occur. CTLA4 conveys a negative, regulatory signal to the T cell when it interacts with CD80/86 compared with the positive signal transmitted by CD28/CD80/86 interactions.

■ Once the TCR/MHC-peptide complex is engaged, engagement of costimulatory molecules (Signal 2) results in a full "immunizing" signal to the T cell with resultant activation.
■ Engagement of CD40/CD40L results in the upregulation of CD80/86 on APCs, thus allowing for more interactions with CD28 on T cells. This interaction results in increased cytokine synthesis and cell proliferation with cytotoxic effector functions.
■ After initial immunizing signals through the CD28/CD80/86 pathway, T cells begin to express another costimulatory molecule (CTLA4 or CD152).
■ This molecule has 100-fold higher avidity for CD80/86 and results in termination of T-cell effector responses. This negative signaling costimulatory pathway has also shed light on how manipulation of this regulatory pathway could be used to regulate T-cell immune responses to allografts.
■ Multiple experimental data[1,13-16] has shown that blockade of the CD28/CD80/86 pathway with the synthetic peptide CTLA4-Ig results in prolonged allograft survival and termination of alloimmune responses.
■ Recent data in human kidney transplantation have shown that a genetically modified CTLA-4 Ig (Belatacept) can prevent allograft rejection and result in long-term rejection-free survival.[17]
■ However, there is concern that costimulatory blockade may not be efficacious in the modification of patients with T-cell memory.[10] The various fates of T cells after activation are shown in Figure 41-5.

## CYTOKINES AND REGULATION OF ALLOIMMUNE RESPONSES

■ The interaction of T cells with APCs is critical for development of allograft-directed immune responses.
■ However, a critical question is how specific effector/regulator cells evolve in this environment. What is traditionally thought of as a productive immune response consists of

T-cell proliferation and differentiation of helper T-cell functions that are graft directed.

- We now know that the regulation and intensity of this response is at least in part dependent on the cytokine environment the T cells are exposed to after activation.
- The original work of Mosmann[18] described two types of T cells (Th1) characterized by interferon-γ/interleukin-2 (IL-2) production and (Th2) characterized by IL-4, IL-5, and IL-13 production that were responsible for humoral immunity and possible suppression of Th1 cells.
- That differential cytokine production by T cells was essential to effector functions was recognized early, but subsequently it was also recognized that a subset of T cells was also responsible for peripheral regulation of Th1/Th2 immune responses and that they preferentially secreted cytokines such as IL-10 and transforming growth factor-β (TGF-β).
- Thus T-cell effectors can be characterized by the types of cytokines they produce after stimulation. Indeed, the responses of activated T cells can be regulated and deviated based on the cytokine milieu encountered. This is shown in Figure 41-6.

## REGULATORY T-CELLS AS POTENTIAL IMMUNOTHERAPY FOR INDUCTION OF TOLERANCE TO ALLOANTIGENS

- Naturally arising CD4+/CD25+ regulatory T cells.
- Regulatory T cells (Treg cells) are produced by the thymus and are responsible for the maintenance of immunologic self-tolerance and negative control of pathologic immune responses.
- Treg cells are fundamental to controlling various immunologic responses, and animal models of adoptive transfer of Tregs can prevent or cure autoimmune diseases and prevent allograft rejecton.[19,20]
- Recently, the identification of the forkhead box P3 (FoxP3+CD4+CD25+) identified a gene that is responsible for Treg activity.
- Of interest is that Tregs can be generated from Tn cells by exposure to a cytokine milieu that includes TGF-β.[20] This

raises the possibility that Tregs could be expanded in vitro and used to treat autoimmune diseases and prevent transplant rejection.

- Although promising, the data from experimental models are limited and as yet have not been successful in preventing rejection of solid organ transplants.[21] This is despite a positive correlation with good long-term allograft outcomes with the presence of increased numbers of Tregs in the circulation of allograft recipients.[22-25]
- Tregs have several modes of action, which are summarized in Figure 41-7.
- Briefly, Tregs may interact with alloreactive Th1 cells and delete them through granzyme and perforin-mediated cytolysis. The interaction of CTLA4 with CD80/86 on APCs induces increased metabolism of tryptophan, an amino acid critical for T-cell growth and function by inducing the enzyme IDO in dendritic cells. This ultimately results in T-cell apoptosis and anergy.
- Tregs can also induce IL-10 production by dendritic cells and regulate APC function by direction secretion of TGF-β. This results in APC dysfunction and T-cell anergy.
- Finally, Tregs can induce the expression B7H4 on APCs, which delivers a negative signal to Th1 cells and results in T-cell cycle arrest.

## HLA ANTIBODIES AND CROSS-MATCH TESTING

- Anti-HLA antibodies are preformed antibodies to HLA antigens.[26-28]
- Renal transplant recipients can develop anti-HLA antibodies as a result of sensitization events that include blood transfusions, previous transplants, pregnancies, and rarely, as a consequence of infections.
- With widespread use of recombinant erythropoietin in patients end-stage renal disease, allosensitization due to blood transfusion has decreased considerably.
- Anti-HLA antibodies bind to HLA antigens expressed on the surface of donor cells, and can cause hyperacute rejection

DIFFERENTIATION OF CD4+ T-CELL SUBSETS

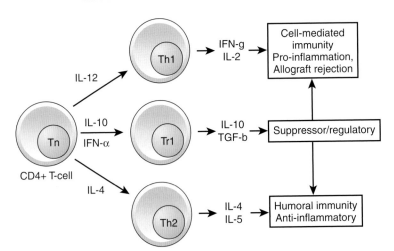

**Figure 41-6:** Differentiation of T-cell subsets depend upon the cytokine exposure initially encountered after activation. Unactivated T cells (Tn) when activated by dendritic cells producing interleukin-12 (IL-12) are deviated to a Th1 or inflammatory cytokine effector pathway. These cells result in allograft rejection. However, if Tn cells are activated in an environment rich in IL-4, they deviate to a Th2 pathway and become responsible for humoral immunity with some anti-inflammatory activity. Of significant interest is the evolution of Tn cells activated with an environment rich in IL-10. These cells develop a Tr or regulatory pathway and can suppress the activity of both Th1 and Th2 cells.

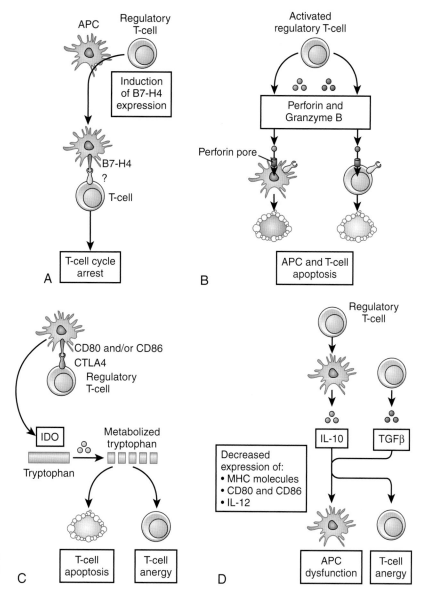

**Figure 41-7:** Mechanisms of action of regulatory T cells. (See text for explanation.)

and immediate graft loss. These antibodies are particularly deleterious if they are directed at HLA class I antigens, and are able to activate the complement cascade by binding to complement proteins.

## Panel Reactive Antibodies

- The anti-HLA antibodies can be detected by testing the transplant recipient's serum against a panel of cells that express potential donor HLA antigens present in the local population.
- The results are expressed as a percentage of donor cells showing a positive test with the recipient's serum. Anti-HLA antibodies determined in this manner are also known as panel reactive antibodies (PRAs), which provide the information on sensitization status and robustness of the immune responses of the transplant candidate.
- The PRA test is performed using the National Institutes of Health recognized complement dependent microlymphocytotoxicity assay (NIH-CDC). The NIH-CDC assay involves determination of the donor's T and B cell lympholysis induced

by anti-HLA antibodies in the recipient's serum in the presence of complement.[26]

- Low-level anti-HLA antibodies can be detected by using more sensitive assays, such as anti-human globulin enhanced NIH-CDC assay, enzyme-linked immunosorbent assay (ELISA), or by flow cytometry using HLA antigen-coated beads.[28] In fact, the HLA antigen-coated beads are the preferred method for determining antibodies to HLA.
- The anti-HLA antibodies can be further characterized in a high-risk or highly sensitized recipient.
- Transplants from donors bearing these HLA antigens should be avoided in such patients. Highly sensitized individuals (PRA > 50%) are more likely to experience acute rejection episodes even when unacceptable antigens are avoided.
- At present, desensitization protocols using intravenous immunoglobulin (IVIG), rituximab, and plasmapheresis have allowed transplantation of such highly-HLA sensitized patients.[29,30] These protocols can reduce antibody titers and inhibit antibody-mediated rejection through mechanisms that are not yet completely understood.

## Cross-match

- Cross-match determines the compatibility between a specific recipient and a donor and is the final pretransplantation immunologic screening step.[26]
- The test involves testing recipient's serum against donor T and B cells to detect any preformed antibodies against donor's lymphocytes. Conventional cross-matching is done by NIH-CDC assay.
- Sometimes, immunoglobulin M (IgM) autoantibodies present in recipient's serum can give a false-positive result in the CDC cross-match test.
- To overcome this, the recipient's serum is pretreated with dithiothreitol (DTT), which disrupts the S-S bonds in IgM autoantibodies and inactivates them. Thus, a negative cross-match with DTT pretreatment is able to differentiate between preformed autoantibodies and alloantibodies.
- A positive T-cell cross-match after DTT treatment is indicative of preformed alloantibodies against donor antigens and is a contraindication to transplantation from that specific donor.
- The sensitivity of the cross-match has now been enhanced many fold by antihuman globulin-enhanced ELISA assay and flow cytometry cross-match techniques. These tests are especially useful for patients undergoing retransplant surgery, as well as for those who are highly sensitized.[29,30]

## IMMUNOSUPPRESSIVE THERAPIES

- Immunosuppressive drugs are used to overcome immunologic barriers to transplantation.[31] The drugs that are used at the time of renal transplantation to suppress unwanted allograft-directed immune responses are referred to as induction agents.
- Those that are used for long-term maintenance of the immunosuppressive state in the recipient are called maintenance immunosuppressives. Because of clinical implications, these two sets of therapies are considered separately.

## Induction Therapies

- Induction agents include polyclonal and monoclonal antibodies, and are also referred to as biologic agents. These therapies target the cell surface molecules of the immune competent cells.
- Polyclonal antibodies include *antithymocyte globulin* raised in horses and rabbits (Thymoglobulin, Genzyme Transplant, Cambridge, MA). Both of these commercially available agents contain antibodies against multiple T-cell surface antigens (CD2, CD3, CD4, CD5, CD8, CD11, CD18, CD28, CD45, and TCR), and cause extensive T-cell depletion.
- Monoclonal antibodies include murine monoclonal *anti-CD3 (OKT-3)* and *anti-IL-2R* antibodies *(dacluzimab and basiliximab)*. OKT3 effaces TCR complex from all T cells, rendering them incapable of recognizing alloantigens. OKT3 is rarely used as an induction agent because of its extensive side effect profile. Anti-IL-2R antibodies bind to the a-chain of IL-2 receptor, making it unavailable for IL-2 binding and subsequent cell division (blocking Signal 3).

## Maintenance Immunosuppressive Drugs

- These are pharmacologic agents capable of acting on targets inside the T cells (see Fig. 41-7) and maintaining a state of immunosuppression for the long-term viability of the allograft.
- These agents include calcineurin inhibitors, such as
- *CsA and tacrolimus (FK506)*, antiproliferative agents such as *mycophenolate mofetil (MMF)*, *azathioprine*, and *sirolimus*, and corticosteroids (prednisone, prednisolone, and methylprednisolone).

## Calcineurin Inhibitors

- *CsA* and *tacrolimus* bind to cyclophilin and FK506-binding proteins (FKBP-13), respectively, and inhibit the activity of the enzyme calcineurin.
- NFAT translocation to the nucleus is consequently blocked, preventing transcription of IL-2 and other cytokine genes.

## Antiproliferative Agents

- *Corticosteroids* act primarily on the APCs and inhibit their ability to produce IL-1 and other cytokines.
- Many cytokine genes, including IL-2, have a glucocorticoid response element (GRE) in the 5' regulatory region that serves as a target for corticosteroid and intracellular glucocorticoid receptor complex.
- Binding of this complex with GRE blocks transcription of cytokines. High-dose methylprednisolone causes lympholysis and therefore, is useful for the treatment of acute rejection (AR).
- *Azathioprine* and *MMF* act as antiproliferative agents by inhibiting de novo purine synthesis required for cell division.
- Mycophenolic acid (MPA), the active metabolite of MMF, is a potent, selective, noncompetitive and reversible inhibitor of inosine monophosphate dehydrogenase, an enzyme required for de novo purine synthesis. MPA inhibits T- and B-lymphocyte proliferation that is critically dependent on de novo purine synthesis.
- Additionally, MPA alters the expression of cell surface adhesion molecules by inhibiting glycosylation of lymphocyte and monocyte glycoproteins.
- *Sirolimus*, previously known as *rapamycin*, acts on the 'molecular target of rapamycin,' and blocks the ability of cells to enter the cell cycle.
- The immune activation cascade and points of action of common immunosuppressive agents is show in Figure 41-8.[31]

## SUMMARY

The evolution of our understanding of basic immunology has contributed greatly to the advancements in human transplantation. At present, there is a sophisticated understanding of T-cell activation and regulation that has led to a more rational approach to development of immunosuppressive/immunoregulatory agents. Advancements in basic immunology continues to hold the promise for advancements in the care and outcomes for transplant patients.

### Brief Illustrative Case

- A 49-year-old woman with sarcoidosis was being managed for severe pulmonary arterial hypertension.
- The pulmonary arterial hypertension was secondary to sarcoid-associated arteriopathy. The patient also had significant cardiac sarcoid involvement.
- Despite active treatment with pulmonary hypertension (PH)-specific therapies (continuous intravenous infusion of treprostinil and oral bosentan), she progressed to severe right-sided heart failure, requiring active intensive care unit management and stabilization.
- The patient was a candidate for combined heart-lung transplantation but was noted to have persistently elevated panel reactive antibody (PRA) tests of 85% or higher. This test indicates the patient has been exposed to HLA of other individuals. This usually occurs as a result of blood transfusions, previous pregnancies, or previous

## SITES OF ACTION OF IMMUNOSUPPRESSIVE DRUGS

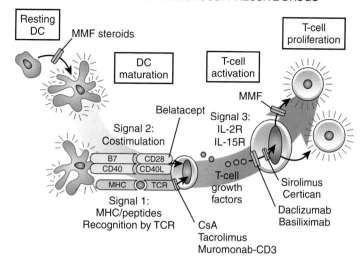

**Figure 41-8:** Immunosuppressive drugs can be categorized by their site or sites of action in the immune activation cascade. Drugs that interfere with Signal 1 include calcineurin inhibitors such as cyclosporine A (CsA) and tacrolimus. Signal 2 inhibitors are not currently available, but one drug (Belatacept) is in phase III trials for kidney transplantation and allows calcineurin-free transplantation. Signal 3 inhibitors include the antiproliferative agents such as rapamycin, mycophenolate mofetil and the IL-2 receptor blockers daclizumab and basiliximab. Understanding the sites of action of particular drugs results in more rational approaches to combination therapy (i.e., combining a Signal 1 blocker with a Signal 3 blocker).

## Brief Illustrative Case—cont'd

transplants. In her case, she had four previous pregnancies and a history of blood transfusions.

- Although actively listed for heart-lung transplantation, the patient was unable to undergo transplant surgery due to persistently positive cross-matches with prospective donors.
- She was deteriorating on the wait list and was referred for desensitization therapy with IVIG and rituximab (anti-CD20, anti-B cell). The patient received two doses of IVIG (2 g/kg per day #0, day #30) and rituximab (1 g day #7 and day #21). Repeat PRAs were checked.
- Approximately 2 months later, the PRA was 35% and later 14%. The patient received a cross-match–negative heart-lung transplant.
- She has subsequently done well without evidence of rejection or infection.

### Key Points

- The evolution of desensitization therapies represents an important new era in transplantation.

- Sensitization to HLA antigens is seen in approximately 30% of patients on the waiting list, and is more common in kidney and heart transplant candidates.
- If patients undergo transplant surgery without desensitization across a positive cross-match barrier, approximately 80% will lose their grafts at 1 year.
- The recognition of the contributions of T cells and B cells to allograft rejection episodes has led to a better understanding of immunologic processes responsible.
- Desensitization therapies including IVIG, rituximab, and plasmaphoresis, often in combination, can offer hope to patients with end stage disease with transplantable thoracic conditions, who would otherwise be denied a lifesaving therapy.

## References

 Interactive references and additional readings for this chapter can be accessed online at *expertconsult.com*.

# THE MEDIASTINUM

## 42 MASSES OF THE ANTERIOR MEDIASTINUM

Alex Hakim, MD, Curtis Sather, MD, Tej Naik, MD,
Robert J. McKenna Jr., MD, and Nader Kamangar, MD, FACP, FCCP

## MASSES OF THE THYMUS

### DEFINITIONS

- **Lymphoid follicular thymic hyperplasia (autoimmune thymitis):** Replacement of the thymic cortex with multiple lymphoid follicles and germinal centers.[1] The tissue retains its shape but may become enlarged.[2] This occurs primarily in myasthenia gravis. This form of hyperplasia can also be associated with systemic lupus erythematosus, thyrotoxicosis, and Addison's disease.[3]
- **True thymic hyperplasia:** Enlargement of the thymus without disruption of normal histological architecture.[4] It is associated with thyrotoxicosis, Graves' disease, acromegaly, and red cell aplasia.[5] Another form of true thymic hyperplasia is thymic rebound. This is the enlargement of the thymus just after the resolution of a stressful event such as chemotherapy.[2]
- **Thymolipoma:** Benign, slow-growing lesion of adipose and lymphoepithelial thymic tissue. These tumors may grow to a very large size.
- **Thymic cysts:** These are fluid-filled cysts that can be congenital or acquired. The acquired form is most common and can develop following radiation for Hodgkin's disease and be of no consequence. However, they may be seen in thymomas, lymphomas, and seminomas; therefore, they require further malignancy workup. They can also be seen in systemic inflammatory diseases such as lupus and Sjögren's syndrome.[2,5] The congenital type of thymic cyst represents a benign remnant of the thymopharyngeal duct.[6]
- **Thymoma:** Thymic neoplasm distinguishes itself from thymic carcinoma both by histology and by its indolent behavior. Once the tumor's surrounding capsule has been traversed, it is referred to as invasive thymoma.[7] This lesion is associated with paraneoplastic syndromes, which include myasthenia gravis, acquired hypogammaglobulinemia, and pure red cell aplasia.
- **Thymic lymphoma:** The thymus is most commonly invaded by the nodular sclerosing type of Hodgkin's lymphoma (HL) than any other type of lymphoma.[7] The non-Hodgkin's lymphoma (NHL) types seen most often are T-cell lymphoblastic lymphoma and primary mediastinal large B-cell lymphoma.[9,10]
- **Thymic carcinoid:** A neuroendocrine malignant disorder that is aggressive but exceedingly rare. It is associated with multiple endocrine neoplasia (MEN) 1 syndrome.

- **Thymic germ cell tumor:** They can be either benign or malignant lesions that originate from mediastinal germ cells. They include benign or malignant teratoma, seminoma, embryonal carcinoma, yolk sac tumor, choriocarcinoma, and mixed types. Seminomas are locally invasive whereas the nonseminomatous malignant germ cell tumors present frequently with distant metastatic lesions.[11]

### EPIDEMIOLOGY

- **Thymic hyperplasia:** 50% to 70% of patients with myasthenia gravis have thymic lymphoid hyperplasia.[12]
- **Thymolipoma** accounts for 1% to 10% of all thymic tumors.[13] It can affect any age group but most commonly young adults.[14]
- **Thymic cysts** are found in 3% of identified anterior mediastinal masses.[15]
- **Thymoma:** Accounts for 20% of all mediastinal tumors and 50% of anterior mediastinal masses. The overall incidence is 0.15 cases per 100,000.[16] The peak incidence is found in the fourth to sixth decades of life and equally in both genders.[17]
  - Although 34% of thymomas are found to directly invade their capsules and grow into surrounding structures and 75% of those lesions involve pleura or pericardium,[7] only 3% of thymomas metastasize outside the chest.[18,19]
  - Ten to fifteen percent of patients with myasthenia gravis are found to have thymomas. Forty percent of thymoma patients have a paraneoplastic condition, of which 20% to 25% is myasthenia gravis.[12] Ten percent of thymoma patients have hypogammaglobulinemia, and 5% to 10% have red cell aplasia.[5,20]
- **Malignant thymoma** is an indolent tumor arising from the thymic epithelial cells located in the anterior mediastinum. These tumor cells spread via regional metastases or invade surrounding structures including the pleural space.
- **Thymic lymphoma:** Of those patients newly diagnosed with Hodgkin's disease, about one third will have thymic enlargement. The thymus may be the primary site of the lymphoma or enlarged secondary to invasion of adjacent lymph nodes.[2] Two percent of patients with NHL will have thymic medullary B-cell lymphoma. It is slightly more common in women, and patients present at a median age of 30 years.[21-23]

■ **Thymic carcinoid:** Rare disorder seen in approximately 3% of patients with multiple endocrine neoplasia type 1 syndrome.[24] It has a high male predominance, and the average patient is between 30 and 40 years of age at the time of diagnosis.[24,25] This tumor is almost never associated with Cushing's syndrome or carcinoid when it is part of the MEN 1 syndrome. However, 30% to 40% of sporadic cases have Cushing's syndrome.[26,27]

■ **Thymic germ cell tumor:** The most common sites for extragonadal germ cell tumors are within or around the thymus. They are usually seen in adolescents or young adults and represent 15% of anterior mediastinal masses.[20] Sixty to eighty percent are benign, but when malignant, 90% are in men.[2,11,28] The most common type is the benign teratoma.[11] Approximately 20% of patients with nonseminomatous germ cell tumors have Klinefelter's syndrome, which is a frequent cause of mortality in these patients.[11,29]

## PATHOLOGY

■ In **true thymic hyperplasia**, the normal thymus architecture is preserved, whereas in **follicular thymic hyperplasia**, there is a replacement with multiple lymphoid follicles and germinal centers.[1,4]

■ **Thymolipoma:** Lesions contain mature adipose cells and normal thymic tissue.[14] Histologically, there are no germinal centers with the frequent presence of cystic degeneration of the Hassall bodies.[30]

■ **Thymic cyst:** Biopsy should show foci of normal tissue, because imaging studies cannot rule out the possibility of malignancy.[31]

■ **Thymoma:** Keratin-containing, p63-positive thymic epithelium characterized by no more than moderate atypia on microscopy.[32,33]

■ **Malignant thymoma:** A tissue sample is required for diagnosis of malignant thymoma and to rule out other possible diagnoses including lymphoma and thymic carcinoma. Peripherally located lesions can be accessed via computed tomography (CT)–guided core biopsy or an anterior mediastinotomy (which provides a larger piece of tissue and higher diagnostic yield), whereas paratracheal tumors may be approached via bronchoscopy or mediastinoscopy. Histolologic features consist of a mixture of keratin-positive neoplastic epithelial cells and lymphocytes subdivided by fibrous bands (Figs. 42-1 through 42-4).

■ **Thymic lymphoma:** HL shows classic Reed-Sternberg cells on microscopy with CD15 and CD30 positivity. Thymic large B-cell lymphoma is a distinct entity of B-cell lymphoma. Microscopy frequently shows mononuclear Reed-Sternberg cell variants, cells with pale "clear" cytoplasms and with clear delicate bands of fibrosis and unlike other B-cell lymphomas, often lacks surface immunoglobulin G (IgG). However, as seen in other B-cell lymphomas, it will demonstrate CD19, CD20, and CD22 positivity.[10,21,22]

■ **Thymic carcinoid:** It is a neuroendocrine tumor histologically similar to atypical bronchial carcinoids. It is characterized by homogenous polygonal cells arranged in a rosette or trabecular pattern lacking lymphocytic and epithelial components.[25,34]

■ **Thymic germ cell tumor:** Benign teratoma contains mature tissue from different cell lines such as fat, cartilage, muscle, and bone.[35] If a teratoma is found to have fetal or neuroendocrine tissue, it is considered a malignant tumor.[36]

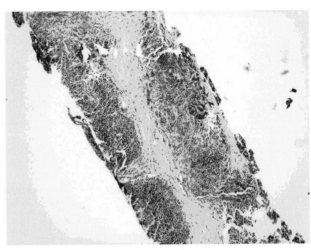

**Figure 42-1:** Histopathologic specimen obtained via computed tomography–guided core pleural biopsy shows a neoplastic proliferation composed of a mixture of lymphocytes and keratin-positive epithelial cells with fibrous bands consistent with thymoma (H&E stain, 10×).

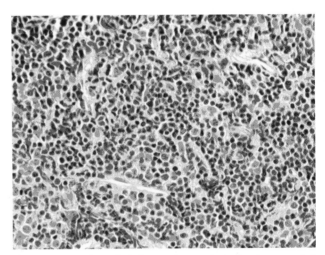

**Figure 42-2:** Histopathologic specimen obtained via computed tomography–guided core pleural biopsy shows a neoplastic proliferation composed of a mixture of lymphocytes and keratin-positive epithelial cells with fibrous bands consistent with thymoma (H&E stain, 100×).

## ANATOMIC CONSIDERATIONS

■ The thymus is a lymphopoietic organ in which T-cell maturation primarily takes place. The size and contour of this gland change dramatically over one's lifetime. At around age 20 years, 80% of the gland has undergone fatty involution, which is complete after the age of 60 years.[1]

■ The thymus, a bilobed organ at the base of the neck, travels into the anterior compartment of the mediastinum. It lies behind the manubrium and the pericardium. The inferior aspect reaches the level of the 4th rib.

■ Ectopic thymus tissue may be found in any of the mediastinal compartments and even the neck.[37] More commonly, a lobe of the thymus can be found posterior to the brachiocephalic vein.

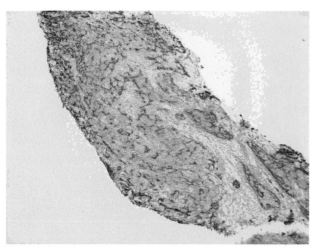

**Figure 42-3:** Histopathologic specimen obtained via computed tomography–guided core pleural biopsy shows a mixture of keratin positive neoplastic epithelial cells and lymphocytes subdivided by fibrous bands consistent with thymoma (Keratin stain, 10×).

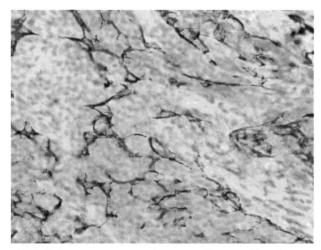

**Figure 42-4:** Histopathological specimen obtained via CT guided core pleural biopsy shows a mixture of keratin positive neoplastic epithelial cells and lymphocytes subdivided by fibrous bands consistent with thymoma (Keratin stain, 10×).

■ The blood supply of the thymus comes primarily from the internal mammary arteries via the anterior intercostal and mediastinal branches. The gland may also receive branches from the inferior thyroid arteries.

## CLINICAL FEATURES

### Clinical Presentation

■ Most thymic masses present as an incidental finding on chest imaging. For example, 90% of thymomas identified in one large study were asymptomatic at the time of diagnosis.[38]

■ Patients may complain of a nonspecific chest fullness or mild pain.

■ If the lesions are large enough to compress central pulmonary structures, they may present as recurrent lung infections or shortness of breath. Dyspnea may again be seen with associated recurrent pulmonary effusions or paralysis of the phrenic nerve due to extension of the tumor into the nerve.

■ Facial plethora may be evident secondary to compression of the superior vena cava.

■ Both **thymoma** and **follicular thymic hyperplasia** are associated with myasthenia gravis.

○ This disorder is characterized by reduction in muscle strength from somatic or autonomic muscles used repeatedly without rest.

○ The most common initial presentation, appearing in 65% of patients,[39] is that of ocular muscle weakness. The patient will note diplopia or the clinician will observe progressive ptosis in a patient asked to stare at an object without blinking.

○ Patients may complain of difficulty swallowing secondary to pharyngeal muscle weakness or dysarthria secondary to weakness in the glossal muscles.

○ In 1% of patients, the initial presentation is respiratory failure.[40]

■ Patients with **invasive thymoma** are typically diagnosed in the fourth or fifth decade of life.

○ They present with constitutional symptoms or symptoms related to tumor compression.

○ In severe cases, malignant thymoma results in superior vena cava syndrome due to local invasion and compression.

■ **Thymic lymphoma:** Owing to the fast growing nature of mediastinal B-cell lymphoma, respiratory symptoms are pronounced at onset, with 30% to 50% presenting with clinical evidence of superior vena cava obstruction. Masses larger than 10 cm at presentation are commonly seen.[21-23] The mass may even be palpable in the supraclavicular fossa.

■ **Thymic carcinoid:** These patients may present with a history of parathyroid, enteropancreatic endocrine tissue (insulinoma) and/or anterior pituitary gland neoplasms as part of the MEN 1 syndrome. The tumor progresses insidiously, and the majority of patients present with an abnormal chest x-ray (CXR), chest CT, or gradual chest discomfort.[34] The rare patients who have clinical carcinoid syndrome will complain of episodic facial flushing accompanied by a presyncopal sensation. They may also complain of frequent diarrhea. Cushing's syndrome is more commonly seen than carcinoid syndrome when the patient does not have MEN 1 syndrome.[41] The presentation of Cushing's syndrome includes progressive obesity with characteristic large fat pads behind the neck and above the clavicles, poorly controlled chronic hypertension, skin atrophy, and purple abdominal striae.

■ **Thymic germ cell tumor:** Patients with benign teratomas can have large mediastinal masses without any symptoms.[11] However, teratomas can cause local injury if they contain active pancreatic tissue producing amylase. In this setting, the patient may present with recurrent effusions, chest pain, tamponade via inflammation of the surrounding tissues, or a cough that may lead to expectoration of the oily contents of the teratoma.[11]

## DIAGNOSTIC STUDIES

### Laboratory Studies

■ Seventy to ninety percent of patients with myasthenia gravis have a positive acetylcholine receptor antibody test, and this test is extremely specific for the disease.[42]

■ In red cell aplasia, the patient has profound anemia with a reticulocyte count of virtually zero.

■ If **thymic carcinoid** is suspected, the patient may have elevated parathyroid levels with hypercalcemia, elevated prolactin, serotonin, gastrin or insulin levels as part of the multiple MEN 1 syndrome.

- When not part of the MEN 1 syndrome, **thymic carcinoid** may cause Cushing's syndrome. This can be diagnosed by showing an elevated 24-hour urinary excretion of cortisol. These patients are also at risk for carcinoid syndrome, the diagnosis of which is achieved through the measurement of 24-hour serotonin (5-hydroxyindoleacetic acid) urinary excretion. This test is 75% sensitive and almost 100% specific.[43]
- More aggressive **thymic germ cell tumors** such as choriocarcinomas, embryonal cell carcinomas, and yolk sac tumors typically express alpha-fetoprotein (AFP) or human chorionic gonadotropin (hCG).[11]

## Imaging Studies

- Positron emission tomography (PET) Scan
  - ○ Not commonly used to classify thymic masses as young adults or people following stressful events can show an increase in fluorodeoxyglucose (FDG) uptake with a normal thymus.[44] The PET scan does not differentiate between thymic hyperplasia and a thymic malignancy. It can be used to look for nodal or distant metastases.[2]
- CT Scan
  - ○ The maximum anteroposterior diameter for a normal thymus is 1.8 cm for people younger than 20 years of age and 1.3 cm in older people.[45]
  - ○ Thymoma
    - Appears as a homogenous, well-defined mass extending to one side of the anterior mediastinum that is usually 5 to 10 cm at the time of diagnosis.[2] They are usually not associated with adenopathy (Fig. 42-5).
    - Thymomas may have areas of calcification and may extend to and even traverse the diaphragm via the retrocrural space.
    - Other radiographic features that are more commonly seen with invasive thymomas include calcification or cystic spaces within the mass and local invasion with pleural effusion and thickening. It is unusual for the disease to present as a massive pleural and mediastinal based mass (Fig. 42-6).
    - In severe cases, a malignant thymoma can invade the superior vena cava (Fig. 42-7).

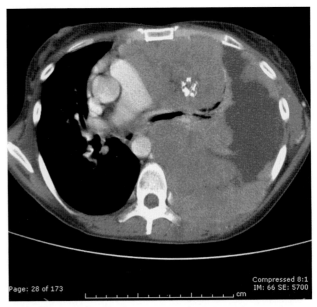

**Figure 42-6:** Contrast-enhanced computed tomography scan shows a large mediastinal- and pleural-based mass with calcification and loculated pleural effusion. Histopathologic analysis demonstrated an invasive thymoma.

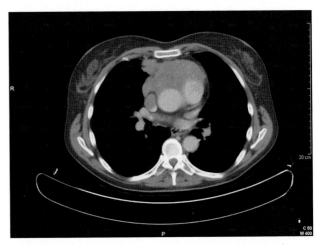

**Figure 42-7:** Contrast-enhanced computed tomography scan shows a homogeneously enhancing anterior mediastinal mass with invasion of the superior vena cava. Histopathologic analysis demonstrated an invasive thymoma.

- The CT scan should be performed with intravenous (IV) contrast (preferably given in an IV in the left arm) to assess the brachiocephalic vessels for surgical consideration.
- The images can show occlusion; however, they are imprecise for distinguishing vessel abutment from invasion.[46]
  - ○ **Thymolipoma:** It appears as a mediastinal mass of fat or soft tissue attenuation connected to the thymus by a small pedicle.[30] This mass is often described as bell shaped. It may also appear as diffuse fatty involvement without a discrete lesion.[2] Thymolipomas may be very large.
  - ○ **Thymic cyst:** Cystic structures with clearly defined walls form classic thymic cysts (Fig. 42-8). Congenital lesions are usually unilocular, whereas acquired lesions are multilocular.[2] Thymic cysts may be associated with thymomas or

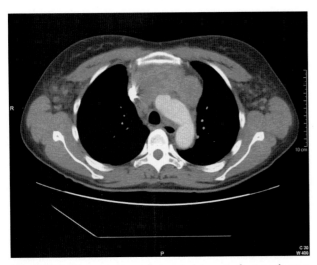

**Figure 42-5:** Contrast-enhanced computed tomography scan shows a partially lobulated, homogeneously enhancing anterior mediastinal mass. Histopathologic analysis demonstrated an invasive thymoma.

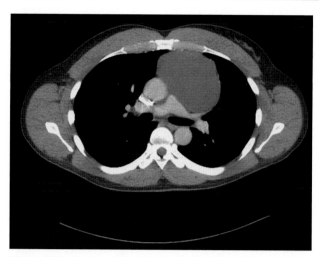

**Figure 42-8:** Contrast-enhanced computed tomography scan shows a homogeneous, smooth anterior mediastinal mass with water density attenuation and well-defined cyst walls. Histopathologic analysis demonstrated a cystic thymoma.

lymphoma. Resection is the only way to absolutely differentiate between a benign cyst versus a cystic thymoma or lymphoma.

○ **Thymic germ cell tumor:** Teratomas usually are well-defined, round lesions with cystic and solid areas. Areas of fat and calcification may be present and represent the different tissue types within.[2,20] Lesions lacking clear margins or distinct tissue types are more likely to be malignant. Teratoma usually contain an oily substance and may contain structures such as teeth.

■ Magnetic resonance imaging (MRI) scan
○ **Thymoma:** The MRI scan may assess invasion better than a CT scan (Fig. 42-9). The thymoma generally has similar signal characteristics to normal thyroid tissue and usually enhances homogenously; however, evidence of cyst formation, hemorrhage, and necrosis may also be seen.[2,5]

■ Nuclear imaging
○ **Octreotide scan:** A radiolabeled somatostatin analogue is administered and has been found to bind to more than

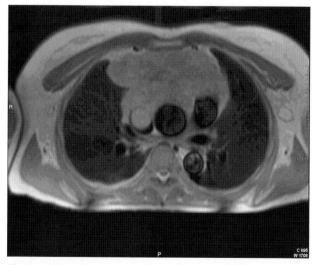

**Figure 42-9:** Magnetic resonance imaging scan showing an anterior mediastinal mass with clear invasion of the superior vena cava. Histopathologic analysis demonstrated an invasive thymoma.

80% of neuroendocrine tumors, such as **thymic carcinoid**, to aid in tumor identification and localization.[47]

■ Other testing
○ **Edrophonium (tensilon) test:** This is the most rapid test for myasthenia gravis in which a cholinesterase inhibitor is administered in a carefully monitored condition to clinically observe for reversal of the characteristic weakness of the disorder. This test is 90% sensitive[48] but may be falsely positive in a number of neuromuscular conditions.
○ **Electromyography (EMG):** Repetitive stimulation electromyography is only 50% sensitive for myasthenia gravis unless single-fiber EMG is used, which boosts the sensitivity to 90%.[49] The single-fiber EMG is a specialized test not commonly available in most hospitals.

## Tissue Diagnosis

■ If tumor markers (β-hCG and alpha-feto protein) are elevated, the diagnosis is mediastinal germ cell tumor so no tissue diagnosis is needed.

■ Otherwise, the appearance of the lesion on CT scan helps if an incisional biopsy or a resection should be performed. A thymectomy should be performed for small, apparently encapsulated lesions. Larger masses with indistinct margins should be biopsied first to determine if the mass is a lymphoma or to diagnose a stage 3 thymoma for neoadjuvant treatment.[46]

■ If a resectable thymoma is suspected, it is usually resected through a median sternotomy.

■ If lymphoma is suspected, an anterior mediastinotomy (Chamberlain procedure) is performed to obtain adequate tissue for diagnosis. This involves a 3- to 4-cm incision over the cartilaginous portion of the second rib. This is usually an outpatient procedure. Intraoperative frozen sections as well as fine-needle aspirations (FNAs) are poor at distinguishing between lymphomas and thymomas.[46,50] The surgeon usually waits till the permanent section slides are available to decide to proceed with thymectomy for thymoma. FNA does not provide enough material for flow cytometry. A core needle biopsy may provide sufficient material to make the diagnosis.[46]

■ Patients in whom lymphoma is suspected should be examined for lymphadenopathy because performing tissue biopsy from an easy-to-access lymph node is far easier than obtaining tissue directly from the thymus.

## *PROGNOSIS*

■ **Thymolipoma:** This tumor is not associated with any malignancy, or immunologic or endocrine disorders. Surgical removal is curative.

■ **Thymoma:** Lesions in which the capsule remains intact (noninvasive thymomas) have an 80% 5-year survival rate. Those lesions that invade beyond the capsule (invasive thymomas) have only a 23% 5-year survival rate.[51] Owing to advancements in the management of myasthenia gravis, this paraneoplastic syndrome does not affect prognosis.[18,33]

■ **Thymic lymphoma:**
○ Primary mediastinal large B-cell lymphoma, unlike diffuse B-cell lymphoma, rarely extends to extrathoracic structures. However, it aggressively invades lung, pericardium and even breast.[52] Rarely, this tumor can involve bone marrow, and a bone marrow biopsy is required for accurate staging.
○ Typical chemotherapy regimens for mediastinal large B-cell lymphoma have an approximate 70% survival rate after 2 years[53]; however, some newer chemotherapy trials have shown initial survival rates of greater than 90%.[21]

○ Bulky tumors (greater than 50% of the transverse diameter of the chest) have a worse prognosis.

○ The most widely recognized predictor of outcome for primary mediastinal B-cell lymphoma is the level of success of the initial round of chemotherapy.[23] Because there is a poor correlation between the size of the residual mediastinal mass post-chemotherapy and the rate of recurrence, nuclear imaging is of great value. A bulky mediastinal mass that remains after a round of therapy can represent simply a collection of fibrotic tissue.[54]

○ There are many other types of thymic lymphomas that are associated with extremely high mortality rates, but they are exceedingly rare.

■ **Thymic carcinoid:** This condition has a poor prognosis, with more than 70% of patients developing metastases within 5 years.[55] However, the tumors may progress slowly so that long-term survival with distant metastases does occur.

■ **Thymic germ cell tumor:** It is very rare for mature teratomas to transform into cancer, and generally resection of teratomas is curative.[11] Malignant germ cell tumors account for 1% to 4% of mediastinal tumors.[11] Among the malignant germ cell tumors, seminomas have a considerably better prognosis because they are very responsive to radiation and chemotherapy. They have a 60% to 80% long-term survival rate.[11,56-58] The nonseminomatous germ cell tumors are much more aggressive, with 85% to 95% presenting with at least one metastasis.[59] Even with aggressive therapy, few of these patients live beyond 1 year and almost no patients have survived beyond 5 years.[11]

## TREATMENT

■ For treatment of myasthenia gravis, in one large study, therapeutic or prophylactic thymectomy has shown no advantage over medical management of the illness alone. This retrospective review of 1976 patients from 1940 to 2000[38] showed that medical management alone produced increasingly better remission rates than a thymectomy. However, certain scenarios did show significant benefit of thymectomy, such as in women who are ventilator dependent. Other series have shown significant benefit to thymectomy, with a 40% complete remission for myasthenia gravis after thymectomy and improvement in another 40%.

■ Thymoma:

○ The Masaoka stage is currently the most widely used staging system for thymomas and helps to determine the management plan (Table 42-1).[60]

■ Stage I malignant thymoma demonstrates encapsulation without microscopic capsular invasion.

■ Stage II disease involves invasion of mediastinum or microscopic capsular invasion.

■ Stage III malignant thymomas show invasion into surrounding structures, including the pericardium, great vessels, and lung.

■ Stage IVA malignant thymoma involves the pleural or the pericardial metastases.

■ Stage IVB disease includes lymphogenous or hematogenous metastases.[60]

■ Chemotherapy and radiation improve survival for patients with stage III or IV thymomas.[61-63] These are typically performed in a neoadjuvant setting.

■ Postoperative radiation for stage II patients is controversial, but a recent meta-analysis showed no difference in prognosis with that of stage I patients, with or without irradiation.

■ Surgery: Complete surgical removal of the tumor, thymus, and surrounding fat is the common practice for stage I to II

### TABLE 42-1 ■ MASAOKA STAGING SYSTEM FOR THYMOMA

| Stage | Characteristics |
|---|---|
| Stage I | Macroscopically encapsulated with no microscopically detectable capsular invasion |
| Stage II | Macroscopic invasion of mediastinal fatty tissue or mediastinal pleura, or microscopic invasion into the capsule |
| Stage III | Macroscopic invasion into surrounding structures (pericardium, great vessels, lung) |
| Stage IV A | Pleural or pericardial dissemination |
| Stage IV B | Lymphogenous or hematogenous metastases |

*From Masaoka A, Monden Y, Nakahara K, et al. Follow-up study of thymomas with special reference to their clinical stages. Cancer 1981;48:2485-2492.*

thymomas. Leaving any residual tissue has been associated with a reoccurrence of myasthenia gravis.[46]

○ Technique

■ Thymectomy may be performed transcervically, with video-assisted thoracic surgery (VATS), or with a median sternotomy. Most surgeons prefer to use a median sternotomy for thymectomy if there is a tumor. VATS can be used if the tumor is small and for thymectomy in myasthenia gravis when there is no tumor. The VATS approaches include right VATS, left VATS, bilateral VATS, and unilateral VATS with a neck incision to facilitate removal of the horns of the thymus.

■ In stages I and II, the goal of the thymectomy is a complete anterior mediastinal exenteration, including the thymus, thymic horns that end on the inferior border of the thyroid, and pericardial fat pad. Basically, all the tissue from the pericardium to the inner table of the sternum and from the diaphragm to the thyroid is resected. Structures invaded by the tumor, such as the pleura, lung, pericardium, and an occluded innominate vein may also be resected.[46] Approximately 30% of what was considered preoperatively to be stage I will be found to have invasive disease.[7]

■ In stages III to IVa, a median sternotomy is used with aggressive resection of any of the invaded structures because a complete removal (R0 resection) may be curative. Such patients may require wedge resections of invaded lung, reconstruction of an invaded superior vena cava, and even sacrificing of an invaded phrenic nerve. Myocardial invasion makes complete resection impossible; however, aggressive debulking may be associated with improved long-term survival.[64]

■ **Thymic lymphoma:** The treatment of HL is complex and outside the scope of this chapter. Mediastinal primary B-cell lymphoma is generally treated with anthracycline-based chemotherapy with frequent restaging because this tumor can progress during treatment. Some sources recommend high-dose chemotherapy, followed by autologous stem cell transplantation because it is tolerated well by the predominantly young patient population. Local radiation is also appropriate following the initial round of chemotherapy in stage I and nonbulky stage II disease.[23] T-cell lymphoblastic lymphoma is a rare tumor type for which the primary therapy also includes chemotherapy and irradiation. The role of surgery for this disease is limited to the initial biopsy for diagnosis or repeat biopsy of a residual mass after treatment to determine if there is scarring or a residual cancer. However, the exact management of this malignancy is still controversial.

- **Thymic carcinoid:** Prophylactic thymectomy is recommended in patients during parathyroidectomy in the setting of the multiple endocrine neoplasia type 1 syndrome due to the high mortality of thyroid carcinoid should it present itself. In addition, thymectomy may remove ectopic parathyroid glands.[25,34] The incidence of an ectopic parathyroid located within thymic tissue ranges from 12% to 39%.[65-68]
- **Thymic germ cell tumor:** Benign teratomas should be completely excised because there is a small risk of malignant transformation. Seminomas are extremely radiosensitive, and local radiation combined with perioperative cisplatin-based chemotherapy has been very effective.[11] Surgical resection of nonseminomatous tumors is challenging and associated with a 4% mortality rate given the extensive invasion at time of diagnosis.[59] Persistent elevation of tumor markers means persistent cancer; however, if the markers normalize and there is a residual mass, the thymus should be resected en bloc to determine if there is residual scar, benign teratoma, or persistent cancer.[69] Analysis of the surgical pathology will help determine the need for additional chemotherapy.
- **Complications**
  - Mortality for thymectomy should be less than 2%, even for patients requiring extensive resections.[46]
  - Rates of injury to the phrenic or recurrent laryngeal nerves in thymectomy has been as much as 2%[55]; however, many trials have shown no such complications.[71-73]
  - The anesthesiologist should take extra consideration in the choice in neuromuscular blockers in the setting of patients with myasthenia gravis.
  - In patients who undergo mediastinal irradiation for thymic tumors, adverse consequences include the following:
    - Pneumonitis, first presenting itself 1 to 3 months after exposure.[74]
    - Cardiac complications include coronary artery disease, pericarditis, cardiomyopathy and valvular heart disease.[75] The risk of cardiovascular death has been shown to be proportional to the amount of radiation exposure in patients who have received mediastinal irradiation for Hodgkin's disease.
    - Exposure of the great vessels to radiation has been known to cause radiation-induced vasculopathy as late as 10 years following the initial insult.[74,76] However, modern irradiation techniques have greatly reduced this risk.
    - Radiation increases the risk of lung cancer by 50%, and the incidence of radiation-induced chest sarcomas is about 0.3%.[77,78]

# LYMPHOMA

## *DEFINITION*

Primary mediastinal lymphoma is a type of solid neoplasm that originates in lymphocytes usually in lymphoid tissue contained within the mediastinum. It is generally a rare entity; however, when it does occur, lymphoma usually occurs in the anterior mediastinum and may be associated with widespread disease. HL comprises the majority of lymphoma in the anterior mediastinum, whereas NHL comprises a smaller percentage.

## *EPIDEMIOLOGY*

- The three most common histological types of mediastinal lymphoma are HL, large B-cell lymphoma, and lymphoblastic lymphoma.[79]
- Primary mediastinal lymphoma is a distinct clinical subset of lymphoma and comprises about 10% of lymphoma in the mediastinum.[80,81]

### Hodgkin's Lymphoma

- Represents 50% to 75% of mediastinal lymphomas
- Has an incidence of approximately 2 to 4 cases per 100,000 people per year[82]
- Shows a bimodal distribution incidence peaking in young adulthood and again after age 50 years.[82]
- For mediastinal-predominant disease, prevalence peaks in young women during the third decade of life, whereas it is unaffected by age in men.[83]
- Of the four subtypes, the nodular sclerosing subtype represents more than two thirds of cases.[84]

### Non-Hodgkin's Lymphoma

- Represents 15% to 25% of mediastinal lymphomas
- The overall incidence of NHL is greatest in those with a mean age of 55 years old.[85]
- Demographically, the incidence is higher in white men
- Large B-cell lymphoma[85,86]
  - Mean age of presentation is 30 to 35 years old.
  - Bimodal age distribution is seen.
    - First peak is seen between 33 and 39 years of age.
      - The female-to-male ratio is 2:1.
      - High frequency of occurrence in the anterior mediastinum
    - Second peak is seen in men at a mean age of 65 years.
- Lymphoblastic lymphoma
  - Generally, a disease of children and adolescent boys
  - Can be seen in all age groups
  - The mean age is 28 years old.[87]

## *PATHOLOGY*

### Hodgkin's Lymphoma

- Nodular sclerosing is the most common subtype.
  - Shows nodular collections of lymphoid tissue
  - Lobules are separated by dense bands of fibrous proliferation.
  - The presence of Reed-Sternberg (RS) cells is pathognomonic for HL
    - The RS cells seen in mediastinal HL often has a lacunar morphology.[88]
      - Show prominent nucleoli, multilobed nuclei on a background of clear cytoplasm
      - Classic RS cells show bilobed nuclei (owl's eyes) with eosinophilic nucleoli

### Diffuse Large B-cell Lymphoma

- Mediastinal large B-cell lymphoma comprises 7% to 10% of all diffuse large B-cell lymphomas and about 2.5% of all NHL.[89,90]
- Thought to arise from medullary B-cells in the thymus.[91-93]
  - Tumor consists of large lymphoid cells with nuclear morphology that may resemble centroblasts, large centrocytes, or multilobed cells.
    - Nuclear pleomorphism can be so prominent that the neoplasm resembles an anaplastic carcinoma or sarcoma.[94]
    - Also seen is diffuse proliferation of large cells with abundant eosinophilic cytoplasm, large vesicular nuclei, and prominent nucleoli.

○ Ten percent of mediastinal B-cell lymphomas exhibit a prominent clearing of the cytoplasm, a variant that has been referred to as primary mediastinal clear cell lymphoma of B-cell origin.[95]
▪ Presence of sclerosing stroma is very characteristic seen in 38% to 100% of cases.[96]
○ This sclerosing stroma of thick hyaline connective tissues can separate the tumor into epithelial nests.
○ This can sometimes mimic the appearance of a seminoma or carcinoma.

### Lymphoblastic Lymphoma
▪ Highly aggressive leukemia/lymphoma[97]
○ Classified by The Revised European American Lymphoma Classification (REAL) classification as a precursor B-lymphoblastic or precursor T-lymphoblastic leukemia/lymphoma.
○ Acute lymphoblastic leukemia (ALL), which is considered to be the leukemic phase of this leukemia/lymphoma.
▪ Characterized by diffuse infiltrate non-cohesive lymphoid cells[98]
○ Cells are of intermediate size and show scanty cytoplasm with very fine nuclear chromatin.
▪ Nucleoli are usually absent, and there are a high number of mitotic figures per high power field.
○ Lack of a dense fibrous stroma and may show a prominent admixture of tingible body macrophages
○ This can give a characteristic "starry sky" appearance on histopathology.

## ANATOMIC CONSIDERATIONS
▪ Knowledge of mediastinal anatomy is important in determining the etiology of masses and the surgical approach.[99]
▪ The mediastinum is generally divided into four compartments (Fig. 42-10).
○ Anterior mediastinum
▪ Anterior border is the sternum
▪ Posterior border is the heart and brachiocephalic vessels
▪ Superior border is the aortic arch
▪ Inferiorly border is the diaphragm
○ Superior mediastinum
▪ Sternum to the vertebral bodies
▪ Top of aortic arch to the thoracic inlet
▪ Note: anterior and superior compartments may be combined into one compartment (anterosuperior compartment)
○ Middle mediastinum
▪ Bounded by the pericardial sac
▪ Superior border is the fourth thoracic vertebrae
○ Posterior mediastinum
▪ Anterior border is the posterior border of the heart and the trachea
▪ Posterior border are the thoracic vertebrae

## CLINICAL FEATURES
### Hodgkin's Lymphoma
▪ A large proportion of patients develop systemic symptoms before the discovery of lymphadenopathy.
○ Typical "B" symptoms of fever, weight loss, and night sweats, and weight loss are common.
▪ Pel-Ebstein fever is the characteristic, although uncommon, intermittent fever associated with HL.
○ Recurs at variable intervals of several days or weeks and lasts for 1 to 2 weeks before waning.[100]

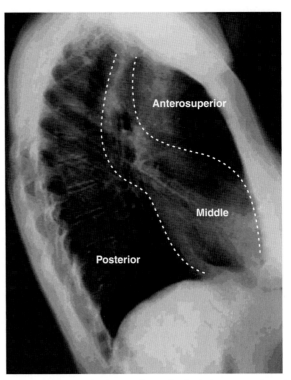

**Figure 42-10:** Lateral chest radiograph depicting anatomic subdivisions of the mediastinum. *(From Townsend CM, Beauchamp RD, Evers BM, Mattos KL, editors. Sabiston textbook of general surgery. 17th ed. New York: Elsevier; 2004.)*

○ Additional symptoms include fatigue, pruritus, and chest pain with injestion of alcohol.
▪ 60% of patients have mediastinal adenopathy at the time of diagnosis.[101]
▪ Common presentation is the incidental finding of a mediastinal mass on a radiograph.
○ These can often be large and asymptomatic.
○ Rarely causes pleural/pericardial effusions
○ Bulky mediastinal disease may cause superior vena cava (SVC) syndrome
○ Can cause symptoms like chest pain, dyspnea, and cough, but these are also uncommon.

### Primary Mediastinal Large B-cell Lymphoma[85]
▪ Frequently present with locally invasive anterior mediastinal mass
▪ Usually originating in the thymus
▪ Presents frequently with airway compromise and SVC syndrome[102]
○ A report of 30 patients showed SVC syndrome was present in 57% of those patients.
○ Eighty percent of patients had radiographic signs of SVC involvement, even without clinical syndrome.
○ Pleural and pericardial effusions were also common.
▪ Relapses tend to be in tissues outside of the lymph nodes.[102]
○ Liver, gastrointestinal tract, kidneys, ovaries, and central nervous system are common sites.

### Lymphoblastic Lymphoma
▪ Can be very aggressive and present very dramatically when mediastinum is involved[103]

○ Mediastinal mass is present in 80% of patients at presentation.
○ Can have common symptoms of cough, dyspnea, and wheezing
○ Tracheal compression causes stridor.
○ SVC syndrome, cardiac tamponade, and tracheal obstruction are more life-threatening presentations that have been known to occur with this type of lymphoma.
■ Generally present with more advanced disease[99]
○ Extranodal involvement
○ Generalized lymphadenopathy

## DIAGNOSTIC STUDIES

### Biopsy

■ Tissue biopsy is necessary for all types of HL and NHL in order to guide management.
■ Mediastinal nodes may be biopsied with mediastinoscopy, mediastinotomy, or endobronchial ultrasound (EBUS). If there is a large anterior mediastinal mass, paralysis with induction of anesthesia may lead to tracheal compression that can occasionally be life-threatening. In these cases, awake intubation may be indicated.
■ Morphology on histologic examination as well as immunophenotyping play key roles in determining treatment.
○ HL[104]
■ Immunohistochemical profile is usually biomarker positive for CD15 and CD30 cells.
■ Important negative biomarkers include LCA (CD45RO) and keratin.
○ The absence of keratin excludes thymoma from the diagnosis.
○ NHL
■ Large B-cell lymphoma[105]
○ Usually express B-cell–associated antigens, which include CD19, CD20, CD22, and CD79a.
○ They are also usually CD45 positive and CD15 negative.
○ Markers such as HMB-45, keratin, and placental alkaline phosphatase (PLAP) should be tested to exclude other possible tumors, i.e., melanoma, thymoma, and seminomas.
○ Rarely are of T-cell origin and show markers consistent with that immunophenotype.
■ Lymphoblastic lymphoma[106]
○ In more than 80% of cases, the cells are of T-cell origin
○ A wide spectrum is seen in terms of differentiation: (1) Early—CD2, CD5, and CD7 positive; CD1, CD3, CD4, and CD8 negative; (2) Intermediate—CD1, CD2, CD5, CD7, CD4 and CD8 positive; CD3 negative; (3) Mature—CD2, CD3, CD5, CD7, CD4 and CD8 positive; (4) Study showed that the majority of a series of 31 T-cell lymphoblastic lymphomas were intermediate (62%); (5) Also showed that terminal deoxynucleotidyl transferase (TdT) was virtually positive in all cases, which can also serve as a marker.

### Imaging Studies

■ CXR study
○ The chest radiograph is abnormal in up to 76% of patients with HL (Table 42-2)
■ Shows enlargement of paratracheal and prevascular lymph nodes[107]
○ Not as helpful in NHL[108]

| Site Involved | Hodgkin's Disease, % (n = 164) | Non-Hodgkin's Disease, % (n = 136) |
|---|---|---|
| Intrathoracic disease (any site) | 67 | 43 |
| Anterior mediastinum | 46 | 13 |
| Tracheobronchial nodes | 45 | 13 |
| Paratracheal nodes | 40 | 13 |
| Hilar nodes | 21 | 8 |
| Subcarinal nodes | 11 | 4 |
| Internal mammary nodes | 7 | 1 |
| Posterior mediastinum | 5 | 11 |
| Lung | 12 | 5 |
| Pleura | 7 | 11 |

**TABLE 42-2 ■ RADIOGRAPHIC DISTRIBUTION OF INTRATHORACIC ABNORMALITIES IN UNTREATED LYMPHOMA (PERCENTAGE OF PATIENTS WITH POSITIVE FINDINGS)**

*Adapted from Filly R, Blank N, Castellino RA. Radiographic distribution of intrathoracic disease in previously untreated patients with Hodgkin's disease and non-Hodgkin's lymphoma. Radiology 1976;120:277-281.*

■ Less than half of all patients with NHL have abnormal chest radiographs.
■ Half of patients have isolated intrathoracic nodal disease that does not involve the paratracheal or prevascular nodes.[109]
■ CT Scan
○ HL
■ Eighty-five percent of patients with newly diagnosed HL have thoracic involvement on chest CT scans[109] (Fig. 42-11).
■ Mediatinal involvement includes[110]
○ Discrete lymph nodes
○ Bulky, matted nodes
○ Discrete or infiltrating thymic mass

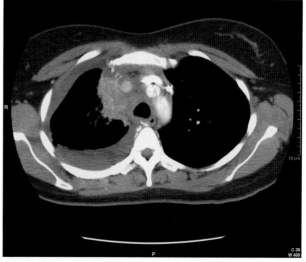

**Figure 42-11:** Contrast-enhanced computed tomography scan shows bulky anterior mediastinal adenopathy with associated loculated pleural effusion. Histopathologic analysis demonstrated nodular sclerosing Hodgkin's lymphoma.

- Typically are homogenous and have the same attenuation as that of soft tissue
- Larger masses with coalescent nodes can demonstrate heterogenous areas, which may represent areas of necrosis and even hemorrhage.
  - NHL[111]
    - Helpful in determining the extent of disease in patients with early-stage disease
    - Helps to determine radiation portals in patients with no other extrathoracic disease
    - Determining recurrence in patients that have already been treated
      - More limited in patients with advanced stage disease that were untreated.
      - Patients with normal chest radiographs that had been treated.
- MRI (not usually used for evaluation of lymphoma)
  - HL[110]
    - Shows a homogenous mass
      - Low signal intensity on T1-weighted imaging
      - High signal intensity on T2-weighted images
      - T2-weighted MRIs can demonstrate increased signal intensity from baseline to help differentiate disease recurrence versus residual fibrotic mass after therapy
  - NHL
    - Has a role in distinguishing residual disease in those patients that have been treated[111]
- Nuclear Imaging[111]
  - PET scanning can be especially useful for staging and disease response for both NHL and HL[112]

## PROGNOSIS

### Hodgkin's Lymphoma

- Staging is usually done clinically according to the Ann Arbor classification,[113] which was subsequently modified at the Cotswold's conference (Table 42-3).[114]

---

**TABLE 42-3 ▪ COTSWOLD MODIFICATION OF ANN ARBOR STAGING OF HODGKIN'S LYMPHOMA AND NON-HODGKIN'S LYMPHOMA**

| Stage | Characteristics |
| --- | --- |
| 1 | Involvement of one lymph node region or lymphoid structure |
| 2 | Two or more lymph node regions on same side of the diaphragm |
| 3 | Lymph nodes on both sides of the diaphragm |
| 4 | Involvement of extra nodal sites |
| Modifications | |
| A | No symptoms |
| B | Fever, night sweats, weight loss >10% in 6 months |
| X | Bulky disease (greater than one third widening of the mediastinum or >10 cm diameter of nodal mass) |
| E | Involvement of single, contiguous, or extra nodal site |

*Adapted from Yung L, Linch D. Hodgkin's lymphoma. Lancet 2003; 361: 943–951.*

---

- Extranodal and bulky disease
  - Extranodal ("e") refers to extranodal contiguous extension (i.e., proximal or contiguous extranodal disease) that can be encompassed within an irradiation field appropriate for nodal disease of the same anatomic extent.
    - The importance of extranodal disease on prognosis is that it shows a striking difference between patients with essentially localized extralymphatic organ involvement, which is contiguous with an involved lymph node region, and disseminated extralymphatic involvement.[115]
  - "X" is used if bulky disease is present.
    - Can have an important role in prognosis and treatment especially with disease in the mediastinum.
    - A node or nodal mass must be 10 cm or greater to be recorded as bulky.
    - Bulky also refers to wide transverse diameter of the mediastinal mass on a standard posteroanterior chest radiogram greater than one third of the maximal diameter of the chest wall at its pleural surfaces, usually at the level of the diaphragm.[116,117]
- There have been numerous studies to identify prognostic factors
  - Distinguishing between favorable and unfavorable especially in early stage (stages I and II) disease.
  - The main prognostic factors
    - Presence of "B" symptoms (designate stage A for absent or B for present)[118]
    - Erythrocyte sedimentation rate (ESR) and both the number of involved sites and the bulk of disease[119]
  - For advanced disease (stages III and IV), International Prognostic Score (IPS),[120] includes the following unfavorable markers:
    - Serum albumin less than 4 g/dL (40 g/L)
    - Hemoglobin less than 10.5 g/dL (105 g/L)
    - Male gender
    - Age older than 45 years
    - Stage IV disease
    - White blood cell count 15,000/μL or more
    - Lymphocyte count less than 600/μL, or less than 8% of the white blood cell count
  - The presence of a greater number of these factors predicted a higher chance of lack of freedom from disease at 5 years.

### NHL

- Ann Arbor staging classification
- Modified for staging of NHL[121]
  - Focuses on number of tumor sites—nodal or extranodal
  - Location
  - Presence or absence of "B" symptoms
- This staging system has been proven to be much less useful for NHL than for HL.
  - NHL frequently metastasizes through hematogenous routes.
- Prognosis is far more dependent on histopathology.
  - Secondarily influenced by clinical parameters, including age, presence of extranodal disease, performance status, and stage (I/II versus III/IV).
- Thus, staging in most cases of NHL as a group focuses more on the identification of early-stage (I/II) and late-stage (III/IV) disease.
  - The following factors are associated with shorter disease free survival and shorter overall survival:
    - Age older than 60
    - Serum lactate dehydrogenase (LDH) concentration greater than normal

- Eastern Cooperative Oncology Group (ECOG) performance status of 2 or more
- Ann Arbor clinical stage III or IV
- More than one involved extranodal disease site.
  - Presence of each factor gives 1 point
    - Low risk—international prognostic index (IPI) score of zero or one
    - Low intermediate risk—IPI score of two
    - High intermediate risk—IPI score of three
    - High risk—IPI score of four or five
  - Five-year overall survivals for scores:
    - of 0 to 1, 73%
    - 2, 51%
    - 3, 43%
    - 4 to 5, 26%,

## TREATMENT

### Hodgkin's Lymphoma

- Chemotherapy either alone or combined with radiotherapy has converted HL from a uniformly fatal disease to one that is curable in approximately 75% of patients worldwide.[122]
- Stage I-II—poor prognosis[123]
  - ESR greater than 50 mm/h
  - ESR greater than 30 mm/h in the presence of B symptoms
  - Mediastinal mass exceeding 0.35 of the intrathoracic diameter at T5/6
  - Four or more sites of disease
- Treatment[123]
  - Doxorubicin, bleomycin, vinblastine, and dacarbazine (ABVD) for three to four cycles.
    - Followed by irradiation to the involved field of 30 Gy (36 Gy in some patients) to the initially involved lymph node site.
  - Alternative is chemotherapy alone for six cycles or radiation therapy alone with larger fields.
  - Lower relapse rate in the first regimen.
- Stage IIIA
  - Combination chemotherapy with total nodal irradiation in patients with non-bulky and limited upper abdominal disease
- Stage IIIB
  - Chemotherapy usually with ABVD is the primary treatment option.
  - There are newer regimens being studied, i.e., the Stanford V protocol.[124,125]
    - Doxorubicin, vinblastine, mechlorethamine, vincristine, bleomycin, etoposide, and prednisone, combined with radiation to bulky lymph node sites 5 cm or more in diameter (Stanford V regimen) in patients with bulky mediastinal stage II, stage III, or stage IV disease.
- Stage IV
  - Chemotherapy with ABVD is the primary modality with nodal irradiation in patients with bulky disease sites.

### NHL

- Mediastinal large B-cell lymphoma[126-134]
  - At present, standard of care is to use combination chemotherapy with cyclophosphamide, doxorubicin, vincristine, and prednisone (CHOP).
  - This is usually used in conjunction with Rituximab (R-CHOP).
  - In limited-stage disease, radiation therapy is usually added.
- Lymphoblastic lymphoma/leukemia[103,106,126-128]
  - Treated in a similar fashion to ALL.

- Induction—patients generally enter complete remission (CR) after this therapy.
- Consolidation—for 4 to 6 months after achievement of CR
- Maintenance—24 to 36 months after finishing consolidation phase,
- Prophylactic central nervous system CNS radiation if CR attained.

## PRIMARY MEDIASTINAL GERM CELL TUMORS

### DEFINITION

- Mediastinal germ cell tumors (GCTs) are a heterogeneous group of benign and malignant neoplasms with histology identical to some neoplasms of the testicle and ovary. They are thought to derive from an interruption of the migration of primitive germ cells from the urogenital ridge to the gonads during early embryogenesis.[135-139]

### EPIDEMIOLOGY

- Although only 2% to 5% of germ cell tumors are located in the mediastinum, these account for 50% to 70% of all extragonadal germ cell tumors.[140,141]
- Germ cell tumors account for 10% to 15% of primary mediastinal tumors,[7] and 10% to 15% of anterior mediastinal masses.[14]
- Usually appear in the third or fourth decade.[142,143]
- Equal frequency in male and female patients.[136,143]
- More than 90% of malignant GCTs occur in men.[136,144]
- Epidemiologic associations with mediastinal GCTs:
  - Twenty percent of patients have Klinefelter's syndrome (unknown if this is causative).[135,145]
  - Hematologic malignancies, especially megakaryoblastic leukemia and malignant histiocytosis.[146,147]
  - Idiopathic thrombocytopenia[148]

### PATHOLOGY

- **Teratoma** is defined as a neoplasm that consists of tissue derived from more than one primitive germ cell layer, at least some of which is foreign to the anatomic site in which it occurs.[136] Ectodermal tissues (skin, hair, tooth-like structures) usually predominate. Mesodermal tissues (fat, cartilage, bone) and endodermal tissues (respiratory and intestinal epithelium) are less common.[149]
  - Teratoma accounts for 45% to 75% of mediastinal GCTs.[150-152]
  - The vast majority are histologically well differentiated and benign.[136]
  - A minority contain fetal or neuroendocrine tissue and are termed "immature."
  - A mature teratoma may rarely contain a malignant component (see Table 42-4 for terminology).[143]
- **Seminoma** is the second most common germ cell tumor of the mediastinum and accounts for 40% of malignant germ cell tumors with a single histology.[153]
  - Histologically, seminoma is composed of nests of clear cells, lymphocytic-predominant inflammatory infiltrate, and thin fibrovascular septae.
  - Histologic features of primary mediastinal and not gonadal seminomas[153]

From Moran CA, Suster S. Primary germ cell tumors of the mediastinum: I. Analysis of 322 cases with special emphasis on teratomatous lesions and a proposal for histopathologic classification and clinical staging. Cancer 1997;80:681-690.

| | |
|---|---|
| **TABLE 42-4 ■ CLASSIFICATION OF GERM CELL TUMORS OF THE MEDIASTINUM** | |

- Teratomatous tumors
  - Mature teratomas (composed of well-differentiated, mature elements)
  - Immature teratomas (with the presence of immature mesenchymal or neuroepithelial tissue)
  - Teratomas with additional malignant components
    - Type I: with another germ cell tumor (seminoma, embryonal carcinoma, yolk sac tumor, and so on)
    - Type II: with a non–germ cell epithelial component (squamous carcinoma, adenocarcinoma, and so on)
    - Type III: with a malignant mesenchymal component (rhabdomyosarcoma, chondrosarcoma, and so on)
    - Type IV: with any combination of the above
- Nonteratomatous tumors
  - Seminomas
  - Yolk sac tumors
  - Embryonal carcinomas
  - Choriocarcinomas
  - Combined nonteratomatous tumors (a combination of any of the above)

From Moran CA, Suster S. Primary germ cell tumors of the mediastinum: I. Analysis of 322 cases with special emphasis on teratomatous lesions and a proposal for histopathologic classification and clinical staging. Cancer 1997;80:681-690.

**TABLE 42-5 ■ CLINICAL STAGING OF MEDIASTINAL GERM CELL TUMORS**

| Stage | Description |
|---|---|
| Stage I | Well-circumscribed tumor with or without focal adhesions to the pleura or pericardium but without microscopic evidence of invasion into adjacent structures |
| Stage II | Tumor confined to the mediastinum with macroscopic and/or microscopic evidence of infiltration into adjacent structures (such as the pleura, pericardium, and great vessels) |
| Stage III | Tumor with metastases |
| IIIA | With metastases to intrathoracic organs (the lymph nodes, lung, etc.) |
| IIIB | With extrathoracic metastases |

From Moran CA, Suster S. Primary germ cell tumors of the mediastinum: I. Analysis of 322 cases with special emphasis on teratomatous lesions and a proposal for histopathologic classification and clinical staging. Cancer 1997;80:681-690.

- Thymic remnants 27%
- Prominent cystic change simulating multilocular thymic cyst 10%
- Positive immunohistochemical staining for CAM 5.2 and broad-spectrum keratins
- **Nonseminomatous germ cell tumors** include malignant tumors of the endodermal sinus, choriocarcinoma, and embryonal carcinoma. About one third have multiple histologic types.[144]
- A classification system has been proposed by Moran and Suster[143] based on the World Health Organization classification of testicular neoplasms, but with additional subdivisions of teratomatous lesions (see Table 42-4).

## CLINICAL FEATURES

### Clinical Presentation

- Benign teratomas are usually asymptomatic and an incidental finding on chest radiograph.
  - Digestive enzymes secreted by pancreatic or intestinal tissue of a teratoma may cause rupture into the bronchi, pleura, pericardium, or lung.[136,149,154]
  - Expectoration of hair (known as trichophytosis) or sebum is very rare, but it is a pathognomonic feature of a ruptured mediastinal teratoma.[149,154]
- Malignant GCTs are usually symptomatic. In 90%, compression or invasion of surrounding mediastinal structures cause chest pain, dyspnea, or cough.[142,144]
- Weight loss and fever are the most common systemic symptoms.
- Physical examination is usually normal, although large tumors may cause decreased breath sounds, dullness to percussion, and SVC syndrome.
  - 10% of patients with seminoma present with SVC syndrome.[155]

- Gynecomastia, related to increased β-hCG and estradiol levels, has been reported.[156]
- Careful physical examination and ultrasound of the testes are routine measures to exclude a testicular primary. There is no role for blind orchiectomy or testicular biopsy in patients in whom these examinations are normal.[136]

### Staging Classification

- A clinical staging scheme has been proposed by Moran and Suster (Table 42-5).[143]

## DIAGNOSTIC STUDIES

### Imaging Studies

- Teratoma
  - In more than 90% of cases, standard chest radiography is abnormal.
  - Typical plain radiographic appearance is a large anterior mediastinal mass with smooth, lobulated, or irregular margins, usually sharply outlined against the adjacent lung (Fig. 42-12).[157,158]
    - Calcification may be present in 20% to 43%.
    - Bone or teeth may rarely be seen; the appearance of teeth is pathognomonic for teratoma.
  - Typical CT appearance is a well-defined encapsulated cystic mass displaying heterogenous attenuation corresponding to a varying combination of soft tissue, fluid, fat, and calcific components (Fig. 42-13).[157]
    - A fat-fluid level, although uncommon, is considered highly specific for the diagnosis of mature teratoma.[159]
  - MRI and ultrasound imaging did not contribute additional information in a series of 66 patients.[157]
- Seminoma
  - Typical plain radiographic appearance is a bulky, well-marginated, lobulated anterior mediastinal mass that may extend to both sides of the midline. Mass effect is often present.[155]
    - Calcification is rare.
  - Typical CT appearance is coarsely lobulated, with homogeneous attenuation enhancing only slightly after administration of contrast.[160]

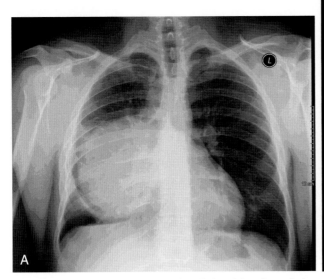

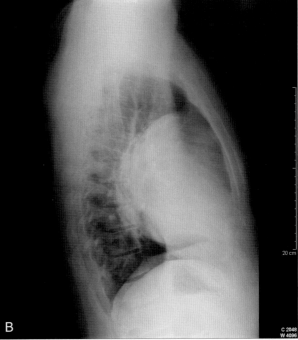

**Figure 42-12:** Posteroanterior (**A**) and lateral chest (**B**) radiograph demonstrates a large anterior mediastinal mass with smooth margins, sharply outlined against the adjacent lung. Histopathologic analysis demonstrated a malignant teratoma.

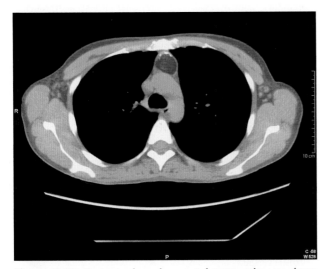

**Figure 42-13:** Contrast-enhanced computed tomography scan shows a well-defined encapsulated cystic mass displaying heterogeneous attenuation corresponding to a varying combination of soft tissue, fluid, fat, and calcific components. Histopathologic analysis demonstrated a teratoma.

■ Extension into the middle and posterior mediastinal compartments can occur, though invasion of adjacent structures is rare.
  ○ Magnetic resonance imaging may play a role in the differentiation between residual neoplasia and fibrosis after treatment.[161]
■ Nonseminatous germ cell tumors
  ○ Typical CXR shows a large, smooth or lobulated anterior mediastinal mass. There may be irregular margins with the adjacent lung parenchyma.[158]

■ Pulmonary metastases may be present.
■ Pleural or pericardial effusion is common.
  ○ Typical CT shows a large mass with heterogeneous attenuation, frequently with large central regions of low attenuation representing areas of hemorrhage or necrosis (Fig. 42-14).[162]
■ Fat planes are typically obliterated.
■ Interface between tumor and adjacent lung may be irregular.
■ Metastases in lung or liver may be seen.

## Laboratory Studies

■ Serologic evaluation for AFP and β-hCG if malignant tumor suspected.[139]
  ○ Elevated AFP is suggestive of an endodermal sinus tumor or embryonal carcinoma and is sufficient, in the presence of a mediastinal mass, to establish the diagnosis.[163,164]
  ○ β-hCG levels may be elevated in 10% of patients with seminoma.[165]

## Tissue Diagnosis

■ If a mass is likely to be benign based on clinical, radiologic, and laboratory data, it can be removed surgically without biopsy.[163]
■ FNA is safe and effective, with a sensitivity of 68% to 83%.[166,167]
■ If FNA is nondiagnostic, an anterior mediastinoscopy (Chamberlain procedure) is usually the best route for tissue diagnosis.[168]
■ Anterior mediastinotomy or VATS may be used for biopsy depending on the anatomic location and radiographic appearance of the mass.[163]

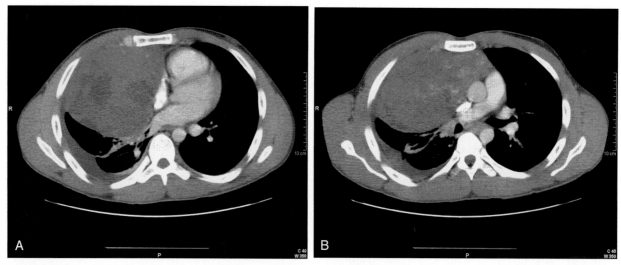

**Figure 42-14:** Contrast-enhanced computed tomography scan shows a large mass with heterogeneous attenuation, frequently with large central regions of low attenuation representing areas of hemorrhage or necrosis. Histopathologic analysis demonstrated a malignant teratoma.

## *PROGNOSIS*

### Teratoma

- Long-term survival is good (64/69, 92.8%).[149]
- Teratoma with malignant components confers a much poorer prognosis (36.7% 2-year survival rate). A sarcomatous component makes the prognosis even worse (84.6% mortality at 1 year).[31]

### Seminoma

- Of the GCTs, seminoma has the best survival (75% at 10 years).[153]
- Chemotherapy alone provides a 90% 5-year survival rate.[169]
- Liver metastases or 2 sites of distant disease are negative prognostic factors.

### Nonseminomatous Germ Cell Tumors

- Primary mediastinal NSGCT has a poorer prognosis than that of a primary gonadal or retroperitoneal location.
- Poor prognostic factors for extragonadal NSGCT include liver, lung, or CNS metastases, and elevation of pretreatment β-hCG.[170]
- Two- and five-year overall survival rates are 65% and 45%, respectively.[170]

## *TREATMENT*

### Teratoma

- Complete surgical excision is curative.
  - Median sternotomy is the most frequently used surgical approach, but thoracotomy may be used.
  - Although these tumors are frequently large, VATS may be possible.[171,172]
  - Dense adhesions with surrounding tissues may complicate resection, and pulmonary resection is often necessary.[173]
  - For 86 patients, Lewis reported a minimal operative mortality before 1952 and zero, thereafter.[149]
- Thorough pathologic examination is necessary to exclude the presence of small foci of immature tissue, other germ cell tumors, or other malignancy.
- There is no role for radiation therapy.

### Seminoma

- Cisplatin-based combination chemotherapy is the treatment of choice.
- Radiation has a higher recurrence rate and a lower survival rate than chemotherapy.
- The management of postchemotherapy residual masses remains controversial. The residual mass is frequently necrotic and only very rarely viable seminoma or mature teratoma.[169]
  - Schultz et al[174] advocate observation of residual masses in cases of pure seminoma, regardless of size, reserving radiotherapy or chemotherapy for those patients who subsequently develop progressive disease.

### Nonseminomatous Germ Cell Tumor

- Cisplatin-based combination chemotherapy is the initial treatment of choice.
- For high-risk disease, consider higher dose chemotherapy with autologous stem cell transplantation rescue,[175] reducing chemotherapy intervals,[176] or alternating cycles of combination chemotherapy.[177]
- Biopsy mass after chemotherapy if markers have normalized. Complete tumor necrosis is infrequent. Surgery for patients in whom tumor markers have not normalized is controversial.[168,178,179]
- Median sternotomy is the most common surgical approach, and most useful for small or medium midline residual masses.
  - Approximately 10% of patients have synchronous pulmonary metastases, and this approach allows for access to both lungs.
- The clamshell incision (transverse sternotomy) allows for superior exposure of larger tumors, especially with hilar involvement lungs, pleural spaces, and mediastinum. This incision, however, is painful.
- A standard posterolateral thoracotomy over the fifth rib may be used for unilateral disease, typically involving the pulmonary hilum.[168]
- Walsh and colleagues[176] described a series of 11 surgical resections of residual mediastinal masses.
  - A severe desmoplastic mediastinal reaction was encountered in all cases.

○ Partial pericardial resection was required in all cases.
○ Resection usually required resection of the thymus and lung.
○ Resection rarely required resection of: inominate vein, SVC, unilateral phrenic nerve, or left recurrent nerve.
■ Operative mortality rate is low; it was 4% in the series of Kesler et al.[178] Most operative mortality occurs in patients requiring major pulmonary resections.
■ If viable tumor is identified in the residual mass, further chemotherapy is recommended.
■ If mature teratoma or complete necrosis is identified, then clinical and radiologic follow-up is satisfactory.[176]

# INTRATHORACIC GOITERS

## DEFINITION

■ An intrathoracic goiter is the caudal extension of enlarging thyroid tissue beyond the thoracic inlet.
■ Contributing factors to this descent of thyroid tissue are gravity on the bulky, enlarged thyroid, negative intrathoracic pressure, and the downward traction from swallowing.[180,181] Its clinical relevance is due to compression or invasion of SVC, trachea, esophagus, carotid artery, recurrent laryngeal nerve, aorta and the cervical sympathetic chain.
■ The commonly used definition for intrathoracic goiter holds that greater than 50% of the thyroid tissue be below the thoracic inlet.[182]

## EPIDEMIOLOGY

■ Eight to twenty percent of cervical goiters enter the thorax[183,184]
■ The incidence of intrathoracic goiters varies from 1 to 2 per 10,000 people.[185]
■ The female-to-male ratio is 2:1 to 3:1.[186,187]
■ Typically discovered in fifth decade of life (range is 15 to 95 years).[186,188,189]
■ Accounts for 15% to 20% of thyroid surgery.[190,191]
■ Accounts for 10% of all mediastinal masses requiring surgical resection.[192]
■ In rare cases (approximately 2%), intrathoracic goiter occurs in ectopic thyroid within the thorax.[180,193]

## PATHOLOGY

■ The majority of intrathoracic goiters are benign, slow-growing lesions.
○ Malignancy is found in 3% to 23% of patients.[194-200]
○ The pathology of thyroid cancer in intrathoracic goiters is similar to the pathology for cervical thyroid.
○ Follicular carcinoma (50%), papillary carcinoma (20%) and medullary carcinoma (15%).[201]

## ANATOMIC CONSIDERATIONS

■ The location for intrathoracic goiter includes anterior mediastinum, posterior mediastinum, and ectopic, and intrathoracic thyroid tissue (primary intrathoracic goiter).
○ Anterior goiters: 80% to 90% of intrathoracic goiters[196,201] and usually leftward as it descends through the thoracic inlet.[183,203]
○ Posterior goiters: 10% to 20% of intrathoracic goiters[198,202] and usually rightward as it descends through the thoracic inlet.[203,204]
  ■ Usually retrotracheal space
  ■ Occasionally retroesophageal

○ Primary intrathoracic goiters: 2% of intrathoracic goiters.[180,193] The tissue originates from the embryonic foregut endoderm separate from the cervical thyroid and draws its blood supply locally.[180,205]

## CLINICAL FEATURES

### Clinical Presentation

■ Common presenting symptoms: Dyspnea (60%–77%), dysphagia (12%–23%), hoarseness (14%–23%), cough, and syncope episodes if the vertebral artery is compressed.[180,187,206]
■ Common presenting signs
○ Short neck
○ Prominent thyroid without palpable inferior margin
○ Venous engorgement, facial flushing
○ Pemberton's sign: stridor with extension of both arms above the head and extension of the neck. 10%[180,187,206]
○ Tracheal deviation[31]
○ Horner's syndrome (rarely)[207,208]
■ Frequently, asymptomatic, radiologic finding.
○ Thirty percent of malignant intrathoracic goiters are asymptomatic.[197,201]
■ Hoarseness suggests malignancy

## DIAGNOSTIC STUDIES

### Laboratory Studies

■ Clinical hyperthyroidism rare.
■ Thyrotoxicosis ranges from 10% to 44%.[190,200]

### Imaging Studies

■ CXR
○ The classic image of a widened mediastinum with tracheal deviation may be the first presentation of the disease, but this test has a sensitivity of only 59% and is very nonspecific.[190]
■ Transcutaneous ultrasound
○ Provides a sensitivity of 77%.[190]
■ CT scan
○ Best imaging modality: 100% sensitivity.[190]
○ Diagnosis: continuity with cervical thyroid.
○ CT findings: encapsulated, lobulated, heterogenous, or smoothly contoured tumor, almost always sharply marginated, and may contain punctate calcifications (Fig. 42-15).[193,203,209]
○ Thyroid tissue shows prolonged enhancement from the iodinated IV contrast.
○ Possible displacement of the hyoid bone, trachea, and larynx (Fig. 42-16). Esophageal displacement is unusual for anterior mediastinal goiters but is seen in almost all posterior mediastinal goiters.[203]
■ Nuclear imaging
○ Not a good study because the intrathoracic portion of the goiter may not have adequate tracer uptake, especially if it has an associated malignancy.
○ Technetium pertechnetate ($^{99m}TcO_4$) commonly used to image the thyroid, cannot be seen behind the increased activity of the great vessels and heart. If nuclear imaging is attempted, iodine-131 should be used because it provides greater penetration to image the intrathoracic goiter owing to its greater thyroid tissue uptake.[203]

### Tissue Diagnosis

■ FNA biopsy cannot be done reliably for intrathoracic goiters because the small sample is not representative of the entire tumor. The goiter may conceal malignant cells that are likely to be missed.[206]

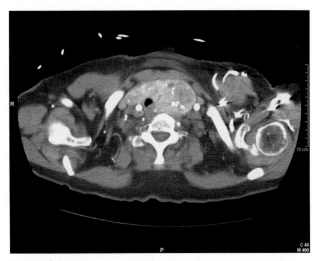

**Figure 42-15:** Contrast-enhanced computed tomography scan shows a sharply marginated, encapsulated and heterogeneous mass containing punctate calcifications. Histopathologic analysis demonstrated a thyroid goiter.

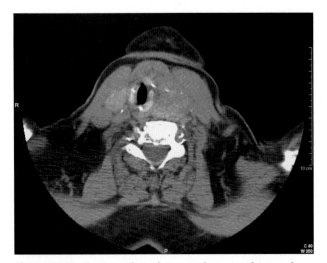

**Figure 42-16:** Contrast-enhanced computed tomography scan shows displacement of the trachea by a thyroid mass. Histopathologic analysis demonstrated a thyroid goiter.

## PROGNOSIS

- Most intrathoracic goiters are benign and have a good prognosis
- Worse prognosis for
- Cancer (difficult to diagnose without resection)
- Catastrophic events:
  ○ Hemorrhage into mediastinum resulting in sudden compression of the trachea and may present as a respiratory emergency.
  ○ Malignant cells cause erosion of the walls of the great vessels, which leads to massive, life-threatening blood loss.
- Catastrophic occurrences are rare.[212]
- Intervention is usually for the morbidity associated with the goiter's mass effect, including choking and gradual respiratory difficulties.

## TREATMENT

- There is no good response to medical only therapy in reducing the size of intrathoracic goiters.[194] Through radiotherapy, radioactive iodine and propylthiouracil help reduce the symptoms of thyrotoxicosis; they do not improve symptoms pertaining to the mass effect of the goiter.[210]

### Surgery

- Technique
  ○ Intrathoracic goiters are usually resected through a cervical incision, with sternotomy needed in only 1.7% to 10%.[180,187,199,200]
  ○ Factors increasing the likelihood of sternotomy: involvement of the posterior mediastinum, extension to aortic arch, recurrent goiter, obstruction of SVC, malignancy with local involvement, CT that suggests the goiter is adherent to surrounding structures, and emergent airway obstruction.[186,190,206,211,212]
  ○ In addition, the longer resection is delayed and the mass permitted to grow, there is a greater likelihood that sternotomy is needed during intervention.[212]
  ○ A primary intrathoracic goiter usually requires sternotomy because its blood supply originates within the thorax and cannot be ligated from a cervical approach.[180,205]
  ○ Cervical approach includes a collar incision, division of the strap muscles, ligation of the middle thyroid vein and inferior thyroid artery, exposure of the recurrent laryngeal nerves, exposure and isolation of the parathyroid glands (or leave small amount of thyroid tissue adjacent to trachea to leave parathyroids intact), and finally, separation and mobilization of the thyroid tissue.
  ○ Morcellation through a cervical incision[182] is to be discouraged because it increases bleeding and may disperse malignant cells throughout the mediastinum. This technique is seldom used today.[205]
  ○ Using smaller caliber endotracheal (ET) tubes and a bronchoscopic device is encouraged during intubation when tracheal compression is suspected.
- Complications
  ○ The mortality rate associated with substernal thyroidectomy is 1.4%, or eight times greater than cervical-only thyroidectomy.[198] Bleeding was the primary cause of mortality.
  ○ Transient hypocalcemia occurs in up to 41% of cases,[190] but chronic hypoparathyroidism occurs in 5.5%.[198]
  ○ Injury to the recurrent laryngeal nerve occurred in 2% to 8% of patients.[187,199,200]
  ○ Tracheomalacia may result from chronic tracheal compression by goiter. This usually does not happen or improves over time. In the short term, a tracheostomy may be needed during the perioperative period.[212] In the long term, tracheoplasty may be required.[213-215]

## SOFT TISSUE TUMORS AND TUMOR-LIKE CONDITIONS

## ANATOMIC CONSIDERATIONS

- Most anterior mediastinal soft tisssue tumors originate in the chest wall and extend locally into the anterior mediastinal compartment.
- Some extend from the middle and posterior compartments.
- Mesenchymal (soft tissue) tumors account for less than 2% of all mediastinal neoplasms.[216]

## TUMORS OF ADIPOSE TISSUE[217]

- Lipomas
  - Pathogenesis:
    - Benign proliferation of adipose tissue
    - Occurs primarily in the chest wall
    - Can arise from primary cardiac sources, although these are usually from subendothelial fat
  - Symptom/findings
    - Usually asymptomatic
    - Generally found incidentally on imaging of the chest.
    - Ill-defined soft, fleshy mass that grows slowly over time.
    - Symptoms, if present, usually are from compression of surrounding structures.
  - Radiographic findings
    - Seen best with CT or MRI, which shows a distinctive fat pattern
  - Diagnosis/treatment:
    - Usually radiographic and by physical examination
    - Excisional biopsy, which is both therapeutic and diagnostic
- Liposarcoma
  - Pathogenesis
    - Malignant mesenchymal tumor of adipose tissue
    - One of the more common mesenchymal tumors seen involving the chest wall and extending into the mediastinum.
    - Generally, an encapsulated structure that is lobulated.
  - Epidemiology:
    - Affects mostly men
    - Generally in the 4th through 6th decades of life
  - Symptom/findings:
    - Usually present as a painless mass or asymptomatic radiologic finding.
    - Extension into the anterior mediastinum may cause local compression of vascular structures.
    - When primarily involving the chest wall, it can present as ill-defined mass arising from the chest.
  - Radiographic findings:
    - Best visualized on CT or MRI with a characteristic appearance.
  - Diagnosis:
    - Tissue biopsy for definitive diagnosis
  - Treatment:
    - Excision with wide margins to prevent recurrence
  - Prognosis:
    - Overall, low recurrence rate. They recur locally or in the lungs.
- Desmoid tumors[217-221]
  - Pathogenesis
    - Slow-growing, benign growth arising from fibrous musculoaponeurotic elements
    - Considered to be a benign fibromatosis
    - Can be either intra-abdominal, that is, those associated with familial adenomatous polyposis (Gardner's syndrome) or extra-abdominal involvement.
    - Those that are extra-abdominal generally affect the shoulder girdle area and less often the chest wall.
  - Epidemiology:
    - They are uncommon
      - 0.03% of all neoplasms
      - Less than 3% of all soft tissue tumors
      - Age range is 15 to 60 years; rare in very young or very elderly.
      - Seen more often in women than in men
      - No known racial predilection
  - Symptoms/findings:
    - Usually seen as a mass on an extremity, chest wall, or shoulder area, which can be painful
    - Usually, asymptomatic, but may cause
      - Paresthesias
      - Neuromuscular weakness
      - Compromise of vascular structures
    - Although benign, these tumors recur locally and are associated with a slightly increased mortality rate.[221,222]
  - Radiographic findings:
    - CT or MRI scan can be used to determine extent of involvement.
      - MRI scan considered superior to evaluate brachial plexus invasion
  - Diagnosis
    - Usually by diagnostic biopsy
      - Favor incisional versus needle biopsy, to obtain a large enough sample to make a definitive diagnosis.
  - Treatment
    - Resection with wide surgical margins
      - Long-term survival does occasionally occur after subtotal excision
      - Local recurrence can be treated with repeat excision[223-225]

## TUMORS OF VASCULAR TISSUE

- Hemangiomas[226-229]
  - Pathogenesis:
    - Benign tumors of the vascular system that originate from endothelial cell
    - Form vascular channels of varying size
    - These tumors tend to be sharply defined but not encapsulated
    - Can form large cavernous hemangiomas that have large frequently cystically dilated spaces that are filled with blood
      - Can contain phleboliths—calcified thrombi.
  - Epidemiology
    - More commonly seen in the middle mediastinum (see Chapter 43)
    - Uncommon benign tumor seen of the media-stinum
      - Less than 0.5% of all mediastinal lesions
      - Rare tumor (only 103 cases of cavernous hemangioma reported in the mediastinum).[228]
    - More recent series of 18 cases of mediastinal hemangioma showed 14 tumors located in the anterior mediastinum and four in the posterior mediastinum.[229]
  - Symptoms/finding:
    - Symptoms are usually due to compression of local structures in the anterior mediastinum.
    - Sometimes found incidentally on routine chest imaging
    - May cause anterior chest pain
  - Radiology:
    - CT with contrast can be diagnostic.
    - Washout of the contrast on subsequent images is slow.
    - This can be helpful in preoperative diagnosis.
  - Treatment:
    - No treatment if asymptomatic
    - Resect if very symptomatic or small, but resection may be a very bloody procedure so should be undertaken with caution.
- Epithelioid hemangioendothelioma[230]
  - Pathogenesis:
    - Low-grade malignant tumor derived from blood vessel or lymphatic components.
    - Considered to be a low-grade angiosarcoma.

- Epidemiology
    - Occurs in adults
    - Mediastinal involvement is uncommon.
    - Occurs more often in women than in men
- Symptoms/findings:
    - Present with local mass effect
    - Usually nonspecific symptoms
- Radiology:
    - Well visualized on CT with contrast enhancement
- Treatment
    - Surgery and sometimes with adjuvant chemotherapy and radiation
- Prognosis
    - High-risk tumors: mitotic activity greater than 3/high power field (hpf) and size larger than 3 cm correlated with the worst prognosis (59%, 5-year survival)
    - Low-risk tumors: (activity less than 3/hpf and size larger than 3 cm) 100% 5-year survival.
- Angiosarcoma[231-233]
    - Pathogenesis:
        - Malignant tumors derived from either blood vessel or lymphatic tissue.
        - No vascular origin in anterior mediastinum.
    - Epidemiology:
        - Middle-aged adults.
    - Symptoms/findings:
        - Dyspnea due to compression of trachea
        - SVC syndrome
    - Diagnosis:
        - Surgical biopsy.
    - Radiology:
        - CT can show a homogenous mass when this tumor is extracardiac
        - Usually heterogenous appearance due to frequent necrosis, hemorrhage, and cyst formation
    - Treatment/prognosis:
        - Prognosis is poor; rarely beyond 3 years
        - Radiation after surgical resection with wide excisional margins.
        - Chemotherapy can sometimes be used to shrink the tumor so that an adequate resection can be done.
- Hemangiopericytoma
    - Usually involve other mediastinal compartments, i.e., the middle mediastinum (see Chapter 43)
- Lymphangioma and lymphangiomatosis
    - Can involve the anterior mediastinum but also seen in other compartments (see Chapter 43)

## TUMORS OF MUSCLE

- Leiomyoma and leiomyosarcoma[231,234,235]
    - Pathogenesis:
        - Benign and malignant tumor arising from smooth muscle tissue
        - One of the more common sarcomas that can affect the lung primarily
        - Usually arises from the esophagus, pulmonary artery, or other mediastinal vasculature
            - Most of these tumors do not involve these structures.
    - Epidemiology
        - Sixth decade
        - Male predominance
    - Symptoms/findings:
        - Symptoms due to local mass effect

- Radiology
    - CT scan: large neoplasms that are often heterogeneous in appearance due to necrosis or hemorrhage within the masses.
    - Leiomyosarcomas of the pulmonary artery frequently grow within the lumen; they can be difficult to distinguish from pulmonary artery thromboses.
        - MRI can be helpful with the use of gadolinium contrast to distinguish when looking at pulmonary artery leiomyosarcomas.
- Prognosis/treatment
    - Surgery
    - For mediastinal leiomyosarcoma, prognosis is worse the larger the tumor size.
        - Owing to higher frequency of local invasion and recurrence
        - Treatment consists of surgical excision along with radiation and chemotherapy
- Rhabdomyoma and rhabdomyosarcoma[217]
    - Pathogenesis
        - Rhabdomyoma—benign tumor arising from striated muscle
        - Rhabdomyosarcoma—malignant mesenchymal tumor arising from striated muscle
        - Can arise anywhere in the anterior mediastinum or by extension from the chest wall
        - Rhabdomyosarcoma is the second most common malignant soft tissue tumor of the chest wall.
    - Epidemiology
        - Occurs in children and young adults.
    - Symptoms/findings:
        - Rhabdomyosarcoma grows rapidly and painlessly.
        - Because of its fast growth, can often cause symptoms by compression of adjacent structures over a relatively short period of time
    - Radiographic finding:
        - MRI can delineate the extent of involvement with high sensitivity
    - Treatment
        - Wide surgical excision if possible is preferable for rhabdomyosarcoma.
        - Adjuvant chemotherapy and radiation confer excellent 5-year survival rates.

## FIBROUS AND FIBROHISTIOCYTIC TUMORS[231,236,237]

- Fibroma and fibrosarcoma
    - Epidemiology:
        - Rare tumors of unknown etiology
        - Fibromas are benign with no malignant potential.
    - Symptoms/findings
        - Dyspnea due to compression of trachea or SVC syndrome
    - Radiology
        - CT and MRI show a solid mass that may be heterogeneous if there is internal necrosis and hemorrhage.
    - Treatment/Prognosis:
        - Treatment is resection.
            - Preoperative chemotherapy may improve resectability.
            - Postoperative radiation therapy for positive surgical margins or if complete resection is not possible.
        - Response to chemotherapy and radiation is poor.
            - Larger masses tend to recur locally.
            - Smaller lesions have a high likelihood of metastases.

- Benign and malignant fibrous histiocytoma[223]
  - Pathogenesis:
    - Malignant fibrous histiocytoma can be classified as
      - Pleomorphic sarcoma
      - Giant cell malignant fibrous histiocytoma (MFH)/undifferentiated pleomorphic sarcoma
      - Inflammatory MFH/undifferentiated pleomorphic sarcoma
  - Epidemiology[224,228]
    - Occurs more often in men than in women
    - Age older than 50 years
    - May be associated with history of radiation
    - Rare tumor in the anterior mediastinum
  - Symptoms/findings
    - Slow-growing, painless, lobulated masses
    - Can be incidental radiologic finding
    - May cause compression of trachea or SVC
  - Diagnosis:
    - Surgical biopsy needed to diagnose
  - Radiographic findings
    - CT scan to define extent of the local tumor and to evaluate for pulmonary metastases
  - Treatment
    - Wide surgical resection
    - Radiation and chemotherapy have little role in the treatment of these types of tumors.[217]

## TUMORS OF BONE AND CARTILAGE

- Osteosarcoma[231,238-242]
  - Pathogenesis
    - Malignant mesenchymal tumor arising in bone.
    - Can occur in areas of pre-existing bony lesion or Paget's disease
    - Can be related to radiation exposure or chemotherapy
    - Extraosseous mediastinal tumors are rare.
  - Epidemiology
    - Osseous osteosarcomas occur in the second and third decades of life.
    - Extraosseous osteosarcomas occur in the fifth decade of life or later.
    - Occurs more often in men than in women.
  - Symptoms/findings
    - Present as a mass, chest wall pain, or both
  - Radiology
    - Usually appear as bone destruction/erosion with an associated soft tissue mass on CXR.
    - CT usually shows a heterogenous mass due to necrosis and hemorrhage.
    - Despite having bone features on histology, ossification on radiology is not always apparent.
  - Diagnosis
    - Requires a biopsy that shows typical histologic features of bone and osteoid matrix, which is definitive
  - Treatment/prognosis
    - Usually treated with preoperative chemotherapy, followed by resection.
    - Postoperative chemotherapy if the tumor exhibits a response to preoperative therapy.
    - Radiation therapy is occasionally used for local control if adequate resection cannot be preformed.
    - Mediastinal osteosarcoma has a poor prognosis.
      - Five-year survival rate of about 15% compared with 60% to 70% in extremity osteosarcomas
    - Metastases develop in about 70% of patients and are associated with a poor prognosis (0% 5-year survival)

- Patients who do not develop metastases have a 5-year survival of more than 50%.
- Chondrosarcoma[243-246]
  - Pathogenesis
    - Rare primary tumor in mediastinum. May start in chest wall and invade mediastinum
  - Epidemiology
    - Wide age range of presentation.
      - Typically 30 to 60 years of age.
      - Slight male predominance.
  - Symptoms/findings
    - Clinically present as masses that can be painless or painful.
  - Radiology
    - CT can show scattered areas of calcification that occur in chondroid matrix.
  - Diagnosis
    - Definitive diagnosis is usually with tissue biopsy which shows characteristic areas of chondroid matrix formation.
  - Treatment/prognosis
    - Wide surgical resection
    - Recurrence is local or pulmonary metastases
      - Synchronous metastatic lesions are usually resected as well.
    - Poor response to chemotherapy and radiation
    - Five-year survival rate is good (>60%) and higher in those patients without metastatic lesions (>80%).
    - Poor prognostic factors include
      - Incomplete resection
      - Metastatic lesions
      - Local recurrence
      - Age older than 50 years

## KEY FACTS

### MASSES OF THE THYMUS

- Thymic masses may be associated with systemic disorders as clinically diverse as myasthenia gravis, carcinoid syndrome, MEN1, red cell aplasia, thyrotoxicosis, Addison's disease, and acromegaly.
- MEN1 should be considered before the resection of parathyroid adenomas, as concomitant prophylactic thymectomy is recommended (because thymic carcinoid frequently develops and has a terrible prognosis).
- The utility of thymectomy in the management of myasthenia gravis remains a controversial subject.

### LYMPHOMA

- The three most common types of mediastinal lymphoma are HL, large B-cell lymphoma (primary mediastinal large B-cell lymphoma), and lymphoblastic lymphoma.
- Primary mediastinal lymphoma is a distinct clinical subset and represents 10% of all mediastinal lymphoma.
- When Hodgkin's disease is identified, the nodular sclerosing subtype is the most common type.
- NHL generally has a poorer prognosis than Hodgkin's disease.
- Prognosis in HL is worse with B-symptoms, multiple sites of disease, and bulky disease.
- Prognosis in NHL is more complicated and depends on individual tumor cell biology.
- Treatment is associated with more success in Hodgkin's disease than that of NHL.

## PRIMARY MEDIASTINAL GERM CELL TUMORS

- GCTs account for 10% to 15% of anterior mediastinal masses.
- Teratoma
  - Accounts for 60% to 70% of GCTs, and is composed of tissue derived from multiple germ cell layers.
  - Usually presents as an incidentally discovered large anterior mediastinal mass in a young adult. Occurs with equal frequency in men and women.
  - Complete surgical excision is curative and prognosis is excellent.
- Primary mediastinal seminoma
  - Typically presents in a young adult man with symptoms related to compression.
  - The prognosis is good with the use of cisplatin-based combination chemotherapy.
- Nonseminomatous germ cell tumors
  - Typically presents in a young adult man with symptoms related to compression; measurement of elevated AFP may assist in diagnosis
  - May be associated with Klinefelter's syndrome or hematologic malignancy
  - The prognosis is poor. The treatment of choice is combination chemotherapy followed by resection of residual mass.

## INTRATHORACIC GOITERS

- Most (>80%) are benign.
- The most common initial presenting symptom is dyspnea.
- CT scan is the diagnostic modality of choice.
- Surgery is indicated to treat symptoms and to rule out malignancy. Most surgical resections (>80%) can be done safely using a cervical incision.

## SOFT TISSUE TUMORS

- Mesenchymal tumors or tumors of soft tissue are rare entities encountered in the mediastinum.
- Can be divided into five separate groups based on origin, those arising from adipose tissue, vascular tissue, muscle, fibrous tissue, and bone and cartilage.
- Most of these tumors arise in the chest wall and grow into the mediastinum.
- A majority of these tumors present in the mediastinum either on incidental imaging or because of local mass effect.
- Treatment is generally resection with chemoradiation in selected cases.

### Brief Illustrative Case

- A previously healthy 27-year-old man presented to his primary care doctor with insidious onset of constant chest pain and cough.
- Physical examination including testicular examination was unremarkable.
- Chest radiograph and subsequent chest CT showed a large lobulated mass with homogeneous attenuation in the anterior mediastinum. There was evidence of mediastinal lymph node involvement.
- Testicular ultrasound was normal, and serum levels of β-hGC and AFP were normal.
- Transthoracic fine CT-guided needle aspiration confirmed the diagnosis of seminoma.
- Chemotherapy with cisplatin, etoposide, and ifosfamide was initiated.
- Resection of residual mass after three cycles of chemotherapy demonstrated only necrotic tissue.
- Serial imaging has shown no evidence of recurrent disease.

### Key Points

- Mediastinal mass in a young man should prompt a thorough physical and ultrasonographic testicular examination and measurement of tumor markers.
- Elevated tumor markers are diagnostic for mediastinal GCTs.
- If markers are not abnormal, anterior mediastinotomy and CT-guided needle aspiration are safe and effective methods for the diagnosis of anterior mediastinal masses.
- Although primary mediastinal seminoma is radiosensitive, cisplatin-based combination chemotherapy is a more effective primary treatment.
- Residual masses should be excised and examined for evidence of vital seminoma or nonseminomatous GCT elements.
- Seminoma carries a relatively good long-term prognosis.

### References

 Interactive references and additional readings for this chapter can be accessed online at *expertconsult.com*.

# 43 MASSES OF THE MIDDLE MEDIASTINUM

John Cho, MD, Dani Hackner, MD, Robert J. McKenna Jr., MD, and Michael I. Lewis, MD

## TERMINOLOGY

- Amyloidosis
- Angioimmunoblastic lymphadenopathy
- Angiomatous lymphoid hamartomas
- Azygos vein varix
- Benign mediastinal lymphadenopathy

- Bronchogenic cyst
- Castleman's disease
- Chylous cysts
- Clear water cyst
- Congenital hernia
- Cystic hygroma
- Diaphragmatic hernias

- Enterogenous cysts
- Esophageal duplication cyst
- Foregut cysts
- Germ cell tumors
- Hemangioma
- Hiatal hernia
- Hodgkin's disease (HD)
- Human herpes virus 8
- Kaposi sarcoma–associated herpesvirus
- Kaposi's sarcoma
- Large B cell lymphoma
- Lymphangioma
- Lymphatic cysts
- Lymphoblastic lymphoma
- Lymphoma
- Malignant hemangiopericytoma
- Metastatic mediastinal lymphadenopathy
- Middle mediastinal mass
- Neurenteric cyst
- Non-Hodgkin's lymphoma (NHL)
- Pancreatic pseudocyst
- Paraganglioma
- Pericardial cyst
- POEMS syndrome
- Reed-Sternberg cells
- Spring water cyst
- Vascular aneurysm
- Vascular hamartoma

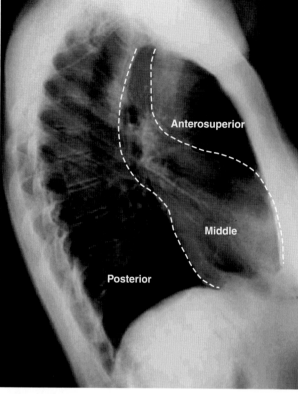

**Figure 43-1:** Figure depicting anatomic subdivision of the middle mediastinum. *(From Townsend CM, Beauchamp RD, Evers BM, Mattos KL, editors. Sabiston textbook of general surgery. 17th ed. New York: Elsevier; 2004.)*

## ANATOMY

The middle mediastinum contains the heart, pericardium, aortic arch and great vessels, trachea, bronchi, upper esophagus, and lymph nodes (Fig. 43-1).

## INTRODUCTION

The majority of the patients with mediastinal masses do not demonstrate clinical symptoms, and the masses are found incidentally on chest radiograph.[1-4] However, some patients exhibit generalized and nonspecific symptoms due to localized compression or invasion of surrounding structures. The masses localized in the middle mediastinum pose a diagnostic challenge because of its relatively inaccessible site with routine clinical testing. Even though the majority of the mediastinal masses are benign (67%), most patients require further diagnostic testing to establish tissue diagnosis. Patient's age, clinical symptoms, and location of the mass determine the likelihood of malignancy.

## SYMPTOMS

Symptoms are related to local compression or invasion of surrounding tissues. Localizing clinical symptoms include cough (60%), chest pain (30%), and dyspnea (16%).[1,5]

## SPECIFIC MASSES OF THE MIDDLE MEDIASTINUM: CYSTS

- **Foregut cysts**[1,2,6-9]
  - ○ Ten to twenty percent of mediastinal masses
  - ○ Twenty percent cannot be classified (indeterminate cysts or nonspecific)
  - ○ Derived from embryonic developmental abnormality
  - ○ Composed of bronchogenic and enterogenous cysts
  - ○ Equal predilection in both sexes except for slightly higher male predominance in neurenteric cysts
- **Bronchogenic cysts**[1,2,5-8,10-16]
  - ○ Pathogenesis
    - Derived from abnormal budding of the ventral foregut during development
    - Respiratory columnar epithelial lining
    - Cysts migrate to atypical locations
    - Arise adjacent to trachea, main bronchi, and carina (85%)
    - Occur in the lung (15%)
    - Located mainly in the middle and posterior mediastinum
    - Other sites include pleura, diaphragm, pericardium, and neck.
    - Cysts contain fluid, mucus, milk of calcium, blood, or purulent material
    - Represents 50% to 60% of mediastinal cysts
  - ○ Demographics
    - Commonly affects adult patients (average age 36)
    - Most common form of foregut cysts
  - ○ Symptoms/findings
    - Forty to sixty-seven percent with symptoms
    - Cough, wheezing, dyspnea, dysphagia, chest pain, or hemoptysis
    - Large cysts may compress airways resulting in airway obstruction
    - Other serious complications include superior vena cava obstruction, extrinsic pulmonary artery stenosis, pericardial tamponade, and severe hemoptysis

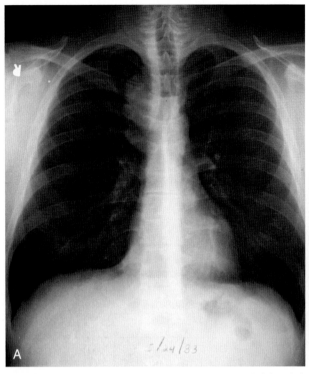
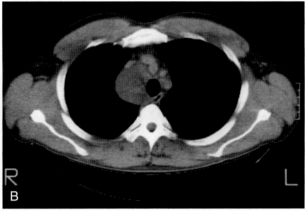

**Figure 43-2:** Bronchogenic cyst depicted in chest radiograph (**A**) and chest CT (**B**).

○ Radiographic findings (Fig. 43-2)
  ■ Well-circumscribed, spherical, mediastinal mass
  ■ Chest computed tomography (CT) scan shows homogenous, nonenhancing mass with variable attenuation.
  ■ Cyst wall contains calcification or enhancement.
  ■ Extension to tracheobronchial tree results in cyst with air-fluid level, air trapping, atelectasis, and tracheal deviation.
  ■ Associated with cartilage in cyst
○ Diagnosis
  ■ Surgical excision
  ■ Thorascopic or bronchoscopic needle aspiration of nonhemorrhagic fluid with mucus and bronchial cells (poor specificity)
○ Treatment
  ■ Symptomatic patients require definitive surgical resection
  ■ Some asymptomatic patients may require complete surgical excision to establish diagnosis and to prevent complication
  ■ Bronchoscopic or thorascopic needle aspiration for patients with high surgical risk
  ■ Risk of recurrence with needle aspiration
■ **Enterogenous cysts**[1,5-7,9,12]
○ Classification
  ■ Esophageal duplication cyst
  ■ Neurenteric cyst
  ■ Accounts for 5% to 10% of cysts
○ Pathogenesis
  ■ Originate from dorsal foregut
  ■ Located in middle or posterior mediastinum
  ■ Cysts contain gastric mucosa, pancreatic tissue, or neural tissue.
  ■ **Esophageal duplication cyst**
    ○ Develops from persistent diverticulum of the dorsal bud of the foregut during early development
    ○ Manifests as paraesophageal tubular lesions

○ Migrates with the lung bud during development and may be located distant from the esophagus
■ **Neurenteric cyst**
  ○ Forms when the foregut and notochord fail to separate
  ○ Contains enteric and neural tissue
  ○ Associated with vertebral anomalies (50%) including scoliosis, anterior spina bifida, vertebral fusion, hemivertebra, and butterfly vertebrae
  ○ Attachment and intraspinal extension to the spine (20%)
○ Demographics
  ■ Discovered during childhood due to tracheobronchial or esophageal compression
  ■ Seventy-five percent of esophageal duplication cyst are discovered by age 1 year owing to acid secretion causing localized symptoms
○ Symptoms/findings
  ■ Mostly asymptomatic but risk of hemorrhage or rupture
  ■ Esophageal duplication cyst
    ○ Associated with congenital gastrointestinal (GI) tract malformations (12%)
  ■ Neurenteric cyst
    ○ Neurologic symptoms due to intraspinal involvement
○ Radiographic findings
  ■ Similar radiographic pattern as bronchogenic cysts
  ■ Rarely see cysts with calcification
  ■ Esophageal duplication cyst
    ○ Adjacent or located within wall of esophagus
    ○ Usually located right side of the esophagus
    ○ Barium esophagram may show extrinsic compression of the esophagus by the cyst
  ■ Neurenteric cyst
    ○ Located mainly in the posterior mediastinum (90%)
    ○ Magnetic resonance imaging (MRI) scan required to exclude intraspinal extension

- Diagnosis
  - Surgical biopsy
  - Classified by histologic features rather than location
  - Enterogenous cysts develop structures of GI tract
- Treatment
  - Surgical excision via video-assisted thoracic surgery
  - Neurenteric cyst excision with excellent prognosis
  - Asymptomatic patients may require complete surgical excision to establish diagnosis and to prevent complication
- **Pericardial cysts**[1,4-9,11,12,17]
  - Pathogenesis
    - Develop from abnormal fusion of the anterior pericardial recesses
    - Attach to diaphragm or anterior pericardium
    - Rarely communicates with the pericardial sac
    - Spring water cysts or clear water cysts
  - Demographics
    - Occurs in 1 in 100,000 patients
    - Discovered during fourth to fifth decades of life
  - Symptom/findings
    - Mostly asymptomatic
    - Chest pain, cough, or dyspnea
  - Radiographic findings (Fig. 43-3)
    - Well-circumscribed, spherical or teardrop-shaped mass
    - Adjacent to the anterior chest wall, diaphragm, and heart
    - With or without calcification within wall of the cyst
    - CT scan of the chest shows nonenhancing, unilocular cystic mass with water attenuation
    - Located in the right costophrenic angle (70%), left costophrenic angle (22%), and other paracardiac location (8%)
  - Diagnosis
    - Radiographic and clinical diagnosis
  - Treatment
    - Percutaneous aspiration of cyst for diagnosis before resection
    - Surgical resection with clinical symptoms
    - Follow clinically and radiologically for asymptomatic patients

## VASCULAR MASSES

- Key points[6,7,11]
  - Ten percent of mediastinal masses
  - Occur in all compartments of mediastinum
  - Obtain CT scan of the chest with contrast, MRI, or angiography
  - Appearance is similar to neoplasm on chest radiograph
- **Paragangliomas**[4,18]
  - Pathogenesis
    - Slow-growing tumors
    - Hypervascular
    - Locally invasive
    - Recurrence rate 55%
    - Metastases 26%
    - Seventy-nine total cases involving anterior and middle mediastinum
  - Symptoms/findings
    - Often asymptomatic
    - Locally compressive symptoms
  - Radiographic findings
    - Enhancing mass
  - Diagnosis
    - Tissue diagnosis
    - Angiographic study reveals feeding vessels from bronchial arteries

- Treatment
  - Preoperative embolization to minimize vascular complications
  - Surgical resection
  - Complete resection difficult given proximity to great vessels, heart, and trachea
  - High local recurrence rate
  - Not responsive to chemotherapy or radiation
- **Malignant hemangiopericytoma**[6,18,19]
  - Pathogenesis
    - Malignant spindle cell cancer
    - Vascular tumor arise from capillaries
    - Arranged in islands separated by thin walled vessels
    - Found in any part of the body
      1. Demographics
    - No sex predilection
    - Any age group
  - Symptoms/findings
    - Most asymptomatic
    - Symptoms related to local compression or metastasis
  - Radiographic findings
    - Well-circumscribed mass
  - Diagnosis
    - Tissue diagnosis
  - Treatment
    - Wide local surgical excision
    - Adjuvant radiation therapy
- **Hemangiomas**[20]
  - Classification
    - Alveolar capillary endothelial cell type
    - Pericytes of Zimmermann type
  - Pathogenesis
    - Derived from capillary endothelium
    - Other types include hemangioblastomas, vascular endotheliomas, capillary hemangiomas, capillary cavernous hemangiomas, and sclerosing hemangiomas
  - Demographics
    - Women older than 30 years of age
  - Symptoms/findings
    - Hemoptysis
  - Radiographic findings
  - Diagnosis
    - Tissue diagnosis
  - Treatment
    - Surgical resection with lobectomy of the lung
- **Systemic venous system**
  - Superior vena cava
  - Azygos vein[21]
    - Giant venous varix of the azygos arch
    - Etiologies include superior vena cava syndrome, Budd-Chiari syndrome, hypervascular tumor, pregnancy, post-traumatic pseudoaneurysm, kinking of the aorta, and portal vein hypertension from liver cirrhosis.
    - Mimics posterior mediastinal mass
    - CT of the chest with intravenous contrast recommended to delineate structures
    - Change in size of mass with position on chest radiograph
    - Mediastinoscopy or percutaneous fine-needle aspiration is contraindicated
  - Hemiazygos
  - Innominate veins
  - Located in the middle or superior mediastinum
- Pulmonary arterial system
  - Pulmonary trunk abnormality
  - Main pulmonary artery abnormality
  - Middle mediastinal or perihilar masses

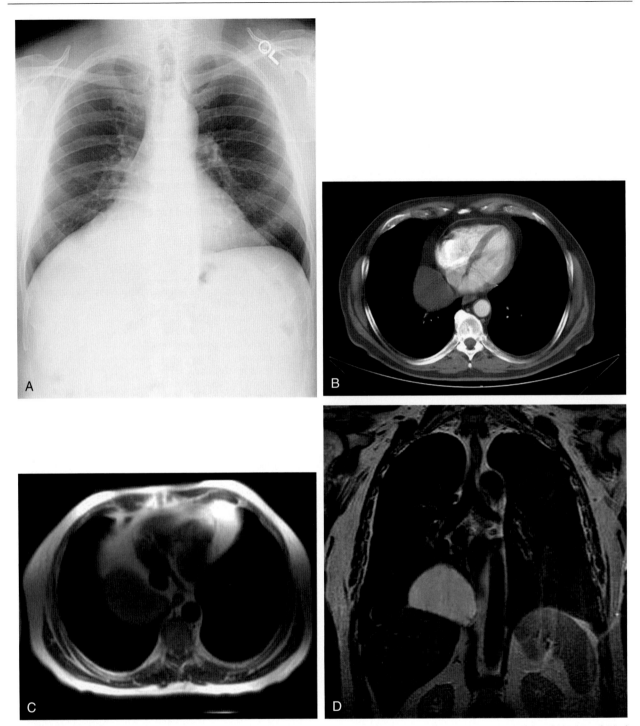

**Figure 43-3:** Pericardial cyst. On plain chest radiograph (**A**) obscuration of the right-sided heart border is evident. On CT (**B**) and MR (**C** and **D**), the cyst is clearly defined.

- Pulmonary venous system
  - Partial anomalous pulmonary venous return
  - Pulmonary vein varix
  - Masses in the middle or superior mediastinum
- Systemic arterial system
  - Innominate arterial aneurysm
    - Appear as curvilinear density above the right clavicle
      1. Aberrant right sublclavian artery
    - Originate from left sided aortic arch
    - Common congenital abnormality of the aortic arch

- Dysphagia lusoria
- Barium esophagram demonstrates anterior displacement of the posterior wall of the esophagus at the level of the aortic arch.
- Aortogram, CT scan, and MRI are diagnostic.
  - Thoracic aortic aneurysm
- Elderly patients with arteriosclerosis and hypertension
- Trauma
- Syphilis
- Cystic medial necrosis

- Peripheral calcification
- Intrinsic pulsations on fluoroscopy
- Angiogram for diagnosis
- MRI scan to evaluate aorta and branching vessels
- Vascular hamartoma, lymphatic type (cystic lymphangiomas)
- See below in lymph node enlargement section under lymphangioma

## LYMPH NODE ENLARGEMENT

- Lymphoma[1,3]
  - Primary mediastinal lymphoma (10%)
  - Usually occurs in anterior mediastinum but may involve middle mediastinum
  - Composed of Hodgkin's disease (HD) and non-Hodgkin's lymphoma (NHD)
- HD[1,2,4,7,11,22]
  - Pathogenesis
    - Large inflammatory cell reaction within fibrotic stroma
    - Enlarged nodes that may undergo necrosis or hemorrhage
    - Produce epithelial-lined cystic areas in the thymus
  - Demographics
    - Fifty percent with mediastinal involvement
    - Bimodal age distribution during early adulthood and age older than 50 years
    - Younger patients (age 29) with mediastinal involvement
    - Both sexes equally affected except for nodular sclerosing HD, which occurs two times more in women.
    - Most common mediastinal lymphoma.
  - Types of HD
    - Nodular sclerosing (66%): mostly affects anterior mediastinum including the thymus
    - Mixed cellularity (25%)
    - Lymphocyte depleted (5%)
    - Diffuse lymphocyte predominant (<3%)
    - Nodular lymphocyte predominant (<3%)
  - Symptoms/findings
    - Constitutional symptoms including fevers, night sweats, and weight loss (20%–30%)
    - Cough, dyspnea, wheezing, chest pain, and dysphagia
    - Pleural effusions, superior vena cava syndrome, and chest wall invasion
    - Cervical or supraclavicular lymphadenopathy
  - Radiographic findings
    - See Table 43-1[23]
    - Abnormal chest radiograph (76%)
    - Bilateral asymmetric nodal disease (90%)
    - CT chest with IV contrast to visualize lymph nodes
    - Prevascular and paratracheal node enlargement
    - Bulky mediastinal lymphadenopathy
    - Multiple, rounded soft tissue masses or infiltrating thymic mass
    - Homogenous soft tissue mass but can have mass with areas of necrosis, hemorrhage and cystic formation
    - Invasion or compression of surrounding structures
    - Nodular sclerosing HD may present with lobulated, anterior, superior mediastinal mass
    - With or without calcification after chemotherapy or radiation therapy
  - Further diagnostic testing
    - Positron emission tomography scan for staging and determine disease progression
    - MRI scan of the chest may be needed to distinguish scar from residual disease

**TABLE 43-1 ■ RADIOGRAPHIC DISTRIBUTION OF INTRATHORACIC ABNORMALITIES IN UNTREATED LYMPHOMA (PERCENTAGE OF PATIENTS WITH POSITIVE FINDINGS)**

| Site Involved | Hodgkin's Disease, % (n = 164) | Non-Hodgkin's Disease, % (n = 136) |
|---|---|---|
| Intrathoracic disease (any site) | 67 | 43 |
| Anterior mediastinum | 46 | 13 |
| Tracheobronchial nodes | 45 | 13 |
| Paratracheal nodes | 40 | 13 |
| Hilar nodes | 21 | 8 |
| Subcarinal nodes | 11 | 4 |
| Internal mammary nodes | 7 | 1 |
| Posterior mediastinum | 5 | 11 |
| Lung | 12 | 5 |
| Pleura | 7 | 11 |

*From Filly R, Blank N, Castellino RA. Radiographic distribution of intrathoracic disease in previously untreated patients with Hodgkin's disease and non-Hodgkin's lymphoma. Radiology 1976;120:277-281.*

  - Diagnosis
    - Tissue needed for diagnosis
    - Mediastinoscopy for paratracheal and subcarinal masses
    - Reed-Sternberg cells pathognomonic for HD
  - Treatment
    - Based on Ann Arbor staging (stages I–IV)
    - Stages I and II receive chemotherapy (ABVD)—epirubicin, bleomycin, vinblastine, and prednisone followed by extended field radiation for bulky disease or disease requiring extensive radiation
    - Stages III and IV are mainly treated with chemotherapy
    - Bone marrow transplant for disease refractory to chemotherapy
- NHL[1,2]
  - Pathogenesis
    - Large B cell lymphoma
      - Rapidly enlarging mass derived from thymus
      - Primarily affects the mediastinum
      - Less involvement of bone marrow and extrathoracic structures
      - Recurrence noted in the liver, kidneys, and brain
      - Flow cytometry and cytogenetics assist in diagnosis
    - Lymphoblastic lymphoma
      - Highly aggressive tumor arising from thymic lymphocytes
      - May involve mediastinum, central nervous system (CNS), gonads, skin, and bone marrow
      - Similar in presentation to T-cell acute lymphoblastic leukemia (ALL)
  - Demographics
    - Represents 15% to 25% of mediastinal lymphoma
    - Highest incidence in white men in their 50s for NHL
    - Younger age group for lymphoblastic lymphoma (10–20 years) and large B cell lymphoma (26 years)
  - Symptoms/findings
    - Chest pain, dysphagia, and hoarseness
    - Cough, wheezing and shortness of breath
    - Constitutional symptoms
    - Superior vena cava syndrome, cardiac tamponade, or tracheal obstruction

○ Radiographic findings
- Abnormal chest radiograph less than 50%
- Intrathoracic nodal disease more than 50%
- Chest CT scan to determine extent of disease
- Involve other sites than paratracheal or prevascular lymph nodes
- Bulky, unencapsulated, invasive masses
- Involve thymus and invade adjacent structures

○ Treatment
- Based on modified Ann Arbor classification and histology
- Indolent disease: palliative local radiation with or without chemotherapy
- Aggressive disease: chemotherapy with or without radiation
- Highly aggressive disease: chemotherapy with or without radiation
- Bone marrow transplant to improve survival
- Large B cell lymphoma–specific treatment
  ○ Treated with chemotherapy and localized radiation
  ○ Bone marrow transplant and high dose chemotherapy for relapse patients
- Lymphoblastic lymphoma–specific treatment
  ○ Treatment similar to ALL with chemotherapy
  ○ Intrathecal chemotherapy needed to prevent CNS relapse
  ○ Mediastinal irradiation and CNS irradiation to prevent relapse
  ○ Bone marrow transplant due to high recurrence rate after treatment

■ **Castleman's disease**[6,24-26]
○ Classification
- Hyaline vascular type (80%–90%)
- Plasma cell type (<10%)
- Multicentric type (<10%)
- See Table 43-2

○ Pathology
- Caused by chronic low grade inflammation, immunodeficiency state, and autoimmunity
- Uncontrolled infection resulting in overproduction of interleukin 6
- Excessive proliferation of B lymphocytes and plasma cells
- Nonmalignant lymph node enlargement with nodal hypervascularity
- In some cases, pathologically similar to HD, drug-induced hypersensitivity reactions, rheumatoid arthritis, Sjögren's syndrome, immunosuppression, and acquired immunodeficiency syndrome (AIDS)
- Hyaline vascular type
  ○ Arranged in concentric, "onion skin" layers with centrally located germinal center
  ○ Presence of numerous capillaries
  ○ Found in conjunction with Kaposi's sarcoma
  ○ Rare progression to malignant lymphoma
  ○ Other sites include lung fissures, central nervous system, orbits, pelvis, neck, muscles, axilla, mesentery, and retroperitoneum
- Plasma cell type
  ○ Prominent germinal center with numerous lymphoid follicles
  ○ Few capillaries present
  ○ Other sites include the mesentery and retroperitoneal space.
  ○ Invade bronchi and cause friable endobronchial lesion
- Multicentric type
  ○ Higher risk in human immunodeficiency virus (HIV)–infected patients

**TABLE 43-2 ■ COMPARISON BETWEEN CLINICAL FEATURES OF LOCALIZED AND MULTICENTRIC CASTLEMAN'S DISEASE**

| Factor | Localized | Multicentric |
|---|---|---|
| Age range (y) | 12–72 | 19–85 |
| Median age (y) | 23.5 | 56 |
| Manifestation | Incidental, "mass effect" | "B" symptoms |
| Histologic features | HV, PC, HV-PC | PC, HV, HV-PC |
| Lymph node | Central | Peripheral |
| Organomegaly | Absent | Yes |
| Premalignant potential | Occasionally | Frequently |
| Clinical course | Benign | Aggressive |
| Treatment | Surgical resection | Chemotherapy |
| Prognosis | Excellent, 100% 5-y survival | Guarded, 26-mo median survival |
| Differential diagnosis | Follicular lymphomas, other causes of adenopathy, AIDS, KS | Follicular lymphomas, AIL, osteosclerotic myeloma, POEMS, AIDS, KS |

AIDS, acquired immunodeficiency syndrome; AIL, angioimmunoblastic lymphadenopathy; HV, hyaline-vascular variant; HV-PC, "mixed" type; KS, Kaposi's sarcoma; PC, plasma cell type; POEMS, polyneuropathy, organomegaly, endocrinopathy, M protein, and skin changes.
*From Shahidi H, Myers JL, Kvale PA. Castleman's disease. Mayo Clin Proc 1995;70:969-977.*

○ Linked with human herpesvirus 8
○ May progress to NHL
○ Associated with Kaposi's sarcoma
○ Similar histologic findings in polyneuropathy, organomegaly, endocrinopathy, monoclonal gammopathy, and skin changes (POEMS) syndrome and osteosclerotic myeloma

○ Demographics
- Young, asymptomatic adults (age < 30) except for multicentric type
- No race or sex predominance

○ Symptoms/findings
- Hyaline vascular type
  ○ Mostly asymptomatic
  ○ Local compressive symptoms including dyspnea and cough
- Plasma cell type
  ○ Constitutional B symptoms (fever, weight loss, and fatigue)
  ○ Anemia and hypergammaglobulinemia
- Multicentric type
  ○ Severe systemic symptoms in older patients (mean age 56)
  ○ Dyspnea and cough
  ○ Constitutional B symptoms
  ○ Symptoms wax and wane within 24 to 48 hours at regular intervals
  ○ Generalized lymphadenopathy
  ○ Hepatosplenomegaly
  ○ Peripheral neuropathy associated with poor prognosis
  ○ Four clinical types: (1) Relapse and remission, (2) stable and persistent, (3) rapidly fatal, and (4) malignant lymphoma transformation

○ Radiographic findings
- Hyaline vascular type
  ○ Large, well-circumscribed lymph node in mediastinum or hilum
  ○ Mostly found in middle and posterior compartment
  ○ With or without calcification
  ○ CT scan reveals homogenous contrast enhancement
  ○ Associated with recurrent pleural effusion
  ○ Arteriography to determine vascularity
- Plasma cell type
  ○ Multiple lymph node enlargement
  ○ CT scan reveals soft tissue mass with mild contrast enhancement
  ○ "Satellite lymphadenopathy"
  ○ Punctate calcification
- Multicentric type
  ○ Peripheral lymph node enlargement
  ○ CT scan with ground glass attenuation
  ○ Reticular-nodular interstitial pattern
  ○ Poorly defined centrilobular nodules
  ○ Bronchoarterial bundle thickening
  ○ Interlobular septal thickening
  ○ Mediastinal lymphadenopathy
  ○ Pleural effusions
○ Diagnosis
- Tissue biopsy
- Clinical staging including CT chest, abdomen, and pelvis
- Skeletal survey
- Gallium scintigraphy
- Serum protein electrophoresis
- Bone marrow biopsy
- Diagnosis of exclusion
○ Treatment
- Hyaline vascular type
  ○ No further treatment required after complete surgical excision
  ○ Preoperative embolization before resection
  ○ Radiation for poor surgical candidates
  ○ Long-term follow-up required

- Plasma cell type
  ○ Surgical resection
  ○ Good outcome with surgery
- Multicentric type
  ○ Immunosuppressive medications with limited benefit
  ○ First-line treatment is with chemotherapy (etoposide, vinblastine, or cyclophosphamide) and steroids
  ○ Initiate highly active antiretroviral therapy treatment for HIV-infected patients
  ○ Limited data on use of anti-CD20 monoclonal antibody (rituximab)
  ○ Undetermined benefit with radiation therapy
  ○ Splenectomy in case of severe pain or peripheral cytopenia
  ○ Poor outcome despite treatment
  ○ Frequent relapse
  ○ Close follow-up due to risk for development of Kaposi's sarcoma and lymphoma
- **Kaposi's sarcoma**[28-30]
  ○ Classification
    - Classic type
    - Endemic type (Africa)
    - Transplantation associated type (iatrogenic)
    - Epidemic type (AIDS associated)
  ○ Pathogenesis
    - Spindle-shaped tumors cells surrounding hyperemic vascular slits
    - Associated with human herpesvirus 8
    - Also known as Kaposi sarcoma–associated herpesvirus
    - Transmitted via bodily fluid (saliva and semen) but remains latent in immunocompetent host
    - Reactivation of virus in immunodeficient state leading to production of interleukin 6 and angiogenesis
    - Herpesvirus 8 also associated with lymphomas and multicentric Castleman's disease
    - Organ transplant–associated Kaposi's sarcoma is more aggressive involving lymph nodes, mucosa, and visceral organs (1%–5%)
    - See Figure 43-4
      1. Demographics

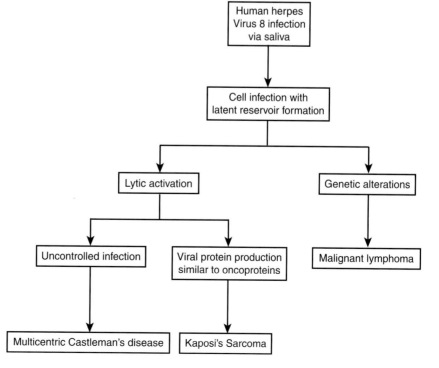

**Figure 43-4:** Figure depicting possible mechanisms whereby Human herpesvirus 8 results in disease processes. *(Adapted from Filly R, Blank N, Castellino RA. Radiographic distribution of intrathoracic disease in previously untreated patients with Hodgkin's disease and non-Hodgkin's lymphoma. Radiology 1976;120:277-281.)*

- Elderly man of Eastern European and Mediterranean origin in classic type
- More common in men than in women (15:1)
- Higher risk in homosexual men
- Increased risk in immunocompromised patients (organ transplant, HIV)
- Most common AIDS-associated cancer in the United States
  ○ Symptoms/clinical findings
    - Most primary infected patients are asymptomatic
    - Multiple purple-blue plaques and nodules on hands, feet, arms, and legs
    - Also involve viscera and mucosa (10%)
    - Lymphadenopathy
    - Lymphedema
  ○ Diagnosis
    - Serologic assays
    - Gold standard method for diagnosis not established
    - Tissue diagnosis
  ○ Treatment
    - Observation for immunocompetent asymptomatic patients
    - Initiate HAART therapy in HIV-infected patients
    - Regression or resolution of disease with reduction or cessation of immunosuppressive treatment (renal transplant)
    - Limited treatment area with single dose of radiation
    - Local injection of interferon alfa
    - Combination treatment with surgery, chemotherapy, and radiation for extensive or recurrent disease
    - Chemotherapeutic agents include etoposide, vinblastine, bleomycin, doxorubicin, paclitaxel, or dacarbazine.
    - Improved response with liposomal doxorubicin
    - Experimental treatments include thalidomide to prevent angiogenesis, retinoic acid to block autocrine growth factors, and human chorionic gonadotropin in men.
- **Lymphangiomas**[1,6,5,11,12,31-36]
  ○ Classification
    - Capillary lymphangiomas (small lymphatics)
    - Cavernous lymphangiomas (larger lymphatics)
    - Cystic lymphangiomas (large macroscopic lymphatics with collagen and smooth muscle)
      1. Pathogenesis
    - Congenital benign tumor
    - Abnormalities of the lymphatic vessel
    - Arise from lymphatic tissue sequestration derived from jugular lymph sac
    - Associated with chromosomal abnormalities
    - Observed with chylothorax and hemangiomas
    - Also known as "cystic hygromas," "lymphatic cysts," or "chylous cysts"
    - Cysts may become infected or hemorrhagic
    - Represents 0.01% to 4.5% of mediastinal tumors
  ○ Demographics
    - 90% identified before the age of 2 for cervicomediastinal cystic hygroma
    - Male-to-female ratio of 1:3
  ○ Symptoms/findings
    - Most asymptomatic
    - Symptoms related to location in the neck and mediastinum
    - Dyspnea, cough, hemoptysis, dysphagia, and chest pain
    - Fever from infected cyst
    - Vocal cord paralysis and stridor
    - Respiratory obstruction
  ○ Radiographic findings
    - Well-circumscribed, homogenous, solitary mass
    - Loculated and cystic

- With or without calcification
- Pleural effusions
- Compression or deviation of trachea, superior vena cava, left innominate vein, or brachiocephalic artery
- Located in cervical region (75%)—children
- Mediastinum (10%)—adults without cervical lymphadenopathy
- Commonly found in anterior and superior mediastinum
- Similar to pericardial cysts in appearance
- Differentiate from pericardial cysts with CT scan of the chest with lymphangiographic contrast
- MRI conclusively demonstrates cystic components and optimal visualization of local invasion.
  ○ Diagnosis
    - Surgical biopsy
    - Histologically similar to pericardial cysts
    - Different location and appearance of the cyst
    - Presence of smooth muscle within the tumor
    - See Table 43-3
  ○ Treatment
    - Surgical excision
    - Radiotherapy in cases complicated by chylothorax
    - High recurrence rate with incomplete excision
    - Limited success with chemotherapy (interferon alfa and cyclophosphamide)
    - Alternative treatments include injection of sclerosing agents such as steroids, hypertonic saline, ethanol, bleomycin, and OK-432
- **Amyloidosis**[37,38]
  ○ Pathogenesis
    - Extracellular deposition of a fibrillary glycoprotein in the tracheobronchial tree, pulmonary parenchyma, or mediastinal lymph nodes
    - Deposits between parenchymal cells, connective tissue, and blood vessel walls cause organ impairment
    - Calcification and ossification
  ○ Symptoms/findings
    - Cough and dyspnea
    - Hemoptysis
    - Recurrent pneumonias
    - Airway obstruction
  ○ Radiographic findings
    - Mediastinal and hilar adenopathy
    - Nodules (solitary or multiple)
      ○ Appear as a mass
      ○ Irregular, poorly defined margins

---

**TABLE 43-3 ■ DIFFERENCE AND SIMILARITIES BETWEEN LYMPHANGIOMA AND PERICARDIAL CYST**

|  | Lymphangioma | Pericardial Cyst |
|---|---|---|
| Location | Middle mediastinum superior portion of anterior mediastinum | Heart Near diaphragm |
| Characteristic | Multilocular | Unilocular |
| Histology | Fluid | Fluid |
| Presence of smooth muscle within tumor | Yes | No |

- ○ Located peripherally and subpleurally
- ○ Cavity formation
- ○ "Stippled or cloudlike" calcification
- ■ Diffuse parenchymal
  - ○ Similar in appearance to pulmonary congestion
- ■ Tracheobronchial (solitary or diffuse)
  - ○ Diffuse infiltration of tracheobronchial tree or mass
  - ○ Involve larynx and subglottic areas
  - ○ Narrowing of the trachea or bronchus
  - ○ Recurrent secondary infiltrations
  - ○ Lobar atelectasis
  - ○ Diffuse calcification of the trachea and bronchi (tracheobronchopathia osteoplastica)
- ■ Cardiac involvement
  - ○ Nonspecific cardiomegaly
  - ○ Pulmonary congestion
    1. Diagnosis
- ■ Tissue required for diagnosis
- ■ Hematoxylin-eosin stain of amorphous acellular eosinophilic deposits with green birefringence with Congo red stain visualized under polarizing microsocope
- ○ Treatment
  - ■ Therapeutic bronchoscopy for removal of obstructing endobronchial lesions
- ■ **Angioimmunoblastic lymphadenopathy**[11,39,40]
  - ○ Pathogenesis
    - ■ Also known as angiomatous lymphoid hamartomas
    - ■ Benign proliferation of immune reactive cells and small blood vessels
    - ■ Hyperimmune response from exposure to medications including penicillin, sulfonamides, aspirin, phenytoin, phenobarbital, and primidone
    - ■ Superficially resembles lymphocytic lymphoma
  - ○ Demographics
    - ■ Mean age of 62 years old
  - ○ Symptoms/findings
    - ■ Cough, dyspnea, and pleuritic chest pain
    - ■ Constitutional B symptoms (fever, night sweats, and weight loss)
    - ■ Pruritus
    - ■ Lymphadenopathy
    - ■ Hepatosplenomeagly
    - ■ Skin rash
    - ■ Hypergammaglobulinemia and eosinophilia
    - ■ With or without Bence Jones proteinuria
    - ■ Similar clinical presentation as HD
  - ○ Radiographic findings
    - ■ Mediastinal or hilar adenopathy (18%)
    - ■ Interstitial pulmonary infiltrates or nodules (15%)
    - ■ Pleural effusions (12%)
  - ○ Diagnosis
    - ■ Lymph node biopsy
    - ■ Small vessel proliferation with hyperplastic endothelium
    - ■ Pleomorphic cellular infiltrates in immunoblasts, lymphocytes, eosinophils, leukocytes, and plasma cells
    - ■ Positive Periodic Acid–Schiff stain
  - ○ Treatment
    - ■ Steroids produce good response (40% remission)
    - ■ Cytotoxic chemotherapy (cyclophosphamide, vincristine)
    - ■ Significant risk of sepsis with steroid and chemotherapy treatment
    - ■ Complete surgical excision
    - ■ Progressive disease with poor prognosis
    - ■ Potential for malignant transformation
      Benign mediastinal lymphadenopathy (granulomatous disease)[3,5,6]

- ○ **Infectious causes**
  - ■ Unilateral and asymmetric lymph node involvement
  - ■ Tuberculosis
    - ○ Tuberculoma
  - ■ Histoplasmosis
  - ■ Coccidioidomycosis
  - ■ Echinococcal cysts
    - ○ Primarily affects the lungs
    - ○ Mediastinal cyst associated with eosinophilia and liver cyst
- ○ **Noninfectious causes**
  - ■ Symmetric and bilateral lymph node involvement
  - ■ Silicosis—"egg shell" calcification
  - ■ Sarcoidosis
  - ■ Reactive hyperplasia—postinfectious reaction or drugs including phenytoin
- ■ **Metastatic mediastinal lymphadenopathy**[3,6,41]
  - ○ Metastasis to mediastinum and hilar lymph nodes
  - ○ Primary lung cancer
  - ○ Breast cancer
  - ○ Renal cell cancer
  - ○ Gastrointestinal cancer
  - ○ Prostate cancer
  - ○ Melanoma
  - ○ **Germ cell tumor**[41] (see Chapter 42)
    - ■ Significant number of testicular nonseminomatous germ cell tumor (NSGCT) with metastases to the mediastinum
    - ■ Metastases via thoracic duct
    - ■ Elevated serum tumor markers correlates with mediastinal metastases
    - ■ Chemotherapy converts some tumors to teratoma or necrotic tissue
    - ■ Surgical resection for metastastic mediastinal disease from residual teratoma or necrotic tissue with favorable long term survival

## MISCELLANEOUS

- ■ **Diaphragmatic hernias**[6]
  - ○ Hiatal hernia
    - ■ Appearance of retrocardiac mass
  - ○ Congenital hernia
    - ■ Herniation of omentum or abdominal wall contents
    - ■ Morgagni hernia—right cardiophrenic angle masses
    - ■ Diagnosis established by gastrointestinal barium or cross sectional imaging
    - ■ Surgical treatment for symptomatic patients
- ■ **Pancreatic pseudocyst**[42,43]
  - ○ Pathogenesis
    - ■ Pancreatitis leading to pseudocyst formation with extension into mediastinum
    - ■ Mostly located in the posterior mediastinum but found in the middle mediastinum
    - ■ Mediastinal extension via diaphragm erosion or esophageal or aortic hiatus
  - ○ Symptoms/findings
    - ■ Local compressive symptoms
    - ■ Dysphagia, dyspnea or chest discomfort
    - ■ Abdominal pain
  - ○ Radiographic findings
    - ■ Retrocardiac density
    - ■ Left-sided or bilateral pleural effusions
    - ■ Diaphragm elevation
    - ■ Subsegmental atelectasis
    - ■ Consolidation (pneumonic or atelectic)

○ Diagnosis
  ■ Usually an incidental finding
  ■ Ultrasound or CT imaging
  ■ Endoscopic retrograde pancreatographic study
○ Treatment
  ■ Observation for asymptomatic patients
  ■ Laparotomy and cystenteric anastomosis for symptomatic patients

## IMAGING STUDIES

■ Plain chest radiograph[4,7,9]
  ○ Initial evaluation of mediastinal mass
■ Chest CT scan
  ○ Optimal evaluation of mediastinum
  ○ Delineate vascular from nonvascular lesions with contrast study
  ○ Plan for diagnostic approach
■ MRI scan
  ○ Equivalent to CT scan for detecting mediastinal lymph nodes and masses
  ○ Cannot differentiate between benign and malignant lymph nodes
  ○ Determine invasion or encasement of major cardiovascular structures
■ Upper extremity venography
■ Esophagogram
  ○ Rule out communication in setting of esophageal duplication cyst

## DIAGNOSIS

■ CT-guided biopsy[4,9]
  ○ Low morbidity with procedure
  ○ Inadequate for diagnosis in certain cases (lymphoma)
  ○ Reliable for diagnosis of germ cell tumors
■ Bronchoscopy
  ○ Paratracheal and subcarinal lymphadenopathy
  ○ History of hemoptysis
  ○ Lobar or segmental atelectasis
■ Surgical procedures
  ○ Thoracotomy or mediastinoscopy to evaluate upper middle mediastinum along trachea to bifurcation (level 2, 4, and 7 lymph nodes).
  ○ Extended mediastinoscopy to evaluate aortopulmonary window lymph nodes (see Chapter 5 on Mediastinoscopy).
  ○ Chamberlain procedure (anterior mediastinotomy) to biopsy para-aortic and aortic pulmonary window nodes (level 6 and 5)

## TREATMENT

■ See earlier discussion for specific disease treatment[4]
■ Hospitalization with urgent surgical consultation for massive hemoptysis or airway compromise

### Brief Illustrative Case

• A 33-year-old woman presented with bulbar signs (dysarthria), ptosis, diplopia and upper limb weakness.
• Electromyogram/nerve stimulation and antibody studies (acetylcholine receptor antibodies) confirmed a diagnosis of myasthenia gravis.

• The patient was initially started on pyridostigmine (Mestinon, Aliso Viejo, CA) therapy and soon thereafter corticosteroids were added.
• Routine and CT imaging studies revealed a middle mediastinal mass (Figs. 43-5 and 43-6).
• Several months later the patient developed acute respiratory failure requiring mechanical ventilation.
• The patient's condition was due to a myasthenic crisis triggered by severe sepsis.
• The patient was given intravenous immunoglobulin, which produced little response. She responded well to plasmaphoresis.
• A subsequent CT of the chest showed a significant reduction in the size of the middle mediastinal mass (Fig. 43-7).

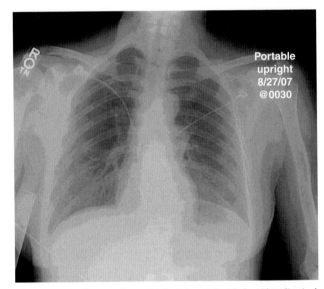

**Figure 43-5:** Chest radiograph depicting left sided midmediastinal mass in patient with myasthenia gravis.

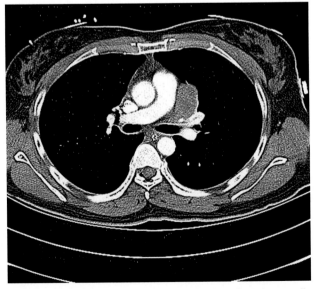

**Figure 43-6:** Computed tomography of the chest depicting a well-defined midmediastinal mass.

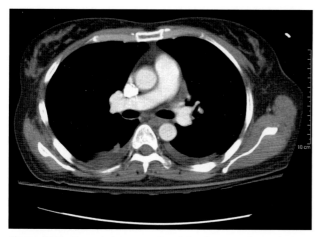

**Figure 43-7:** Computed tomography of the chest several months later depicting a marked reduction in the size of the midmediastinal mass depicted in Figure 43-6.

- Once fully recovered, the patient underwent thymectomy/mass removal via a median sternotomy approach.
- Pathology revealed an invasive thymoma with invasion into the capsule and lymphatics and reactive hyperplasia (Fig. 43-8).

**Key Points**

- The above-mentioned clinical description is fairly typical for myasthenia.
- Thymoma usually is located in the anterior mediastinum, but several reports of middle mediastinal location have been reported.
- Seventy-five percent of patients with myasthenia have some form of thymic abnormality.

*(Continued)*

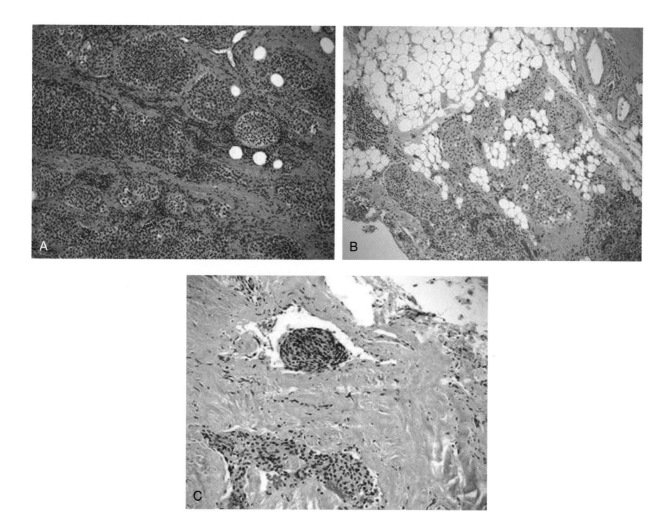

**Figure 43-8:** Pathology from thymectomy: (**A**) AB type thymoma, (**B**) invasion into extracapsular fat, and (**C**) invasion into lymphatics.

## References

 Interactive references and additional readings for this chapter can be accessed online at *expertconsult.com*.

# 44 POSTERIOR MEDIASTINAL MASSES

Dani Hackner, MD, Robert J. McKenna Jr., MD, and Michael I. Lewis, MD

## TERMINOLOGY

- The *posterior mediastinum* is bounded by the pleura laterally and is posterior to the pericardium. It includes the thoracic spine and the paraspinal gutters.

## ANATOMY

Depending on the classification used, the posterior compartment of the mediastinum includes the following structures found from the posterior pericardium to and including the thoracic spine and para-spinal gutters (Fig. 44-1).

- Vertebral bodies
- Sympathetic chains
- Descending aorta
- Esophagus
- Azygous and hemiazygous veins
- Thoracic duct
- Posterior mediastinal lymph nodes
- Lower portion of the vagus nerve
- Fat

## INTRODUCTION TO THE POSTERIOR MEDIASTINUM

- This section describes masses in the posterior mediastinum, with special emphasis on the more commonly encountered lesions (Table 44-1).
- The differential diagnosis of posterior mediastinal masses spans multiple disciplines.
  - Hematology/oncology
  - Infectious diseases
  - Neurology
  - Neurosurgery
  - Pulmonology
  - Rheumatology
  - Thoracic surgery
  - Other specialties
- The aim of this chapter is to enable the clinician to provide a rational differential diagnosis for posterior mediastinal masses and to initiate an appropriate workup.

## PRINCIPLES OF WORKUP

- Demographics[1]
  - This chapter identifies differences between pediatric and adult populations.
- Symptoms and signs
  - Incidental findings (asymptomatic)
  - Constitutional or systemic features (such as fever and weight loss)
  - Cough
  - Site-specific symptoms such as chest or back pain
  - Neurologic symptoms and signs
  - Other disease-specific features
- Imaging
  - Plain radiographs
    - May show features of a mass compatible with a posterior mediastinal location
    - May include alterations of visibility of mediastinal structures or displacement of mediastinal lines/interfaces (e.g., paraspinal lines)
  - *Computed tomography (CT) scan* is key to demonstrate the presence of a mass, along with its characteristics and location.
  - *Magnetic resonance imaging (MRI) scan* is better than CT scan for assessment of the extension of neurogenic tumors into neural foramina or cord compression.
  - Other imaging studies, including *positron emission tomography (PET)* or *other radionuclide* studies, are rarely indicated.

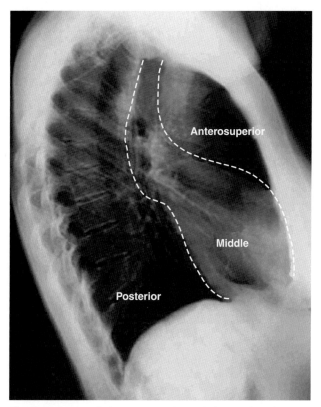

**Figure 44-1:** Lateral chest x-ray study marked to outline the three mediastinal compartments. *(From Townsend CM, Beauchamp RD, Evers BM, Mattos KL, editors. Sabiston Textbook of General Surgery. 17th ed. New York: Elsevier; 2004.)*

- Biochemical markers
  - ○ Tumor markers
  - ○ Urinary catecholamines for paraganglionic masses
- Tissue diagnosis
  - ○ The utility of fine-needle biopsy is unclear and likely not helpful for most posterior mediastinal masses. May be used to aspirate presumed benign cystic lesions (e.g., pericardial cyst). However, these are rarely posterior mediastinal in location.
  - ○ Complete surgical excision of a localized mass usually confirms the presence of a benign lesion.
  - ○ Limited surgical biopsy via thoracoscopy or open approaches may be warranted for workup of complex cases, especially when the primary treatment is not surgical. Examples include lymphoma or germ cell tumors that are not easily biopsied in a less invasive fashion. Such lesions are rare in the posterior mediastinum.[2]

## SPECIFIC MASSES OF THE POSTERIOR MEDIASTINUM

- **Neurogenic tumors**[1-7]
  - ○ Derived from neural crest tissue
  - ○ Asymptomatic tumors are often detected as an incidental finding on an unrelated imaging test.
  - ○ Three quarters of neurogenic tumors are benign.
  - ○ Neurogenic tumors make up 20% adult mediastinal tumors.[1,3]
  - ○ Neurogenic tumors make up 25% to 35% of pediatric mediastinal tumors.[1,3]
  - ○ Neurogenic tumors make up 75% of primary posterior mediastinal tumors.[1,3]
  - ○ Nearly all mediastinal neurogenic tumors are located in the posterior mediastinum (90%–95%).
  - ○ Nerve sheath tumors are more common in adults and are usually benign.
  - ○ Ganglion tumors are more common in children and often are malignant.
  - ○ In adults, the ratio of schwannomas to neurofibromas is 3:1 to 4:1.

## TABLE 44-1 ■ POSTERIOR MEDIASTINAL MASSES

**Neurogenic Tumors**

Nerve sheath tumors
   Schwannoma (neurilemmoma)
   Neurofibroma
   Malignant nerve sheath tumors
Autonomic ganglion cell tumors
   Ganglioneuroma
   Ganglioneuroblastoma
   Neuroblastoma
Paraganglionic tumors
   Paragangliomas
   Pheochromocytoma
   Chemodectoma

**Infectious Paraspinal Masses**

Infectious paraspinal abscess
   Tuberculosis (Pott's disease)
   Pyogenic bacterial infections
   Fungal infections

**Hematologic Disorders**

Extramedullary hematopoiesis

**Mediastinal Cysts**

Lateral thoracic meningocele

**Esophageal Masses**

Benign esophageal tumors
Malignant esophageal tumors
Esophageal duplication cyst
Esophageal disorders
   Hernia (e.g., Bochdalek diaphragmatic hernia)
   Achalasia

**Rare Presentations of Posterior Mediastinal Masses**

Sarcomas (osteosarcoma, chondrosarcoma)
Other mesenchymal tumors (lipomas, fibromas,
   xanthogranulomas, leiomyomas, mesenchymomas,
   mesotheliomas, benign fibrous tumors)
Carcinoma: metastatic; rare primary
Lymphoma and other lymph node disorders
Germ cell tumors
Hemangioma
Lymphangioma
Thoracic duct cyst
Vascular (aortic aneurysm; dilated azygous or hemiazygous
   vein; varices)

## Nerve Sheath–Related Tumors

- **Schwannomas (neurilemmomas)**
  - Pathology
    - Arise from the nerve sheath of spinal nerve roots of the intercostals or sympathetic nerves
    - Found in any thoracic location
    - They are rarely malignant.
    - May erode bone locally and compress nerves
    - Generally appear as a lobulated mass encapsulated and containing varying numbers of Schwann cells and myxoid tissue.
    - May exhibit cystic degeneration or hemorrhage
    - Fibroblasts and mast cells are often contained in the tumor mass.
  - Demographics
    - Affect men and women equally
    - Age: 30 to 50 years
  - Clinical features
    - Majority of schwannomas are asymptomatic
    - Compression symptoms can occur including
      - Pain (more typical in malignant tumors)
      - Paresthesias
      - Neurologic deficits (e.g., with intraspinal extension)
  - Imaging
    - Spherical, with smooth or lobulated borders
    - Variable size, but potentially large when asymptomatic
    - May extend horizontally along nerve axis
    - May span one to two rib spaces
    - May erode adjacent ribs or vertebra
    - Variable appearance on CT scans
      - May show reduced attenuation more consistent with fat or fluid
      - Occasionally show punctuate calcifications (10%)
      - May have contrast enhancement
    - MRI scan with gadolinium (T1 and T2) may be useful to evaluate neural foramina extension.
      - When extending into the spinal canal Schwannomas form a dumbbell or hourglass shape in less than 10% of cases (Figs. 44-2 and 44-3).[9]

- Management
  - Such tumors often require combined thoracic surgical and neurosurgical intervention because removal of only the thoracic component of the tumor can compress the spine and cause paralysis (see later).

- **Neurofibromas**
  - Pathology
    - Nonencapsulated
    - Well-marginated and lobulated like schwannomas
    - Homogenous collection of myelinated and/or unmyelinated nerve elements, nerve sheath cells, fibroblasts, and matrix
    - May exhibit cystic degeneration
    - One variant, plexiform neurofibroma, may involve entire nerve trunks or plexi.
    - Risk of malignant transformation
      - Five percent of lesions undergo malignant transformation in adults.
      - Much higher malignant transformation rates in children[3,10]
  - Demographics
    - Equal male-to-female ratio
    - Usually present in 3rd to 4th decades
    - Thirty to forty-five percent of cases occurring in the setting of neurofibromatosis.[1,3]
  - Clinical features
    - Commonly asymptomatic
    - May exhibit features of neurofibromatosis (see below)
    - Multiple neurofibromas or a single plexiform lesion are criteria for neurofibromatosis, a common disease.[11]
    - Pain at presentation increases the likelihood of malignant transformation.
    - Compressive symptoms can be observed, as in cases of schwannomas.
    - Recurrence and malignancy rates are higher in the setting of neurofibromatosis (10% lifetime hazard).[12]
  - Imaging
    - Similar to schwannoma

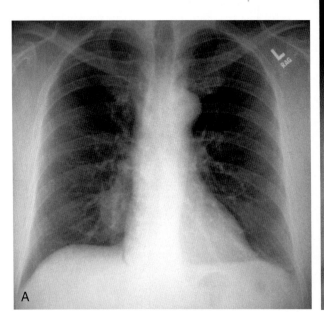
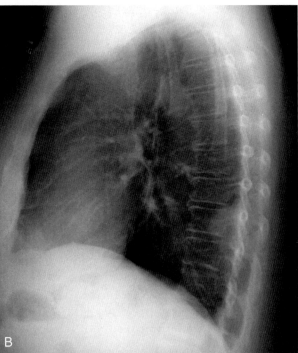

**Figure 44-2:** Posteroanterior (**A**) and lateral chest radiograph (**B**) showing posterior mediastinal mass (nerve sheath tumor; schwannoma).

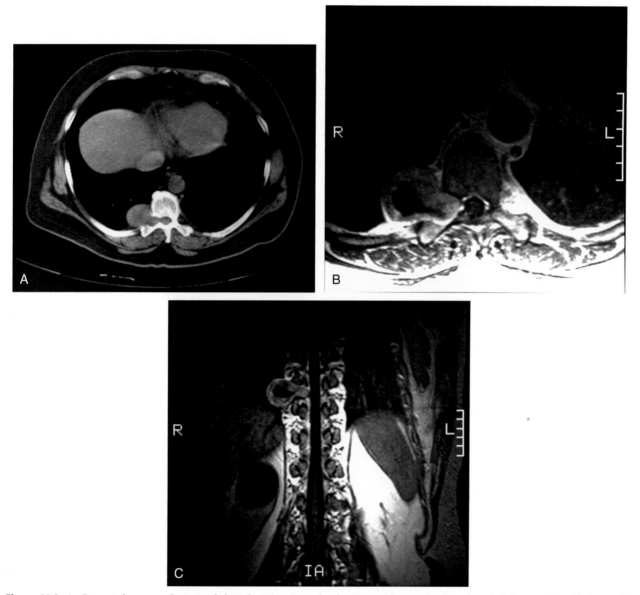

**Figure 44-3:** **A,** Computed tomography scan of chest depicting nerve sheath tumor with extension into the spinal foramen (dumbbell tumor). **B,** Transaxial magnetic resonance imaging (MRI) scan depicting the same. **C,** MRI coronal view with clear depiction of dumbbell shape and intraspinal extension.

- In comparison with schwannoma, neurofibromas are less commonly calcified and more homogeneous in contrast enhancement
- Malignant degeneration may be associated with pulmonary nodules or with pleural effusion.
  ○ Neurofibromatosis
  - Neurofibromatosis 1 (NF1) accounts for 85% of cases.
  - Autosomal dominant genetic disorder
  - 1:3000 individuals
  - Fifty percent are familial; 50% are acquired mutations.
  - Clinical criteria include
    ○ Café-au-lait macules
    ○ Neurofibromas
    ○ Axillary/inguinal freckling
    ○ Optic gliomas
    ○ Lisch nodules (iris hamartomas)
    ○ Sphenoid dysplasia or thinning of long bone cortex
    ○ Pseudarthroses
    ○ First-degree relative with NF1

- Share abnormalities of chromosome 17q11
- Meningiomas, neurilemmomas, and neurosarcomas (in children) have been associated with neurofibromatosis.
- Treatment considerations of nerve sheath tumors
  ○ Prognosis
    - For benign neurogenic tumors, prognosis with surgery is excellent.
    - By contrast, the outcome remains poor with malignant tumors, despite aggressive treatment measures.
  ○ Surgical removal is routinely recommended.[4]
    - Tumors will slowly increase in size, with resultant compressive or neurologic signs and symptoms.
    - Surgical removal can rule out malignancy.
  ○ Video-assisted thoracic surgery (VATS) has replaced the posterolateral thoracotomy approach as the preferred operative approach.[13-18]
  ○ Relative contraindications to VATS[16]
    - Tumors greater than 6 cm in size
    - Paragangliomas, owing to their vascularity

○ Dumbbell tumors may be amenable to a combined approach.[16-19]
  ▪ Posterior laminectomy, initially
  ▪ Thoracoscopic resection, subsequently
○ Invasion of foramina or vertebral body[20]
  ▪ En bloc resection may be feasible in some cases
○ Plexiform neurofibromas
  ▪ Frequently infiltrate or invade a trunk or nerve plexus.
  ▪ Complete excision is not usually possible.
○ Malignant nerve sheath tumors
  ▪ Complete surgical removal is the procedure of choice.
  ▪ For unresectable or incomplete resections, chemotherapy and radiotherapy are considerations, although response rates are not high.[3]
  ▪ Prognosis is poor.
○ Surgical complications[4]
  ▪ Partial sympathectomy
  ▪ Horner's syndrome
  ▪ Paraplegia
  ▪ Recurrent laryngeal nerve injury

▪ **Malignant tumors of nerve sheath origin.**[21]
  ○ Pathology
    ▪ Spindle cell sarcomas
      ○ Malignant neurofibroma
      ○ Neurogenic fibrosarcoma
      ○ Rare, malignant schwannoma
    ▪ May arise from neurofibromas
      ○ 50% associated with NF1
      ○ Sporadic or associated with risk factors such as radiation
      ○ Originate in isolated or plexigenic neurofibroma
    ▪ Usually cellular, high-grade sarcomas
  ○ Demographics
    ▪ Male and female equal prevalence
    ▪ 3rd to 5th decades
  ○ Clinical features
    ▪ Signs of neurofibromatosis may be present.
    ▪ More likely to have symptoms and signs of nerve or vertebral compression
    ▪ Metastases most frequently to the lung
  ○ Imaging
    ▪ Often large in size (e.g., >5 cm) but well circumscribed
    ▪ CT appearance
      ○ Heterogeneous appearance
      ○ Necrosis and/or hemorrhage are characteristic of malignant lesions.
      ○ Compression/invasion of adjacent structures may be noted.
  ○ Treatment[21]
    ▪ Complete surgical excision with wide tumor free margins is the treatment of choice.
    ▪ When complete excision is not possible
      ○ Simple excision
      ○ High-dose radiation
      ○ The role of chemotherapy has not been well defined.
    ▪ Adjuvant chemotherapy may not add benefit.
    ▪ Survival is poor.
      ○ Less than 35% 5-year survival

## SYMPATHETIC GANGLION TUMORS

▪ General considerations
  ○ Rare tumors
  ○ Subtypes
    ▪ Neuroblastoma (more than 95% of cases)
    ▪ Ganglioneuroblastoma
    ▪ Paraganglioma (often considered with above)

○ Range in behavior
  ▪ Benign (ganglioneuroma)
  ▪ Aggressive (metastatic neuroblastoma)
  ▪ Sympathetic ganglion cell tumors may represent a continuum.
○ Origins
  ▪ Neuronal primordial neural crest cells
  ▪ Adrenals (50% neuroblastoma)
○ In general, rare tumors

▪ **Neuroblastoma**[22-26]
  ○ Pathology
    ▪ Nonencapsulated elongated mass with varying degree of necrosis, cystic degeneration, and hemorrhage
    ▪ Sheets of small round cells
    ▪ Locally invasive or metastatic, or both
  ○ Demographics
    ▪ Children younger than 5 years; most younger than 3 years
    ▪ No gender bias
  ○ Clinical features
    ▪ General malaise and weight loss
    ▪ Symptoms attributable to metastatic disease in two thirds
    ▪ Pain
    ▪ Neurologic deficits, weakness, paralysis, ataxia
    ▪ Horner's syndrome
      ○ Ptosis, pupillary miosis, and facial anhidrosis
      ○ Arises from injury to stellate ganglion and T1
      ○ This affects the oculosympathetic pathway
      ○ May result from tumor compression or infiltration
    ▪ Respiratory compromise
    ▪ Paraneoplastic syndrome
      ○ Catecholamines (hypertension, flushing)
      ○ Vasoactive intestinal peptide (abdominal pain and watery diarrhea)
      ○ Psoclonus-polymyoclonus ataxia (cerebellar and truncal ataxia, and bouncing eye movements)
  ○ Imaging
    ▪ Typically elongated heterogeneous paraspinal mass (necrosis and hemorrhage)
    ▪ Often extends across midline
    ▪ Local compression/invasion
    ▪ Calcification usually evident: more than 85% on CT; 10% plain films; fine
    ▪ MRI scan again modality of choice for intraspinal extension
  ○ Treatment is determined by disease stage.
    ▪ Stage 1: Complete macroscopic removal of tumor is indicated for limited disease
    ▪ Stage 2: (local invasion) surgery plus postoperative chemotherapy and radiation
    ▪ Stage 3: (extension across the midline plus regional lymph node involvement) surgery plus postoperative chemotherapy and radiation
    ▪ Stage 4 (metastatic disease): chemotherapy and radiation. Surgery is controversial and may have limited value if a good response to chemotherapy.
  ○ In high-risk cases, surgery, chemotherapy, and blood stem cell transplantation have been performed.
  ○ Prognosis
    ▪ Poor prognostic features include
      ○ Late stage
      ○ Older patient
      ○ Poorly differentiated
      ○ Large tumor size
      ○ Extrathoracic origin
    ▪ Stages
      ○ Stages 1, 2, and 4S (stage 1 or 2 with metastasis to liver, skin or bone marrow): 75% to 90% 3-year event-free survival (EFS)

○ Stage 3: younger than 1 year of age; similar to stage 1 and 2; older than 1 year of age: 50% 3-year EFS
○ Stage 4: younger than 1 year of age: 60% to 75% 3-year EFS; older than 1 year of age: 15% 3-year EFS

■ **Ganglioneuromas**[22]
○ Pathology
■ Encapsulated
■ Clusters of ganglion cells and matrix
○ Demographics
■ Afflicted children older than 3 years of age; adolescents and adults in the second to third decade
■ No gender bias
○ Clinical features
■ Asymptomatic in 50%
■ Symptoms associated with local compression or intra spinal extension possible
○ Imaging
■ Typically elongated, well-marginated tumors that extend vertically along the anterolateral aspect of the spin. May extend across three to five vertebrae.
■ Coarse calcification may be evident
■ Benign pressure erosion of vertebrae may be evident
■ MRI scan modality of choice for intraspinal extension
○ Treatment
■ Complete surgical resection
■ Tumors with intraspinal extension require combined thoracic and neurosurgical procedures.
■ Prognosis excellent with surgical resection alone

■ **Ganglioneuroblastomas**[22]
○ Pathology
■ Exhibit histologic features of ganglioneuroma and neuroblastoma
■ Falls between ganglioneuromas and neuroblastoma in terms of differentiation and invasiveness.
■ Varying admixture of ganglion and neuroblast cells
○ Demographics
■ Presents mainly in children younger than 10 years of age
■ No gender bias
■ Least common neurogenic tumor
○ Clinical features
■ Can be asymptomatic
■ Symptoms due to compression, intraspinal extension, or local invasion
■ Can exhibit metastatic disease
○ Imaging
■ Typically elongated and extend vertically
■ Coarse calcification may be evident
■ Again, MRI scan is the modality of choice for intraspinal extension.
○ Treatment
■ Therapy is often based on histologic pattern.
■ Some subtypes have promising prognosis with surgical resection.
■ Others require chemotherapy based on histology, age, and stage of disease.[23,24]

■ **Paraganglionic tumors**
○ Pathology
■ Vascular tumors arising from aorticosympathetic para-ganglia and vagus nerve.
■ Histology shows amine precursor uptake and decarboxyl-ation (APUD) cells and vascular spaces
■ Rare tumors, often termed extra-adrenal pheochromo-cytomas.
■ Usually occur in paravertebral sulcus but may be found in the brachial arch of the middle mediastinum.
■ Ten percent of patients have multiple paragangliomas.

○ Demographics
■ Uncommon in children; usually appear 2nd to 3rd decade.[27]
■ Male-to-female ratio is 2:1.
■ Infrequent chemodectomas are reported in patients older than 40.
○ Clinical
■ Can present with symptoms and signs of catecholamine excess (e.g., flushing, headaches, hypertension refractory to medical management, anxiety, etc.). Incidence of 48% in a case series of 31 patients[27]
■ Locally invasive with neurologic signs in 5 of 31 patients[27]
■ Metastatic disease in 2 of 31 patients[27]
■ As many as 50% hereditary lesions associated with[28]
○ Familial paraganglioma
○ NF1 or von Hippel–Lindau disease.
○ Carney's triad (paraganglioma, pulmonary chondroma, and gastric leiomyoscarcoma).[3]
○ Multiple endocrine neoplasia (MEN) type 2 syndrome
○ Imaging/investigations
■ *CT and MR:* avid homogeneous contrast enhancement
■ *PET:* may show uptake
■ *I[123] metaiodobenzylguanidine (MIBG) radionuclide scan:* MIBG radionuclide study is positive in 70% of patients.
■ *Biochemical:* document catecholamine and fractionated metanephrine hypersecretion before imaging[28]
○ Treatment
■ Complete surgical excision, usually by thoracotomy
○ These are bloody tumors, and there may be less manipulation with an open procedure.
○ The aim is to release less catecholamines and maintain better hemodynamic control
■ Need preoperative catecholamine blockage
○ Alpha blockade with phenoxybenzamine is the first-line treatment, although few controlled trials have been reported.[29]
○ Nonselective beta blockade for epinephrine secreting tumors only after alpha blockade
○ Beta blockade without alpha blockade runs risk of accelerated hypertension due to unopposed alpha as well as beta-blocker related vasospasm
■ Locally invasive and metastatic disease
○ I 131 MIBG with or without combination chemo-therapy[30]

## OTHER EXTRADURAL TUMORS

■ Metastatic disease
○ Most spinal malignancies are located extradurally.
○ These are usually metastatic[10]
■ In metastatic cancer, vertebral metastases are commonly found at autopsy.
■ Prostate, breast and lung cancer are common cancers metastasizing to the vertebra.
○ Most of these tumors arise from the vertebral body.
○ Symptoms usually result from epidural extension.[31,32]
■ Constant pain
■ Night-time awakenings
■ Distal sensory deficits
■ Muscular weakness
■ Paralysis
○ Extradural tumors can cause spinal cord compression by intradural invasion.

- Sarcomas
  - Most arise from mesenchymal components and erode into bone.
    - Osteosarcoma
      - Ten to fifteen percent of sarcomas in general
      - Can be seen in 1% of patients with Paget's disease.[18]
    - Chondrosarcoma
      - Most common malignant tumor of the chest wall
      - Twenty percent of all bone tumors
      - Seen in third and fourth decades
      - May represent malignant conversion of benign tumors[33]
      - More typically found in the anterior costochondral region
    - Ewing's sarcoma (ES)[34,35]
      - Rare in this anatomic location; typically extremities
      - Fewer than 5% of cases in adults older than 40
      - Part of Ewing's sarcoma family of tumors (EFT); neuroectodermal origin likely, related to neuroblastoma
      - Arise from spine, paravertebral area, or even chest wall; extraosseous ES more typically found in these regions
      - Generally, treatment is chemotherapy.
    - Leiomyosarcoma—rare
    - Chordoma
      - Rare
      - Originate from primitive notochord
      - Highly resistant to radiation
      - Notable for recurrence at surgical sites.[36]
- Primary carcinoma
  - Accounts for a minority of mediastinal masses
  - Large cell, undifferentiated tumors are most common but still rare presentation

## PRIMARY CYST

- Lateral thoracic meningocele
  - Rare
  - Cyst containing cerebrospinal fluid and neural tissue that herniates through spinal foramina. Wall of cyst is made of dural tissue.[1,37]
  - Majority associated with neurofibromatosis. May also be associated with spinal trauma
  - Demographics: fourth to fifth decade; no gender bias
  - Clinical: asymptomatic or radicular intercostal pain
  - CT and MRI imaging modalities of choice. Well-circumscribed, 2- to 3-cm, fluid-containing mass. May note evidence of bony erosion and widening of spinal foramina
  - Surgical resection required in symptomatic cases
- Other mediastinal cysts
  - Paravertebral, thin-walled cysts are benign.
  - Often present as an incidental finding during workup for another disease.
  - Cysts may be found during workup for back pain, but the pain is almost always unrelated to the cyst and removal of the cyst will not relieve the pain.
  - Generally, resection is not indicated.
  - See Chapter 43 on Masses of the Middle Mediastinum.

## EXTRAMEDULLARY HEMATOPOIESIS

- Extramedullary hematopoiesis is a compensatory adaptation to chronic severe anemias[38]
- Most common predisposing conditions
  - Thalassemia
  - Chronic hemolytic anemias
  - Sickle cell anemia
  - Congenital spherocytic anemia
  - Myelofibrosis
  - Gauchers
- Lobulated paraspinal masses containing hematopoietic tissue
  - Mostly asymmetric
- Most commonly multiple and bilateral but can be unilateral. Usually below mid-thoracic region
- Imaging
  - CT
    - Lobulated
    - No calcification
    - Enhances with contrast
    - No evidence of bony compression sequelae (Fig. 44-4)
  - Technetium sulfur colloid scan
    - Can be used to support diagnosis (Fig. 44-5)
- Clinical
  - Can cause spinal cord compression
- Treatment
  - Responsive to low levels of radiation therapy.
  - Can suppress hematopoietic stimulus with transfusion and hydroxyurea.[39,40]
  - Resection is often contraindicated because patients need this source of red blood cells.
  - The only indication for surgery is emergency decompression of cord compression unresponsive to above approaches or emergency time constraints.

## INFECTIOUS ETIOLOGIES

- Osteomyelitis and paraspinal abscess
  - Bacterial
    - *Staphylococcus aureus* (more than 50% of all cases)
    - Less common bacteria
      - Enteric gram-negative bacilli
      - *Pseudomonas aeruginosa*
      - Group B streptococci
      - Group G streptococci.
    - Fungal
    - Candidal
    - Endemic fungal organisms
    - Mycobacterial (tuberculosis)

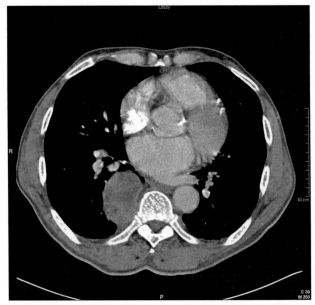

**Figure 44-4:** Extramedullary hematopoiesis exhibiting smooth paravertebral mass in a patient with thalassemia.

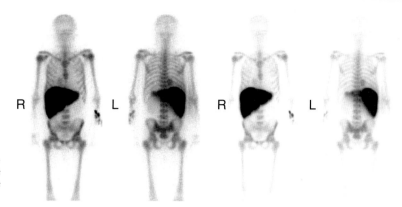

**Figure 44-5:** Technetium sulfur colloid scan showing prominent uptake in the mass shown above (same patient).

○ Osteomyelitis risk factors
  ■ Intravenous drug use
  ■ Endocarditis
  ■ Prior surgery and infected hardware
  ■ Diabetes
  ■ Immunosuppression
  ■ Prior radiation to spine
  ■ Corticosteroid therapy

## VASCULAR ETIOLOGIES

■ Thoracic aortic aneurysm
  ○ As opposed to the fusiform aneurysms, the saccular type can appear as a localized distension of wall.
  ○ Aortic aneurysms occur most commonly in the sixth and seventh decade of life.
  ○ The male-to-female ratio is 3:1.
  ○ Risk factors: hypertension, atherosclerosis (hyperlipidemia), age, Marfan's syndrome, Ehlers-Danlos syndrome, other aortic aneurysms.
  ○ See vascular section in Chapter 43 (Masses of the Middle Mediastinum) for more details.
■ Pseudoaneurysm
  ○ False aneurysm of aorta
  ○ Collection of tissue outside the aortic wall
  ○ Usually secondary to a rupture and contained bleed
■ Azygous and hemiazygous veins
  ○ Benign enlargement of these veins may be seen on imaging
  ○ Also may be enlarged in superior vena cava (SVC) syndrome due to recruitment
  ○ Transudative pleural effusions associated with occlusions
  ○ Lung cancer may involve these vessels in T3 disease.

## ESOPHAGEAL LESIONS

See Chapters 56 and 57 on malignant and benign esophageal disease.

## POSTERIOR MEDIASTINAL LYMPH NODES

See disorders of lymph nodes in Chapters 42 and 43 for details on these disorders.

## KEYS TO WORKUP

### Vertebral Disease

■ Perform malignancy risk assessment
  ○ Age older than 50
  ○ Prior malignancy

○ Unexplained weight loss
○ Pain over 1 month's duration (when associated with back pain)
■ Take history of
  ○ Infection
  ○ Intravenous drug use
  ○ Associated rheumatologic conditions or family history
  ○ Trauma
■ Examine for evidence of
  ○ Point tenderness
  ○ Neurologic impairment
    ■ Dermatomal sensory deficits
  ○ Severe kyphoscoliosis
■ Additional disease evident on imaging
  ○ Thoracic disc disease
  ○ Diffuse idiopathic skeletal hyperostosis (ankylosing hyperostosis or Forestier's disease)
  ○ Ankylosing spondylitis
  ○ Pott's disease (tuberculosis)
  ○ Syndesmophytes of reactive arthritis (formerly Reiter's syndrome)

### Neurologic Disease

■ Neurogenic tumors are most common of posterior mediastinal tumors.
  ○ Twenty percent of mediastinal tumors
■ Most neurogenic tumors are benign
■ Most present with nonspecific symptoms
  ○ Chest-specific chest pain
  ○ Unexplained weight loss
  ○ Rib pain (compression of intercostals)
■ Tumors may extend into middle mediastinum
  ○ Affecting trachea
  ○ Obstructing bronchi
■ When nerve sheath tumor is encountered, review criteria for von Recklinghausen's disease (NF1).
  ○ Diagnosed with two or more of the following:
    ■ Six or more café-au-lait macules with greatest diameter smaller than 5 mm in prepubertal and larger than 15 mm in postpubertal individuals
    ■ Two or more neurofibromas of any type
      ○ One plexiform neurofibroma
    ■ Axillary/Inguinal Freckling
    ■ Optic glioma
    ■ Two or more Lisch nodules (iris hamartomas)
    ■ A distinctive bony lesion
      ○ Sphenoid dysplasia
      ○ Thinning of the long bone cortex
    ■ A first-degree relative (parent, sibling, or offspring) with NF1
  ○ Risk of malignancy will affect followup and patient counseling

## Brief Illustrative Case

- Mrs. G., a 79-year-old woman, presented with dysphagia, anemia, and tarry stools.
- Physical examination revealed a pale woman in no acute distress.
  - Neck examination revealed thyromegaly.
  - Chest examination revealed dullness at the right base.
  - Abdominal examination revealed tenderness in the epigastrium.
- Laboratories/Studies
  - The patient was anemic (hemoglobin 10 g/dL).
  - A chest x-ray study revealed cardiomegaly and opacification of cardiac borders.
  - A CT scan showed a large hiatal hernia, small, right pleural effusion, and large posterior mediastinal mass (Fig. 44-6).
- Upper endoscopy for ongoing bleeding.
  - At 32 to 40 cm: subtotal obstruction of esophagus.
  - A 4-cm, submucosal mass appeared umbilicated.
  - Locally treated with epinephrine and biopsied.
- F18-deoxyglucose-PET study
  - Revealed intense increased activity (maximum SUV = 5.1) in the posterior mediastinal area in the region of the GE junction.
  - Findings consistent with neoplastic lesion.
  - No other focal areas of increased activity were seen in the remaining mediastinum, hilar regions, lung, or neck.
- Preoperative pulmonary function studies
  - Suggested patient could tolerate further surgical workup.
- Surgical workup
  - Flexible esophagogastroduodenoscopy, exploratory celiotomy with transhiatal esophagectomy with gastric pull-up pyloroplasty.
  - Followed by feeding jejunostomy.
  - The procedure identified an 8-cm tumor nearly obstructing the distal esophagus and extending into the posterior mediastinum.
- Frozen section confirmed the presence of a mesenchymal tumor with surgical margins free of disease.
- Thyroid isthmus biopsy was taken at the same time, later revealing follicular type papillary carcinoma of the thyroid.
- Mediastinal mass histopathology
  - Focal, poorly differentiated malignant neoplasm.
  - The tumor lacked histologic features of a typical squamous carcinoma or adenocarcinoma.
  - The results of the immunostains effectively excluded malignant lymphoma, malignant melanoma, or poorly differentiated neuroendocrine neoplasm.
  - Vimentin (a mesenchymal marker) suggested a mesenchymal neoplasm with aberrant keratin expression.
  - Final pathology classified it as a malignant gastrointestinal stromal tumor (GIST) involving the distal esophagus and proximal stomach with CD34 and CD117 immunoreactivity.

## Key Points

- With the history of dysphagia and the presence of a posterior mediastinal mass, a primary esophageal mass needs to be considered. Extrinsic compression of the esophagus could also produce dysphagia, however.
- GIST tumor of the esophagus is distinctly rare.[41]
  - GISTs are the most common mesenchymal tumors of the gastrointestinal tract.
    - Ten to twenty cases per 1 million population
    - One third are malignant.
    - Formerly called leiomyomas or leiomyosarcomas
    - KIT oncogene malignant transformation
      - Most patients have KIT mutation.
      - Imatinib mesylate, a tyrosine kinase inhibitor
        - Significantly improves the outcome for metastatic and unresectable GISTs
  - Workup
    - Contrast-enhanced CT first-line evaluation tool
    - Functional imaging with 18F-fluorodeoxyglucose positron emission tomography (FDG-PET) or diagnosis and follow-up
      - 80% of patients will demonstrate imatinib response on PET images
  - Biopsy
    - Percutaneous route is not recommended
      - The tumors are often fragile
      - Risk of intratumoral hemorrhage or necrosis
    - Endoscopic techniques recommended
  - Primary operative approach: complete surgical resection without disruption of tumor
    - Achieved in 40% to 60% of GIST
    - Wide margins generally not indicated
    - Lymphadenectomy generally not indicated
    - Often protrude displacing surrounding structures.

## References

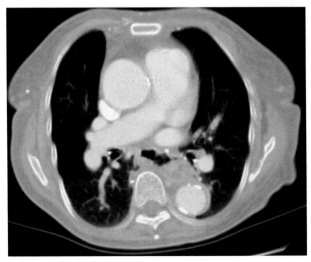

**Figure 44-6:** Computed tomography scan of the chest depicting posterior mediastinal mass inseparable from the esophagus.

 Interactive references and additional readings for this chapter can be accessed online at *expertconsult.com*.

# OTHER MEDIASTINAL DISORDERS: FIBROSING MEDIASTINITIS, ACUTE MEDIASTINITIS, AND MEDIASTINAL HEMORRHAGE

Atikun Limsukon, MD and Michael I. Lewis, MD

## FIBROSING MEDIASTINITIS

### TERMINOLOGY

- Fibrosing mediastinitis
- Sclerosing mediastinitis
- Mediastinal fibrosis
- Idiopathic fibroinflammatory lesions of the mediastinum

### INTRODUCTION

- Fibrosing mediastinitis (FM) is a rare, benign, gradually progressive fibroinflammatory reaction occurring in any compartment of the mediastinum but most commonly in the middle mediastinum, especially around the right paratracheal and subcarinal region or diffusely.[1,2]
- The pathogenesis is unclear.
- Affected patients usually present with signs and symptoms related to obstruction or compression of the mediastinal structures such as the superior vena cava (SVC), pulmonary arteries and veins, airways, or esophagus.
- The heart, coronary artery, and the aorta and its branches are much less frequently involved.

### EPIDEMIOLOGY

- Most affected patients are relatively young at presentation, although the disease can be found over a very wide range of ages.
- Men and women are affected in roughly equal proportion.[1]
- One series suggested a predilection for blacks.[3]
- Reported from many areas of the world but most of series are from North America and Europe.

### ETIOLOGY AND PATHOGENESIS

- The etiology of this disease entity is unclear, thus Flieder and colleagues[3] proposed the term *idiopathic fibroinflammatory lesions of the mediastinum* in 1999. Most of the cases in North America are strongly associated with *Histoplasma capsulatum* infection, whereas series from Europe are more often associated with tuberculosis.[2,4-14]
- Other infectious and noninfectious etiologic associations with FM have been reported anecdotally. These include
  - Aspergillosis, mucormycosis, blastomycosis, cryptococcosis, actinomycosis, syphilis, *Wuchereria bancrofti* infestation.[15-19]
  - Behçet's disease, Langerhans' cell histiocytosis, radiation therapy, silicosis, traumatic mediastinal hemorrhage, and the drug methysergide maleate.[16,20-23]

- The association of the FM and histoplasmosis in North America is based on several observations[1]:
  - Most disease occurrences are in the endemic area of *H. capsulatum* infection.
  - Many affected patients have positive skin tests for *H. capsulatum* antigen as well as residual granulomatous inflammation, or the *H. capsulatum* organism is occasionally identified in the histopathologic specimens.
  - Note: definitive histopathologic diagnosis of the infection is absent in most cases.
- The pathogenesis of the FM was not extensively studied owing to the rarity of the disease and the limited experience.[5,12,14,24-27]
- The most generally accepted hypothesis is the delayed-type hypersensitivity reaction to the fungal, mycobacterial, or other unknown antigens.[5]
- The relationship between FM and the granulomatous mediastinitis is also controversial. It is debated whether they are the different spectrums of the same disease or totally distinct and separate entities. The granulomatous mediastinitis tends to be more focal and less symptomatic compared with diffused FM.
- In 180 patients, Schowengerdt and colleagues[13] could establish a definitive diagnosis in 33 of 103 patients categorized in the granulomatous mediastinitis group but in only 3 of 77 patients in the mediastinal fibrosis category.
- In rare instances, the development of FM and retroperitoneal fibrosis or other fibrotic disorders (Riedel's thyroiditis, sclerosing cholangitis, sclerosing cervicitis, orbital pseudotumor, ligneous perityphlitis of the cecum, and keloids) were present in the same patient or in other family members.[28-38] This led to the term *familial fibrosing multifocal* fibrosclerosis, which was proposed by Comings and colleagues.[39]

### PATHOLOGY

- The gross pathologic characteristic of the FM is the ill-defined soft tissue mass that is composed of dense, white fibrous tissue involving the mediastinum either locally or diffusely.[1]
- Classic histopathologic features are an abundance of paucicellular, hyaline, fibrous tissue replacing the normal adipose tissue.[1]
- Flieder and colleagues[3] described three histopathologic spectrums that may help predict the outcome following the medical treatment:
  - Stage I: edematous fibromyxoid tissue with numerous spindle cells, eosinophils, mast cells, lymphocytes, plasma cells, and thin-walled blood vessels.
  - Stage II: thick glassy bands of haphazardly arranged collagen with focal interstitial spindle cells, lymphocytes, and plasma cells.

○ Stage III: dense paucicellular collagen, with scattered lymphoid follicles and occasional dystrophic calcification are the main characteristics.

## CLINICAL FEATURES

■ Patients can be asymptomatic but usually present with wide variety of symptoms and signs secondary to the obstruction or compression of the vital mediastinal structures as shown in Table 45-1.
■ The most common complaints are cough, hemoptysis, dyspnea, chest pain, and recurrent pulmonary infection.[1-3,6,7,16,40]
■ The incidence of SVC syndrome varies among series.
■ Patients can also present with dysphagia or bleeding esophageal varices.[10]
■ Involvement of pulmonary vein can lead to pseudomitral stenosis syndrome with pulmonary venous hypertension and recurrent hemoptysis. Complicating pulmonary edema can occur unilaterally or bilaterally depending on which side and which pulmonary vein is involved. Pulmonary venous infarction can also occur.[41-44]
■ Progressive obstruction of the main pulmonary arteries can result in pulmonary hypertension, cor pulmonale, and right-sided heart failure.[41,45]
■ Other clinical features include hoarseness from compression or entrapment of the recurrent laryngeal nerve, diaphragmatic paralysis from phrenic nerve involvement, tachycardia from compression of the vagus nerve, or Horner's syndrome from compression of the autonomic ganglion or nerve involvement.[13]
■ Finally, patients may present with only nonspecific constitutional symptoms as fever and weight loss.

## RADIOLOGIC FEATURES

■ Chest radiograph: usually abnormal and varies depending on whether the disease is localized or diffuse.[1]
■ The abnormal findings are composed of
   ○ Mediastinal widening
   ○ Hilar mass
   ○ Calcification
   ○ Lung parenchymal opacities
   ○ Pleural effusion
   ○ Airway narrowing
   ○ Note: changes on plain radiograph can be subtle

■ Computed tomography (CT) imaging: This method provides far greater information and is the imaging procedure of choice.
   ○ The CT findings[40,46-55] of FM may include the following:
      ■ A well defined mass
      ■ A diffuse infiltrating soft tissue density that obliterates mediastinal fat and encases or compresses the great vessels, tracheobronchial tree, or esophagus (Fig. 45-1)
      ■ A stippled or dense calcification throughout the lesion, which is also a common feature, especially in the focal pattern
   ○ Contrast-enhanced CT is useful in cases of suspected SVC or pulmonary vessel obstruction.
   ○ The pulmonary parenchymal abnormalities are secondary to pulmonary veno-occlusion and include ground-glass attenuation, interlobular septal thickening, or pleural effusion, as well as a wedge-shaped, homogenous consolidative process suggestive of a pulmonary infarct.
   ○ Two- or three-dimensional reconstruction images are helpful for the surgical or local therapy planning.
■ MR imaging[1,46,47,56]:
   ○ Typically, the lesion appears as an infiltrative area or mass with heterogeneous intermediate and low signal intensity on T1- and T2-weighted images.
   ○ The addition of the gadolinium can enhance the more active inflammatory areas and thus creates more heterogeneity. Low signal intensity represents areas of more mature fibrous tissue with less cellular components or calcification.
■ Positron emission tomography scans for FM are sparse with contradicting results.[57]
■ In summary, the CT scan is usually sufficient to suggest the diagnosis of FM, with magnetic resonance imaging (MRI) providing more information for noncalcified areas on CT (low signal intensity suggests the more mature fibrous tissue).

## TISSUE DIAGNOSIS

■ Surgical biopsy specimens obtained through mediastinoscopy, or more likely mediastinotomy, are usually required for the definitive diagnosis and for ruling out other neoplasms associated with extensive fibrosis in which the biopsy samples obtained with a percutaneous needle technique may be insufficient.[1,16,58]
■ Examples of these tumors are sclerosing non-Hodgkin's lymphoma, nodular sclerosis variant of Hodgkin's disease, or metastatic disease with prominent fibrogenic response.[1]

| Study | Cough | Dyspnea | Chest Pain | Hemoptysis | SVC Syndrome | Dysphagia | Pneumonia | Fever | Weight Loss |
|---|---|---|---|---|---|---|---|---|---|
| Loyd et al[2] (n = 52) | 41 | 32 | 23 | 31 | 6 | 2 | 23 | 19 | 10 |
| Urschel et al[7] (n = 22) | – | 14 | – | – | 59 | 14 | – | – | – |
| Mathisen et al[6] (n = 20) | – | 40 | – | 30 | 10 | – | 25 | – | – |
| Sherrick et al[40] (n = 33) | 45 | 42 | 27 | 27 | 39 | 6 | 27 | – | – |
| Mole et al[16] (n = 18) | – | 66 | 22 | 33 | – | 10 | – | – | – |
| Flieder et al[3] (n = 28) | 43 | 25 | 21 | 14 | 18 | – | – | 18 | 14 |

TABLE 45-1 ■ CLINICAL FEATURES OF FIBROSING MEDIASTINITIS

SVC, superior vena cava.

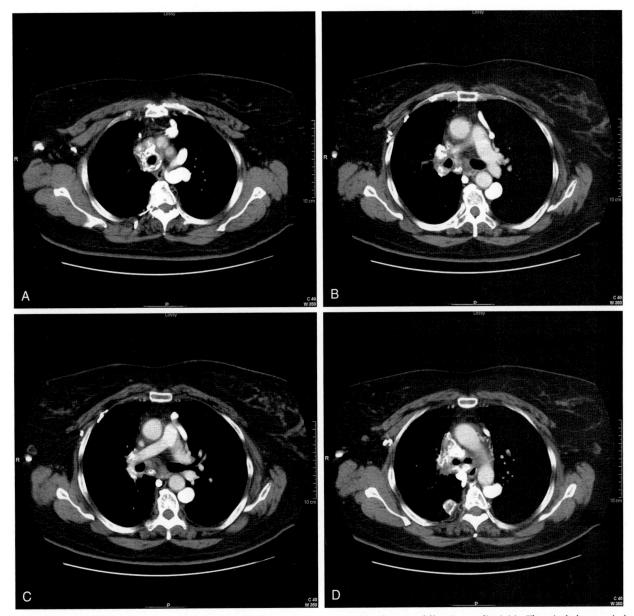

**Figure 45-1:** Serial axial CT mediastinal images (**A** to **D**) demonstrating some unique features of fibrosing mediastinitis. These include extensively infiltrating masses with prominent calcification; involvement in several locations (pretracheal, around the superior vena cava [SVC], retrotracheal extending into the right hilum, subcarinal areas); SVC obstruction with extensive development of collateral vessels from the azygous and hemiazygous system. Not shown: focal areas of geographic perfusion (compatible with focal air trapping due to airways obstruction).

## TREATMENT

- At present, there is no definitive treatment for this disease entity.
- There are limited and variable data on the use of systemic antifungal agents or corticosteroids in the setting of *H. capsulatum* infection and its inflammatory sequelae. Most of the available data are based on either case reports or small series, with no published randomized controlled trials.[6,7,58-60]
- Surgical treatment approaches are limited. Palliative resection may result in symptomatic amelioration in cases of localized disease.[4,6,58] A complete resection is rarely possible. There have been attempts at extensive vascular or airway reconstruction. For SVC syndrome, bypass grafting may be feasible in rare circumstances.[11,16,61] Overall, the results have been disappointing and associated with high morbidity and mortality.
- More recently, less invasive palliative approaches[62-64] have been used. These include
  - Endovascular stents used for SVC obstruction (see Chapter 28 on SVC Syndrome) or pulmonary vessel involvement.
  - Balloon dilatation and endobronchial stent placement.

## PROGNOSIS

- The FM often has an unpredictable course. Despite being a benign disorder, the clinical impact of the condition is often devastating.

- Loyd and colleagues[2] reported a mortality rate of greater than 30%. By contrast, Mole and associates[16] reported that 10 of 18 patients were alive up to 15 years after diagnosis, with only two deaths from malignancy and six lost to follow-up.
- Involvement of the pulmonary vessels, development of pulmonary hypertension and right-sided heart failure are associated with poor outcome and attributable mortality.

## ACUTE MEDIASTINITIS

### TERMINOLOGY

- Acute mediastinitis
- Descending (necrotizing) mediastinitis
- Postoperative mediastinitis

### INTRODUCTION

- Acute infections of the mediastinum are relatively uncommon, and most are reported after cardiothoracic surgeries.[65-68]
- Other etiologies[69-84] include
  - Infections of the head and neck, which cause descending (necrotizing) mediastinitis through the fascial planes
  - Esophageal perforation from endoscopic procedures, neoplasm, or after forceful vomiting (Boerhaave's syndrome)
  - Tracheobronchial perforation followed intubation or trauma
  - Direct extension of infections from adjacent tissues such as the retropharyngeal space, bones and joints, lymph nodes, pericardium, lungs, or pleura.
  - Rarely, it can occur after hematogenous spread of extrathoracic infection, such as septic arthritis.
- It is a life-threatening condition if it is not detected early or if treatment is suboptimal.

### ANATOMIC CONSIDERATIONS

- The mediastinum is bordered by the thoracic inlet superiorly, diaphragm inferiorly, parietal pleura laterally, sternum anteriorly and vertebral column posteriorly.
- The anterior mediastinal structures include the aortic arch and branches, great veins, lymphatics, and the thymus gland.
- The middle mediastinum contains the heart and pericardium, trachea, bronchi and hila of both lungs, the lymph nodes, and the phrenic nerves.
- The posterior mediastinum includes the esophagus, the descending aorta, the azygos vein, the thoracic duct, the vagus and sympathetic nerves, and the lymph nodes.
- The *three major fascial pathways of the deep neck*, along which oropharyngeal infections can spread to the mediastinum, are the pretracheal, lateral pharyngeal (perivascular) and retropharyngeal spaces.[69]
- The *pretracheal space* is limited superiorly by thyroid cartilage and ends in the mediastinum at the level of carina.
- The *lateralpharyngeal (perivascular) space* extends from the base of skull to the aortic arch and drains into the middle mediastinum. This space contains the carotid artery, the internal jugular vein and the vagus nerve.
- The *retropharyngeal space*, also called the *prevertebral* or *retrovisceral* space, starts at the C6 level of the spine and continues as far as the level of T1 and from that point onward, the so-called *danger space* begins. This danger space is patent to the diaphragm.

## EPIDEMIOLOGY AND CLASSIFICATION

- As mentioned earlier, acute mediastinitis is usually a complication of cardiac surgical procedures. In one large retrospective series of 10,713 patients,[66] the overall rate was 1.1%. In other series, acute mediastinitis was reported in 1% to 3%.[85-89]
- The host risk factors that contribute to the postoperative mediastinitis[65,90] include
  - Obesity
  - Diabetes mellitus
  - The use of bilateral internal mammary arteries
  - Advanced age, female sex
  - Chronic lung disease, active smoking
  - Prolonged mechanical ventilation
  - The use of steroids
  - Preoperative hospital stay longer than 5 days.
- Descending necrotizing mediastinitis (DNM)[69]
  - Mainly affects young adults
  - The median age is 36 years, and 86% of the patients are men.
  - Most common cause of DNM is odontogenic infection, especially of the second and third lower molars. This accounts for 40% to 60% of the cases. Retropharyngeal abscess and peritonsillar abscess makes up another 25%.
  - Less common causes include cervical lymphadenitis, traumatic endotracheal intubation, clavicular osteomyelitis, external trauma, intravenous drug abuse, parotitis, and thyroiditis.
  - Gravity and the negative intrathoracic pressure during inspiration help facilitate the drainage of pus from orocervical spaces into the mediastinum.
- Conditions like diabetes, alcoholism, neoplasm, and radionecrosis are risk factors for developing DNM.[91,92]
- Endo and coworkers[93] classified DNM into three groups based on the magnitude of infection as noted on CT. In the type I or focal type, the infection is limited in the superior mediastinal space above the tracheal bifurcation. The infection extends diffusely into the inferior anterior mediastinum and the inferior posterior mediastinum in type IIA and type IIB respectively.

## MICROBIOLOGY

- The most commonly isolated pathogens in acute mediastinitis following cardiac procedures are *Staphylococcus epidermidis* and *Staphylococcus aureus*. However, other gram-positive and gram-negative bacteria are also found in much lesser percentage.[66]
- The microorganisms causing DNM or acute mediastinitis after perforation of the esophagus are different. They involved aerobes and anaerobes, and often, mixed infection. The major bacteria recovered from infections originating from the oral flora are group A streptococci and oral anaerobic bacteria such as *Prevotella* and *Porphyromonas* spp, *Fusobacterium* spp, and *Peptostreptococcus* spp. Infections caused by *Bacteroides fragilis* were also reported.[82,94-96]

## CLINICAL FEATURES

- Depending on the location of the infection, clinical syndromes range from subacute to acute devastating forms.
- Chills, fever, tachycardia, dyspnea, and nonproductive cough are the most common symptoms associated with mediastinitis.[81,95]

- Retrosternal pain that radiates to the neck may be present if the upper mediastinum is involved, whereas pain from posterior mediastinal involvement may originate from the interscapular region and radiates around the chest.[81]
- Dysphagia, odynophagia, dysphonia, regurgitation, and cervical skin edema might also appear in the case of DNM. Subcutaneous emphysema is seen when there is a perforation of the upper aerodigestive tract.[69]
- In postoperative mediastinitis, most patients present within 2 weeks of surgery with evidence of increasing sternal pain, a draining wound site, and progressive redness.[82,97]
- When the infection is advanced, the patients may present with severe sepsis and signs of tissue hypoperfusion.
- Hamman's sign, which is a crunching sound auscultated over the precordium during systole, is due to the presence of air and fluid churning in the mediastinum.
- The diagnostic criteria for DNM proposed by Estrera and associates[98] are:
  - Evidence of oropharyngeal infection
  - Radiographic characteristics of mediastinitis
  - Intraoperative (or postmortem) documentation of mediastinal infection
  - Establishment of a relationship between oropharyngeal and mediastinal processes.

## RADIOLOGIC FEATURES

- Radiographic abnormalities of acute mediastinitis include widening of mediastinum, associated pleural disease, diffuse or focal ectopic gas bubbles within the mediastinum, focal mediastinal soft tissue masses, and mediastinal air-fluid levels. However, it is not possible to precisely characterize mediastinal infection and mediastinal abscess on the basis of chest radiography alone.[69,76,77,81,99]
- As mentioned earlier, the CT scan is crucial both for diagnosis and planning of treatment approaches (Fig. 45-2). The

contrast-enhanced CT scan findings can demonstrate fluid collections, extraluminal air, obliteration of normal mediastinal fatty planes, and air-fluid levels within the mediastinum or in the soft tissues of the neck. Extraluminal air is an important CT scan finding of esophageal perforation and is present in 92% of cases. Extravasation of ingested contrast material into the mediastinum can also be detected in esophageal perforation. The CT scan is also useful in monitoring the clinical course (Fig. 45-3) and outcome following the treatment.
- MRI usually does not provide more information in the diagnosis of acute mediastinitis, provided a good quality contrast-enhanced CT scan is available.

## DIAGNOSIS

- Besides the suggestive clinical presentation and imaging studies, the definitive diagnosis requires Gram's stain and cultures.
- The biologic material can be obtained by mediastinoscopy, subxiphoid aspiration,[100] or during definitive operative procedures.

## TREATMENT

- The treatment of acute mediastinitis often requires both antibiotics and surgical procedures, along with the supportive measures.
- Maintaining the airway, monitoring vital signs, and administering parenteral fluids are essential.
- The surgical procedures include correction of perforations, débridement of the infected wound, drainage of cervical or mediastinal collections, excision of chronic lesions, and mediastinal irrigation.
- Broad-spectrum antibiotics should be initiated as soon as possible before the surgery, once there is a clinical suspicion. Empirical regimens should include agents effective against anaerobes in the case of DNM or perforation of the esophagus. Piperazillin-tazobactam plus vancomycin is a good choice for the empiric treatment while awaiting culture results. Alternatives include clindamycin plus a third-generation cephalosporin or fluoroquinolone in penicillin-allergic patients. Carbapenems and metronidazole are also suggested.[69,100]
- After obtaining the culture results, antibiotics can be tailored. The duration of the antibiotics can vary from weeks to months. Oral antibiotics are usually continued when the patient is discharged from the hospital.
- Four different surgical approaches have been described.[91,100-103] The decision depends on the extent of infection.
  - Transcervical: usually sufficient for type I DNM; it is less invasive but may not reach deep regions.
  - Posterolateral thoracotomy: indicated for type IIA and type IIB, easiest to access mediastinal structures and also allows decortication in cases of concurrent empyema.
  - Median sternotomy: easiest for bilateral collections but also carry the risk of the sternal osteomyelitis and dehiscence.
  - Transthoracic:
    - Subxiphoid approach: useful in cases of anterior mediastinal collections; can be used in combination with transcervical approach
    - Clamshell incision (bilateral thoracotomy plus median sternotomy): excellent exposure but very invasive and carries a high risk of damaging the phrenic nerves
- Video-assisted thoracoscopy (VATS) has been reported, but its use remains limited. Early stages of infection or posterior mediastinal collections are ideal for a VATS approach.[84,104]

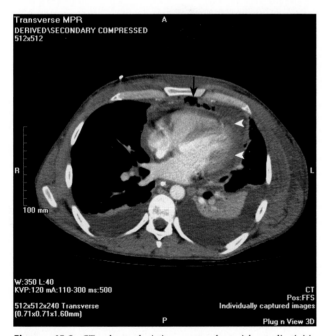

**Figure 45-2:** CT chest depicting acute bacterial mediastinitis complicating esophageal rupture. Note mediastinal fluid and air collection (*large arrow*) as well as pericardial fluid collection (*small arrows*). (From Dawes L. http://radpod.org/about-me. [with permission].)

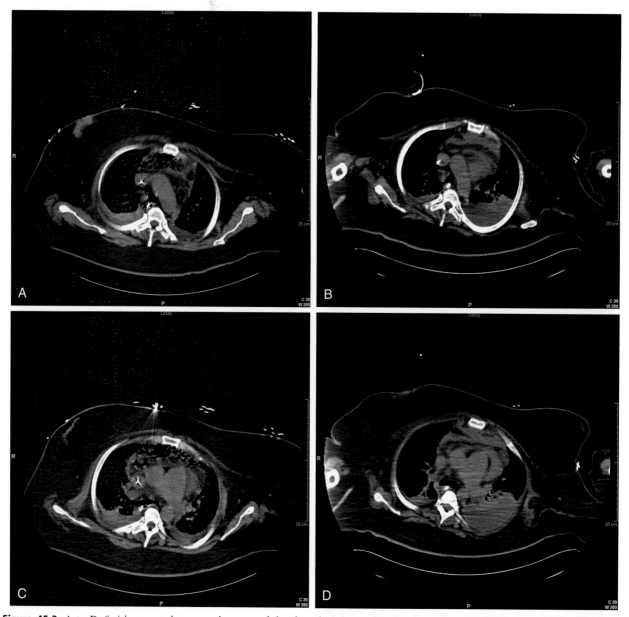

**Figure 45-3:** **A** to **D,** Serial computed tomography scans of the chest depicting evolving acute mediastinitis over a 2-week period. Although mediastinal air (**A** and **C**) decreases over time, significant infiltration of mediastinal fat is clearly evident (**B** and **D**).

- Regardless of the surgical approaches, irrigation and continuous drainage must be performed. It is also possible for continuous irrigation with antimicrobial solutions. The median time for keeping the drain is approximately 3 weeks.[100,105]
- CT scans should be performed serially following the intervention.
- Second operations are essential for persistent or recurrent, nondrained collections, to prevent further clinical deterioration.

## COMPLICATIONS AND PROGNOSIS

- The outcome depends on many factors including the degree of infection, and the underlying disease, or comorbidities. Overall, prognosis is generally poor, with high mortality rates reported (about 50%) for DNM,[69] less for esophageal rupture (10%–40%) and after cardiac surgery (20%–40%).[106]

- The key factors for improving the clinical course are early detection and readily available aggressive multimodality therapy.
- The main complication of acute mediastinitis is sepsis. Other complications include pneumoperitoneum, pneumothorax, pleural effusion or empyema, thrombosis of the internal jugular veins, carotid pseudoaneurysm, aortopulmonary fistula, aspiration pneumonia, epidural abscess, and adult respiratory distress syndrome.[69,78,80]

## CONTROVERSIAL AREAS

- The following controversial areas need further study to determine the best approaches to treatment:
  - ○ The optimal surgical approach
  - ○ The indication for tracheostomy

- ○ The role of hyperbaric oxygen
- ○ Defining optimal conditions for a VATS approach
- ○ The duration of antibiotics
- ○ The ideal time for wound closure

# MEDIASTINAL HEMORRHAGE

## TERMINOLOGY

- Mediastinal hemorrhage
- Mediastinal hematoma
- Hemomediastinum

## CAUSES

- Noniatrogenic traumatic injuries, including blunt and penetrating injuries of chest. Deceleration and traction stresses are also classic mechanisms of the thoracic aortic injury. Nonpenetrating injuries are usually high impact and severe in nature, such as those associated with motor vehicle accidents or falls from a height.[107-110]

- Note: Horizontal deceleration creates shearing forces at the aortic isthmus, the junction between the relatively mobile aortic arch and the fixed descending aorta. Vertical deceleration displaces the heart caudally and into the left pleural cavity, and acutely strains the ascending aorta or the innominate artery. Sudden extension of the neck or traction on the shoulder can overstretch the arch vessels and produce tears of the intima, disruption of the media, or complete rupture of the arterial wall.[107]

- Iatrogenic causes of mediastinal hemorrhage are usually complications of cardiothoracic surgery (most common), aortography or cardiac catheterization, central venous catheterization (Fig. 45-4), intra-aortic balloon pump insertion, endoscopic procedures or transthoracic needle aspiration or biopsy of a mediastinal mass.[111-115]

- Spontaneous mediastinal hemorrhage is rarer and can occur in the following circumstances:
  - ○ Abnormal clotting or fibrinolysis associated with hemodialysis, anticoagulant or fibrinolytic therapy, or hemophilia, which can be congenital or acquired factor deficiency.[116,117]
  - ○ Hemomediastinum secondary to hemorrhage into mediastinal glands, cysts, or tumors such as thymoma or germ cells tumor.[118,119]

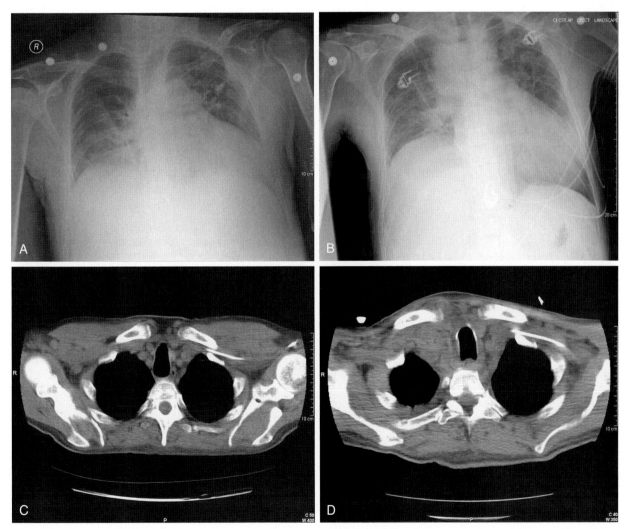

**Figure 45-4:** Chest radiographs (**A** and **B**) before and following acute mediastinal hemorrhage. Chest computed tomography scans (**C** and **D**) also depicting images taken before and following acute mediastinal hemorrhage that complicated a percutaneous central line insertion.

○ Idiopathic hemomediastinum occurring after a sudden increase in intrathoracic pressure, during coughing, sneezing or vomiting, or sudden sustained hypertension.

○ Spontaneous rupture of the thoracic aortic aneurysm or aneurysm of other vessels in the mediastinum.[120]

○ Necrotizing infection such as anthrax or suppurative mediastinitis.[121,122]

## CLINICAL FEATURES

■ Clinical manifestations depends on the etiology. Mediastinal hemorrhage itself can cause chest pain, dyspnea, hemodynamic instability, or symptoms and signs resulting from compression of other structures such as diminished peripheral pulse, upper airway obstruction. With massive extravasation of blood, this can be rapidly fatal.[107,115,117] Compression of the heart by mediastinal clot can produce an atypical tamponade-like condition.

■ Specific signs of an injury to the thoracic aorta are rarely present. Pseudocoarctation or decreased blood pressure in the left arm occurs in only 5% of patients with rupture of the aortic isthmus.

■ Clinical signs of injury to an arch artery are more common and include cervical or supraclavicular hematomas, bruits, and diminished peripheral pulses.

■ Coma or stroke-like symptoms may occur in cases of rupture of a common carotid artery.

## DIAGNOSTIC MODALITIES AND RADIOLOGIC FEATURES

■ Conventional chest radiography is essential for screening and typically shows symmetric uniform widening of the mediastinum. Local accumulation of blood, such as a hematoma, can be manifested by a homogeneous focal opacity that may project to one or both sides of the mediastinum and may be situated in any compartment (see Fig. 45-4A and B). Abnormal contour of the aortic arch, obscuration of aortopulmonary window, deviation of the trachea and main bronchus, or widening of paratracheal stripe could suggest rupture of the thoracic aorta or its branches.[99]

■ Contrast-enhanced chest CT, ideally multidetector CT, is a very powerful tool for demonstrating hemomediastinum and the possible underlying cause. The extravasation of the contrast-enhanced material is a direct sign. Indirectly, approximately 90% of acute hematomas are associated with localized areas of high attenuation as a result of high attenuation of clotted blood. These high-attenuated areas persist for about 72 hours, then gradually decrease secondary to lysis of the blood (see Fig. 45-4C and D).[99,108,110,120]

■ Transesophageal echocardiography is another highly sensitive and specific method to detect hemomediastinum related to thoracic aortic injury. It also allows quantitative assessment of traumatic hemomediastinum and can assist in the diagnosis of atypical tamponade. Further evaluation by aortography may be necessary.[123,124]

## MANAGEMENT

■ The management of mediastinal hemorrhage is mainly focused at the underlying cause and also depends on the severity, location, and the local effect of the hematoma itself.

■ The optimal management of mediastinal hematoma is to exclude catastrophic aortic disease. Once excluded, surgical intervention may be necessary to determine the etiology, manage ongoing bleeding, and ameliorate the effects of clot compression.

■ Small hematomas have been documented to resolve spontaneously with conservative treatment and correction of the coagulopathy.

■ Surgical evacuation is recommended for large hematomas, which can cause significant morbidity by causing compression of the heart, vessels or airways.[125]

---

### Brief Illustrative Case

• Twenty-three-year-old woman, who was born and grew up in Ohio.

• Presented with chronic cough and abnormal chest radiograph.

• Mild weight loss (10 lbs) noted over several months with intermittent low-grade fever.

• Physical examination was unremarkable.

• Chest CT (Fig. 45-5A and B) revealed a soft tissue mass in anterior and midmediastinal regions.

• VATS biopsy revealed chronic inflammation, fibrosis, and necrotizing granuloma formation. (Fig. 45-6A-C). Special stain (GMS) demonstrated fungal yeast forms compatible with histoplasmosis (see Fig. 45-6D).

### Key Points

• In the United States, histoplamosis is endemic within the Ohio and Mississippi River Valleys.

• The diagnosis is compatible with histoplasma associated mediastinal granuloma (epithelioid granulomas with caseous necrosis), although fibrosis is also evident.

• According to the latest Infectious Diseases Society of America guidelines,[126] with mediastinal granuloma, treatment is usually not recommended unless patient symptomatic. With mediastinal fibrosis, antifungal treatment is not recommended.

• Palliative stenting of vascular and other structures indicated in patients with symptomatic compression. Surgical management of mediastinal fibrosis is generally not recommended.

• In the above-mentioned patient, a 3-month course of itraconazole (200 mg daily) was proposed in view of her symptomatic state. There was no evidence of vascular, airway or other structure compression. Close follow-up was indicated.

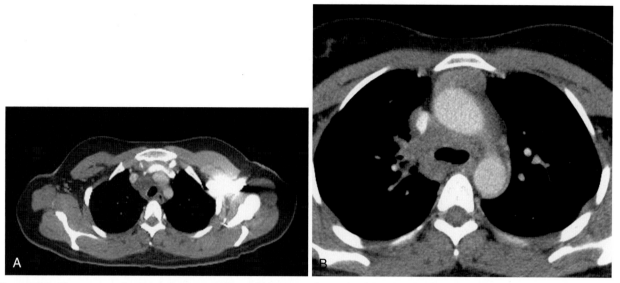

**Figure 45-5:** Chest computed tomography scan revealing soft tissue mass in anterior (**A**) and midmediastinal (**B**) regions.

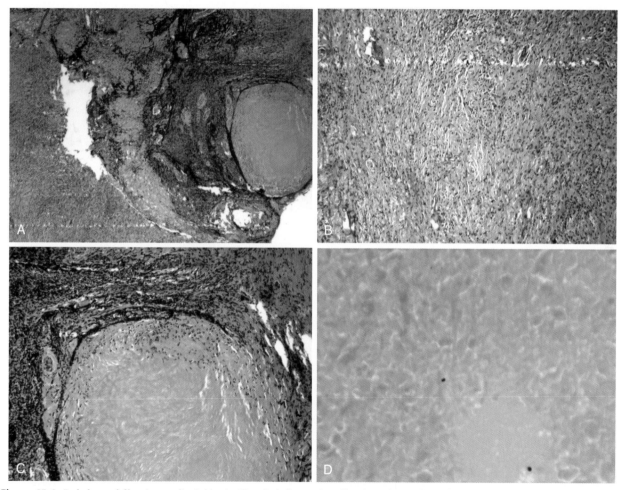

**Figure 45-6:** Pathology of fibrosing mediastinitis. **A,** Chronic inflammation, fibrosis, and granuloma formation. **B,** Chronic lymphadenitis and mediastinitis. **C,** Epithelioid granuloma with necrosis. **D,** Special stain (GMS) demonstrating fungal yeast forms compatible with histoplasmosis.

# References

 Interactive references and additional readings for this chapter can be accessed online at *expertconsult.com.*

# DISEASES OF THE PLEURA

## 46 TUBE THORACOSTOMY

### Alden M. Parsons, MD and Richard H. Feins, MD

## TERMINOLOGY

- Tube thoracostomy

## DEFINITION

A thoracostomy tube refers to a drainage tube placed percutaneously into the pleural space for drainage of intrapleural air or fluid.

## HISTORY

- Hippocrates was the first to describe drainage of the pleural space with metal tubes for empyema drainage.
- Playfair was the first to use an underwater seal with a drainage tube in 1872.
- Hewitt described closed drainage of empyemas in 1876, but it was not commonly employed until 1917 to drain postinfluenza epidemic empyemas.
- The use of chest tubes postoperatively for thoracic procedures was not common until reported by Lilienthal in 1922.

## INDICATIONS

Chest tubes are used to drain the pleural space in both emergent and non-emergent settings (also see Chapters 47 and 49 on pleural effusions and pneumothorax).[1] A variety of conditions can require drainage including pneumothorax (air), hydrothorax (fluid), hemothorax (blood), chylothorax (lymph), and (empyema or infection). Placement of a chest tube is indicated either acutely, when a patient is experiencing respiratory distress or is septic, or subacutely, when the patient is not in any distress, but the lung is prevented from fully expanding.

- Pneumothorax
  - ○ **Tension pneumothorax:** Ideally, there should never be an x-ray study documenting a tension pneumothorax. This is a clinical diagnosis based on respiratory distress with or without hemodynamic compromise and unilaterally decreased breath sounds. Tracheal deviation may be present, but it is often difficult to confirm. In this scenario, if the patient is truly unstable and a tension pneumothorax is suspected, needle decompression should be performed promptly with

a large-bore angiocath in the second intercostal space anteriorly followed by a chest tube.
  - ○ **Nontension pneumothorax:** A stable pneumothorax may at times be just closely followed with serial imaging if the patient is not in distress, has a relatively small space (<5 cm down from the chest apex), is reliable, and has been stable for at least several hours. Should it increase in size or should the patient develop respiratory distress, a chest tube should be placed. Usually a chest tube placed for air should be in the anterolateral fourth or fifth intercostal space and directed anteriorly.
- **Hydrothorax:** The character of the intrapleural fluid determines the management course. Intrapleural fluid may be serous, serosanguineous, purulent, or bloody.
  - ○ **Pleural effusion:** Serous or serosanguineous fluid may be either exudative or transudative. **Transudative** effusions result from increased hydrostatic pressure within the capillaries or decreased oncotic pressure related to an underlying process such as congestive heart failure or cirrhosis. **Exudative** effusions result from increased permeability of the capillary membrane from a process such as an infection or malignancy. Ordinarily, exudative effusions require chest tube drainage, whereas transudative effusions can be managed by treating the underlying causative medical condition.
    - Exudative
    - **Malignant:** effusions that have been confirmed to be related to a malignancy by positive cytology may be drained by a chest tube but are likely to recur unless treated by pleurodesis.
    - **Infectious:** effusions confirmed to be infectious by the presence of organisms on Gram's stain, positive culture, or pH less than 7.0, should be drained by chest tube placement.
    - **Transudative:** Pleural effusions that do not satisfy Light's criteria for exudative effusions are deemed to be related to an underlying medical condition predisposing to volume overload, such as congestive heart failure, cirrhosis, or renal failure.
- **Hemothorax:** Bloody pleural fluid is considered to be a hemothorax if the hematocrit is greater than 50% of that of the peripheral blood.
  - ○ **Traumatic:** Post-traumatic hemothorax should be drained with a large-bore chest tube. Undrained blood in the chest will develop into a fibrothorax and result in

underexpansion of the lung. A well-placed chest tube will drain early hemithorax, but an undrained clot may require the addition of intrapleural fibrinolytics or decortication for resolution.

■ **Empyema:** Pleural fluid may be classified as exudative or infectious based on the above-mentioned criteria, but an empyema is a true abscess of the chest. It is purulent intrapleural fluid that is loculated, and it does not change position with repositioning of the patient. Patients may have spiking fevers and sepsis if it is undrained. Proper chest tube positioning for empyema drainage may be curative if all of the pus is drained.

## PROCEDURE

■ What size?[1-3]
  ○ The choice of size depends on the indication for the drainage. For a hemothorax or empyema, a large-bore tube (i.e., at least 28 Fr) is needed. For a pneumothorax, a smaller (i.e., 24–28 Fr.) tube is adequate.
■ Where does it go?
  ○ The indication for the chest tube determines the location for the insertion. Most often, a tube is placed one to two intercostal spaces below the nipple in the anterior axillary line. For fluid drainage, the tube should be directed posteriorly. For air, it will be most effective if it is directed anteroapically.
■ What do I need?
  ○ A nurse to administer narcotics (although most of the time, you can perform the procedure with local anesthetic only), thoracostomy tray, chest tube, 4 × 4s, betadine, 0 silk, cloth tape, sterile towels, sterile gown/gloves/mask, chest drainage system, suction, 20 mL of 1% lidocaine (this is the most important part of pain control). A functioning intravenous needle should be in place as patients can develop hypotension from a vagal response during tube placement or lung re-expansion.
■ Where do I start?
  ○ Position patient so that correct side is close to edge of bed, with the arm above the head. Place something under the patient to elevate the side for the tube at a 45-degree angle. Prep a wide area with betadine or chlorhexidine.
  ○ First, anesthetize a small area with local anesthetic. Prior to making an incision, aspirate with a 22-gauge needle in the interspace where you intend to enter the pleura. This maneuver confirms that a tube in that location will provide the desired drainage of air or fluid.
  ○ The periosteum, interspace, and pleura are liberally anesthetized with local anesthetic, and then a small (~1.5 cm in length) incision is made in the anterior axillary line over about the sixth rib.
  ○ Before tunneling, place your sutures so you can secure the tube once it is in the chest. We generally place one 2-0 silk stitch at the edge of the incision to hold the tube in place and a second stitch directly in the middle of the incision to be tied after the tube is removed. This latter stitch can have its end knotted together and then be wrapped around the tube while the tube is in place. Placing the sutures at this point in the procedure (before the tube is placed) gives additional time for the local anesthetic to take effect and makes tying the tube in after placement more convenient.
  ○ Next, using a sharp Kelly clamp, bluntly dissect over the rib in the intercostal space to be accessed. You should hug the top of the rib. The neurovascular bundle runs on the inferior posterior surface of ribs, so it is critical to stay on the top of the rib. An intercostal artery injury during chest tube

placement will lead to a significant hemothorax and likely require surgery for evacuation.
■ Handheld ultrasound guidance
  ○ At times either the fluid or the air in the chest can be minimal and loculated, so the chest tube must be directed exactly into the desired space. In these circumstances, the surgeon can use a handheld ultrasound to locate the space and help guide a drainage tube into it. Smaller percutaneous tubes (pigtail catheters) or guidewire directed larger tubes are best used (Fig. 46-1).
    ■ Penetrating the pleura should not require force if spreading of the intercostal muscles is adequate. Selecting one spot and spreading the intercostal tissue slowly, repeatedly, and completely will allow entry into the pleura without pain or undue force. When the pleura is opened, there should be either a rush of air or fluid.
    ■ Open the jaws of the Kelly clamp widely in the pleura to make the chest tube hole big enough for the tube. If needed, a finger may be passed into the thorax to confirm an intrapleural location and to feel for adhesions that can be gently lysed, as needed.
    ■ The tube can be guided into the pleural cavity with a Kelly clamp or by using a trocar chest tube. Make sure the last hole of the tube is all the way into the chest cavity. If there is resistance to insertion of the chest tube, do not force it—you may be in the fissure. Pull back and redirect the tube. It is a good idea to have a Kelly clamp occluding the other end of the tube as it is being placed to keep the fluid from excessive soiling. This should not be done if the tube is being placed for pneumothorax. You will notice condensation in the tube as the pneumothorax escapes through the tube.
    ■ Secure the tube with the 2.0 silk suture. Make sure the incision is occluded to minimize drainage around the tube or air into the chest. Wrap the second stitch around the tube for use after the tube is removed.
    ■ After it is secured, hook the tube to the collection system but do not place to suction initially. Tape the tubing connection with thin strips of cloth tape in an H shape so that you can still visualize the connection. Tape the entrance site with cloth tape to create a seal. Create a mesentery of tape for the floundering remainder of the tube.
    ■ Note: If the tube is placed for a large pleural effusion, place a partial occluding clamp on the tube to drain the chest slowly. Do not put to suction immediately. Rapid draining is painful and can cause hemodynamic or respiratory complications or re-expansion pulmonary edema.

## SELDINGER TECHNIQUE

■ Fully equipped commercial chest tube kits are available.[4]
■ Following a 2-cm incision, an introducer needle is introduced into the pleural space with aspiration of air or fluid as described earlier.
■ A guidewire is inserted through the needle introducer and directed to a desired position (e.g., apical for pneumothorax).
■ Dilators of increasing size passed over the guidewire to form a tract for the chest tube.
■ After the chest tube and its accompanying dilator are passed into the pleural space, the guidewire and dilator are removed.
■ Cautions regarding the Seldinger technique:
  ○ Does not permit appreciation of adhesions
  ○ Presence of adhesions may facilitate lung parenchymal puncture
  ○ Should be attempted only with obvious separation of lung and parietal pleura on imaging studies.

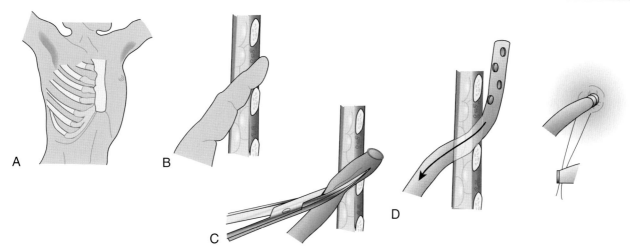

**Figure 46-1: A** to **D,** Technique of tube thoracostomy placement.

## IMAGE-GUIDED DRAINAGE

- Computed tomography (CT)–guided drainage with minitube insertion such as a pig-tail catheter now employed in selected patients[5-7]
- Not indicated to drain blood or viscous fluids

## PULLING CHEST TUBES

This seems obvious, but if it is not done right, there is potential to re-introduce air into the pleural space.[8] When a chest tube is removed, the incision for the chest tube can be closed with either a suture that was placed at the time of the chest tube incision or with an occlusive dressing.

- What do I need?
  - You will need a suture removal kit, gauze with petroleum jelly, a 4 inch × 4 inch gauze pad, and a roll of wide cloth tape.
- Important points
  - The goal of chest tube removal is to get the chest tube out without allowing air to be sucked into the chest. There are varying opinions as to how to achieve this. Some believe that the tube should be removed at full inspiration when there is little chance that the patient could inhale more. Although this may be true, it does create the paradox of removing the tube when the negative chest pressure is greatest. Others believe that the tube should be pulled at end expiration, when the negative intrapleural pressure is lowest. Unfortunately, it is at this point that the patient, having no alternative, is most likely to suck air into the chest with deep inspiration. For the past 3 decades, we have asked the patient to simply blow out hard and pulled the tube at mid-forced expiration. This technique allows the tube to be removed in a much more gentle way and has not resulted in any air being introduced. The tube should be pulled quickly. Do not let it linger partially removed, with air holes of the chest tube simultaneously inside and outside the chest.
  - Editor's note: It likely makes no difference when in the respiratory cycle that a chest tube is removed. Chest tube removal is easiest with a previously placed suture. The suture is pulled to close the hole as the tube is removed. With a suture in place, timing of the respiratory cycle makes no difference.

- Procedure
  - Remove the chest tube dressing, then cut the suture holding the tube in place. Hold the pursestring suture up as the chest tube is quickly pulled in a downward direction. Quickly tie the stitch without allowing it to relax. Cover the chest tube site with an occlusion dressing. If there is no closure stitch available, then cover the chest tube incision with petroleum jelly or iodoform gauze and a 4 inch × 4 inch gauze pad, as the tube is pulled.

## MANAGEMENT

- **Drainage system:** Management of a chest tube requires an understanding of the pressures within the chest. During normal inspiration, the intrathoracic pressure is negative. To allow air or fluid to drain from the chest, a drain placed into the pleural space needs either a one way valve that prevents air from being sucked into the chest or needs suction on the drain to overcome the negative pressure within the chest.[1,2,9]
- Originally, this was accomplished by placing the end of the tube 2 cm under the water level in a bottle. Unfortunately, as fluid drained from the chest into the bottle, drainage into the bottle became more difficult as the end of the tube was progressively further below the surface of the water. This means that progressively more pressure is needed for fluid to drain into the bottle. These bottles would have to be periodically emptied and returned to keep the tube 2 cm below the surface of the water.
- The next improvement in the system was to add a second bottle in parallel to collect the fluid, while keeping the waterseal at 2 cm.
- Finally, a third bottle in parallel was added to put suction on the system. The amount of suction was determined by the level of water in the third bottle and was usually set at 20 cm of water.
- That three-bottle system is the basis for the commercially available plastic chest drainage systems which provide waterseal (one-way valve), fluid collection, and suction (Figs. 46-2 and 46-3).
- **Persistent air leak**
  - The traditional belief is that an air leak from the visceral surface of the lung should heal with adequate apposition of the pleural surfaces. That has been shown to not always be the case. With severely emphysematous lung or other

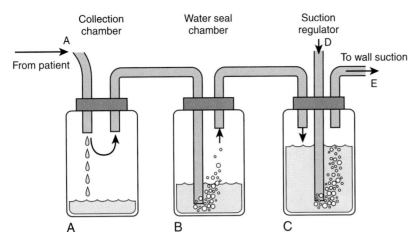

Collection chamber    Water seal chamber    Suction regulator

A    From patient

To wall suction    E

A    B    C

**Figure  46-2:** Concept of tube thoracostomy drainage system.

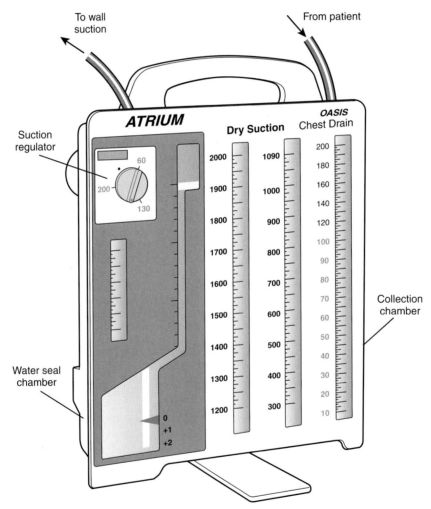

To wall suction

From patient

Suction regulator

*ATRIUM*    **Dry Suction**    *OASIS* Chest Drain

Collection chamber

Water seal chamber

0
+1
+2

**Figure 46-3:** Current chest tube collection systems.

pathology, the leak may heal slowly or occasionally require reoperation. Alternatively, the chest tube may remain in place for an extended period. A Heimlich valve (a one-way valve placed at the end of a chest tube) may be an option for some patients to go home with a chest tube in place until the air leak resolves.

- Fluid output
  ○ Thoracic surgeons remove the chest tubes when the air leak has sealed and the fluid drainage is low enough in a 24-hour period. There is a wide variation in the definition of "low enough." The number varies from 200 to 450 mL. The trend has been to remove the tubes with greater amounts of drainage. Removal with lower volumes is especially important for patients with poor pulmonary function or when the tube was placed for empyema.
- Underwater seal versus negative pressure[9]
  ○ Several recent prospective, randomized trials have evaluated optimal treatment practices for air leaks.[9]

○ In general, chest tube duration was longer if the chest drainage system was placed on suction compared with no suction.

○ **Exceptions:** Expanding pneumothorax, worsening hypoxemia, large air leaks, significant volumes of chest tube drainage, and significant subcutaneous emphysema. (In these cases, modest levels of negative pressure could be applied, e.g., –10 to –20 cm $H_2O$)

■ Question of prophylactic antibiotics
  ○ There is no evidence-based medicine to support the use of prophylactic antibiotics for a chest tube.

## COMMON PROBLEMS WITH CHEST TUBE MANAGEMENT

### Differential Diagnosis and Solutions

■ New-onset large air leak
  ○ May indicate that the connection between the chest tube and the chest drainage system has become loose, so check the connection.
  ○ May indicate that the chest tube has come out partly or completely from the chest. Check that there are no chest tube holes outside the chest. If so, the tube should be replaced.
■ No output
  ○ The tube needs to be checked to make sure that it is not kinked, blocked by blood clot, or blocked by talc.
  ○ Management is to relieve the obstruction by stripping the tube, unkinking the tube, placing a new tube, and rarely, passing an embolectomy catheter into the tube to remove the material that has blocked the tube.
■ Fluid backs up in a chest tube attached to a Heimlich valve
  ○ This usually means that the chest tube is ready for removal. When the air leak stops, fluid does not pass as well through the tube. It almost never means that the tube needs to be stripped of the material in the tube.
■ Subcutaneous emphysema
  ○ The sudden onset of subcutaneous emphysema could indicate that the chest tube is kinked (in a patient with an air leak), a chest tube hole is outside of the patient's body, a large air leak has developed, patient has a significant pneumothorax, or the water level in the water seal or suction chambers in the chest drainage system are low.
  ○ Management: Order a chest x-ray study, unkink the chest tube, make sure that the dressing change did not result in kinking of the tube, place an additional chest tube as needed, place the chest drainage system on suction, and fill the water levels of the chest drainage system as needed to the proper levels.

## COMPLICATIONS

■ Bleeding[10-18]
  ○ Chest tube insertion can cause bleeding if the insertion process injures an intercostal vessel, lung parenchyma, or intra-abdominal structure (liver or spleen, if the tube or needle for local anesthesia transverses the diaphragm).
  ○ Hints to reduce risk
    ■ Study the chest x-ray study or CT scan to determine the optimal level for insertion.
    ■ If a patient is on the ventilator, stop the ventilator briefly as the tube is actually inserted.
    ■ Pass the tube over the top of a rib, not under a rib, where the vessels are located.

■ Lung injury
  ○ Chest tube insertion can injure the lung, especially if a trocar tube is used
  ○ Hints to reduce risk:
    ■ As noted earlier, briefly stop the ventilator as the tube is actually being inserted.
    ■ A trocar tube is very helpful for getting the chest tube in the correct location, but it can be dangerous if used improperly. Do not advance the tube if there is resistance.
■ Vasovagal response
■ Pain
  ○ Pain during insertion of a chest tube should be minimal.
  ○ Hints to reduce pain:
    ■ Generous use of local anesthesia in the skin, the intercostal space, and the pleura. Do not waste local anesthesia in the fat, where there are no pain fibers.
    ■ Technique with the Kelly clamp is very important. The process should be advance, spread, pull out, and close the clamp. If this is done several times with slow progress to create a tract for the tube, the process usually is not very painful for patients.
  ○ Pain following insertion of the chest tube is common and should be managed with analgesics as needed.
■ Re-expansion edema (see Fig. 47-4 in Pleural Effusion chapter)
■ Malposition[15]
  ○ Most prevalent with emergency placement of a chest tube (15%–26% versus 1% with elective placement).[15-18]
  ○ CT is superior in detecting malposition. Only 30% of cases malposition were diagnosed on plain chest radiograph.[15]
  ○ Malposition sites include extrathoracic, intrafissural, and intraparenchymal. The latter two most commonly missed on plain chest radiographs.
  ○ Malposition more common with lateral versus ventral insertion sites.
■ Rarely reported complications:
  ○ Right atrial perforation
  ○ Right ventricular perforation
  ○ Right ventricular compression with pseudotamponade
  ○ Mediastinal injury and bleeding
  ○ Pulmonary artery perforation
  ○ Contralateral hemothorax or pneumothorax
  ○ Chest tube–associated necrotizing fasciitis
  ○ Liver injury

### Brief Illustrative Case 1

- *History:* A 32-year-old man with 1-day history of progressive mild shortness of breath. He also has very mild chest pain on the right side with inspiration.
- *Examination:* Vitals: tachycardia (100-105 beats/min); BP 110/60; respirations 16/min; temp: 98.8° F, $SPO_2$ 99% room air. Very tall and thin. Breath sounds on the right side are slightly diminished at the apex.
- *Blood tests:* Complete blood count and electrolytes—normal.
- *Imaging:* Posteroanterior and lateral chest x-ray study reveals a right pneumothorax. Airspace is about 30% of the space in the right hemithorax.
- *Management of spontaneous pneumothorax:* 28 French right chest tube on –20 mm Hg wall suction until air leak resolves.

*(Continued)*

## Brief Illustrative Case 1—cont'd

### Key Points

- Most commonly, patients presenting with a spontaneous pneumothorax are tall, thin men.
- First occurrence is treated with a chest tube and usually is the definitive management.
- For the second occurrence, the usual recommendation is an apical blebectomy and mechanical pleurodesis.

## Brief Illustrative Case 2

- *History:* 65-year-old man with 10-day history of progressive shortness of breath. He has a history of known NSCLC with a malignant pleural effusion.
- *Examination:* Vitals: tachycardia (115/min); BP 140/60; respirations 22/min; temp: 98.8° F, SPO$_2$ 91% on 6L NC O$_2$. Breath sounds are not present on the left side.
- *Blood tests:* Complete blood count and electrolytes—normal.
- *Imaging:* Chest x-ray study reveals complete white out of left hemithorax. Contrast CT scan of the chest reveals a very large left dependent pleural effusion, an infrahilar mass and pleural nodules.

- *Diagnosis/Pathology:* Pleural fluid cytology positive for malignant cells.
- *Management of malignant pleural effusion:* Tube thoracostomy placement. Drainage of the fluid should be followed by additional imaging to determine whether the lung will re-expand to the chest wall. If this is the case, the patient may benefit from talc pleurodesis. If it does not re-expand, placement of a tunnelled indwelling drainage catheter may be indicated.

### Key Points

- Confirm cytology before definitively treating a malignant pleural effusion.
- Whether the lung re-expands dictates further course of management.
- If the patient is symptomatic, drain the effusion with a chest tube then determine further management. If the effusion is large, drain the effusion slowly (<500 mL/h) to avoid hemodynamic consequences.

## References

 Interactive references and additional readings for this chapter can be accessed online at *expertconsult.com*.

---

# 47 PLEURAL EFFUSIONS AND COMPLICATIONS

Benjamin E. Haithcock, MD, Michael I. Lewis, MD, Robert J. McKenna Jr., MD, and Richard H. Feins, MD

## DEFINITION

The accumulation of pleural fluid due to an imbalance in hydrostatic and oncotic pressure or increased permeability.

## ETIOLOGY

- The pleural space exists between the parietal and visceral pleura. This space has a small amount of fluid, the purpose of which is to lubricate the parietal and visceral pleura to assist with lung mechanics.
- The amount of pleural fluid within each pleural space at any given time is <1 ml.[1] The rate of pleural fluid production is approximately 0.01 mL/kg/h. The route of pleural fluid egress is through parietal pleural lymphatics normally at a rate 28 times faster than production.[2]
- In diseased states, either the egress or production of pleural fluid results in pathologic states of pleural fluid accumulation. There are several factors that can cause an increase in pleural fluid.[3]

  ○ Increase in hydrostatic pressure (i.e., congestive heart failure)
  ○ Decrease in oncotic pressure (i.e., malnourished patients)
  ○ Increase in the space available for pleural fluid accumulation (lung collapse)
  ○ Increase in the permeability of the microvascular circulation secondary to inflammatory mediators
  ○ Inadequate egress of pleural fluid through lymphatics secondary to obstruction from tumor or fibrosis
  ○ Transdiaphragmic movement of ascitic fluid into the pleural space
  ○ Increased production of fluid by intrathoracic malignancy

## CLINICAL FEATURES

- An extensive history including prior surgery, medications, connective tissue disorders, past hospitalization, and social history can assist with focusing the differential diagnosis in a patient presenting with a pleural effusion.

- Dyspnea is the predominant complaint and is more prominent with activity.
- Other symptoms include cough and chest pressure.
- Physical examination findings include
  - Decreased breath sounds on the affected side
  - Dullness to percussion
  - Decreased fremitus.

## DIAGNOSIS

- Imaging studies
  - Plain chest radiographs.
    - There is typically blunting of the costophrenic angle, and when apparent, a meniscus on the chest x-ray study signifying a pleural effusion.
    - Chest x-ray is not helpful in diagnosing pleural effusions until the amount in the thoracic space exceeds 500 mL.[4]
    - To determine how loculated the effusion appears, a decubitus film is helpful to visualize the fluid layering on the lateral chest wall or mediastinum.
    - Pleural effusions in conjunction with other radiographic findings can help with determining the etiology of the effusion.
    - Complete opacification of the hemithorax with contralateral shift of the mediastinum is usually the result of malignancy, or other cause of a massive effusion.
    - Bilateral effusion in the presence of a large cardiac silhouette is typically suggestive of congestive heart failure being the cause of the effusions. Other etiologies for bilateral effusions with a normal cardiac silhouette include systemic illnesses such as lupus erythematosus, renal failure, or cirrhosis.
  - Ultrasound
    - This can detect effusions as small as 50 mL.
    - This mode of imaging helps to determine whether the fluid is loculated and assist with localization of the fluid for thoracentesis.[5]
  - Computer tomography
    - This mode of imaging may be helpful in determining the etiology of the pleural effusion, assessing if the effusion is loculated, and assisting with treatment plans (Fig. 47-1).

- Thoracentesis
  - The initial step in evaluating the patient with a pleural effusion is determining if the effusion is transudative or exudative.
  - **Transudate pleural effusion** usually results from an increase in hydrostatic pressure or a decrease in oncotic pressure (Table 47-1).
  - **Exudative effusion** results from an increase in permeability (Table 47-2).
  - This procedure can be both diagnostic and therapeutic (Figs. 47-2 and 47-3).
  - This will assist in determining the characteristics of the effusion (transudate versus exudates) and will determine if the lung will re-expand and replace the space initially occupied by the pleural effusion.
  - There are no absolute contraindications for thoracentesis.
  - Relative contraindications are coagulopathy, an uncooperative patient, and cutaneous disease such as herpes zoster infection at the needle entry site.[6]
  - Not all pleural effusions need to be analyzed if the etiology of the effusion is known (e.g., postsurgical changes after thoracic or abdominal surgery or related to congestive heart failure). But if the cause or etiology is unclear, diagnostic thoracentesis should be performed.
  - Diagnostic thoracentesis should be performed when a clinically suspected pleural effusion has been confirmed on chest x-ray study and remains undiagnosed.
  - Therapeutic thoracentesis is performed to relieve symptoms associated with large pleural effusions such as dyspnea.
  - Lung volumes increase by about one third of the volume of fluid withdrawn, but arterial blood gases usually show little change.[7]
  - Chest x-ray study should be performed following successful and unsuccessful thoracentesis.
- Complications associated with thoracentesis include
  - Pneumothorax
    - The incidence of pneumothorax varies between 3% and 20%.[8] Thoracentesis can be performed on patients receiving artificial ventilation. The incidence of pneumothorax in this patient population has been reported to be 6%.[9]

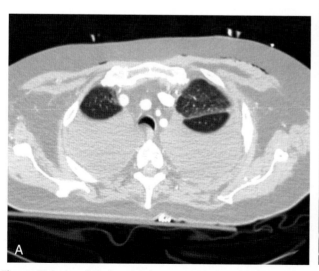
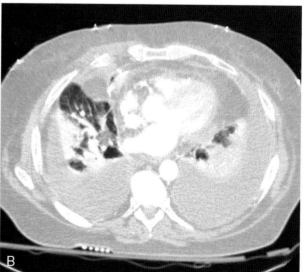

**Figure 47-1: A** and **B,** Computed tomography scan evaluation of patient after double lung transplant with large bilateral pleural effusions and compressive atelectasis.

| TABLE 47-1 ▪ CAUSES OF TRANSUDATIVE EFFUSIONS |
| --- |
| Congestive heart failure |
| Cirrhosis |
| Nephrotic syndrome |
| Peritoneal dialysis |
| Atelectasis |
| Myxedema |
| Pulmonary edema |
| Hypoalbuminemia |
| Constrictive pericarditis |
| Malignancy |
| Sarcoidosis |
| Pulmonary embolism |

- Pneumothorax following ultrasound-guided thoracentesis may be due to the generation of nonuniform pressure gradients over the visceral pleura, producing stress failure and microfistulae. This scenario would occur particularly if the lung cannot conform to a new geometric chest configuration with large volume drainage.[10] Thus, in some cases, pneumothorax may be unavoidable and unrelated to inadvertent lung puncture.
  ○ Pain at the site of the procedure
  ○ Vasovagal reaction
  ○ Re-expansion pulmonary edema
    - Rare complication. Reported in 1% to 2% of patients[11,12]; likely less
    - More likely to occur with prolonged lung collapse

- Pathogenesis is not well characterized. Edema fluid analysis compatible with permeability edema. Mechanical stress failure of alveolar-capillary membranes due to high negative pleural pressures or reperfusion, or both, are likely mechanisms.
- Clinical features include acute dyspnea, cough, pink frothy sputum (sometimes copious), signs of respiratory distress, and cyanosis, which can progress over several hours to 1 to 2 days.
- Chest x-ray study shows unilateral pulmonary edema; can be bilateral on occasion (Fig. 47-4).[13]
- Treatment: supportive
- Prevention: Do not remove >1 liter of fluid unless monitoring pleural pressures. With chest tube insertion, connect to underwater-seal, not negative pressure.
- Outcome: up to 20% mortality rate reported,[13] but the rate is likely lower with current treatment approaches for adult respiratory distress syndrome.
  ○ Subcutaneous hematoma
  ○ Pleural infection.

## EVALUATION OF PLEURAL EFFUSIONS

- Before sending the pleural effusion to the laboratory for evaluation, the bedside visual inspection of the fluid may assist in determining a diagnosis.
  ○ Grossly bloody effusions: trauma or malignancy
  ○ Whitish fluid/milky: chylothorax or pseudochylous effusion
  ○ Foul odor and/or pus: empyema
  ○ Food particles within the fluid: esophageal rupture.
  ○ Brown/"anchovy paste": amebic liver abscess with rupture into pleural cavity

| TABLE 47-2 ▪ CAUSES OF EXUDATIVE PLEURAL EFFUSIONS | |
| --- | --- |
| **Malignancy** | **Other** |
| Lung | Pulmonary embolism |
| Lymphoma | Dressler's syndrome |
| Mesothelioma | Asbestos |
| Metastatic disease | Uremia |
| | Trapped lung |
| **Infectious** | Radiation therapy |
| Parapneumonic condition | Meig's syndrome |
| Tuberculosis | Trauma |
| Fungal infection | |
| Viral infection | **Lymphatic Disease** |
| Parasitic | Chylothorax |
| Abdominal abscess | Lymphangioleiomyomatosis |
| Hepatitis | Yellow nail syndrome |
| **Noninfectious Gastrointestinal** | **Drug Induced** |
| Pancreatitis | Drug-induced lupus erythematosus |
| Esophageal rupture | Nitrofurantoin |
| Abdominal surgery | Dantrolene |
| Variceal sclerotherapy | Amiodarone |
| | Methysergide |
| **Collagen Vascular Disease** | Procarbazine |
| Lupus erythematosus | Practolol |
| Rheumatoid arthritis | Bromocriptine |
| Wegener's granulomatosis | Minoxidil |
| Churg-Strauss syndrome | Bleomycin |
| Familial Mediterranean fever | Methotrexate |
| Sjögren's syndrome | Methysergide |
| Immunoblastic lymphadenopathy | Mitomycin |

*Adapted from Bartter T, Santarelli R, Akers SM, Pratter MR. The evaluation of pleural effusion. Chest 1994;106:1209-1214 (with permission).*

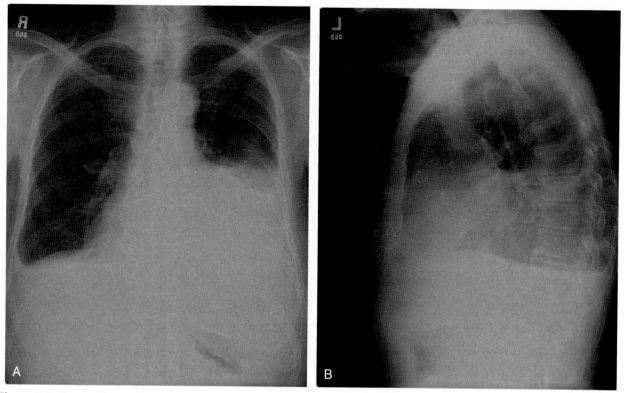

**Figure 47-2:** **A** and **B**, Patient after coronary artery bypass graft surgery with moderate-size left pleural effusion.

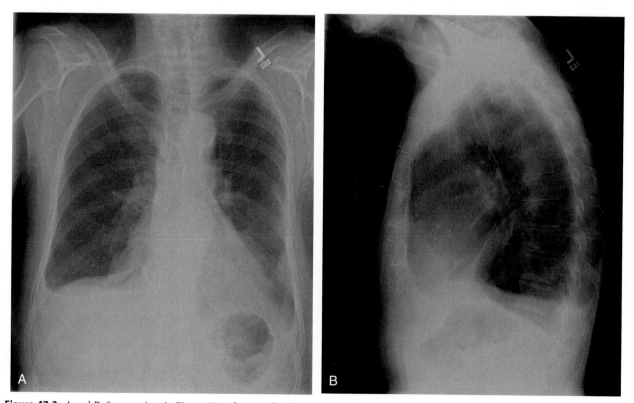

**Figure 47-3:** **A** and **B**, Same patient in Figure 47-2 after complete thoracentesis and medical therapy of heart failure.

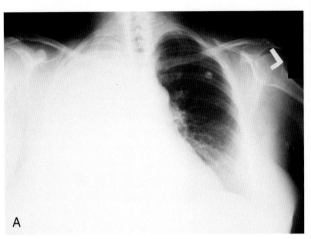
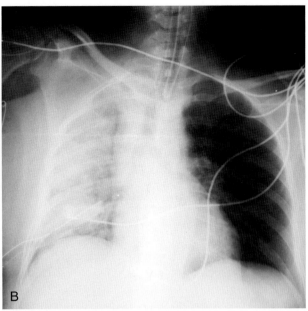

**Figure 47-4:** Chest x-ray study depicting re-expansion pulmonary edema (**A**) following large volume pleural fluid removal. The patient is now intubated. (**B**, Baseline film showing large pleural effusion.)

    ○ Yellow/green with or without debris: rheumatoid arthritis
    ○ Black: Aspergillus niger empyema
    ○ Viscous: mesothelioma
    ○ Ammonia odor: urinothorax
■ **Light's criteria** is still the standard with which other diagnostic tests are compared to evaluate pleural fluid.[14] Performed by simultaneously measuring the lactate dehydrogenase levels (LDH) and protein in the serum and pleural fluid.
    ○ **Exudate.** One or more of the following
      ■ Pleural fluid/serum LDH greater than 0.6
      ■ Pleural fluid/serum protein greater than 0.5

      ■ Pleural fluid LDH greater than two thirds of upper normal limits for serum
      ■ A pleural fluid/serum cholesterol greater than 0.3 is a new addition.
    ○ **Transudate.** None of the above-mentioned criteria are met.
■ **Other studies** ordered at the time of the thoracentesis include (Table 47-3):
    ○ pH
      ■ Decreased pH (<7.20) in pleural effusions is related to increased acid production by cells and organisms and due to impaired efflux from the pleural space due to

## TABLE 47-3 ■ EXUDATIVE PLEURAL FLUID ANALYSIS

| | |
|---|---|
| **Low Glucose (<60)**<br>Complicated parapneumonic effusion<br>Rheumatoid<br>Malignant<br>Tuberculous | Pulmonary embolism<br>Hemothorax<br><br>**Elevated Lymphocytes**<br>Lymphoma |
| **Low pH (<7.2)**<br>Empyema<br>Complicated parapneumonic effusion<br>Rheumatoid<br>Malignant<br>Tuberculous<br>Esophageal rupture | Other malignancy<br>Chronic infection<br>  Tuberculosis<br>  Fungi<br>Postpericardiotomy syndrome<br>Sarcoidosis<br><br>**Eosinophils** |
| **Elevated Amylase**<br>Esophageal rupture<br>Pancreatitis<br>Malignancy | Hemothorax<br>Pneumothorax<br>Thoracentesis<br>Parasitic disease<br>Pulmonary infarction<br>Drug induced |
| **Elevated RBCs (>100,000/mm³)**<br>Trauma<br>Malignancy | Asbestos<br>Malignancy |

RBCs, red blood cells.
*Adapted from Bartter T, Santarelli R, Akers SM, Pratter MR. The evaluation of pleural effusion. Chest 1994;106:1209-1214 (with permission).*

pleuritis or pleural effusions.[15] Causes include complicated parapneumonic effusion and empyema, effusions associated with esophageal rupture, malignant effusions; occasionally, rheumatoid and tuberculous effusions.

- ○ Glucose
  - ▪ Decreased glucose (<60 mg/dl) is due to decreased transport of glucose from the blood to the pleural fluid (impact on glucose transporters), as well as increased utilization by polymorphonuclear leukocytes, malignant cells, and bacteria.[16] The differential diagnosis of low glucose, low pH effusions are seen in Table 47-4.
- ○ Cell count and differential
  - ▪ Leukocyte count: greater than 50,000/μL complicated parapneumonic effusion/empyema; greater than 10,000/μL indicates significant inflammation; transudates usually less than 1000/μL
  - ▪ Lymphocye-predominant: tuberculosis (also absence of reactive mesothelial cells); lymphoma main considerations
  - ▪ Eosinophils: mainly associated with hemothorax, prior thoracentesis, pneumothorax, pulmonary infarction and parasitic disease. Note: more than 30% is idiopathic.
  - ▪ Basophils: more than 10% can occur with leukemia
  - ▪ Plasma cells: myeloma and related conditions
- ○ Cytology
- ○ When appropriate, also include
  - ▪ Gram's stain and culture
  - ▪ Triglycerides and cholesterol if chylothorax or pseudochylous effusion suspected
  - ▪ Amylase (and serum amylase) if pancreatitis, pancreatic pseudocyst, malignancy, and esophageal rupture are considered.
  - ▪ Antinuclear antibody (ANA), rheumatoid factor, lupus erythematosis (LE) cells
- ▪ Transudate effusion
  - ○ Secondary to imbalances in the hydrostatic or oncotic pressures, or a movement of fluid from the peritoneal cavity.
  - ○ The most common etiology is congestive heart failure, with the other etiologies being those seen in Table 47-1.
- ▪ Exudate effusion
  - ○ The differential diagnosis of exudative effusion is significantly larger than that of transudate effusion, as seen in Table 47-2.
  - ○ Table 47-4 narrows the differential diagnosis based on characteristics from the pleural effusion analysis.

## PARAPNEUMONIC EFFUSION AND EMPYEMA

- ▪ Definition, incidence and importance:
  - ○ Parapneumonic effusion is an effusion accompanying pneumonia and is not limited solely to bacterial pathogens (can include atypical and viral pneumonias).[17]
  - ○ Occurs in 20% to 57% of hospitalized patients with bacterial pneumonia.[17,18]

### TABLE 47-4 ▪ CAUSES OF LOW GLUCOSE, LOW pH EFFUSIONS

Rheumatoid pleurisy
Empyema
Esophageal rupture
Malignancy
Tuberculosis
Lupus pleuritis

- ○ Presence of a parapneumonic effusion is associated with higher mortality rates for pneumonia. It can become complicated, increasing morbidity, added interventions, hospital stay, costs, and the mortality rate.[17]
- ○ Can progress very rapidly and become loculated very quickly, so diagnosis and drainage is very important.
- ○ An empyema is classically defined by the presence of pus on aspiration of the pleural space. The presence of organisms on Gram's stain of aspirated pleural fluid has also been included in the definition.
- ▪ Pathogenetic classification and risk stratification[17-20]
  - ○ Divided into three stages
  - ○ The stages represent a continuum, with no well-defined temporal sequences (i.e., patient, clinical setting, organism specific).
  - ○ **Stage 1: Uncomplicated parapneumonic effusion** due to movement of fluid from the lung, together with increased permeability of pleural capillaries in the presence of limited capacity to efficiently resorb the fluid. The fluid is exudative, sterile, and free flowing, and resolves with resolution of the pneumonia.
  - ○ **Stage 2: Complicated parapneumonic effusion** due to fibroproliferation, resulting in loculations, bacterial invasion, influx of neutrophils, pleural fluid acidosis (pH, 7.2), low glucose (<60 mg/dL) and higher LDH (3 times upper limit of normal serum value).
  - ○ Negative bacterial studies in the presence of a complicated parapneumonic effusion are common and can be due to: antibiotic therapy, sampling error due to a missing infected loculation, clearance of organisms from pleural space,[21] and the presence of fastidious organisms that are difficult to culture, such as anaerobes.
  - ○ Loculations and visceral peel are flimsy and easily lysed.
  - ○ **Stage 3: Empyema:** Fulfills above-mentioned definition. Associated with progressive locuation and the proliferation of fibroblasts, resulting in visceral and parietal pleural peel that can prevent full lung expansion (trapped lung).
  - ○ *Risk Stratification for parapneumonic effusion and empyema:* An evidence-based approach was developed by the American College of Chest Physicians (ACCP) Concensus Panel.[18] This is depicted in Table 47-5.
- ▪ Bacteriology of complicated parapneumonic effusion and empyema
  - ○ Commonly mixed infection, particularly in advanced stages
  - ○ Anaerobes implicated in a third to three quarters[22,23]
  - ○ Other organisms: *Staphylococcus aureus*/methicillin-resistant *S. aureus* (MRSA) can complicate up to 20% of complicated parapneumonic effusions; pneumococcus, 1% to 5%. Other organisms include aerobic gram-negative bacteria, such as *Klebsiella pneumoniae* (alcoholism and diabetes increase risk) and *Streptococcus milleri*.
- ▪ Imaging
  - ○ Chest x-ray study: decubitus films can delineate if fluid is free flowing.
  - ○ Contrast computed tomography (CT) imaging is the procedure of choice. Best modalilty to define loculations, pleural peel, lung parenchymal, and other abnormalities (Fig. 47-5).
- ▪ Treatment
  - ○ **Guidelines for drainage:** depicted in Table 47-5 (ACCP Concensus[18]). Note: only about 10% of parapneumonic effusions require some type of drainage procedure.[17]
  - ○ **Uncomplicated parapneumonic effusion:** Does not require drainage procedures. Empiric antibiotic choices depend on the clinical setting, with tailoring depending on cultures. Any change in clinical status should prompt a red flag, because rapid progression can occur in less than 24 hours.

## TABLE 47-5 ■ CATEGORIZING RISK FOR POOR OUTCOME IN PATIENTS WITH PARAPNEUMONIC EFFUSIONS

| Pleural Space Anatomy | | | Pleural Fluid Bacteriology | | | Pleural Fluid Chemistry | | Category | Risk of Poor Outcome | Drain |
|---|---|---|---|---|---|---|---|---|---|---|
| A0 | Minimal, free-flowing (<10 mm on lateral decubitus film) | AND | Bx | Culture and Gram's AND stain results unknown | AND | Cx | pH unknown | 1 | Very low | No |
| A1 | Small to moderate free-flowing effusion (>10 mm and <1/2 hemithorax) | AND | B0 | Neg culture and Gram's stain | OR | C0 | pH ≥ 7.20 | 2 | Moderate | No |
| A2 | Large, free-flowing (≥ 1/2 hemithorax) loculated effusion, or effusion with thickened parietal pleura | OR | B1 | Positive culture or Gram's stain | OR | C1 | pH < 7.20 | 3 | Moderate | Yes |
| | | | B2 | pus | | | | 4 | High | Yes |

From Colice GL, Curtis A, Deslauriers J, Heffner J, Light R, Littenberg B, et al. *Medical and surgical treatment of parapneumonic effusions: An evidence based guideline. Chest 2000;118:1158-1171 (with permission).*

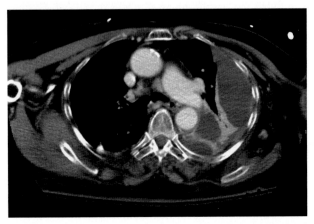

**Figure 47-5:** Computed tomography scan depicting loculated empyema.

- **Complicated parapneumonic effusion and empyema:**
  - Drainage approaches are driven by clinical circumstances.
  - Tube thoracoscopy:
    - This together with antibiotics is the most common method employed.
    - Should be placed in the most dependent portion.
    - Chest tube size is controversial. Traditionally, large caliber tube is used. Small size chest tubes, including pigtail catheters, can be successfully used with both good[24] and poor success rates[25] reported.
    - Postprocedure imaging is important to assess residual disease and likelihood of success.
    - Improvement in clinical status should be evident within 24 hours.
    - Inadequate drainage, residual loculations, peel, and poor clinical improvement indicates the need for further treatment measures.
    - If radiologic imaging does not show adequate drainage, then further intervention should be prompt.
  - Intrapleural fibrinolytic therapy
    - Considered with poor drainage and presence of loculations.
    - Uncontrolled case series reported positive results for streptokinase, urokinase, and tissue plasminogen activator (see excellent review by Light[17] for details).
    - Several small controlled studies suggested higher clinical responses and less referral to surgery (see the review by Light[17] for details).
    - However, a large randomized, double-blind, multicenter study (n = 427) comparing streptokinase and placebo was negative.[26] Fibrinolytic therapy conferred no benefit with regard to surgical referral (27%–31%), length of stay, or mortality rate. A recent meta-analysis drew similar conclusions.[27]
    - Use of fibrinolytic therapy should probably be limited to circumstances in which thoracic surgical intervention is not readily available in stable patients or when patients are not considered operative candidates.
    - The combination of intrapleural DNase and fibrinolytic therapy needs further study.
- Video-assisted thoracic surgery (VATS)
  - Indicated with poor drainage or the presence of loculations
  - Several studies suggest superiority of VATS to fibrinolytic therapy.[28-31]
  - Several recent studies employing VATS reported good success with a median need for chest tube drainage of 3 to 7 days.[32-35]
  - A recent study evaluated VATS in 234 patients with complicated parapneumonic effusion and empyema.[36] Successful treatment was reported in 86% of cases. Open decortication or repeat procedure was required in only 40 patients.
  - Most thoracic surgeons are comfortable with VATS treatment of stage 1 and 2 empyema. Some surgeons successfully treat stage 3 empyema with VATS
- Decortication
  - Refers to removal of fibrous peel from visceral and parietal pleura, which limits full lung expansion
  - Can be performed by VATS or via thoracotomy
  - The procedure is performed with the goal of breaking up all loculations, draining all areas of fluid, allowing the lung to expand fully (remove any pleural peel), allowing the diaphragm to be fully mobile (remove any peel on the diaphragm that prevents mobility of the diaphragm), and removing visceral pleural peel if it is constricting the hemithorax and preventing expansion of the chest wall.

■ Open thoracostomy
  ○ Previously considered with multiloculated empyema. VATS employed currently, if medically feasible.
  ○ Involves rib resection and chest tube drainage with gradual withdrawal of the chest tube over several months, as the empyema cavity closes.
■ Special circumstances:
  ○ Trapped lung
    ■ In some cases, the lung cannot be decorticated, so the lung remains trapped. The ideal treatment of an empyema is decortication and full expansion of the lung.
    ■ When there is a residual pleural space, drainage is needed. This can be with a chest tube that is cut off and slowly advanced out of the chest over several weeks (short tube).
    ■ Alternatively, a pleurocutaneous flap (Eloesser flap) can be created (see Chapter 49 on Bronchopleural Fistula).
  ○ Postpneumonectomy empyema
    ■ Occurs mainly following pneumonectomy (5%–10%) but can occur following lobectomy.[37]
    ■ Majority (>80%) occur in the context of a bronchopleural fistula (see Chapter 49 on Bronchopleural Fistula).
    ■ Divided into early and late
    ■ Initial management is chest tube drainage and antibiotics.
    ■ Good success with pleural space irrigation, bronchial stump closure, and obliteration of the pleural space with an antibiotic solution was effective for early postpneumonectomy empyema.[38]
    ■ Traditional approach: open pleural drainage, serial débridement, open pleural packing, closure of bronchopleural fistula, and chest closure following antibiotic installation (Claggett procedure) is also successful.[39]
    ■ Key management is prevention.
    ■ The mortality (12%) and morbidity rates with postpneumonectomy empyema are high.
  ○ Pediatric parapneumonic effusion and empyema
    ■ Parapneumonic empyema occurs in 1 in 150 hospitalized children with pneumonia.[40]
    ■ Bacteriology differs in children with lower incidence of anaerobic infections. Offending organisms may also reflect an underlying disease state (e.g., *S. aureus*/MRSA or pseudomonas infection in children with cystic fibrosis).
    ■ Treatment approaches: in general, similar to the principles described earlier.
    ■ A recent large meta-analysis of operative (including VATS) versus nonoperative therapy for pediatric empyema[41] was conducted. It reported a lower in-hospital mortality rate, reintervention rate, length of stay, chest tube time, and duration of antibiotic therapy with an operative approach compared with antibiotic and thoracentesis/chest tube drainage alone.
    ■ There is no consensus regarding timing of surgical intervention. It seems logical to use intervention earlier than later. Prospective trials are needed.

## Thorascopy for Exudative Pleural Effusion

■ Evaluation of an exudative pleural effusion is usually diagnostic in 74% of cases or clinically useful information is obtained.[42]
■ If after evaluation of the pleural fluid and an etiology of the exudative pleural effusion remains unclear, then a second thoracentesis is warranted to increase the yield of a diagnosis.[43]

■ Patients with continued undiagnosed exudative pleural effusions who have pulmonary abnormalities either clinically or radiographically should undergo bronchoscopy.
■ If after the above-mentioned studies conclude with an undiagnosed exudative pleural effusion, the patient should undergo thorascopy.
  ○ Thorascopy will determine the etiology of the exudative pleural effusion in more than 90% of the cases.[44]
  ○ During the procedure, a third pleural fluid evaluation is performed, as well as pleural biopsies and evaluation of the visceral and parietal surfaces of the lung, chest wall and mediastinum.

## *CHYLOTHORAX*

**Definition**: Chylothorax is the accumulation of chyle in the pleural space due to the disruption of the thoracic duct or one or more of its tributaries. Chyle is a milky opalescent fluid containing chylomicrons and very low density lipoproteins (formed from dietary long-chain triglycerides) and cells.[45]

## Functional Anatomy of the Thoracic Duct

■ Chyle (formed from dietary long chain triglycerides) is secreted into the intestinal lacteals and then transported to the cisterna chili located anterior to L2 and posterior and right of the abdominal aorta.[45,46]
■ Coalescence of lymphatic vessels then forms the thoracic duct, which ascends through the diaphragmatic esophageal hiatus into the thorax.
■ The thoracic duct then ascends in the posterior mediastinum along the right anterolateral surface of the thoracic aorta. It is positioned in close proximity to the azygous vein, descending aorta, esophagus, and peri-cardium.
■ At T4 to T6, the thoracic duct crosses to the left and ascends between the aortic arch and left subclavian artery.
■ The thoracic duct continues past the thoracic inlet and arches above the clavicle to drain into the left subclavian vein or internal jugular vein.
■ Multiple anatomic variations exist at all levels.

## Normal Physiology

■ Daily production of chyle is 1.5 to 2.5 liters.
■ A high level of fat ingestion, especially long-chain triglycerides, increases production of chyle and lymphatic flow.
■ Chyle contains a significant number of lymphocytes (several thousand per cubic millimeter)
■ Protein content is about 3g/dL
■ Electrolyte content mirrors that of serum.

## Causes

■ The epidemiology may be changing.
  ○ Light[46] reviewed 143 cases from five case series between 1964 and 1981. Tumors accounted for 54% of the total with lymphoma, accounting for 40% of the total (75% of tumors). Trauma (mainly surgical) accounted for 25% of the cases. Idiopathic accounted for 10%.
  ○ A recent case series from the Mayo Clinic (1980–2000) reported on 203 cases.[47] Lymphoma accounted for only 11% of cases, whereas trauma (including surgical) accounted for close to 50%. Idiopathic causes accounted for 6%.
■ Table 47-6 is a comprehensive list of common and uncommon reported causes of chylothorax.

---

### TABLE 47-6 ■ ETIOLOGY OF CHYLOTHORAX

**Tumors**

Hematologic
  Lymphoma
  Chronic lymphatic leukemia
  Acute lymphoblastic leukemia
  Myeloma
Epithelial
  Lung cancer
  Carcinoid tumor
  Metastatic (stomach, prostate)
Other
  Kaposi's sarcoma
  Neurogenic tumors
  Lymphangioma (posterior mediastinal)

**Trauma**

Surgical
  Cardiac:
    Congenital heart disease (e.g., Fontan procedure);
      incidence 3.8%[54]
    Heart transplant
    Coronary artery bypass surgery
    Valve replacement
  Thoracic:
    Surgery for lung cancer
    Mediastinal node dissection for lung cancer
    Left sided sleeve resection
  Esophageal:
    Esophagectomy
    Transhiatal approach
  Neck:
    Left radical neck dissection

Bilateral neck surgery
Cervical node dissection
  Kidney:
    Nephrectomy
  Spine:
    Thoracolumbar surgery
  Other trauma
    Penetrating injury
    Blunt
    High pressure injury:
      Childbirth
      Weight lifting
      Severe emesis or coughing

**Congenital and Idiopathic (Includes Congenital Lymphatic Disorders)**

**Miscellaneous Medical**

Vascular
  Left subclavian thrombosis
  Superior vena cava thrombosis
  Extramedullary hematopoiesis
Lymphangioleiomyomatosis and tuberous sclerosis
Postradiation
Chylous ascites
Other:
  Tuberculosis
  Sarcoidosis
  Beçhet's disease
  Gorham's (massive osteolysis) syndrome
  Hypothyroidism

---

## Clinical Details

- Dyspnea is the most common presenting symptom. Present in 57% of a recent large cohort with chylothorax.[47]
- Nontraumatic causes often have a more insidious course.
- Symptoms and signs associated with the underlying condition, such as B symptoms of lymphoma, may be present.
- Have a high index of suspicion, especially in the right clinical setting.

## Diagnosis

- Milky opalescent pleural fluid. Note: If the patient is to have nothing by mouth or is on a low-fat diet, the pleural fluid may not be milky in up to 40% of patients.[48]
- **Pleural fluid analysis:** Pleural fluid triglyceride level greater than 110 mg/dL and ratio of pleural fluid to serum cholesterol ratio less than 1 is sufficient for diagnosis.

## Complications

- Malnutrition due to significant loss of proteins[49]
- Metabolic aberrations due to loss of fluid and electrolytes
- Immune impairment due to
  - Loss of lymphocytes and generation of lymphopenia (impaired cell mediated immunity)
  - Loss of immunoglobulins (impaired humoral immunity)
- Predisposition to infection, including opportunistic
- Respiratory distress, including tension chylothorax[50]
- Local complications including development of adhesions, loculation, organization, and empyema. However, these complications are uncommon because the effusions are usually free flowing and the presence of lymphocytes may offset infection.

## Treatment

- Nonoperative approaches[45,46,49,51-54]
  - Treatment of underlying disease
  - Nutritional: reduce production and flow of chyle
    - The patient usually receives nothing by mouth.
    - Medium-chain triglyceride diet
    - Total parenteral nutrition
    - Nutritional approaches alone are rarely completely effective.
  - Therapeutic thoracentesis
    - Palliative when the patient is dyspneic
  - Tube thoracostomy with or without chemical pleurodesis[53]
  - Octreotide
    - Mechanism unknown but likely an effect in reducing lymphatic flow[55]
    - Shown to be safe and effective in patients of all ages and etiologies
    - High-dose therapy (80–100 µg/day) with up-titration is recommended.[56]
    - Duration of therapy to obtain clinical response not determined and variable
  - Percutaneous thoracic duct embolization[57]
    - Large retroperitoneal channel (>2 mm) identified on lymphangiogram and cannulated. Catherization and embolic occlusion of the thoracic duct performed under fluoroscopy
    - A recent series reported a 65% cure rate in 60 patients with high-output chylothorax that was not controlled by nonsurgical means.
    - Few radiologists are able to perform this procedure.

- Operative approaches
  - ○ **Indications:** when conservative management fails or is suboptimal
  - ○ **Thoracic duct closure**
    - Can be clipped or ligated
    - VATS is well suited and is the procedure of choice for this condition, making thoracotomy a less desirable approach.[51,52]
  - ○ Surgical pleurodesis: via talc poudrage
  - ○ Chylothorax following esophagectomy[58]:
    - Associated with high morbidity and mortality
    - Need high index of suspicion
    - Early surgical intervention needed if conservative approaches fail to rapidly reduce lymphatic flow
    - Type of surgery dictated by initial approach to esophagectomy
    - Duct or nodal basin needs to be clipped and talc pleurodesis considered
    - Surgery has a low failure rate
  - ○ Pleuroperitoneal shunt:
    - Chylous ascites a contraindication
    - Prevents malnutrition

## *PSEUDOCHYLOTHORAX*

- Definition: A milky non-chylous effusion.[59]
- Causes
  - ○ Usually seen with chronic effusions
  - ○ Tuberculosis accounts for the majority of cases (54%). Seen particularly in those patients with prior collapse therapy. Effusion is usually sterile.
  - ○ Rheumatoid arthritis
- Diagnosis:
  - ○ Elevated pleural fluid cholesterol (>200 mg/dL)
  - ○ Pleural fluid sediment can show cholesterol crystals
- Clinical
  - ○ Usually unilateral
  - ○ Long-standing effusions (>5 years)
  - ○ Associated with pleural thickening
  - ○ Dyspnea on effort
- Treatment
  - ○ Rule out active tuberculosis
  - ○ Therapeutic thoracentesis
  - ○ With significant symptoms, need for frequent pleural taps; with trapped lung, may consider decortication, provided lung parenchyma viable

## *MALIGNANT PLEURAL EFFUSION*

- The etiology of malignant pleural effusions is due to a variety of factors (Table 47-7).
  - ○ The main cause is lymphatic obstruction. Can occur peripherally within the pulmonary parenchyma or centrally within the mediastinal lymph nodes.
  - ○ Tumor invasion of the pleura either seeds the mesothelial surface or invades the subserosal layer.
  - ○ The neoplasms that more commonly cause malignant effusions are listed in Table 47-7.
- Diagnosis is usually performed with thoracentesis.
- In about 50% of pleural effusions in patients without a known cancer, the initial thoracentesis is diagnostic, and if not, a repeated thoracentesis raises the diagnostic sensitivity of cytologic examination from 50% to 65%.[60]

### TABLE 47-7 ■ MALIGNANT PLEURAL EFFUSIONS: ETIOLOGY

| Anatomic Location | Percentage |
| --- | --- |
| Lung | 35 |
| Breast | 23 |
| Lymphoma/leukemia | 10 |
| Adenocarcinoma—primary unknown | 12 |
| Reproductive tract | 6 |
| Gastrointestinal tract | 5 |
| Genitourinary tract | 3 |
| Primary unknown | 3 |
| Other | 5 |

*Adapted from Hausheer FH, Yarbro JW: Diagnosis and treatment of malignant pleural effusion. Semin Oncol 12:54, 1985.*

- ○ The addition of a closed pleural biopsy may improve the cytologic yield; generally, not greatly due to sampling error.[60,61]
- Most malignant pleural effusions are exudative by Light's criteria.
- If diagnosis remains a challenge despite thoracentesis, then thorascopy with pleural biopsy is indicated.
- A small number of patients who have pleural effusion associated with a malignancy will not have malignant cells on cytologic examination of the thoracentesis specimen or from the pleural biopsy. These effusions are due to the underlying malignancy but not due to direct pleural involvement; these effusions are termed *paramalignant effusions*. The etiology of these effusions may be related to the direct local effects of the tumor causing lymphatic obstruction or to bronchial obstruction, leading to pneumonitis or atelectasis.[62]

### Management of Malignant Pleural Effusions

- Recognizing that the majority of patients who develop malignant pleural effusions are not curable, the treatment is then tailored toward achieving the most effective palliation (Fig. 47-6).

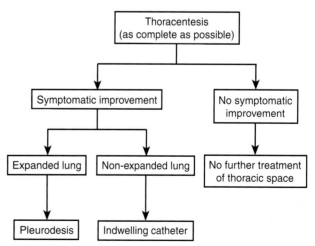

**Figure 47-6:** Decision schema for the treatment of malignant pleural effusions.

- Some malignant effusions are chemosensitive (lymphoma and small cell lung cancer), and chemotherapy alone, after complete drainage by thoracentesis, may control the effusion. When this is not possible, local therapy to the pleural is then warranted.
- **Thoracentesis**. Only relieves the symptoms acutely. The mean time to fluid reaccumulation is as short as 4 days, with a 98% recurrence rate at 30 days.[63]
- **Pleurodesis**. Control of pleural fluid reaccumulation by agents that sclerose the pleural space to achieve a visceropatietal pleural symphysis.
  ○ Beneficial in 70% to 90% of all patients with malignant pleural effusion.
  ○ Compared with other agents, sterilized talc appears to be the most attractive sclerosing agent due to its cost, effectiveness, and less treatment-associated side effects compared with other agents.[64]
  ○ Various other agents, including tetracycline and bleomycin, have been used with variable results.
  ○ Two methods exist for chemical pleurodesis
    ■ Talc slurry
      ○ Tube thoracostomy for drainage
      ○ Lung re-expansion confirmed by chest x-ray study
      ○ Four to five grams sterile talc suspended in 120 mL of normal saline instilled into chest through chest tube
      ○ Chest tube clamped for 2 hours, with patient position changed every half hour
      ○ Chest tube removed after 48 hours if 24-hour drainage is less than 200 mL.
    ■ Thoracoscopic pleurodesis
      ○ Thorascopic evacuation of effusion under direct vision and, if needed, lysis of adhesions to facilitate lung expansion
      ○ Confirmation of lung re-expansion
      ○ Insufflation of 4 to 5 g aerolisized talc
      ○ Tube thoracostomy
      ○ Remove chest tube after 48 hours, when 24-hour drainage is less than 200 mL.
    ■ Advantages
      ○ Effusion treated usually within 3 to 5 days
    ■ Disadvantages
      ○ Requires hospitalization
      ○ Small but real incidence of talc injury to lung
      ○ Possible re-expansion pulmonary edema
- Chronic indwelling pleural catheter.
  ○ Demonstrated to be safe and effective in managing the pleural effusion.[65] Catheters are especially useful when pleurodesis is not possible because of entrapment of the lung from the malignant pleural process.
    ■ Special catheter placed into chest, and chest drained
    ■ Chest drained at home with special suction bottles
    ■ Frequency depends on volume drained and symptoms. May be every day or less often as volume decreases.
    ■ Can be removed if no fluid accumulation for 2 weeks with high likelihood of fluid not recurring
  ○ Advantages
    ■ Can be placed as outpatient
    ■ Less chance of re-expansion pulmonary edema
    ■ Trapped lung may expand with the introduction of a pleural catheter
  ○ Disadvantages
    ■ Requires weeks or months of treatment by drainage
    ■ Catheter and bottles expensive
    ■ Possible risk of infection especially if undergoing chemotherapy

## TRAPPED LUNG SYNDROME

- Definition[66,67]
  ○ Inability of the lung to expand due to a visceral pleural restrictive process
  ○ Absence of an active acute process
  ○ Chronic and stable
  ○ Note: many *acute processes* can produce a thoracic restrictive process and a trapped lung, such as complicated parapneumonic effusions and empyema. These conditions produce acute or subacute signs and symptoms, and are different from the trapped lung syndrome. (See conditions listed earlier.)
- Causes[68,69]
  ○ Coronary artery bypass surgery
  ○ Postcardiac injury syndrome
  ○ Hemothorax
  ○ Tuberculous pleurisy
  ○ Empyema
  ○ Rheumatoid pleural disease
  ○ Systemic lupus pleural disease
  ○ Uremic pleuritis
  ○ Drug-associated pleural disease
  ○ Asbestos pleural thickening
- Clinical
  ○ Diagnosis often delayed for years
  ○ Can be asymptomatic
  ○ Dyspnea on effort
  ○ Reduced thoracic excursion and diminished intensity of breath sounds are subtle and often over-looked.
- Diagnosis
  ○ Clinical suspicion
  ○ Inability of the lung to expand fully after drainage.
  ○ Exclusion of other processes, such as congestive heart failure
  ○ Restrictive ventilatory defect on pulmonary function studies
  ○ Pleural fluid analysis: rule out an active inflammatory or malignant condition.
  ○ Pleural manometry[66,69]: measurement of pleural space elastance (i.e., pleural pressure change for a given volume of pleural fluid removal). The upper limit of the normal range is 14.5 cm $H_2O$/liter. Values greater than 15.5 cm $H_2O$/L compatible with trapped lung. Values can exceed 100 cm $H_2O$/L.
  ○ Air-contrast CT has been suggested as a means of detecting visceral pleural peel that is usually relatively thin in these patients (<3 mm)
- Treatment principles
  ○ Treat only symptomatic patients.
  ○ Decortication is the treatment of choice.

## FIBROTHORAX

- This refers to an exuberant deposition of thick fibrous tissue on the visceral pleura.[70]
- The causes are similar to those listed earlier for the trapped lung syndrome. However, mainly seen after poorly evacuated hemothorax, empyema and tuberculosis.
- Calcification of the pleural peel is common (Fig. 47-7).
- Produces restrictive ventilatory defect of varying degree. Can be more severe than anticipated based on the imaging.
- Treatment: decortication in symptomatic patients with (1) stable chronic disease and (2) no severe underlying lung disease.

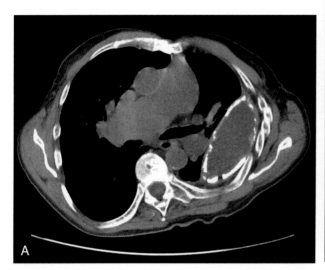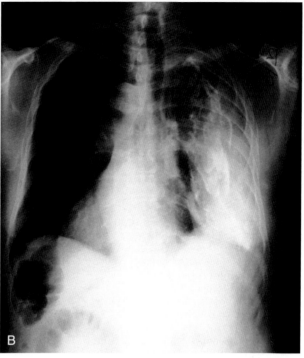

**Figure 47-7: A,** Computed tomography scan depicting fibrothorax secondary to tuberculosis. **B,** Chest x-ray study depicting fibrothorax secondary to remote empyema.

## Brief Illustrative Case

- A 42-year-old woman with a history of chronic alcohol abuse and recent binging presented to the emergency department complaining of fever, sweats, severe left pleuritic chest pain, and dyspnea.
- About 10 days earlier, she had presented to an urgent care center with cough, sputum production, and a low-grade fever. She was given a course of azithromycin. Although she exhibited some clinical response initially, hectic fevers and progressive severe chest pain ensued
- Examination revealed a fever of 102.7° F, heart rate of 108 per minute and respirations of 30 per minute. She had poor dentition and gingivitis. Chest examination revealed dullness to percussion at the left base with bronchial breath sounds and a pleural rub. She exhibited tenderness with the percussive maneuvers.
- Blood work revealed a leukocytosis of 22,000 per microliter and a left shift.
- Because the chest radiograph suggested the presence of pleural fluid loculations, a CT scan was obtained for better imaging. This demonstrated complex loculations on the left (see Fig. 47-5).
- A diagnostic thoracentesis using ultrasound guidance revealed cloudy pleural fluid. The fluid was clearly exudative (LDH 1010 with serum LDH of 214; protein 5.9 g/dL). The glucose was less than 5 mg/dL and the pH 6.89. Total white blood cell count was 19,000 with predominant neutrophils. Gram's stain: gram-positive cocci.
- Broad-spectrum antibiotics, including MRSA and anaerobic cover, was instituted.

- The patient was taken to surgery. A VATS approach was undertaken, with removal of purulent fluid, breakdown of loculations, and decortication of pleural peel. Chest tube drainage continued postoperatively for several days. The patient improved dramatically and was discharged home to complete antibiotic course.
- Culture of pleural fluid grew MRSA.

### Key Points

- The patient fulfilled criteria for *category 3* complicated parapneumonic effusion and needed urgent drainage.
- In this setting, chest tube only with or without fibrinolytic therapy would likely incur a high failure rate; hence, urgent VATS.
- The history of heavy alcohol intake raises suspicions for various organisms: anaerobes (gingivitis and risk of aspiration), *K. pneumoniae* and *S. aureus*.
- MRSA infection is increasingly being seen in the community, even in normal hosts.[71,72]
- In this patient, mixed aerobic and anaerobic infection is likely. Anaerobes are notoriously difficult to culture unless specific provisions are undertaken in the microbiology laboratory.

## References

 Interactive references and additional readings for this chapter can be accessed online at *expertconsult.com*.

## TYPES OF PLEURAL MASSES

- Mesothelioma
- Solitary Fibrous Tumor of the Pleura
- Other Rarer Pleural Masses (Table 48-1)

## MALIGNANT PLEURAL MESOTHELIOMA

- Epidemiology[1-5]
  - Rare and very aggressive, primary malignant pleural tumor
  - Originates from the mesothelial cells that line the parietal and visceral pleura
  - Usually diagnosed in the fifth to seventh decades of life
  - Strong male predominance (80%)[6]
  - 2500 cases per year in the United States
    - 2000 cases in men
    - 500 cases in women
  - Incidence: 15 cases per million population[6]
  - Incidence rising in the United States, particularly in men aged 75 years or older
  - Incidence rising in Europe, with 5000 dying in 1998 and 9000 projected to die by 2018
  - Occupational exposure to asbestos is the main risk factor
    - Association between lung cancer and asbestos exposure first established in 1955[7]
    - 80% patients with mesothelioma have asbestos exposure
    - Only 10% of those with asbestos exposure develop mesothelioma
    - Latency period between exposure and death is generally between 25 to 49 years[8]
  - Human simian virus (SV)-40 may play a role because human mesothelial cells are highly susceptible to infection by the virus.[9-11] SV-40 may have contaminated vaccines in the 1960s.
  - Smoking and asbestos have synergistic effect in lung cancer development, but there is no known association of smoking and mesothelioma development.[5]
- Clinical features
  - Symptoms[12,13]
    - Dyspnea and nonpleuritic chest wall pain (60%) are most common.
    - Patients can be asymptomatic.
    - Typically, progressive shortness of breath, chest pain, anorexia and weight loss as disease advances.
  - Signs
    - Ipsilateral dullness to percussion, decreased breath sounds on affected side, decreased chest wall excursion at base of hemithorax, physical distortion of the ribcage with diseased side smaller than the contralateral hemithorax.
    - Ninety percent have unilateral pleural effusion.[14]
    - Clubbing occurs in less than 1%.[6]
    - Advanced disease almost always due to local invasion of chest wall, pericardium, or diaphragm. Distal metastases are rare.
    - Invasion of contralateral lung or peritoneal cavity occurs in 10% to 20% cases.[15]
    - Local invasion can rarely lead to dysphagia, Horner's syndrome, superior vena cava syndrome, spinal cord compression, cardiac tamponade, vocal cord paralysis, or diaphragm paralysis.[3]
  - Prognosis
    - Median survival from the onset of symptoms without therapy is generally 6 months; with single-modality therapy, survival can be increased to 9 to 12 months.[12,16-18]
    - Death is usually secondary to respiratory failure, cachexia, or infection.
    - Poor prognostic factors[16,17,19]
      - LDH level greater than 500
      - Poor performance status
      - Chest pain
      - Platelet count greater than 400,000
      - Nonepithelial histology
      - Age older than 75 years
      - Male gender
  - Pathophysiology[5,14]
    - Asbestos fibers
    - Serpentine asbestos fibers are large, curly, and not able to travel to distal airways.
    - Amphibole asbestos fibers are narrow and straight and travel to distal pulmonary airways and are clearly associated with mesothelioma formation.
      - Asbestos miners
      - Shipyard workers
      - Naval veterans serving on World War II era ships
      - Insulation in cold environments
      - Family members of workers with heavy exposure (from clothing)
  - Pathology—three types
    - Epithelial
      - Fifty percent of cases
      - More favorable prognosis
    - Sarcomatoid
      - Fifteen percent of cases
      - More aggressive course, worse prognosis
    - Mixed
      - Thirty-five percent of cases
      - Because sarcomatoid element is aggressive, similar prognosis to pure sarcomatoid variant

### TABLE 48-1 ■ CLASSIFICATION OF PLEURAL MASSES

| Benign | Malignant |
| --- | --- |
| Solitary fibrous tumor of the pleura | Mesothelioma |
| Pleural lipoma | Angiosarcoma |
| Angiomas | Synovial sarcoma of the pleura |
| Fibroma | Primary pleural lymphoma |
| Neurofibroma | Ectopic pleural thymoma |
| Calcifying fibrous pseudotumor of the pleura | Metastasis |

- Vimentin negative
- Cytokeratin positive
- Diagnosis
  - Chest x-ray study (CXR) typically shows unilateral pleural thickening, pleural mass, pleural effusion, and basilar atelectasis (Fig. 48-1). Plaques are signs of asbestos exposure but may not be a precursor to mesothelioma[6]
  - Computed tomography (CT) scan of the chest[20,21]
    - Unilateral pleural effusion (74%)
    - Thickened irregular pleural based masses (92%)
    - Chest wall invasion (18%)
- Pleural plaques (20%)
- Differential diagnosis includes
  - Fibrothorax
  - Rheumatologic causes
  - Adenocarcinoma
  - Magnetic resonance imaging (MRI) helpful in determining extent of local invasion into mediastinum, chest wall, or diaphragm[21]
  - Echocardiography used to assess pericardial involvement, pulmonary hypertension, and baseline ejection fraction[5]

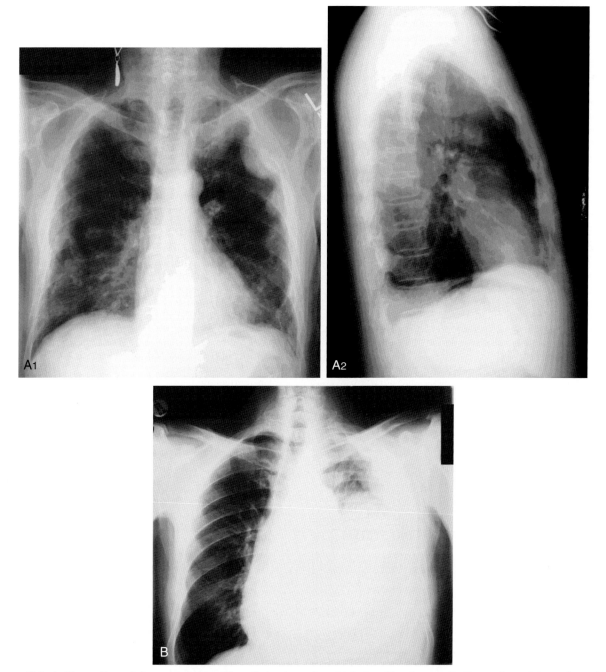

**Figure 48-1:** **A,** Chest radiograph (posteroanterior and lateral) showing unilateral left pleural based masses. **B,** Chest radiograph in another patient showing advanced mesothelioma. Still evident are large pleura-based masses on the left, together with extensive opacification due to tumor encasement. This patient had significant chest wall pain and dyspnea, and the latter was due to thoracic restriction by the tumor.

○ Positron emission tomography (PET) scan can help rule out extrathoracic disease that would preclude surgical intervention. Mesothelioma is frequently not intense in tracer uptake.

○ Serum markers may be helpful in near future.
  ■ Serum mesothelin–related protein is elevated in 84% of patients with malignant mesothelioma and is elevated in less than 2% of patients with other pleural diseases.[22]
  ■ Serum mesothelin–related protein levels increase with mesothelioma progression and decrease with tumor resection, making it perhaps useful in monitoring disease recurrence.

○ Thoracentesis is frequent initial diagnositic step for unilateral pleural effusion.
  ■ Unreliable because fluid cytology can be negative (pleural biopsy preferred). Also, very difficult to distinguish mesothelioma from sarcomas and adenocarcinomas based on fluid cytology alone.

○ CT-guided pleural biopsy[23]
  ■ Sixty percent yield (single attempt) to 85% yield (multiple attempts)

○ Thorascopy-guided pleural biopsy (best workup)[24-26]
  ■ Greater than 90% yield
  ■ Rare complications include bleeding, infection, air leak
  ■ Forty percent chance of seeding tumor at the port sites
  ■ Port should be placed in line of posterolateral thoracotomy incision. If patient seeks multimodality therapy (i.e., chemotherapy, radiation, and surgery), this location will facilitate wide local excision of the port site during surgical therapy.

○ Open thoracotomy and pleural biopsy is discouraged.

■ Staging
  ○ Butchardt: earliest system, now rarely used (Table 48-2)[5]
  ○ Brigham and Women's system (Table 48-3)[5]
  ○ TNM staging, International Mesothelioma Interest Group (Table 48-4)[5,27]

■ Treatment
  ○ The key is to use a multimodality approach.
  ○ Single modality (i.e., surgery alone, chemotherapy alone, radiation alone) palliates symptoms but does not significantly affect survival.
  ○ Surgery
    ■ Thoracoscopy and pleurodesis for diagnosis and palliation
    ■ Pleurectomy
      ○ Removal of visceral and parietal pleura of entire ipsilateral lung
      ○ May include removal of ipsilateral pericardium and diaphragm.

### TABLE 48-2 ■ BUTCHART STAGING SYSTEM

| Stage | Description |
|---|---|
| I | Tumor confined within the pleural envelope |
| II | Invading chest wall or mediastinal structures |
| III | Invading through the diaphragm or into contralateral pleura |
| IV | Distant metastases |

*From Butchart EG, Ashcroft T, Barnsley WC, et al. Pleuropneumonectomy in the management of diffuse malignant mesothelioma of the pleura. Thorax 1976;31:15-24.*

### TABLE 48-3 ■ REVISED STAGING SYSTEM FOR MALIGNANT PLEURAL MESOTHELIOMA

| Stage | Description |
|---|---|
| I | Disease completely resected within the capsule of the parietal pleura without adenopathy: ipsilateral pleura, lung, pericardium, diaphragm, or chest wall limited to previous biopsy sites |
| II | All of stage I with positive margins and/or intrapleural adenopathy |
| III | Local extension of disease into the chest wall or mediastinum; heart, or through diaphragm, peritoneum or with extrapleural lymph node involvement |
| IV | Distant metastatic disease |

■ Extrapleural pneumonectomy (EPP) (Fig. 48-2)[28]
  ○ Most aggressive
  ○ En bloc resection of lung, pericardium, ipsilateral diaphragm, and visceral and parietal pleura, with reconstruction of the diaphragm and pericardium
  ○ Major operation associated with high morbidity and mortality rates. Appropriate for young patients with low comorbidity and preserved functional status.
  ○ Consider referral to major center with extensive experience.
  ■ Surgery alone does not improve survival, but multimodality approach has produced positive results.[29]

○ Radiation
  ■ To encompass all disease in the unilateral hemithorax requires a prohibitively large radiation field.
  ■ There is no survival advantage to radiation alone.[30,31]
  ■ After EPP, patients can receive higher doses safely because there is no longer an ipsilateral lung to suffer postradiation pneumonitis.
  ■ Intensity-modulated radiotherapy is a successful fractionation method, which is used after surgical resection to control local recurrence.[32] This is especially aimed at the fields of highest risk of recurrence, such as the base of the hemithorax.

○ Chemotherapy
  ■ Chemotherapy alone is only palliative.
  ■ Single-agent response rates are less than 20%.[33]
  ■ Platinum analogues, taxanes, and gemcitabine combination therapies have better response rates.[33,34]

○ Trimodality therapy
  ■ Brigham and Women's experience
    ○ EPP and adjuvant chemotherapy (carboplatin/paclitaxel): (1) Overall 2-year survival is greater than 38%; (2) overall 5-year survival is greater than 16%.
    ○ Subset of patients: epithelial histology, no nodes, clear margins: (1) 2-year survival is greater than 68%; (2) 5-year survival is greater than 46%.
    ○ Addition of intraoperative heated chemotherapy: (1) 1-hour lavage of cisplatin at 42° C; (2) dose-limiting renal toxicity at 250 mg/m$^2$; (3) dose response for long-term survival; (4) epithelial tumors and high-dose cisplatin produced 26-month median survival.[35]

○ Novel agents
  ■ Pemetrexed[36-41]
    ○ Inhibitor of thymidylate synthase and dihydrofolate reductase
    ○ In a trial with 448 patients comparing pemetrexed and cisplatin, median survival was 12.1 months and 9.3 months, respectively, and response rate of 41%.[42]

**TABLE 48-4 ▪ TNM STAGING SYSTEM AND TNM STAGE GROUPING**

| Stage | Description |
| --- | --- |
| **The TNM Staging System** | |
| T1 | Tumor involves ipsilateral parietal pleura, with (T1b) or without (T1a) focal involvement of visceral pleura |
| T2 | Confluent visceral pleural tumor, invasion of diaphragm muscle, and/or invasion of lung parenchyma |
| T3 | Invasion into endothoracic fascia or mediastinal fat, a single focus invading chest wall, soft tissue and/or nontransmural involvement of the pericardium |
| T4 | Diffuse/multifocal chest wall soft tissue invasion, rib involvement, transdiaphragmatic invasion, invasion of mediastinal organs, direct extension to contralateral pleura, invasion of spine, extension through pericardium, malignant pericardial effusion, invasion of myocardium or brachial plexus. |
| N0 | No regional lymph node metastases. |
| N1 | Metastases in ipsilateral bronchopulmonary or hilar lymph node. |
| N2 | Metastases in subcarinal and/or ipsilateral internal mammary or mediastinal lymph nodes |
| N3 | Metastases in contralateral mediastinal, internal mammary or hilar lymph nodes, and/or ipsilateral or contralateral supraclavicular or scalene lymph nodes |
| M0 | No distant blood-borne metastases |
| M1 | 1 or more distant blood-borne metastases |

| **TNM Stage Grouping** | | | |
| --- | --- | --- | --- |
| I | T1 | N0 | M0 |
| II | T2 | N0 | M0 |
| III | T1, T2 | N1 | M0 |
| | T1, T2 | N2 | M0 |
| | T3 | N0-2 | M0 |
| IV | T4 | N0-3 | M0 |
| | T1-4 | N3 | M0 |
| | T1-4 | N0-3 | M1 |

*From International Mesothelioma Interest Group. A proposed new international TNM staging system for malignant pleural mesothelioma. Chest 1995;108:1122-1128.*

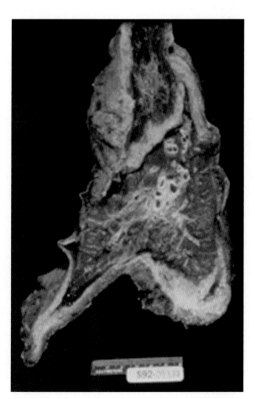

**Figure 48-2:** Gross pathology specimen following extrapleural pneumonectomy.

- Bevacizumab (antivascular endothelial growth factor antibody)[41,43]
- Imatinib (Gleevec, Novartis, Basel, Switzerland) blocks platelet-derived growth factor pathway.
- Gefitinib (Iressa, AstraZeneca, Wilmington, DE) blocks epidermal growth factor pathway.
  ○ Palliation
  - Radiation for reducing chest wall pain and dyspnea symptoms
  - Surgical pleurodesis or pleural catheter to reduce pleural effusion symptoms
  - Chemotherapy benefit demonstrated in overall quality of life.

## SOLITARY FIBROUS TUMOR OF THE PLEURA

- Rare tumor, with only about 800 cases reported in the literature[44,45]
- Localized tumor of the pleura as opposed to the diffuse nature of mesothelioma
- Appears to arise from the submesothelial mesenchymal layer
- Other names
  ○ Localized pleural mesothelioma
  ○ Pleural fibroma
  ○ Localized fibrous mesothelioma
  ○ Submesothelial fibroma
  ○ Localized fibrous tumor
- Occurs predominately in the sixth or seventh decades of life[46]
- Equal male-to-female ratio

- No genetic predisposition
- No relationship to exposure to asbestos, smoking, or any environmental substance
- Eighty percent benign
- Twenty percent malignant
- Clinical features
  - Symptoms[46-49]
    - Patients with benign tumors have symptoms 54% to 67% of the time.
    - Patients with malignant tumors have symptoms more than 75% of the time.
    - Cough, chest pain, dyspnea and fever are the most common symptoms.
    - Hypertrophic pulmonary osteoarthropathy.[50]
      - Most common paraneoplastic syndrome with solitary fibrous tumors
      - Reported in up to 22% of patients
      - Bilateral arthritic symptoms of stiffness, swelling, arthralgia of joints
      - Clubbing, gynecomastia, or galactorrhea have also been reported.
      - Symptoms improve dramatically after tumor removal within days or hours

- Symptomatic hypoglycemia[46,50]
  - Incidence is approximately 3% to 4%
  - Secondary to insulin-like growth factors produced by tumor
  - Resolves rapidly after tumor removal
  - Signs
    - Clubbing is the most frequent (2%–19%)
  - Pathology[45,51,52]
    - Can arise from either parietal or visceral pleura
    - Vimentin positive
    - Cytokeratin negative
    - Mesothelioma is vimentin negative and cytokeratin positive
    - Benign solitary fibrous tumors have few mitoses per high powered field (HPF) (<4 per HPF), uniform elongated spindle cells in a patternless pattern and normal nuclei (Fig. 48-3)
    - Malignant solitary fibrous tumors show increased cellularity, overlapping nuclei, cellular pleomorphism, and high mitotic count (>4 per HPF)
- Diagnosis[53]
  - Chest radiograph shows solitary mass in chest along the periphery of the lung.

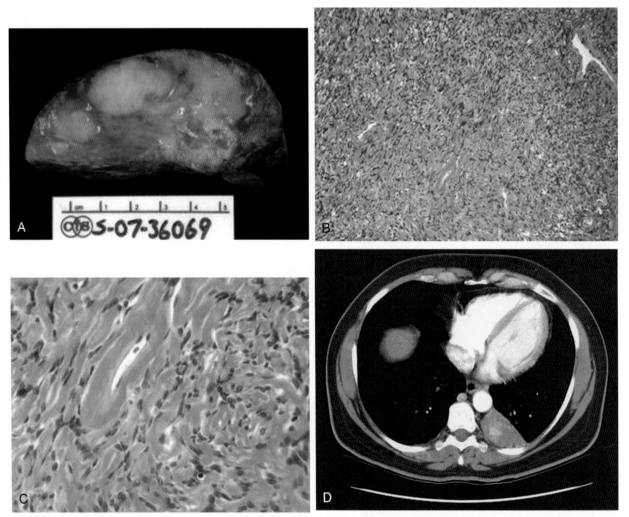

**Figure 48-3: A,** Gross pathology specimen following video-assisted thoracic surgery resection of solitary fibrous tumor of the pleura. **B** and **C,** Histology from above-mentioned case showing spindle cells with *patternless pattern*. **D,** Computed tomography scan of the chest of above-mentioned case showing pleural mass on left with variable attenuation.

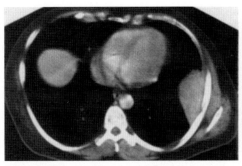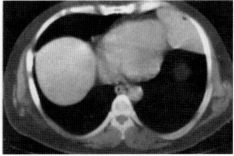

**Figure 48-4:** Computed tomography scan of the chest demonstrating solitary fibrous tumor of the pleura. The tumor was pedunculated, allowing movement in different body positions. In the left panel, the patient is supine, and in the right panel, the patient is prone. *(From Lewis MI, et al. The case of the moving intrathoracic mass. Chest 1985;88:897-898, with permission.)*

- ○ Chest CT scan
  - ■ Fifty percent pedunculated. (With a long stalk, the tumor mass moves with a change in body position [Fig. 48-4].)
  - ■ Twenty-six percent have calcifications
  - ■ Six to thirty-seven percent have a small pleural effusion
  - ○ Controversy regarding the need to biopsy the mass before resection[45,46,54,55]
    - ■ Slow growth on follow-up scans
    - ■ Recognized due to unique appearance at thoraco-scopy
- ■ Treatment[45-49] Note: see video of video-assisted thoracic surgery resection
  - ○ Surgical excision while preserving as much normal lung as possible
  - ○ Pedunculated visceral pleural masses require only small margin of normal lung tissue.
  - ○ Sessile masses may require major lung resection such as lobectomy or segmentectomy
  - ○ En bloc chest wall resection may be required in malignant invasive cases
  - ○ If complete surgical resection is performed, adjuvant therapy is not required.
  - ○ Single or multiple rib resection may be necessary in parietal-based benign tumors.
  - ○ Postoperative radiation for patients with incomplete resection
  - ○ Recurrent disease should be surgically resected as primary treatment
  - ○ Recurrence rates
    - ■ Benign penduculated    = 2%
    - ■ Benign sessile         = 8%
    - ■ Malignant penduculated = 14%
    - ■ Malignant sessile      = 63% (30% mortality)

## OTHER PLEURAL MASSES

- ■ Metastasis[56]
  - ○ Forty percent lung cancer
  - ○ Twenty percent breast cancer
  - ○ Ten percent lymphoma
  - ○ Others include colon, melanoma, thyroid, adenocarcinoma of unknown primary, and sarcomas.
- ■ Pleural lipoma[57]
  - ○ Most common benign tumors of the chest wall
- ■ Calcifying fibrous pseudotumor of the pleura[58]
  - ○ Uncommon benign lesion
  - ○ Childhood fibrous tumor with psammoma bodies

- ○ Usually presents in young adults in the extremities without lung involvement
- ○ Pleural location is very rare
- ○ Painless, slow-growing masses
- ○ Treatment is simple local excision
- ■ Ectopic pleural thymoma[59]
  - ○ Extremely rare, with only eight cases reported in the literature
  - ○ Treatment is surgical excision.
- ■ Synovial sarcoma of the pleura[60]
  - ○ Patients present with dyspnea and chest pain.
  - ○ Pleural effusions and pleural-based masses are seen on CXR.
  - ○ CT scan shows soft tissue mass. Can show intratumoral calcifications in 20% to 30% despite the malignant nature
  - ○ Treatment is surgical resection, radiation, and chemotherapy.
  - ○ Favorable prognosis when tumor is smaller than 5 cm, low mitotic rate, absence of necrosis, and complete resection.
  - ○ Metastasis occurs in 50%.
  - ○ Five-year survival rate is 36% to 76%; 10-year survival rate is 20% to 63%.
- ■ Primary pleural lymphoma[61]
  - ○ Extremely rare
  - ○ Long-standing pleural inflammation is an important etiologic factor

### Brief Illustrative Case

- *History*: A 53-year-old man with right-sided pleuritic chest pain and shortness of breath worsening over several months. Currently has dyspnea on walking 100 feet on a flat surface. No prior smoking history and remote exposure (>30 years) to asbestos as shipyard worker.
- *Physical examination*: Afebrile, and normal vital signs. Slightly diminished breath sounds at the right base, no masses, and no clubbing. He has decreased tactile fremitus and positive egophony over the right base of the chest. He has decreased chest wall excursion on the right.
- *Laboratory tests*: Complete blood count and electrolytes normal.

*(Continued)*

## Brief Illustrative Case—cont'd

- *Imaging*: CXR showed a small right pleural effusion and pleural opacity. CT scan (Fig. 48-5) showed unilateral pleural thickening in the right hemithorax. Chest MRI scan showed no invasion through the pericardium. Cardiac echo showed a normal ejection fraction and no evidence of pulmonary hypertension. PET scan showed no extrathoracic disease.
- *Diagnosis/Pathology*: The patient underwent a right-sided thorascopic pleural biopsy through a single port in the sixth intercostal space, midaxillary line. This confirmed epithelioid mesothelioma. He was deemed an appropriate surgical candidate after preoperative evaluation and workup, which included a negative cervical mediastinoscopy.
- *Treatment*: He underwent an extrapleural pneumonectomy with intraoperative heated chemotherapy and reconstruction of the diaphragm and pericardium with Gore-Tex patch. He was discharged home without complications after 7 days. He had an impaired functional status for 8 weeks but then regained his stamina and independence. His final pathology revealed epithelioid mesothelioma with no invasion into chest wall, diaphragm, pericardium, or lymph nodes. He began adjuvant chemotherapy and radiation after full recovery.

### Key Points

- Typical symptoms, signs, and occupational exposure history for patient presenting with mesothelioma.
- Long latency period of exposure to development of mesothelioma is characteristic.
- Subtle physical examination findings are common.
- Chest radiography and CT scan of the chest show classic unilateral pleural abnormalities.

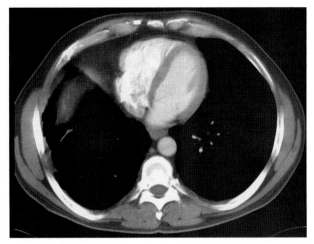

**Figure 48-5:** Computed tomography of the chest showing unilateral pleural thickening in the right hemithorax.

- Pathologic diagnosis was definitively made by thorascopic biopsy. The biopsy site was placed so a wide local excision of the port site could be performed during surgical therapy.
- If detected at an early stage and aggressively treated surgically, cure is possible but is not typical for most patients who present with mesothelioma.

### References

 Interactive references and additional readings for this chapter can be accessed online at *expertconsult.com*.

# 49 PNEUMOTHORAX AND BRONCHOPLEURAL FISTULA

Michael E. Halkos, MD and Joseph I. Miller Jr., MD

## PNEUMOTHORAX

### DEFINITIONS

- A **pneumothorax** is a condition in which air has entered and becomes entrapped within the pleural space.
- A **spontaneous pneumothorax** is either primary or secondary and occurs because of parenchymal (lung) disruption.
- An **acquired pneumothorax** most often is iatrogenic in nature but can also occur secondary to blunt or penetrating trauma.
- **Tension pneumothorax** is a condition in which increasing positive pleural pressure leads to hemodynamic compromise as a result of severe hypoxemia, impaired venous return, and occlusive mechanical shift and compression.

## ETIOLOGY

The more common causes of pneumothorax are listed in Table 49-1. Spontaneous primary pneumothorax is most commonly caused by the rupture of an apical subpleural bleb in patients without clinically apparent underlying lung disease. Spontaneous secondary pneumothoraces occur in patients with known underlying parenchymal disorders, such as bullous disease related to chronic obstructive pulmonary disease (COPD), malignancy, or as a sequelae of infectious disorders. Acquired pneumothorax occurs most commonly in a hospital setting secondary to complications of central venous access, pacemaker insertion, lung biopsy, thoracentesis, mechanical ventilation, or thoracic and abdominal operations. Traumatic pneumothorax is also secondary and associated with blunt and penetrating thoracic injuries.

| TABLE 49-1 ■ CLASSIFICATION OF PNEUMOTHORAX |
| --- |

**Spontaneous**

Primary
    Subpleural apical bleb rupture
Secondary
    COPD—bullous disease
    Esophageal rupture
    Infection—pneumonia, lung abscess
    Catamenial
    Malignancy—lung cancer, metastatic sarcoma
        AIDS—pneumocystis pneumonia
        Interstitial lung disorders

**Acquired**

Iatrogenic
    Transbronchial or transthoracic needle biopsy
    Subclavian or internal jugular venous access
    Percutaneous pacemaker insertion
    Thoracentesis
    Laparoscopic (foregut) surgery
    Barotrauma
Traumatic
    Penetrating trauma
        Stab or gunshot wounds
    Blunt trauma
        Motor vehicle collisions
        Falls
        Contact sports-related injuries

AIDS, acquired immunodeficiency syndrome; COPD, chronic obstructive pulmonary disease.

## *KEY FACTS*

### Spontaneous Primary Pneumothorax

- Occurs more commonly in men with a male-to-female ratio of 6:1. Often taller and thinner individuals. A familial tendency has been described.
- More common in smokers than non-smokers.[1]
- Tends to occur in late adolescence or early adulthood in patients with excellent pulmonary reserve.
- May be secondary to a Valsalva maneuver, such as a severe coughing spell, straining, or with physical activity (rare presentation, however).
- Etiology obscure but may be associated with distal airway inflammation and obstruction and bronchial abnormalities.[2,3] Small airway inflammation associated with smoking may contribute. Bronchial abnormalities include smaller than usual bronchial dimensions, and anatomic variations including missing bronchi or accessory airways. Broad swings in atmospheric pressure can result in bleb overdistension and rupture. In addition, in taller individuals, base-to-apex pleural pressure gradients are greater, with apical blebs subjected to increased distending forces (Fig. 49-1).
- The chief physiologic consequence is a reduction in vital capacity and hypoxemia. In young healthy individuals, this is usually well tolerated. The larger the pneumothorax, the more severe the impact on gas exchange. Hypoxemia is due to shunt and low V/Q units.
- Is associated with a 30% recurrence rate when managed by observation, needle aspiration, or chest tube drainage.[1,4,5]

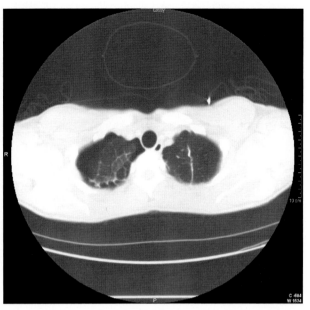

**Figure 49-1:** Computed tomography scan of the chest demonstrating significant and numerous blebs at both apices of the lungs (R > L), with an accompanying pneumothorax on the right side.

### Spontaneous Secondary Pneumothorax

- Occurs in patients with underlying lung disorders and poor pulmonary reserve.
- When associated with bullous disease from emphysema or in patients with cystic fibrosis, it is usually poorly tolerated by patients, even with small pneumothoraces.
- May be the primary manifestation of a ruptured esophagus.
- May be associated with metastatic cancer, especially sarcoma, or may rarely be a primary manifestation of lung cancer.[6]
- Occasionally develops in patients with acquired immunodeficiency syndrome in association with *Pneumocystis* pneumonia (Fig. 49-2).[7] Microscopically, extensive tissue necrosis

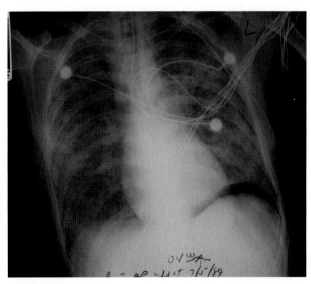

**Figure 49-2:** Chest x-ray study in a patient with *Pneumocystis* pneumonia with residual subpulmonic pneumothorax who is on mechanical ventilation.

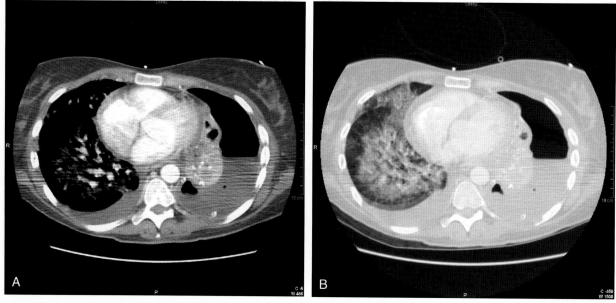

**Figure 49-3:** Computed tomography scans of the chest demonstrating a left-sided pyopneumothorax in a patient with severe bilateral bacterial pneumonia and adult respiratory distress syndrome.

is evident. Similarly, spontaneous secondary pneumothorax can complicate any cause of necrotizing pneumonia (Fig. 49-3).

■ **Catamenial pneumothorax** is defined as a spontaneous pneumothorax occurring within 72 hours before or after the onset of menses. The pathogenesis is not entirely clear, with evidence in some patients of intrathoracic endometriosis or diaphragm defects, or both. However, this is not universally identified in women with catamenial pneumothorax.[8,9] (See later for more details.)

## Acquired Iatrogenic Pneumothorax

■ Commonly associated with complications secondary to placement of subclavian or jugular venous central lines, percutaneous pacemaker insertion via the subclavian vein, or with thoracentesis in which the underlying lung is punctured with a needle allowing air to escape into the pleural space. Pneumothorax following ultrasound-assisted thoracentesis with good visualization may relate to uneven pleural pressure gradients developed as the lung re-expands in an uneven fashion.

■ May occur secondary to barotrauma associated with alveolar overdistension and rupture. Air dissects into the perivascular adventitia and then tracks along the perivascular bundles into the mediastinum, producing a pneumomediastinum. The gas may decompress to other areas (e.g., fascial planes of the neck), but if decompression is inadequate, the pressure rises with rupture of the mediastinal parietal pleura and production of a pneumothorax. Risk factors for barotrauma include high positive end expiratory pressure (PEEP), high tidal volume ventilation, and high peak and mean inspiratory pressures. Patient factors include disease setting such as acute lung injury/adult respiratory distress syndrome (ARDS), emphysema (alveolar overdistension at lower pressures), status asthmaticus, pulmonary fibrosis, necrotizing pneumonia and so on.

■ May also occur after transthoracic needle biopsy or transbronchial lung biopsy.

■ Occurs in the operative setting during open or laparoscopic abdominal procedures involving the diaphragmatic hiatus (Nissen fundoplication, Heller myotomy, paraesophageal hernia repair, or gastric bypass surgery).

## Acquired Traumatic Pneumothorax

■ May occur secondary to blunt or penetrating injuries.

■ With blunt injuries associated with rib fractures, fractured segments can violate parietal pleura and puncture underlying lung parenchyma.

■ Can also occur in high-speed collisions without obvious signs of trauma because of parenchymal disruption associated with high intrathoracic pressure at the moment of impact or from shearing injuries related to sudden deceleration. (Sudden nonuniform increase in alveolar pressures, overdistension and membrane shearing injury)

## Tension Pneumothorax

■ May occur with any of the aforementioned etiologies.

■ In this case, intrapleural pressure exceeds atmospheric pressure during expiration. It likely occurs secondary to a one-way valve effect, whereby gas enters the pleural space during inspiration with no return flow during expiration, producing increasing positive pleural pressure (Fig. 49-4).

■ The key pathophysiologic events include severe hypoxemia, which occurs early and precedes hypotension. The latter is due to impaired venous return because of increased resistance, as well as occlusive mechanical compression (late event), which decrease stroke volume and cardiac output, despite compensatory tachycardia.

■ This condition is a true emergency and is associated with rapid clinical deterioration that requires prompt needle or tube decompression.

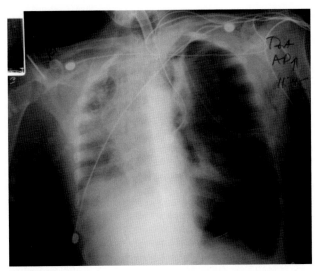

**Figure 49-4:** Chest x-ray study in a patient with left-sided tension pneumothorax. Note: Marked expansion of the left hemithorax (also wide rib spaces and downward displacement of the left hemidiaphragm), together with marked shift of the heart and mediastinum to the right.

## CLINICAL FEATURES

### Symptoms
- Sudden onset of chest pain, dyspnea, and cough ranging from mild to severe without a precipitating event

### Signs
- With a small pneumothorax, clinical findings may be absent.
- With moderate to large pneumothorax
  - Decreased breath sounds over ipsilateral hemithorax
  - Hyperresonance to percussion over ipsilateral hemithorax
  - Hypoxia
- With tension pneumothorax, physical findings are accentuated and include
  - Hypotension and tachycardia
- Absent breath sounds and hyperresonance to percussion over the ipsilateral hemithorax
- Tracheal deviation towards the contralateral side.
- Hypoxia
- Note: in patients on mechanical ventilation, an abrupt increase in peak and plateau pressures (volume-cycled ventilation) or abrupt fall in expired tidal volume (pressure preset ventilation) may be observed.

## DIAGNOSIS

- The chest radiograph is the standard modality for establishing the diagnosis.
- Should be obtained as an upright, expiratory position.
- Supine films can easily obscure the diagnosis because air will not be visualized in the apex in this position.
- Lateral films can also assist in the diagnosis by evaluating the anterior and posterior aspects of the chest.
- In patients with signs or symptoms of tension pneumothorax or in patients with impending cardiovascular collapse, prompt needle or chest tube decompression of the suspected side can be both diagnostic and therapeutic and should be instituted without any delay for diagnostic imaging.

- Computed tomography (CT) obtained for other reasons may identify a pneumothorax (occult pneumothorax) that is not evident on plain chest films but should not be routinely employed as a diagnostic modality for primary spontaneous pneumothorax.
- Although some physicians use a chest CT scan to look for blebs in cases of spontaneous pneumothorax, the American College of Chest Physicians consensus is that a chest CT scan is not routinely recommended.

## TREATMENT

### Spontaneous Primary Pneumothorax
#### Treatment Options
- Observation (inpatient versus outpatient) (Fig. 49-5)
- Needle aspiration
- Tube thoracostomy
- Thoracoscopy
- Thoracotomy

## CONSIDERATIONS

- Age
- Clinical condition
- Size of pneumothorax[10]
  - Small (<3 cm or <20%)
  - Large (≥3 cm or ≥20%)

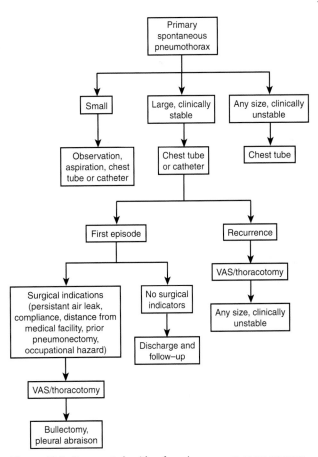

**Figure 49-5:** Treatment algorithm for primary spontaneous pneumothorax.

- Duration of symptoms
- Patient compliance (social situation)
- Proximity to emergency services
- Occupation or hobby (pilot, scuba diver, athlete)

## First Episode

- Clinically stable patients with small pneumothoraces can be treated on an outpatient basis with a catheter and a Heimlich valve, observed in the emergency department, or as an inpatient and discharged home within 6 to 24 hours if repeat chest radiograph excludes enlargement of pneumothorax.[11] We prefer to proceed with either percutaneous catheter or chest tube placement in all but the smallest of pneumothoraces to allow for complete lung re-expansion, but we acknowledge that practice patterns vary widely.
- Clinically stable patients with large pneumothoraces should undergo an intervention to remove air from the pleural space and reexpand the lung. Options include needle aspiration or chest tube insertion with attachment to 20-cm suction or waterseal.[11-13] Controversy exists in the literature regarding the ideal treatment and this also is influenced by practice patterns among individual physicians. We prefer chest tube placement for large pneumothoraces.
- In clinically unstable patients, regardless of pneumothorax size, tube thoracostomy should be the treatment of choice.
- Chest tubes can be removed after the lung has expanded, the pneumothorax has resolved, and the air leak has subsided.
- Patients can be discharged and followed-up as outpatients.
- Consider early surgical intervention for patients with occupational or lifestyle hazards[14] (Table 49-2). Although some physicians perform a pleurodesis through a chest tube, that is not a common practice and there is no convincing literature to support that practice.

## Recurrent Primary Spontaneous Pneumothorax

- Recurrent pneumothorax occurs in approximately 30% of patients, regardless of initial treatment (observation, simple aspiration, catheter, or chest tube management) and usually warrants surgical intervention.[1,4,5]
- Goals of surgery
  - Find and remove offending agent (bleb/bullae)
  - Minimize recurrence with pleural abrasion to create pleural symphysis
- Options
- Video-assisted thoracoscopic surgery (VATS)
- Thoracotomy
  - Limited axillary thoracotomy
  - Traditional posterolateral thoracotomy
- Chemical pleurodesis
  - Should be reserved for patients unwilling to consent to a surgical procedure, those with associated malignancy, and those deemed unfit for surgery

---

### TABLE 49-2 ■ SURGICAL INDICATIONS

Persistent air leak for >5 days
Recurrent spontaneous pneumothorax
Patients with prior pneumonectomy
Patients with occupational hazards or leisure pursuits in which a recurrence may pose excessive risk
Bilateral pneumothoraces
Long-distance from medical facilities

---

- Complicates future surgical intervention secondary to adhesion formation
- Is associated with a higher failure rate compared with surgery (10%–20% versus 0–5%)[15]
- Techniques
  - Patients with apical bullae visualized at surgery should undergo bullectomy, most commonly performed using stapling techniques.
  - Intraoperative pleurodesis should also be performed with parietal pleural abrasion (using a dry gauze or electrocautery scratch pad) to encourage adhesion formation between the visceral and parietal pleura.
  - We recommend against the *routine* use of chemical pleurodesis (talc or doxycycline) in benign disease.
  - Concerns about acute lung injury with use of talc pleurodesis have been reported as case reports (see review by Kennedy and Sahn[16] for details).
  - Several large case series have published on the successful use of talc pleurodesis for primary spontaneous pneumothorax.[17-21] These reported no cases of acute respiratory complications, 95% or greater success rate in several large series, preserved lung function on long-term follow-up, and feasibility of repeat VATS talc insufflation after prior talc pleurodesis.[17-21]
  - In patients in whom no bleb is found, pleurectomy or talc pleurodesis may be considered.
- Recommendations
  - Surgical approaches via thoracoscopy or thoracotomy have yielded excellent long-term results, with success rates of 95% to 100%.[5,15,22]
  - Either approach provides acceptable visualization although thoracoscopic approaches have been associated with less postoperative pain, shorter recovery and hospitalization time, and improved cosmesis.[15]
  - A limited axillary thoracotomy through a 5- to 6-cm incision provides excellent visualization and is an acceptable alternative to thoracosopy with equivalent morbidity.[23]
  - Mechanical pleurodesis and resection of apical blebs/bullae, if present, is the current standard.

## Secondary Spontaneous Pneumothorax

- In general, patients have underlying lung disease, limited pulmonary reserve, and associated comorbidities that are likely to influence treatment decisions.
- Usually require more early and aggressive intervention (Fig. 49-6)
- Clinically stable patients with small pneumothoraces should be hospitalized and can be treated with observation or chest tube placement depending on their course and symptoms.[11] We prefer to manage patients with secondary pneumothorax with a chest tube because of associated comorbidities, underlying lung disease, and the limited cardiopulmonary reserve of these patients in the event of progression of the pneumothorax.
- All patients with large pneumothoraces or those who are clinically unstable should be treated with chest tube placement.
- Computed tomography of the chest is a useful adjunct to plain radiographs to provide additional diagnostic information about underlying pulmonary or chest wall pathology (bullous disease, malignancy, infection).
- In patients who are suitable for operation, surgical intervention via thoracoscopy or limited thoracotomy is usually indicated to provide diagnostic information (biopsy) as well as to treat the underlying disorder (bullectomy).[22] Mechanical or chemical pleurodesis is an important adjunct to encourage adhesion formation and prevent recurrence.

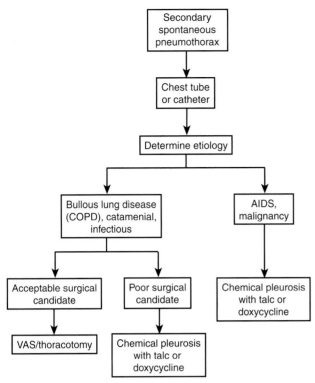

**Figure 49-6:** Treatment algorithm for secondary spontaneous pneumothorax.

- In patients deemed high-risk or those unfit for surgery and general anesthesia, chemical pleurodesis through a previously placed chest tube can be used to minimize recurrence, albeit not as effectively as surgical approaches.[11]
- Owing to the presence of underlying thoracic pathology, surgical intervention is not as effective for secondary pneumothorax compared with primary pneumothorax, yet it remains the best treatment option for these patients.

## *SPECIFIC CONDITIONS*

### Chronic Obstructive Pulmonary Disease

- Patients with COPD usually have underlying bullous disease that can be effectively treated with bullectomy and intraoperative pleurodesis.
- Chemical pleurodesis through the chest tube is a viable option for patients who are not candidates for surgery.

### Acquired Immunodeficiency Syndrome

- Most patients have evidence of active infection with *Pneumocystis carinii*.[7]
- Persistent air leak or recurrent pneumothorax is frequent.
- Mortality is more common in these patients.
- Patients suitable for operation should undergo thoracoscopy or limited thoracotomy to identify and seal air leaks in addition to mechanical or chemical pleurodesis.
- Treatment with tube thoracostomy alone associated with high recurrence rate.
- Treatment with chemical pleurodesis more effective than chest tube drainage alone but not as effective as surgery. However, this remains a viable option for these high-risk patients.[7]

## Catamenial Pneumothorax

- Definition:
  - Recurrent pneumothorax occurring within 72 hours before or after the onset of menses[8,24]
  - Some authors have restricted the definition to within 24 hours before menstruation and 72 hours after.[25]
- Pathogenesis[8,9,25-29]
  - Usually attributed to intrathoracic endometriosis.
  - Note: intrathoracic endometriosis is not always found; however, it was present in 64% of cases in a recent large series.[25]
  - Several mechanisms have been proposed to account for extrapelvic endometrial tissue:
    - Transabdominal migration of endometrial tissue following retrograde menstruation. Preferential flow of air and endometrial tissue along the right paracolic gutter may explain right-sided predominance of the condition.
    - Endometrial implantation in ectopic sites via hematogenous or lymphatic passage.
  - Several mechanisms proposed to account for catamenial pneumothorax:
    - Transabdominal influx of air from the pelvis across diaphragm defects. Loss of cervical mucus during menses may facilitate passage of environmental air across the peritoneal cavity. Diaphragm defects are likely acquired by sloughing of diaphragmatic foci of endometriosis.
    - Sloughing of visceral pleural foci of endometrial deposits.
    - Air trapping and rupture of alveoli due to high levels of prostaglandin $F_2$-alpha inducing bronchiolar constriction
    - Rupture of apical blebs
- Clinical details:
  - Accounts for 1% to 5% of spontaneous pneumothorax in women[24,25]
  - Intermenstrual spontaneous pneumothorax in women, in whom intrathoracic endometriosis is found at surgery, has been reported.[25]
  - Mean age 32 to 37 years; range 19 to 54 years[8]
  - Pelvic endometriosis found in about two thirds of cases
  - Dyspnea and chest pain most common presenting symptoms
  - Right sided in more than 95%
  - Serosanguineous pleural effusion is rare.[25]
- Treatment Approaches:
  - Surgical
    - Findings: diaphragm perforations, nodules or both in 38% to 79%; apical blebs/bulla in 30% to 50%; visceral pleural brown nodules in 30% to 50%; parietal pleural brown nodules in 10%[9,25,29-31]
    - **VATS** is approach of choice[25,29]
    - **Surgical treatments** include[25,29,30]
      - Resection of endometrial diaphragm deposits and repair of existing or surgical defects (mesh; plication)
      - Apical resection of blebs
      - Resection of endometrial pleural deposits
      - Pleurodesis: although mechanical pleurodesis (abrasion) is commonly employed and effective for the usual cases of primary spontaneous pneumothorax, it has a high recurrence rate for catamenial pneumothorax
      - Pleurectomy and talc insufflation are the treatments of choice for catamenial pneumothorax
  - **Medical**[25,29,30]
    - Hormonal approaches include
      - Gonadotropin-releasing hormone agonists (medical treatment of choice)
      - Oral contraception
      - Bilateral salpingo-oophorectomy
    - Can be used before and following surgery

○ Combined approach
  ■ Surgery together with prolonged hormonal therapy should be the standard approach.
■ Outcome:
  ○ Despite surgery and prolonged hormonal therapy, a high relapse rate exists (32%–40%)[25,30]
  ○ Talc pleurodesis appears to significantly reduce recurrences.[25]

## Malignancy

■ Careful assessment of patients with a history of malignancy, especially sarcoma, should be performed to identify patients with metastatic pulmonary disease who present with pneumothorax.

## Esophageal Rupture

■ Any patient with a history of recent esophageal manipulation (endoscopy, transesophageal echocardiography) who later presents with pneumothorax, with or without an effusion, should be evaluated with a gastrograffin swallow to rule out perforation.
■ Patients with pneumothorax and effusion with a history of esophageal disease (benign or malignant), history of violent wretching (Boorhaave's syndrome), or signs of sepsis should also undergo a gastrograffin swallow.

## Acquired Pneumothorax
### Iatrogenic

■ Common complication of central venous access procedures, transthoracic lung biopsy, and thoracentesis.
■ Small pneumothoraces in clinically stable patients with minimal symptoms can be observed.
■ Large pneumothoraces, those associated with clinical instability, or those occurring in critically ill or ventilated patients should be managed with tube or catheter thoracostomy.
■ Associated with barotrauma secondary to mechanical ventilation.
  ○ Higher incidence with high tidal volume ventilation, elevated positive end expiratory and peak inspiratory pressures, and pressure control ventilation.[32]
■ Occurs in approximately 5% to 7% patients with ARDS.[33]
■ Potentially life-threatening complication that warrants chest tube placement in all cases.

### Traumatic
#### Blunt Trauma

■ May occur from direct parenchymal injury as a result of rib fractures
■ May also occur from parenchymal rupture secondary to a sudden increase in intrathoracic pressure during impact
■ Large air leaks should raise suspicion for tracheobronchial injuries.
■ Large pneumothoraces or those occurring in hemodynamically unstable or multiply-injured patients should be managed with chest tube decompression.
■ Occult pneumothoraces are defined as those discovered on chest CT that are not evident on plain radiographs. Although these can be managed expectantly, we prefer chest tube placement in ventilated patients even if otherwise clinically stable.[34]
■ In the presence of hemothorax, all patients with pneumothorax should be managed with large-bore (>28 F) chest tube drainage.

#### Penetrating Trauma

■ Occurs secondary to parenchymal disruption from penetrating injuries
■ Requires chest tube drainage in most cases

# BRONCHOPLEURAL FISTULA
## DEFINITION

■ A bronchopleural fistula is a communication between the pleural space and the bronchial tree (Fig. 49-7).
■ A postresectional bronchopleural fistula is a rare but dreaded complication of pulmonary resection.

## ETIOLOGY

■ Can occur as a complication of lung resection or secondary to bronchial or parenchymal disorders (Table 49-3)
■ Most common cause is a postresectional bronchopleural fistula
■ Both local and systemic factors increase the risk of developing postresectional bronchopleural fistula (Table 49-4).

## KEY FACTS

■ Occurs as a complication of pneumonectomy in 2% to 20% of patients[35-40]
■ Occurs as a complication of lobectomy in less than 1% of cases.[41]

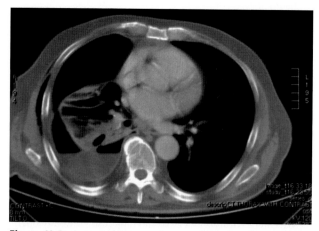

**Figure 49-7:** Computed tomography scan of the chest from a patient with a bronchopleural fistula, complicating rupture of a coccidioidal cyst. Significant lung destruction/bronchiectasis is present on the right side as well.

---

### TABLE 49-3 ■ ETIOLOGY OF BRONCHOPLEURAL FISTULA

Postresectional
Idiopathic
Necrotizing lung infections
Persistent spontaneous pneumothorax
Thoracic trauma
Adult respiratory distress syndrome
Tuberculosis
Postprocedural (lung biopsy, bronchoscopy)

| TABLE 49-4 ■ **RISK FACTORS FOR POSTRESECTIONAL BRONCHOPLEURAL FISTULA** |
| --- |

**Technical Factors**

Right pneumonectomy versus left
Completion pneumonectomy
Long bronchial stump
Residual cancer at bronchial margin
Extensive bronchial devascularization
Surgeon experience
Intraoperative contamination of postresectional space
Poor closure of stump

**Preoperative Risk Factors**

Poorly controlled diabetes mellitus
Preexisting infection (obstructive pneumonia, preexisting
    empyema)
Steroid dependence
Malnutrition
Older age
Induction chemotherapy and radiation therapy
COPD
Resection for infectious or inflammatory conditions
    versus malignancy

**Postoperative Risk Factors**

Postoperative mechanical ventilation
Pulmonary infections
Empyema

COPD, chronic obstructive pulmonary disease.

- Higher incidence after right pneumonectomy (8%–13%) compared with left pneumonectomy (1%–5%)[38,42]
- Occurs more commonly after right pneumonectomy because
  - In most cases, the right main bronchus vascular supply is provided by one bronchial artery compared with two bronchial arteries for the left main stem bronchus, making it more susceptible to devascularization during dissection.
  - The left main bronchus retracts underneath the aortic arch after pneumonectomy and is better protected by mediastinal tissues.
- May be prevented in higher risk patients by reinforcing bronchial stump with pedicled flap of muscle, omentum, or pericardium.[43,44]
- More devastating complication when it occurs after pneumonectomy compared with lesser lung resections.
- A long bronchial stump may increase the risk for postresectional bronchopleural fistula because of excess pooling of contaminated secretions and subsequent stump breakdown.
- Residual carcinoma at the bronchial stump margin will inhibit bronchial healing and may predispose to the development of bronchopleural fistula. All attempts should be made to obtain negative margins but not at the expense of extending resection too close to tracheal bifurcation.
- Preoperative infections including obstructive pneumonia should be adequately treated before resection to minimize potential intraoperative contamination of the pleural space.
- Controversy exists regarding the ideal method of bronchial stump closure (hand-sewn versus stapled).
- Important technical considerations include a tension-free closure, avoidance of extensive devascularization, and good mucosal approximation.

- Adequate control of diabetes mellitus, minimizing steroid use (if possible), and optimizing nutritional status reduces the incidence of postresectional bronchopleural fistula.
- Mechanical ventilation places additional stress on the bronchial stump after resection and should be avoided, if possible, in the postoperative period. In cases in which mechanical ventilation is mandatory, minimizing airway pressure, PEEP, and tidal volumes is essential.
- Patients with preoperative risk factors (induction therapy, comorbidities) should have the bronchial stump reinforced with pedicled flaps of muscle, omentum, pericardium, or pleura (see later for details).[43,44]
- Postresectional bronchopleural fistulas are associated with mortalities of 20% to 50%.[45,46]
- Death usually occurs in the postoperative period secondary to respiratory failure, recurrence of cancer, or hemorrhage.

## PRESENTATION AND DIAGNOSIS

- Bronchopleural fistulas can present early in the postoperative period (1–2 days) or several months after pulmonary resection.
- Clinical manifestations include
  - Fever
  - Cough productive of purulent or serosanguinous sputum, especially when the patient is in the lateral decubitus position with the operated side up
  - Purulent chest tube drainage
  - Persistent large air leak
  - Sudden increase in the size of an air leak
  - Presence of an empyema
  - Respiratory insufficiency
  - Subcutaneous emphysema
  - Radiographic appearance of increasing air-fluid level or increasing residual intrapleural space
  - Development of tension pneumothorax
- Early fistulas are usually associated with dehiscence of the bronchial stump after pneumonectomy or lobectomy.
- Late-occurring fistulas are usually associated with rupture on an empyema through the bronchial stump or by failure of healing of the stump.
- Diagnosis can be confirmed with bronchoscopy, which should include careful inspection of the bronchial stump as well as obtaining cultures and assessing the contralateral bronchus.
- Chest CT is also indicated to identify and characterize the empyema cavity and assess the severity of coexisting lung disease.

## PRINCIPLES OF MANAGEMENT

- When a bronchopleural fistula is suspected, the immediate action should be to make sure that the patient does not lie in a position with the fistula up because that could lead to pus going from that side of the chest into the bronchus and then to contaminate the opposite lung.
- Pulmonary flooding can be controlled with positioning the patient with the affected side down and airway control using a dual lumen endotracheal tube, if necessary.
- The initial management strategy also focuses on adequate drainage of all air-filled and fluid-filled spaces.
- This can be accomplished with bedside placement of chest tubes or CT-directed placement of chest catheters.
- All fluid should be cultured and appropriate antibiotic therapy instituted and tailored to culture results.

- Control of sepsis with adequate drainage and antibiotic therapy.
- Optimization of nutritional status
- Thorough assessment of clinical condition and pulmonary reserve
- Thorough assessment to rule out recurrent malignancy
- Small occult fistulas can be managed conservatively if the patient's clinical condition is stable (asymptomatic or minimally symptomatic) and the pleural space is well drained.[41,47]
- Almost all large fistulas require surgical management.
- Early fistulas (up to 7–14 days) usually require prompt return to the operating room for reclosure of the bronchial stump with reinforcement by pedicled flaps.
- Fistulas occurring later in the postoperative course can usually be surgically managed after the clinical condition improves and sepsis is controlled (weeks to months later).

## Endoscopic Management

- Small fistulas in stable patients can be treated endoscopically after drainage of the pleural space has been achieved, sepsis is controlled, and optimization of comorbidities has been accomplished.
- Endoscopic application of sealants can be directly applied through the bronchoscope after the bronchopleural fistula has been confirmed.[48]
- Peripheral fistulas tend to be more amenable to this technique compared with more centrally located fistulas (postpneumonectomy).
- Use of sealants including fibrin glue, cyanoacrylate glue, albumin-glutaraldehyde tissue adhesive, and gel foam have been described.[48]
- Randomized controlled trials demonstrating the efficacy of this technique are lacking, and most reports are anecdotal.
- Success is variable but may be a viable option for patients unable to tolerate thoracotomy.
- Does not prohibit future surgical attempts if unsuccessful.

## Surgical Management

- Principles of management include drainage and débridement of infected pleural space, reclosure of bronchial stump reinforced with pedicled flaps, and obliteration of residual pleural space.
- This can be accomplished in a one- or two-stage procedure. A one-stage procedure is indicated when the bronchopleural fistula occurs within the first few days after the operation. If the fistula occurs later, or if an empyema is present, then a two-stage approach is used.
- A variety of pedicled flaps have been used (Table 49-5).

### TABLE 49-5 ■ OPTIONS FOR PEDICLED FLAPS

Extrathoracic skeletal muscle
   Serratus anterior
   Latissimus dorsi
   Pectoralis major
   Intercostal
   Rectus abdominus
Pericardium
Pericardiophrenic fat pad
Diaphragm
Omentum
Thymus

- Transsternal transpericardial closure is a good approach when the bronchial stump is long enough. A median sternotomy avoids the contaminated pleural cavity and avoids trying to dissect through dense adhesions in the mediastinum.

## Techniques
### Single-Stage Procedure
- Reopening original thoracotomy incision
- Wide débridement of empyema cavity
- Identification of fistula and closure if technically feasible
- Omental or pedicled muscle flap used to reinforce closure of stump
- Residual space obliterated with pedicled muscle flaps

### Two-Stage Procedure (Modified Clagett Technique)
#### FIRST STAGE
- Reopening original thoracotomy incision and leaving it open (Fig. 49-8)[47,49]
- Identification and closure of fistula
- Transposition of a pedicled extrathoracic skeletal muscle flap to reinforce closure
- Thorough débridement of pleural cavity
- Thoracotomy wound is packed with moist dressings

#### SECOND STAGE
- When the pleural space is clean, the cavity is completely filled with an antibiotic solution (0.5 g neomycin, 0.1 g polymyxin B sulfate, 80 mg gentamicin per liter of saline).
- Chest wall is closed in multiple layers.

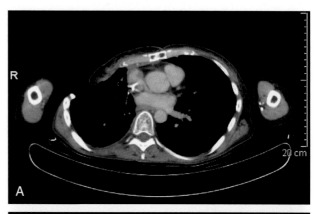

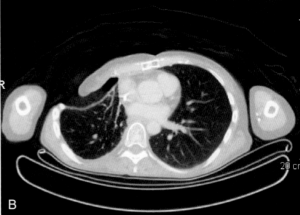

**Figure 49-8:** Computed tomography scans of the chest showing features of an Eloeser flap procedure.

## *SUMMARY*

- Bronchopleural fistula is a dreaded complication of pulmonary resection.
- Higher incidence with pneumonectomy (right > left) compared with lobectomy or wedge resection.
- Prevention is best accomplished with adequate preoperative control of comorbidities (infection, diabetes), meticulous surgical technique, and using pedicled flaps to reinforce bronchial stump in patients at higher risk for postresectional bronchopleural fistula.
- Usually requires surgical intervention except in those cases of occult or small fistulas.
- Mortality, although improving, remains high.

### Brief Illustrative Case

- A 31-year-old man.
- Presented with acute shortness of breath and right chest pain following exercise.
- Multiple prior episodes of similar right chest pain, which resolved spontaneously and did not reach medical attention.
- History of asthma, but currently asymptomatic requiring only rare use of rescue bronchodilators.
- Family history of spontaneous pneumothorax: both father and brother.
- On arrival to the Emergency Department, the patient exhibited tachycardia and tachypnea. SpO$_2$ was 84% on room air. The patient was hemodynamically stable. Examination of the chest revealed significantly diminished intensity of breath sounds on the right. He had a tall thin lanky appearance.

- A chest x-ray study revealed a 60% right-sided pneumothorax (Fig. 49-9A)
- A small-caliber (20 French) chest tube was inserted with relief of symptoms, re-expansion of the lung, and minimal air leak that rapidly resolved.
- A follow up CT of the chest revealed bilateral apical blebs (see Fig. 49-9B).
- The patient underwent VATS resection of right-sided apical blebs and mechanical pleurodesis with no recurrence after more than 1 year of follow-up.

### Key Points

- The family history of primary spontaneous pneumothorax is intriguing. No clear clinical features of Marfan's syndrome (despite lanky appearance) or Ehlers-Danlos syndrome were evident.
- Pneumothorax following exercise is well described, albeit unusual.
- The repeated history of chest pain on the right was interpreted as compatible recurrent primary spontaneous pneumothoraces (strong inference).
- The decision to proceed to surgery was based on the above-mentioned inferences and the serious current clinical presentation. The likelihood of significant relapse was high.
- A standard approach was employed, that is, bleb resection and mechanical pleurodesis via VATS.
- An excellent American College of Chest Physicians Consensus Statement on Primary Spontaneous Pneumothorax is available.[11]

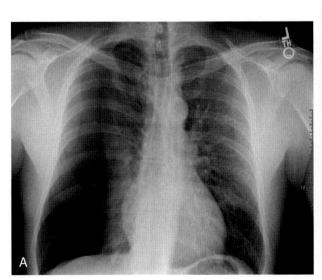
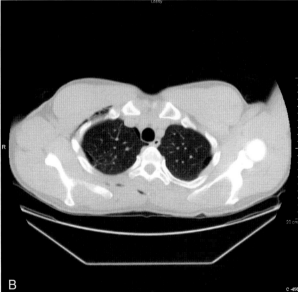

**Figure 49-9:** **A,** Chest x-ray study showing a 60% right-sided pneumothorax. **B,** Computed tomography of the chest showing bilateral apical blebs.

## References

Interactive references and additional readings for this chapter can be accessed online at *expertconsult.com*.

# DISEASES OF THE CHEST WALL AND DIAPHRAGM

## 50 CHEST WALL

Francis C. Nichols, MD

## *CHEST WALL TUMORS*

### Introduction

- Tumors of the chest wall include a wide variety of bone and soft tissue diseases (Tables 50-1 and 50-2):
  - Primary benign and malignant neoplasms of the bony skeleton and soft tissue
  - Neoplasms that invade the chest wall from adjacent structures such as the lung, pleura, mediastinum, and breast
  - Postradiation-induced chest wall neoplasms, which are frequently necrotic
  - Non-neoplastic benign disorders
- Thoracic surgeons are frequently asked to evaluate and manage patients with chest wall neoplasms for
  - Establishment of diagnosis
  - Treatment for cure
  - Management of necrotic, foul-smelling ulcerated tumors
- From a practical standpoint, wide surgical resection is the preferred treatment for the majority of chest wall tumors.[1-4] The following items are important to successful surgical resection:
  - Establishment of a correct diagnosis
  - Ability to reconstruct large chest wall defects

### Incidence

- Primary chest wall tumors including both bony and soft tissue neoplasms comprise approximately 5% of all thoracic tumors and 1% to 2% of all primary tumors found in the body.[5] The incidence of malignancy in primary chest wall tumors varies ranging from 50% to 80%. The malignancy rate is higher for soft tissue neoplasms compared with bony or cartilaginous tumors.
  - In a Mayo Clinic series of 100 consecutive patients having chest wall resection for tumor Pairolero and Arnold[3] found
    - Local invasion from adjacent tumors in 24%
    - Metastatic lesions in 32%
    - Primary chest wall tumors in 44%
  - In a 20-year experience involving 317 patients with resected chest wall tumors, Martini and colleagues[6] from Memorial Sloan-Kettering Cancer Center found:

- Primary lung cancer in 127 patients (40%)
- Metastatic carcinoma (breast, kidney, colon, other) or sarcoma in 107 patients (34%)
- Primary chest wall sarcoma in 83 patients (26%)
- The most common primary malignant chest wall tumors the thoracic surgeon is asked to manage are chondrosarcoma, Ewing's sarcoma, liposarcoma, malignant fibrous histiocytoma, osteosarcoma, and rhabdomyosarcoma.
- The most common benign chest wall tumors the thoracic surgeon is asked to manage are chondroma, desmoids, fibrous dysplasia, and osteochondroma.
  - Desmoids are controversial tumors that are considered to be benign by some because of their microscopic features and the fact that they do not distantly metastasize.[7,8] However, others consider desmoids low-grade fibrosarcomas because of their locoregional extension and propensity for recurrence.[9]
- Any portion of the thoracic skeleton (clavicles, ribs, sternum, and scapula) may be involved with primary or metastatic chest wall tumors.
  - The most common site of involvement is the ribs.
  - In a review of 11,087 Mayo Clinic cases, Unni and coworkers[10] found primary neoplasms of the sternum, clavicle, and scapula were rare, but when present, the overwhelming majority were malignant.

### Clinical Presentation

- In general, patients with benign chest wall tumors are 14 years younger (average age 26 years) when compared with patients with malignant tumors (average age 40 years).[11]
- The male-to-female ratio for chest wall tumors is approximately 2:1, except for desmoids, which in some series have a 1:2 female-to-male ratio.[11]
- Chest wall tumors commonly present as asymptomatic, slowly enlarging masses.
  - Some are incidental findings on chest imaging obtained for unrelated reasons.
  - Presenting symptoms are chest wall masses (70%) and pain (25-50%).[12,13]
    - As they grow, nearly all malignant chest wall tumors become painful compared with only two thirds of benign tumors.

## TABLE 50-1 ■ CLASSIFICATION OF CHEST WALL TUMORS

Primary chest wall neoplasms
  Malignant
  Benign
Metastatic chest wall neoplasms
  Carcinoma
  Sarcoma
Adjacent neoplasms with local chest wall invasion
  Breast
  Pleura
  Lung
Benign non-neoplastic disorders
  Cyst
  Inflammation

*Adapted from Pairolero PC: Tumors of the chest wall. In Niederhuber JE, editor: Current Therapy in Oncology. New York: Mosby, 1993. p. 218-221.*

## TABLE 50-2 ■ PRIMARY CHEST WALL TUMORS

**Malignant**
Bone and Cartilage
  Askin's tumor
  Chondrosarcoma
  Ewing's sarcoma
  Lymphoma
  Myeloma
  Osteogenic sarcoma
Soft Tissue
  Hemangiosarcoma
  Leiomyosarcoma
  Liposarcoma
  Lymphangiosarcoma
  Malignant fibrous histiocytoma
  Neurofibrosarcoma
  Rhabdomyosarcoma

**Benign**
Bone and Cartilage
  Aneurysmal bone cyst
  Chondroma
  Chondroblastoma
  Eosinophilic granuloma
  Fibrous dysplasia
  Giant cell tumor
  Osteoblastoma
  Osteochondroma
Soft Tissue
  Desmoid
  Fibroma
  Hemangioma
  Lipoma
  Lymphangioma
  Neurilemoma

- The pain is initially generalized, and many patients have a history of treatment for musculoskeletal complaints or neuritis.
  - Fatigue, fever, weight loss, lymphadenopathy, brachial plexus neuropathy, leukocytosis, and eosinophilia may be present.

## Diagnosis

- Successful treatment requires early diagnosis and, in many cases, surgical resection with appropriate reconstruction.
- The diagnostic evaluation should include
  - Careful history and physical examination with particular attention to personal histories of malignancy, ionizing radiation, and trauma (Figs. 50-1A and B)
  - Laboratory tests include liver function tests and alkaline phosphatase levels.
  - Conventional x-ray studies of the involved area may be useful, and if possible, comparison with prior studies may help in assessing the rate of growth (Figs. 50-2 and 50-3).
  - Computed tomographic (CT) scans help in the delineation of soft tissue, bony, pleural, mediastinal, and pulmonary involvement. CT is superior to magnetic resonance imaging (MRI) in the assessment of calcification (Fig. 50-4) and possible pulmonary metastases. Although MRI is not routinely obtained, it can be used selectively and is helpful in delineating blood vessels, nerves, and spinal cord involvement.
  - Although CT and MRI are capable aiding in the differentiation of chest wall neoplasms, their sensitivity and specificity are not accurate enough to eliminate the need for tissue diagnosis.
  - Whether or not to biopsy a chest wall tumor depends upon the clinical presentation and suspected histo-pathology.
    - Biopsy techniques include
      - Fine-needle aspiration (FNA), which often yields a cytology specimen not sufficient for the diagnosis of primary chest wall neoplasms.
      - Core needle biopsy, which yields a specimen that maintains the neoplasm's architecture and in recent years has demonstrated an accuracy of 92% to 96%[14,15]
      - Excisional biopsy, which if performed, should include a minimum 1-cm margin. Excisional biopsy may be appropriate for small 1- to 5-cm neoplasms. The location of the excisional biopsy must not interfere with possible future wide surgical resection. Chest wall closure for these small neoplasms is usually straightforward and does not require skeletal reconstruction. For benign neoplasms, no further treatment is needed. For malignant neoplasms, the treatment may be chemotherapy, radiation therapy, wide surgical resection, or a combination of all three.[16-18]
      - Incisional biopsies should be approached cautiously because of the concern over local tumor spread and the possibility of underdiagnosis.[11,17-19] Incisional biopsies may be appropriate when a needle biopsy is nondiagnostic, when metastatic disease from a known distant primary is suspected, or for larger (>5 cm) primary neoplasms. Incisional biopsies must be via small, carefully oriented incisions placed so that definitive wide resection if eventually required is not compromised. Skin flaps should not be raised, the pleura not broached, and the capsule of the mass closed following biopsy.
- If the chest wall mass is suspected of being infectious, then FNA may be helpful in establishing a diagnosis.
- Chest wall tumors suspected of being metastatic from a known primary elsewhere can be accurately diagnosed by FNA, core needle, or incisional or excisional biopsy techniques.
  - In our practice, core needle and incisional biopsies are not routinely performed for suspected primary benign or malignant chest wall neoplasms.

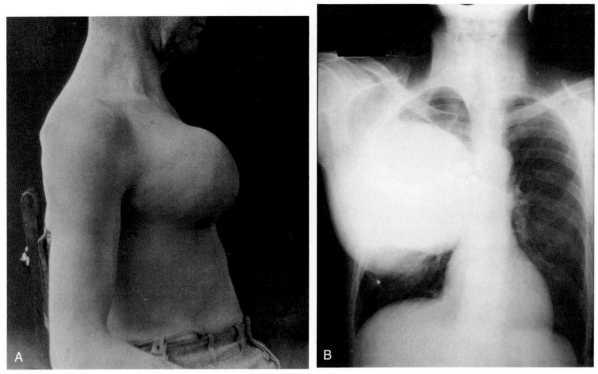

**Figure 50-1: A,** A 56-year-old gentleman with a giant chondrosarcoma arising from the right anterior upper costochondral arch. He had a distant history of significant right chest wall trauma. **B,** Chest x-ray study.

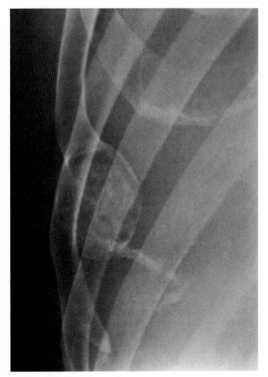

**Figure 50-2:** Fifty-three year old gentleman with chondrosarcoma of the right anterior sixth rib. The mass had been present for 18 months without pain. *(Reproduced from McAfee MK, Pairolero PC, Bergstralh EJ, Piehler JM, Unni KK, McLeod RA, et al. Chondrosarcoma of the chest wall: factors affecting survival. Ann Thorac Surg 1985;40:535-540, with permission.)*

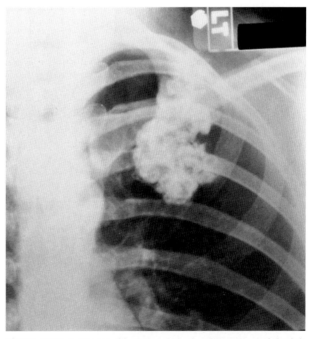

**Figure 50-3:** A 32-year-old woman with chondrosarcoma of the left anterior first rib. The mass had been present with pain for 2 months. *(Reproduced from McAfee MK, Pairolero PC, Bergstralh EJ, Piehler JM, Unni KK, McLeod RA, et al. Chondrosarcoma of the chest wall: factors affecting survival. Ann Thorac Surg 1985;40:535-540, with permission.)*

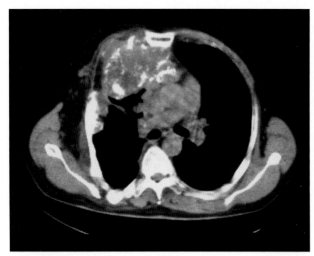

**Figure 50-4:** Computerized tomography of a 52-year-old gentleman with a right anterior chest wall chondrosarcoma. Of note is the destruction of the bony cortex and calcific stippling throughout the neoplasm.

- Needle and incisional biopsies may underdiagnose certain low-grade malignancies such as chondrosarcoma, misleading the surgeon not to perform wide resection, which, in turn, compromises the patient's opportunity for cure.
  - The author, Pairolero, and Unni believe that chest wall neoplasms suspected of being metastatic from a known primary elsewhere can be accurately diagnosed with FNA, core needle, or incisional biopsies (Peter C. Pairolero, MD, and K. Krishnan Unni, MD, personal communication, 2008).
  - The author and Pairolero believe that either benign or malignant primary neoplasms are preferably diagnosed with an excisional biopsy, which includes a minimum 1 cm margin (Peter C. Pairolero, MD, personal communication, 2008).[16,17] The location of the excisional biopsy should not interfere with subsequent treatment. Excisional biopsy results in
    - Excision of the entire mass, thus providing adequate tissue to firmly establish the tumor's histopathology
      - At Mayo Clinic Rochester, frozen section gives us an immediate, accurate and definitive diagnosis in greater than 90% of bone tumors (K. Krishnan Unni, MD, personal communication, 2008).[10]
      - Histopathologically proven benign neoplasms need no further treatment.
      - If the neoplasm is best treated by chemotherapy, radiation, or both, then no additional surgical resection is required.
      - If frozen section diagnosis cannot be established at the time of excisional biopsy then the chest wound should be closed. If malignancy is eventually diagnosed that is best treated by wide resection, then subsequent wide resection including en bloc resection of the entire biopsy site (skin, subcutaneous tissue, and muscle) is performed (Peter C. Pairolero, MD, personal communication, 2008).[16,17]
  - At the University of Texas M.D. Anderson Cancer Center, core needle biopsies are attempted in all patients, and there have been no incisional biopsies required for the diagnosis of chest wall neoplasms since the late 1980s.[19]

## Pathology
### Benign Bone/Cartilage Tumors

- Osteochondroma
  - Most common benign bone neoplasm, representing almost 50% of all benign rib tumors[10]
  - Begins in childhood and grows until skeletal maturity is reached. Affects men 3 times more frequently than women
  - Most patients are asymptomatic; however, pain may indicate malignant degeneration.
  - Arises from the bony cortex in the metaphyseal portion of the rib and looks like bony protuberance on a stalk with a cartilaginous rim
  - Radiographically stippled calcifications may be seen within the tumor as well as a calcified rim.
  - Treatment of choice is resection.
  - Complete surgical resection is recommended in children after puberty and in adults. In children before puberty, osteochondromas should be resected for pain or increasing size.
- Chondroma
  - Fifteen percent of all benign rib neoplasms
  - Can occur at any age, with both sexes equally affected
  - Presents as an asymptomatic, occasionally slightly painful anterior costochondral junction mass
  - Radiographically seen as an expansile mass with thinning of the cortex
  - Grossly it is a lobulated mass, and microscopically lobules of hyaline cartilage are seen.
  - Cannot clinically or radiographically differentiate a chondroma from a low-grade chondrosarcoma. Microscopic differentiation may also be very difficult
  - All chondromas must be considered malignant and thus managed with wide excision of 2 to 4 cm.
- Fibrous dysplasia
  - A cystic, non-neoplastic lesion probably representing a developmental bony abnormality characterized by fibrous replacement of the medullary cavity of the rib.
  - Usually presents as a slowly enlarging, solitary, nonpainful mass in the posterolateral rib cage.
  - Both sexes are equally affected.
  - Radiographically it has a characteristic appearance consisting of an expansile lesion with thinning of the bony cortex and a central ground-glass appearance. Microscopically, bony trabeculations, fibrous tissue, and occasional calcification are seen.
  - Although treatment can be conservative, resection is often undertaken for painful, enlarging lesions, and to rule out malignancy. Resection is curative.
- Eosinophilic granuloma
  - A disease of the lymphoreticular system and not a true neoplasm
  - May be solitary or multifocal and is the unifying feature of the conditions designated as histiocytosis X (eosinophilic granulomas, Letterer-Siwe disease, and Hans-Schüller-Christian disease).
  - Occurs in young to middle-aged adults, with peak incidence of 5 to 15 years
  - Most commonly found in the skull, but rib involvement is seen in 10% to 20% of afflicted patients.
  - Presentation is often pain limited to the involved bone or bones, but patients with Letterer-Siwe and Hans-Schüller-Christian disease may have systemic findings including fever, malaise, weight loss, lymphadenopathy, and splenomegaly, anemia, eosinophilia, and leukocytosis.
  - Radiographically an expansile rib lesion is seen with periosteal new bone formation. Uneven destruction of the bony cortex results in endosteal scalloping.

○ Microscopically there are eosinophils, giant cells, Langerhans cells, and neutrophils.

○ In patients with eosinophilic granuloma alone, excision is diagnostic and curative if the lesion is solitary. For patients with multiple eosinophilic granulomas, the treatment is low-dose radiation therapy (300 to 600 cGY). For Letterer-Siwe and Hans-Schüller-Christian disease, systemic treatments including chemotherapy and corticosteroids are used.

### Benign Soft Tissue Tumors

▪ A variety of benign neoplasms of the chest wall have been reported. These include fibromas, hemangiomas, lipomas, lymphangiomas, and neurogenic tumors. Malignant degeneration is rare, and all can be treated by local excision.

▪ Desmoid

○ Desmoid tumors are rare soft tissue tumors whose etiology is not completely understood and have a propensity for local recurrence.[20]

○ Forty percent occur in the shoulder and chest wall regions.[17]

○ Thirty-three percent of patients with Gardner's syndrome have desmoid tumors, and 2% of patients with desmoids have Gardner's syndrome.[21]

○ Most commonly occur between adolescence and 40 years of age, and are only rarely seen in infants and the elderly.

○ Reported to be associated with a history of trauma and estrogen-induced growth.

○ Initial presentation is a poorly circumscribed mass with little or no pain. With growth of the tumor, pain may occur. Desmoids located in the shoulder region cause entrapment of the brachial plexus, resulting in paresthesias, hyperesthesia, and motor weakness. This also limits the margin of resection and increases the risk of local recurrence.

○ They originate in muscle and fascia extending along tissue planes often with finger-like projections into the surrounding tissues (Fig. 50-5).

○ Microscopically, there is a uniform bland spreading pattern of fibroblasts without mitoses or necrosis but infiltration of the surrounding tissues occurs. Some pathologists consider these benign fibromatosis and others low-grade fibrosarcoma.[7-9]

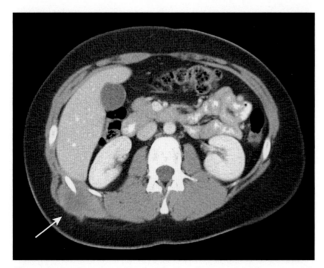

**Figure 50-5:** Computerized tomography of a 19-year-old woman with a right posterolateral lower chest wall desmoid (*arrow*).

○ Treatment is wide surgical resection.

▪ We reported on 53 patients who underwent resection of chest wall desmoid tumors.[20] Five-year overall probability of developing a recurrence was 37.5%. Recurrence occurred in eight of nine patients (89%), with positive resection margins and eight of 44 (18%) with negative margins. Factors adversely affecting the rate of postoperative recurrence were the need for reoperation, positive resection margins, proximity to the brachial plexus, and postoperative radiotherapy. Importantly, patients who had postoperative radiotherapy were more likely to have undergone an incomplete resection. None of our patients who had negative surgical margins and subsequently had postoperative radiotherapy had recurrent tumor, which is in contrast to almost 33% of patients who did not have radiotherapy and had recurrence. Importantly, however, whether postoperative radiation therapy is beneficial in all patients who have complete resection of their desmoid cannot be determined from our nonrandomized data.[20] Others have demonstrated radiotherapy to be of benefit in patients with gross residual disease or recurrence.[22,23]

○ Tamoxifen has been reported to decrease both the size and symptoms of desmoid tumors and may be of benefit in patients not capable of having surgical resection.[24]

### Malignant Bone/Cartilage Tumors

▪ Chondrosarcoma

○ Accounts for 30% of all primary chest wall bony neoplasm and occurs most frequently in the anterior chest wall, with 75% arising in the costochondral arches or sternum.[17]

○ More common in men

○ Most common in middle age

▪ In the Mayo Clinic series by McAfee and colleagues,[25] the median age was 54 years, and ranged from 17 to 78 years.

○ Cause is unknown.

▪ Malignant degeneration of benign cartilaginous tumors has been reported.

▪ Association with severe crushing ipsilateral chest wall trauma was found in 12.5% of patients in McAfee's series.[25]

○ Presentation commonly is a slowly enlarging, painful mass.

○ Radiographically there is a lobulated mass arising in the medullary portion of the rib or sternum with cortical destruction. A stippled calcification pattern is most common (see Fig. 50-4).

○ Because the majority of chondrosarcomas are well differentiated, differentiation from chondroma is difficult, and misdiagnosis of chondroma is common. A definitive diagnosis can only be made pathologically, and it is for this reason that excisional biopsy is recommended.

○ Pairolero[17] states that from a practical standpoint, all tumors arising within costal cartilage should be considered malignant and, thus, treated by wide resection.

○ Natural history is one of slow growth, local recurrence, and if untreated, late metastases.

○ Treatment is complete wide resection because these tumors are not sensitive to chemotherapy or radiation.[12,25,26]

▪ Surgical resection margins should be 4 cm in all directions

▪ Wide resection results in cure in nearly all patients. The 10-year survival rate for patients with chondrosarcoma treated by wide resection was 96%, local excision 65%, and palliative excision 14% ($P < 0.0001$) (Fig. 50-6).

▪ Although in McAfee's series[25] tumor diameter, grade, location, and date of surgical resection all effected

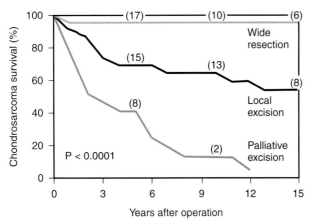

**Figure 50-6:** Survival of 72 patients with chondrosarcoma classified by the extent of resection. Zero time on the abscissa represents the day of resection. The numbers in parentheses are the number of patients alive at 5, 10, and 15 years. *(Reproduced from McAfee MK, Pairolero PC, Bergstralh EJ, Piehler JM, Unni KK, McLeod RA, et al: Chondrosarcoma of the chest wall: factors affecting survival. Ann Thorac Surg 1985;40:535-540, with permission.)*

survival, a more recent review from our institution showed that the only prognostic factor was the surgical margin.[26]

■ Osteosarcoma
  ○ Osteosarcoma is the most frequent bone tumor; however, chest wall osteosarcomas are less common than chondrosarcomas, constituting 6% of all primary malignant chest wall bone neoplasms.[27]
  ○ They are a more malignant tumor with a worse prognosis than chondrosarcoma.
  ○ Occur most commonly between ages of 10 and 25 years and after age 40.[11]
  ○ There is an association between osteosarcomas and prior radiation therapy, Paget's disease, and chemotherapy. Souba and colleagues found that the mean latency period from radiation therapy was 13 years and the prognosis for radiation-induced sarcomas of the chest wall is very poor.[28,29]
  ○ Frequently presents as a rapidly enlarging painful mass.
  ○ Serum alkaline phosphatase levels and lactate dehydrogenase levels may be elevated and correlate with decreased survival.[30]
  ○ Radiographically osteosarcomas can be large, lobulated, and extend through cortical bone into adjacent soft tissues (Fig. 50-7). Calcifications may occur producing a sunburst appearance.
  ○ Treatment is neoadjuvant chemotherapy in order to shrink the tumor before resection.
    ■ The combination chemotherapy of cisplatin, doxorubicin, and high-dose methotrexate is most common.
    ■ Surgical resection consists of wide resection of the tumor, including the entire involved bone (rib or sternum) and adjacent soft tissues.
    ■ Radiation therapy has not been of benefit.
    ■ With the addition of multidrug neoadjuvant chemotherapy, 5-year disease-free survival rates have improved from 20% with surgery alone to greater than 50%.[11]
■ Ewing's sarcoma
  ○ Account for 12% of all primary chest wall bony neoplasms.
  ○ Sixty-six percent of all Ewing's sarcomas occur in persons younger than 20 years of age; however, it is rare in infants.[10]
  ○ Presentation commonly is a progressively painful enlarging mass. Fever, malaise, anemia, leukocytosis, and an elevated erythrocyte sedimentation rate may be present.

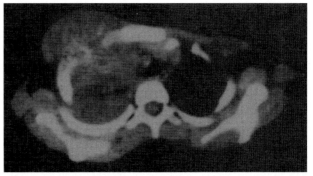

**Figure 50-7:** Computerized tomography of an osteosarcoma of the right third rib with bone destruction. *(Reproduced from Graeber GM, Jones DR, Pairolero PC: Chest wall and sternum: primary neoplasms. In Pearson FG, Cooper JD, Deslauriers J, Ginsberg RJ, Hiebert CA, Patterson GA, Urschel HC Jr, editors. Thoracic Surgery. 2nd ed. Philadelphia: Churchill Livingstone; 2002. p. 1417-1430, with permission.)*

  ○ Radiographically, an onion-skin appearance of the bone caused by elevation of the periosteum and multiple layers of new subperiosteal bone formation may be seen, but this is not pathognomonic. These features can be seen in osteosarcoma, osteomyelitis, and other bone tumors.
  ○ Usually, Ewing's sarcoma is confined to one rib; however, involvement of multiple ribs does occur (Fig. 50-8).
  ○ In the series by Burt and colleagues,[31] 23% of patients had synchronous metastases at initial presentation. Of the patients who presented with only local disease, 71% developed distant metastases.
  ○ Treatment is systemic chemotherapy, followed by resection or radiation therapy to the primary site.
    ■ Doxorubicin, dactinomycin, cyclophosphamide, and vincristine in combination are the most frequently used chemotherapeutic agents.
    ■ Using combined-modality therapy, 5-year event-free survival rates of 62% to 68% have been reported.[32,33]
    ■ In patients with distant metastatic disease, survival is extremely poor.

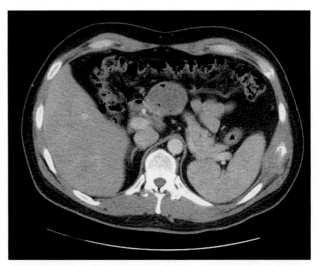

**Figure 50-8:** Computerized tomography of a 28-year-old gentleman with a left posterolateral chest wall Ewing's sarcoma. Of note is the destruction of the left ninth rib and the surrounding soft tissue mass.

### Malignant Soft Tissue Tumors

- Malignant fibrous histiocytoma
  - Most common primary chest wall neoplasm the thoracic surgeon is asked to evaluate.[3,12]
  - Usually occurs between the ages of 50 and 70 years, and is rare in childhood.
  - Sixty-six occur in men.
  - Presentation most commonly is a painless slowly enlarging mass.
  - Grossly, it tends to be a lobulated mass, which spreads along fascial planes or between muscle fibers.
  - Treatment is wide resection.
    - It is unresponsive to chemotherapy and radiation therapy
    - Five-year survival is approximately 38% (Fig. 50-9).
- Rhabdomyosarcoma
  - Second most common soft tissue chest wall neoplasm, seen most frequently in children and young adults.
  - Presentation is a rapidly enlarging mass intimately associated with striated muscle fibers. Despite rapid growth, rhabdomyosarcomas are usually not painful.
  - Treatment is wide resection, followed by radiation therapy and multidrug chemotherapy.
    - Five-year survival is 70% (Fig. 50-9).

## Metastatic Chest Wall Tumors

- Approximately 33% of all chest wall neoplasms are due to metastatic disease.[3,6]
- Because this represents disseminated disease, the majority of patients cannot be cured by surgical resection.
- However, surgical resection can be considered in carefully selected patients.
  - Curative resection can be considered in patients in whom
    - There is local-regional control of the primary site
    - The chest wall is the sole site of metastatic disease
    - Complete resection with negative resection margins is possible
    - The patient can tolerate the surgical procedure
  - Palliative resection can be considered in carefully selected patients to control pain, ulceration, and infection resulting from the metastatic tumor.

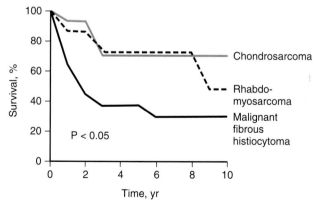

**Figure 50-9:** Survival (death from any cause) for patients with chondrosarcoma, malignant fibrous histiocytoma, and rhabdomyosarcoma. Zero time on the abscissa represents the day of chest wall resection. (*Reproduced from King RM, Pairolero PC, Trastek VF, Piehler JM, Payne WS, Bernatz PE. Primary chest wall tumors: factors affecting survival. Ann Thorac Surg 1986;41:597-601, with permission.*)

- With a median follow-up of 31.5 months, Pairolero and Arnold[3] reported that 41% of patients were alive. Similarly, Martini and colleagues[6] found the 5-year survival for chest wall metastasectomy excluding lung and breast cancers to be 20%.

## Chest Wall Tumor Summary

- Early diagnosis and, when appropriate, aggressive surgical resection and reconstruction are critical to successful treatment of primary chest wall tumors.
- For certain tumors (e.g., osteosarcoma and Ewing's sarcoma), combined-modality therapy including neoadjuvant and adjuvant chemotherapy, radiation therapy, and wide surgical resection may be appropriate.
- With current surgical and reconstructive techniques, wide resection of these tumors can be accomplished with low morbidity and mortality.[1-4,17]

## CHEST WALL AND STERNAL INFECTIONS

### Introduction

- Chest wall infections may be classified as primary, that is spontaneously arising, or secondary (e.g., postoperative, postradiotherapy) infections.
  - In the United States and other industrialized nations, the majority of chest wall infections are secondary.
  - Regardless of whether the tumor is primary or secondary, treatment similarities exist, ranging from careful observation to radical débridement with complex reconstruction.
- Sternotomy wound infection following cardiac surgery is the most common, with a reported incidence of 0.25% to 6.4%.[34]
- Other secondary infections include
  - Thoracotomy wound infection
  - Costochondritis
  - Gangrene (necrotizing soft tissue infections)
  - Osteomyelitis
    - Rib
    - Sternoclavicular joint
  - Radionecrosis of the chest wall

### Sternal Wound Infections

- In 100 consecutive patients, Pairolero and associates[35] showed that 92% of sternal wound infections were secondary to cardiac surgery and the remaining 8% secondary to other mediastinal diseases, primarily cancer.
- Incidence of sternal wound infections following coronary bypass
  - Superficial sternal wound infections range from 1.6% to 6.4%.[34]
  - Deep sternal wound infections range from 0.25% to 2.7%.[34]
- Risk factors include[34,36,37]
  - Age older than 75 years
  - Female gender
  - Body Mass Index (BMI) greater than 30 kg/m$^2$
  - Diabetes
  - New York Heart Association class greater than 3
  - Transfusion with more than 4 units of red blood cells or more than 2 units of platelets, or both
  - Use of bilateral internal mammary arteries
  - Chronic obstructive pulmonary disease
  - Immunosuppression
  - Renal failure
  - History of radiation therapy

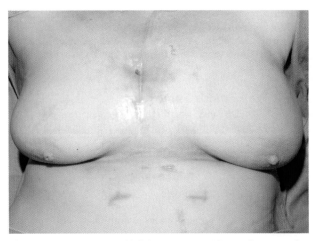

**Figure 50-10:** A 66-year-old diabetic woman with a Body Mass Index (BMI) of 37 kg/m² 3 months following five-vessel coronary artery bypass grafting using the left internal mammary artery and four vein grafts. Note the sternal wound erythema with draining sinus tract.

■ Presentation may include
  ○ Fever, chest pain, serosanguineous wound drainage, sternal instability, and leukocytosis (Fig. 50-10).
  ○ In some deep-seated, smoldering infections, these classic findings may be absent and the diagnosis more difficult.
    ■ CT scans may demonstrate sternal periosteal reaction, adjacent soft tissue inflammation, and retrosternal fluid collections.[38]
      ○ CT sensitivity is almost 100%, but specificity ranges from 33% to 100%.[39]
    ■ Radiolabeled leukocyte scans using indium 111 or technetium 99m-labeled monoclonal granulocyte antibody scintigraphy have also been used with high levels of accuracy.
■ Classification
  ○ The clinical classification of infected sternotomy wounds by Pairolero and Arnold is of great practical significance (Table 50-3).[35,40]
■ Treatment
  ○ Left untreated, these infections can extend to aortic and cardiac suture lines, prosthetic grafts, and intracardiac prostheses resulting in death.
  ○ Treatment of infected sternotomy wounds continues to generate controversy, especially with regard to the extent of débridement necessary
  ○ Following the classification of infected sternotomy wounds outlined in Table 50-3, treatments include
    ■ **Type I (minor débridement required):** Under general anesthesia, the sternotomy is reopened; subcutaneous and mediastinal spaces are inspected, débrided, and irrigated. Because the mediastinum is still soft and pliable, the residual mediastinal space is easily obliterated by mediastinal drains and the sternum can be reclosed using a parasternal weave.[41,42] Antibiotics are limited to the perioperative period unless cultures dictate otherwise. Most Type I sternal infections are appropriately handled by the operating cardiac surgeon.
    ■ **Type II (some sterna débridement required):** Similar to Type I infections, these are best inspected in the operating room. The sternotomy is reopened and the subcutaneous and mediastinal spaces explored. All necrotic tissue including soft tissue, bone, and cartilage

## TABLE 50-3 ■ CLASSIFICATION OF INFECTED STERNOTOMY WOUNDS

**Type I:** Sternal wound separation with or without sternal instability
  Occurs within days of sternotomy
  Serosanguineous drainage present
  Cellulitis, pus, chondritis, osteomyelitis absent
  Mediastinum soft and pliable
  Cultures usually negative

**Type II:** Fulminant mediastinitis
  Occurs within the first few weeks of sternotomy
  Skin cellulitis, purulent drainage, mediastinal suppuration present
  Osteomyelitis frequent
  Costochondritis rare
  Obvious communication with sternum and mediastinum
  Cultures usually positive for staphylococcal species

**Type III:** Late chronically infected sternotomy wounds
  Occurs months to years later
  Chronically draining sinus tract
  Localized skin cellulitis
  Mediastinitis rare
  Osteomyelitis, costochondritis, or retained foreign body always present
  Cultures often positive

*From Pairolero PC, Arnold PG, Harris JB. Long-term results of pectoralis major muscle transposition for infected sternotomy wounds. Ann Surg 1991; 213:583-590; and Pairolero PC, Arnold PG. Management of infected median sternotomy wounds (editorial). Ann Thorac Surg 1986;42:1-2.*

should be excised. Any exposed cartilage needs to be resected back to normal rib. All exposed foreign material including sternal wires, pledgets, and sutures are removed. The wound is usually kept open and treated intraoperatively with every day to every other day wound débridements, pulse irrigation, and antibiotic soaked gauze dressing changes. For the gauze, the authors use an antibiotic solution called débridement antibiotic solution (DABS) consisting of 20 mg gentamicin and 5000 units of polymixin B in 1000 mL of 0.9% sodium chloride solution. The wound is closed when there is no further evidence of drainage; all nonviable bone, periosteum, cartilage, and perichondrium has been resected; and the wound is clean with healthy granulation tissue. After several initial débridements, application of a vacuum-assisted wound closure (VAC) device may speed this portion of wound healing. Our preferred method of wound closure is transposition of the pectoralis major muscles with obliteration of the mediastinal space. The overlying skin and subcutaneous tissues are then reapproximated with polypropylene suture. If the pectoralis major muscles are not available, then secondary choices for transposition are the rectus abdominus muscle or omentum.
    ■ **Type III (major débridement required):** Treatment often requires wide resection of all infected bone and necrotic tissue. This often requires total sternectomy. Sinus tracts often extend down to retained infected mediastinal foreign bodies, which must be removed. All affected cartilages require resection back to healthy rib. Similar to type II sternal infections, these wounds are left open and require serial débridements. When healthy granulation tissue is present and clean, wound closure is accomplished

with pectoralis major muscle, rectus abdominus muscle, or omental transposition. If the skin and subcutaneous tissues cannot be reapproximated, skin grafting is required (Fig. 50-11).

- Results of treatment
  - Pairolero and associates[35] reported on 100 consecutive patients undergoing repair of infected sternotomy wounds.
    - Median number of operations was 4 (range, 1 to 11)
    - Wound closure was performed at a median of 14 days (range, 2 to 192 days) following initial débridement
    - Mechanical ventilation beyond postoperative day 2 was necessary in 30 patients.
    - Hospitalization ranged from 7 to 210 days (median 26.5 days).
    - Fifty-nine complications occurred in 42 patients.

- The mortality rate was 2%.
- Follow-up ranged from 1.3 to 13.5 years (median, 4.2 years)
- Recurrent infection developed in 26% and was most commonly related to incomplete removal of nonviable tissue. The majority of these wounds were ultimately successfully closed; however, interestingly the recurrence rate following both the second and third surgical attempts to heal the wounds was 28% and 25%, respectively.

## Thoracotomy Wound Infections

- Occasionally occurs following thoracotomy
- Treatment is opening the wound, culturing, débridement and packing, and antimicrobial therapy. Use of VAC may speed wound healing.

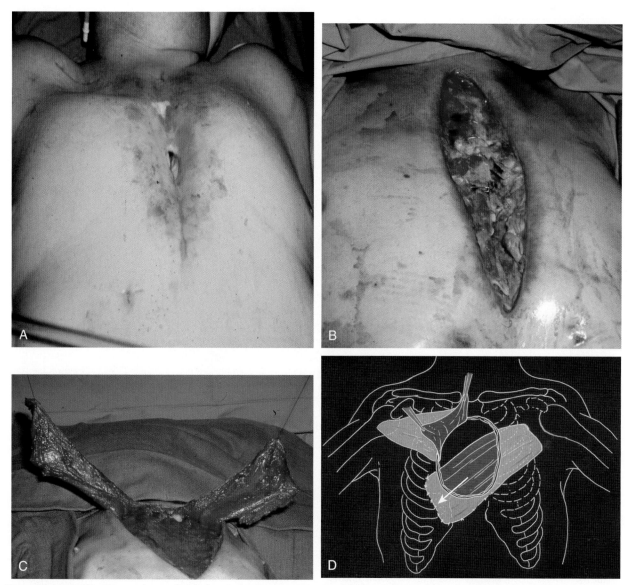

**Figure 50-11: A,** Type III sternal wound with chronic draining sinus tract. **B,** After reopening of the skin and subcutaneous tissue, there was obvious necrotic soft tissue, sternum, and cartilage. **C,** Serial operations were performed in which all necrotic tissue including soft tissue, the entire sternum and all exposed cartilages were resected with eventually good granulation tissue forming. It was then that both pectoralis major muscles were elevated including their detachment of their humeral attachments; **D,** Diagram depicting how the pectoralis major muscles are advanced over each other.

*(Continued)*

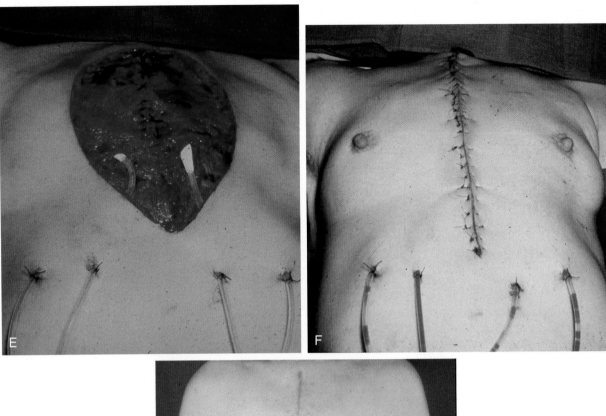

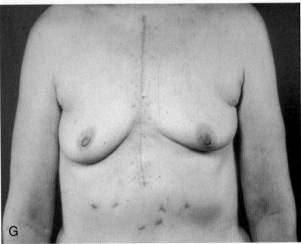

**Figure 50-11—cont'd: E,** The pectoralis major muscles have been overlapped and sutured in place obliterating the mediastinal dead space. Also, drains are placed above and below the muscle flaps. **F,** Skin flaps were elevated and closed with interrupted polypropylene suture. **G,** Wound appearance several months following closure. *(Courtesy of Peter C. Pairolero.)*

## Costochondritis

- Most commonly follows median sternotomy, thoracoabdominal incisions, or chest wall trauma
  - May appear weeks or longer even years after an uneventful procedure
- Presentation may include malaise, fever, wound erythema, swelling, purulent drainage through wound sinus tracts.
- Treatment is wide débridement of the affected areas. Necrotic cartilages need to be excised in their entirety from the sternum to the more lateral osseous rib. If the resulting surgical wound is large, soft tissue reconstruction with muscle flaps or omentum may be necessary. If all necrotic cartilage is excised, the results are good.

## Gangrene (Necrotizing Soft Tissue Infections)

- Rare, but can be highly lethal.[43]
- In the chest, the usual cause is a thoracic surgical procedure, such as chest tube placement for empyema or treatment of esophageal perforation.
  - Excessive dissection of the chest wall soft tissues while placing a chest tube or during thoracotomy for empyema may predispose to this condition.
- May result from head and neck infections or dental procedures
- Causative bacteria include *Clostridium perfringes, Bacteroides melaninogenicus,* Group A streptococcus, and Group C streptococcus, and it may also be polymicrobial.

- Clinical features are similar to necrotizing soft tissue infections in other anatomic locations
  - Skin blisters and crepitus
  - Foul smelling wound discharge
  - Excessive pain that is sometimes out of proportion to the skin findings
  - Rapid clinical deterioration
- Diagnosis is often late
- Treatment is radical débridement of all involved necrotic tissue, antibiotic therapy, ongoing serial chest wall débridement as necessary, and eventual delayed wound closure using tissue flaps that are available. In these cases, many of the first-line muscle flaps commonly used for closure may have been sacrificed during the initial débridements, and alternative flaps such as omentum may be necessary (Fig. 50-12).

## Osteomyelitis

- Rib osteomyelitis
  - Presentation is commonly localized rib pain, and there may be signs and symptoms of a localized inflammatory process. Occasionally, a draining sinus tract may be present.
  - Although not necessary for diagnosis, a CT scan may help in assessing for associated intrathoracic pathology.
  - Treatment is excision of all diseased bone, and occasionally, this requires serial extensive débridements with soft tissue reconstruction.
- Sternoclavicular joint
  - These are rare infections.
  - We identified 26 patients over a 13-year period.[44]
  - All patients had symptoms, which included pain, swelling, fever, and erythema.
  - Twelve patients had history of infection in other areas, five suffered trauma, and in one patient, an ipsilateral central line
  - CT of the chest may show swelling, bone destruction, abscess formation or a mass.
  - Wound cultures are commonly positive, with the most common organism being *Staphylococcus aureus*.
  - Treatment should be aggressive surgical management. It is our preference to resect the sternoclavicular joint and aggressively débride all surrounding soft tissues. The wound is most commonly left open and undergoes serial débridements. Once healthy granulation tissue forms, closure is accomplished with pectoralis major muscle transposition, elevation of skin flaps, and skin closure. Antibiotic therapy is directed by wound culture results.

## Radionecrosis

- The radiated wound has been recognized as a challenging problem by surgeons for more than 50 years.
  - Chest wall reconstructive problems associated with radiation therapy are some of the most awesome defects reconstructive surgeons face.[2]
  - Complications of wound healing are commonplace and solutions for reconstruction limited.
- Incidence ranges from 10% to 24% in several large chest wall resection and reconstruction series.[2,45,46]
  - Median time from last course of radiation to the first day of surgical débridement was 5.6 years (range, 2 months to 33 years).[47]
- Inadequate resection of radiation-damaged tissue is the main reason for failure.
- Arnold and Pairolero[2] stress that resection of virtually all tissue that can be closed safely with tissue transposition is critical to success.

- For tissue transposition, it is best to use nonirradiated tissue if at all possible. When irradiated muscles are transposed, total muscle necrosis is a very real possibility.[2,47]
- A 79-year-old woman afflicted with radiation necrosis of her left chest wall is shown in Figure 50-13.

## CHEST WALL RECONSTRUCTION

### Introduction

- Defects of the chest wall occur almost always as a result of neoplasm, infection, radiation, or trauma.
  - Approximately 25% of our patients requiring chest wall reconstruction have multiple combinations of these requiring significant preoperative planning and a secondary plan for closure should initial reconstructive efforts fail.
- The defect caused by chest wall resection results in the loss of the adjacent skeleton and often the overlying soft tissue.
- Partial- or full-thickness defects may occur with infection, radiation necrosis, or trauma.
- Over the past 40 years, numerous authors have made significant contributions confirming that aggressive chest wall surgical resection with dependable reconstruction is appropriate for managing the above-mentioned problems.[1-4,35,40,45-50]
- The use of musculocutaneous flaps has been considered one of the milestones in reconstructive surgery.
- It is strongly believed by the author and others that chest wall resection and reconstruction must include
  - Resection of all devitalized tissue
  - Restoration of chest wall rigidity if the defect is large enough so as to prevent flail, although Larsen reported a small series of patients whose preoperative and postoperative pulmonary function were unchanged after chest wall reconstruction with a myocutaneous flap, but without an additional prosthesis for rigidity.[51]
  - Coverage of the defect with healthy tissue to seal the pleural cavity, protect underlying organs, and prevent infection
  - These important items are most safely accomplished by the joint efforts of a thoracic surgeon and a plastic surgeon.[1,2]

### Considerations for Reconstruction

- Skeletal reconstruction
  - The ability to close large chest wall defects is the primary consideration in the surgical treatment of most chest wall disorders.
  - Chest wall reconstruction involves consideration of many factors (Table 50-4).
  - Reconstruction of the chest wall is controversial
    - Defects smaller than 5 cm in greatest diameter anywhere on the chest wall do not require reconstruction
    - Posterior defects less than 10 cm in size do not require reconstruction, provided the scapula covers the defect
    - When required, stabilization of the bony thorax can be accomplished with a variety of materials: 2-mm thick polytetrafluoroethylene soft-tissue patch (PTFE) (Gore-Tex) (W.L. Gore & Associates, Inc, Flagstaff, AZ), single knitted Marlex mesh (Davol and Bard, Cranston, RI), Dexon mesh, Vicryl mesh, double-knitted Prolene mesh (Ethicon Inc, Somerville, NJ), and methylmethacrylate.
      - Advantages of PTFE include its rigidity in all directions and its impermeability to both air and water.
      - Neither Marlex nor Prolene mesh are impermeable to air and water.
      - We have not used methylmethacrylate, and in 500 chest wall reconstructions, Arnold and Pairolero used

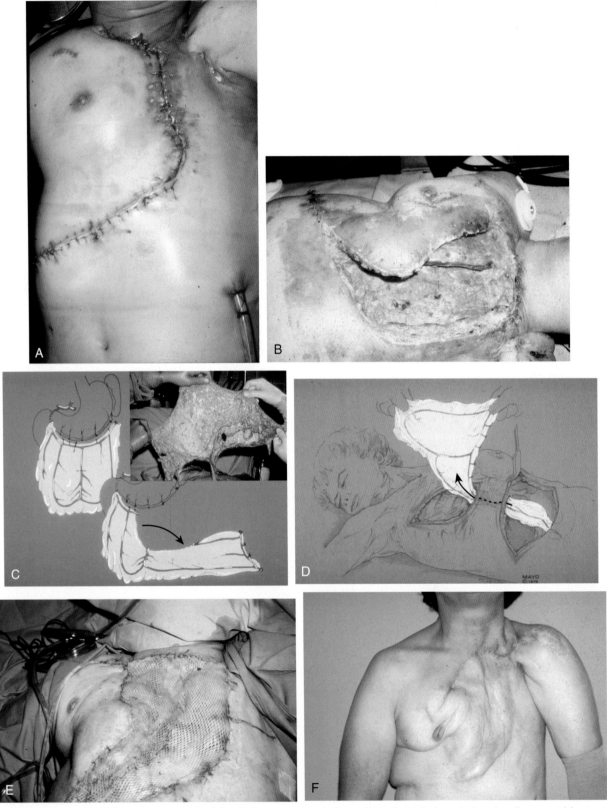

**Figure 50-12:** **A,** 62-year-old woman 20 years after left radical mastectomy and chest wall irradiation had a radiation ulcer that was widely resected with right pectoralis major transposition and primary closure, and she is now transferred to us with evidence of necrotizing soft tissue infection. **B,** Intraoperative view at the time of the full-thickness chest wall débridement. The patient underwent serial intraoperative débridements for 1 week. **C,** Diagram depicting the harvesting of the omentum based on the right gastroepiploic artery, with inset showing an intraoperative photograph of the completely mobilized omentum. **D,** Diagram depicting the transfer of the omentum through a defect created in the diaphragm; **E,** the omentum adequately covered the anterior chest wall defect, and 96 hours following omental transposition, a split-thickness skin graft was applied over the omental graft. **F,** Completely healed wound 24 months later. *(Courtesy of Peter C. Pairolero, MD.)*

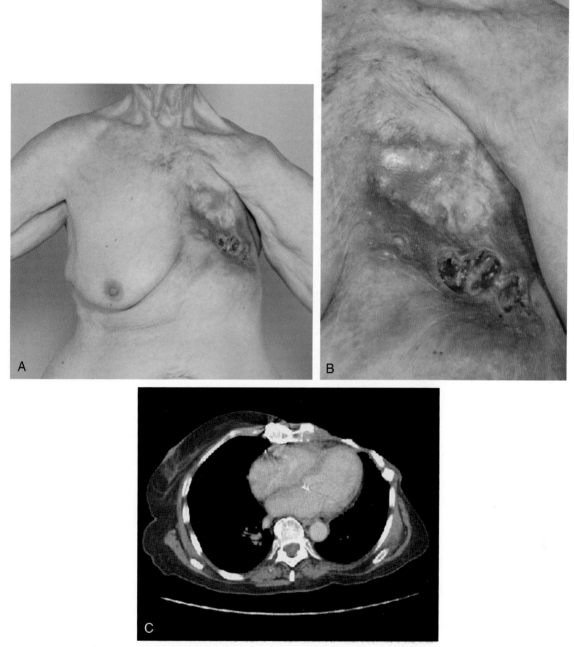

**Figure 50-13:** **A,** 79-year old woman with radionecrosis of the left anterior chest wall. Thirty years previously, she underwent left radical mastectomy and chest wall irradiation. Thirteen years previously, she had coronary bypass surgery via a median sternotomy. She has had 12-year history of a nonhealing progressive left chest wall ulceration. **B,** Close-up of the radionecrosis. **C,** Computed tomography scan showing bone mottling, irregularity, and sclerosis related to chronic osteoradionecrosis.

*(Continued on page 462.)*

it only once.[2] Nonetheless, others have used this with success.[45,46,50]

○ Deschamps and colleagues[52] retrospectively reviewed 197 patients who underwent chest wall resection and either PTFE or Prolene mesh reconstruction. A well-healed asymptomatic wound was obtained in 127 patients (71%). Little difference was found between reconstruction with PTFE or Prolene mesh, and they believed that the decision of which prosthesis to use could be the surgeon's preference.

▪ Soft tissue reconstruction
  ○ Both muscle and omentum can be used to reconstruct soft tissue chest wall defects (Figs. 50-14 and 50-15)
    ▪ Muscles include pectoralis major, latissimus dorsi, rectus abdominus, serratus anterior, external oblique, and trapezius
    ▪ Muscle can be transposed as muscle alone or as a musculocutaneous flap.
    ▪ In our practice, omentum is most commonly used as a back-up for failed muscle transpositions.

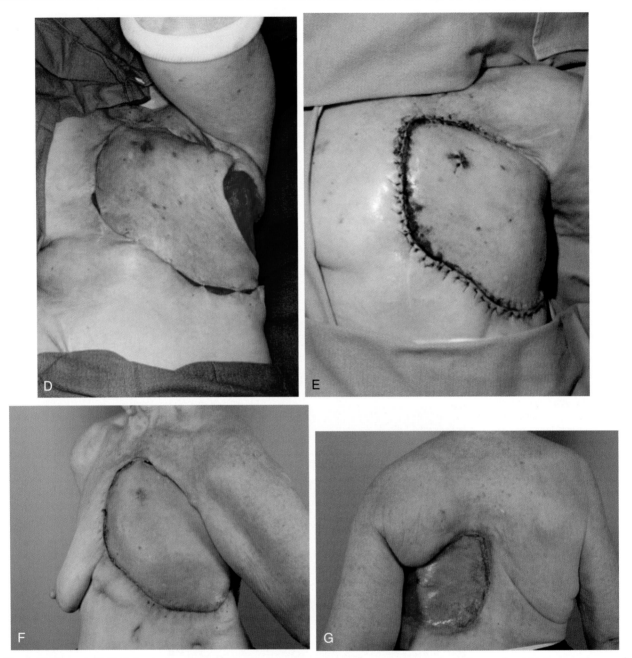

**Figure 50-13—cont'd: D,** Following resection of all irradiated anterior chest wall bone, cartilage, and soft tissue and serial intraoperative wound débridements and pack changes, a left latissimus dorsi myocutaneous flap was transposed to cover the anterior chest wall defect, the posterior donor site was initially treated with a vacuum-assist closure device. **E,** Latissimus dorsi myocutaneous flap sutured in place with interrupted absorbable monofilament suture. **F and G,** Healing latissimus dorsi myocutaneous flap and skin grafted donor site 6 weeks postoperatively.

- Clinical experience.
  - In Arnold and Pairolero's[2] report of 500 consecutive chest wall reconstruction patients
    - Patients underwent an average of 2.3 operations and were hospitalized an average of 21 days
    - The mortality rate was 3.0% (15 patients)
    - Average follow-up was 57 months, and 8% had an excellent result with a healed, asymptomatic chest wall
  - Deschamps and colleagues[52] found the morbidity rate of chest wall reconstruction to be 46.2%. Most common were respiratory complications in 24.4% of patients with seroma and wound infections occurring in 7.1% and 4.6% of patients, respectively.

## *THORACOPLASTY*

### Introduction

- Thoracoplasty is a surgical technique initially designed to permanently collapse tuberculous cavities by resection of ribs from the chest wall.
  - Thoracoplasty began in 1885 with de Cerenville, who resected short segments of two or more ribs anteriorly, resulting in collapse of the anterior chest wall.
  - In 1890, Shede described the resection of multiple ribs, parietal pleura, periosteum, intercostal muscles, and the neurovascular bundles, leaving only the extrathoracic muscles and skin to collapse.[53]

| TABLE 50-4 ▪ **CONSIDERATIONS FOR CHEST WALL RECONSTRUCTION** |
| --- |
| Location of the defect |
| Size of the defect |
| Full or partial thickness defect |
| Duration of the defect |
| Local tissue conditions |
|    Infection |
|    Radiation |
|    Residual neoplasm |
|    Prior resection and reconstruction |
| Patient condition |
|    Debility |
|    Nutritional status |
|    Immunosuppression |
| Job and lifestyle requirements |
| Prognosis |

- The process was mutilating and resulted in an unstable chest wall
  - In 1937, Alexander described the three-stage, 10- or 11-rib thoracoplasty. In the first stage, the posterior segments of the first through third ribs and sometimes portions of their transverse processes were resected. The periosteum was left in situ, resulting in new bone formation that maintained the long-term collapse of the lung. The second and third stages removed additional ribs at 3-week intervals.
    - The operative mortality rate was 10%, but cavity closure was successful in 93% of treated patients.

- Most thoracoplasties produce some degree of chest wall and shoulder deformity (Fig. 50-16).
  - Scoliosis may develop
  - Restriction of shoulder motion may occur
  - Some patients develop progressive respiratory failure

## Current Use

- At present, thoracoplasty is seldom used because of the advent of better ways to obliterate the pleural space.
  - Decortication may be successful in re-expanding residual lung.
  - Open drainage can be obtained by making a U-shaped chest wall opening over the empyema space as described by Samuel Robinson in 1915 and was later popularized by Eloesser.[54-56]
  - Transposition of extrathoracic muscles can be performed to obliterate the open pleural space.[57,58]
  - For postpneumonectomy empyema, the Clagett procedure may be appropriate. This consists of open pleural drainage, followed by serial pleural cavity débridements and gauze packing, and finally, when clean, filling the residual pleural cavity with antibiotic solution and then closing the wound as much as possible in layers, with the skin closed in a watertight fashion.[59]
    - Satisfactory results with the Clagett procedure are justification by Pairolero for using this technique in the treatment of persistent nonpneumonectomy empyema with a 67% success rate for control of the empyema and without evidence of bronchopleural fistula (BPF).[60] The success rate is the same for a redo procedure.

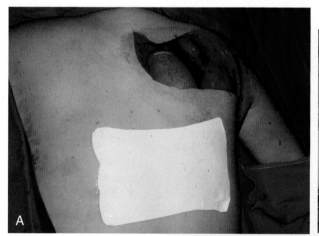

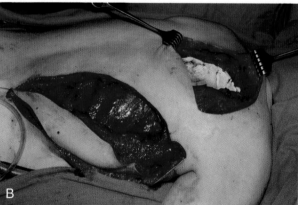

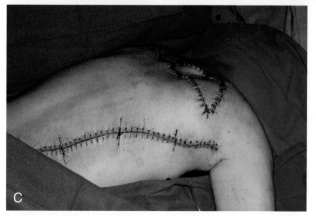

**Figure 50-14: A,** A 48-year-old man with a posterior chest wall mass after wide resection. **B,** A 2-mm thick Gore-Tex soft tissue patch reconstruction and mobilization of the right latissimus dorsi musculocutaneous flap. **C,** Completed reconstruction, which, in this case, included primary closure of the donor site. *(Courtesy of Peter C. Pairolero, MD.)*

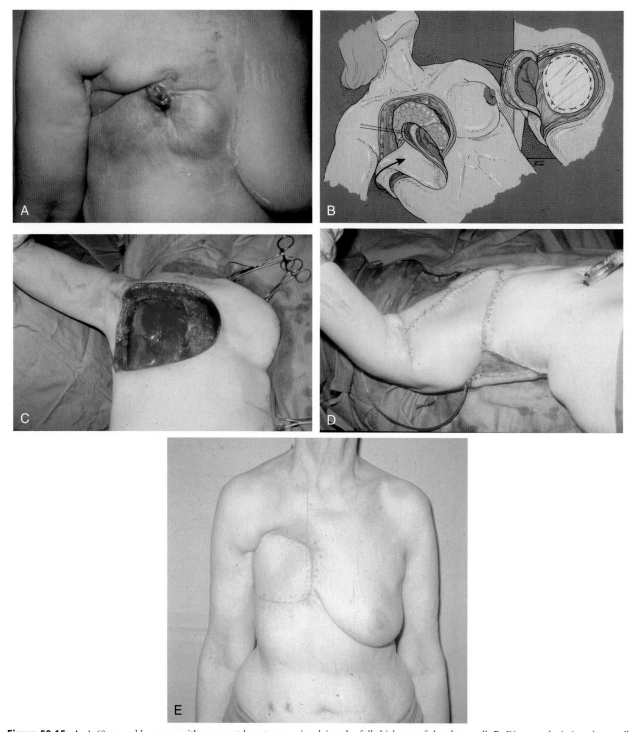

**Figure 50-15: A,** A 60-year-old woman with recurrent breast cancer involving the full thickness of the chest wall. **B,** Diagram depicting chest wall resection, Gore-Tex soft tissue patch reconstruction, and latissimus dorsi musculocutaneous flap. **C,** Chest wall defect following wide resection. **D,** Completed reconstruction with skin grafting of a portion of the donor site. **E,** Chest wall appearance 4 months following resection and reconstruction. *(Courtesy of Peter C. Pairolero, MD.)*

## Management of the Chronically Infected Pleural Space

- Goals of therapy are to protect the patient's life by obtaining a healed chest wall and without evidence of infection
- Table 50-5 outlines considerations that help determine which technique of management is the best option for an individual patient

- Our preferred approach is the modified Clagett procedure (Fig. 50-17).[61,62]
  - Operative management is guided by the presence or absence of a BPF.
  - If necessary, a chest tube is initially placed to protect the contralateral lung from contamination.

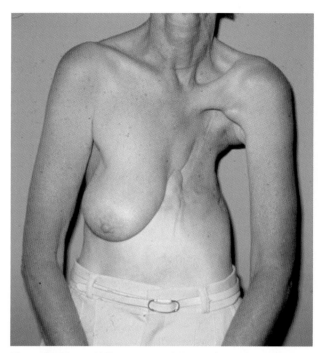

**Figure 50-16:** A middle-age woman following thoracoplasty. Although the patient's chest wall is healed, note the developing scoliosis and marked chest wall deformity. (*Courtesy of Peter C. Pairolero, MD.*)

**TABLE 50-5 ▪ CONSIDERATIONS FOR THE TREATMENT OF CHRONICALLY INFECTED PLEURAL SPACES**

Is the patient in good health?
Can the entrapped lung expand?
Is a bronchopleural fistula present?
Are local muscles available for intrathoracic transposition?

○ The first-stage of the Clagett procedure is
  ▪ Contralateral lung protection with a double-lumen endotracheal tube
  ▪ Evacuation of the pleural contents, débridement, and inspection for a BPF.
    ○ The chest cavity is filled with saline and observed for bubbles escaping from the ipsilateral bronchus.
○ If BPF is not present,
  ▪ The chest is débrided and packed with antibiotic soaked gauze.
    ○ The antibiotic solution is DABS, which contains 20 mg gentamicin and 5000 units of polymixin B in 1000 mL of 0.9% sodium chloride.
  ▪ Further débridement and wound packing occurs every 48 hours.
  ▪ When granulation tissue forms, the pack changes occur several times per day at the patient's bedside.
  ▪ Pulse irrigation is used as needed.

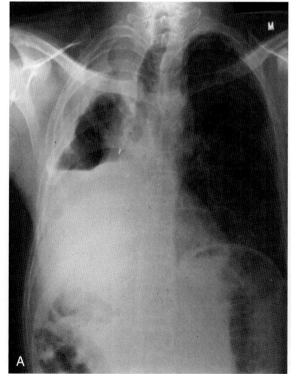

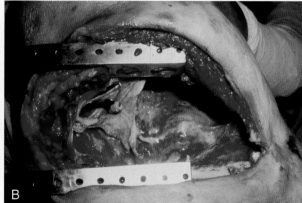

**Figure 50-17: A,** A 51-year-old gentleman 8 years after a right pneumonectomy now has a symptomatic bronchopleural fistula. Note the air fluid level on the chest x-ray study. **B,** The right side of the chest was reopened through the initial thoracotomy incision, purulent debris was encountered, the chest cavity was decorticated.

*(Continued)*

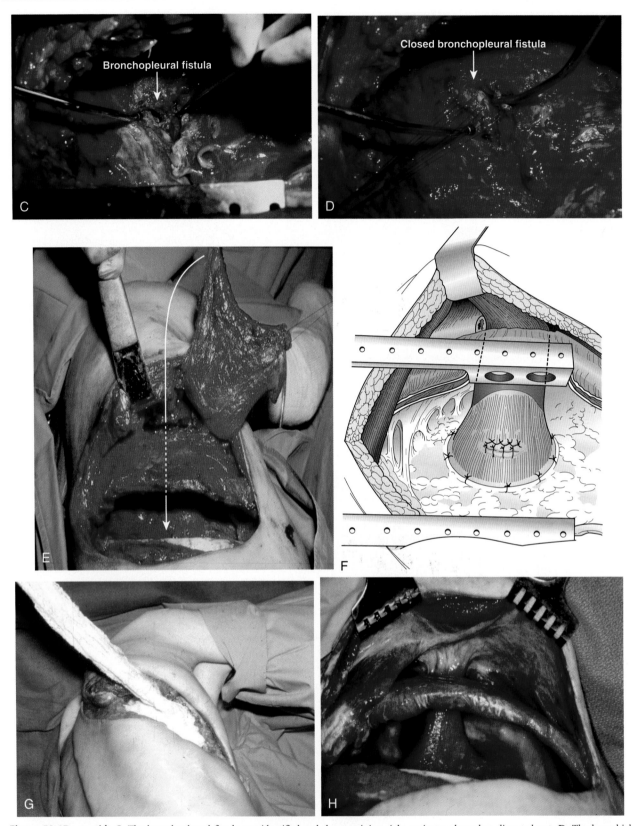

**Figure 50-17—cont'd: C,** The bronchopleural fistula was identified and the remaining right mainstem bronchus dissected out. **D,** The bronchial stump was closed with interrupted 3-0 polypropylene suture, and the chest was then packed with antibiotic soaked gauze. **E,** Forty-eight hours later, the serratus anterior muscle was mobilized, a portion of the right third rib resected, and the serratus muscle then brought into the chest through the bed of the partially resected third rib. The muscle was secured to the right main stem bronchial stump and surrounding mediastinal tissue with interrupted 3-0 polypropylene suture. **F,** Diagram depicting the serratus anterior muscle covering the closed bronchial stump. **G,** The patient undergoes chest cavity débridements and pack changes with antibiotic soaked gauze every other day. **H,** The serratus anterior muscle grows into place and the chest cavity becomes replaced with healthy granulation tissue.

*(Continued)*

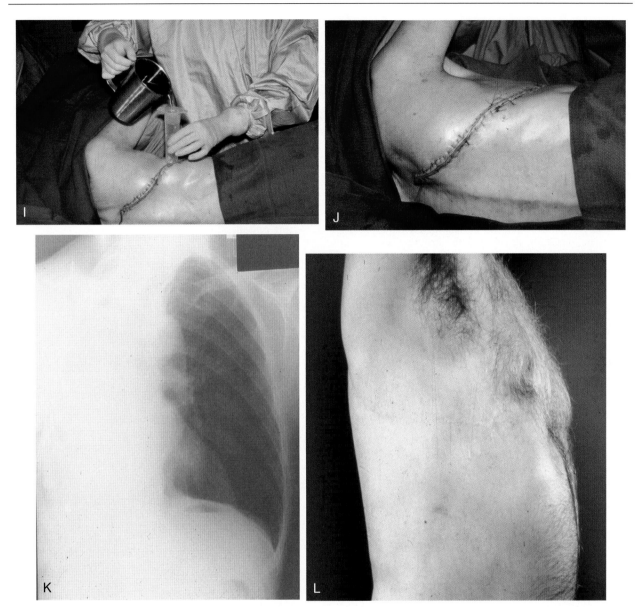

**Figure 50-17—cont'd: I,** The wound is closed in layers, and the skin is closed with a watertight closure using polypropylene suture. Before placing the last stitch, the chest cavity is filled with antibiotic solution. **J,** The final skin closure. **K,** The healed chest wound 2 years later. **L,** A chest x-ray study 2 years later now showing complete opacification of the right hemithorax.

- When healthy granulation tissue is present throughout the pleural cavity with no evidence of exudates, the chest wound is filled with DABS and then closed in layers, with the skin having a watertight closure.
○ If BPF is present
  - The bronchial stump is dissected free and closed with polypropylene suture
  - The reclosed stump is reinforced with intrathoracic transposition of an extraskeletal muscle, most commonly the serratus anterior.
  - In some cases with a long residual bronchial stump, the stump can be closed through a median sternotomy. This means that the bronchial stump is closed in a clean, uninfected field.
  - If there was insufficient bronchial stump to close, then the transposed muscle is sutured directly to the perimeter of the fistula.

- The chest cavity is then filled with gauze soaked in DABS and managed in the fashion outlined earlier.
○ In our recently published series involving 84 patients with postpneumonectomy empyema and the use of the modified Clagett procedure
  - The operative mortality rate was 7.1%.
  - The BPF, if present, eventually remained closed in all patients.
  - Overall, 89% of patients had a healed chest wound without evidence of recurrent infection.

## References

 Interactive references and additional readings for this chapter can be accessed online at *expertconsult.com.*

# DIAPHRAGM DISORDERS: PARALYSIS, HERNIA, EVENTRATION

Michael I. Lewis, MD

## DIAPHRAGM PARALYSIS

### Functional Anatomy of the Diaphragm and Other Respiratory Muscles

- *Primary inspiratory muscles* are those respiratory muscles that are phasically recruited with each ventilatory effort, under resting conditions. In humans, the diaphragm, parasternal intercostals, and scalene muscles are considered primary.[1,2]
- The *diaphragm* is responsible for expanding the lower chest cage. The costal portion is opposed to the lower six ribs, producing a zone of apposition occupying about 30% of the total surface area of the rib cage.
- *Diaphragm action* on the lower rib cage is mediated by two mechanisms:
  - *Appositional action*: with contraction, the diaphragm descends meeting abdominal resistance to its excursion. Abdominal pressure rises, which is transmitted through the zone of apposition to expand the lower rib cage (Fig. 51-1).
  - *Insertional action*: the alignment of costal diaphragm fibers are such that with abdominal resistance to excursion, the vector of the forces generated by contraction is oriented cranially, such that the ribs are pulled up and out (Fig. 51-2).
- *Abnormal geometric configuration* of the chest cage affects diaphragm function. For example, with hyperinflation, the diaphragm becomes flatter and shorter, reducing its force, generating potential by reducing or eliminating its appositional action and altering its insertional action such that fiber orientation and direction of force vectors are altered to produce in extreme cases, ribcage paradox (i.e., inward movement of the rib cage).
- The diaphragm is *innervated* by the right and left phrenic nerves, which arise from cervical roots 3, 4, and 5.
- *Other primary inspiratory muscles*: the parasternal intercostals are the interchondral portion of the internal intercostals and produce cranial motion of the ribs and an increased anteroposterior dimension of the upper rib cage. They are innervated by the intercostal nerves. The scalene neck muscles increase the anteroposterior and transverse diameters of the upper rib cage and elevate the sternum. They are innervated by cervical nerves C4–C8.
- *Accessory respiratory muscles* are those recruited under conditions of increased demand (e.g., load, chemical drive, and exercise). These include the external intercostals and levator costae, which generally function as reserve inspiratory muscle groups, the sternocleidomastoids (inspiratory, innervated by the X1 cranial nerves), and the internal interosseous intercostals, which generally subserve an expiratory function.
- *Expiratory muscles*: the abdominal muscles are silent at rest but exert phasic expiratory influences on the chest cage under conditions of increased ventilatory demand. In addition, they subserve an important functional role in the act of coughing. They are innervated by branches of T7 to T12.

### Introduction to Diaphragm Paralysis

- Paralysis or severe weakness of the diaphragm can be either unilateral or bilateral.
- Paralysis can occur as an isolated phenomenon or as part of a more generalized neuromuscular disorder.
- The impact on ventilatory function depends on the degree of weakness, the extent of muscle involvement (bilateral more than unilateral), the rapidity of onset, the extent of other inspiratory muscle weakness, and comorbidities (particularly cardiac, pulmonary, or chest wall abnormalities).[3]

### Clinical Features

- *Orthopnea* is a classic symptom of bilateral diaphragm paralysis and occurs rapidly with supine posture. It may be seen with acute presentations of unilateral diaphragm paralysis.[4]
- *Exertional dyspnea* may be seen in patients with both bilateral and unilateral paralysis,[5-7] culminating in reduced exercise tolerance.
- *Immersion dyspnea* in water is another symptom of bilateral diaphragm paralysis.[8,9] This occurs when the water is at the level of the lower ribcage.
- *Abdominal paradox* (inward inspiratory motion of the abdomen) while supine is a key sign of bilateral diaphragm paralysis.[10] The sign is less evident with lesser degrees of weakness and may be absent with maximum transdiaphragmatic pressure ($Pdi_{max}$) greater than 30 $cmH_2O$.[11] Abdominal paradox may also be noted with unilateral diaphragm paralysis.[12]
- In general, inspiratory muscle strength of patients with unilateral diaphragm paralysis is most decreased in those with associated cardiopulmonary disease.[12]
- *Sleep-disordered breathing and nocturnal hypoventilation* may occur with diaphragm paralysis. This condition is most commonly noted in patients in whom weakness of other inspiratory muscles is also present.[5]
- *Arm elevation* may result in increased metabolic and ventilatory cost, producing dyspnea.[13]

### Diagnostic Tests

- **Imaging:**
  - *Chest x-ray study* shows elevated hemidiaphragm with unilateral diaphragm paralysis or the appearance of small lung volumes and basilar subsegmental atelectasis in the case of bilateral diaphragm paralysis, which can be misinterpreted as poor inspiratory effort. Note: An elevated hemidiaphragm lacks specificity for unilateral diaphragm paralysis (44%) with sensitivity and negative predictive values of 90% and 93%, respectively.[14]
  - *Fluoroscopy*, demonstrating paradoxical motion of a hemidiaphragm when supine following a vigorous sniff, is useful with unilateral paralysis.[15] However, with bilateral paralysis, the patient is unable to lie supine and the test lacks sensitivity. In the upright posture, expiratory muscle recruitment elevates the flaccid diaphragm, which then descends

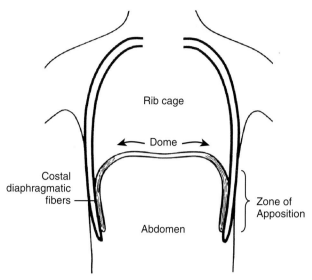

**Figure 51-1:** Figure demonstrating *appositional action of the diaphragm.* Note: the zone of apposition of the costal diaphragm with the lower six ribs is well depicted. With diaphragm contraction, the muscle moves down like a piston and meets resistance from the relatively incompressible abdominal contents. Intra-abdominal pressure rises, which is transmitted through the zone of apposition, to expand the lower rib cage. *(From De Troyer Estenne M. Functional anatomy of the respiratory muscles. Clin Chest Med 1988;9:175-193, with permission.)*

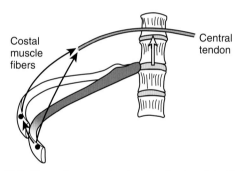

**Figure 51-2:** Figure demonstrating *insertional action of the diaphragm.* Note: the orientation of diaphragm muscle fibers are such that with contraction, the main vector of the forces generated, pulls the lower ribs up and out, to assist with expansion of the lower rib cage. *(From De Troyer Estenne M. Functional anatomy of the respiratory muscles. Clin Chest Med 1988;9:175-193, with permission.)*

passively at the onset of inspiration as abdominal muscles relax.

○ *Ultrasound* can assess both diaphragm motion[16] as well as diaphragm muscle morphometry.[17,18] Ultrasound can determine diaphragm atrophy with paralysis (thickness at zone of opposition with chest wall at a functional residual capacity [FRC] <2 mm and <20% increase in thickness during inspiration).[19] M-mode ultrasound was also useful in assessing diaphragm motion in a large cohort of pediatric patients[20] and can be employed serially at the bedside.

▪ **Pulmonary function studies**
○ Table 51-1 depicts pulmonary function in patients with bilateral[5] and recent unilateral diaphragm weakness or paralysis.[7]
○ Although the vital capacity (VC) may be influenced by inspiratory and muscle strength, other factors such as compliance of the lungs or chest wall and airway closure may also contribute.[21,22]

○ Thus, the VC exhibits poor specificity in the diagnosis of respiratory muscle weakness and is considered to be less sensitive than maximum mouth pressures in the presence of mild respiratory muscle weakness.[23] Serial measurements in the intensive care unit (ICU) offer more reliable data and trends.
○ An exaggerated fall in VC when supine is a useful test.[5]
▪ *Arterial blood gases*
○ Awake arterial blood gases are relatively insensitive indices of respiratory muscle weakness until late and severe impairment of respiratory muscles is present.
○ In patients with chronic myopathies and no lung disease per se, awake hypercapnia was unlikely, until respiratory muscle strength was reduced to less than 40% of predicted and the VC to less than 50%.[24]
○ Borderline hypercapnia may rapidly change to overt respiratory failure when even mild changes in load or ventilatory drive ensue.
▪ Measurement of respiratory muscle pressures in the workup of diaphragm dysfunction
○ *Maximum inspiratory mouth pressure (PI_{max})*
  ▪ *Global test of inspiratory muscle strength.* Reflects the pressure generated by the inspiratory muscles (P mus) plus the passive elastic recoil pressure of the respiratory system (lung and chest wall; Prs). At FRC, Prs = 0, whereas at residual volume (RV), Prs can be considerable (e.g., −30 cmH₂O). Thus, measure $PI_{max}$ at FRC rather than at RV.
  ▪ *Normal values* are depicted in Table 51-2.
  ▪ *Major disadvantage*: test is effort dependent and requires patient motivation, cooperation, and coordination.[25-31] In the presence of intrinsic positive end-expiratory pressure (PEEP), the pressure generated by the inspiratory muscles will be underestimated.
○ *Maximal esophageal (Pes) and nasal (Pnas, sn) pressures:*
  ▪ Also global inspiratory measures but less variances. Requires insertion of an esophageal balloon catheter or nasal catheter.
  ▪ In nonintubated patients, Pes following a maximum sniff may be easier to perform.[32]
  ▪ Pnas, sn, using a catheter wedged in one nostril, may represent a relatively noninvasive measure mirroring Pes measurements.[33] Pnas, sn tends to underestimate Pes, sn in patients with lung disease (e.g., chronic obstructive pulmonary disease [COPD]).[34]
○ *Pdi*
  ▪ Measured as the difference between gastric pressure (Pga) and Pes (i.e., Pdi = Pga − Pes). Is a measure of *diaphragm strength.*
  ▪ *Maximal Pdi (Pdi_{max})* may be achieved using different techniques: a maximal static inspiratory effort (Mueller maneuver),[35] a Mueller maneuver combined with an abdominal expulsive effort,[30] and a maximal sniff (sniff Pdi).[28]
  ▪ Such efforts require patient motivation, cooperation, and coordination, which may be difficult to achieve in critically ill patients. (See Table 51-2 for normal values.)
  ▪ Phrenic nerve stimulation at FRC provides an objective, reproducible nonvolitional test.
  ▪ This can be achieved using either *electrical stimulation* (surface or needle electrodes)[36] or magnetic stimulation in which rapidly changing magnetic fields produce brief electric fields within conducting tissues.
  ▪ Although *cervical magnetic stimulation* produces bilateral phrenic stimulation, it requires the stimulating coil to be positioned behind the neck, making this technically challenging in ICU patients, who are commonly supine.[37]

### TABLE 51-1 ■ PULMONARY FUNCTION WITH DIAPHRAGM PARALYSIS

| | VC (L) (% pred) | Supine fall in VC (%) | TLC (% pred) | RV (% pred) |
|---|---|---|---|---|
| Bilateral[5] | 2.1 + 0.7 (48) | 37 + 9 | 67 + 11 | 104 + 23 |
| Unilateral[7] | 2.9 + 0.9 (76) | 11.8 + 8.1 | 88 + 17 | 108 + 23 |

Values are means ± SD.
RV, residual volume; TLC, total lung capacity; VC, vital capacity.

### TABLE 51-2 ■ NORMAL VALUES FOR TESTS OF RESPIRATORY MUSCLE PERFORMANCE

| Test | | Male | Female | Reference |
|---|---|---|---|---|
| *$PI_{max}$ | (tube MP) | −123 ± 21 | −87 ± 15 | 25 |
| ($cmH_2O$) | (flanged MP) | −106 ± 30 | −73 ± 21 | 27 |
| *$PE_{max}$ | (tube MP) | 232 ± 42 | 152 ± 56 | 26 |
| ($cmH_2O$) | (flanged MP) | 148 ± 34 | 93 ± 16 | 27 |
| Sniff Pes | | −105 ± 25 | −89 ± 21 | 28 |
| ($cmH_2O$) | | | | |
| Sniff Pdi | | 145 ± 24 | 121 ± 25 | 28 |
| ($cmH_2O$) | | | | |
| Maximum Static Pdi (Mueller) ($cmH_2O$) | | 108 ± 30 | 65 ± 31 | 28 |
| Pdi (combined Mueller/expulsive technique) ($cmH_2O$) | | 180 ± 14 | | 29 |
| UMS-Tw-Pdi ($cmH_2O$) | | 16 ± 3 (left; <10 abnormal) | | 29 |
| | | 12 ± 4 (right; <6 abnormal) | | |
| BAMPS-Tw-Pdi | | 27.6 ± 1.6 (male and female; | | 38 |
| ($cmH_2O$) | | < 20 abnormal) | | |

BAMPS, bilateral anterior magnetic phrenic stimulation; UMS-Tw-Pdi, unilateral magnetic stimulation, twitch Pdi.
*Normal values in the elderly and in children are available.[25,27]

*Unilateral or bilateral anterior magnetic stimulation* approaches to stimulate the phrenic nerves are better suited to the ICU environment (Fig. 51-3).[29,30,38]

■ Electrical or magnetic phrenic nerve stimulation uses single supramaximal stimuli to produce a twitch (Tw) Pdi. In general, bilateral phrenic nerve Tw-Pdis are about a quarter of the $Pdi_{max}$ achieved by maximum voluntary effort (see Table 51-2).[39]

○ *Data with diaphragm paralysis:*
  ■ Table 51-3 summarizes mean respiratory pressures generated in patients with bilateral severe diaphragm weakness/paralysis[5] or hemidiaphragm paralysis.[7]
  ■ Typical tracings of pressure deflections for Pdi and its components (gastric and esophageal pressures) following a sniff maneuver in a patient with bilateral diaphragm weakness and a control subject are depicted in Figure 51-4.
  ■ The ratio of △ Pga to △ Pes is normally less than −1. With diaphragm paralysis, other chest and neck inspiratory muscles are recruited such that the ratio approaches +1. This index, which correlates with $Pdi_{max}$, may, thus, be a useful index of diaphragm weakness.[40]

○ *Nerve conduction and electrophysiology:*
  ■ *Phrenic nerve conduction time* (PNCT) may also be measured following unilateral phrenic nerve stimulation (normal in adults: 6–8 ms).[41] In general, marked prolongation of PNCT suggests a demyelinating process, whereas preserved PNCT coupled with reduced

amplitude of the compound action potential suggests axonal damage.[41]
  ■ Although surface and needle electrodes have been used, the recent use of esophageal electrodes offers precise and reproducible measurement of PNCT and amplitude of the diaphragm compound action potential.[42,43]

## Causes of Diaphragm Paralysis

A comprehensive classification of diaphragm paralysis is provided in Table 51-4.[44-51]

## Specific Conditions

■ **Phrenic nerve injury after cardiac surgery:**
  ○ Phrenic nerve injury occurs because of phrenic nerve cooling when ice slush is placed around the heart for cooling. Complete phrenic nerve conduction block has been well documented with cooling in dogs,[52] and more recently, changes in the evoked electromyographic (EMG) response of the diaphragm have been demonstrated in patients undergoing cardiac surgery using bilateral magnetic phrenic stimulation.[53] Note: The latter occurred with mild degrees of hypothermia (31°C).[53]
  ○ Internal mammary harvesting may also increase the risk of phrenic injury.[54]
  ○ Traction and vascular compromise of the phrenic nerve may contribute to injury.

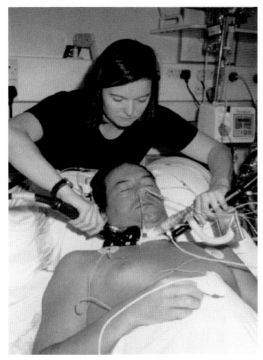

**Figure 51-3:** Bilateral anterior magnetic stimulation of phrenic nerves. *(From Polkey MI, Moxham J. Clinical aspects of respiratory muscle dysfunction in the critically ill. Chest 2001;119:926-939, with permission.)*

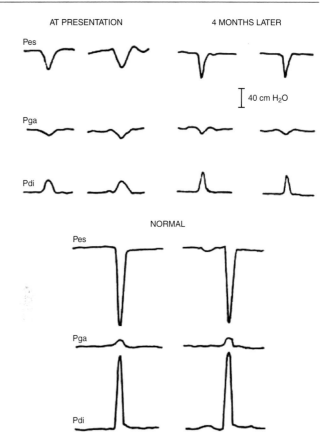

**Figure 51-4:** Serial measurement of maximum transdiaphragmatic pressures (Pdi) in a patient with severe diaphragm weakness compared to a normal subject. *(From Spiteri MA, Mier AK, Pantin CF, Green M. Bilateral diaphragm weakness. Thorax 1985;40:631-632, with permission.)*

○ The incidence of phrenic injury following cardiac surgery has decreased with the introduction of preventive measures, including insulation. Prior incidence has been reported as 10% to 36%.[55-58]

○ Diehl and coworkers[59] reported the prevalence of clinically significant diaphragm dysfunction to be 2.1% (ice slush) and 0.5% (with insulation). In general, bilateral diaphragm paralysis is rare (<5% of cases with phrenic injury).[60]

○ A low incidence has recently been described in children (0.28% bilateral diaphragm paralysis).[61]

○ Phrenic dysfunction has also been described after heart-lung and lung transplantation.[62]

○ The clinical presentation of diaphragm paralysis may be acute or subacute and may contribute to significant morbidity and/or mortality (see clinical features discussed earlier).[59,63]

○ The majority of affected patients recover function. With injury limited to the myelin sheath, recovery by 12 weeks is expected.[64] With accompanying axonal damage, recovery is further delayed and full recovery can take 1 to 2 years.[57,64] About 30% of patients fail to fully recover diaphragm function.[65]

○ Supportive ventilatory measures may be required in the acute or symptomatic chronic dysfunction. In the latter scenario, diaphragm plication (either unilateral or bilateral) is a therapeutic option (see discussion of treatment later).

## TABLE 51-3 ■ RESPIRATORY MUSCLE PRESSURES WITH DIAPHRAGM PARALYSIS

| | PI$_{max}$ (% pred) | PE$_{max}$ (% pred) | Pdi$_{max}$ (Mueller) | Pdi$_{max}$ (Sniff) | TwPdi |
|---|---|---|---|---|---|
| **Bilateral** | 4.0 ± 18 (43) | 135 ± 51 (98) | 11 ± 8 | 13 ± 6 | 0.8 ± 2 |
| **Unilateral** | 49 ± 9 (62) | 112 ± 53 (95) | * | 62 ± 13:   1.2 ± 1.6 (affected) | |
| | | | | 11.1 ± 3.5 (normal) | |

Values are means ± SD.
Pdi, transdiaphragmatic pressure; PI$_{max}$, maximum inspiratory mouth pressure; PE$_{max}$, maximum expiratory mouth pressure; Tw, twitch.
*Maximum static values variable and depend on gender.
*Data from Laroche CM, Carroll N, Moxham J, Green M. Clinical significance of severe isolated diaphragm weakness. Am Rev Respir Dis 1988;138: 862-866; and Laroche CM, Mier AK, Moxham J, Green M. Diaphragm strength in patients with recent hemidiaphragm paralysis. Thorax 1988;43:170-174.*

### TABLE 51-4 ■ ETIOLOGY OF DIAPHRAGM PARALYSIS

| | |
|---|---|
| Spinal cord | Charcot-Marie-Tooth disease |
|   High cervical cord trans-section/injury | Acute porphyria |
|   Multiple sclerosis | Collagen vascular and vasculitic |
| Motor neurons |   Systemic lupus erythematosis |
|   Amyotrophic lateral sclerosis |   Wegener's granulomatosis |
|   Postpolio syndrome | Radiation injury |
|   Spinal muscular atrophy | Neuralgic amyotrophy |
| Cervical nerve roots | Diabetes |
|   Cervical spondylosis | Idiopathic |
|   Complication of spinal surgery | Diaphragm myopathy |
|   Chiropractic manipulation |   Dystrophy |
| Phrenic nerves |     Limble girdle |
|   Trauma |   Collagen vascular disorders |
|     Blunt; sharp |     Systemic lupus erythematosis |
|     Surgical |     Dermatomyositis |
|       Cooling (cardiac surgery) |     Systemic sclerosis |
|       Transection or stretch injury |     Mixed connective tissue disease |
|       Cervical manipulation |   Endocrine |
|       Birth injury (forceps, etc.) |     Hypothyroidism |
|       Radiofrequency ablation |     Hyperthyroidism |
|   Infective |     Glucocorticoid excess (Cushing's disease, |
|     Herpes zoster |       iatrogenic administration) |
|       Lyme disease |   Critical illness |
|       Lymph node compression |     Critical illness myopathy |
|   Neoplastic |   Nutrition/metabolic |
|     Tumor compression |     Anorexia nervosa |
|     Lymph node compression |     Electrolyte deficiency |
|     Paraneoplastic |     Periodic paralysis |
|   Polyneuropathy |   Acid maltase deficiency |
|     Gullain-Barré syndrome and associated conditions |   Amyloidosis |
|     Chronic inflammatory polyneuropathy |   Idiopathic |
|     Critical illness polyneuropathy | |

*Adapted from Mistry S, Lewis MI. Neuromuscular respiratory failure in the ICU: an overview. In: Mohsenifar Z, SooHoo GW, editors. Practical pulmonary and critical care medicine: disease management. Vol 214. Philadelphia: Taylor and Francis; 2006. p. 221-285.*

■ **Neuralgic amyotrophy:**
- ○ Neuralgic amyotrophy is an idiopathic inflammatory condition affecting the bronchial plexus, which may lead to unilateral or bilateral diaphragm paralysis.[66,67]
- ○ Patients may present with dyspnea (particularly with exercise or with immersion) after a prodromal flulike illness in which neck and shoulder pain are prominent.[68]
- ○ Nocturnal desaturation and obstructive sleep apnea have been described,[66] possibly related to involvement of upper airway muscles.[69]
- ○ Upper limb weakness/paralysis resolves within 3 years in most cases.[68]
- ○ Long-term recovery of diaphragm strength was delayed and generally took greater than 3 years.[70]
- ○ No specific therapy is available. In patients with delayed recovery (>2–3 years), diaphragm plication can be considered.[70]

■ **Systemic lupus erythematosis (SLE)**
- ○ The mechanisms responsible for producing the shrinking lung syndrome in patients with SLE are not well understood.
- ○ Pathogenic mechanisms include (1) demyelinating phrenic neuropathy, which may be responsive to corticosteroid therapy,[71] (2) diaphragm myopathy,[72] and (3) chest wall restriction rather than diaphragm weakness per se.[73] Diaphragm fiber atrophy and fibrosis have been described in an autopsy study.[74]

■ **Spinal cord trauma**
- ○ Complete cord injury at levels C1–C3: produce bilateral diaphragm paralysis as well as paralysis of other primary inspiratory and expiratory muscles.

- ○ Complete cord injury at levels C3–C5: produce variable loss of diaphragm force–generating ability, as well as paralysis of other primary inspiratory and expiratory muscles.
- ○ Complete cord injury at levels C6–C8: diaphragm and neck accessory muscles intact.
- ○ A recent study revealed the following on hospital discharge or transfer[75]: 100% ventilator dependence with complete cord injury of C4 and higher; 56% with C5 injury; 15% with C6 injury.
- ○ Need for long-term mechanical support depends on complete versus partial spinal cord injury, the level of the injury, resolution of edema and inflammation with apparent descent of the injury level, onset of muscle spasticity and rib cage stiffening, age, comorbidities and complications.

## Treatment of Diaphragm Paralysis

■ **Diaphragm plication:**
- ○ Surgical plication of the diaphragm is a technique in which sutures are placed in the paralyzed hemidiaphragm in order to render it taut, thus preventing it from being sucked up into the thorax with inspiration.[76] On chest x-ray study, the diaphragm is usually elevated to halfway up the chest cavity. Plication puts the diaphragm back in its normal position.
- ○ This procedure is mostly performed in patients with symptomatic unilateral diaphragm paralysis.[76,77] This procedure should not be performed until enough time has passed to allow a phrenic nerve to recover function (usually 1 year). Note: bilateral diaphragm plication has been used in selected cases with good long-term success.[78]

○ The procedure can be performed using a video-assisted thorascopic approach,[79,80] conventional posterolateral thoracotomy, or via a laparoscopic approach.[81]

○ Diaphragm plication has been associated with improved gas exchange, chest mechanics (including supine VC), respiratory muscle function (including $Pdi_{max}$), exercise performance, symptoms, and social well-being.[77-84]

○ In children, diaphragm plication may also facilitate weaning from mechanical ventilation.[82,85]

○ Sustained long-term effects (up to 10 years) have been reported.[77,83]

○ Abdominal compartment syndrome has been reported as a rare complication of diaphragm placation.[86]

▪ **Diaphragm pacing**

○ This technique may be considered in patients with high cervical spinal cord injuries (above C3), that is, high quadriplegia.[87,88] Advantages: independence from mechanical ventilation, the ability to speak, normalized gas exchange, reduced infections, and improved quality of life.

○ Major prerequisites: intact lower phrenic motor neurons, normal cognitive function and absence of recovery of diaphragm function after a period of at least 4 months.

○ If the phrenic nerve is not functional, an intercostal nerve is grafted to the phrenic nerve. The pacing wires are attached to the intercostal nerve. This procedure is successful in 50% of cases. Re-enervation of the phrenic nerve takes 6 months, so there is a considerable delay before success can be determined.

○ Diaphragm pacing electrodes can be inserted around phrenic nerve trunks in the neck (cervical approach) or in the chest (standard thoracotomy or thoracoscopic approach).[89]

○ There is also increasing experience with intramuscular implantation of pacing electrodes into the diaphragm laparoscopically.[90,91]

○ Once electrodes are inserted, conditioning regimens of gradually increasing periods of diaphragm pacing are required for up to 9 months before full uninterrupted pacing.[92]

○ Long-term favorable results have been reported in patients with quadriplegia, who have been fully paced for a mean period of 14.8 years.[93]

○ Combined intercostal and diaphragm pacing has recently been described in ventilator-dependent patients due to spinal cord injury.[94]

▪ **Ventilatory support**

○ Acute bilateral diaphragm paralysis with or without associated pulmonary complications or other inspiratory muscle involvement may require intubation and full mechanical ventilation.

○ Prolonged continuous or intermittent mechanical ventilatory requirements necessitate tracheostomy and positive pressure ventilation.

○ Symptomatic patients with isolated bilateral diaphragm paralysis may be managed with noninvasive positive pressure ventilatory support (nocturnal + intermittent daytime).[95]

○ Other noninvasive devices used include the pneumobelt, rocking bed, and negative pressure devices (cuirass, pneumo-wrap).[84]

## DIAPHRAGM HERNIA

*Congenital or developmental defects of the diaphragm* are rarely diagnosed in adulthood. When the defects are diagnosed, they are discovered either incidentally or because of some morbid, usually acute complication. Such events are often misdiagnosed because they are rarely considered in the differential diagnosis. These will be briefly considered.

### Bochdalek Hernia
#### Definition

▪ Failure of the posterolateral region of the diaphragm to close or fuse (i.e., persistence of posterolateral pleuroperitoneal foramen), producing a defect through which abdominal contents can heriate into the thorax (Fig. 51-5).[96]

#### Clinical Features

▪ Pediatric data[97-99]

○ 0.3 cases per 1000 live births; more common in boys

○ Eighty-five percent occur on the left side.

○ Herniated abdominal contents compress the developing lung, resulting in lung hypoplasia, the degree of which impacts on morbidity of survivors.

○ Associated with other congenital abnormalities (cardiac, genitourinary, skeletal, neural) in a third of cases

○ Herniated viscera include colon (70%), gastric (43%), spleen (28%), duodenum/pancreas (11%), liver (7%), omentum (6%), kidney (4%), retroperitoneal fat (3%).

○ Usually presents in the first 24 hours with severe respiratory distress requiring complex ventilatory support and surgical intervention

○ Survivors may suffer recurrent infections, development of bronchitis or bronchiectasis, obstructive or restrictive ventilatory defects, and airway hyper-reactivity.

▪ Adult data[100-102]

○ Rare; 5% of all adult diaphragm hernias, although true prevalence not known

○ Sixty-six percent on the left; right side, 33%; bilateral in 15%

○ Can be an incidental finding

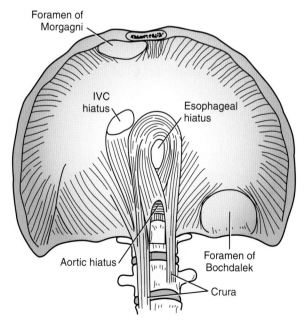

**Figure 51-5:** Schematic demonstrating classic locations for Bochdalek and Morgagni hernias. *(From Naunheim KS. Adult presentation of unusual diaphragmatic hernias. Chest Surg Clin N Am 1998;8:359-369, with permission.)*

○ Acute presentation in adulthood is usually related to gastrointestinal (GI) problems[100-104]: small and large bowel obstruction with or without strangulation (incarceration), gastric obstruction, and volvulus, resulting in an atypical presentation of an acute abdomen (nausea, emesis, chest and abdominal pain, and constipation).

○ Respiratory presentations include: acute dyspnea, respiratory failure and adult respiratory distress syndrome. Separating these symptoms from complications of associated sepsis (acute abdomen) is difficult.

○ Pregnancy may precipitate herniation of abdominal viscera due to progressive mechanical factors.[105]

### Imaging

▪ *Chest x-ray study:* appearance depends on hernia contents and whether gas is present in herniated bowel. A lateral radiograph may also be helpful in delineating a posterior defect/herniated contents

▪ *Computed tomography (CT)* with multiplanar images (with or without the use of oral contrast) is the *procedure of choice* to demonstate the posteromedial defect and herniated contents

▪ *Magnetic resonance imaging (MRI)* can yield similar data to those of CT imaging

### Treatment

▪ **Surgical repair:** should be considered even in asymptomatic cases with large defects, to offset complications

▪ **Approach:** either transthoracic (thoracotomy or video-assisted thoracic surgery [VATS])[106] or transabdominal (laparotomy or laparoscopy[107]). Principles include full reduction of hernia contents and repair of the defect with prosthetic mesh or if small by direct suture closure

▪ **Outcome:** mortality with elective surgery low (3%), but rises significantly with complications (>30%)

## Morgagni Hernia
### Definition

▪ Failure of the anterior parasternal region of the diaphragm to close or fuse producing a defect (Larrey's space), through which abdominal contents can heriate into the thorax[108]

### Clinical Features

▪ Pediatric data
○ Usually not diagnosed in children.
○ Several case series described (see Table 1 of reference #108 for summary)

▪ Adult data[101,108]
○ Rare 2% of all adult diaphragm herniae. Incidence increases with age and obesity.
○ See Table 2 of reference #108 for summary of adult case series
○ Most commonly on the right side (rarely bilateral)
○ Contents: omentum, colon, stomach, liver
○ Can be an incidental finding
○ May complain of nonspecific retrosternal discomfort
○ Acute presentation, usually GI related: small and large bowel obstruction with or without strangulation, gastric obstruction, volvulus.

### Imaging

▪ *Chest x-ray study:* right-sided anterior parasternal or retrosternal mass. Images may reflect bowel contents (Fig. 51-6A and B). Lateral radiograph may be helpful (see Fig. 51-6B). With gastric volvulus, may note a double-bubble sign with air fluid levels both above and below the diaphragm.

▪ *CT* with multiplanar images (with or without use of oral contrast) can clearly demonstrate the defect and herniated contents

▪ *MRI* can yield data similar to those of CT imaging

▪ *A barium enema* can demonstrate colonic herniation

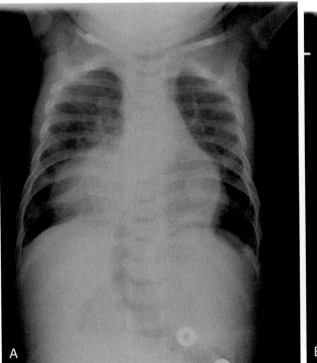
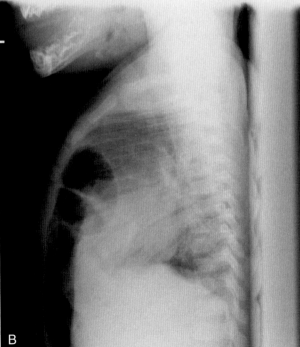

**Figure 51-6:** Posteroanterior bowel protruding through the hernia in anterior location (**B**) into the chest, with shift of the heart to the right (**A**), simulating a mass. *(Courtesy MedPix and James M. Grimson MD.)*

## Treatment

- **Surgical repair:** indicated even in asymptomatic cases to offset complications. If small and contains only omentum, surgery usually reserved with recurrent symptoms.
- **Approach**[108]: either thoracic (thoracotomy or VATS)[109] or abdominal (laparotomy or laparoscopy[107,108]). In the case of large hernias, a transthoracic approach may be favored to allow for visualization and protection of the phrenic nerve with the repair. Principles include full reduction of hernia contents and repair of the defect with synthetic mesh. With small defects, primary suture repair is possible. It remains controversial whether to remove the associated hernia sac.

## DIAPHRAGM EVENTRATION

**Definition:** Nonparalytic thinning and weakness of a sizable portion of the hemidiaphragm, resulting in partial permanent elevation of that portion of the diaphragm[110,111]

## Clinical Features

- Usually unilateral; occasionally bilateral.
- Can be congenital[112]
- Mostly acquired. More common in women; incidence increases with age, particularly in those older than 60 years of age
- Mostly asymptomatic
- Can be associated with dyspnea on effort, recurrent chest infections, atelectasis
- Rupture, either spontaneous or iatrogenic, is a rare major complication

## Imaging

- *Chest x-ray study:* (Fig. 51-7)
  - Best seen on lateral x-ray study, where a two-humped diaphragm is noted.
  - Elevated diaphragm in a recent series: 7.5 +/− 1.8 cm in the frontal view[113]
- *Fluoroscopy and ultrasound:* sniff test shows normal motion.

- *CT and MRI*
  - Clearly shows elevated portion of the diaphragm anteriorly
  - Can demonstrate thinned but intact diaphragm muscle
  - Compressive atelectasis and ipsilateral volume loss may be evident
- **Note:** differential diagnosis includes hemidiaphragm paralysis, diaphragm hernias, subpulmonic effusion, and other causes of diaphragm displacement

## Treatment

- No treatment is required for most cases.
- In symptomatic cases or following complications, diaphragm plication is effective.
- Plication can be performed by VATS.[113-115]

---

### Brief Illustrative Case

- A 57-year-old woman presented with increasing dyspnea on effort over the preceding 10-week period. She also complained of neck and right shoulder pain.
- History of SLE for more than 20 years that was currently quiescent on minimal dose steroids.
- No chest pain. No constitutional symptoms.
- Examination revealed the following: Normal vital signs. Chest: few crackles at the right base. Normal abdominal excursion. Mild weakness around the right shoulder girdle.
- Pulmonary function tests revealed a FVC of 1.85 L (62%), which fell to 1.57 L in the supine position (−15%).
- Chest x-ray study: significantly elevated right hemidiaphragm with associated mild subsegmental atelectasis (Fig. 51-8). (Not noted on prior chest radiographs)

*(Continued)*

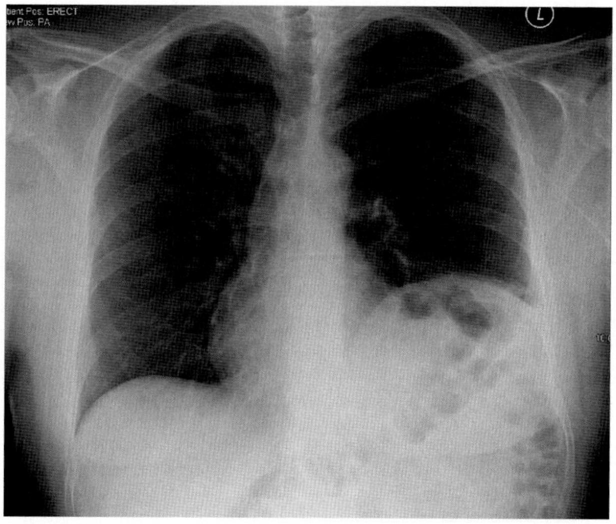

---

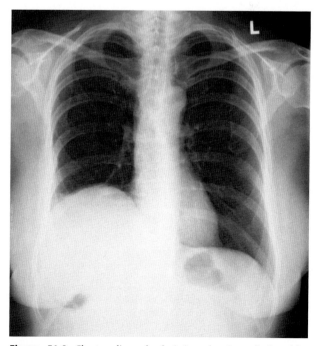

**Figure 51-7:** Chest radiograph depicting eventration of the left hemidiaphragm. Note: Loops of bowel filling subdiaphragmatic space. Unilateral phrenic nerve stimulation revealed normal results for both right and left hemidiaphragms.

**Figure 51-8:** Chest radiograph depicting elevation of the right hemidiaphragm, together with mild subsegmental atelectasis.

## Brief Illustrative Case—cont'd

- Sniff fluoroscopy: paradoxical upward motion of the right hemidiaphragm
- CT chest: elevated right hemidiaphragm; no mass lesions or other abnormalities along the course of the right phrenic nerve.
- MRI of cervical spine and brachial plexus: mild cervical spondylitis C5/6 and C6/7. Normal brachial plexus area.
- Phrenic nerve stimulation: no response on the right; normal left. (No generalized process noted on EMG examination.)

### Key Points

- The patient has clinical evidence of right hemidiaphragm paralysis.
- Likely etiologic considerations include diaphragm involvement due to lupus (vanishing lung syndrome), cervical spondylosis, neuralgic amyotrophy, and idiopathic. Phrenic nerve compression or invasion by a malignant tumor (the most common cause [25%–33%] of unilateral diaphragm paralysis was excluded).
- Vanishing lung syndrome: Rare complication. Usually bilateral. Patient's lupus quiescent both clinically and serologically. May respond to steroid therapy in only a minority of cases.

- Cervical spondylosis: Rare cause. Neck and shoulder pain common. Nerve root compression can result in radicular pain. Muscle atrophy (small muscles of hand) and sensory symptoms in a dermatomal distribution may be present. Cord compression can result in signs of a myelopathy. The distribution and mild nature of cervical disk disease and spondylitic bar formation make this diagnosis unlikely.
- Neuralgic amyotrophy: The presenting symptoms and clinical features are compatible but not diagnostic.
- Often in cases such as these, no firm diagnosis is found despite extensive investigation.
- Therapeutic considerations: Symptomatic therapy. If right hemidiaphragm paralysis is persistent and symptomatic (>1 year), unilateral diaphragm plication could be considered.
- Unilateral diaphragm plication would be expected to produce sustained improvements in pulmonary function studies. FVC: +11.8%; forced expiratory volume in 1 second ($FEV_1$): +15.4%; FRC: +26%; total lung capacity (TLC): +13.3%

## References

Interactive references and additional readings for this chapter can be accessed online at *expertconsult.com*.

# PULMONARY VASCULAR CONDITIONS

## 52 CLINICAL FEATURES AND EVALUATION OF CHRONIC THROMBOEMBOLIC PULMONARY HYPERTENSION

Peter F. Fedullo, MD and William R. Auger, MD

### TERMINOLOGY

- Chronic thromboembolic pulmonary hypertension (CTEPH)
- Pulmonary thromboendarterectomy (PTE)
- Pulmonary arterial hypertension (PAH)

### DEFINITION

CTEPH refers to a variant of secondary PAH characterized by chronic thromboembolic obstruction of the pulmonary arteries. The obstruction may be at any level in the pulmonary arterial system, but only those involving the main, lobar or segmental arteries are amenable to surgical correction.[1,2]

### ETIOLOGY

CTEPH represents an alternate outcome following a single or recurrent episode of acute pulmonary embolism and must be differentiated from in situ PAH, which can occur in the setting of established PAH or parenchymal lung disease.[3]

### ETIOLOGY—KEY FACTS

- Incomplete anatomic recovery following an acute pulmonary embolic event occurs more commonly than was previously recognized.[4,5]
- Estimates of the incidence of CTEPH following acute pulmonary embolism range from 0.5% to 3.8%.[6-8]
- A history of acute venous thromboembolism is not present in approximately 30% of patients presenting with CTEPH.
- Factors that appear to predispose to the development of CTEPH include recurrent embolic events and single events in which more than 50% of the pulmonary vascular bed is occluded.[7,9]

- Thrombophilic states associated with CTEPH include the presence of a lupus anticoagulant, elevated levels of antiphospholipid antibodies, and elevated levels of factor VIII.[10-13]
- Deficiencies of protein C, protein S, antithrombin III, or the presence of factor V Leiden mutation do not appear to be associated with a higher risk of CTEPH.

### CLINICAL FEATURES—SIGNS AND SYMPTOMS

- The symptoms and signs of CTEPH are similar to those of other forms of pulmonary hypertension, depend on the severity of the disease at presentation, and include
  - Exertional dyspnea
  - Fatigue
  - Exertional chest pain
  - Exertional presyncope or syncope
  - Lower extremity edema
  - Right ventricular lift
  - Jugular venous distension
  - Tricuspid or pulmonic regurgitation
- A unique physical finding in 30% of patients with CTEPH is the presence of flow bruits over the lung fields,[14] a finding not encountered in patients with small vessel variants of PAH such as idiopathic PAH.

### DIAGNOSIS

Unlike other variants of PAH, CTEPH is potentially amenable to surgical correction. The primary purpose of the diagnostic evaluation is to quantify the degree of pulmonary hypertension, to establish its etiology, and if major vessel thromboembolic disease is present, to determine whether it is amenable to surgical intervention.[15]

## IMAGING STUDIES

- Chest Radiograph
  - Abnormal in majority
  - Clues: enlarged central pulmonary arteries, asymmetric size of central pulmonary arteries, right ventricular enlargement, areas of parenchymal hypolucency, and peripheral scars consistent with prior infarction.[16]
- Ventilation-perfusion (V/Q) scan
  - Most useful imaging modality to separate large vessel variants of PAH (CTEPH) from small vessel variants such as idiopathic (primary) PAH.[17,18]
  - The V/Q scan in CTEPH is characterized by the presence of segmental or larger mismatched defects (Fig. 52-1), whereas in small vessel variants, the scan is either normal or demonstrates subsegmental defects.
  - Other pulmonary hypertensive disorders that may be associated with segmental or larger perfusion defects include pulmonary veno-occlusive disease, fibrosing mediastinitis, pulmonary artery sarcoma, and large vessel pulmonary vasculitis.[19-21]
  - The abnormalities appearing on the V/Q scan in patients with CTEPH can understate the actual degree of chronic thromboembolic obstruction. Even a single mismatched segmental defect should raise the suspicion of CTEPH.[22]
- Computed tomographic (CT) scan
  - Imaging may demonstrate a mosaic pattern of perfusion, enlargement of the right ventricle or main pulmonary arteries, and peripheral scars consistent with prior infarction.[23-25]
  - Contrast imaging may demonstrate filling defects within the main pulmonary arteries and the presence of bronchial artery collateral vessels.
  - The absence of computed tomographic findings does not completely exclude the possibility of CTEPH.
  - Useful in evaluating the pulmonary parenchyma in patients with coexisting obstructive or restrictive disease.
  - Useful in evaluating the mediastinum when external compression of the pulmonary arteries is suspected (e.g., fibrosing mediastinitis, adenopathy, or malignancy).[26]
- Magnetic resonance angiography (MRA)
  - Emerging technique in the preoperative evaluation of CTEPH.[27-29]
  - Useful in patients with contrast allergy.
  - Does not provide essential hemodynamic data necessary to determine operability and operative risk.
- Echocardiography[30,31]
  - Often the first technique to confirm the presence of resting pulmonary hypertension
  - May demonstrate enlargement of the right atrium and right ventricle, and flattening of the interventricular septum
  - Can provide an estimate of pulmonary artery pressure
  - Using contrast enhancement, can detect the presence of atrial or ventricular level shunts
  - Can provide useful information regarding the status of valvular structures and the left ventricle
- Right heart catheterization with conventional pulmonary angiography
  - At most centers, remains the gold standard for diagnosis[32]
  - Provides essential hemodynamic data
  - More sensitive than CT and MRA in evaluating the segmental pulmonary vessels
  - The angiographic appearance of chronic thromboembolic disease is distinct from that of acute thromboembolic disease and is characterized by the presence of pouch defects; pulmonary arterial webs and bands; complete vascular obstruction at the main, lobar, or segmental level; abrupt vessel narrowing; and intimal irregularities (Fig. 52-2).[33]

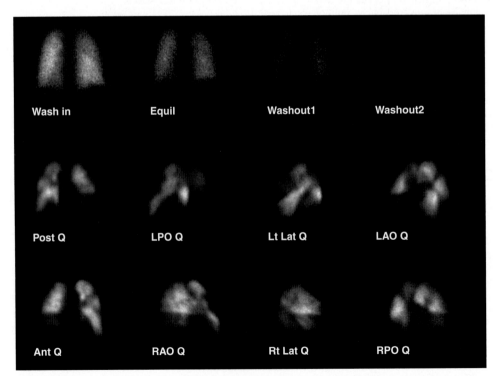

**Figure 52-1:** Lung ventilation-perfusion study in patient with chronic thromboembolic pulmonary hypertension. Large unmatched perfusion defects are seen in both lower lobes.

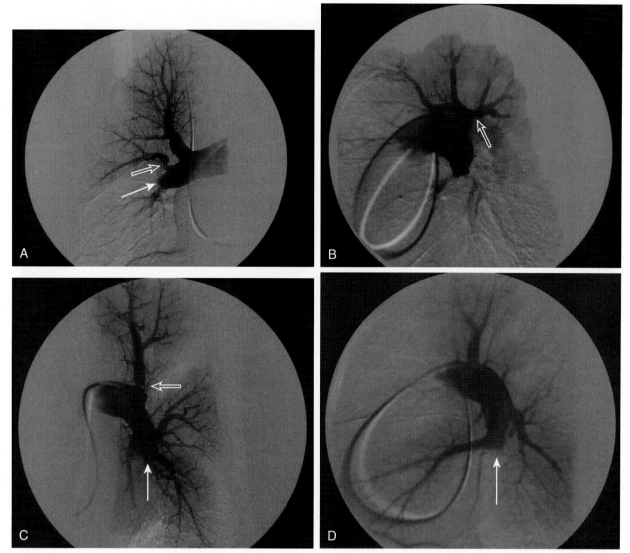

**Figure 52-2: A,** The right pulmonary arteriogram of the patient whose V/Q scan is depicted in Figure 52-1. The solid arrow highlights an angiographic "pouch" occlusion of the right interlobar vessel. The presence of organized thromboembolic disease is also evident by "web" narrowing of the proximal anterior upper lobe artery (*open arrow*). **B,** The lateral right pulmonary arteriogram in the same patient shows another "web" narrowing (*open arrow*) of the proximal posterior upper lobe vessel not appreciated on the anteroposterior films. **C** and **D,** The left pulmonary arteriogram reveals a "pouch defect" in the proximal upper lobe artery (*open arrow*). This is accompanied by an angiographic "web" in the proximal apical artery; the other vessels leading to the upper lobe appear to be occluded. There's a rounded appearance (*solid arrow*) to the distal descending pulmonary artery, with a paucity of vasculature to the lower lobe. The lateral view (**D**) shows a patent lingular artery and superior segmental artery, right lower lobe. This view reveals that the posterior-lateral and anterior-medial vessels to the lower lobe are occluded.

## ADJUNCTIVE STUDIES

- Pulmonary function testing
  - ○ Recommended preoperatively to exclude the possibility of a significant coexisting obstructive or restrictive ventilatory defect
  - ○ Commonly demonstrates a mild restrictive defect thought secondary to areas of pulmonary infarction.[34]
  - ○ Severe reduction (<50%) of the diffusing capacity for carbon monoxide is unusual and should raise the possibility of other disease processes such as pulmonary veno-occlusive disease, interstitial lung disease, or emphysema.[35]
- Arterial blood gas analysis
  - ○ The resting arterial $PO_2$ may be within normal limits. However, the alveolar-arterial oxygen gradient is typically widened and the majority of patients have a decrease in the arterial $PO_2$ with exercise
  - ○ Hypoxemia is related to ventilation-perfusion mismatch, reduction in cardiac ouput, and right-to-left shunting in the presence of a patent foramen ovale.[36]
- Pulmonary angioscopy
  - ○ May be a useful adjunct in a select group of patients.
  - ○ Allows visualization of pulmonary arterial walls to confirm presence of chronic thromboembolic disease and help determine if amenable to surgical intervention.
  - ○ May demonstrate webs, bands, intimal pitting, partial recanalization, masslike chronic embolic material. (Fig. 52-3)
- Coronary angiography
  - ○ Patients with coronary risk factors who are deemed candidates for PTE should undergo coronary angiography before the procedure.

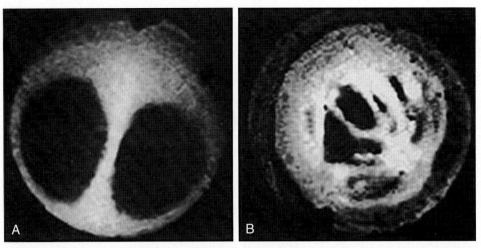

**Figure 52-3: A,** Angioscopic view of a vessel bifurcation in a pulmonary artery free of chronic thrombus, revealing a smooth vascular intima. **B,** Appearance of organized thrombus through a pulmonary angioscope. Note: Recannalization and web formation. *(From Fedullo PF, Auger WR, Channick RN, Kerr KM, Rubin LJ. Chronic thromboembolic pulmonary hypertension. Clin Chest Med 2001;22:561-581, with permission.)*

○ Coronary artery bypass grafting can be performed at the time of thromboendarterectomy
■ Inferior vena cava filter placement
  ○ An inferior vena caval filter is recommended before PTE to protect the patient from embolic recurrence during the early, high-risk postoperative period, when anticoagulation may not be feasible and over the long-term in the event anticoagulant therapy needs to be interrupted.

## SURGICAL SELECTION

The decision to proceed to surgery involves an interplay among anatomic variables (the extent and proximal location of the pulmonary vascular obstruction), hemodynamic variables (the severity of the pulmonary hypertension and the function of the right ventricle), and patient variables (coexisting disease processes that may increase perioperative risk).

■ Patients undergoing surgery, with rare exceptions, have a resting pulmonary vascular resistance in excess of 300 dynes/sec/cm$^{-5}$ (approximately 4 Wood units)
■ The majority of operated patients have a pulmonary vascular resistance in the range of 800 to 1200 dynes/sec/cm$^{-5}$ (10–15 Wood units)
■ Patients who fall into the lower range of pulmonary hemodynamic impairment include those with involvement of a single main pulmonary artery, those with unusually vigorous lifestyle expectations, and those who live at high altitude.
■ Current surgical techniques allow removal of obstructing thrombi whose most proximal location is at the level of the segmental pulmonary arteries.
■ The most complex aspect of the evaluation process, one that requires a considerable experiential base, is determining whether the degree of pulmonary hypertension is consistent with the extent of accessible thromboembolic material and estimating the hemodynamic and symptomatic improvement that might be achieved with surgical intervention.
■ Advanced age or the presence of comorbid disease processes do not represent absolute contraindications to PTE, although they do influence risk assessment, which must be understood and accepted by the patient before surgery.

## SURGICAL TREATMENT

PTE represents the therapeutic modality of choice. This procedure, which must be distinguished from pulmonary embolectomy for hemodynamically massive acute pulmonary embolism, involves cardiopulmonary bypass, deep hypothermia, and periods of complete circulatory arrest.[2,37-39]

Figure 52-4 depicts chronic thromboembolic material removed at the time of surgery from patient depicted in Figures 52-1 and 52-2.

■ Indications:
  ○ Primary modality for patients who meet operative criteria (see Surgical Selection)
■ Postoperative complications[40]
  ○ Similar to those associated with other open heart, bypass procedures including wound infections, atrial and ventricular arrhythmias, bleeding, and delirium.

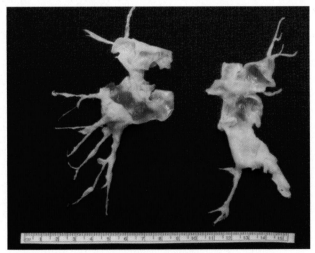

**Figure 52-4:** The chronic thromboembolic material removed at the time of surgery in this patient. (Same patient as in Figure 52-1.)

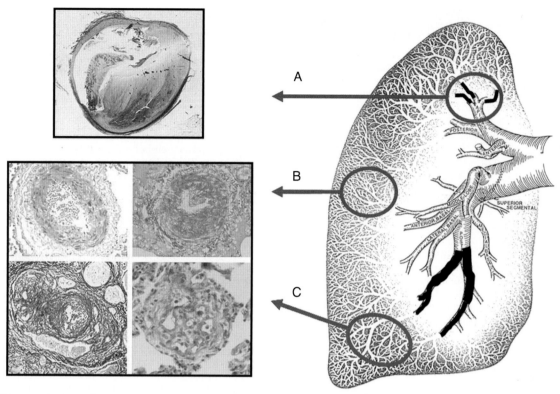

**Figure 52-5:** Mechanisms of small vessel involvement in CTEPH: **A,** Obstruction of subsegmental arteries not amenable to surgery. **B,** Pulmonary arteriopathy in microvasculature not distal to proximal obstructive disease (changes are similar to those noted in pulmonary arterial hypertension of varying etiology). **C,** Pulmonary arteriopathy in small vessels distal to partially or completely obstructed large proximal elastic vessels. *(From Galie N, Kim NHS. Pulmonary microvascular disease in chronic thromboembolic pulmonary hypertension. Proc Am Thorac Soc 2006;3:571-576, with permission.)*

○ Reperfusion pulmonary edema (a localized form of high-permeability, neutrophil-mediated acute lung injury).[41] Occurring to a variable extent in 30% to 40% of patients undergoing PTE, it is limited to those areas of the lung served by pulmonary arteries from which proximal thromboembolic obstruction has been removed. Therapy is supportive until the process resolves.

○ Persistent pulmonary hypertension (defined as a postoperative pulmonary vascular resistance greater than 500 dynes/sec/cm$^{-5}$). Occurring in approximately 15% of patients undergoing the procedure, it remains a major cause of postoperative morbidity and mortality.

○ Overall mortality rates in programs experienced in the diagnosis and management of this disease have fallen in the range of 4% to 8%. Mortality rates are considerably lower in patients with preserved right ventricular function and less severe pulmonary hypertension (PVR < 1000 dynes/sec/cm$^{-5}$).[40,42-44]

■ Efficacy and long-term outcome:

○ A rapid and sustained improvement in pulmonary hypertension, cardiac output, and functional status can be expected postoperatively.[45-47]

○ Patients with residual postoperative pulmonary hypertension may experience subsequent hemodynamic and functional decline and require careful follow-up and consideration of medical management.

○ Pulmonary microvascular disease

○ Pulmonary microvascular disease may be a major factor contributing to progression of pulmonary hypertension in patients with untreated CTEPH, inoperable status

(10%–30%) or persistent postoperative pulmonary hypertension (10%).[48]

○ As illustrated in Figure 52-5, distal small vessel vasculopathy may occur in a number of different settings, such as (1) obstruction of small subsegmental elastic pulmonary arteries, (2) pulmonary arteriopathy occurring distal to nonobstructed proximal vessels, or (3) arteriopathy in microvessels distal to partially or completely obstructed vessels.[48]

○ Preoperative partitioning of PVR to determine upstream resistance (from analysis of the pulmonary artery occlusion pressure waveform; R$up$) has been evaluated as an experimental tool to assist in identifying patients at risk for persistent pulmonary hypertension following PTE.[49] In this study, an estimated R$up$ of less than 60% conferred the highest risk.[49]

## MEDICAL TREATMENT

The long-term efficacy of medical therapy in this disease process remains to be determined. Preliminary data suggest that medical therapy may benefit patients not considered candidates for thromboendarterectomy due either to the distal nature of their embolic disease or to comorbid conditions. Medical therapy may also benefit patients with persistent pulmonary hypertension following thromboendarterectomy. Therapies demonstrated to be effective include the endothelin receptor antagonist bosentan, the phosphodiesterase-5 inhibitor sildenafil, and intravenous epoprostenol.[50-54]

## Brief Illustrative Case

- *History:* A 62-year-old woman with a 15-month history of exertional dyspnea and chest pain. Dyspnea was first noted following an open cholecystectomy complicated by what was believed to be hospital-acquired pneumonia and has slowly progressed to the point where the patient experiences dyspnea while performing normal daily activities (New York Hospital Association Class III). Past medical history is otherwise negative, and there is no history of thromboembolic disease. Family history is strongly positive for coronary artery disease.
- *Examination:* Vitals: resting tachycardia (104/minute); BP = 124/70; RR 16/min at rest; $SPO_2$ = 93% at rest, 86% with exercise. Flow murmur auscultated over right posterior hemithorax. RV tap with prominent P2 component of second heart sound. Trace pedal edema.
- *Blood tests:* Complete blood count and electrolytes were normal.
- *Imaging:* Chest radiograph: enlarged central pulmonary arteries; V/Q scan: multiple bilateral segmental mismatched defects.
- *Echocardiogram:* moderate right atrial and right ventricular enlargement, severe tricuspid regurgitation, estimated pulmonary artery systolic pressure 84 mm Hg, contrast study positive for atrial level shunt.
- *Right heart catheterization:* PA pressure = 94/32 with a mean pressure of 53, PCWP = 10 mm Hg, cardiac output = 3.6 L/min; PVR = 965 $dynes/sec/cm^{-5}$
- *Pulmonary angiography:* Evidence of chronic thromboembolic disease involving the segmental right upper lobe arteries, complete obstruction of the right lower lobe artery, and segmental defects involving the inferior lingula and the left lower lobe arteries.
- *Coronary angiogram:* 85% proximal stenosis of the left anterior descending artery.
- *Management:* PTE and a coronary bypass graft were performed. A small patent foramen ovale was also closed at the time of the procedure. Tricuspid valve replacement was not performed. Postoperative PVR was 360 $dynes/sec/cm^{-5}$. Chest radiograph disclosed an alveolar filling process involving predominantly the right lower lobe lingual, and extubation was delayed 72 hours due to poor oxygenation. The patient was discharged on the 10th postoperative day on full-dose warfarin, low-dose aspirin, and a statin. Echocardiogram before discharge revealed only mild right atrial and right ventricular enlargement, an estimated pulmonary artery systolic pressure of 40 mm Hg, and trace tricuspid regurgitation. Follow-up evaluation was scheduled in 1 to 2 months to determine whether the addition of medical therapy was indicated.

### Key Points

- Typical presentation of CTEPH. A documented history of acute pulmonary embolism is not necessary.
- Pulmonary flow murmurs, although not unique to CTEPH, can suggest the diagnosis.
- The finding of segmental mismatched defects on V/Q scan excludes small vessel variants of PAH.
- Exertional chest pain usually occurs late in the course of CTEPH. The patient is postmenopausal and provided a strong family history of coronary artery disease. Coronary angiography revealed a critical coronary artery stenosis, and bypass grafting was performed at the time of PTE.
- Closure of a patent foramen ovale is undertaken in approximately 25% to 30% of patients undergoing PTE.
- Even in the setting of severe preoperative tricuspid regurgitation, tricuspid valve replacement is rarely necessary owing to reduction in right ventricular size and tricuspid annulus diameter following PTE.
- Postoperative chest radiograph and gas exchange were consistent with mild reperfusion pulmonary edema.
- Early postoperative pulmonary vascular resistance, although substantially improved, remained elevated. However, this may have been the result of reperfusion lung injury and its associated hypoxemia. The predischarge echocardiogram appeared substantially more optimistic in terms of the hemodynamic outcome. Follow-up evaluation is advised with consideration of medical therapy if the pulmonary vascular resistance remains substantially elevated.

## References

 Interactive references and additional readings for this chapter can be accessed online at *expertconsult.com*.

# 53 CHRONIC THROMBOEMBOLIC PULMONARY HYPERTENSION AND PULMONARY THROMBOENDARTERECTOMY

Michael M. Madani, MD, FACS, and
Stuart W. Jamieson, MB, FRCS, FACS

## TERMINOLOGY

- Chronic thromboembolic pulmonary hypertension (CTEPH)
- Pulmonary hypertension secondary to chronic pulmonary emboli
- Pulmonary thromboendarterectomy (PTE)
- Pulmonary endarterectomy (PEA)

## DEFINITION

Pulmonary hypertension and subsequent right-sided heart failure as a result of chronic thromboembolic disease is a relatively uncommon condition, occurring in 1% to 5% of adult patients who survive an acute pulmonary embolic event.[1,2] The unresolved thromboembolic material undergoes chronic fibrotic changes and causes an obstructive lesion that is unresponsive to any medical therapy. The signs and symptoms are related to those of pulmonary hypertension and the subsequent right-sided heart failure. Once chronic pulmonary hypertension develops, the prognosis is poor, and this prognosis is even worse in patients without an intracardiac shunt. The survival of patients with chronic thromboembolic pulmonary hypertension is inversely related to the magnitude of pulmonary artery systolic pressure and pulmonary vascular resistance.[3] When the mean pulmonary artery pressure in patients with thromboembolic disease exceeds 50 mm Hg, the 5-year mortality rate approaches 90%.[4]

## ETIOLOGY

The etiology of chronic thromboembolic pulmonary hypertension is related to the same causative factors as those for deep venous thrombosis and acute pulmonary embolism (PE). One or more elements of Virchow's triad (venous stasis, hypercoagulable state, and intimal injury) are typically present. Although a good portion of patients have no history of deep venous thrombosis (DVT) or PEs, approximately 20% have an underlying hypercoagulopathy. The thromboembolic material within the pulmonary vascular tree generally resolves in time in the majority of patients suffering from acute PE. However, in a certain group of patients, the embolic material persists and eventually transforms into fibrotic obstruction of the pulmonary vasculature.

### Key Facts

- Chronic thromboembolic pulmonary hypertension seems to be an extension of the etiologic factors and natural history of acute PE.
- Benign DVT and venous thromboembolic events (TEs) are the major causes in chronic obstruction of the pulmonary vasculature.
- Hypercoagulable conditions or abnormal fibrinolytic pathways predisposing patients to DVT or venous TE are vague and present in only a subgroup of patients.
- The presence of a lupus anticoagulant or anticardiolipin antibodies can be established in about 10% to 24% of patients with chronic thromboembolic disease.[5,6]
- Protein C, protein S, and antithrombin III deficiencies appear in less than 5% of the patients.[7]
- Factor V Leiden is present in 4% to 6.5% of the patients with CTEPH.[6,8]
- In patients who survive an acute PE, approximately 20% to 50% have unresolved thromboembolic material.
- Approximately 4% to 5% of patients with unresolved pulmonary emboli will develop chronic pulmonary hypertension.
- Other causes
  - Intravascular devices
    - Increasing incidence of placement.
    - Indwelling venous catheters.
    - Pacemaker leads
    - Implantable defibrillator leads
    - Ventriculoatrial (VA) shunts in patients with a history of hydrocephalus
      - Generally, patients with indwelling catheters and intravascular devices have recurrent small thromboemboli.
      - These typically get lodged in the segmental and subsegmental branches of the pulmonary vascular tree, making surgical removal somewhat more challenging.
  - Unilateral disease
    - In rare patients, the disease is confined to one side only (Fig. 53-1).
    - These seem to be in a different category than the patients with typical CTEPH.
    - Typically these patients are women and the disease is confined to the left side only
    - There is no history of DVT or PE, nor is there history of hypercoagulopathy
    - There seems to be an underlying pulmonary vasculopathy related to the left side with subsequent thrombosis
    - In a subgroup of these patients, there will be no reperfusion to the affected lung despite complete endarterectomy
  - Secondary thrombosis
    - In rare cases, the clot within the pulmonary vasculature is secondary to other underlying conditions such as
      - Pulmonary vasculitis
      - Sarcoidosis
      - Fibrosing mediastinitis
  - Tumors
    - Rarely, the cause of chronic pulmonary obstruction and pulmonary hypertension is not related to clot and is secondary to a sarcoma (Fig. 53-2).

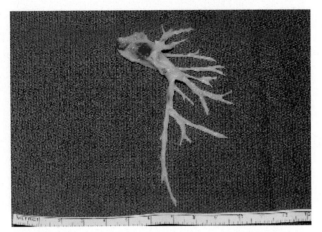

**Figure 53-1:** Specimen removed from a patient with unilateral disease. Note that the disease is more common in women and typically seen in the left lung.

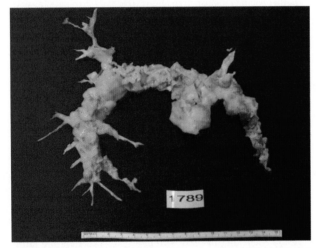

**Figure 53-2:** Specimen removed from a patient with advanced pulmonary sarcoma involving both right and left lungs. Note the gelatinous and glistening appearance of the tumor.

- Pulmonary sarcomas are rare, although their exact incidence is unknown.
- Tumors generally arise from the main pulmonary artery at the supravalvular level but may be valvar or at the subvalvular/right ventricular outflow tract level.
- Prognosis is poor; however, long-term survival with aggressive removal of the tumor and reconstruction of the remaining pulmonary arteries, pulmonary valve, and right ventricular outflow tract (if involved) is rarely possible.

## CLINICAL FEATURES

- There are no *specific* signs or symptoms for chronic thromboembolic pulmonary hypertension.
- **Symptoms**
    ○ The most common symptom associated with CTEPH, as with all other causes of pulmonary hypertension and right-sided heart failure, is exertional dyspnea.
    ○ Dyspnea is out of proportion to any abnormalities found on clinical examination.

○ As with complaints of easy fatigability, dyspnea that initially occurs only with exertion is often attributed to anxiety or being out of shape.
○ Syncope or presyncope (light-headedness during exertion) is another common symptom of pulmonary hypertension. Generally, it occurs in patients with more advanced disease and higher pulmonary arterial pressures.
○ Nonspecific chest pains or tightness occur in approximately 50% of patients with more severe pulmonary hypertension.
○ Hemoptysis can occur in all forms of pulmonary hypertension and probably results from abnormally dilated vessels that are distended by increased intravascular pressures.
○ Peripheral edema, early satiety, and epigastric or right upper quadrant fullness or discomfort develop as the right heart failure progresses.
○ Some patients with chronic pulmonary thromboembolic disease present after a small acute pulmonary embolus that may produce acute symptoms of right heart failure.

- Signs and physical examination
    ○ The physical signs of pulmonary hypertension are the same regardless of the underlying pathophysiology.
    ○ Initially, the jugular venous pulse is characterized by a large A-wave. As the right side of the heart fails, the V-wave becomes predominant as tricuspid regurgitation progresses.
    ○ The right ventricle is usually palpable near the lower left sternal border.
    ○ Pulmonary valve closure may be audible in the left second intercostal space.
    ○ Occasional patients with advanced disease are hypoxic and slightly cyanotic. Clubbing is an uncommon finding.
    ○ The second heart sound is often narrowly split and varies normally with respiration; P2 is accentuated. A sharp systolic ejection click may be heard over the pulmonary artery.
    ○ As the right side of the heart fails, a right atrial gallop usually is present, and tricuspid insufficiency develops.
    ○ Because of the large pressure gradient across the tricuspid valve in pulmonary hypertension, the murmur is high pitched and may not exhibit respiratory variation. These findings are quite different from those usually observed in tricuspid valvular disease.
    ○ A murmur of pulmonic regurgitation may also be detected.
    ○ A specific auscultatory finding to CTEPH is a loud flow murmur heard over the back. This is thought to be related to flow through large bronchial collaterals or flow through stenosed pulmonary vessels.

## DIAGNOSIS

To ensure the diagnosis in patients with right-sided heart failure as a result of chronic pulmonary thromboembolism, a standardized evaluation is recommended for all patients who present with unexplained pulmonary hypertension. This workup includes a variety of imaging studies, as well as right-heart catheterization.

- Electrocardiogram
    ○ The electrocardiogram demonstrates findings of right ventricular hypertrophy.
    ○ Right axis deviation
    ○ Dominant R-wave in V1
- Pulmonary function tests
    ○ Pulmonary function tests are necessary to exclude obstructive or restrictive intrinsic pulmonary parenchymal disease as the cause for the hypertension.
- Echocardiogram
    ○ Perhaps the most useful screening test is a two-dimensional surface echocardiography with Doppler imaging.

○ The standard echo helps to define the presence and severity of right-sided heart failure, tricuspid regurgitation, and severity of pulmonary hypertension.

○ In addition, it is also helpful to rule out certain other causes, such as Eisenmenger's syndrome.

○ Demonstrates right-sided chamber enlargement and right ventricular hypertrophy.

○ The main pulmonary artery is usually enlarged.

○ The intraventricular septum may appear flattened and often exhibits paradoxical motion, with encroachment of the right ventricular septum into the left ventricle in systole.

○ Varying degrees of tricuspid regurgitation are usually present.

○ Continuous wave Doppler scanning of the tricuspid regurgitation jet is helpful in the estimation of the pulmonary artery systolic pressure.

○ Because exercise characteristically increases the pulmonary hypertension, echocardiography with exercise should always be applied whenever the disease is suspected but when the resting echocardiogram demonstrates only subtle abnormalities.

▪ Radiologic studies:

○ Plain chest radiograph

  ▪ May be normal even in patients with severe pulmonary hypertension.

  ▪ May show either apparent vessel cutoffs of the lobar or segmental pulmonary arteries or regions of oligemia, suggesting vascular occlusion.

  ▪ Central pulmonary arteries are generally enlarged, and the right ventricle may also be enlarged without any enlargement of the left atrium or ventricle.

○ Ventilation/perfusion scan

  ▪ The ventilation/perfusion lung scan is the fundamental test for establishing the diagnosis of unresolved pulmonary thromboembolism.

  ▪ An entirely normal lung scan excludes the diagnosis of both acute or chronic, unresolved thrombo-embolism.

  ▪ The usual lung scan pattern in most patients with primary pulmonary hypertension either is relatively normal or shows a diffuse nonuniform perfusion.

  ▪ When subsegmental or larger perfusion defects are noted on the scan, even when matched with ventilatory defects, pulmonary angiography is appropriate to confirm or rule out thromboembolic disease.

○ Computed tomography (CT) scan

  ▪ In recent years higher resolution helical CT scans of the chest have been used more frequently in diagnosis of pulmonary thromboembolic disease.

  ▪ The presence of large clots in lobar or segmental vessels generally confirms the diagnosis (Fig. 53-3).

  ▪ Evidence of organized thrombus lining the pulmonary vessels in an eccentric fashion

  ▪ Enlargement of the right ventricle and the central arteries

  ▪ Variation in size of segmental arteries

  ▪ Parenchymal changes characteristic of pulmonary infarction.

  ▪ CT scans can be helpful in differentiating thromboembolic disease from other causes such as mediastinal fibrosis, lymph nodes, or tumors.

○ Pulmonary angiogram

  ▪ Still the gold standard for diagnosis of CTEPH, although more and more centers are relying on the diagnostic power and the noninvasive nature of high-resolution CT scans and magnetic resonance imaging (MRI) scans.

  ▪ Combined with right-sided heart catheterization, this method allows measurements of hemodynamic numbers and calculation of pulmonary vascular resistance.

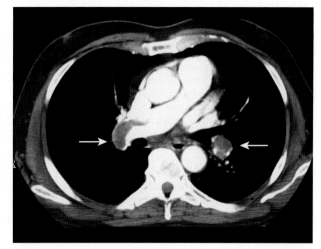

**Figure 53-3:** Computed tomography scan of a patient with significant proximal pulmonary thromboembolic disease. Please note the arrows indicating presence of clot in pulmonary arteries bilaterally.

▪ Organized thromboembolic lesions do not have the appearance of the intravascular filling defects seen with acute pulmonary emboli.

▪ Experience is essential for the proper interpretation of pulmonary angiograms in patients with unresolved, chronic embolic disease.

▪ Organized thrombi appear as unusual filling defects, webs, or bands, or completely thrombosed vessels that may resemble congenital absence of the vessel (Fig. 53-4).

▪ Patients older than 45 years of age undergo coronary arteriography and other cardiac investigation as necessary.

## TREATMENT

### Medical Treatment

▪ There is no curative role for medical management of CTEPH patients.

▪ Medical therapy in CTEPH is palliative at best.

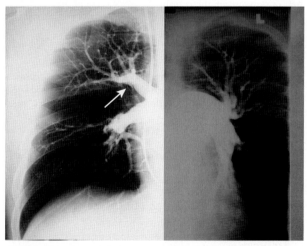

**Figure 53-4:** Right and left pulmonary angiograms demonstrate enlarged pulmonary arteries, poststenotic dilatation of vessels, lack of filling to the periphery in many areas, and abrupt cut-offs of branches. The arrow points to intraluminal filling defects representative of a web or band.

- There are a number of pulmonary vasodilators that are now available for the treatment of the pulmonary hypertension and right-sided heart failure, but considering the fact that the primary pathology in this disease is the physical obstruction of pulmonary vasculature, it is not surprising that their effects are minimal and only transient at best.
- Right ventricular failure may show some improvement with combination of diuretics and vasodilators, but will not resolve until the obstruction is removed.
- The prognosis is unaffected by medical therapy and remains poor.
- Chronic anticoagulation represents the mainstay of the medical regimen.
- Anticoagulation is primarily used to prevent future embolic episodes, but it also serves to limit the development of thrombus in regions of low flow within the pulmonary vasculature.
- Inferior vena caval filters are used routinely to prevent recurrent embolization.

## Surgical Treatment

Pulmonary thromboendarterectomy is the treatment of choice for patients with CTEPH. It is a technically demanding operation that is performed only in select centers around the world. Proper patient selection, meticulous surgical technique, and vigilant postoperative management have contributed to the success of this operation. A true endarterectomy (not an embolectomy) of all affected parts of the lung is essential to clear all affected areas of the pulmonary vasculature. It is clear that PEA relieves pulmonary hypertension by improving lung ventilation/perfusion match and, in turn, improving right ventricular function and tricuspid regurgitation, limiting retrograde extension of clot obstruction, and preventing arteriopathic changes in the remaining patent small pulmonary vessels.[9,10] After operation, once the pulmonary hypertension has resolved, the right ventricle will regress to a normal size and improve its overall function.

Although there have been other reports of surgical treatment of CTEPH, most of the surgical experience in PEA has been reported from the University of California, San Diego (UCSD) Medical Center.[11,12] With our growing experience now accounting for more than 2300 of these procedures, we have established that there are certain principles of this procedure that must be adhered to. Although an endarterectomy is possible even if one deviates from these principles, a successful and complete endarterectomy is not, and such outcomes are questionable.

## Surgical Principles

- PTE is mainstay of treatment in patients with CTEPH.
- Because of the bronchial circulation, pulmonary embolization seldom results in tissue necrosis. Therefore, surgical endarterectomy will allow distal pulmonary tissue to be used once more in gas exchange.
- The surgical approach must be bilateral through a median sternotomy.
  - For pulmonary hypertension to be a major factor, both pulmonary arteries must be substantially involved.
  - It is extremely rare to have unilateral disease as the result of thromboembolism.
  - The only practical approach to both pulmonary arteries is through a median sternotomy incision.
  - A median sternotomy incision, apart from providing bilateral access, avoids entry into the pulmonary vasculature through the pericardium,
  - It also allows the ready institution of cardiopulmonary bypass.

- A unilateral approach through a thoracotomy ignores the disease on the contralateral side, subjects the patient to hemodynamic jeopardy during the clamping of the pulmonary artery, and does not allow good visibility because of the continued presence of bronchial blood flow. Such an approach is outdated and dangerous.
  - In addition, collateral channels develop in chronic thrombotic hypertension not only through the bronchial arteries but also from diaphragmatic, intercostal, and pleural vessels. Therefore, the dissection of the lung in the pleural space via a thoracotomy incision can be extremely bloody.
- Cardiopulmonary bypass is an essential part of this operation.
  - It is integral to ensure cardiovascular stability during the procedure.
  - Cardiopulmonary bypass allows the patient to be cooled in preparation of circulatory arrest, and it is used for rewarming the patient after endarterectomy.
- Complete circulatory arrest under profound hypothermia is necessary for a complete endarterectomy.
  - Thorough endarterectomy is possible only under a bloodless field, so the surgeon can define an adequate endarterectomy plane and then can follow the PEA specimen deep into the subsegmental vessels.
  - Because of the copious bronchial blood flow usually present in these patients, periods of circulatory arrest are necessary to ensure perfect visibility.
  - Although an endarterectomy is possible without circulatory arrest, a complete endarterectomy is not.
  - Surgeons claiming success with a complete endarterectomy without circulatory arrest are likely to leave behind distal disease in the subsegmental branches without recognizing it.
  - The procedure is initiated without circulatory arrest, and depending on the collateral flow through the bronchial arteries and other channels, a variable amount of dissection is possible before the circulation has to be stopped but never a complete dissection.
  - The circulatory arrest periods are typically limited to 20 minutes, with restoration of flow between each arrest.
  - With experience, a complete endarterectomy usually can be performed within a single period of circulatory arrest on each side.
- Developing and recognizing the correct endarterectomy plane is crucial.
  - Another principle of this operation relies mainly on the experience of the operator in recognizing the true endarterectomy plane of the media.
  - The specimen is then followed distally methodically to the feathered tail end in each branch.
  - A plane that is too shallow can leave disease behind and result in residual pulmonary hypertension.
  - A plane too deep can cause a tear in the distal pulmonary arteries with disastrous outcome and uncontrollable massive hemoptysis.
- It is essential to appreciate that the removal of visible thrombus is largely incidental to this operation. Indeed, in most patients, no free thrombus is present; and on initial direct examination, the pulmonary vascular bed may appear normal.
- The early literature on this procedure indicates that thrombectomy was often performed without endarterectomy, and in these cases, the pulmonary artery pressures did not improve, often with the resultant death of the patient.
- Once a complete endarterectomy is performed, the circulation is restarted and the patient is gradually rewarmed to normal body temperature and is taken off cardiopulmonary bypass.

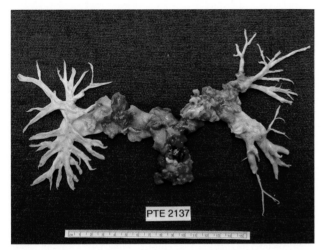

**Figure 53-5:** Type I disease. Surgical specimen removed from a patient showing evidence of some fresh and some old thrombus in the main and both right and left pulmonary arteries. Note that simple removal of the gross disease initially encountered on pulmonary arteriotomy will not be therapeutic, and any meaningful outcome involves a full endarterectomy into all the distal segments.

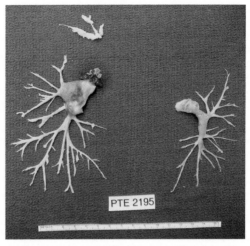

**Figure 53-6:** Specimen removed in a patient with type II disease. Both pulmonary arteries have evidence of chronic thromboembolic material. Note the distal tails of the specimen in each branch. Full resolution of pulmonary hypertension is dependent on complete removal of all the distal tails.

■ Thromboembolic disease classification: There are four broad types of pulmonary occlusive disease related to thrombus that can be appreciated, and we use the following classification[12]:

○ Type I:
- Approximately 20% of cases of thromboembolic pulmonary hypertension (Fig. 53-5)
- It refers to the situation in which major vessel clot is present and readily visible on the opening of the pulmonary arteries.

○ Type II:
- Approximately 60% of cases (Fig. 53-6)
- No major vessel thrombus can be appreciated.
- Thickened intima can be seen, occasionally with webs.
- The endarterectomy plane is raised in the main, lobar, or segmental vessels.

○ Type III:
- Approximately 20% of cases (Fig. 53-7)
- Presents the most challenging surgical situation.
- The disease is very distal and confined to the segmental and subsegmental branches.
- Type III disease is most often associated with presumed repetitive thrombi from indwelling catheters (such as pacemaker wires) or ventriculoatrial shunts.

○ Type IV:
- The disease does not represent primary thromboembolic pulmonary hypertension and is inoperable.
- In this entity there is intrinsic small vessel disease, although secondary thrombus may occur as a result of stasis.
- Small vessel disease may be unrelated to thromboembolic events (primary pulmonary hypertension) or occur in relation to thromboembolic hypertension as a result of a high-flow or high-pressure state in previously unaffected vessels similar to the generation of Eisenmenger's syndrome.
- We believe that there may also be sympathetic cross-talk from an affected contralateral side or stenotic areas in the same lung.

■ Postoperative management
○ Meticulous management of patients following pulmonary thromboendarterectomy is absolutely essential.
○ A complete understanding of the physiologic changes that occur postoperatively is necessary to achieve successful outcome.

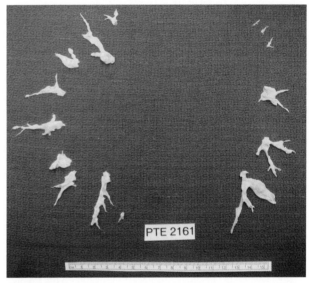

**Figure 53-7:** Specimen removed from a patient with type III disease. Note that the disease is distal, and the plane was raised at each segmental level.

○ Most aspects of management involving these patients are very similar to other patients undergoing cardiac surgery involving cardiopulmonary bypass.
○ Complications are also similar to other cardiac surgery patients and may include arrhythmias, coagulation disorders, bleeding, wound infections, nosocomial pneumonias, and rare delirium.
○ Cerebrovascular accidents and myocardial infarctions are extremely rare despite the use of circulatory arrest.
○ All patients are mechanically ventilated overnight, and all patients are subjected to a maintained diuresis, with the goal of reaching the patient's preoperative weight within 24 hours.
○ The electrocardiogram, systemic and pulmonary arterial and central venous pressures, temperature, urine output, arterial oxygen saturation, chest tube drainage, and fluid balance are monitored.

○ A pulse oximeter is used to continuously monitor peripheral oxygen saturation.

○ In addition, higher minute ventilation is often required early after the operation to compensate for the temporary metabolic acidosis that develops after the long period of circulatory arrest, hypothermia, and cardiopulmonary bypass.

○ Tidal volumes higher than those normally recommended after cardiac surgery are therefore generally used to obtain optimal gas exchange. The maximum inspiratory pressure is maintained below 30 cm of water, if possible.

○ Management of cardiac arrhythmias and output, and treatment of wound bleeding are identical to other open heart operations.

○ Diuresis
  ■ Patients have considerable positive fluid balance after operation.
  ■ After hypothermic circulatory arrest, patients initiate an early spontaneous aggressive diuresis for unknown reasons, which may, in part, be related to the increased cardiac output related to a now lower PVR level, and improved RV function.
  ■ This should be augmented with diuretics, however, with the aim of returning the patient to the preoperative fluid balance within 24 hours of operation.
  ■ Because of the increased cardiac output, some degree of systemic hypotension is readily tolerated.
  ■ Fluid administration is minimized.
  ■ The patient's hematocrit level should be maintained above 30% to increase oxygen-carrying capacity and mitigate against the pulmonary reperfusion phenomenon.

○ Arrhythmias
  ■ The development of atrial arrhythmias, at approximately 10%, is no more common than that encountered in patients who undergo other types of nonvalvular heart surgery.
  ■ Atrial arrhythmias are managed in a fashion similar to that of other cardiac procedures.

○ Transfusion
  ■ Despite the requirement for the maintenance of an adequate hematocrit level, with careful blood conservation techniques used during operation, transfusion is required in a minority of patients.

○ Inferior vena cava filter and anticoagulation
  ■ A Greenfield filter is usually inserted before the operation, to minimize recurrent PE after PEA.
  ■ Postoperative venous thrombosis prophylaxis with intermittent pneumatic compression devices is used.
  ■ The use of subcutaneous heparin is begun on the evening of surgery.
  ■ Anticoagulation with warfarin is begun as soon as the pacing wires and mediastinal drainage tubes are removed, with a target International Normalized Ratio (INR) of 2.5 to 3.
  ■ In patients with hypercoagulopathy a more aggressive anticoagulation protocol is used in the immediate postoperative period:
    ○ Generally, a heparin drip is started once the chest tube output is less than 50 mL/h for at least 2 consecutive hours
    ○ A target partial thromboplastin time (PTT) of about 60 to 70 is then used

## COMPLICATIONS

Patients are subject to all complications associated with open heart and major lung surgery (e.g., arrhythmias, atelectasis, wound infection, pneumonia, mediastinal bleeding) but also may develop complications specific to this operation. These include persistent pulmonary hypertension and reperfusion pulmonary response.

■ Persistent pulmonary hypertension
  ○ In a few patients, an immediately normal pulmonary vascular tone is not achieved, but an additional substantial reduction may occur over the next few days.
  ○ In such patients, it is usual to see a large pulmonary artery pulse pressure; the low diastolic pressure indicating good runoff, yet persistent pulmonary arterial inflexibility still resulting in a high systolic pressure.
  ○ There are a few patients in whom the pulmonary artery pressures does not resolve substantially, mainly because of misdiagnosis in ther original condition, such as in type IV patients.
  ○ We do operate on some patients with severe pulmonary hypertension but equivocal embolic disease. Despite the considerable risk of attempted endarterectomy in these patients, because transplantation is the only other avenue of therapy, there may be a point when it is unlikely that a patient will survive until a donor is found.
  ○ In our most recent 500 patients, more than one third of perioperative deaths were directly attributable to the problem of inadequate relief of pulmonary artery hypertension.
  ○ This was a diagnostic rather than an operative technical problem.
  ○ Attempts at pharmacologic manipulation of high residual PVR levels with sodium nitroprusside, epoprostenol sodium, or inhaled nitric oxide are generally not effective.
  ○ Because the residual hypertensive defect is fixed, it is not appropriate to use mechanical circulatory support or extracorporeal membrane oxygenation in these patients if they deteriorate subsequently.

■ The reperfusion response or reperfusion injury
  ○ Reperfusion response or reperfusion injury is defined as a radiologic opacity seen in the lungs usually within 72 hours of PEA. Therefore, this unfortunately loose definition may encompass many causes, such as fluid overload and infection (Fig. 53-8).

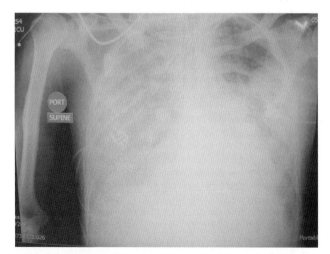

**Figure 53-8:** Postoperative chest radiograph of a patient with significant bilateral pulmonary reperfusion injury. Patient had undergone successful bilateral pulmonary thromboendarterectomy with excellent hemodynamic outcome and lung function. He was extubated on first postoperative day with minimal oxygen requirements, but on third postoperative day, he developed reperfusion edema and required intubation shortly afterward. The chest radiograph was taken 1 week after surgery at the height of reperfusion injury and before recovery.

- ○ It seems to be a form of high-permeability, neutrophil-mediated lung damage.
- ○ It generally leads to prolonged mechanical ventilation (over 2 days).
- ○ True reperfusion injury that directly adversely affects the clinical course of the patient now occurs in approximately 10% of patients.
- ○ In its most dramatic form, it occurs soon after operation (within a few hours) and is associated with profound desaturation.
- ○ Edema-like fluid, sometimes with a bloody tinge, is suctioned from the endotracheal tube.[13]
- ○ However, frank blood from the endotracheal tube signifies a mechanical violation of the blood airway barrier has occurred at operation and stems from a technical error. This complication should be managed, if possible, by identification of the affected area by bronchoscopy and balloon occlusion of the affected lobe until coagulation can be normalized.
- ○ The reperfusion phenomenon is often encountered in patients after a seemingly technically perfect operation with complete resolution of high pulmonary artery pressures.
  - ■ In these cases, the response may be one of reactive hyperemia, after the revascularization of segments of the pulmonary arterial bed that have long experienced no flow.
  - ■ Other contributing factors may include perioperative pulmonary ischemia and conditions associated with high permeability lung injury in the area of the now denuded endothelium.
- ○ Fortunately, the incidence of this complication is much less common now in our series, probably as a result of the more complete and expeditious removal of the endarterectomy specimen that has come with the large experience over the last decade.
- ■ Management of the reperfusion response
  - ○ Early measures should be taken to minimize the development of pulmonary edema with diuresis, maintenance of the hematocrit levels, and the early use of peak end-expiratory pressure.
  - ○ Once a capillary leak has been established, treatment is supportive because reperfusion pulmonary edema will eventually resolve if satisfactory hemodynamics and oxygenation can be maintained.
  - ○ Careful management of ventilation and fluid balance is required.
  - ○ The hematocrit is kept high (>28%), and the patient undergoes aggressive diuresis, even if this requires ultrafiltration.
  - ○ The patient's ventilatory status may be dramatically position sensitive. The $FiO_2$ level is kept as low as is compatible with an oxygen saturation of 90%.
  - ○ A careful titration of positive end-expiratory pressure is carried out, with a progressive transition from volume-limited to pressure-limited inverse ratio ventilation and the acceptance of moderate hypercapnia.
  - ○ The use of steroids is discouraged because they are generally ineffective and may lead to infection.
  - ○ Infrequently, inhaled nitric oxide at 20 to 40 parts per million can improve the gas exchange.
  - ○ Extracorporeal perfusion support
    - ■ On occasion we have used extracorporeal perfusion support (extracorporeal membrane oxygenator or extracorporeal carbon dioxide removal) until ventilation can be resumed satisfactorily, usually after 7 to 10 days.[14]
    - ■ Use of perfusion support is limited to patients who have benefited from hemodynamic improvement, but are suffering from significant reperfusion response.
    - ■ Extracorporeal devices should not be used if there is no evidence or hope of subsequent hemodynamic improvement, because it carries a mortality rate close to 100%, and will not play a role in improving irreversible pulmonary pressures.
- ■ Delirium
  - ○ Early in the PEA experience (before 1990), there was a substantial incidence of postoperative delirium.
  - ○ A study of 28 patients who underwent PEA showed that 77% experienced the development of this complication.[15,16]
  - ○ Delirium appeared to be related to an accumulated duration of circulatory arrest time of more than 55 minutes.
  - ○ The incidence fell to 11% with significantly shorter periods of arrest time.[15-17]
  - ○ With the more expeditious operation that has come with our increased experience, postoperative confusion is now encountered no more commonly than with ordinary open heart surgery.
- ■ Pericardial effusion
  - ○ Encountered more frequently in these patients than other routine cardiac surgery patients.
  - ○ Probably secondary to the lymphatic tissue that is encountered during the dissection of the hilum and the mobilization of the superior vena cava.
  - ○ Also combined with the diminution of cardiac size that occurs immediately after the operation.
  - ○ Another contributing factor is the aggressive anticoagulation regimen postoperatively.
  - ○ It is now our practice to either create a posterior pericardial window at the end of the operation, or place a posterior pericardial drain, which we usually keep longer.
  - ○ These techniques have essentially eliminated the problem, and in general, it is much easier to treat the pleural effusion on the left side in the occasional patient who may develop this complication.

## *RESULTS*

- ■ For the last 1000 patients in our series at UCSD, the mortality rate has been in the range of 4%.
- ■ Hemodynamic response is usually instant.
- ■ Long-term follow-up shows that the hemodynamic benefits are permanent and sustained.
- ■ Right-sided heart remodeling results in the resumption of tricuspid competence.
- ■ In experienced hands, there is no disease that is too distal or surgically inaccessible.
- ■ There is no degree of right-sided heart failure or pulmonary hypertension or high pulmonary vascular resistance that is considered inoperable.
- ■ The most valuable assessment of likely outcome is to match the pulmonary vascular resistance with the degree of angiographic occlusion on angiogram. Discordance between these two may be related to secondary or Eisenmenger-like changes in the remaining open pulmonary vascular bed.
- ■ Such discordance should not prevent operation but may mean that complete resolution of pulmonary hypertension may not occur.

Brief Illustrative Case (See Chapter 52)

## **References**

 Interactive references and additional readings for this chapter can be accessed online at *expertconsult.com*.

# THORACIC TRAUMA

## 54 INITIAL TRAUMA MANAGEMENT

Tina T. Ng, MD and Daniel R. Margulies, MD

## KEY WORDS

- Advanced Trauma Life Support (ATLS)
- Rapid sequence intubation
- Glasgow Coma Scale (GCS)

## INTRODUCTION

- Trauma is a public health issue and one of the leading causes of morbidity and mortality.
- Trauma mortality has a trimodal distribution.[1]
- Seconds to minutes after injury:
  - Major injury to aorta, heart, brain stem, or spinal cord, or acute respiratory distress usually contributes to death during the first mortality peak.
  - These patients are unlikely to be salvageable.
- Minutes to the few hours after injury (the so-called golden hour):
  - Death during the second peak is likely due to epidural or subdural hematoma, hemopneumothorax, severe liver or spleen injury, pelvic fractures, or injuries involving major hemorrhage.
  - The main objective of ATLS protocol is to reduce mortality during this critical period.
- Days to weeks after injury:
  - Death during the third peak usually stems from multisystem organ failure and infection. Not infrequently, withdrawal of care is selected because of a poor prognosis such as after severe head trauma.

## INITIAL ASSESSMENT

ATLS outlines the correct prioritization of diagnostic and therapeutic interventions. The surgeon plays a key role in the proper evaluation and resuscitation. The primary survey constitutes the **ABCDE** of trauma care:

- **A**irway maintenance with cervical spine precaution
- **B**reathing
- **C**irculation
- **D**isability
- **E**xposure and environmental control

## AIRWAY

- The first priority is establishment of airway patency and air exchange.
  - Assessment includes inspecting the oropharynx for foreign body obstruction, observing chest wall movements, and listening for breath sounds at the patient's nose, mouth, and chest, and palpation.
  - Maxillofacial trauma can produce fracture and dislocation, leading to airway obstruction. Neck and laryngeal trauma can cause significant disruption and hemorrhage, thereby compromising the airway.
- Maneuvers such as repositioning the head and mandible (chin lift and jaw thrust), and removing foreign objects from oropharynx can help establish airway patency.
- Cervical spine precaution is critically important. Cervical spine injury is assumed in any patient with multisystem injuries or altered level of consciousness.
  - Inline cervical spine immobilization techniques must be used to protect spine and spinal cord.
- Patients with an altered level of consciousness may not be able to protect their airway.
- Should there be any doubt about a patient's ability to maintain airway patency, establishing definitive airway control is necessary (Table 54-1).
- Rapid-sequence intubation is a technique of administering fast-acting anesthetic agent, followed by neuromuscular blocker, thereby allowing efficient airway establishment. The combination of etomidate and succinylcholine is frequently used.
- Endotracheal intubation:
  - Orotracheal intubation: frequently used technique for airway establishment
  - Nasotracheal intubation: contraindicated in the apneic patient
- Surgical airway: indicated in the patient with significant maxillofacial injury, anatomically distorted injury, or in whom endotracheal intubation cannot be performed
  - Cricothyroidotomy: the preferred method of surgical airway whereby an endotracheal tube or tracheostomy tube is inserted through the cricothyroid membrane
  - Tracheostomy: indicated in patients with severe laryngeal trauma or patients younger than 12 years of age

| TABLE 54-1 ■ INDICATIONS FOR ESTABLISHING DEFINITIVE AIRWAY | |
|---|---|
| **Need for Airway Patency** | **Need for Ventilation** |
| Altered mental status (GCS score < 8) | Apnea |
| Severe maxillofacial injuries | Respiratory distress and inadequate air exchange |
| Risk for aspiration | Severe head injury with need for hyperventilation |
|   Severe orophayngeal bleeding | |
|   Vomiting | |
| Risk for airway obstruction | |
|   Expanding neck hematoma | |
|   Laryngeal injury | |
|   Tracheal injury | |

GCS, Glasgow Coma Scale.

## BREATHING

- After establishing airway control, adequate gas exchange and ventilation are assessed.
- Evaluation of the patient's breathing involves three elements:
  ○ Inspection of chest wall movement and chest injuries.
  ○ Auscultation for equal and symmetric breath sounds.
  ○ Palpation to detect chest injuries.
- Plain chest radiograph (CXR), pulse oximetry, and arterial blood gas are useful diagnostic tools.
- Life-threatening thoracic injuries, such as hemopneumothorax or tension pneumothorax, should be recognized and managed immediately on recognition. Refer to Chapter 55 for a detailed discussion of thoracic injuries.

## CIRCULATION

- After airway and breathing are evaluated, the circulatory system is assessed. The aim is to evaluate the patient's hemodynamic status and to control hemorrhage.
- Hypotension is frequently secondary to hypovolemia. Assessment of the patient's volume status involves several clinical factors.
  ○ Level of consciousness:
    ■ Hypovolemia can lead to impaired cerebral perfusion, resulting in altered level of consciousness.

○ Skin color and capillary refill
○ Pulse: assess for symmetry, rate, regularity, and quality
○ Urinary output: Foley catheter should be placed for accurate assessment of urine output.
- Intravenous lines should be placed to permit fluid resuscitation.
  ○ Placement of at least two large-bore (16-gauge or larger) catheters in peripheral veins is necessary.
  ○ If peripheral lines cannot be established, central lines should be placed. Femoral access is preferred over subclavian vein. Saphenous vein cutdown is an alternate route. In small children, intraosseous infusion is the preferred route.
- Fluid resuscitation begins with 1-liter bolus of lactated Ringer's or normal saline solution for an adult or 20 ml/kg for a child.
- Blood transfusion should be considered if the patient does not respond to fluid bolus adequately.
- Determine response to bolus therapy by frequent assessment of the above-mentioned clinical factors.[2]
  ○ The patient's response to bolus therapy and clinical presentation reflect the degree of hemorrhage (Table 54-2).
- The surgeon must recognize and treat life-threatening thoracic injuries, such as pericardial tamponade. Refer to Chapter 55 for a detailed discussion of thoracic injuries.

## DISABILITY

- The patient's neurologic status should be rapidly assessed. Four elements are evaluated[3]:
  ○ GCS
    ■ Assess the patient's eye opening, response to verbal stimuli, and response to painful stimuli (Table 54-3)
  ○ Pupillary response
    ■ Assess pupil diameter and reaction to light.
  ○ Lateralizing signs
  ○ Spinal cord injury level
- Note that the patient's neurologic status can be influenced by sedatives or neuromuscular blockers.

## EXPOSURE/ENVIRONMENTAL CONTROL

- The patient should be completely undressed so that a full assessment of injuries can be performed.
- After thorough evaluation, the patient should be covered with blankets.
  ○ Hypothermia can be prevented with warm blankets, external warming devices, and infusion of warm intravenous fluids.

| TABLE 54-2 ■ CLASSES OF HEMORRHAGE | | | | |
|---|---|---|---|---|
| | **Class I** | **Class II** | **Class III** | **Class IV** |
| Blood loss (mL) | <750 | 750–1500 | 1500–2000 | >2000 |
| Blood loss (percentage of blood volume) | <15% | 15–30% | 30–40% | >40% |
| Pulse rate | <100 | >100 | >120 | >140 |
| Blood pressure | Normal | Normal | Decreased | Decreased |
| Pulse pressure (mm Hg) | Normal or increased | Decreased | Decreased | Decreased |
| Respiratory rate | 14–20 | 20–30 | 30–40 | >35 |
| Urine output (mL/h) | >30 | 20–30 | 5–15 | Negligible |
| Mental status | Slightly anxious | Mildly anxious | Anxious, confused | Confused, lethargic |

## TABLE 54-3 ■ GLASGOW COMA SCALE

| Feature | Score |
| --- | --- |
| **Eye Opening** | |
| Spontaneous | 4 |
| To verbal stimulus | 3 |
| To painful stimulus | 2 |
| Eyes close | 1 |
| **Best Verbal Response** | |
| Oriented and appropriate | 5 |
| Confused | 4 |
| Inappropriate words | 3 |
| Inappropriate sounds | 2 |
| No sound | 1 |
| **Best Motor Response** | |
| Obeys commands | 6 |
| Localizes painful stimulus, purposeful movement | 5 |
| Withdraws from pain | 4 |
| Flexion (decorticate posture) | 3 |
| Extension (decerebrate posture) | 2 |
| No response | 1 |
| **Total GCS** | 3–15 |

GCS, Glasgow Coma Score.

## CONCLUSION

■ The ATLS protocol aims to reduce trauma mortality during the golden hour.

■ The primary survey is a systemic approach to identifying life-threatening injuries.

■ The trauma surgeon plays a key role in implementing the correct sequence of diagnostic studies and therapeutic interventions. Life-threatening injuries must be recognized and treated immediately upon recognition.

### Brief Illustrative Case

• A 25-year-old man sustained multiple gunshot wounds at a drive-by shooting scene.

#### Primary Survey

• Airway:
  • Airway appeared clear and patent.
  • Patient appeared alert and awake to protect his airway.
  • Patient had a cervical collar to stabilize his cervical spine, pending further evaluation for clearance.
• Breathing:
  • On examination, he had diminished breath sounds in the left chest and moderate subcutaneous emphysema involving bilateral chest. One bullet entrance wound was found in the left posterior chest, and one bullet entrance wound found in the left lower leg. No corresponding exit wound was seen.
  • He maintained adequate saturations on nasal cannula.
  • He was mildly tachypneic. No use of accessory respiratory muscles was present.
  • Initial plain chest radiograph revealed bilateral subcutaneous emphysema, pneumomediastinum,

right upper lobe and left lower lobe pulmonary contusions. There was also a left pleural effusion (Fig. 54-1).
  • Given the suspicion of a left pneumohemothorax, a left tube thoracostomy was performed.
• Circulation:
  • Patient's systolic blood pressure maintained above 100 mm Hg. He was mildly tachycardic (100–110 min) but had palpable 2+ radial and femoral pulses. Capillary refill was less than 2 seconds.
  • Adequate IV accesses in bilateral antecubital fossae were obtained. Normal saline intravenous fluids were started.
  • A Foley catheter was placed, and the initial urine output was approximately 30 mL.
  • Patient remained alert and following commands, implying adequate cerebral perfusion.
• Disability:
  • Patient's GCS score was 15.
  • Patient's pupils were 3 mm and briskly reactive to light.
  • Patient moved all extremities with grossly intact strength and motor function. There were no lateralizing signs or evidence to suggest spinal cord injury.
• Exposure/environmental control:
  • Patient was completely undressed, and all apparent injuries were identified.
  • Patient was warmed with blankets and kept on warm intravenous fluids.

#### Secondary Survey

• Further diagnostic studies were indicated given the severity of the injury.
• *Computed tomography of the chest* confirmed the suspicion of a left pneumohemothorax and also revealed a right pneumohemothorax. Lacerations and pulmonary contusions were identified in the left lower lobe and

*(Continued)*

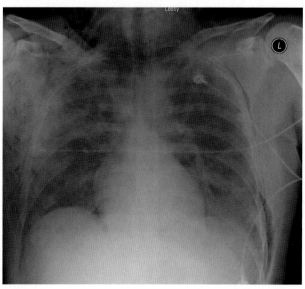

**Figure 54-1:** A plain chest radiograph showing bilateral subcutaneous emphysema, pneumomediastinum, bilateral pulmonary contusions, and left pleural effusion.

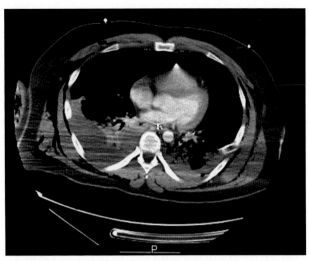

**Figure 54-2:** Computed tomography of the chest demonstrated bilateral pneumohemothoraces, left chest tube, pulmonary contusions and lacerations, bilateral lower lobes collapse, and pneumomediastinum.

### Brief Illustrative Case—cont'd

posterior segment of the right upper lobe. There is also collapse of right and left lower lobes secondary to a transmediastinal bullet (Fig. 54-2).

• Pneumomediastinum was seen in the prevertebral soft tissues of the mid thoracic spine along the suspected course of the bullet tract, and hence, an esophageal injury was suspected.

• An *esophogram* was performed, and no esophageal injury was detected (Fig. 54-3).

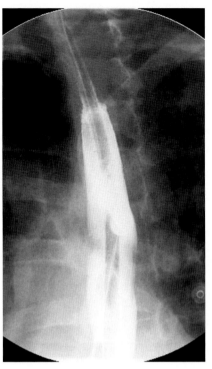

**Figure 54-3:** The absence of contrast leak on esophogram ruled out esophageal perforation.

### References

Interactive references and additional readings for this chapter can be accessed online at *expertconsult.com*.

# 55 MANAGEMENT OF THORACIC TRAUMA

John D. Symbas, MD, Tina T. Ng, MD, Daniel R. Margulies, MD, and Panagiotis N. Symbas, MD

## TERMINOLOGY

▪ Thoracic trauma
▪ Trauma to the chest
▪ Penetrating and blunt trauma to the thorax

## DEFINITION

Thoracic trauma encompasses the sequalae secondary to trauma to all of the thoracic organs: heart, great vessels, lungs, airways, esophagus, diaphragm, and chest wall.

## KEY WORDS

▪ Simple pneumothorax
▪ Tension pneumothorax
▪ Open pneumothorax
▪ Hemothorax
▪ Flail chest
▪ Rib fracture
▪ Pulmonary contusion and penetrating lung parenchymal injury
▪ Cardiac tamponade
▪ Blunt and penetrating cardiac injuries
▪ Traumatic aortic disruption

- Tracheobronchial injury
- Esophageal injury
- Traumatic diaphragmatic injury
- Transmediastinal penetrating injury
- Subcutaneous emphysema
- Emergency thoracotomy
- Video-assisted thoracic surgery (VATS)

# EPIDEMIOLOGY

- Thoracic injuries account for approximately 20% to 25% of trauma mortality, second to head and spinal injuries.[1-5]
- It is the leading cause of death in young people of the industrialized nations, as well as the number one cause for prolonged hospitalization and loss of working days.
- Most thoracic trauma can be treated with airway control, needle/tube thoracostomy, respiratory support, and analgesia.
- Less than 10% of blunt trauma and 15% to 30% of penetrating trauma require operative intervention.[6]

# PATHOPHYSIOLOGY

- Chest trauma leads to hypoxia, hypercapnia, and metabolic acidosis.[6]
  - ○ Hypoxia is due to inadequate oxygen delivery from airway obstruction, hypovolemia, pulmonary ventilation/perfusion mismatch, or intrathoracic pressure changes.
  - ○ Hypercapnia is due to hypoventilation, which is often associated with altered mental status from head injuries or exogenous intoxication. It can also stem from chest wall dysfunction.
  - ○ Acidosis is secondary to tissue hypoperfusion.
- Penetrating thoracic trauma occurs when an object or projectile causes anatomic disruption, frequently leading to hemorrhage.[7]
- Three types of force lead to blunt thoracic trauma[8]:
  - ○ Thoracic compression
    - ▪ Rib fractures occur when applied pressure overcomes thoracic cage strength.
  - ○ Shearing forces
    - ▪ Bell clanger effect: aortic transection occurs when rapid acceleration or deceleration exceeds the tensile strength of the attached tissue, leading to tear or rupture.
  - ○ Explosions
    - ▪ Blast pressure wave creates a pressure differential, transmitting force to the lung.
    - ▪ Blast injury can produce subcutaneous emphysema.

# INITIAL ASSESSMENT

- The primary survey as outlined by Advanced Trauma Life Support (ATLS) dictates the initial management of chest trauma patients.[6]
  - ○ The first priority is establishment of airway patency and air exchange.
  - ○ Assessment includes inspecting the oropharynx for foreign body obstruction, observing chest wall movements, palpation, and listening for breath sounds at the patient's nose, mouth, and chest.
  - ○ Maxillofacial trauma can produce fracture and dislocation, leading to airway obstruction.
  - ○ Neck and laryngeal trauma can cause significant disruption and hemorrhage, thereby compromising the airway.
    - ▪ The triad of symptoms for laryngeal injury is hoarseness, subcutaneous emphysema, and palpable fractures.
  - ○ Maneuvers such as repositioning the head and mandible (chin lift and jaw thrust), and removing foreign objects from the oropharynx can help clear airway.
  - ○ Patients with more severe injuries may require establishment of definite airway, either by endotracheal (nasal or oral) intubation or by a surgical airway (cricothyroidotomy).
- The secondary survey is a systematic examination that incorporates ancillary tools to identify other life-threatening chest injuries.
  - ○ Plain chest radiograph (CXR), arterial blood gas (ABG) measurement, pulse oximetry monitoring, and electrocardiographic (ECG) monitoring are useful diagnostic modalities.
  - ○ Other tools include ultrasound, computed tomography (CT) of the chest, bronchoscopy, esophagography, and angiography.
  - ○ Diagnosis of chest injuries ultimately relies on a high index of suspicion.

# ETIOLOGY—KEY FACTS

## Penetrating Trauma

Most penetrating thoracic injuries are due to missile or knife wounds, but the intrathoracic organs are occasionally punctured by a bony fragment resulting from nonpenetrating trauma.

Penetrating injuries of the chest may cause one or more of the following clinical conditions[2]:

- Sucking wound of the chest
- Hemothorax or hemopneumothorax
- Tension pneumothorax
- Penetrating wound of the lung
- Penetrating wound of the trachea or bronchus
- Penetrating wound of the esophagus or diaphragm
- Penetrating wound of the heart
- Penetrating wound of the great vessels

## Blunt Trauma

The vast majority of blunt injuries to the thorax are due to vehicular accidents, although other forms of trauma from various sports or falls may also cause such injury. Blunt traumatic injury to the chest may result in a variety of clinical conditions[2]:

- Sucking wound of the chest
- Tension pneumothorax
- Rupture of the airways
- Rupture of the diaphragm
- Rupture of the aorta
- Rupture or contusion of the heart

# SPECIFIC CONDITIONS

## Pneumothorax

**Definition:** A pneumothorax is defined as a condition in which air leaks into the pleural cavity; the normally negative intrathoracic pressure becomes more positive. Air in the potential space collapses the lung, thereby creating a ventilation/perfusion mismatch.[9]

- Pneumothorax can be due to blunt chest injury causing rib fractures and lung laceration or penetrating chest trauma.

### Simple Pneumothorax

- Decreased lung volume without mediastinal shift or hypotension
- Clinical features:
  - ○ Decreased breath sounds, hyperresonance to percussion, depressed lung expansion during inspiration
- Diagnostic investigations:
  - ○ Plain chest radiograph shows decreased lung volume, a visceral pleural line and air in the pleural cavity (Fig. 55-1).
- Treatment: tube thoracostomy in the fourth or fifth intercostal space, anterior to midaxillary line.

### Tension Pneumothorax

- Accumulation of air from lung or airway injuries into the pleural space under pressure.
- One-way-valve air leak results in air being forced into the pleural space without outlet to escape so complete lung collapse occurs.
- Complete lung collapse causes tracheal deviation and mediastinal shift that compresses the opposite lung and compromises venous return.
- The resulting impaired cardiac output leads to hypotension and hypoxia.
- A simple pneumothorax can become a tension pneumothorax if it is not managed initially or if positive pressure ventilation is applied. All patients with pneumothorax should undergo tube thoracostomy before administration of mechanical ventilation.
- Patients suspected to have tension pneumothorax should be diagnosed clinically and not radiographically. A plain chest radiograph is depicted in Figure 55-2.
- Clinical features:
  - ○ Tachypnea, dyspnea, tracheal deviation, distended neck veins, unilateral absence of breath sounds, hypotension, diaphoresis, and cyanosis.
  - ○ Displacement of the maximum cardiac impulse.
- Treatment:
  - ○ Immediate decompression with needle thoracostomy in the second intercostal space in the midclavicular line converts the injury into a simple pneumothorax.
  - ○ Definite treatment with tube thoracostomy in the fourth or fifth intercostal space, anterior to midaxillary line.

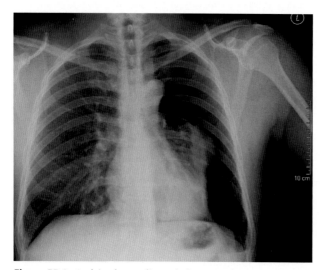

**Figure 55-1:** A plain chest radiograph demonstrating a complete left pneumothorax.

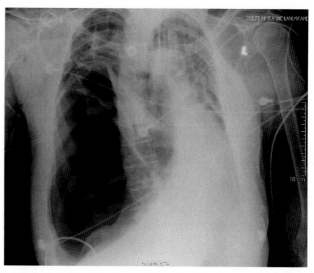

**Figure 55-2:** A plain chest radiograph showing a right tension pneumothorax with tracheal deviation (and endotracheal tube) and mediastinal shift to the left chest.

### Open Pneumothorax (Sucking Chest Wound)

- Trauma creating significant chest wall defect greater than two thirds of the tracheal diameter such that air preferentially enters the chest defect. Rapid equilibration between the atmospheric pressure and intrathoracic pressure leads to lung collapse.
- Air enters through an open wound of the chest wall into the pleural space during inspiration and leaves during expiration.
- Clinical features:
  - ○ Sucking wound is diagnosed from the noise of the air entering and leaving the pleural space through the chest wall defect.
  - ○ Hypoxia, hypercapnia, hypotension, and circulatory failure.
- Treatment:
  - ○ Application of sterile occlusive dressing taped on three sides creates a flutter-valve effect, which allows air escape from the pleural space during expiration.[2]
  - ○ Tube thoracostomy in an area remote from wound. A large-bore (>28 French tube) is usually placed.
  - ○ Definitive surgical closure of chest wall defect.

## Hemothorax

- Chest trauma disrupting lung parenchymal or surrounding vessels, leading to blood accumulation in the pleural cavity
- Massive hemothorax:
  - ○ Rapid accumulation of more than 1500 mL of blood into chest cavity causes lung collapse, leading to hypoxia
  - ○ Etiology of fluid accumulation may come from three sources:
    - Major vascular injury
    - Direct lung parenchymal injury
    - Chest wall injury (intercostal vessels).
- Clinical features:
  - ○ Hypotension, decreased/absence of breath sounds, dullness to percussion.
  - ○ Flat neck veins due to hypovolemia.
  - ○ Distended neck veins if associated with tension pneumothorax.

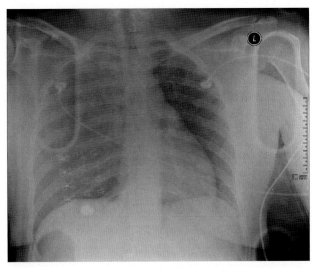

**Figure 55-3:** A plain chest radiograph showing a large right hemothorax. (Bullet is lodged in the liver.)

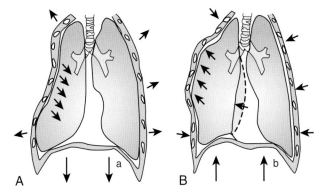

**Figure 55-4:** Two views of flail chest, showing paradoxical movement of the "floating" section of chest wall and paradoxical airflow in the affected lung on inspiration (**A**) and expiration (**B**).

- Diagnostic investigations:
  - ◦ Plain chest radiograph shows large pleural fluid or opacification of hemithorax (Fig. 55-3).
- Treatment:
  - ◦ Decompression of chest cavity with tube thoracostomy in the fourth or fifth intercostal space, anterior to midaxillary line. The chest tube (usually >28 French tube) should be connected to a collecting chamber capable for autotransfusion.
  - ◦ Restoration of lost blood volume with rapid crystalloid infusion and blood transfusion.
  - ◦ Initial chest tube output of at least 1500 mL, followed by continuous blood loss of 200 to 300 mL/h and persistent blood transfusion requirements indicate need for operative intervention for hemorrhage control.
    - An operation is also indicated for the following reasons:
    - Incomplete expansion of the lung
    - Retained hemothorax: (1) Plain chest radiographs should be performed to follow the chest cavity after a chest tube has been inserted for chest trauma; (2) Medical treatment to dissolve the retained clots is not effective, so surgical drainage is indicated because retained blood in the chest leads to chronically trapped lung.

## Flail Chest

- Chest wall segment lacks bony continuity with the rest of the thoracic cage.
  - ◦ Multiple rib fractures: two or more ribs fractures in two or more consecutive ribs.
  - ◦ Costochondral separation.[9]
- Clinical features:
  - ◦ Paradoxical chest wall motion: inward with inhalation and outward with exhalation (Fig. 55-4)
  - ◦ Associated pulmonary contusion and bony pain lead to respiratory failure.
- Diagnostic investigations:
  - ◦ Plain chest radiograph shows rib fractures and pulmonary contusions. There may be a hemothorax or pneumothorax
- Treatment:
  - ◦ Maintenance of ventilation:
    - Patients without respiratory distress can be managed with analgesia only.

- Patients displaying respiratory distress should be intubated promptly. Patients who were intubated earlier had a lower mortality rate than those from whom intubation was withheld for 24 hours until clinical signs of respiratory compromise.[8]
  - ◦ Respiratory distress associated with a flail chest is usually caused by an underlying pulmonary contusion, not by the flail motion of the chest.
  - ◦ Overhydration should be avoided because it can impair respiratory function.
  - ◦ Operative intervention may be considered to ameliorate pain control, to restore lung volume loss, and to assist with wean from mechanical ventilator support.[10-12]

## Rib Fracture

- The most common injuries in chest trauma. Ribs 4 to 10 are commonly fractured.
- Upper ribs (1 to 3) are well protected; such fractures may be associated with major vascular injuries.
- Middle ribs (4 to 8) are often accompanied with pneumothorax, hemothorax, pulmonary contusion, or flail chest.
- Lower ribs (9 to 12) are associated with hepatic and/or splenic injuries.
- Rib fractures are less common in pediatrics as their ribs are more pliable.
- Clinical features:
  - ◦ Pain on inspiration leads to poor ventilation and build-up of respiratory secretion, possibly infectious complications.
  - ◦ Tenderness to palpation
  - ◦ Visible or palpable chest deformity
  - ◦ Crepitus
- Diagnostic investigations:
  - ◦ Plain chest radiograph identifies rib fractures and other associated injuries.
  - ◦ Chest CT can identify rib fractures not seen on chest radiograph.
- Treatment:
  - ◦ Pain management and pulmonary toilet:
    - Oral or intravenous narcotics
    - Oral or intravenous nonsteroidal anti-inflammatory agents
    - Intercostal nerve blocks with local anesthetics
    - Epidural analgesia has been shown to be an independent predictor of decreased mortality or pulmonary complications.[13]
- Prognosis:
  - ◦ Outcome is associated with the number of ribs fractured and the extent of underlying pulmonary contusion.

## Pulmonary Parenchymal Injury: Contusion, Laceration and Pseudocyst

- Definitions
  - **Contusion:** Trauma causing lung edema and hemorrhage without major parenchymal disruption.
  - **Lung laceration:** Trauma resulting in parenchymal disruption, often with space generation due to retractive forces acting on the surrounding lung parenchyma
  - **Traumatic pulmonary pseudocyst:** a trauma-induced pneumatocele associated with parenchymal laceration
- Mechanisms of injury
  - Blunt chest trauma with transmission of large compressive forces can result in both contusion and laceration
  - Penetrating parenchymal injury
    - Knife, bullet, and other penetrating objects
    - Rib fracture penetrating injury
- Clinical features:
  - Often associated with rib fractures and accounts for the major factor contributing to morbidity with flail chest.
  - Pulmonary contusion:
    - Can lead to poor respiratory compliance, ventilation-perfusion mismatches, shunt and hypoxia
    - An important cause of acute lung injury and acute respiratory distress syndrome (ARDS)
    - Can be complicated by infection
    - Major contusion can cause bronchial hemorrhage, leading to airway obstruction.
  - Lung laceration:
    - Can be associated with parenchymal ecchymosis or alveolar hemorrhage
    - Patients may present with features that are similar to pulmonary contusion.
    - Traumatic pulmonary pseudocysts are filled with air but can contain blood.
    - Hemopneumothorax may complicate penetrating lung laceration.
- Diagnostic investigations:
  - Plain chest radiograph:
    - Shows localized infiltrate underneath the contused chest wall region (Fig. 55-5).

- Note: contracoup contusions can be seen with major blunt trauma, especially in the presence of compliant chest walls, as noted in pediatric patients.
- Hematomas (single or multiple) appear as dense opacities.
- Pneumatoceles can be single or multiple
  - Chest CT:
    - Is a more sensitive modality for detecting pulmonary contusion.[8]
    - Note: contusions are not limited by anatomic boundaries.
    - Paravertebral lacerations/hematomas can occur secondary to compressive forces acting on the lung together with limited lung excursion due to the rigid bony spine posteriorly.
    - CT is useful for delineating other associated thoracic trauma issues or sequelae (e.g., atelectasis) that may obscure or make difficult, interpretation on the plain radiograph.
- Treatment:
  - Pulmonary contusion:
    - Pain management control
    - Pulmonary toilet and supplemental oxygen
    - Ventilatory support for respiratory failure due to ARDS or other mechanisms (The greater the area of contusion, the higher the risk for acute lung injury.)
    - Bronchoscopy can be useful for evaluating airways for suspected injury or obstruction.
    - Uncomplicated contusion usually resolves over 7 to 10 days.
  - Lung parenchymal injury:
    - Similar measures to contusion listed above
    - Lung parenchymal injury often requires only chest tube drainage for bleeding from the lung.
    - Persistent bleeding for the lung parenchyma requires surgical intervention.
    - A tractotomy (placing a cutting stapler into a tract and firing the stapler to open the lung parenchyma to expose the source of the bleeding may be necessary).
    - If a section of the lung has been destroyed or if the bleeding cannot be stopped, then resection (lobectomy or pneumonectomy) may be required.
    - Uncomplicated pulmonary ecchymosis usually takes longer than uncomplicated contusion to resolve. Residual scarring may be evident.

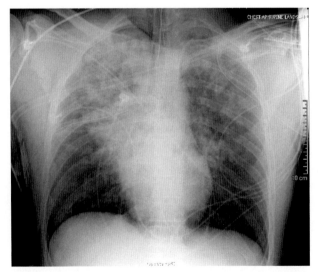

**Figure 55-5:** A plain chest radiograph showing bilateral pulmonary contusion. Rib fractures lie posteriorly. An endotracheal tube, nasogastric tube, and right-sided chest tube are also present.

## Cardiac Tamponade

- Leakage of blood into pericardial sac impairs venous filling and restricts cardiac activity.[14]
- Clinical features:
  - **Beck's triad:** distended neck veins, muffled cardiac sounds, hypotension.
  - **Pulsus paradoxus:** decrease in systolic pressure with spontaneous inspiration.
  - **Kussmaul's sign:** increase in venous pressure with spontaneous inspiration.
- Diagnostic investigations:
  - Transthoracic echocardiogram.
  - Echocardiogram findings:
    - Right atrial collapse with expiration
    - Right ventricular collapse with expiration
    - Minimal to no changes in inferior vena cava dimensions with respiration due to high back pressure
    - Left atrial compression
    - Note: with a naïve pericardium, a moderate or large amount of fluid is not a prerequisite. Thus, tamponade can occur with a small amount of blood in the pericardial space.
  - Subxyphoid pericardial window.
  - Pericardiocentesis to detect pericardial fluid.

■ Treatment:
  ○ Pericardiocentesis can be a temporary therapeutic measure.
  ○ Emergent median sternotomy or open thoracotomy to assess and repair cardiac injury.

## Blunt Cardiac Injury
### Cardiac Chamber Rupture
■ Most cardiac chamber injuries are fatal.
■ Those who present to the hospital often have pericardial tamponade.
  ○ Emergency department ultrasound is useful in diagnosis.
■ Emergent operative intervention is often mandated.

### Valvular Disruption
■ Valvular injury after blunt chest trauma is rare.
■ Clinical features:
  ○ Aortic insufficiency, heart murmur, apical displacement or thrill, pericardial effusion.
■ Diagnostic investigations:
  ○ Plain chest radiograph shows chamber enlargement, mediastinal hemorrhage, left pleural cap.
  ○ Electrocardiogram demonstrates sustained dysrhythmia, Q-waves, ST or T wave abnormalities, frequent ectopic beats.
  ○ Echocardiogram is modality of choice for detecting valvular disruption.
■ Treatment:
  ○ Operative intervention: valve reconstruction or replacement.

### Myocardial Contusion
■ Injury to myocardium frequently results from severe blunt chest trauma.
  ○ Caused by various types of blunt trauma to the chest, the most common of all is the steering wheel injury suffered in road collisions.
■ Associated with rib fractures or pulmonary contusion.
■ Clinical features:
  ○ The vast majority of the patients with contusion to the heart have no cardiac symptoms.
  ○ The symptomatic patient may complain of chest pain or of shortness of breath.[15-17]
■ Diagnostic investigations:
  ○ Elevated serum troponin level, elevated serum level of MB band of creatinine kinase.[18]
  ○ ECG demonstrates ST- or T-wave changes, right bundle branch block, supraventricular arrhythmia, ventricular arrhythmia.
  ○ ECG may show wall motion abnormality.
■ Treatment:
  ○ Close monitoring in telemetry or intensive care unit setting for arrhythmia.

## Penetrating Cardiac Injury
■ The clinical manifestations are usually dependent on the site and size of the cardiac injury and the state of the pericardial wound.
  ○ When the pericardial wound remains open and allows free drainage of the intrapericardial blood, the cardiac wound presents with symptoms and signs of hemorrhage and hemothorax.
  ○ When the pericardial wound is obliterated, cardiac tamponade ensues.
■ Gunshot wounds typically carry a higher mortality rate than stab wounds.
  ○ Emergency department ECG is useful for rapid diagnosis.

| TABLE 55-1 ■ **GOALS OF EMERGENCY THORACOTOMY** | |
|---|---|
| **Maneuver** | **Rationale for Maneuver** |
| Release of pericardial tamponade | Allow venous filling and restoration of cardiac output |
| Direct control of cardiac or vascular hemorrhage | Stop blood loss and restore cardiac volume |
| Allow open cardiac massage | Closed cardiac massage for cardiac arrest or PEA is not adequate for patients in extremis |
| Cross-clamping of descending aorta | Redirects limited blood supply to brain and augments diastolic filling of coronary vessels |

PEA, pulseless electrical activity.

■ Usually necessitate immediate operative intervention for repair
  ○ Emergency thoracotomy may be indicated. (Refer to indications and rationale for emergency thoracotomy in Table 55-1)
■ After cardiac repair, diagnostic assessment of cardiac valve and coronary vessels is necessary.

## Traumatic Aortic Disruption
■ Complete aortic disruption injuries are generally fatal at the scene.
■ Incomplete aortic tear from rapid acceleration/deceleration injury most commonly occurs at the insertion of ligamentum arteriosum (Fig. 55-6).
  ○ The intact adventitial layer contains the mediastinal hematoma and temporarily prevents massive hemorrhage.
■ Clinical features:
  ○ Chest pain, particularly midscapular pain
  ○ Midscapular or precordial murmur

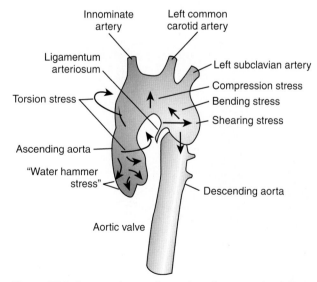

**Figure 55-6:** Forces acting on the aortic wall as a result of blunt thoracic trauma that may cause rupture of the aorta at different sites. (*From Symbas P. Traumatic injuries of the heart and great vessels. Springfield, IL: Charles C Thomas; 1971. p. 153, courtesy of Charles C Thomas, Publisher, Springfield, IL.*)

○ Increased pulse amplitude and hypertension of upper extremities

○ Rarely anuria or loss of function of the lower limbs may be present.[19-22]

○ Aortic rupture usually occurs just distal to the take off of the left subclavian artery and has an 80% mortality rate at the scene of the trauma.

▪ Diagnostic investigations:

○ Plain chest radiograph:

▪ Widened mediastinum (Fig. 55-7)

▪ Fractures of first rib, second rib, or scapula

▪ Deviation of trachea to the right

▪ Depression of the left main stem bronchus.

▪ Deviation of the esophagus (nasogastric tube) to the right

▪ Obliteration of the aortic knob

▪ Obliteration of space between pulmonary artery and aorta (obscured anteroposterior window).

▪ Presence of pleural or apical cap

▪ Left hemothorax

▪ Widened paratracheal stripe or paraspinal interfaces

○ Helical contrast-enhanced chest CT may definitely diagnose thoracic aortic injuries or may provide indeterminate findings that warrant further studies.[23]

○ Aortography can diagnose aortic rupture when chest CT is indeterminate (Fig. 55-8).

○ Transesophageal echocardiography is a less invasive diagnostic tool that supplements aortography.[24]

▪ Treatment:

○ Strict blood pressure control and avoiding hypertension are imperative.

▪ Generally maintain mean systemic blood pressure at less than 70 mm mercury.[2,21-22]

○ Timely intervention either by open repair (resection with placement of interposition synthetic graft) or endovascular technique (stenting)

○ Optimal timing of traumatic aortic injury must be coordinated with treatment of other injuries.

○ Surgical repair of rupture with cardiopulmonary bypass.

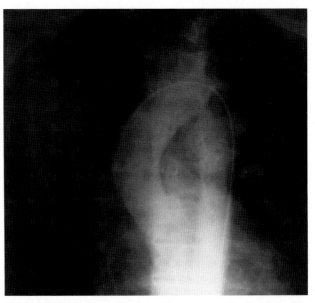

**Figure 55-8:** Aortagram showing a false aneurysm distal to the origin of left subclavian artery.

## Tracheobronchial Injury

▪ Tracheobronchial injuries are rare and are typically fatal at the scene.

▪ Possible scenarios:

○ Direct airway compression with a closed glottis.

○ Rapid deceleration leading to tracheal laceration or right main stem bronchus avulsion from the carina.

▪ Clinical features[25,26]:

○ Subcutaneous emphysema, hemoptysis, tension pneumothorax.

○ Pneumothorax with persistent large air leak after tube thoracostomy.

▪ Diagnostic investigations:

○ Plain chest radiography or CT scan: may show abnormal mediastinal shadow, pneumomediastinum, subcutaneous emphysema, pneumothorax.

○ Bronchoscopy

▪ Treatment:

○ Maintenance of airway patency; main stem intubation on the unaffected side may be necessary.

○ Small injuries may heal spontaneously.

○ Large injuries require operative repair.

## Esophageal Injury

▪ Suspect esophageal injury in patients with penetrating injuries transversing the mediastinum through wounds near the posterior midline.

▪ Penetrating esophageal injury is more common and can occur at any level.

▪ Esophageal injury from blunt trauma is usually due to abrupt intraesophageal pressure increase from insult to upper abdomen; similar to Boerhaave's syndrome.

▪ Clinical features:

○ Subcutaneous emphysema[27]

○ Left pneumothorax or hemothorax without rib fracture.

○ Severe insult to epigastrium and with pain out of proportion to injury.

○ Particulate matter from chest tube output.

○ Chest tube that bubbles during inspiration and expiration.

○ Mediastinal air or empyema.

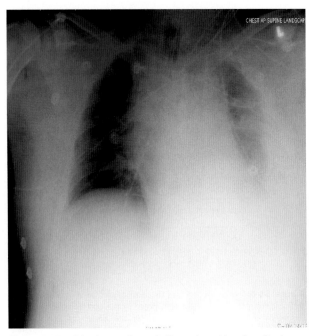

**Figure 55-7:** Plain chest radiograph illustrating widened mediastinum.

- Diagnostic investigations:
  - Chest tube output with amylase level higher than serum amylase level.
  - Osmolyte swallow study (aspiration of gastrograffin may cause fatal ARDS)
  - Esophagoscopy
- Treatment:
  - Drainage of pleural cavity and mediastinum with direct esophageal repair via thoracotomy or VATS.
  - Surgical repair of the injury and wide drainage of adjacent area. This usually involves a two-layer repair of the esophagus. Initially, the muscle layers must be opened to fully expose the mucosal injury. After the mucosal injury has been repaired, then the muscle layers are closed. If an esophageal injury is suspected preoperatively, an intercostal muscle flap should be created in the process of making the thoracotomy incision. This flap can then be used to cover the esophageal repair.
  - If the esophagus cannot be repaired, it will repair itself and the patency of the esophageal lumen will be restored because the staples will retract.
  - If the tissues of the esophagus are too inflamed for a repair or if the pleural cavity is too inflamed for the esophageal leak, the alternative to that approach is esophageal exclusion. This involved an end cervical esophagostomy, stapling the gastroesophageal junction, and placement of a gastrostomy tube. Eventually, when the patient has recovered in a few months, the patient will require a colon interposition or gastric pullup to restore esophageal continuity.
  - Tube thoracostomy is connected to 14 to 20 cm $H_2O$ suction.[2,27]

## Traumatic Diaphragmatic Injury
- Blunt trauma can cause large diaphragmatic lacerations with visceral organ herniation.
- Penetrating trauma produces small perforations, with no immediate herniation.
- Frequently occurs on the left side; the liver shields the right hemidiaphragm.
- Diagnostic investigations:
  - Plain chest radiograph:
    - Abnormal or elevated appearance of hemidia-phragm
    - Acute gastric dilatation
    - Presence of nasogastric tube in the left chest
    - Appearance of air-fluid chest contents simulating loculated pneumohemothorax
  - Upper gastrointestinal contrast study is used when injury is not apparent on plain chest radiograph.
  - Chest CT.[23]
- Thoracoscopy or laparoscopy, or both, are useful in identifying injury.
  - Caution should be taken when performing laparoscopy because gas from pneumoperitoneum can create or worsen pneumothorax.
- Treatment:
  - Operative repair.

## Transmediastinal Penetrating Injury
- Potential serious injuries to the heart, great vessels, tracheobronchial tree, or esophagus.
- Hemodynamically unstable patients mandate exploratory thoracotomy.
- Hemodynamically stable patients should undergo complete evaluation to rule out possible vascular, tracheobronchial, or esophageal injury and to direct operative treatment.

- Diagnostic investigations:
  - A plain chest radiograph can identify entrance wound in one hemithorax and exit wound in opposite hemithorax.
  - Contrast-enhanced chest CT is used as screening tool to establish projectile trajectory and to identify other injuries.
  - Angiography evaluates great vessels.
  - Esophagram and esophagoscopy.
  - Bronchoscopy examines tracheobronchial tree.
  - Hemodynamically stable patients should undergo complete evaluation to rule out possible vascular, tracheobronchial, or esophageal injury and to direct operative treatment.
  - Echocardiography.

## Subcutaneous Emphysema
- Associated with injury to airway, tracheobronchial tree, or lung.
- By itself of minimal clinical significance. May be clue to other serious injury
- Can decompress with introduction of several subcutaneous small bore cannulae at strategic sites, including eyelids, subclavicular regions, and so on.

## *EMERGENCY THORACOTOMY*
- An established procedure in the management of life-threatening chest trauma.[7]
  - Goals of emergency thoracotomy (see Table 55-1)
    - Release of pericardial tamponade.
    - Direct control of cardiac or vascular hemorrhage.
    - Allow open cardiac massage.
    - Cross-clamping of descending aorta.
- Survival rates after emergency thoracotomy are 9% to 12% for penetrating thoracic trauma and 1% to 2% for blunt thoracic trauma.
- Indications:
  - Penetrating thoracic trauma: loss of pulse/pressure during transport or in the emergency room.
  - Blunt thoracic trauma: loss of pulse/pressure in the emergency room.
- Because the patient requires immediate operative repair after emergency thoracotomy, surgeon presence is required.

## *VIDEO-ASSISTED THORACIC SURGERY*
- Minimally invasive modality for management of thoracic injuries.
- Often a good approach if the patient is stable. If the bleeding is from an intercostal artery or a simple lung parenchymal injury, then the problem can be corrected with video-assisted thoracic surgery (VATS).
- Reduced pain and morbidity and shorter postoperative recovery time compared with open thoracotomy.[28,29]
- Post-traumatic empyema that once required open thoracotomy can now be treated with VATS.[30]
- VATS is also useful for evaluating retained hemothorax, thereby reducing restrictive lung disease as a long-term sequela.
- Diaphragmatic injury is underappreciated and can be diagnosed with VATS.
- VATS has proven to be a safe technique to management of various thoracic injuries in hemodynamically stable patients.[31]

## *CONCLUSIONS*
- Thoracic injuries remain a major cause of morbidity and mortality in trauma patients.
- Diagnosis relies on a high level of suspicion.

■ Most injuries can be treated nonoperatively.
■ Early recognition and timely management of thoracic trauma are essential and may be life-saving.

## Brief Illustrative Case

• A 25-year-old man was involved in a motor vehicle collision. He was an unrestrained passenger who was ejected from the vehicle.
• He presented with poor respiratory effort and nasal voice.
• On examination, he had significant subcutaneous emphysema (right more than left) and markedly decreased breath sounds in right chest.
• A right thoracostomy was performed immediately, and the patient was intubated. Subsequently, a left chest tube was inserted.
• A chest radiograph is depicted in Figure 55-9.
• The amount of subcutaneous emphysema worsened.
• The right chest tube revealed a large continuous air leak and drainage of a moderate amount of serosanguinous fluid. No air leak and minimal fluid drainage was evident on the left.
• Chest CT revealed bilateral extensive bilateral subcutaneous emphysema (right more than left) together with extensive mediastinal air. Bibasilar pulmonary contusions (left more than right) were also observed (Fig. 55-10).
• Bronchoscopy showed a right middle lobe bronchial laceration. There was blood in the airway.
• The patient was immediately taken to the operating room. A double-lumen endotracheal tube was positioned.
• At thoracoscopy, the bronchial tear was visualized and sutured with resolution of the air leak.
• A decision was made to proceed to VATS right middle lobectomy.

### Key Points

• Massive subcutaneous emphysema can be a clue to tracheobronchial trauma
• Other clues include pneumothoraces and mediastinal air collections as noted in this patient
• In the above-mentioned patient, the greatest clue was the presence of a large continuous air leak despite chest tube drainage and lung expansion
• Although repair of a major airway tear is usually sufficient, in this case, right middle lobectomy was undertaken. The *rationale* was that the right middle lobe orifice was even more narrow than usual following repair. Thus, there was concern for impaired clearance of secretions leading over time to the potential for recurrent pneumonia in this young man. It was believed to be safer to perform a right middle lobectomy in this patient (with presumed normal baseline lung function before the accident) to offset future pulmonary complications.

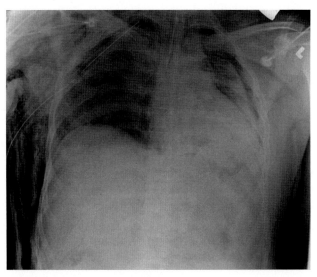

**Figure 55-9:** A plain chest radiograph demonstrating significant subcutaneous emphysema involving bilateral chest walls. An endotracheal tube and a right-sided chest tube are also present. (This patient with a traumatic right tracheobronchial injury also sustained a left pneumothorax.)

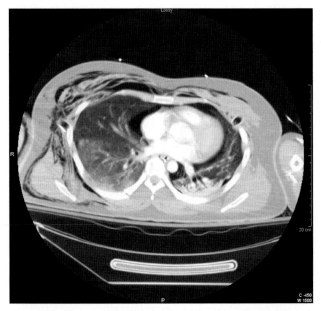

**Figure 55-10:** Computed tomography of the chest showing bilateral extensive bilateral subcutaneous emphysema (right more than left), together with extensive mediastinal air. Bibasilar pulmonary contusions (left more than right) are also evident.

## References

 Interactive references and additional readings for this chapter can be accessed online at *expertconsult.com*.

# DISORDERS OF THE ESOPHAGUS

## 56 CARCINOMA OF THE ESOPHAGUS

David Tom Cooke, MD and Allan Pickens, MD

### TERMINOLOGY

- Carcinoma of the esophagus
- Esophageal cancer
- Esophageal malignancy

### INTRODUCTION AND DEFINITION

Carcinoma of the esophagus is a growing problem in the United States, where an estimated 16,470 new cases and 14,755 deaths were predicted for 2008.[1] Eighty percent of primary tumors of the esophagus are malignant.[2] Histology includes squamous cell carcinoma, adenocarcinoma, anaplastic small cell (oat cell) carcinoma, adenoid cystic carcinoma, carcinosarcoma, lymphoma, leiomyosarcoma, and melanoma (Table 56-1). The most common esophageal cancer worldwide is squamous cell carcinoma, especially in certain endemic areas such as Asia, eastern and southern Africa, and the Middle East.[3] The most common histology in the nonendemic areas, especially the United States, is adenocarcinoma. Adenocarcinoma accounts for more than 50% of esophageal malignancies, and the incidence is rising; the rate of the second highest esophageal malignancy, squamous cell carcinoma, is steadily decreasing. In the United States, carcinoma of the esophagus is the seventh leading cause of cancer death in men.[4]

### ETIOLOGY

There are clear and numerous risk factors for squamous cell carcinoma[5] and only a few identifiable risk factors for adenocarcinoma.

- **Squamous cell carcinoma:** Most commonly occurs in the proximal two thirds of the esophagus.
  - Carcinogens:
    - Nitrosamines:
      - Associated with cured meats and pickled foods.
    - Tobacco
  - Nutritional factors
    - Alcohol
    - Vitamin Deficiencies

- Anemia
- Previous gastric surgery
  - Premalignant lesion
    - Leukoplakia
    - Previous head and neck malignancy
    - Previous external beam irradiation
  - Injury or chronic irritation
    - A result of chronic stasis injury
      - Achalasia
      - Esophageal diverticula
      - Plummer-Vinson syndrome
    - Chronic irritation
      - Ingestion of hot foods and beverages
      - Caustic burn injury

- **Adenocarcinoma:** Smoking and obesity are thought to be risk factors for adenocarcinoma. Barrett's metaplasia and gastroesophageal reflux disease (GERD) are clear risk factors. Adenocarcinoma most commonly occurs in the distal two thirds of the esophagus.
  - GERD
    - GERD causes Barrett's metaplasia. In a nationwide Swedish case-controlled study, patients with long-term symptomatic GERD had a 43 times increased risk of developing adenocarcinoma of the esophagus compared with asymptomatic controls.[6]
  - Barrett's metaplasia[7,8]
    - Characterized by the change of nonkeratinizing stratified squamous esophageal epithelium to gastric or intestinal type columnar epithelium with goblet cells, beginning at the esophagogastric junction (EGJ) and extending proximally.
    - Barrett's metaplasia leads to a 30 to 40 times increased risk of developing adenocarcinoma.
    - Barrett's metaplasia should be suspected when a patient with long-standing heartburn has resolution of his or her symptoms. Barrett's metaplasia is an acid-insensitive lesion.
    - All patients with Barrett's metaplasia should undergo an indefinite surveillance program.
      - Adenocarcinoma occurs in 2% of all patients with Barrett's metaplasia without dysplasia, 7% of patients with low-grade dysplasia, and 22% of patients with high-grade dysplasia.

## TABLE 56-1 ■ MALIGNANT ESOPHAGEAL TUMORS

| Histology | Incidence in the United States |
|---|---|
| **A. Primary Tumors** | |
| Adenocarcinoma | >95% |
| Squamous cell carcinoma | |
| **B. Unusual Primary Tumors** | |
| Adenocarcinoma variants | |
|     Adenoid cystic carcinoma (cylindroma) | |
|     Mucoepidermoid carcinoma | |
|     Adenoacanthoma | |
|     Choriocarcinoma | |
| Squamous cell variants | |
|     Verrucous carcinoma | |
|     Polypoid carcinoma (pseudosarcoma) | |
| Small cell carcinoma | |
| Melanoma | |
| Lymphoma | 1–2% |
| Mesenchymal Tumors | |
|     Leiomyosarcoma | |
|     Rhabdomyosarcoma | |
|     Fibrosarcoma | |
|     Chondrosarcoma | |
|     Osteosarcoma | |
|     Liposarcoma | |
|     Kaposi's sarcoma | |
| **C. Secondary Tumors** | |
| Metastatic cancer | |
|     Breast, lung, stomach | |

○ Surveillance program consists of flexible endoscopy every 2 years, with brushings and four quadrant biopsies every 2 cm of involved mucosa.

○ On endoscopy, Barrett's metaplasia appears as salmon-colored tonguelike projections into normal-appearing mucosa (Fig. 56-1).

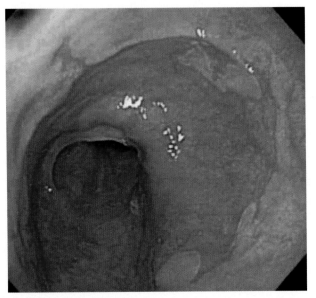

**Figure 56-1:** Esophageal endoscopy showing salmon-colored Barrett's intestinal metaplasia, surrounded by pink, normal-appearing esophageal mucosa.

## CLINICAL FEATURES

### Symptoms and Signs

Most patients with carcinoma of the esophagus present with dysphagia. Dysphagia may start with solids and progresses to liquids. Patient can often point to the exact site of their obstruction.

- Other symptoms include
  - ○ Weight loss
  - ○ Odynophagia
  - ○ Chronic anemia from a friable lesion
  - ○ Hematemesis
  - ○ Recurrent pneumonias
    - ■ From aspiration or a malignant tracheoesophageal fistula
  - ○ Hoarseness
    - ■ From direct invasion of the recurrent laryngeal nerve.
  - ○ Horner's syndrome.
    - ■ Invasion of the stellate ganglia.

## DIAGNOSIS

The diagnosis of esophageal cancer can be made in 95% of patients using a combination of barium swallow and flexible endoscopy with brushings for cytology and biopsy of suspicious lesions. Barium swallow may identify strictures or other filling defects (Fig. 56-2). Flexible endoscopy may identify malignant-appearing strictures or fungating, ulcerative, or infiltrative masses (Fig. 56-3).

## STAGING

The TNM classification of the American Joint Committee of Cancer (Table 56-2) is used to define staging of carcinoma of the esophagus, where T is depth of tumor penetration, N is

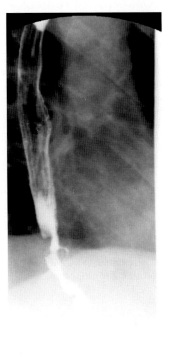

**Figure 56-2:** Barium esophagram demonstrating distal esophageal narrowing and intraluminal defect.

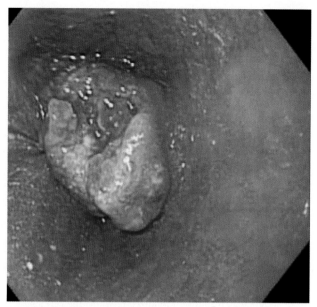

**Figure 56-3:** Esophageal endoscopy showing an esophagogastric junction mass. Biopsy proved adenocarcinoma.

## TABLE 56-2 ■ TNM STAGING FOR CARCINOMA OF THE ESOPHAGUS

**Primary Tumor (T)**

| | |
|---|---|
| TX: | Primary tumor cannot be assessed |
| T0: | No evidence of primary tumor |
| Tis: | Carcinoma in situ |
| T1: | Tumor invades lamina propria or submucosa |
| T2: | Tumor invades muscularis propria |
| T3: | Tumor invades adventitia |
| T4: | Tumor invades adjacent structures |

**Regional Lymph Nodes (N)**

| | |
|---|---|
| NX: | Regional lymph nodes cannot be assessed |
| N0: | No regional lymph node metastasis |
| N1: | Regional lymph node metastasis |

**Distant Metastasis (M)**

| | |
|---|---|
| MX: | Distant metastasis cannot be assessed |
| M0: | No distant metastasis |
| M1: | Distant metastasis |
| | Tumors of the lower thoracic esophagus |
| |    M1a: Metastasis in the celiac lymph nodes |
| |    M1b: Other distant metastasis |
| | Tumors of the midthoracic esophagus |
| |    M1a: Not applicable |
| |    M1b: Nonregional lymph nodes and/or other distant metastasis |
| | Tumors of the upper thoracic esophagus |
| |    M1a: Metastasis in cervical nodes |
| |    M1b: Other distant metastasis |

**Stage**

| | |
|---|---|
| 0 | TisN0M0 |
| 1 | T1N0M0 |
| IIA | T2N0M0 |
| | T3N0M0 |
| IIB | T2N1M0 |
| | T1N1M0 |
| III | T3N1M0 |
| | T4AnyNM0 |

lymph node involvement and M is nonregional nodal and distant organ metastasis.[9] At the time of diagnosis, 50% of patients have disease that has advanced beyond locoregional limits, and 80% of resected specimens have regional lymph node metastasis.[4]

- Tumor depth of penetration (T)
  - T1 lesions invade through the lamina propria into the submucosa.
  - T2 lesions infiltrate the muscularis propria.
  - T3 lesions grow into the surrounding adventitia.
  - T4 lesions grow into surrounding structures such as the carina and pericardium.
- Lymph node involvement (N)
  - EGJ lymph nodes are left gastric, subcarinal, and intrathoracic paraesophageal lymph nodes.
    - For intra-abdominal esophageal tumors, celiac nodes can be swept with the specimen.
  - Intrathoracic esophageal regional lymph nodes are subcarinal and intrathoracic paraesophageal nodes.
  - Cervical esophageal regional lymph nodes are the internal jugular, scalene and cervical paraesophageal lymph nodes.
- Metastatic disease (M)
  - M1a refers to nonregional nodal metastasis. M1a staging for upper thoracic esophageal tumors are the cervical lymph nodes. M1a staging for lower thoracic esophageal tumors are the celiac axis lymph nodes. M1a staging for midthoracic esophageal tumors are nonapplicable because nonregional nodal metastasis carries the same prognosis as distant (M1b) metastasis.
  - **Staging imaging studies:** Important staging studies must include chest and abdominal computed tomography (CT) scan with oral and intravenous contrast, endoscopic ultrasound (EUS), and positron emission tomography (PET) with 18F-deoxyglucose (FDG).
  - CT scan
    - Useful for defining the locoregional spread of the primary tumor, invasion of adjacent structures, and distant organ metastasis.
  - EUS with fine-needle aspiration (FNA)
    - Study of choice for determining T stage of primary tumor.
    - EUS also identifies regional lymph nodes, which can be biopsied by FNA.
      - Biopsy of nodes near the primary tumor may lead to false-positive results.
    - Five sonographic layers corresponding to the mucosa (first two layers), submucosa, muscularis propria, and the adventitia.
    - Tumors and lymph nodes appear as hypoechoic lesions.
    - Combined CT and EUS demonstrate an accuracy of 79% for staging the primary tumor and 82% for staging regional lymph nodes.[10]
  - PET scan
    - Useful in staging nodal metastasis and distant organ metastasis.
    - PET has a sensitivity of 78% for detecting distant nodal and other metastatic disease.[11]

## TREATMENT

The gold standard treatment for esophageal cancer is surgical resection. Some patients are candidates for preoperative neoadjuvant chemoradiotherapy, or postoperative adjuvant chemoradiotherapy. For patients who are unable to undergo resection for cure, there are a number of palliative options.

- Resectable disease is defined as T1–T3 or resectable T4, N0-1, or stage IVA.[12]
  - Resectable T4: Invasion of pleura, diaphragm, or pericardium.
  - Unresectable T4: Adherence to the aorta and other great vessels, heart, or trachea.
- In addition to preoperative staging, patients who are candidates for resection should have drawn a complete blood count and complete metabolic panel, including liver function tests.
- Patients who are anemic may need a blood transfusion. Patients who are malnourished may require preoperative placement of a Dobboff nasogastric feeding tube (Tyco Healthcare/Kendall, Mansfield, MA) or feeding jejunostomy for enteric tube feeds before surgery.
- A feeding gastrostomy tube should be avoided to protect the stomach as a potential conduit.
- Lesions found during staging suspicious for metastatic disease should be biopsied.
- If the primary tumor is at or above the carina and there is no evidence of M1 disease, a bronchoscopy should be performed to rule out bronchial invasion.
- **Chemoradiotherapy**—Patients who can medically tolerate an operation and have resectable disease may undergo three types of treatment: (1) Neoadjuvant chemoradiotherapy, followed by surgery; (2) esophagectomy, followed by adjuvant chemoradiotherapy, if applicable; (3) definitive chemoradiotherapy.
  - **Neoadjuvant chemoradiotherapy**—Early studies have suggested a survival advantage for patients receiving neoadjuvant therapy with 5-flurouracil (FU) and cisplatin plus 40 Gy of external-beam irradiation.[13] Meta-analysis studies suggest that neoadjuvant chemoradiotherapy plus surgery may downstage tumor, and reduce the 3-year mortality and locoregional recurrence rates. However, the rate of postoperative mortality may be increased.[14,15]
    - At the University of Michigan, we recommend neoadjuvant chemoradiation for any medically fit patient who is younger than 75 years of age with stage II to III carcinoma of the esophagus.
      - University of Michigan regimen: 3 weeks of cisplatin and 5-FU or taxol with concurrent 45 Gy radiation therapy, 3 to 4 weeks of rest, followed by surgery.
  - **Adjuvant chemoradiotherapy**—The decision for postoperative chemoradiotherapy (5-FU–based chemotherapy/radiation therapy) is determined by the surgical staging of the disease as well as histology.[12]
    - Completely resected squamous cell carcinoma can be observed.
    - Stage I (T1N0) adenocarcinoma can also be observed.
    - Patients with T2N0 adenocarcinoma can be observed unless the tumor demonstrates unfavorable histology, which includes:
      - Poorly differentiated adenocarcinoma
      - Neurovascular invasion
      - Lymphovascular invasion
    - Patients with T3 disease or greater should receive postoperative chemoradiotherapy.
- **Surgical resection**—There are multiple surgical techniques for esophageal resection and reconstruction. These techniques can be divided between those that do not require a thoracotomy, specifically the transhiatal esophagectomy (THE), and those that require a thoracotomy, such as the Ivor Lewis and McKeown or three-hole esophagectomy. Each technique has its advantages and disadvantages. In addition, there are newer minimally invasive techniques for esophageal resection. All of the above-mentioned techniques require the stomach, colon, or small bowel as conduits to replace the resected esophagus.

- The stomach is the standard conduit. Previous gastric surgery may preclude the use of the stomach; however, the stomach can often be mobilized and used effectively after previous gastrostomy tubes and anti-reflux surgery.
- The left or right colon can be used if the stomach is not an option. The vascular pedicle is derived from the left or right colic arteries.
- Jejunal free grafts can be used, but the results are inferior to colon interposition grafts.[16]
  - **THE**[17-19]—THE is performed in three phases (Fig. 56-4)
    - Abdominal phase: Performed through an upper midline incision. The stomach is inspected and mobilized by ligating the short gastric, left gastroepiploic, and left gastric arteries. The duodenum is mobilized with a Kocher maneuver, and a pyloromyotomy is performed. The esophageal hiatus is widened, and the distal esophagus is mobilized with sharp and blunt dissection.
    - Cervical phase: A neck incision is made at the anterior border of the sternocleidomastoid muscle and carried down to the prevertebral fascia with blunt dissection. The middle thyroid vein and inferior thyroid artery are ligated without consequence. From the neck, the superior esophagus is bluntly mobilized down to the carina.
    - Mediastinal phase: The posterior mediastinum is further mobilized with blunt dissection with the surgeon's hand. The cervical esophagus is divided with a stapler, and the thoracic esophagus is delivered into the abdomen. The proximal stomach is divided with a 4 cm margin. The gastric conduit is delivered through the posterior mediastinum to the neck. A feeding jejunostomy is fashioned, and the abdomen is closed. After a side-to-side stapled cervical esophagogastric anastomosis, the neck is closed over a drain.
    - The average THE postoperative course involves a 7- to 10-day hospital stay. Most patients can be extubated in the operating room and admitted to a monitored floor bed. This outcome is very dependent on good preoperative instruction and conditioning. Patients must be motivated to perform incentive spirometry and ambulate during the early postoperative course. Epidural anesthesia is vital to good postoperative performance. Postoperative ileus rarely lasts beyond 48 hours; thus, a jejunostomy tube feeding is started at 30 mL/h on postoperative day 3. If low rate tube feeding is tolerated for 12 hours, then tube feeding is advanced to the goal rate. The nasogastric tube (NGT) is also removed on postoperative day 3 if drainage is less than 100 mL per 8-hour shift. A liquid diet is started on postoperative day 4 and advanced as tolerated to a soft diet. Because patients swallow saliva across the cervical anastomosis, there is no need to restrict oral intake until barium swallow is completed. Routinely, a barium swallow is performed on postoperative day 7 to document that the anastomosis is intact. At least 1 week is usually required for patients to adjust to the initial retrosternal fullness, early satiety, or postvagotomy cramping, and diarrhea that may occur. Each of these postesophagectomy conditions can frequently be corrected with dietary behavior modifications such as eating frequent small meals, avoiding foods that are high in fat or simple sugars, and avoiding meals just before sleep.
    - The NGT is removed on postoperative day 3, a liquid diet is started on postoperative day 4, and a barium swallow is performed on day 7.
    - Advantages:
      - No thoracotomy
      - Cervical anastomosis: low morbid consequence of esophageal leak

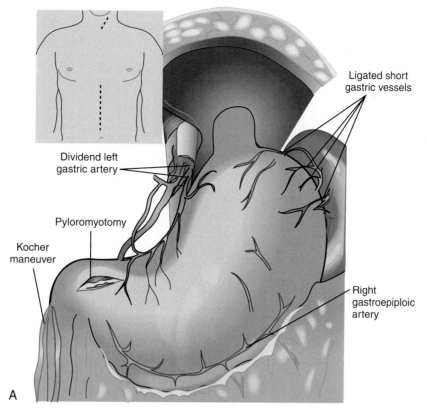

**Figure 56-4: A,** Gastric mobilization, showing ligated short gastric, left gastroepiploic and left gastric arteries, pyloromyotomy, and completed Kocher maneuver.

*(Continued on page 508.)*

- ○ Minimal postoperative reflux
- ○ Easy vertical margins
- ■ Disadvantages and potential complications:
  - ○ Pneumonia (2%)
  - ○ Bleeding
  - ○ Recurrent laryngeal nerve injury (<1%)
  - ○ Chylothorax (<1%)
  - ○ Tracheal/bronchial injury (<1%)
- ○ **Ivor Lewis esophagectomy** (transthoracic esophagectomy [TTE]) - Performed in two phases
  - ■ Abdominal phase: Mobilization of the stomach and distal esophagus identical to THE. A pyloromyotomy may or may not be performed. A whole stomach conduit that has not been tubularized may be more susceptible to gastric outlet obstruction if a drainage procedure, such as pyloromyotomy, is not performed.[20] But this assertion is controversial.
  - ■ Thoracic phase: A right posterolateral thoracotomy is performed, and the remainder of the esophagus is mobilized. The azygous vein is divided and the thoracic duct is often divided prophylatically as it enters through the hiatus to prevent chylothorax. The mobilized stomach is brought into the chest through the esophageal hiatus, the proximal stomach is divided with a stapler, and the fundus is anastomosed to the proximal thoracic esophagus.
  - ■ Advantages
    - ○ Lower leak rate than cervical anastomosis
    - ○ Vocal cord paralysis is rare (incidence)
  - ■ Disadvantages and potential complications
    - ○ The patient must be repositioned and prepped for the thoracic phase.

- ○ Anastomotic leak can cause severe mediastinitis, with a mortality between 8.5% and 60%.[21,22]
- ○ Chylothorax
- ○ Pulmonary complications
- ○ Bleeding
- ○ Comparing TTE with THE, meta-analysis reveals that TTE has significantly higher rates of in-hospital mortality, operative blood loss, pulmonary complications, and chylothorax, and longer hospital stays.[23] THE demonstrates a higher anastomotic leak rate and a higher incidence of vocal cord paralysis.
- ○ In a randomized study comparing TTE with THE, TTE demonstrated a trend toward a higher rate of 5-year disease-free survival, but this was not statistically significant.[24]
- ○ **McKeown esophagectomy** (three-hole esophagectomy)
  - ■ Abdominal and thoracic mobilization is performed similar to Ivor Lewis esophagectomy, but the esophagogastric anastomosis is placed in the left neck, as seen in THE. At the University of Michigan, we perform a McKeown esophagectomy if the tumor is too difficult to mobilize via a blunt mediastinal dissection.
- ○ **Minimally invasive esophagectomy**[25,26]
  - ■ Total laparoscopic THE: The stomach and distal two thirds of the esophagus are mobilized laparoscopically. Vessels are divided using the LigaSure (Valleylab, Boulder, CO) or a harmonic scalpel. The proximal esophagus is bluntly mobilized via a left cervical incision, and an esophagogastric anastomosis is fashioned in the left neck, as previously described.
  - ■ Combined thorascopic/laparoscopic esophagectomy: Similar to the McKeown esophagectomy, but the thoracic and abdominal phases are performed thorascopically and

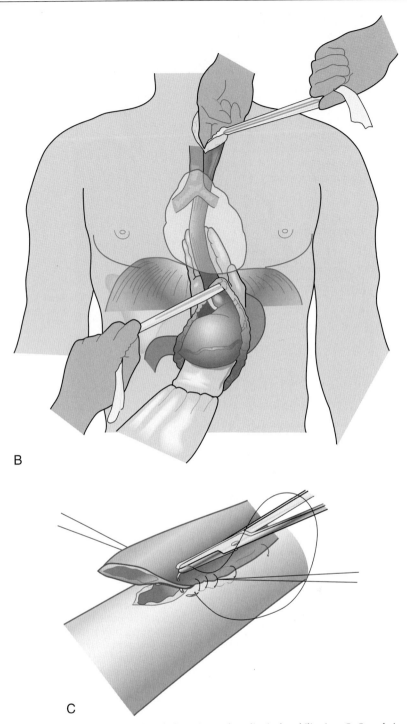

B

C

**Figure 56-4—cont'd: B,** Figure demonstrating completed neck dissection and mediastinal mobilization. **C,** Completion of cervical esophagogastric anastomosis. *(Adapted from Orringer MB. General thoracic surgery: Transhiatal esophagectomy without thoracotomy. J Oper Techn Thorac Cardiovasc Surg 2005;3:63-83.)*

laparoscopically respectively. The esophagogastric anastomosis is performed in the neck.

○ **Esophagectomy complications**[27]

■ Intraoperative esophagectomy complications include pneumothorax, tracheal tear, and hemorrhage.

■ Pneumothorax occurs in two thirds of transhiatal esophagectomies. Visual inspection or palpation should be performed to identify pleural entry. Chest tubes should be placed immediately to drain any accumulating fluid or air.

■ Tracheal tears may range from small, linear tears to major tracheal disruptions. Tracheal disruptions generally occur with densely adherent or invading tumors. Tracheal tears are denoted by a rush of air from the mediastinum with ventilation. If a tracheal tear occurs, the endotracheal tube cuff should be advanced into the distal trachea or left main bronchus by manual or bronchoscopic guidance. After removal of the esophagus, primary tracheal repair should be performed.

- Major hemorrhage generally involves greater that 1 liter of blood loss. Aortic esophageal arteries branch into small capillaries before they reach the wall of the esophagus; thus, most of these vessels thrombose with arterial contraction. Direct pressure from packs facilitates this hemostasis. Occasionally, larger vessels require direct ligation by a transhiatal or transthoracic approach.
- Postoperative esophagectomy complications generally occur within the first 10 days and include hoarseness, supraventricular tachyarrhythmias, sympathetic pleural effusions, chylothorax, and anastomotic disruption.
  - Hoarseness occurs due to recurrent laryngeal nerve injury. Impaired cricopharyngeal motor function may result in cervical dysphagia and aspiration that can cause severe pneumonia. Most immobilized vocal cords realign eventually, but cord injection with paraffin or fat is sometimes necessary to reduce aspiration risk. It is best to avoid traumatic retraction on the nerve to prevent injury.
  - Supraventricular tachyarrhythmias occur in many patients following chest surgery. The arrhythmia is often transient and can be controlled with electrolyte replacement and drug therapy (calcium channel blockers, beta blockers). Cardioversion is rarely needed.
  - Sympathetic pleural effusions are treated with thoracentesis or chest tube drainage when symptomatic.
  - Chylothorax results from thoracic duct injury. The diagnosis may not be apparent until the patient begins enteral or oral intake of fat. Excessive or milky chest tube drainage is typical. Triglyceride and chylomicron content of the fluid can confirm the diagnosis. Conservative management with non-fat enteral tube feeding or intravenous hyperalimentation controls most chyle leaks. Attempts at conservative management should not be extended much beyond 2 weeks due to nutritional and immune factor loss. Direct ligation at the site of thoracic duct injury or mass ligation at the diaphragm level may be necessary.
  - Cervical anastomotic leak can occur with any form of esophagectomy. If a patient develops a persistently elevated temperature following esophagectomy, the anastomosis must be evaluated. Water-soluble contrast (Gastrografin, Bracco Diagnostics, Inc, Princeton, NJ) is used to identify possible leaks; if water-soluble contrast does not reveal a leak, dilute barium sulfate is used because barium sulfate better defines mucosal detail. Cervical anastomotic leaks are treated by opening the cervical incision and performing frequent dressing changes. Intrathoracic anastomotic leaks require tube drainage. Patients who remain febrile require surgical drainage and possible takedown of the anastomosis. All anastomotic leaks should be dilated early because strictures develop due to edema and fibrosis.

## Postoperative Care

Postoperative care is directed at pulmonary toilet and observation for potential postoperative complications. About 50% of patients experience some type of complication after esophagectomy.

- Respiratory care
  - Note: non-invasive positive pressure ventilation is *contraindicated*, as this may compromise surgical connections.
  - Early ambulation and pulmonary toilet to minimize the risk of atelectasis or pneumonia.
  - Head of the bed should be elevated to reduce the risk of aspiration.

- Maintain optimal perfusion
  - Need to keep the patient well hydrated to ensure that the stomach or colonic interposition is optimally perfused.
  - Approaches vary across centers, from careful clinical observation and fluid replacement (e.g., ensure adequate hourly urine output, etc.) to the above and low dose dopamine infusion or even the further addition of a nitroglycerin infusion to that of dopamine perioperatively.
- Diet after esophagectomy
  - Evaluate the patients for possible recurrent laryngeal injury because that leads to aspiration. Speech therapy evaluation for patients with vocal cord paralysis to perform a swallowing evaluation. Liquids are more likely to pass through the cords into the trachea than solid food.
  - When the patients start eating, esophageal soft diet may be safer than liquids.
- Tube feedings
  - Jejunal feedings are much safer than total parenteral nutrition. They cannot be bolused like gastric feedings can.
  - When patients are discharged after an esophagectomy, they usually have anorexia and early satiety so that they eat only about 500 calories per day.
  - Jejunal feedings are started on the first postoperative day and are progressively increased so that intravenous fluid can be discontinued by the third or fourth postoperative day.
  - When the patients start eating, feedings are continued for 10 to 12 hours overnight while the patients sleep.
  - When the patients are discharged from the hospital, they continue feedings until patients can maintain their weight without the feedings (usually about 6 weeks), so discharge planning begins a few days after the operation to arrange for home health care.
  - The jejunostomy is removed in the office when it is no longer required.
  - Sometimes before the tube is scheduled to be removed, it may fall out. Patients are instructed to clean the tube and immediately replace the tube before the tube tract closes.
- Care of incisions
  - Abdominal and thoracic incisions rarely become infected.
  - Cervical incision rarely becomes infected. If there is erythema in the cervical incision, generally means that there is an anastomotic leak.
  - The incision is opened and packed. Esophageal dilations are begun.
  - The leak usually heals in 1 to 2 weeks. The patient can still eat unless there is a large output through the neck incision.
- **Palliation**
  - **Nd:YAG Laser Therapy**[28]—Uses 1065 nm light to burn tumor.
    - Useful for small tumors <5 cm in size.
    - Improvements in dysphagia symptoms last 8 to 32 weeks.
    - 1% to 6% perforation rate.
  - **Photodynamic therapy**[29]—The patient is administered 2 mg/kg of the photosensitizer sodium porfimer, which is preferentially taken up by tumor. After 48 hours, the tumor is exposed to 300 to 400 joules/cm of tumor of 630-nm light. Excited porfimer releases tumorcidal oxygen-free radicals.
    - Improvements in dysphagia last up to 11 weeks.
    - Useful in treating stent occlusion.
    - <5% perforation rate.
    - May see skin injury from exposure to sunlight.
  - **Brachytherapy**[30]—Local catheter release of radioisotopes such as iridium 192.
    - Median dysphagia-free survival of 10 months.
    - Risk of stricture and fistula formation.

○ **Esophageal stents**[30,31]—Plastic and self-expanding metal stents (SEMS), are deployed via flexible endoscopy with use of fluoroscopy.

■ Plastic stents
  ○ Removable stents
  ○ Have a high rate of migration
■ SEMS
  ○ Made of nonferrous metals such as nickel/titanium alloy (nitinol).
  ○ Can be covered with polyurethane or silicone.
  ○ Metal stents are permanent
  ○ 95% of patients experience short-term relief of dysphagia.
  ○ Covered stents are effective in sealing tracheoesophageal fistulas.
  ○ Complications include stent occlusion and migration.

## Brief Illustrative Case

• *History:* A 44-year-old man with a 1-year history of dysphagia to solids and progressing to liquids. In addition the patient had a 20-pound unintentional weight loss over the course of a year. The patient's past medical history includes long-standing gastroesophageal reflux.
• *Examination:* Vitals: Afebrile and vital signs within normal limits. No palpable lymphadenopathy.
• *Blood tests:* Complete blood count and electrolytes—normal; liver function tests: normal.
• *Imaging:* Barium swallow revealed high-grade narrowing of the distal esophagus (see Fig. 56-2). A contrast CT scan of the chest, abdomen and pelvis revealed a thickened distal esophagus with subcentimeter distal paraesophageal lymph nodes.
• *Esophagoscopy/EUS:* Esophagoscopy demonstrated a 5-cm fungating mass near the esophagogastric junction (see Fig. 56-3). EUS demonstrated T3N1Mx (Mx = metastasis unknown) disease (Fig. 56-5).
• *PET scanning:* PET scanning illustrated FDG uptake only in the area of the distal esophagus, with no evidence of local or distant metastasis (Fig. 56-6).
• *Diagnosis/Pathology:* Biopsy and brushings at the time of the endoscopy revealed poorly differentiated adenocarcinoma. Staging demonstrates radiographically T3N1M0 (stage III) carcinoma of the esophagus.
• *Management of carcinoma of the esophagus:* The patient was referred for neoadjuvant chemoradiation, which included cisplatin and taxol therapy and a total dose of 45 GY in 1.5-Gy fractions given twice a day. Restaging with barium swallow and contrast CT scan revealed diminishment in size of the esophageal mass, and no additional lesions. After standard pre-operative assessment, the patient underwent a THE.

### Key Points

• Common presentation of carcinoma of the esophagus.
• The barium swallow raises the suspicion of malignancy.
• Endoscopic biopsy provides diagnosis of adenocarcinoma.
• CT, PET, and EUS provide preoperative staging.

• Stage III disease is amendable to neoadjuvant chemoradiotherapy.
• THE is an effective surgical approach even after preoperative chemoradiotherapy.

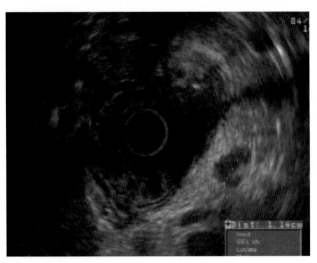

**Figure 56-5:** Endoscopic ultrasound demonstrates paraesophageal lymph node (*green line*).

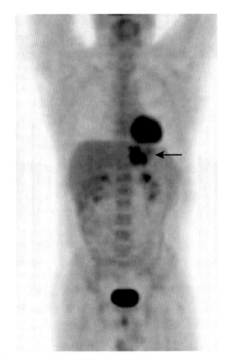

**Figure 56-6:** Positron emission tomography scan demonstrates metabolically active distal esophagus (*arrow*) and no metastatic disease.

## References

 Interactive references and additional readings for this chapter can be accessed online at *expertconsult.com.*

# 57 BENIGN ESOPHAGEAL DISEASE

## Harmik J. Soukiasian, MD and James D. Luketich, MD

## ESOPHAGEAL STRICTURE

There are two benign disease processes that may result in esophageal strictures:

- Extrinsic disease
- Intrinsic disease

The etiology of these strictures may be elucidated based on the patient's symptoms, physical examination, contrast radiographic imaging, endoscopy, and pathology.

Strictures may be further classified as[1]

- Simple
  - Esophageal lumen permits passage of endoscope
  - Straight
  - Short (<2 cm)
- Complex
  - Too narrow to allow for easy passage of the endoscope
  - Angulated stricture
  - Irregular

## BENIGN ETIOLOGIES OF ESOPHAGEAL STRICTURE

### General Causes
- Peptic stricture
- Schatzki's ring
- Motility disorder of esophagus
- Autoimmune
- Immunocompromised state
- Graft versus host disease
- Collagen vascular disease
- Crohn's disease
- Infectious esophagitis
- Hiatal hernia
- Caustic
- Congenital, iatrogenic
- Medication related
- Prior photodynamic therapy (PDT)
- Foreign body reaction
- Radiation therapy
- Malignancy
- Idiopathic

### Peptic Stricture
The most common cause of benign esophageal stricture and accounts for approximately 75% of all benign esophageal strictures.

## ETIOLOGY

- The primary inciting factor is exposure of the esophagus to acid resulting in collagen deposition and eventually a fibrous esophageal stricture.[2-4]
- Dysfunctional or impaired lower esophageal sphincter (LES)

- LES pressure usually less than 8 mm
- Impaired esophageal motility, with decreased clearance[5]
- Association with hiatal hernia exists.
- Alkaline reflux may play a role.
- Approximately 70% of all esophageal strictures are peptic strictures secondary to reflux.[6-9]
- Use of proton pump inhibitors (PPIs) has decreased the need for dilatation as well as the risk of recurrence.[6,10-13]

## CLINICAL FEATURES

- Progressive dysphagia to solids is very common. It is believed that dysphagia is the best predictor of esophageal stricture.[6]
- Food impaction
- Weight loss
- Heartburn
- Chest pain
- Pulmonary symptoms
  - Adult onset asthma, usually secondary to aspiration
  - Chronic cough
- Stricture diameter is only partially responsible for symptoms of dysphagia. Esophagitis has an equal or greater impact on the level of dysphagia a patient feels.[14]
- When the luminal diameter is less than 5 mm, then luminal diameter will be the determinant for the degree of dysphagia.[14]

## DIAGNOSIS

Diagnosis and cause should be established because treatment depends on etiology. Dysphagia is the most common symptom. Frequently, patients will describe a progression of dysphagia from solids to liquids. The presence of dysphagia should prompt an investigative workup to find the cause behind it.[1]

### Imaging Studies
- Esophagram
  - Very sensitive test to detect luminal narrowing
  - Provides information about the location, diameter, contour, length, size and complexity of the lesion.
  - May help identify malignancy
  - May show associated abnormalities that may impact the choice of therapeutic intervention.
  - Findings on barium swallow can help guide future endoscopic evaluation (Fig. 57-1A and B).
- Computed tomography scan (CT)
  - CT is helpful in evaluation of strictures due to malignancy.
  - Can help with determining the size of the lesion
  - Helpful in the evaluation of extraluminal spread or invasion of neighboring structures by malignancy
  - Useful in evaluating metastatic spread
- Esophagogastroduodenoscopy (EGD)
  - EGD is useful in identifying stricture.
  - Evaluating for evidence of esophagitis
  - Identify possible malignant lesion
  - Obtain tissue for pathologic examination

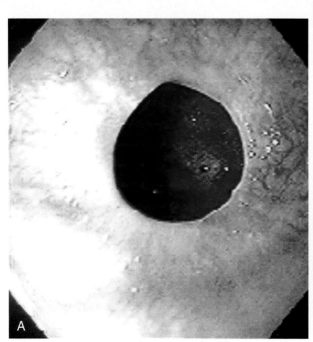

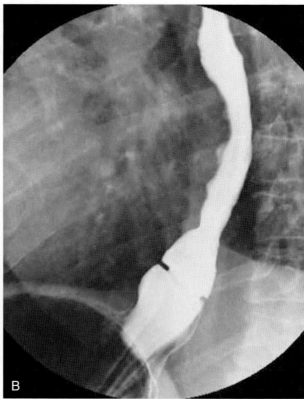

**Figure 57-1:** **A,** Schatzki's ring. **B,** Barium esophagram with Schatzki's ring.

■ Endoscopic ultrasound (EUS)
  ○ EUS most useful in cases of malignancy
  ○ Very accurate in determining depth of invasion and nodal involvement
  ○ EUS has a sensitivity of 93% and a specificity of 100% when combined with fine-needle aspiration for regional nodal staging.[15]
■ Esophageal manometry
  ○ Useful in evaluating patients with suspected esophageal dysmotility
  ○ Information about the patient's esophageal motility can help guide planning for those who will undergo possible antireflux surgery.
  ■ 24-hour pH
  ○ Helpful in identifying patients with acid reflux who may benefit from PPIs
  ○ Can help identify patients who may benefit from an antireflux procedure

### Treatment

The goal of treatment is to relieve the dysphagia. Initial therapy is usually esophageal dilatation, but concomitant implementation of medical therapy is essential to promote healing as well as decrease the chance of recurrence. Esophageal resection may be necessary for patients refractory to the above treatments.[1,7]

■ Medical therapy
  ○ Treatment with PPIs is very beneficial.
  ○ Studies have demonstrated that the use of PPIs has decreased the need for dilatation as well as the risk of recurrence and need for repeat dilation.[6,10,12]

■ Dilatation
  ○ Esophageal dilation dates back to the 16th century. During that time, wax fashioned in the shape of a wand was used to dilate the esophagus. The current word bougie was derived from an Algerian city named Boujiyah, which was the main site for candle trade during medieval times.
  ○ Both balloon and mechanical (bougie type) dilators are used.
  ○ Balloon dilator
    ■ Passed and used under direct visualization by the endoscope
    ■ Not reusable
    ■ Fluoroscopy not mandatory
  ○ Mechanical dilators include
    ■ Maloney
      ○ Flexible rubber dilators weighted with mercury
      ○ Indicated for uncomplicated strictures
      ○ Not wire guided
      ○ Diameter of stricture greater than 10 mm
    ■ Savary—Gilliard dilators
      ○ Wire guided, flexible polyvinyl chloride
      ○ Fluoroscopy guided
      ○ Radio-opaque at the base of the taper
      ○ Indicated for more complex strictures: (1) irregular, (2) long, (3) tight
    ■ American dilation system
      ○ Wire guided, flexible poly-vinyl chloride
      ○ Fluoroscopy guided
      ○ Short, less tapered
      ○ Impregnated with barium so they are radio-opaque throughout the length of the dilator.
      ○ Indicated for more complex strictures: (1) Irregular, (2) long, (3) tight

○ Risk of perforation ranges 0.1% to 0.4%

○ No clear difference in perforation rates between mechanical and balloon dilators[16-20]

○ The choice of which type of dilator to use is dependent mostly on the characteristics of the stricture and endoscopist's preference.[21]

○ Balloon dilators are not reusable, whereas mechanical dilators can be reused.

○ A postdilation luminal diameter of at least 12 mm is required to relieve symptoms of dysphagia

○ Most patients experience relief after successful dilatation up to 40 to 54 French, some will even attempt to dilate up to 60 French.

○ Dilation is tailored specifically for each patient based on findings, technical difficulty during the procedure, and symptomatic response of the patient to level of dilatation.

○ Thirty to forty percent of patients with benign strictures have recurrence within 1 year of dilation, even with the aid of concomitant acid suppression.

○ Refractory strictures most commonly occur in patients with stricture secondary to caustic ingestion or radiation[1,2,12,22,23]

▪ Steroid injection

○ Steroid injection into the stricture may reduce stricture recurrence.

○ May be effective for patients[24-27]

▪ Requiring frequent dilations

▪ Poor symptomatic relief from dilation

▪ Both Long strictures and short strictures

▪ Stent: There exist both metal and nonmetal stents, as well as covered and noncover stents.

○ Stents are commonly used in patients with dysphagia secondary to malignancy.

○ Stents are both permanent and removable.

○ Indications:

▪ Recurrent stricture after repeated dilations

▪ Recurrent stricture after steroid injection

▪ Patients with inoperable malignancy

▪ Recurrent stricture after nonsurgical treatment

▪ Esophageal fistula

▪ Surgery: Reserved for those patients with strictures refractory to the above-mentioned interventions

○ Benign dilatable strictures

▪ Esophageal sparing operation

▪ Anti-reflux procedure

○ With or without esophageal-lengthening procedure, as indicated (Collis)

○ Stricture not dilatable

▪ Esophageal resection may be needed

## BARRETT'S ESOPHAGUS

▪ Replacement of the normal esophageal squamous mucosa with columnar epithelium containing goblet cells (metaplasia).

▪ Found in 7% to 10% of patients with chronic, severe gastroesophageal reflux disease (GERD)

▪ Barrett's esophagus predisposes patients to the development of mucosal dysplasia and, ultimately, adenocarcinoma; therefore, the condition should be considered a premalignant (50- to 100-fold increased risk of cancer compared with the general population).[28]

▪ The frequency of Barrett's esophagus has quadrupled over the past few decades, most likely due to improved diagnostic capability with the expansion of flexible endoscopy.

▪ The risk of developing adenocarcinoma in patients with Barrett's esophagus has been estimated to be 0.5% per year (Fig. 57-2A and B).[29]

## CLINICAL FEATURES

▪ Risk factors for the development of Barrett's esophagus are[30,31]

○ Male sex

○ Smoking history

○ Obesity

○ White ethnicity

○ Age older than 50 years

○ Greater than 5-year history of reflux symptoms

▪ Esophageal motility in Barrett's esophagus

○ Weak lower esophageal sphincter allowing for pathologic reflux to occur.

○ Esophageal peristalsis is often impaired, exacerbating the delay in acid clearance from the distal esophagus.

▪ Chronic inflammation and fibrosis may lead to esophageal stricture, frequently at the proximal end of the involved segment.

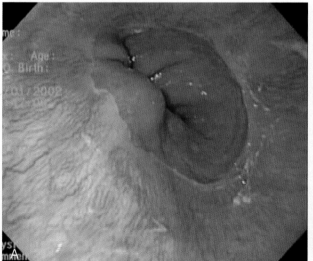
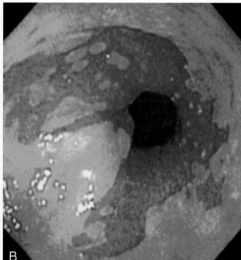

**Figure 57-2: A,** Normal gastroesophageal junction. **B,** Barrett's esophagus.

## SIGNS AND SYMPTOMS

- Most patients with Barrett's esophagus have a history of heartburn and acid regurgitation.
- Less frequent symptoms include
  ○ Dysphagia
  ○ Chest pain
  ○ Hematemesis
  ○ Melena
  ○ Cough
  ○ Wheezing
- Only 4% to 10% of patients with such clinical symptoms, however, have Barrett's esophagus.
- No symptoms are specific for Barrett's esophagus[31,32]

## PATHOPHYSIOLOGY

It is believed that Barrett's esophagus may progress from metaplasia to dysplasia and eventually to carcinoma.

- Barrett's esophagus usually arises in the setting of chronic gastroesophageal reflux, with the incidence increasing proportionally to the degree of acid exposure.
- Bile reflux is very closely associated with Barrett's esophagus.
- In Barrett's esophagus, the squamous epithelium in the distal portion of the esophagus is replaced by a columnar epithelium, which contains goblet cells.
- The cuboidal cell population located at the true gastroesophageal junction is postulated to be the cell of origin of the metaplastic epithelium with the aberrant proliferation of these cells accounting for the development of intestinal metaplasia.[33]
  ○ This cell exhibits markers of both squamous and columnar epithelia, and is abundant in microvilli and secretory vesicles.
- Evidence that Barrett's metaplasia can progress from dysplasia to carcinoma is as follows[34]:
  ○ Metaplastic and dysplastic epithelium are often found adjacent to each other in pathologic specimens.
  ○ The progression from metaplasia to low-grade dysplasia then high-grade dysplasia and, ultimately, to carcinoma has been described.
- *Helicobacter pylori* does not infect the esophagus and is not associated with an increased risk of Barrett's esophagus or the development of esophageal adenocarcinoma.[35]
  ○ Postulated inverse relation between strains of *H. pylori* infection and the risk of esophageal/gastric cardia adenocarcinoma
  ○ It is postulated that *H. pylori* may actually protect the esophagus by decreasing gastric acidity and, hence, the effects of acid reflux.

## DIAGNOSIS

The diagnosis of Barrett's esophagus is suggested by finding abnormal columnar epithelium lining the distal esophagus on endoscopy; however, this finding must be confirmed by biopsy showing intestinal metaplasia, usually with the hallmark presence of mucin-producing goblet cells.

- One must remember that shorter segments or even just tongues of columnar epithelium may be associated with adenocarcinoma of the gastroesophageal junction.[36]
  ○ Traditionally, the diagnosis of Barrett's esophagus was based on the finding of long segments ($\geq$3 cm) of columnar epithelium, but intestinal metaplasia has been identified by

short segments of columnar epithelium, even in the absence of GERD
- Barrett's esophagus is classified as follows[37]:
  ○ **Long-segment Barrett's esophagus** ($\geq$3 cm of specialized intestinal metaplasia)
  ○ **Short-segment Barrett's esophagus** ($\leq$3 cm of specialized intestinal metaplasia)
  ○ Same management for both

## TREATMENT OF GASTROESOPHAGEAL REFLUX

The goal of therapy for GERD is to ameliorate or eliminate the signs and symptoms of GERD and to prevent the development of complications from this disease. Medical treatment has been $H_2$-receptor antagonists or more recently PPIs. Surgical treatment is gastric fundoplication, which effectively reduces or eliminates reflux symptoms. Both treatments are effective in reducing acid reflux symptoms (>90% symptomatic improvement). Despite the effectiveness in the control of symptoms, neither medical nor surgical antireflux therapy has been definitively proven to decrease the risk of esophageal adenocarcinoma.[38]

- Antisecretory therapy[39]
  ○ Goal is acid suppression.
  ○ Should be based on the severity of the associated esophagitis
  ○ Control the reflux in the hope of preventing its deleterious effects
  ○ Allows for more reliable pathologic evaluation of epithelium in looking for dysplasia by decreasing the amount of esophagitis in the field
  ○ Currently, PPIs are frequently prescribed as the first line of therapy.
- pH studies may demonstrate continued reflux even when symptoms resolve.
- Despite twice-a-day administration of PPIs, up to 80% of patients continue to demonstrate nocturnal gastric acid reflux.[40]
- Aggressive use of PPIs has been shown to promote partial regression of esophageal intestinal metaplasia. In a study of patients with Barrett's esophagus and acid reflux, the use of acid suppression with PPI (omeprazole 40 mg) twice a day was compared with H2-blockers (ranitidine 150 mg) twice daily.[41,42]
  ○ The PPI (omeprazole) treatment reduced reflux in 99% of patients.
  ○ Although small, a statistically significant regression in the length and area of Barrett's was achieved.
  ○ These findings do not necessarily translate into a decreased risk of cancer.
  ○ Therefore, the need for continued surveillance is unchanged.
- There are some data that suggest that the use of antisecretory medical therapy on a long-term chronic basis may actually increase the chance of developing cancer. Furthermore, achlorhydria is believed to be a risk factor for the development of adenocarcinoma of the stomach secondary to the propagation of bacteria that produce carcinogenic compounds which flourish with achlorhydria.[43]
- Is Barrett's esophagus better treated with surgery than with medical treatment?
  ○ To date, no randomized trial has definitively answered this question.[44,45]
  ○ Some studies have shown that control of reflux by fundoplication can result in regression of Barrett's esophagus.

○ Additionally, several large nonrandomized series have seen a reduction in the overall risk of cancer progression.[46]

○ In a study of endoscopic surveillance for Barrett's esophagus, no patients who underwent Nissen fundoplication developed dysplasia or adenocarcinoma, whereas some patients in the medically treated group developed low-grade dysplasia, high-grade dysplasia, and some even progressed to adenocarcinoma with medical treatment alone.[47]

○ Five-year follow-up after fundoplication for Barrett's esophagus showed[48]

■ Regression from low-grade dysplasia to nondysplastic Barrett's epithelium in 44% of patients.

■ No development of high-grade dysplasia or carcinoma during 410 patient-years of follow-up.

○ Failure of surgical therapy is due to[49]

■ Technical error in wrap construction, especially in re-operative cases.

■ Failure to recognize and identify the presence of a shortened esophagus.

■ DeMeester and colleagues[50] showed a high rate of regression of low-grade dysplasia after an adequate fundoplication. That is not typically seen with maximal medical therapy regimens. Intestinal metaplasia of the esophagus is unlikely to regress after antireflux surgery, although intestinal metaplasia confined to the cardia may regress.

## Conclusions Regarding Surgery for Barrett's Esophagus

■ Surgical correction of the lower esophageal sphincter mechanism may offer the best long-term results in the treatment of patients with Barrett's esophagus and minimize the risk of progression to cancer.

■ Fundoplication can be performed using minimally invasive techniques.

■ Fundoplication is safe and effective with long-lasting results.

■ This approach should be strongly considered in patients with Barrett's esophagus.

## SURVEILLANCE

■ Patients with either long-segment or short-segment Barrett's esophagus require regular endoscopic surveillance.

■ The objective is to identify any dysplastic changes, progression of dysplasia, or progression to adenocarcinoma. Biopsy results may reveal

○ No dysplasia

○ Inclusive biopsies

○ Low-grade dysplasia

○ High-grade dysplasia

○ Invasive adenocarcinoma.

■ High-grade dysplasia is characterized pathologically by enlarged pleomorphic nuclei, loss of nuclear polarity, decreased or absent mucus production, and abnormal glandular architecture.

■ When this process penetrates and extends beyond the basement membrane, it is classified as adenocarcinoma.

■ Among patients with Barrett's esophagus,

○ Approximately 15% to 25% have low-grade dysplasia.

○ Five to ten percent have high-grade dysplasia.

○ Approximately 5% to 10% of patients will progress from metaplasia to dysplasia per year, and 1% will progress to adenocarcinoma.

■ Dysplasia exhibits no gross distinctive features that can be identified visually; therefore, multiple random biopsies from the affected Barrett's segment should be obtained.

■ One third to one half of patients diagnosed with high-grade dysplasia on biopsy already have an invasive malignancy if a resection is performed.[51]

○ There should be high suspicion of an underlying cancer if a nodularity or stricture is present in patients with high-grade dysplasia

■ Although the natural history of dysplasia in general is not well understood, high-grade dysplasia is known to be associated with the development of adenocarcinoma.[52,53]

○ Ten to twenty-eight percent of patients progress from high-grade dysplasia to adenocarcinoma within 5 years.

■ Unsuspected cancer was found in 33% to 45% of patients with Barrett's esophagus who underwent esophagectomy for high-grade dysplasia without preoperative evidence of carcinoma.[54,55]

■ Thus, in patients with high-grade dysplasia, endoscopic surveillance is performed every 3 to 6 months.

■ Performing four-quadrant biopsies taken at 1-cm intervals to help maximize the sensitivity for the detection of early cancers.

■ Surveillance is controversial because no randomized trial has proven that surveillance improves survival.

## TREATMENT OPTIONS FOR DYSPLASIA

■ High-grade dysplasia has three potential treatment options: (1) intensive surveillance (as described above); (2) endoscopic ablative therapy; (3) esophagectomy.

■ Endoscopic ablative therapies:

○ Employ thermal or photochemical energy to destroy the metaplastic esophageal epithelium.

○ The esophageal columnar epithelium may be removed with the aid of

■ Laser coagulation

■ Electrocautery

■ Heater probe

■ Radiofrequency ablation

■ Argon beam coagulator

■ PDT

■ Endoscopic mucosal resection (EMR)

○ Barrett's esophagus is generally a localized, superficial process for which ablative modalities may represent a potentially viable treatment modality.

○ Because early carcinoma identified in high-grade dysplasia is typically intramucosal (>90%), so local ablative therapy may be reasonable.

■ EMR is an option in patients with neoplastic lesions smaller than 2 cm in diameter and with no sign of submucosal infiltration, positive lymph nodes, or distant metastasis.

■ EMR allows for (Fig. 57-3A and B)[56]:

○ Complete resection of affected area

○ Preserves architecture of resected specimen

○ Enhanced staging (EUS)

○ Ninety percent local remission

○ Positive deep margins and submucosal invasion require surgical resection.

○ Relatively new and controversial procedure

■ PDT

○ Low-grade dysplasia[57]

■ In a prospective, double-blind, randomized placebo-controlled study of PDT for the treatment of Barrett's esophagus with dysplasia, 18 patients with low-grade dysplasia were randomized to 5-aminolevulinic–induced PDT versus follow-up.

■ In the treatment group, no residual dysplasia was seen within the treatment area of any patient in the PDT group.

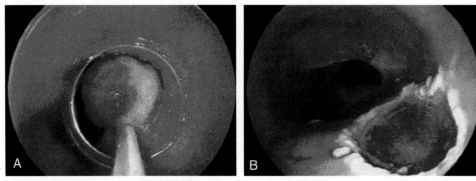

**Figure 57-3: A,** Endoscopic mucosal resection (EMR). **B,** Esophageal bed after EMR.

- In the placebo group, persistent low-grade dysplasia was found in 12 of 18 patients ($P < 0.001$).
- There were no short- or long-term major side effects, and the effects of treatment were maintained for up to 24 months.
○ High-grade dysplasia[58]
- The majority of patients demonstrate squamous re-epithelialization, with no evidence of residual dysplasia.
- Minor side effects were frequent
- Esophageal strictures developed in approximately one third of patients.
- Esophagectomy
○ Ablative therapies demonstrate promise in patients unfit for esophagectomy
○ However, ablative therapies may not eradicate all of the tissue capable of neoplastic progression, and carcinoma has been reported to develop deep to the superficial layers ablated by the phototherapy.
○ Therefore, endoscopic ablative therapies should, at present, be considered only when surgical options are not possible.
○ Esophagectomy is the only therapy guaranteed to prevent the progression of dysplasia to cancer.
○ Almost 40% of patients with high-grade dysplasia are found to be harboring carcinoma in the resected specimen. Fortunately, cancers found at this stage are highly curable, with 5-year survival rates for patients with high-grade dysplasia exceeding 90%.
○ However, surgery does have risk. Operative mortality rates of 3% to 12% have been reported, but centers with high volume and extensive experience in esophageal resection have minimized the rates of morbidity and mortality, hence improving the risk/benefit ratio.[59]
○ Minimally invasive esophagectomy has been developed as a safe and feasible alternative to the traditional open techniques and represents an ideal approach for this lesion and may help minimize the morbidity associated with esophageal resection. This is further aided by the mucosal localization of disease in Barrett's esophagus, making the operation technically easier to accomplish.[60-62]

## Guidelines

- The most comprehensive recommendations are derived from the American College of Gastroenterology Updated guidelines are available for the diagnosis, surveillance, and therapy of Barrett's esophagus.[63]
○ Treatment of GERD in patients with Barrett's esophagus should be the same as in patients without Barrett's esophagus.
○ With the diagnosis of Barrett's, patients should have surveillance endoscopy with biopsy at intervals based on the presence or absence of dysplasia as well as the grade of dysplasia.
- Without dysplasia, patients should undergo endoscopy every 2 to 3 years.
- In the management of low-grade dysplasia, patients should undergo endoscopy at 6 months, at 1 year, and then yearly if there is no progression
- In high-grade dysplasia, confirmation of the pathology should be obtained from an experienced independent pathologist.
○ Once confirmed, patients should undergo either esophagectomy or intensive endoscopic surveillance (every 3 months).
- The International Society for Diseases of the Esophagus as well as the consensus panel of the Society for Surgery of the Alimentary Tract, the American Gastroenterological Association, and the American Society for Gastrointestinal Endoscopy for the management of Barrett's esophagus all advocate[64,65] esophagectomy for fit patients with high-grade dysplasia.

## SUMMARY

- Barrett's esophagus is defined by replacement of the normal esophageal squamous mucosa with columnar intestinal metaplasia of the distal esophagus, and carries a 50- to 100-fold increased risk of esophageal adenocarcinoma compared with the general population.
- Risk factors for Barrett's include
○ Male sex
○ Smoking history
○ Obesity
○ White ethnicity
○ Age older than 50 years
○ History of reflux symptoms for more than 5 years.
- For Barrett's with either no dysplasia or low-grade dysplasia, a fundoplication may be considered. Fundoplication is safe and effective, and can be performed with lasting results using minimally invasive techniques.
- Medical or surgical antireflux therapy may improve and ameliorate symptoms, but no randomized trials have proved that they reduce the risk of developing esophageal adenocarcinoma.
- Random sampling of esophageal tissue for dysplasia remains a clinical standard for Barrett's esophagus.
- No studies have established that endoscopic screening or surveillance programs decrease the rates of death from cancer.
- Patients with Barrett's esophagus and high-grade dysplasia, who are fit, should undergo esophagectomy, to help prevent the risk of developing esophageal carcinoma.

- Endoscopic ablative approaches may represent a reasonable therapeutic alternative for patients who are in poor health or too old, or those who refuse esophagectomy.

# ESOPHAGEAL DIVERTICULA

A diverticulum is an outpouching or sac arising from the wall of the esophagus that can contain one or more layers of the wall. Diverticula can be classified based on histology, etiology, and location[66-68]:

## HISTOLOGY

- Three general types of diverticula exist, which are differentiated by the number of intestinal wall layers involved.
  - True diverticula
    - Contain all layers of the wall
  - False diverticula (pseudodiverticula)
    - Contain only mucosa and submucosa
  - Intramural diverticula (pseudodiverticula)
    - Outpouching within the submucosal layer secondary to dilated submucosal excretory ducts

## ETIOLOGY

- Acquired
  - Pulsion diverticula[69-72]
    - Secondary to increased intraluminal pressure at a weak point in the wall of the esophagus secondary to either anatomic or functional disturbance. There is frequent association with esophageal motility disorders such as diffuse esophageal spasm and achalasia.
      - Zenker's diverticulum
      - Epiphrenic diverticulum
  - Traction diverticula[73]
    - Secondary to extraluminal traction or pulling on the outside wall of the esophagus secondary to an inflammatory process and fibrosis such as histoplasmosis or tuberculosis
      - Midthoracic to parabronchial location
  - Intramural diverticula (pseudodiverticula)[67,68]
    - Esophageal submucosal glands, which are in communication with the esophageal lumen, become dilated.
    - Associated with inflammation and thickening of the esophagus, but the pathogenesis of this process is uncertain.
    - Possible etiology may be dilation of the submucosal glands secondary to obstruction by inflammation and debris.
    - Stasis and inflammation may also play a role in this disease.
    - Very often, there is associated esophageal dysmotility or strictures within the body of the esophagus.
    - May be a connection with history of corrosive esophageal injury
- Congenital
  - Present at birth

## LOCATION

- Pharyngeal
  - Zenker's diverticulum[74,75]
    - Acquired pulsion diverticula of the hypopharynx
    - Occur between the inferior pharyngeal constrictors and the cricopharyngeus
      - Killian's triangle
      - Discoordination between swallowing and relaxation of the cricopharyngeus (upper esophageal sphincter)
      - Fibrosis of cricopharyngeus over time and decreased upper esophageal sphincter compliance
      - Results in increased intraluminal pressure during swallowing
      - Results in herniation of mucosa through a weak area in the posterior wall of the hypopharynx in Killian's triangle.
- Body
  - Midthoracic-parabronchial[76]
    - Usually a traction diverticulum
    - May be congenital
    - In some instances, it may be associated with esophageal motility disorder, such as diffuse esophageal spasm and achalasia.
    - Rarely may occur in the setting of esophageal stricture
  - Epiphrenic
    - Usually a pulsion diverticulum of the distal 10 cm of the esophagus.
  - Esophageal intramural diverticula (pseudodiverticulosis)
    - Very rare condition
    - Numerous small outpouchings form in the wall of the esophagus.
    - May range in number from just a few to hundreds of pseudodiverticula.
    - The disease can have segmental distribution or diffusely involve the esophagus

## DIAGNOSIS

- Pharyngeal—Zenker's diverticulum
  - Clinical features
    - Aspiration pneumonia
    - Halitosis
    - Regurgitation
    - Dysphagia, ranging from globus sensation to obstruction
    - Bleeding
    - Perforation
    - May develop carcinoma within the pouch
  - Physical findings
    - Neck mass if the diverticulum is large
  - Imaging
    - Barium swallow
      - Visualized in the neck or cervical region
      - Lateral views demonstrate the extent of the Zenker's diverticulum
    - Computed tomography (CT) scan
      - May show air- or fluid-filled structure in communication with esophageal lumen
      - Allows for evaluation of surrounding structures in relation to the diverticulum
  - Procedures
    - EGD
      - Endoscopy is not always necessary in Zenker's diverticulum if the diagnosis has already been made by barium swallow.
      - If EGD is to be done, caution is warranted. (1) The true esophageal lumen is smaller than the lumen of the Zenker's diverticulum. (2) To decrease the risk of injury and possible perforation the scope should only be inserted gently and guided in under direct visualization.
- Midthoracic—Parabronchial
  - Clinical features
    - Usually asymptomatic

- Dysphagia is the most common symptom, but it is often due to an underlying motility disorder rather than the diverticulum itself.
- Regurgitation
- Aspiration pneumonia
- May develop obstruction
- Bezoar formation has been described
- May develop carcinoma within the pouch
  ○ Physical findings
  - Often normal
  ○ Imaging
  - Barium swallow
    ○ Visualized in the chest
    ○ Usually small in size
    ○ Pouch usually has a broad base with a wide-mouthed pouch.
    ○ Usually located near the tracheal bifurcation
  - CT scan may be performed.
    ○ Will show air- or fluid-filled structure in communication with esophageal lumen
    ○ Allows for identification of enlarged or calcified mediastinal nodes
    ○ Allows for evaluation of surrounding mediastinal structures in relation to the diverticulum
  ○ Procedures
  - EGD
    ○ Allows for visual inspection of the esophagus
    ○ Will help in identifying any erosion or other endoluminal pathology that may be associated with or the cause of the diverticulum.
    ○ Helpful in evaluation of the pouch and ruling out a carcinoma within the diverticulum
  - Esophageal manometry
    ○ Helpful in diagnosing an esophageal motility disorder that may be present. (1) Esophageal motility disorder may be the underlying cause of the diverticulum. (2) Manometry is useful in planning for surgical intervention
- Epiphrenic
  ○ Clinical features
  - Usually asymptomatic
  - Dysphagia is the most common symptom, but it is often due to an underlying motility disorder, rather than the diverticulum itself.
  - Regurgitation
  - Aspiration pneumonia
  - May develop obstruction
  - Bezoar formation has been described
  - May develop carcinoma within the pouch
  ○ Physical findings
  - Often normal
  ○ Imaging
  - Barium swallow
    ○ Visualized near the diaphragm
    ○ Usually a large globular pouch
    ○ May see abnormal esophageal contractions (Fig. 57-4)
  - CT scan may be performed
    ○ Will show air- or fluid-filled structure in communication with esophageal lumen
    ○ Allows for evaluation of surrounding structures in relation to the diverticulum
  ○ Procedures
  - EGD
    ○ Allows for visual inspection of the esophagus
    ○ Will help in identifying any erosion or other endoluminal pathology that may be associated with or the cause of the diverticulum.

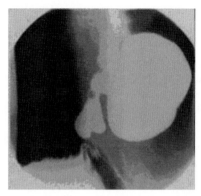

**Figure 57-4:** Epiphrenic diverticulum.

    ○ Helpful in evaluation of the pouch and ruling out a carcinoma within the diverticulum
  - Esophageal manometry
    ○ Helpful in diagnosing an esophageal motility disorder that may be present. (1) Esophageal motility disorder may be the underlying cause of the diverticulum. (2) Manometry is useful in planning for surgical intervention
- Intramural pseudodiverticulosis[77,78]
  ○ Clinical features
  - Dysphagia is the most common symptom.
  - May have esophageal dysmotility
  - May be associated with esophageal stricture
  ○ Physical findings
  - Often normal
  ○ Imaging
  - Barium swallow
    ○ May be segmental or diffusely distributed throughout the esophagus
    ○ Will see numerous small diverticula lining the esophageal wall
  ○ Procedures
  - EGD
    ○ Openings of the small diverticula are usually not visible on endoscopy.

## TREATMENT

- Zenker's diverticulum[79-85]
  ○ Usual treatment is surgical
  ○ The cricopharyngeus must be addressed during the time of operation. That is why a diverticulectomy alone is not performed, because the underlying problem will not be addressed.
  ○ Surgical options include
  - Diverticulectomy: Diverticular resection, as well as a concomitant cricopharyngeal myotomy
  - Diverticulopexy: Diverticular suspension, as well as a concomitant cricopharyngeal myotomy.
  - For very small diverticula, one option may be a cricopharyngeal myotomy alone.
  - Transoral approach using a rigid scope and a cutting-stapling device to divide the common wall between the esophagus and diverticulum as well as the cricopharyngeus.
  - Some have described a diverticulectomy performed with the use of a flexible endoscope to cut the common wall between the esophagus and diverticulum.

- Patients with Zenker's diverticulum and concomitant GERD warrant surgical intervention. Some advocate a combined procedure combining an antireflux procedure combined with an operation addressing the diverticulum. The goal of this approach is to prevent the possibility of regurgitation and aspiration postoperatively.
- Midthoracic and epiphrenic diverticula
  - Midthoracic or epiphrenic diverticula that are asymptomatic do not need to be treated.
  - Surgical intervention is mostly reserved for patients who are symptomatic and should be aimed at the underlying esophageal motility disorder or stricture.[86-88]
    - The more common complaints being dysphagia, regurgitation, weight loss, chest pain, and heartburn.
    - An open transthoracic approach is the traditional operative choice.
    - A linear stapling device is used for excision of the sac, with the staple line running parallel to the long axis of the esophagus to reduce tension, risk of leak, and subsequent diverticulization.
    - Any underlying esophageal motor disorder or reflux must be addressed with an extended myotomy, diverticulectomy, and an antireflux procedure, which is also required to address the underlying motility disorder.
    - The mortality and leak rates for open surgery have ranged from 0 to 11% and 6% to 18%, respectively.
    - Recent reports have demonstrated the technical feasibility of minimally invasive diverticulectomy, with two larger series reporting a mortality of 5% to 7.7% and a leak rate of 20% to 23.3%.[89,90]
      - Owing to the challenging nature of the operation as well as a potentially increased leak rate, it is advisable that the minimally invasive technique be considered only in centers with extensive experience in minimally invasive esophageal surgery, especially in cases in which the diverticulum is large.

# CONGENITAL ESOPHAGEAL DUPLICATION AND DUPLICATION CYST

## ETIOLOGY

- Originate from the primitive foregut
  - The defect responsible for esophageal cysts is the failure of proper development of the posterior division of the primitive foregut.
- Esophageal cysts are the second most common benign lesion of the esophagus.
- Account for up to 20% of benign esophageal lesions.
- The cysts are composed of
  - Acquired epithelial cysts
    - A minority of the cysts.
  - Congenital foregut cyst[91,92]
    - Represent majority of cases
    - Lined by squamous, respiratory, or columnar epithelium; may contain smooth muscle, cartilage, or fat
  - Esophageal duplication cyst[92-96]
    - A type of congenital foregut cyst
    - Lined by squamous epithelium
    - May contain gastric mucosa
    - Can be attached either to the esophagus or to the tracheobronchial tree.
    - Develop independently from the native esophagus
    - Usually does not have continuity with the native esophagus

- May be associated with other congenital malformations[95,96]
  - Vertebral abnormalities
  - Spinal cord abnormalities
  - Tracheoesophageal fistula
  - Esophageal atresia distal to the duplication
  - Other gastrointestinal duplications, more often small bowel.

## CLINICAL FEATURES

- Most are diagnosed in childhood, because most children are symptomatic
- May present in the first year of life with respiratory compromise secondary to mass effect from the cyst
- Cysts may become symptomatic in adulthood
  - Usually located in the right posterior mediastinum.
  - Chest pain or chest discomfort is most common.
  - Cough, stridor, tachypnea and other respiratory complaints due to compression from mass
  - Hematemesis can occur if there is gastric epithelium within the cyst.
  - Dysphagia may occur.
  - Cardiac arrhythmias may occur due to compression.
  - Other complications may include[96,97]
    - Infarction
    - Rupture
    - Dysplasia and malignant degeneration

## DIAGNOSIS

- History and appropriate imaging usually result in the diagnosis.
- Imaging
  - Chest x-ray study
    - May demonstrate a soft tissue mass or a cystic structure within the mediastinum with possible shift.
  - Barium swallow[97]:
    - May show esophageal compression.
    - May detect tubular esophageal duplication if it has a communication with the esophagus.
    - It may miss an esophageal cyst with no communication with the esophageal lumen.
  - CT
    - The study of choice
    - Allows for diagnosis
    - Usually identify a cystic fluid-filled mass intimately related to the esophagus
    - Helps aid in operative preparation, by delineating the anatomy of the mass and its surrounding structures before surgical resection (Fig. 57-5).

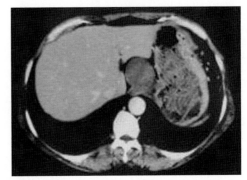

**Figure 57-5:** Esophageal duplication cyst.

○ Technetium scan
  ▪ The addition of a nuclear (technetium) scan may help identify ectopic gastric mucosa within the cyst.
○ Magnetic resonance imaging
  ▪ May be helpful in diagnosing esophageal cysts.
○ Endoscopy demonstrates extrinsic compression with intact mucosa.
○ Endoscopic ultrasonography reveals a cystic, filled structure in connection with the esophagus.
▪ Procedures
  ○ Esophagoscopy:
    ▪ Need to rule out intraluminal pathology
    ▪ If any lesion or abnormality is seen, it should be biopsied to evaluate for possible malignancy.
  ○ EUS
    ▪ Help delineate the intramural or extraesophageal extent of the cyst.
    ▪ Distinguish between solid and cystic masses

## TREATMENT

▪ Removal of all discovered cysts is advocated, because most will eventually be symptomatic by adulthood
▪ Definitive treatment involves complete surgical resection of the duplication, even for asymptomatic cysts.[98]
▪ Simple cysts may be enucleated
▪ Duplications need to be excised.
▪ Traditionally, a posterolateral thoracotomy was employed for access to the lesion.
▪ At present, with the advent of minimally invasive techniques, the use of video-assisted thoracoscopic surgery has become the procedure of choice in the approach to these lesions.
▪ Transesophageal endoscopic drainage has been described, but this procedure does not address the lining of the cyst and the recurrence rate is high.[99]

### Brief Illustrative Case

- *History:* A 55-year-old slightly obese man with complaints of cough in the mornings and reflux.
- *Examination:* In no acute distress. Abdomen is rotund. Lungs are clear to auscultation.
- *Medication:* PPI for 8 weeks.
- *Imaging:* Barium swallow reveals no abnormalities, lesions, or obstruction.
- *Studies:*
  - Endoscopy reveals Barrett's esophagus.
  - Twenty-four-hour PH study is positive and reveals continued acid reflux.
  - Esophageal manometry reveals normal esophageal motility and a decreased LES pressure.
- *Diagnosis/Pathology:* —Biopsy confirms Barrett's with no dysplasia.
- *Management of GERD:* The most comprehensive recommendations are derived from the American College of Gastroenterology Updated guidelines for the diagnosis, surveillance and therapy of Barrett's esophagus.[63]
  - Treatment of GERD in patients with Barrett's esophagus should be the same as in patients without Barrett's esophagus.

- With the diagnosis of Barrett's esophagus, patients should have surveillance endoscopy, with biopsy at intervals based on the presence or absence of dysplasia as well as the grade of dysplasia.
- The International Society for Diseases of the Esophagus as well as the consensus panel of the Society for Surgery of the Alimentary Tract, the American Gastroenterological Association, and the American Society for Gastrointestinal Endoscopy for the management of Barrett's esophagus all advocate[64,65] esophagectomy for fit patients with high-grade dysplasia.

### Key Points

- Barrett's esophagus is defined by replacement of the normal esophageal squamous mucosa with columnar intestinal metaplasia of the distal esophagus, and carries a 50-100–fold increased risk of esophageal adenocarcinoma compared with the general population.
- Risk factors for Barrett's include
  - Male sex
  - Smoking history
  - Obesity
  - White ethnicity
  - Age older than 50
  - A history of reflux symptoms lasting more than 5 years.
- For Barrett's esophagus with either no dysplasia or low-grade dysplasia, a fundoplication may be considered. Fundoplication is safe and effective, and can be performed with lasting results using minimally invasive techniques.
- Medical or surgical antireflux therapy may improve and ameliorate symptoms, but no randomized trials have proven that they reduce the risk of developing esophageal adenocarcinoma.
- Random sampling of esophageal tissue for dysplasia remains a clinical standard for Barrett's esophagus.
- No studies have established that endoscopic screening or surveillance programs decrease the rates of death from cancer.
- Patients with Barrett's esophagus and high-grade dysplasia, who are fit, should undergo esophagectomy to help prevent the risk of developing esophageal carcinoma.
- Endoscopic ablative approaches may represent a reasonable therapeutic alternative for patients who are in poor health, too old or those who refuse esophagectomy.

## References

 Interactive references and additional readings for this chapter can be accessed online at *expertconsult.com*.

# 58 MANAGEMENT OF ESOPHAGEAL PERFORATION

Harmik J. Soukiasian, MD and James D. Luketich, MD

## INTRODUCTION

Esophageal perforation is a dangerous problem with a high mortality rate (9%–36%), as reviewed by Bufkin and associates.[1] Early diagnosis and management is key to improved outcomes. Thus, it is important to appreciate those circumstances in which esophageal perforation might occur and to have a high index of suspicion in such instances.

## CAUSES

Usually results from some form of trauma

- **Forceful retching or vomiting (Boerhaave's syndrome).**
- **Penetrating trauma**
- **Foreign body ingestion**
  - Usually, ingested foreign objects that are smaller than 2 cm pass through the normal adult esophagus without causing perforation.[2]
  - Eighty to ninety percent of ingested foreign objects pass through the esophagus and eventually the rest of the gastrointestinal tract without the need for intervention.
  - The remainder of these patients who do mandate intervention most often are treated with endoscopic techniques, with less than 1% needing to go for surgery.[3]
- **Chemical or caustic perforation: three phases[4,5]:**
  Initial phase
  - Inflammation, edema, and necrosis occurring days after injury.
  - Next, there is sloughing of the esophagus and development of mucosal ulceration
  Second phase
  - Esophageal wall is weakest and prone to perforation.
  - Granulation tissue
  - Collagen deposition
  - Re-epithelization lasting about 3 weeks to 4 weeks
  Third phase[6,7]
  - Damaged and destroyed esophageal submucosa and muscularis are replaced with scar tissue.
  - Stricture formation

  Mechanism of injury:

  Alkaline
  - More esophageal than gastric injury. Produces liquefactive necrosis, resulting in a deep injury
  - Induces pylorospasm, thus resulting in reflux back into the esophagus
  - Cricopharyngeal muscle spasm also occurs and forces the refluxate back into the stomach.
  - Hence, alkali causes both esophageal and gastric burns.
  Acid
  - More gastric than esophageal injury; produces coagulative necrosis, and forms an eschar, which, in turn, limits tissue penetration

  - Acid passes through the esophagus faster than alkaline substances.
  - Acid will also trigger pylorospasm, pooling the acid in the distal antrum and producing severe gastritis.
  - May progress to full-thickness gastric necrosis and perforation within 24 hours to 48 hours.
- **Iatrogenic[8]**
  - Traumatic intubation
  - Nasogastric tube placement
  - Following endoscopic procedures
    - Esophagogastroduodenoscopy
    - Dilation
    - Transesophageal Echo (TEE)
    - Sclerotherapy
    - Endoscopic retrograde cholangiopancreatography
  - Postoperatively following surgery
    - Any esophageal operation
      - Myotomy or achalasia
      - Esophageal leiomyoma enucleation
      - Collis gastroplasty
      - Esophageal diverticula
    - Fundoplication
    - Vagotomy
    - Hiatal hernia repair
    - Lung transplantation
    - Pneumonectomy
    - Thyroid resection
    - Tracheostomy
    - Thoracic aneurysm repair
    - Mediastinoscopy
    - Cervical spine surgery

### Clinical Features
- The primary symptoms include[9]
  - Acute chest pain—the most common symptom (71%)
  - Fever (51%)
  - Dyspnea or shortness of breath (24%)
  - Crepitus (22%)
  - Dysphagia
  - Odynophagia
  - Epigastric pain
  - Productive cough
- The clinical presentation in delayed presentations may be more advanced, with the patient showing signs of toxicity and shock.

## DIAGNOSIS
### Chest Radiography
**Radiography** is essential in the diagnosis of esophageal perforation.[10,11]

### Cervical Esophageal Perforation
- Lateral neck radiograph is recommended as it may demonstrate air in the prevertebral facial planes.

## *Thoracic and Abdominal Esophageal Perforation*

- Posterior and lateral chest radiographs as well as upright abdominal films are recommended (Figs. 58-1 and 58-2). **Radiographic findings** include
  - ○ Pneumomediastinum—generally takes 1 hour or more after injury to be readily identified on CXR.[10]
  - ○ Subcutaneous emphysema
  - ○ Mediastinal air-fluid levels or pleural effusions
    - ■ Effusion is generally on the right with perforation of the midesophagus.
    - ■ Effusion is generally on the left with perforation of the distal esophagus.
  - ○ Hydropneumothorax
  - ○ Mediastinal widening

## Computed Tomography

**Computed tomography (CT) scanning** is also valuable in defining the extent of the infective process and allows a serial measure of progress in therapy.[12-14] **CT findings** include

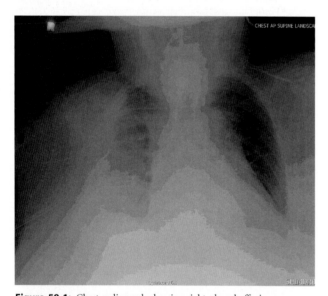

**Figure 58-1:** Chest radiograph showing right pleural effusion.

- Pneumomediastinum
- Extraluminal air
- Esophageal thickening
- Pleural effusion
- If prolonged, an abscess cavity may be present.
- Communication of the esophagus with pleural cavity or an adjacent mediastinal air-fluid collection

## Esophagoscopy/Endoscopy

**Esophagography** aids in diagnosing as well as localizing the leak (Fig. 58-3).

- Has a false-negative rate of 10%.[15]
- Esophageal perforation may be preceded by inflammation and edema, and hence, have no evidence of extravasation. However, the leak may later develop as the esophageal wall breaks down and perforates.
- Rigid esophagoscopy
- Flexible esophagoscopy
  - ○ Although esophagography is effective at detecting perforation, there still exists the risk of converting a mucosal or submucosal injury into a perforation during air insufflation. Based on this problem, some authors advise against the use of esophagoscopy in the diagnosis of esophageal injuries.[16]

## *MANAGEMENT*

- The **usual therapy** includes
  - ○ Broad-spectrum antibiotics
  - ○ Early, aggressive surgical intervention
    - ■ Drainage, débridement and control of the perforation site to prevent or treat sepsis.
- Several **surgical approaches** are available for the management of esophageal perforation. The options include
  - ○ Débridement and primary closure
    - ■ Possible use of autogenous tissue flap reinforcement.
  - ○ Placement of an esophageal T-tube
  - ○ Exclusion-diversion
  - ○ Mediastinal drainage and esophagectomy.
- The **choice of approach** is based on
  - ○ Cause and duration of the perforation
  - ○ Degree of surrounding tissue inflammation and injury
  - ○ Clinical condition of the patient

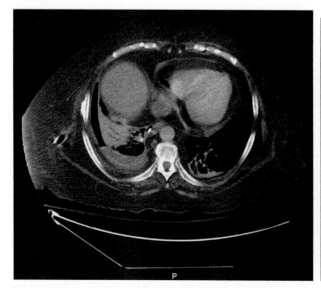

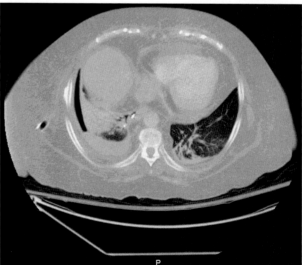

**Figure 58-2:** Computed tomography scan reveals pleural effusion and pneumothorax in a patient with esophageal perforation.

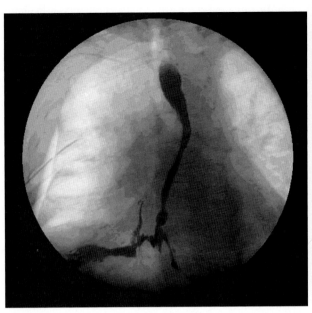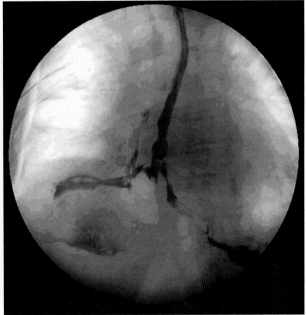

**Figure 58-3:** Esophagram showing esophageal perforation with extravasation of dye into the right side of the chest.

- As expertise is gained in video-assisted esophageal surgery, minimally invasive surgical approaches to esophageal perforations and leaks have been developed and have become the preferred approach in many situations. Nguyen and coauthors[17] summarize the main goals in the minimally invasive approach to esophageal perforations, which are the same principles held with open repair,[18,19] namely
  - ○ Identification of the esophageal perforation
  - ○ Débridement of ischemic and necrotic tissue
  - ○ Myotomy with exposure and identification of mucosal edges of the defect
  - ○ If possible, closure of defect in two layers
  - ○ Control of the leak (primary closure or T-tube placement)
  - ○ Wide drainage of the mediastinum
- In upper esophageal injuries
  - ○ Usually occur secondary to trauma (gunshot wounds, difficult intubations) or may occur post-operatively following an esophagectomy
  - ○ Aided by gravity, as well as negative intrathoracic pressures, organisms and pus may rapidly accumulate in the deep cervical and mediastinal fascial planes, accounting for mortality rates as high as 30% to 40%.
  - ○ Transcervical drainage is a highly effective means of controlling hypopharyngeal and proximal esophageal perforations.
  - ○ This approach allows adequate exposure to control and repair perforations and leaks extending into the upper mediastinum down to the level of the carina.
  - ○ Transcervical drainage is also useful in treating descending cervical mediastinitis, which may be odontogenic, peritonsillar, cervicofacial, or esophageal in origin, as discussed by Kiernan[20] and Wheatley[21] and their associates.
  - ○ Esophageal leaks after esophagectomy may be managed in most instances by opening the neck incision and packing the wound.
  - ○ Cervical exploration through this wound allows access to the upper mediastinum, facilitating assessment of the leak, the condition of the gastric tube, and esophagogastric anastomosis.

- ○ It also permits adequate exposure for débridement and drain placement.
- Mid-distal esophageal perforations
  - ○ Typically require transthoracic drainage
  - ○ Some authors advocate the routine use of thoracotomy to provide maximal exposure in order to carry out a thorough débridement, repair, or drainage.
  - ○ Increasingly, thoracoscopy is being used in place of thoracotomy when conditions are favorable for video-assisted thoracic surgery (VATS), as reviewed by Chung and colleagues.[22]
  - ○ Scott and Rosin[23] were the first to report a minimally invasive repair of esophageal rupture secondary to Boerhaave's syndrome.
  - ○ The usual thoracoscopic approach employs three to four trocars positioned conventionally via a right-sided approach through the chest.
  - ○ A left-sided VATS, as described by Ikeda and coworkers,[24] or transabdominal approach, as advocated by Landen and coauthors,[25] can be employed in distal esophageal perforations, or when the leak is demonstrated by esophagram to extend into the left chest.

## Surgical Management
- The initial step is retraction of the lung and evacuation of fibrinous debris and purulent exudates.
- Intraoperative endoscopy is performed to assist in identifying the site of perforation.
- The suspected region can be submerged under irrigation during endoscopic insufflation to pinpoint the precise location of perforation.
- Once identified, the devitalized margins of the perforation are débrided,
- Myotomy with exposure and identification of mucosal edges of the defect
- A decision is made whether to attempt a primary closure, depending on the degree of surrounding tissue injury as well as the clinical condition of the patient.

- If the defect is small (<1 cm) and surrounded by viable tissue, a primary closure can be performed with interrupted sutures in two layers.
- An important caveat to remember in delayed presentation (i.e., those presenting after 24 hours of perforation), is that the leak rate after repair remains very high.
  - Even with the use of reinforced primary esophageal repair, an esophageal leak can occur in 83% of these patients.[26]
- In the case of larger injuries or perforations surrounded by severely inflamed tissue in which repair is not possible, or in hemodynamically unstable patients who cannot tolerate definitive esophageal repair, wide drainage is performed with placement of a T-tube to control the leak.
- Wide defects may allow direct placement of a T-tube through the perforation site.
- For smaller holes, a loop wire can be inserted transthoracically through the perforation defect. Endoscopy is performed to retrieve the loop wire, which is then brought back through the mouth. The end of a T-tube is sutured to the loop wire, and the wire or T-tube is pulled transorally down the esophagus and out through the chest, with the T-tube tip positioned intraluminally at the perforation site. Final positioning of the T-tube can be confirmed by endoscopy.
- Jackson-Pratt drains as well as a 28 to 32 French chest tube are positioned strategically to provide wide drainage of the mediastinum and chest.
- Identification and elimination of any distal obstruction, such as a stricture.
- There are **unusual and rare circumstances** encountered during esophageal perforation that call for creative and safe surgical approaches to this serious problem.
  - Perforations involving an esophageal diverticulum can be managed by minimally invasive diverticulectomy and drainage, as reported by Tinoco and colleagues.[27]
- Perforation of the distal esophagus after esophageal dilatation for achalasia can occur with a frequency of 0 to 15%.
  - The location of the perforation is typically the left posterior esophagus.
  - Full-thickness perforations tend to begin within a centimeter of the squamocolumnar junction, and extend proximally from a few millimeters to as much as 10 cm.
  - These perforations can usually be repaired using a thoracoscopic or transabdominal laparoscopic technique with suture closure of the perforation, contralateral Heller myotomy, and Toupet posterior fundoplication, as summarized by Nathanson and associates[28] and Bell.[29]
  - A contralateral myotomy is performed extending 5 cm along the length of the esophagus and extending 1 cm onto the surface of the stomach, with care taken to spare the vagus nerves.
  - A posterior fundoplication is then performed in the manner of Toupet, suturing the edges of the myotomy to the edges of the plicated stomach over a length of 4 cm.
    - This technique has the advantage of covering the closed esophageal perforation with a gastric serosal patch, while at the same time treating the underlying motility disorder.
  - A closed suction drain is placed into the mediastinum.
- Early recognition, and prompt surgical intervention allow primary closure in the majority of circumstances without the need for muscular flaps or esophageal exclusion.
  - Although the most common surgical approach is transthoracic, the excellent visualization of the distal 6 to 7 cm of thoracic esophagus is amenable to a transabdominal laparoscopic approach, as advocated by Swanstrom and Pennings.[30,31]

- Definitive treatment of achalasia is obtained by performance of a myotomy with a fundoplication to help diminish the risk of postmyotomy reflux.
- A transthoracic approach should probably be used if the tear extends more than 5 cm proximally, or if there is gross extravasation of contrast into the left pleural space, as summarized by Laisaar.[32]
- The location of the tear on the circumference of the esophagus is not a significant issue in deciding on this approach, because adequate visualization of the entire circumference of the esophagus is possible by gentle rotation.
- Advantages of a minimally invasive approach include
  - Excellent, magnified view of the entire thoracic cavity
  - Ability to achieve adequate débridement and drainage of the mediastinum and pleura, as summarized by Roberts and coworkers.[33]
  - Using VATS, either primary closure or an esophageal T-tube with drainage can be used to control the esophageal leak in the same manner as is done with open thoracotomy.
  - If any difficulties arise, it is always possible to convert to open thoracostomy.
  - By avoiding thoracotomy, however, the patient experiences less postoperative pain, a decrease in wound-related complications and a faster postoperative recovery.

## Nonoperative Management

- Considered in highly selected, healthy, nontoxic patients with well-contained perforation and minimal to no mediastinal contamination. Management consists of[34,35]:
  - Keeping the patient on nothing by mouth (NPO)
  - Antibiotics
  - Total parenteral nutrition (TPN)
  - Drainage of fluid collections
- It must be stressed that up to 20% of patients undergoing nonoperative management require surgical intervention within 24 hours,[34] and lack of improvement or worsening and deterioration requires timely surgical intervention.

### Esophageal Stent

Management of early esophageal perforation using esophageal stents is an emerging modality. It has also been used in the management of esophageal perforation due to TEE and endoscopic instrumentation such as esophageal dilation, postoperative leak, foreign body ingestion, and Boerhaave's syndrome.[36-41]

## CONCLUSIONS

- Esophageal perforation is a very serious and potentially fatal problem.
- A high index of suspicion as well as diligence in the workup of patients who may have esophageal perforation is crucial.
- Early diagnosis and treatment is paramount, because there is a worsening prognosis and outcomes with delay and eventual onset of sepsis and shock.
- With early diagnosis of an esophageal leak surgical therapy, abiding by the principles of early repair, tissue reinforcement, and drainage of fluid collections, antibiotics and TPN should be instituted as soon as possible in cases of open unconfined esophageal leakage.
- In a delayed presentation of esophageal perforation or in cases of patient instability, wide drainage remains the mainstay of treatment.

■ In other cases of esophageal perforation where the indications for immediate repair may not be as clean cut, such as in contained leaks in healthy nontoxic patients, there may be other options available on an individual patient-to-patient basis.

## Brief Illustrative Case

- *History:* A 55-year-old woman with a history of distal esophageal stricture. Patient has required repeated dilations in the past. Her last dilatation was 24 hours ago, which was an outpatient procedure. Patient now returns to the emergency department reporting shortness of breath, chest pain, and fever.
- *Examination:* Patient is pale and diaphoretic. Abdomen is benign. Lungs sounds slightly diminished on the left with rhonchi. Right side is clear to auscultation.
- *Medication:* Steroids for arthritis.
- *Imaging:*
  - Chest radiograph reveals left pleural effusion
  - Esophagram reveals extravasation of dye into the left chest
  - CT scan reveals consolidation of the lower lobe, a small pneumothorax, and pleural effusion
- *Studies:*
  - Endoscopy reveals esophageal perforation 3 cm proximal to the gastroesophageal junction
  - *Diagnosis/Pathology:* Esophageal perforation.
- *Management:*
  - This patient was resuscitated with intravenous fluids.
  - Antimicrobial therapy was instituted.
  - Patient was emergently taken to the operating room.
  - Both the esophagus and injury point were evaluated.
  - There was severe stricturing distal to the point of injury. Additionally, there were severe reactive changes in the area of injury.
  - The injury was a 4 cm rent in the esophagus with jagged and devitalized edges.
  - A decision was made to perform an esophagectomy and gastric pull-up with drainage of the area as well as placement of a feeding jejunostomy. This is not a common surgical management strategy with esophageal perforation. The rationale for esophagectomy was multifactorial:

- The patient's long history of severe symptomatic esophageal stricture, which had worsened over time and had become less responsive to dilatational therapy.
- The size and severity of the injury also compounded the problem in that the esophagus was injured beyond the point of repair or possibility of recovery.
- An inflamed esophagus.
- It was felt that the safest course of action for the patient would be esophagectomy with drainage.
- Feeding jejunostomy was placed to aid in alimentation.
- The patient did well, survived, and was discharged home.

## Key Points

- Esophageal perforation is a very serious and potentially fatal problem.
- A high index of suspicion as well as diligence in the workup of patients who may have esophageal perforation is crucial.
- Early diagnosis and treatment is paramount, because there is worsening prognosis and outcomes with delay and eventual onset of sepsis and shock.
- With early diagnosis of an esophageal leak, surgical therapy, abiding by the principles of early repair, tissue reinforcement, drainage of fluid collections, antibiotics and TPN, should be instituted as soon as possible in cases of open unconfined esophageal leakage.
- In the delayed presentation of esophageal perforation or in cases of patient instability, wide drainage remains the mainstay of treatment.
- In other cases of esophageal perforation in which the indications for immediate repair may not be as clean cut, such as in contained leaks in healthy non-toxic patients, there may be other options available on an individual patient-to-patient basis.

## References

 Interactive references and additional readings for this chapter can be accessed online at *expertconsult.com*.

# INDEX

*Note: Page numbers followed by f refer to figures; those followed by t refer to tables.*